Textbook of Biochemistry

THIRD EDITION

Textbook of Biochemistry

THIRD EDITION

Harbans Lal PhD, FIAO, FACBI
Sr. Professor, Department of Biochemistry
Maharaja Agrasen Medical College, Agroha, Hisar
Former
Sr. Professor, Department of Biochemistry, Post Graduate Institute of Medical Sciences
Pt. BD Sharma University of Health Sciences, Rohtak
Visiting Professor, Department of Biosciences, MD University, Rohtak
WHO Fellow and Visiting Assistant Professor, Louisiana State University Medical Centre, New Orleans, USA

Late **Rajesh Pandey** MD
Ex-Professor and Head, Department of Biochemistry
Maharishi Markandeshwar Institute of Medical Sciences and Research
Mullana, Ambala (Haryana)

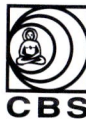

CBS Publishers & Distributors Pvt Ltd

New Delhi • Bengaluru • Chennai • Kochi • Kolkata • Mumbai
Hyderabad • Nagpur • Patna • Pune • Vijayawada

Disclaimer

Science and technology are constantly changing fields. New research and experience broaden the scope of information and knowledge. The authors have tried their best in giving information available to them while preparing the material for this book. Although all efforts have been made to ensure optimum accuracy of the material, yet it is quite possible some errors might have been left uncorrected. The publisher, the printer and the authors will not be held responsible for any inadvertent errors, omissions or inaccuracies.

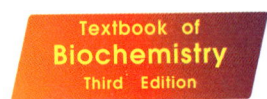

ISBN: 978-93-85915-79-6

Copyright © Harbans Lal

Third Edition: 2017

First Edition: 2004
  Reprint: 2008, 2010
Second Edition: 2011
  Reprint: 2014

Published by Satish Kumar Jain and produced by Varun Jain for
CBS Publishers & Distributors Pvt Ltd
4819/XI Prahlad Street, 24 Ansari Road, Daryaganj, New Delhi 110 002, India.
Ph: 23289259, 23266861, 23266867   Fax: 011-23243014   Website: www.cbspd.com
    e-mail: delhi@cbspd.com; cbspubs@airtelmail.in.
Corporate Office: 204 FIE, Industrial Area, Patparganj, Delhi 110 092
Ph: 4934 4934   Fax: 4934 4935   e-mail: publishing@cbspd.com; publicity@cbspd.com

Branches

- **Bengaluru:** Seema House 2975, 17th Cross, K.R. Road, Banasankari 2nd Stage, Bengaluru 560 070, Karnataka
  Ph: +91-80-26771678/79   Fax: +91-80-26771680   e-mail: bangalore@cbspd.com
- **Chennai:** 7, Subbaraya Street, Shenoy Nagar, Chennai 600 030, Tamil Nadu
  Ph: +91-44-26680620, 26681266   Fax: +91-44-42032115   e-mail: chennai@cbspd.com
- **Kochi:** Ashana House, 39/1904, AM Thomas Road, Valanjambalam,
  Eranakulam 682 018, Kochi, Kerala
  Ph: +91-484-4059061-62-64-65   Fax: +91-484-4059065   e-mail: kochi@cbspd.com
- **Kolkata:** 6/B, Ground Floor, Rameswar Shaw Road, Kolkata 700 014, West Bengal
  Ph: +91-33-2289-1126, 1127, 1128,   e-mail: Kolkata@cbspd.com
- **Mumbai:** 83-C, Dr E Moses Road, Worli, Mumbai-400018, Maharashtra
  Ph: +91-22-24902340/41   Fax: +91-22-24902342   e-mail: mumbai@cbspd.com

Representatives

- **Hyderabad** 0-9885175004   • **Nagpur** 0-9021734563   • **Patna** 0-9334159340
- **Pune** 0-9623451994   • **Vijayawada** 0-9000660880

Printed at Rashtriya Printers Delhi-110095

to

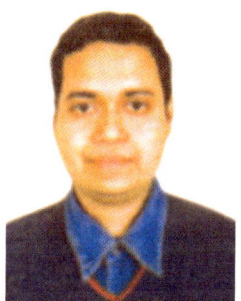

Foreword

It is a pleasure to write a brief introduction to *Textbook of Biochemistry* written by Dr Harbans Lal, Professor of Biochemistry, Pt. BD Sharma Postgraduate Institute of Medical Sciences, Rohtak (Haryana).

Biochemistry deals with the chemistry of life and living processes. The scope of biochemistry is as vast as life itself. It is the most rapidly developing branch of science as it gives an understanding of the functioning of the living body at the cellular and molecular level.

The book written by Dr Harbans Lal will be warmly welcomed both by the students as well as the teachers of various medical institutions in the country, for it is written with clarity and in a simple comprehensive style.

The book is mainly based on the MBBS curriculum; however, recent advances have been covered in almost all the chapters. It gives a thorough understanding of the health and disease status in the human body.

I congratulate Dr Harbans Lal for the enormous efforts he has made in compiling this textbook which will be very useful to the medical students in particular as well as the teaching faculty of various scientific institutions of our country.

Kiranjeet Kaur MD
Professor and Head
Department of Biochemistry
and
Principal
Government Medical College
Patiala

Preface to the Third Edition

The encouraging response to the second edition *Textbook of Biochemistry* inspired me to bring out the third edition. Like the previous editions, I have endeavored to convey knowledge of time-old principles of biochemistry supplemented with modern developments, in a simple, precise and lucid manner. The contents have been organized into various sections and the chapters are updated with multiple choice questions, new figures, tables and applied biochemistry in the form of 'chemistry to clinics'. In all, more than 120 new colored figures have been incorporated. A new chapter on radioisotopes has been added. Some of the shortcomings in the previous edition as pointed out by the students have been rectified. Still, a few lacunas may have remained.

I acknowledge the entire team of CBS Publishers & Distributors, New Delhi, for their efforts. I expect that the book will be appreciated by the students and colleagues alike. Comments and constructive criticism are welcome in order to improve further.

Harbans Lal
hl.biopgimsr@gmail.com

Preface to the First Edition

The appreciative response of my fellow teachers and students from various colleges throughout the country, to my previous publication, *Textbook of Biochemistry for Dental Students*, encouraged me to write this book.

Biochemistry is the chemistry of the living matter in its different phases of activity, from the smallest micro-organisms to the most complex and highly evolved human beings. The subject has made a great advances worldwide, backed by intensive research and application.

The purpose of introducing this book *Textbook of Biochemistry* is to convey a knowledge of modern biochemistry to the readers in a simple, precise and lucid manner. The text of the book has been supplemented with the self-explanatory flowcharts, diagrams and tables. Some of the important aspects of clinical relevance/application too have been highlighted in colored boxes for a better understanding of the subject. It is intended that the book will meet the requirement of the students who are to take a basic course in biochemistry, particularly those studying biochemistry in relation to medicine.

This book would never have been accomplished without the encouragement and support of my sincere friends and associates. To each one of them, I extend my most earnest thanks. I am highly indebted to Prof SK Aggarwal, MMES Medical College, Maulana (Haryana), and Dr Vijay Shanker, Associate Professor of Biochemistry, PGIMS, Rohtak, for giving their valuable suggestions. I am also grateful to Dr Rajesh Pandey, Research Associate, Department of Biochemistry, PGI, Chandigarh, for his encouragement and help. I also tender my thanks to Dr Manju Pahwa, Lecturer, and Dr Ashuma Sachdeva; Dr Anjali Singh; Dr Deepa Rao; Dr Richa; Dr Anuj; Dr Munish; Dr Parul and Dr Ekta, Residents, Department of Biochemistry, PGIMS, Rohtak, for their help in completion of the book. My appreciation also extends to Mr SK Jain and his team from CBS Publishers & Distributors, New Delhi, for bringing out this book.

Every care has been taken in preparing the text of this book, however, there could have been a few short-coming oversights. To overcome the same, I welcome comments, criticism along with useful suggestions from the students and faculty for the improvement of this book.

Nov. 2003
Rohtak (Haryana)

Harbans Lal

Contents

Section 1: General Biochemistry

Section 2: Metabolism and Endocrinology

Section 3: Molecular Biology

Section 4: Nutrition

Section 5: Immunity and Defence

Section 6: Special Topics and Clinical Chemistry

1

General Biochemistry

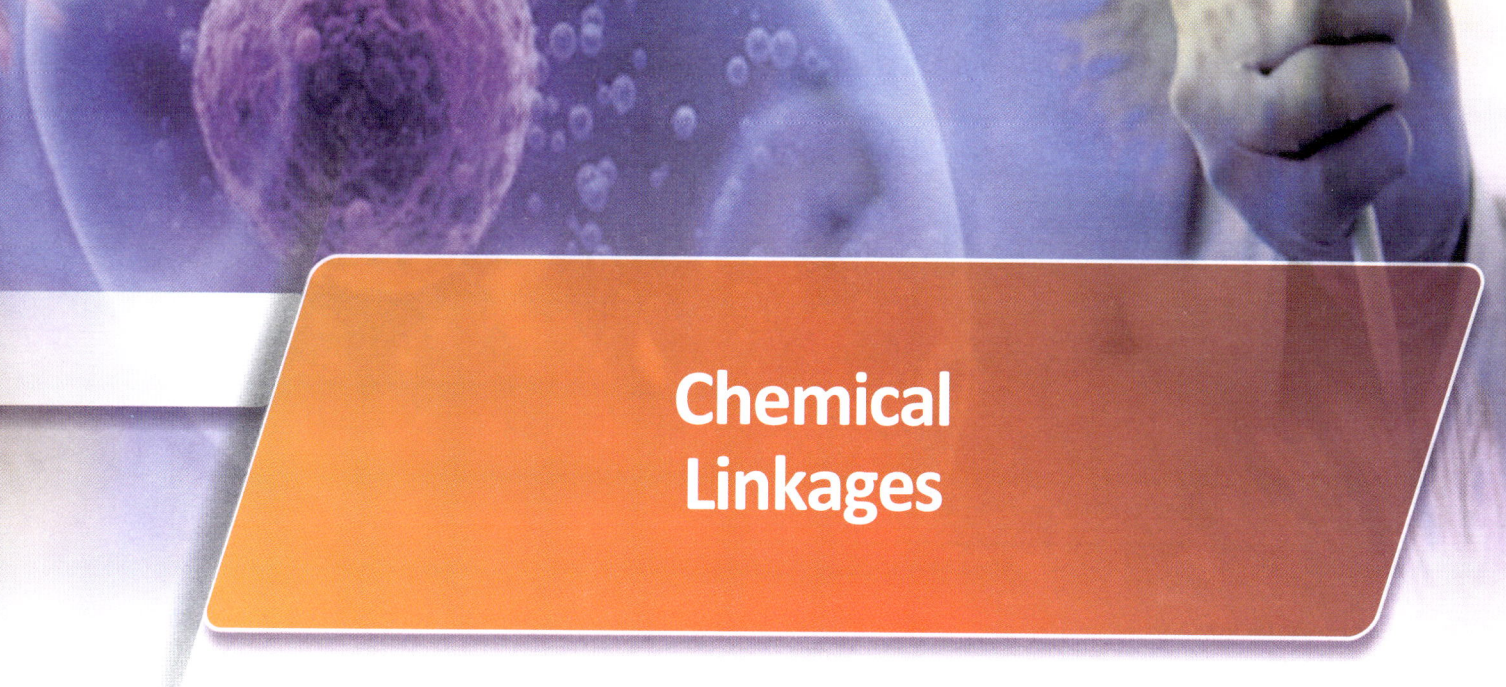

Chemical Linkages

A basic knowledge of the various chemical linkages would be helpful in understanding the structural aspects of biomolecules, biochemical reactions and their related disorders discussed in the subsequent chapters. Linkages or bonds are, broadly speaking, either weak bonds or strong bonds.

WEAK BONDS

Weak bonds include ionic bonds, hydrophobic interactions and van der Waals forces.

Ionic Bonds

The outer electron(s) of an atom may interact with those of other atoms, resulting in chemical bonds or chemical linkages. In ionic bonds, electrons are actually transferred from one atom to another. Such atoms or aggregates of atoms are called ions. The atom gaining electron(s) becomes a negatively charged **anion** because it has more number of negative electrons than the number of positive protons. Similarly, the atom losing electron(s) becomes a positively charged **cation** because it has more number of positive protons than the number of negative electrons. Since oppositely charged ions attract one another, they can be held together to form electrically neutral ionic compounds. Such attractions are called **electrostatic attractions or ionic attractions or ionic bonds** (Fig. 1.1).

Hydrophobic Interactions

These interactions arise because water molecules prefer to interact with each other rather than with non-polar molecules. Hence, non-polar molecules are forced to redistribute from a dispersed state in water into an aggregated organic phase surrounded by water. This phenomenon is important in the spontaneous assembly of biological membranes.

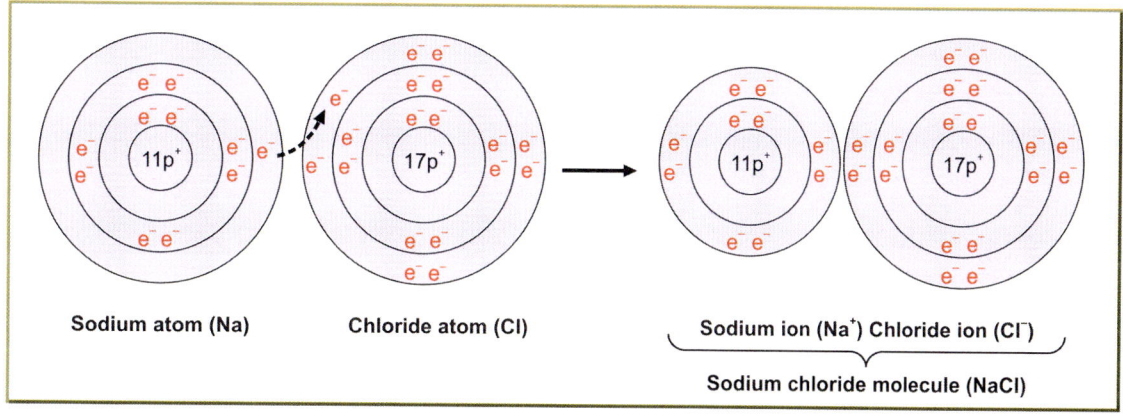

Fig. 1.1: Formation of ionic/electrostatic bond.

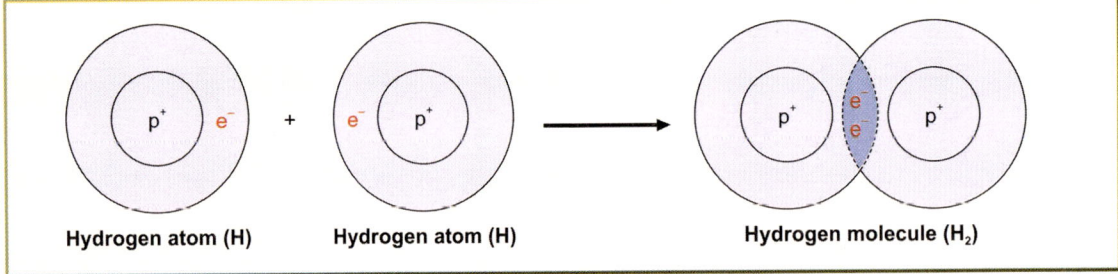

Fig. 1.2: Formation of non-polar covalent bond.

van der Waals Forces

These forces result from induced electrical attractions between closely approaching atoms or molecules. The attraction exists between the positively charged nuclei of a given atom and the electrons of neighboring atoms, hence van der Waals forces operate over **very short distances**.

STRONG BONDS

Strong bonds include covalent bonds, polar and non-polar bonds, and hydrogen bonds.

Covalent Bonds

Instead of transfer of electrons as discussed above, if two or more atoms share electrons in their outer energy level, covalent bonds are formed. In a hydrogen molecule (H_2), the two H atoms share one pair of electrons located in the region between the two nuclei (Fig. 1.2).

The attraction between the electrons in the middle and the protons in the two nuclei holds the molecule strongly together by a single covalent bond. When two pairs of electrons are shared, a double bond is formed, e.g. oxygen (O_2). When three pairs of electrons are shared, a triple bond is formed, e.g. nitrogen (N_2).

Polar and Non-polar Bonds

When the **shared electrons are attracted equally** to both atoms as in case of H_2, a **non-polar covalent bond** is formed. On the other hand, if **one atom attracts the shared electrons more strongly** than the other, the bond is a **polar covalent bond** and the resulting molecule is a polar molecule with positive and negative regions. **Water (H_2O) is a polar molecule** because oxygen attracts the shared electrons more strongly and becomes somewhat negative whereas the hydrogen regions become somewhat positive (Fig. 1.3).

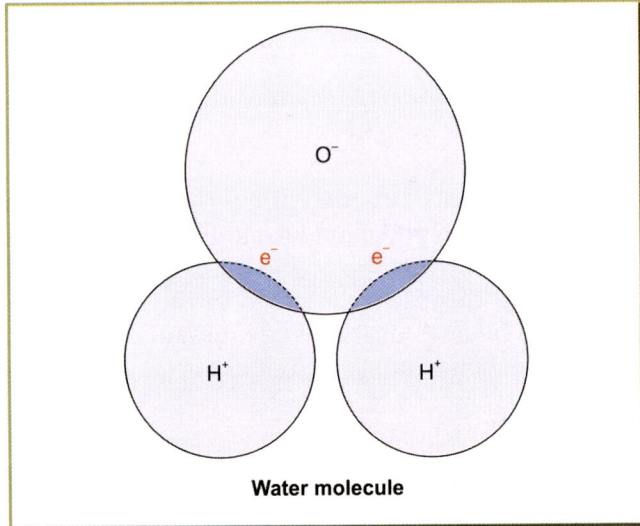

Fig. 1.3: Formation of polar covalent bond.

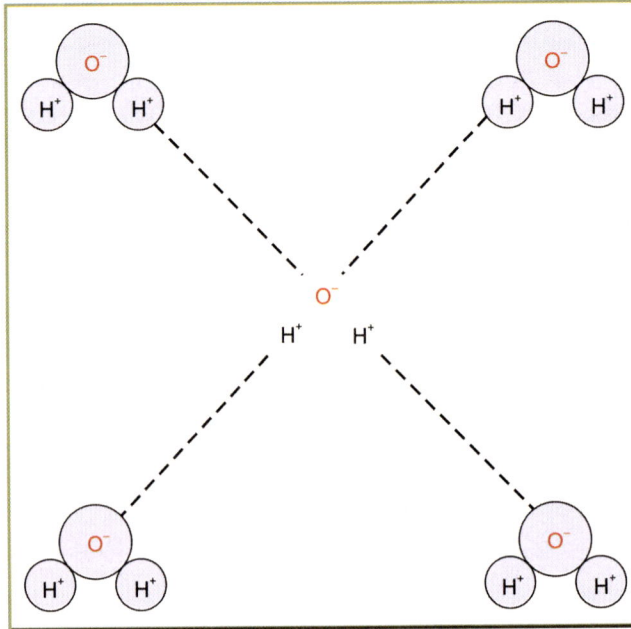

Fig. 1.4: Formation of hydrogen bonds.

Polar bonds allow water to dissolve many molecules that are crucial to life.

Hydrogen Bonds

The oppositely charged regions of different polar molecules can also attract one another. Such a bond, commonly between hydrogen and either oxygen or nitrogen, is called a hydrogen bond. They are weak bonds but since they are present in large numbers, they provide strength and stability to important biomolecules, e.g. water (Fig. 1.4), proteins and nucleic acids.

Chemical linkages are required to form and stabilize various biomolecules which eventually determine the overall molecular and cellular organization (Chapter 2).

SOME IMPORTANT QUESTIONS

1. Differentiate between weak bonds and strong bonds.
2. Write notes on:
   i. Ionic bonds
   ii. van der Waals forces
   iii. Covalent bonds
   iv. Hydrogen bonds

MULTIPLE CHOICE QUESTIONS

1. **The following is chemically a strong linkage:**
   A. Ionic bond
   B. Covalent bond
   C. Hydrophobic interaction
   D. van der Waals forces

2. **van der Waals forces operate over:**
   A. Very short distances
   B. Very long distances
   C. Either of the above
   D. Intermediate distances

3. **Water is a polar molecule because:**
   A. Oxygen repels the shared electrons more strongly
   B. Oxygen attracts the unshared electrons more strongly
   C. Oxygen repels the unshared electrons more strongly
   D. Oxygen attracts the shared electrons more strongly

4. **Hydrogen bonds provide strength and stability to:**
   A. Water   B. Nucleic acids
   C. Proteins   D. All of the above

5. **Hydrophobic interactions arise because:**
   A. Water molecules prefer to interact with each other
   B. Water molecules interact with nonpolar molecules
   C. Nonpolar molecules interact with each other
   D. Water molecules interact with other polar molecules

Structure and Functions of the Cell and Subcellular Entities

MOLECULAR ORGANIZATION

Simple precursors or raw materials such as CO_2, H_2O, NH_3, N_2 and NO_3^- and their derivatives like pyruvate, citrate, succinate, 3-phosphoglycerate, etc. (commonly referred to as metabolites) are required to synthesize basic structural molecules known as building blocks. These include:

- Monosaccharides (Chapter 4)
- Fatty acids and glycerol (Chapter 5)
- Amino acids (Chapter 6)
- Nucleotides (Chapter 7)

Building blocks, either through polymerization or other chemical means, form macromolecules such as polysaccharides, lipids, proteins and nucleic acids. Interaction among macromolecules results in supramolecular complexes, e.g. multienzyme complexes, cytoskeleton, ribosomes, etc. An orderly assembly of such complexes forms various membrane-bound organelles or non-membranous entities (subcellular fractions), all of which are defined within a physical boundary to form a cell (Fig. 2.1).

THE CELL

The cell is a structural and functional unit of life. All animals and plants are made up of a large number of such units, in a manner to the utilization of bricks in the construction of a building. Living cells are divided into two groups, i.e. the prokaryotic cells and the eukaryotic cells. As their name suggests (pro = prior to; karyot = nucleus; eu = true), the fundamental difference between them is the absence or presence of a true nucleus.

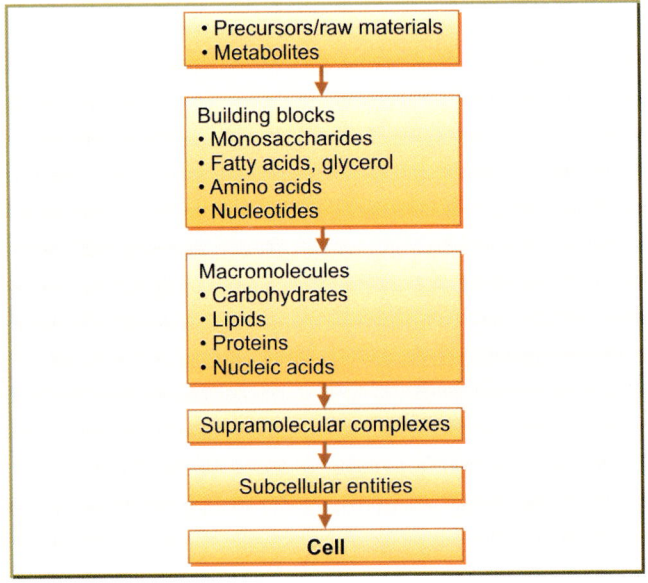

Fig. 2.1: Hierarchy of molecular organization.

Prokaryotic Cells

The simplest form of the cell is a prokaryotic cell. Prokaryotes, e.g. bacteria are unicellular and have one of the three basic shapes, viz. spheroidal (cocci), rodlike (bacilli) and helically-coiled (spirella).

A prokaryotic cell is small (1 to 10 nm), relatively simple in structure and has only a single membrane called cell membrane which is usually surrounded by a rigid cell wall of characteristic structure. There may or may not be a surrounding capsule. Besides, there is a single chromosome comprised of a molecule of double helical DNA which is densely coiled to form a nuclear zone. Reproduction is by asexual division. The

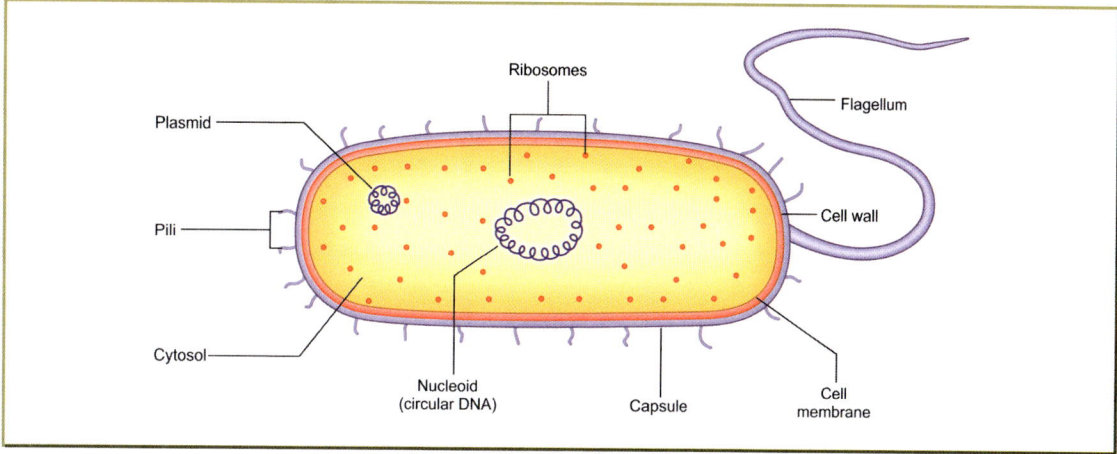

Fig. 2.2: A prokaryotic cell.

best characterised prokaryotic cell is *Escherichia coli*. Some prokaryotes possess pili and flagella for adhesion and movement respectively (Fig. 2.2).

Eukaryotic Cells

Animals, plant, fungi and protozoa are called eukaryotes which may be unicellular as well as multicellular. Eukaryotic cells are one to ten thousand times larger and are more complex in structure than the prokaryotic cells. They may vary from one tissue to another with respect to its function, e.g. the liver parenchymal cell, adipose cell, nerve cell, renal tubular cell, white blood cell, etc.

Generally, a eukaryotic cell has a well-defined membrane-bound nucleus containing several chromosomes. Their chromosomes undergo replication of DNA during mitosis and get separated into daughter chromosomes, i.e. these cells reproduce by cell division.

A typical eukaryotic cell contains various organelles such as a nucleus, endoplasmic reticulum, Golgi apparatus, mitochondria, etc. (Fig. 2.3).

Major differences between prokaryotic and eukaryotic cell structure are given in Table 2.1.

SUBCELLULAR ENTITIES: CELL ORGANELLES AND SUBCELLULAR FRACTIONS

An **organelle** is defined as a subcellular membranous entity which can be isolated by high speed centrifugation. On the other hand, non-membranous entities such as ribosomes, cytoskeleton and cytosol are not subcellular organelles and are better designated as **subcellular fractions**.

Subcellular Fractionation

Functions of different subcellular entities can be studied after their separation and isolation from the cell. The various steps include:

1. *Preparation of tissue homogenate:* The cells are disrupted under mild conditions, e.g. the tissue may be grinded in a pestle and mortar or is homogenized by using a homogenizer. In a homogenizer, a manually operated or motor driven pestle is rotated within a glass tube containing a small piece of the tissue in some suitable solution (an isotonic medium such as 0.25 M sucrose solution, adjusted to pH 7.4, between 0 and 4° C, is commonly used to avoid loss of biological activities). Mechanical force disrupts cells and causes liberation of the cellular constituents into the medium. This is called **tissue homogenate**. Besides homogenization, use of a detergent or osmotic shock can also disrupt plasma membrane.

2. *Differential centrifugation:* Due to the differences in their size and density, various cellular fractions can be separated by centrifugation at variable speeds and timings:
   i. *Low speed centrifugation:* The homogenate is first centrifuged at low speed to separate nuclear fraction which contains the nuclei and the unruptured cells.
   ii. *Intermediate speed centrifugation:* The **supernatant** is thereafter again centrifuged at an

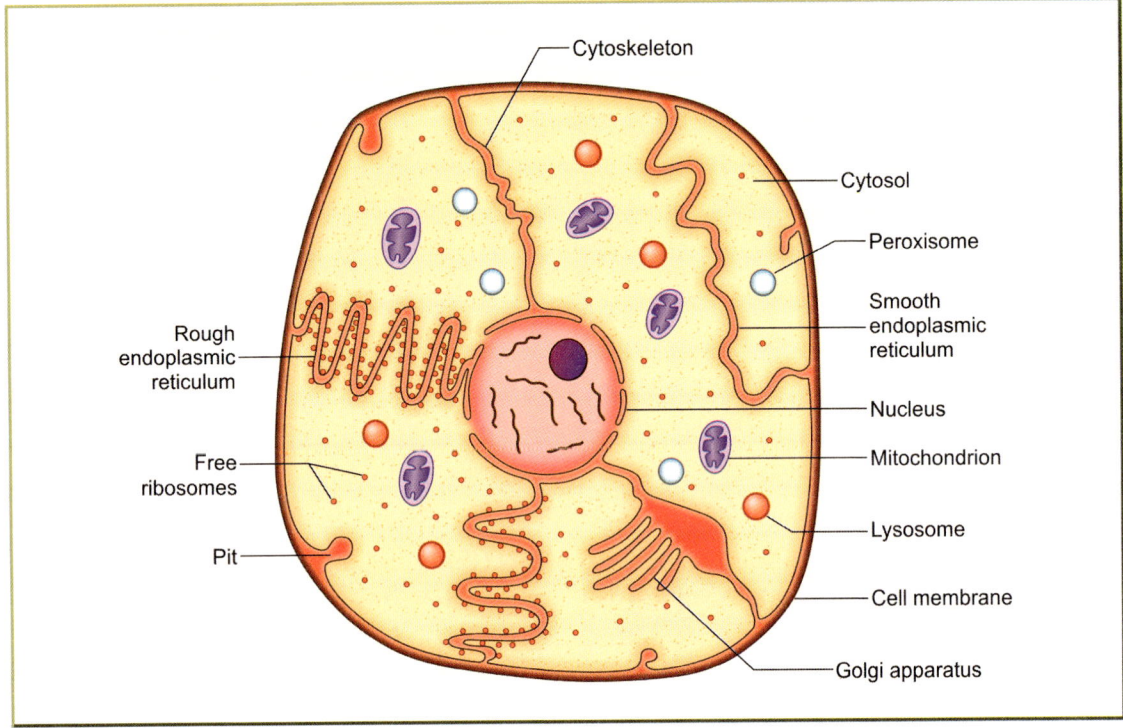

Fig. 2.3: A eukaryotic cell.

Labels in figure: Cytoskeleton, Cytosol, Peroxisome, Smooth endoplasmic reticulum, Nucleus, Mitochondrion, Lysosome, Cell membrane, Golgi apparatus, Rough endoplasmic reticulum, Free ribosomes, Pit

intermediate speed to get mitochondrial fraction, which contains mitochondria, lysosomes and peroxisomes.

iii. *High speed centrifugation (ultracentrifugation):* High speed centrifugation of the left-over supernatant gives the microsomal fraction. The microsomal fraction contains free ribosomes, fragments of the endoplasmic reticulum and the plasma membrane. Therefore, 'endoplasmic reticulum' and 'microsomes' are not synonymous. The former is a distinct organelle in an intact cell whereas the latter contains fragments of the endoplasmic reticulum obtained by ultracentrifugation in a laboratory.

The supernatant, after separation of the microsomal fraction, is a clear solution which corresponds to the cell-sap or cytosol and contains free ribosomes and soluble molecules. It is thus possible to isolate each organelle from most organs and cells in a relatively pure form, by various modifications of this general procedure, i.e. differential centrifugation (Fig. 2.4).

Table 2.1: Major differences between prokaryotic and eukaryotic cell structure

Parameters	Prokaryotic cells	Eukaryotic cells
Cell size	Smaller	Larger
Overall organization	Simple	Complex
Boundary	Cell membrane and cell wall sometimes surrounded by a capsule	Cell membrane
Subcellular entities	Few	Many
Nucleus	Single DNA double helix in a poorly defined region called nucleoid	Well defined nucleus with a membrane and multiple DNA double helices organized into chromatin
Reproduction	Asexual	Sexual
Examples	Bacteria, blue-green algae	Plant and animal cells

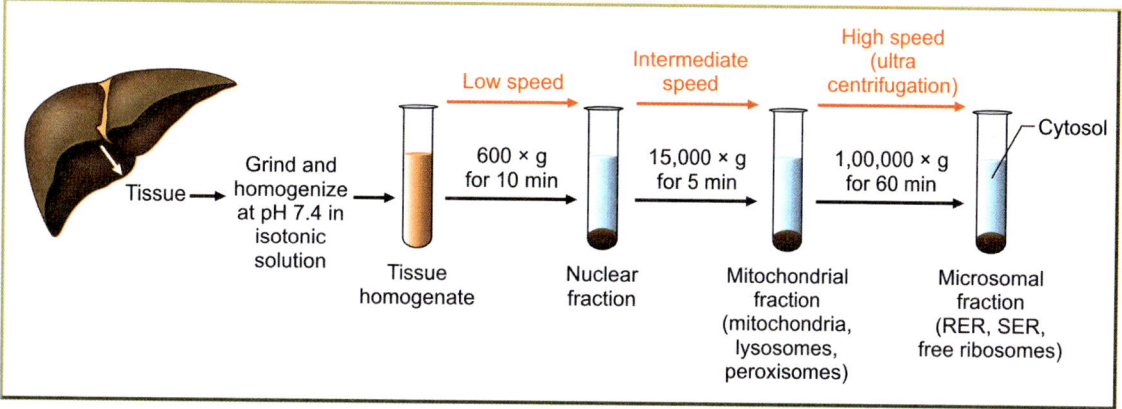

Fig. 2.4: Separation of subcellular fractions by differential centrifugation.

3. *Identification of subcellular entities:* Each entity can be assessed by the measurement of some suitable marker (which is an enzyme or chemical constituent of the particular fraction), either by the use of an electron microscope or by its biochemical estimation. Various intracellular organelles/subcellular fractions, their functions and markers are given in Table 2.2.

Structure and Functions of Subcellular Entities

The Nucleus

The nucleus is the largest component of the cell, containing DNA organized into separate chromosomes, and is surrounded by a membrane called nuclear membrane.

The nuclear membrane or nucleolemma consists of two layers which are separated by an intermembrane space termed perinuclear space (cisterns). The outer membrane though is continuous with the endoplasmic reticulum but the two layers of the nuclear membrane are fused together at several places producing nuclear pores for the exchange of materials between the nucleus and the cytoplasm. The nucleus is filled with nucleoplasm which has a discrete body called nucleolus and a thread-like structure called chromatin (Fig. 2.5).

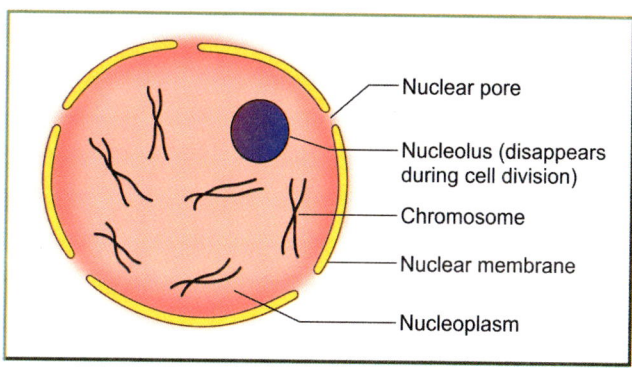

Fig. 2.5: The nucleus.

Table 2.2: Subcellular entities, their functions and biochemical markers

Subcellular entity	Function	Biochemical marker
Cell membrane	Transport across cell membrane, bears receptor and enzymes, cell-cell recognition	Na$^+$/K$^+$-ATPase
Nucleus	DNA replication, cell division, control of RNA and protein synthesis	DNA polymerase
Endoplasmic reticulum	Protein synthesis, lipid metabolism, xenobiotic metabolism	Glucose-6-phosphatase
Golgi apparatus	Post-translational modification of proteins and their sorting	Galactosyl transferase
Mitochondria	ATP synthesis, fatty acid oxidation, Krebs cycle, cytosolic Ca^{2+} regulation	Succinate dehydrogenase, glutamate dehydrogenase
Lysosomes	Intracellular digestion and detoxification	Acid phosphatase
Peroxisomes	Fatty acid oxidation, detoxification of H$_2$O$_2$	Catalase, uric acid oxidase
Cytoplasm	Glycolysis, fatty acid synthesis, bears the cytoskeleton	Lactate dehydrogenase

Nucleolus: The number of nucleoli may vary from one cell type to another. The genes for three of the four ribosomal RNA molecules are located in the nucleolus. Nucleoli are rich in RNA and disappear during cell division.

Chromatin: It contains most of the cellular DNA in association with basic proteins termed histones. At the time of cell division, the chromatin is organized into small thread-like structures called **chromosomes**. Human somatic cell contains 23 pairs of chromosomes. Important functions of nucleus include:

- Control of cell-division (DNA replication).
- Protein synthesis (by controlling the synthesis of RNA).

The regulation of DNA synthesis and other functions of the nucleus are severely disturbed in some pathological conditions, such as cancer.

DNA and **DNA polymerase** are the markers of the nucleus.

The Endoplasmic Reticulum

Endoplasmic reticulum is a system of membranes (lipid bilayer structures) with a network of vesicular spaces. This network is present throughout the cytoplasmic matrix and grows by its own synthesis. These membranes run parallel to each other creating channels which are called cisternae. The interior of the endoplasmic reticulum thus is well connected with perinuclear spaces and through pores on the cell surface, with the extracellular space. Cisternae have a role in the exchange of materials between the cell and the extracellular fluid.

The surface of the endoplasmic reticulum may or may not bear ribosomes. Accordingly, endoplasmic reticulum is of two types:

- *Rough endoplasmic reticulum (RER):* It is also called as the granular type of endoplasmic reticulum since it has small granules attached to it. These granules are termed as ribosomes.

- *Smooth endoplasmic reticulum (SER):* It is also called as the agranular type of endoplasmic reticulum since it consists of the membranous structure only and does not contain ribosomes on its outer surface. The SER has enzymes for the biosynthesis of lipids and glycoproteins. Further, SER are very important in hepatocytes where these are primarily concerned with oxidative metabolism

and for the detoxification of many drugs and other toxic organic molecules.

Glucose-6-phosphatase is a marker enzyme for the endoplasmic reticulum.

The Ribosomes

Ribosomes consist of ribonucleoprotein particles of two sizes, i.e. 50S and 30S in prokaryotes or 60S and 40S in eukaryotes. Because of their high RNA content, ribosomes are the site of protein synthesis. Ribosomes on the RER are associated with the synthesis of proteins for export from the cell. Free ribosomes on the other hand are present in the cytoplasm and synthesize proteins for use within the cell.

RNA is used as a marker for the ribosomes.

The Golgi Apparatus

The Golgi apparatus is a smooth membrane system with vacuoles. It is rich in lipids and is considered to be the site where secretions from other organelles are brought and assembled. The newly synthesized proteins are also transferred from RER and stored in the Golgi apparatus temporarily. Some of the synthesized proteins also undergo post-translational modifications within the Golgi apparatus and thereafter are transported to different destinations. The Golgi apparatus is thus especially active in cells which produce proteins for export. They form secretory granules for the proteins after their synthesis on the ribosomes.

Galactosyl transferase is a marker enzyme for the Golgi apparatus.

Endoplasmic reticulum with Golgi apparatus has a role in the formation of other cellular organelles, such as lysosomes and peroxisomes.

The Mitochondria

The mitochondria are the major organelle of a eukaryotic cell lacking any direct structural relationship with other organelles and contain their own DNA (Fig. 2.6). A mitochondrion produces energy in the form of ATP for the cellular functions and is thus called as a **power house** of the cell. Thus, depending upon energy requirement of the cell, mitochondria may vary in size, shape and number, from cell to cell. Besides producing energy, mitochondria also help to control the level of calcium

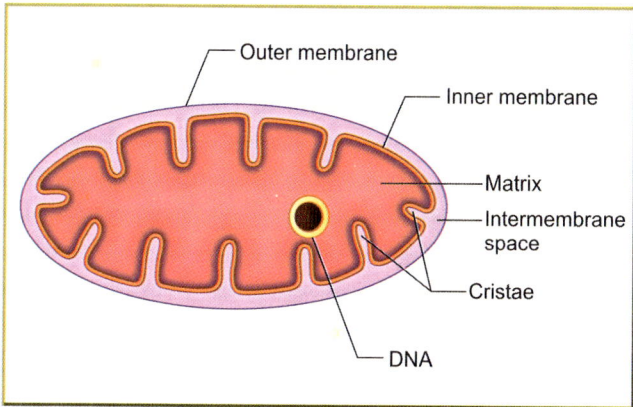

Fig. 2.6: A mitochondrion.

in the cytoplasm. Most of the cells contain several hundred mitochondria.

Mitochondrial membrane: It is a double-layered structure where the two layers are separated from each other by 50–100 Å intermembrane space. Several enzymes especially those involved in the nucleotide metabolism are located here.

- The **outer membrane** of the mitochondria has a smooth structure. It is composed of both lipids and proteins and is freely permeable to most of the small molecules. Several enzymes involved in lipid metabolism such as the enzymes for fatty acid elongation, glycerol phosphate acyltransferase and phospholipase A are associated with the outer membrane of the mitochondria.
- The **inner membrane** of the mitochondria has a denser structure. It has more proteins than lipids. The inner membrane has extensive irregular folding called cristae. Cytochromes, the enzymes of electron transport chain and flavoproteins are localized within the inner membrane of the mitochondria.

Matrix: The intra-mitochondrial space (enclosed within the inner membrane) is called the mitochondrial matrix. This chamber contains enzymes for β-oxidation of fatty acids, for citric acid cycle and glutamate dehydrogenase. In addition, mitochondria also have DNA, referred to as mtDNA.

Succinate dehydrogenase and **glutamate dehydrogenase** are marker enzymes for mitochondria.

Mitochondrial DNA: Mitochondria are the only cellular organelles that contain their own chromosomal DNA (mtDNA), which is maternally inherited. Human mtDNA is a small double-stranded circular

molecule (about 16,000 base pairs), encoding 13 polypeptides that are integrated into the inner mitochondrial membrane along with other polypeptides encoded by nuclear genes. In addition, it encodes 2 rRNAs and 22 tRNAs that are used in protein synthesis within the organelle. mtDNA differs from nuclear DNA in several aspects.

Nuclear DNA versus mitochondrial DNA: In contrast to nuclear DNA, the mtDNA is exposed to high levels of mutagenic free radicals and is not protected by the usual DNA repair mechanisms. This results in mutations in mtDNA that affect mitochondrial structure and function, leading to various muscular and neurological disorders (Chemistry to Clinics 2.1). A comparison between nuclear DNA and mtDNA is given in Table 2.3.

The Lysosomes

The lysosomes are small sac-like organelles surrounded by a membrane. These are intermediary in size between the mitochondria and the microsomes. Lysosomes are rich in all types of hydrolases, such as for carbohydrates, lipids, proteins and nucleic acids since digestion of these macromolecules takes place within the lysosomes. Release of lysosomal enzymes as well as absence of lysosomal enzymes is of clinical importance (Chemistry to Clinics 2.2 and 2.3).

Acid phosphatase is a marker enzyme of the lysosomes.

Age-related pigments: Any foreign particle which enters the cell is completely destroyed by the

Table 2.3: Comparison between nuclear DNA and mitochondrial DNA (mtDNA)

Parameters	Nuclear DNA	mtDNA
Location	Nucleoplasm	Mitochondrial matrix
Inheritance	Both paternal and maternal	Maternal
Shape	Linear	Circular
Base pairs	3×10^9	16×10^3
Introns	Present	Absent
Histones	Present	Absent
Encoded proteins	Used within the cell as well as exported	Used within mitochondria
Repair mechanisms	Well developed	Poorly developed
Mutation rate	Low	High

Chemistry to Clinics 2.2: Suicide Bags

Various hydrolases are enclosed in the lysosomal membrane in such a way that they are not able to result in lysis of their own cells. However, a disruption of the lysosomal membrane leads to the release of lysosomal enzymes. This in turn causes digestion of cellular components leading to their release from the cell. This process is called autolysis. Due to this specific role of lysosomes these are also called suicide bags. Lysosomal enzymes play key roles in phagocytosis, acute and chronic inflammation such as arthritis.

Chemistry to Clinics 2.3: Lysosomal Storage Disorders

Absence of the specific lysosomal enzyme is seen in a number of genetic disorders. This in turn results in accumulation of various cellular components which cannot be digested (hydrolysed) due to inherited deficiency of the lysosomal enzyme. Lysosomes of the affected individuals become enlarged with the undigested material and thus interfere in normal cellular processes. Various such lysosomal disorders are known:

- *Lysosomal acid lipase deficiency:* It results in Wolman's disease in infants, and cholesterol ester storage disease in adults. There is accumulation of triacylglycerol and cholesterol esters in tissues, particularly in the liver.
- *Maltase deficiency:* It results in glycogen storage disease type II.
- *α-Iduronidase deficiency:* It results in Hurler's syndrome with accumulation of glycosaminoglycans.

lysosomal enzymes. The lysosomes are normally active after their fusion with a vacuole. These vacuoles may contain ingested foreign particles, such as dead bacteria and result in their lysis (the process is called heterophagy). Further, in these vacuoles, the destruction of redundant/damaged cellular components such as mitochondria also occurs (the process is called autophagy). If not destroyed, indigestible material gets accumulated in the vesicles which are referred to as residual bodies that may be removed by exocytosis. The residual bodies containing a high concentration of lipids are designated as lipofuscin. Since these residual bodies accumulate in cells of the older individuals, these are also called age-related pigments.

The Peroxisomes

Certain oxidative enzymes, e.g. uric acid oxidase, D-amino acid oxidase and catalase are associated with special organelles called peroxisomes or microbodies. The major function of the peroxisomes is in hepatocytes where these are involved in the oxidation of fatty acids by a modified α-oxidation pathway. Besides, peroxisomes also represent a very primitive cellular organelle which provides protection to the cell from the toxicity of hydrogen peroxide (H_2O_2).

Catalase and **uric acid oxidase** are marker enzymes of the peroxisomes.

Absence of functional peroxisomes results in **Zellweger syndrome**, a rare autosomal recessive disease characterized by abnormalities of several organs due to the decreased levels of plasmalogens.

The Cytosol

The cytosol or cell-sap is a structureless material filling the cell (aqueous matrix) in which all the cellular organelles float. It is a colloidal solution of proteins containing nearly 70% water. Besides proteins, the cytosolic fraction also contains various enzymes for glycolysis, gluconeogenesis and HMP shunt, and a variety of organic as well as inorganic substances such as glucose, potassium and magnesium.

The cytosol is in contact with all the cellular organelles and is an important vehicle for the transport of metabolites from one organelle to the other.

The cytosol of all eukaryotic cells also contains a network of fibres collectively called as the **cytoskeleton** which includes microtubules, intermediate filaments and microfilaments (Chapter 35).

Lactate dehydrogenase is a marker enzyme of the cytosol fraction of the cell.

The Plasma Membrane

Plasma membrane or cell membrane is the outer membrane of the cell. It is in contact with the extracellular matrix. Structure and functions of the cell membrane are described separately (Chapter 3).

STEM CELLS

Cell potency: Stem cells are the **master cells** and potential building blocks of the body because they can change into and thus create all other tissues, organs and systems in the body (Fig. 2.7). This 'changing' is known as differentiation. Thus, 'multipotent' stem cells become 'committed' stem cells once they follow a particular line of differentiation (Table 2.4).

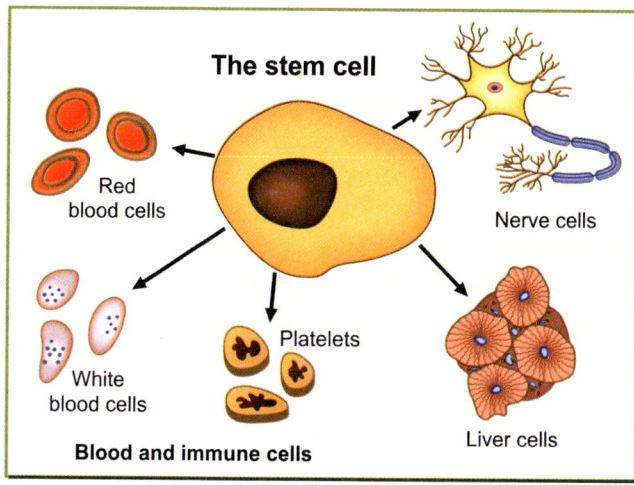

Fig. 2.7: Examples of cells derived from stem cells.

Table 2.4: Stem cell potency

Totipotent stem cells: The zygote and cells derived from it during the first 4 days of conception; give rise to all cell types and even whole organism.

Pluripotent stem cells: Cells of the inner cell mass after 4 days of conception; give rise to all cell types except placenta; cannot form the whole organism.

Multipotent stem cells: Form several cell types restricted to a particular tissue/organ, e.g. hemopoietic stem cells in the bone marrow (forming RBC, WBC and platelets), neuronal stem cells (forming various cells of the nervous system).

Unipotent/committed stem cells: Form a specific cell type, e.g. erythroid progenitor cells, myeloid progenitor cells.

Availability: Stem cells are found in the bone marrow and peripheral blood of adults and the umbilical cord blood of newborn infants. The cord blood cells are preferred because the baby's blood cells have not yet developed their typical set of antigens and because umbilical cord blood lacks well-developed immune cells that usually cause graft-versus-host disease.

In addition to cells with blood-forming potential, few mesenchymal stem cells are also found in bone marrow. These cells can give rise to a large number of tissue cells, such as bone, cartilage, fat and connective tissue cells. However, such adult stem cells may be obtained from any tissue, are capable of self-renewal and are multipotent with the potential to form all cell types in the concerned tissue. Thus, **adult stem cells** are 'undifferentiated cells' in a 'differentiated tissue'.

Stem cell therapy: The possibilities for stem cell therapy are unlimited, once we understand how to control their differentiation into all types of tissue cells:

- The major clinical use of stem cells to date has been to restore a patient's hemopoietic system that has been completely disrupted by radiation or chemotherapy for treatment of leukemia and solid tumors (Chemistry to Clinics 2.4).
- Based on the same principle, patients with AIDS could be supported by periodic infusions of T cell precursors.
- Infusions of neutrophil progenitors would help patients with cancer to recover from aggressive cancer therapy.
- Patients with certain anemias would benefit from infusions of red cell progenitors.
- Platelet progenitors may be used in patients with inborn or acquired thrombocytopenia.
- Treatment of some of the most common degenerative diseases such as Alzheimer's disease, Parkinson's disease, muscular dystrophy, spinal cord injury, stroke, and various liver and cardiac diseases.

Chemistry to Clinics 2.4: Stem Cell-based Hematotherapy

Traditionally, in bone marrow transplantation, the entire hematopoietic system of the recipient, including the most primitive multipotent stem cells, is ablated and restored with cells from the donor. However, using stem cell-based 'hematotherapy' (Fig. 2.8), only the specific committed stem cells are transplanted that develop along specific lineages into the mature cells that are nonfunctional in a patient with a particular disease. The healthy portion of the patient's hemopoietic system is thus kept intact.

2

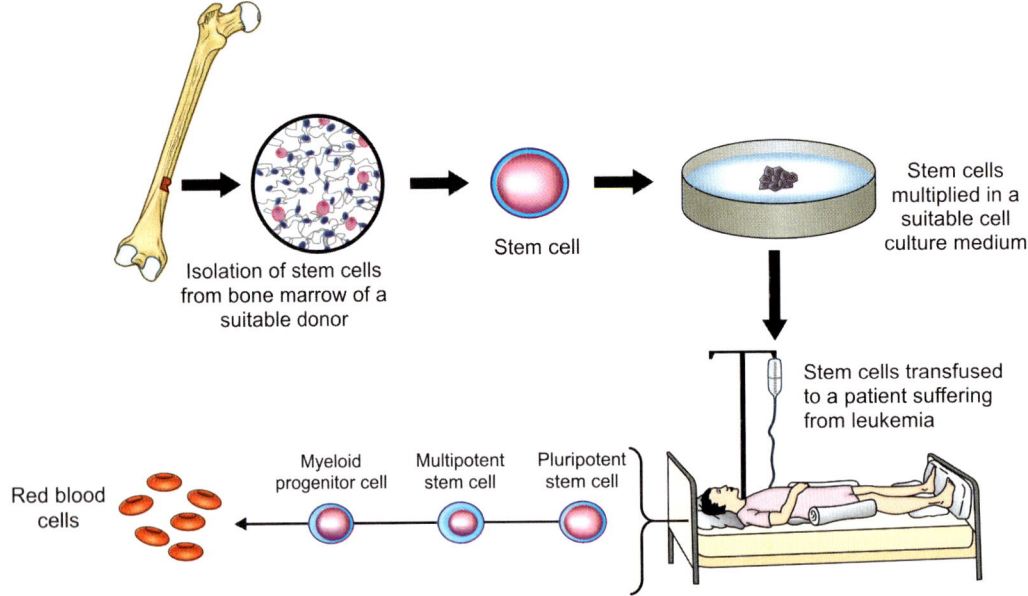

Fig. 2.8: A patient received treatment for leukemia (tumor of white blood cells) due to which his red blood cell count dropped resulting in severe anemia. By selecting a suitable donor and using **stem cell-based hematotherapy,** the red blood cells are restored.

Role of molecular biology: The clinical potential of stem cell therapy can be enhanced by combining traditional stem cell harvesting methods with modern molecular biology methods. Therapeutic cloning might enable the creation of embryonic stem cells that are genetically identical to the patients' cells. Embryonic stem cells are highly desirable to work with because they have the capacity to become any mature cell (totipotency). Existing stem cells can be genetically manipulated by replacing a defective or missing gene.

Demerits of stem cell therapy: One limitation for the use of stem cells lies in the problem of avoiding tumor growth because stem cells are naturally programmed to divide. Additionally, the benefits of stem cell therapy must be carefully balanced with ethical and social concerns.

SOME IMPORTANT QUESTIONS

1. **Describe structure, functions, isolation and biochemical markers of various subcellular entities of a eukaryotic cell.**

2. **Explain:**
   i. Mitochondria as a power house of the cell.
   ii. Functions of the rough endoplasmic reticulum.
   iii. Difference between nuclear and mitochondrial DNA.
   iv. Molecular organization.

3. **Write notes on:**
   i. The nucleus
   ii. Ribosomes
   iii. The Golgi apparatus
   iv. Matrix

   v. Suicide bags
   vi. Age-pigments
   vii. Lysosomal disorders

4. **Biomedical importance of stem cells.**

MULTIPLE CHOICE QUESTIONS

1. **The following is not a true organelle:**
   A. Ribosome
   B. Mitochondrion
   C. Lysosome
   D. Nucleus

2. **Galactosyltransferase is the biomarker for the following subcellular entity:**
   A. Cell membrane
   B. Cytoplasm
   C. Golgi apparatus
   D. Endoplasmic reticulum

3. **Glucose-6-phosphatase is the biomarker for the following subcellular entity:**
   A. Cell membrane
   B. Cytoplasm
   C. Golgi apparatus
   D. Endoplasmic reticulum

4. **Protein synthesis occurs in:**
   A. Ribosomes only
   B. Mitochondria only
   C. Ribosomes and mitochondria
   D. Smooth endoplasmic reticulum and mitochondria

5. **Protein sorting occurs in:**
   A. Golgi apparatus
   B. Endoplasmic reticulum
   C. Cell membrane
   D. Mitochondria

6. **Mitochondrial DNA is:**
   A. Paternally inherited and more prone to mutations than nuclear DNA
   B. Paternally inherited and less prone to mutations than nuclear DNA
   C. Maternally inherited and more prone to mutations than nuclear DNA
   D. Maternally inherited and less prone to mutations than nuclear DNA

7. **Membrane folds called cristae are associated with:**
   A. Outer nuclear membrane
   B. Inner nuclear membrane
   C. Outer mitochondrial membrane
   D. Inner mitochondrial membrane

8. **'Suicide bags' refer to:**
   A. Lysosomes   B. Peroxisomes
   C. Ribosomes   D. Nucleus

9. **Zellweger syndrome is due to absence or loss of functions of:**
   A. Lysosomes
   B. Peroxisomes
   C. Ribosomes
   D. Endoplasmic reticulum

10. **The ideal source for obtaining stem cells is:**
    A. Adult peripheral blood
    B. Adult bone marrow
    C. Neonatal peripheral blood
    D. Umbilical cord blood

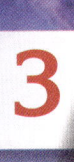

Biological Membranes and Translocation Systems

3

All living cells are surrounded by a highly viscous yet flexible structure called **cell membrane** which, in animal cells, is also called as the **plasma membrane**. In addition to the cell membrane, eukaryotic cells also contain internal membrane systems (nuclear membrane, mitochondrial membrane, lysosomal membrane, etc.) which form specialized compartments within the cell. Cell membrane and other membranes are collectively referred to as **biological membranes** that determine which substances are to enter or exit from the enclosed region.

COMPOSITION OF A BIOLOGICAL MEMBRANE

Biological membranes are composed of lipids, proteins and carbohydrates. Different membranes within the cell and between cells, however, have different composition (Fig. 3.1).

Lipids

Lipids form >50% of the total membrane constituents. Membrane lipids comprise both hydrophobic as well as hydrophilic regions, and thus are termed as **amphipathic** molecules. Lipids have a polar head group and a nonpolar tail (Fig. 3.2). Fatty acids present in the tail are both saturated as well as unsaturated.

Phospholipids form the major proportion of the lipid component of cell membranes (Fig. 3.3). Besides, **free/unesterified cholesterol** is also present.

There are also qualitative differences between the classes of lipids and the individual lipids in different membranes within the cell as well as between the cells, e.g. plasma membrane has higher concentration of cholesterol and sphingolipids while intracellular membranes primarily contain glycerophospholipids with little sphingolipids or cholesterol.

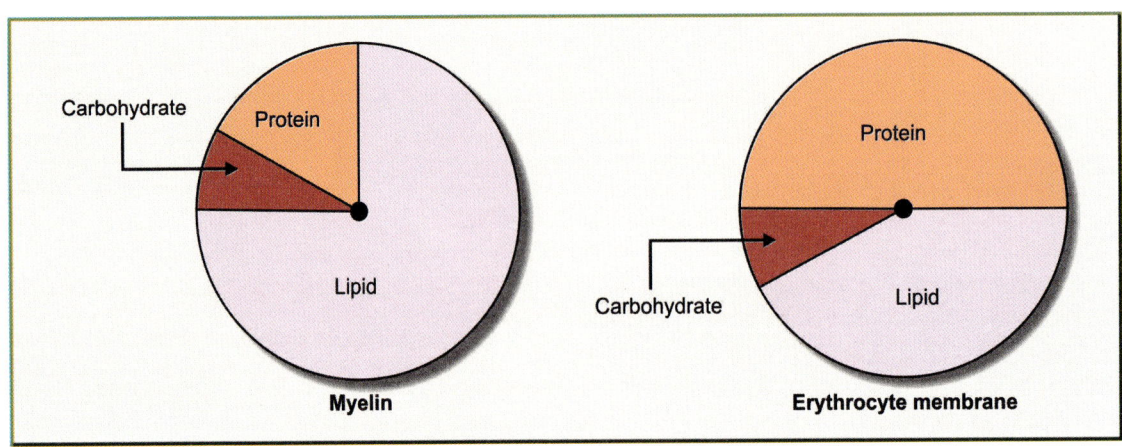

Fig. 3.1: Composition of biological membranes.

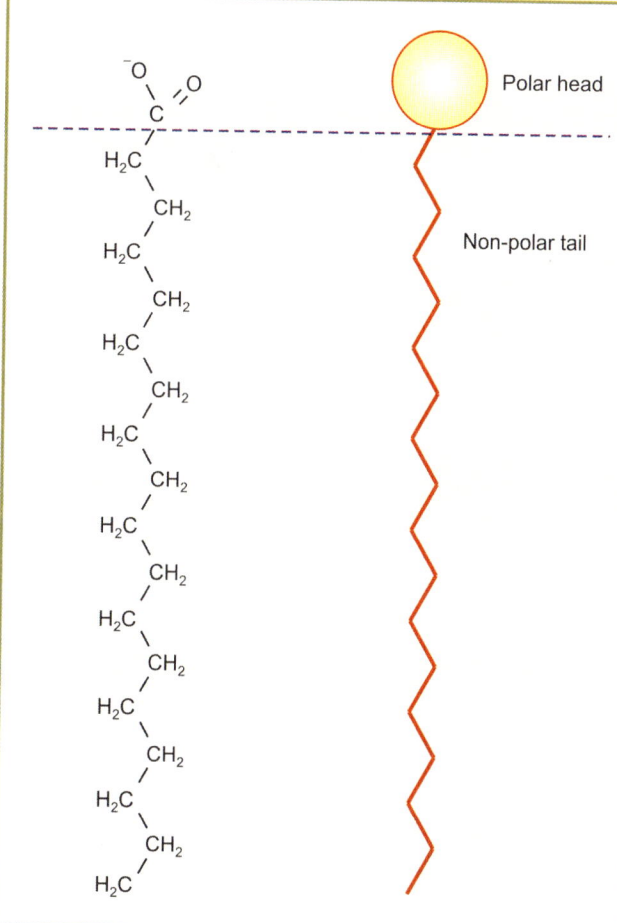

Fig. 3.2: A fatty acid.

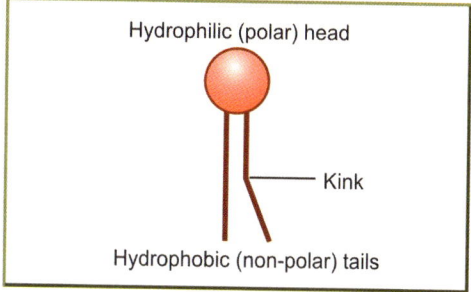

Fig. 3.3: A phospholipid.

In an aqueous solution, amphiphilic molecules form structurally ordered aggregates, such as micelles and bilayers, which form the structural basis of biological membranes.

Micelles: A micelle is a spheroidal aggregate where a large number of amphiphilic molecules, e.g. soaps and detergents, are arranged in such a way that their

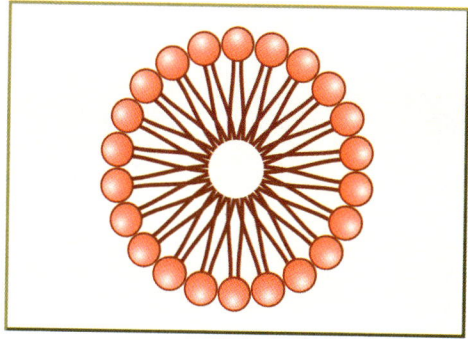

Fig. 3.4: A micelle.

hydrophilic groups (at the globular surface) interact with the aqueous solvent while the hydrophobic groups are associated at the centre, i.e. away from the solvent (Fig. 3.4). Micelles are formed when the cross-section of the hydrophilic head group exceeds that of the hydrophobic tails. This molecular arrangement eliminates unfavourable contact between water and hydrophobic tails of amphiphiles.

Lipid bilayers: Bilayers are formed when the cross-section of the hydrophilic head group of amphiphilic lipids equals that of the hydrophobic tails. Lipid bilayers are the key structures in biological membranes. A lipid bilayer exists as a sheet, i.e. an expanded planer-aggregate, in which hydrophobic regions of phospholipids are protected from the aqueous environment while the hydrophilic regions are immersed in water (Fig. 3.5).

These are extremely stable structures which are held together by noncovalent interactions of the hydrocarbon chains and ionic interactions of the charged head groups with water. Lipophilic molecules such as cholesterol intercalate between fatty acyl residues of phospholipids and have minimal contact with the aqueous phase.

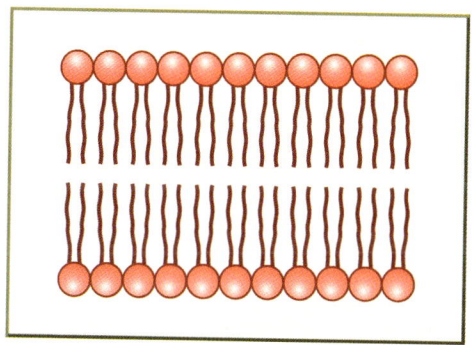

Fig. 3.5: A lipid bilayer.

3

A lipid bilayer when closes on itself and forms a spherical vesicle which separates the external environment from the internal compartment is called a liposome.

Preparation: A variety of techniques have been devised for the synthesis of liposomes in a laboratory. These can be prepared by using synthetic phospholipids or lipids extracted from natural membranes suspended in an aqueous solvent and subjected to very high frequency ultrasonic waves.

Types: Depending on the preparation technique employed, liposomes may either be bound by a single lipid bilayer (**unilamellar liposomes**) or may consist of more than one concentric lipid layers alternating with aqueous layers (**multilamellar liposomes**) (Fig. 3.6).

Properties
1. Closed, self-sealing, solvent-filled vesicles formed from a suspension of phospholipids (glycerophospholipids or sphingomyelins) with or without cholesterol.
2. Usually have a diameter of 20–200 nm, and in a given preparation, are uniform in size.
3. Non-toxic.
4. Biodegradable.

Significance
1. The outer structures of liposomes are similar to a biological membrane. Thus, liposomes serve as models of biological membranes.
2. When administered intravenously, liposomes are absorbed by many cells through fusion with the plasma membrane. This has a profound clinical application because the technique can be used to deliver those compounds to a patient which cannot be absorbed when administered orally. Thus, they are used as vehicles for drug delivery, e.g. liposomal Amphotericin B is commercially available for the treatment of systemic fungal infections in immunocompromised patients. Liposomes have also been prepared with enzymes and DNA.
3. A major problem associated with liposomes is their nonspecific uptake by the reticuloendothelial system following intravenous administration. This can be circumvented by a two-fold strategy: firstly, by coating them with specific ligands so that they are targeted to the tissue bearing the cognate receptors, and secondly, by incorporating polyethylene glycol in the bilayer which avoids uptake by the reticuloendothelial system. Such liposomes act as 'homing devices' for the encapsulated molecules including drug(s). It also minimizes the side effects of the drug(s).

Liposomes are a special type of vesicles surrounded by lipid bilayer and are of clinical significance (Chemistry to Clinics 3.1).

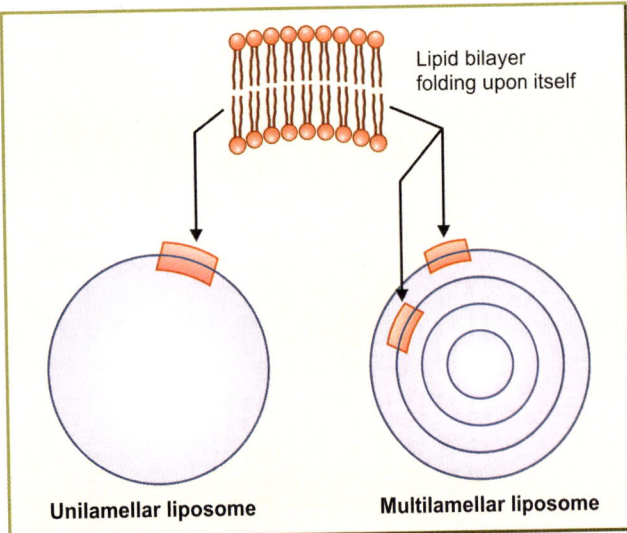

Fig. 3.6: Liposomes.

Proteins

Proteins form another major portion of the membrane and play several roles such as the structural components, transport systems, enzymes and recognition sites for hormones. Protein concentration varies from about 20% in the myelin sheath to about 80% in the inner membrane of the mitochondria.

Membrane proteins are classified by their mode of interaction with the membrane, as integral membrane proteins, peripheral membrane proteins and lipid-linked proteins (Fig. 3.7).

Integral membrane proteins: These proteins have the following characteristics:
- Span the cell membrane from one side to the other.
- Also called **transmembrane proteins** or **intrinsic proteins**.
- Amphiphilic molecules tightly bound to the membrane by hydrophobic interactions.
- Some proteins contain α-helical structure consisting primarily of hydrophobic amino acids. This, in

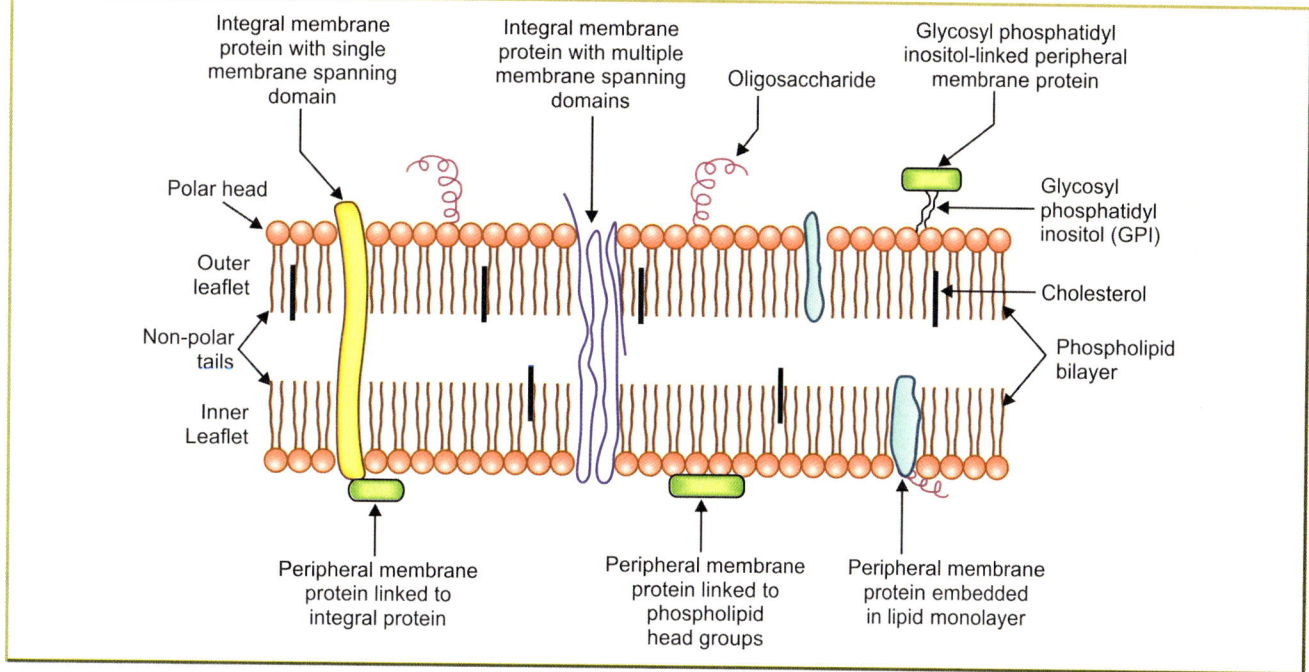

Fig. 3.7: Fluid-mosaic model of biological membrane.

turn, forms a transmembrane sequence which has three domains, i.e. a sequence exterior to the cell containing the $-NH_2$ terminal end, a transmembrane sequence and a sequence extending into the cell with the $-COOH$ terminal end.

- Can be separated from the membrane only by drastic treatment with certain agents that disrupt membranes, such as organic solvents or detergents.
- *Example:* **Glycophorin A**, which spans the erythrocyte membrane.

Peripheral membrane proteins: These proteins have the following characteristics:

- Proteins which are embedded on any one side of the membrane.
- Also called **extrinsic proteins**.
- Immersed in the membrane only partially and are weakly bound to the hydrophilic region of the specific integral proteins.
- May have various modes of attachment: Some bind to integral proteins, such as an antigen. On the other hand, some peripheral proteins such as cytochrome b_5, have sequences of hydrophobic amino acids at one end of the peptide chain which serve as an anchor in the membrane lipid.

- Can be released by relatively mild procedures that leave the membrane intact, such as by treatment with a salt solution of high ionic strength or by extremes of pH.
- *Example:* **Cytochrome c**, in the outer surface of the inner mitochondrial membrane.

Lipid-linked proteins: These proteins have the following characteristics:

- Membrane-associated proteins containing covalently attached lipids.
- Lipids anchor proteins to the membrane and thus mediate protein-protein interaction or modify structure and activity of the protein to which these are attached.
- Removal of the lipid fraction from these proteolipids leads to denaturation of the membrane proteins and loss of their biological functions.
- *Example:* **Lipophilin** present in the myelin.

Carbohydrates

Some of the membrane proteins and lipids bear short chains of carbohydrates (oligosaccharides), covalently attached either to a protein (**glycoprotein**) or to a lipid **(glycolipid)** (Fig. 3.7). Carbohydrate content of biological membranes varies between 3 and 10%. Oligosaccharide chains are normally located on the outer surface of the membrane or on the terminal side of the endoplasmic reticulum.

STRUCTURE OF A BIOLOGICAL MEMBRANE: FLUID-MOSAIC MODEL

As described above, the **lipid bilayer** forms the structural basis of a biological membrane. Some proteins span the lipid bilayer whereas others are only immersed partially. This is called as the **fluid-mosaic model** because the membrane is **fluid** in consistency, consisting of a **mosaic** of proteins and lipids which are **free to drift** about in the plane of the membrane (Fig. 3.7). The model has the following characteristics:

- Sheet-like structure forming a closed boundary; thickness ≈ 7–10 nm.
- Non-covalent, asymmetric assemblies of amphiphilic lipids and proteins.
- Electrically polarized (inside negative with respect to outside).
- Membrane fluidity is regulated by:
  i. The presence of unsaturated fatty acids. Since *cis*-double bonds cause fatty acyl chains to bend (i.e. form kink), the membrane thus becomes less tightly packed and therefore is more fluid in nature (Figs 3.3. and 3.7).
  ii. *The degree of unsaturation of fatty acids:* Higher the unsaturation more is the fluidity.
  iii. Ca^{2+} (increased Ca^{2+} decreases membrane fluidity).
  iv. Cholesterol content of the biomembrane.

Cholesterol and membrane fluidity: Cholesterol is made up of three basic chemical parts that interact with the biological membrane:

1. The steroid nucleus which intercalates between phospholipid hydrocarbon tails.
2. A long hydrocarbon chain located in the non-polar core.
3. The hydroxyl group that interacts with the polar head groups of phospholipids.

At high temperature, cholesterol prevents lateral movement of phospholipid hydrocarbon tails thereby preventing an abnormal rise in membrane fluidity. At low temperature, it prevents the close packaging

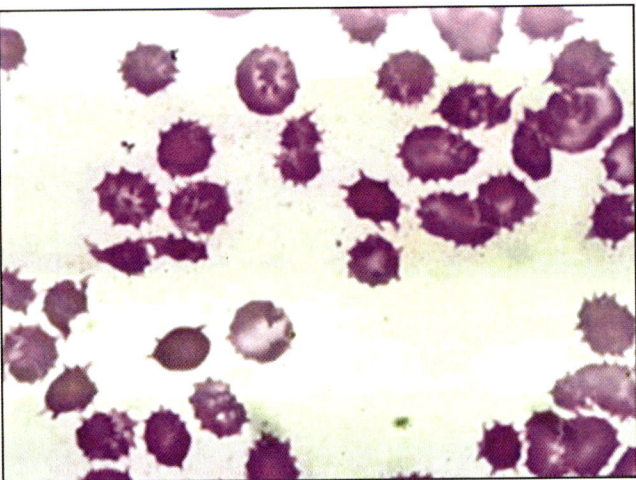

Fig. 3.8: Spur cells or acanthocytes: Red blood cells with multiple irregularly distributed, thorn-like spicules often with drumstick ends, projecting from the cell membrane. These biomembranes have an abnormally high cholesterol content derived from cholesterol-rich plasma lipoproteins.

of the same hydrocarbon tails thereby preventing an abnormal fall in membrane fluidity. Hence, it is aptly said that **cholesterol 'modulates' membrane fluidity**. Abnormally high membrane cholesterol is observed in **spur cells** (Fig. 3.8).

FUNCTIONS OF A BIOLOGICAL MEMBRANE

1. *Compartmentalization:* It separates two different microenvironments, e.g. the cell membrane separates the intracellular compartment from the extracellular matrix or extracellular fluid.
2. *Cell shape:* Plasma membrane proteins have a structural role, i.e. maintain shape of the cell and define its boundaries.
3. *Cell movement:* Specific arrangement of plasma membrane proteins is critical in controlling the movements of some cells, e.g. movement of neutrophils from the intravascular to the extra-vascular compartment requires a change in cell shape as well as movement, known as diapedesis.
4. *Enzymes:* Many of the membrane proteins are enzymes and are located either within or on the cell membrane. The inner mitochondrial membrane is essential for localization and correct orientation of the respiratory enzymes within it for their maximum efficiency. The membrane of the endoplasmic reticulum plays an important role in localizing lipophilic substrates for their oxidation by the enzymes present therein.

5. *Receptor molecules:* Membrane proteins act as recognition sites, such as hormone receptors for insulin or glucagon or immunoreceptors present on B lymphocytes for the recognition and response to foreign antigens, etc.

6. *Translocation of substances:* Membrane proteins regulate translocation of molecules, such as amino acids, glucose and various ions.

7. *Signal transduction:* Various membrane proteins help in the transmission of signals, such as transmission of nerve impulses.

MEMBRANE TRANSLOCATION

'Translocation' versus 'transport': As a general rule, the term 'translocation' should be used to describe any type of transmembrane movement irrespective of the size of the substance to be moved. Further, it may or may not require a 'helper', located in the membrane itself. However, when such a helper or 'transporter' is required, the process should be called 'transport'.

MEMBRANE TRANSLOCATION SYSTEMS

The translocation may or may not require the formation of a membrane-bound vesicle; accordingly, the translocation may be **vesicular or non-vesicular** (Fig. 3.9).

Functional Mechanisms of Translocation

Translocation of a substance across the cell membrane can be described, in a functional sense, according to the number of molecules transported and the direction of their movement (Fig. 3.10):

Uniport: The process which allows the movement of one type of molecules in only one direction, e.g. glucose uptake in erythrocytes.

Cotransport: The process where transfer of one solute depends upon the simultaneous or sequential transfer of the other. It includes:

- *Symport:* Two types of molecules when move in the same direction, it is called as symport, e.g. the Na^+ glucose transporter-1 (SGLT1) or the Na^+ amino acid transporter in the cells lining the small intestine and proximal renal tubules.

- *Antiport:* Two types of molecules when move in the opposite direction, it is called as antiport, e.g. the Na^+-K^+ antiport, the Na^+-Ca^{2+} transporter and the Cl^-–HCO_3^- antiport.

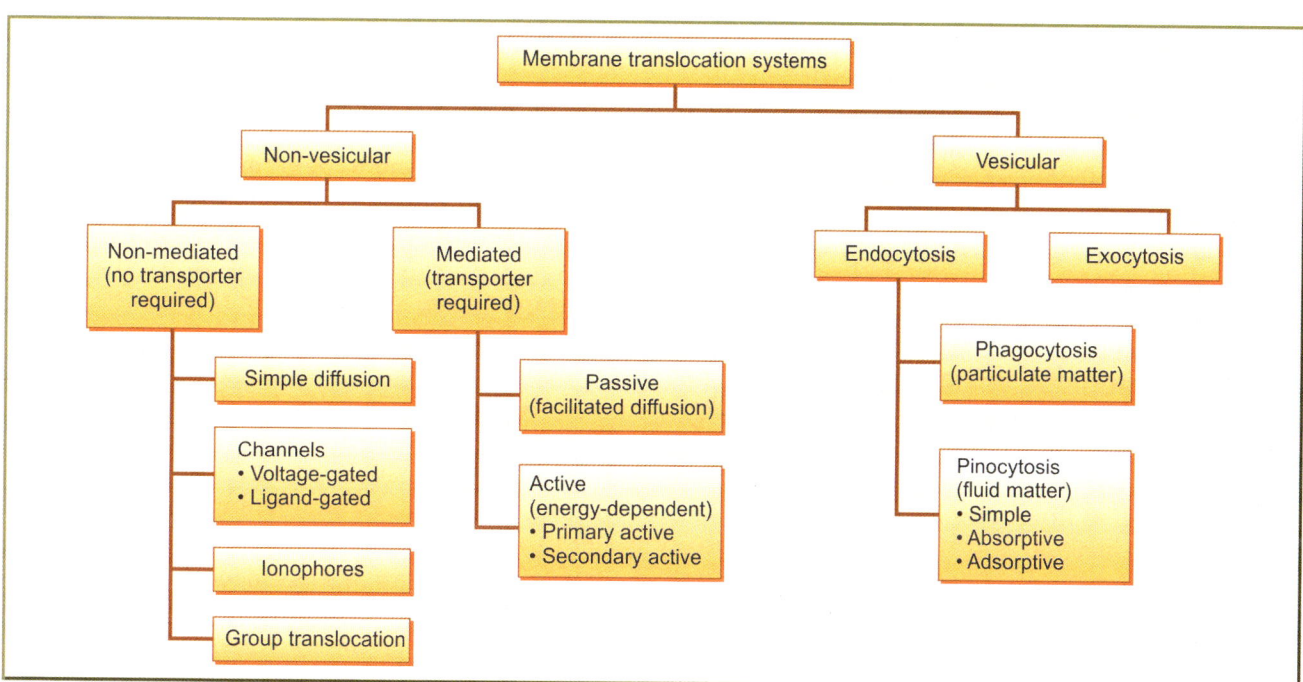

Fig. 3.9: Membrane translocation systems.

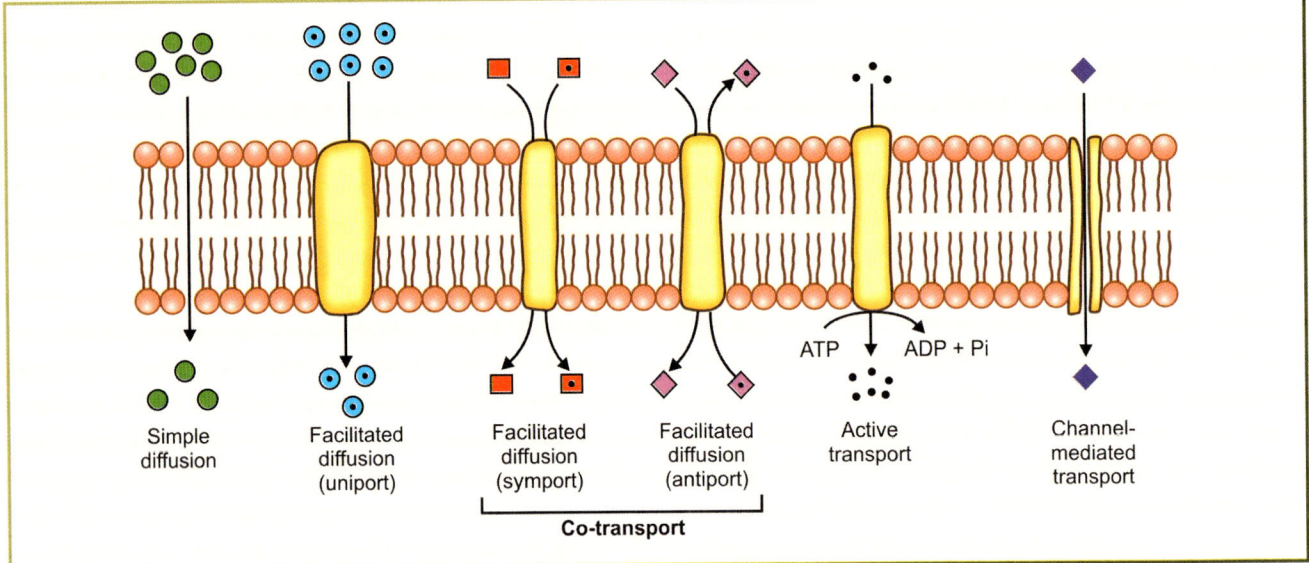

Fig. 3.10: Types of membrane translocation.

NON-VESICULAR TRANSLOCATION SYSTEMS

These are of two types, i.e. the non-mediated translocation system and the mediated translocation system (Fig. 3.9).

NON-MEDIATED TRANSLOCATION

- Some solutes (O_2, N_2, CO_2, NO, urea, etc.) move across the cell membrane by diffusing down an electrochemical gradient and do not require metabolic energy. This, passive non-mediated translocation is called **simple diffusion**.
- It is limited by the thermal agitation of the specific molecule, by the concentration gradient across the membrane, and by its solubility in the hydrophobic core of the membrane bilayer. Electrolytes, since are poorly soluble in lipids, acquire a shell of water by electrostatic interaction. The size of the shell is directly proportional to the charge density of the electrolytes. For example, electrolytes with a large charge density have a larger shell of hydration and thus a slower diffusion rate.
- The direction of flow is always **from a higher to a lower concentration** and the net movement of a molecule from one side to the other continues until concentration on each side is at chemical equilibrium.
- Diffusion of a substance may also occur through membrane channels or pores.

Channels

- Pore-like structures **formed by integral membrane proteins**.
- Permit rapid movement of specific ions or molecules from one side of membrane to the other (Fig. 3.10).
- The permeability of a channel depends upon the size, the extent of hydration, and the charge density on the ion.
- Specific channels exist for Na^+, K^+, Ca^{2+}, Cl^-, etc. These channels are **very selective** and permit the passage of only one type of ions.
- Channels are opened transiently, i.e. they are gated. The channel opening and closing involves a change in the voltage/membrane potential (**voltage-gated channel**) or the binding of a chemical agent (**ligand-gated channel**) (Table 3.1).
- Sometimes, one ion can regulate the activity of the other ion, e.g. a decrease in Ca^{2+} ion concentration in the extracellular fluid increases membrane permeability and diffusion of Na^+. This, in turn, depolarizes the membrane and triggers nerve discharge.
- A number of pharmacologic agents that modulate these channels are used therapeutically.
- Mutations in genes encoding polypeptide constituents of ion channel may lead to certain diseases termed as **channelopathies**, e.g.

Table 3.1: Types of ion channels

Channel	Responsive factor
Voltage-gated	Change in membrane potential, e.g. Na^+, K^+ and Ca^{2+} channels in the heart
Ligand-gated	• A specific extracellular molecule, such as acetylcholine for the acetylcholine receptor channel of the neuromuscular junction.
	• A specific intracellular molecule, e.g. cAMP for Ca^{2+} channels in myocytes.

Chemisty to Clinics 3.2: Channelopathies

1. *Myasthenia gravis:* It is an acquired autoimmune disease characterized by muscle weakness due to decreased neuromuscular signal transmission. Autoantibodies against acetylcholine receptors accelerate their turnover and reduce their number. Acetylcholinesterase-inhibitor drugs are given to enhance the stay of acetylcholine at the neuromuscular junction. Ultimately, the patients require the removal of the culprit antibodies from the plasma at regular intervals, a process called 'plasmapheresis'.

2. *Cystic fibrosis:* It though is a multiorgan disease but its gene product is a cystic fibrosis transmembrane conductance regulator (CFTR), which is a cAMP-dependent Cl^- channel. Patients have reduced membrane permeability which impairs fluid and electrolyte secretion and leads to luminal dehydration.

myasthenia gravis and cystic fibrosis (Chemistry to Clinics 3.2).

Movement of water across biological membranes— aquaporins: Water can move rapidly in and out of cells, but the partition coefficient of water into lipids is low; therefore, the permeability of the membrane lipid bilayer for water is also low. Specific membrane proteins that function as water channels explain the rapid movement of water across the plasma membrane. These water channels are small (M_r nearly 30 kDa), integral membrane proteins known as **aquaporins** (**AQP**). Many different forms have been discovered so far; at least six forms are expressed in cells in the kidneys (Chemistry to Clinics 3.3) and seven forms in the gastrointestinal tract, tissues in which water movement across plasma membranes is particularly rapid.

Ionophores

Besides channels, the other transmembrane route for the non-mediated translocation is through ionophores, whose features include:

Chemistry to Clinics 3.3: Nephrogenic Diabetes Insipidus

In the kidneys, aquaporin-2 (AQP2) channels are abundant in the distal and collecting tubules and are the target of the hormone arginine vasopressin, also known as antidiuretic hormone (ADH). This hormone increases water transport in the tubules by stimulating the insertion of AQP2 proteins into the apical plasma membrane. AQP2 plays a critical role in inherited and acquired disorders of water reabsorption by the kidney. For example, diabetes insipidus is a condition in which the kidney loses its ability to reabsorb water properly, resulting in excessive loss of water and excretion of a large volume of very dilute urine (polyuria). Although inherited forms of diabetes insipidus are relatively rare, it can develop in patients receiving chronic lithium therapy for psychiatric disorders, giving rise to the term lithium-induced polyuria. Both of these conditions are associated with a decrease in the number of AQP2 proteins in the collecting ducts of the kidney and are therefore called nephrogenic diabetes insipidus.

- These are small organic molecules such as antibiotics which are synthesized by some bacteria and function as shuttles.
- Ionophores **increase permeability of the membrane to a particular ion** by binding the ion, diffusing it through the membrane and releasing it on the other side. To ensure the net transport, uncomplexed ionophores return to the original side of the membrane and are ready to repeat the process.
- Because of their ability to complex specific ions and facilitate their transport, ionophores contain hydrophilic centres for ion-binding and are surrounded by peripheral hydrophobic regions. This allows the molecules to dissolve effectively in the membrane and diffuse through it. The net diffusion of a substance thus depends upon:
  1. Its concentration gradient across the membrane.
  2. The electric potential across the membrane.
  3. The permeability coefficient of the substance for the membrane.
  4. The hydrostatic pressure gradient across the membrane, and
  5. Temperature.
- Each ionophore, e.g. valinomycin or nigericin has definite ion specificity. **Valinomycin** translocates K^+ by an electronegative import mechanism. **Nigericin** is an electrically neutral antiporter which translocates K^+ in exchange for H^+ across the membrane.

Group Translocation

Principle: Group translocation involves chemical modification of the transported substrate. The **γ-glutamyl cycle (Meister cycle)** transports **amino acids** across the plasma membrane. During the translocation, the substrate (amino acid) undergoes alteration and is released into the cell as a different molecule.

Mechanism: The pathway involves the membrane-bound enzyme γ-glutamyl transpeptidase (γ-GT). The amino acid transported is the substrate to which the γ-glutamyl residue of glutathione (GSH), a tripeptide, is transferred. This leads to the formation of a dipeptide containing γ-glutamyl residue of GSH with the transported amino acid. The dipeptide, γ-glutamyl amino acid, is transported into the cell and the complex is then hydrolyzed by a separate cytosolic enzyme to liberate the free amino acid. Glutamate is released as 5-oxoproline while cysteinylglycine is cleaved to its component amino acids (Fig. 3.11).

Salient Features

- Group translocation is especially active in renal epithelial cells, liver and enterocytes.
- All amino acids except proline can be transported by group translocation.
- Rapid process.
- High capacity.

- *Energetically expensive:* The energy for the transport comes from the hydrolysis of a peptide bond in GSH. For the system to continue, GSH must be resynthesized which requires 3 molecules of ATP. Hence, for each amino acid translocated across the membrane, 3 ATP are used.

CARRIER-MEDIATED TRANSPORT

Molecules that cannot freely diffuse through the membrane by themselves, need to be transported in association with specific carrier molecules/transport proteins.

Salient Features of a Transport Protein

- Carrier molecules (variously designated as carriers, permeases, porters, **translocases or transporters**), behave much like enzymes.
- Have a high degree of **structural stereospecificity** for the substances to be transported.
- Demonstrate **saturation kinetics**, i.e. when binding sites on all the transport proteins are occupied, the system is saturated and the rate of transport reaches a plateau.
- Can be **inhibited** by both competitive and noncompetitive inhibitors. The inhibition can prevent transport by blocking the binding sites or by interacting with the transport protein and altering its conformation so that it becomes non-functional.

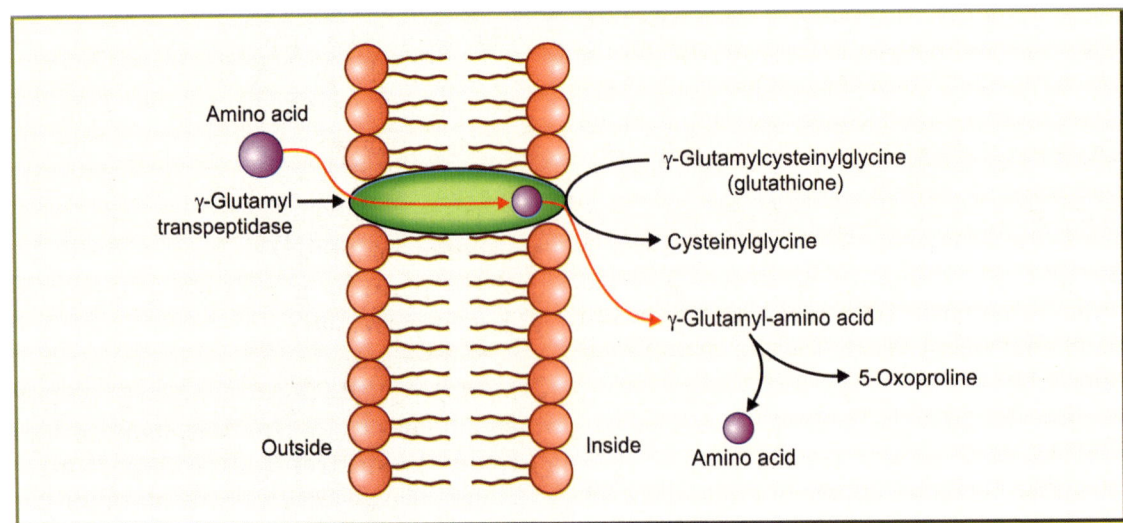

Fig. 3.11: Group translocation (γ-glutamyl cycle).

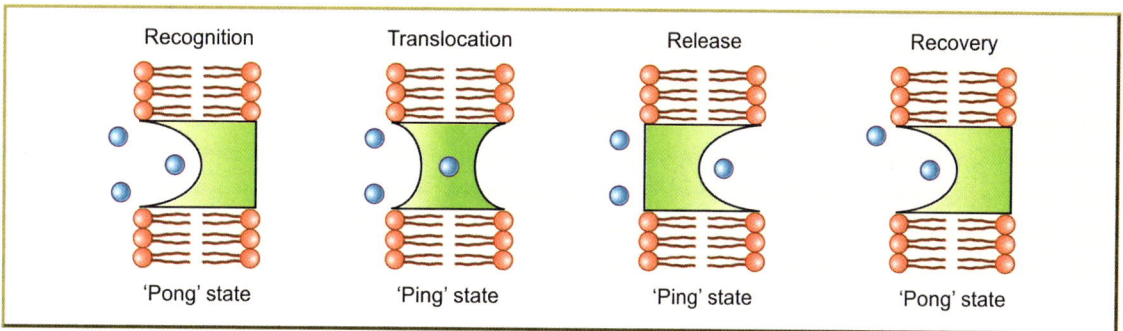

Fig. 3.12: 'Ping-pong' model for mediated membrane translocation.

- All cell membranes contain highly specific transporters for the movement of ions (Na^+, K^+, Cl^-, HCO_3^-, etc.) as well as organic compounds (such as amino acids and sugars).
- The transport of a solute molecule mediated by a transport protein has four aspects, explained by a **'ping-pong' mechanism** (Fig. 3.12):
  1. *Recognition:* Transport proteins have receptor sites to which the solute attaches. The transporter thus recognizes an appropriate solute from the aqueous environment for its translocation across the membrane.
  2. *Translocation:* After binding of the solute with the transporter protein, there occurs a conformational change in the transporter protein which translocates (moves) the solute molecule to the opposite side of the membrane.
  3. *Release:* A change in the conformation of the transporter protein decreases affinity of the solute and release it to the new environment.
  4. *Recovery:* After release of the solute, the transport protein reverts to its original conformation to accept another solute molecule, i.e. the transporter is recovered in its original conformation.
- Carrier-mediated transport includes (Fig. 3.9):
  1. **Passive transport** (passive mediated transport) or **facilitated diffusion**.
  2. Active transport.

Polarized epithelial cell: Before discussing the details of carrier-mediated transport, it is useful to understand the concept of polarized epithelial cells (Fig. 3.13) lining the **small intestine** and the **renal tubules**. Epithelial cells occur in layers or sheets that allow the directional movement of solutes not only across the plasma membrane but also from one side of the cell layer to the other. Such regulated movement is achieved because the plasma membranes of epithelial cells have **two distinct regions** with different morphologies and different transport systems. These regions are the **apical membrane** facing the lumen, and the **basolateral membrane** facing the blood supply. The polarized organization of the cells is maintained by the presence of **tight junctions** at the areas of contact between adjacent cells. Tight junctions prevent proteins on the apical membrane from migrating to the basolateral membrane and vice versa. Thus, the entry and exit steps for solutes can be localized to opposite sides of the cell. This is the key to transcellular transport across epithelial cells.

PASSIVE MEDIATED-TRANSPORT/ FACILITATED DIFFUSION

- Passive mediated-transport, also referred to as facilitated diffusion, leads to the translocation of solutes through membrane transport proteins **without the expenditure of metabolic energy**.
- The process can operate either unidirectionally or bidirectionally and the net flux across the membrane occur down a concentration gradient, i.e. the molecules flow from a higher to the lower concentration.
- 'Ping-pong' mechanism explains facilitated diffusion of molecules across the biological membrane with the help of a transport protein which exists in two principal conformations (Fig. 3.12).
- Several hormones (such as insulin, glucocorticoids, growth hormone, etc.) regulate facilitated

3

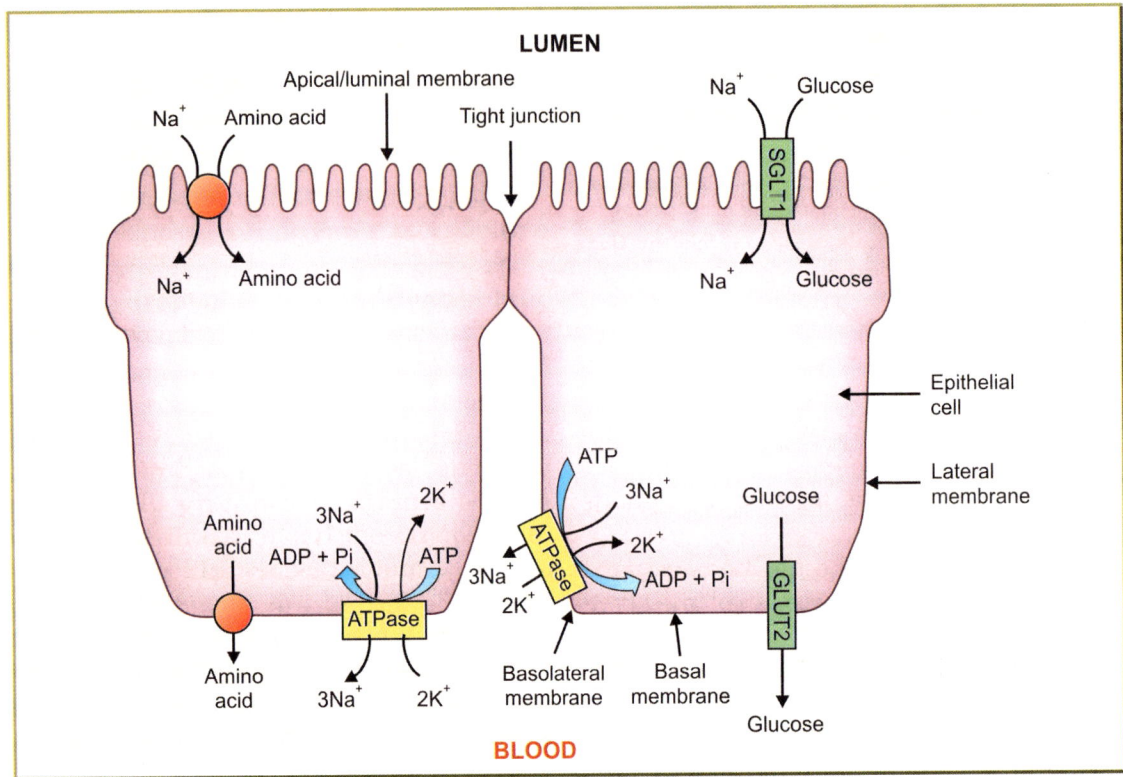

Fig. 3.13: Polarized epithelial cells of the small intestine with important membrane transport systems.

diffusion by changing the number of transport proteins available.

- Examples of the transport proteins which mediate facilitated diffusion include:

  1. *Glucose transporters (GLUT):* A group of transport proteins present in the plasma membrane of mammalian cells for the transport of D-glucose, e.g. GLUT1, GLUT2, etc. These are referred to as glucose permeases. They translocate several D-sugars by a uniport mechanism.

  2. *Cl^-/HCO_3^- exchanger:* It is an anion exchanger protein for the antiport movement of Cl^- and HCO_3^- in RBC membrane.

  3. *ATP-ADP translocase:* An antiport for the exchange of anions (ADP^{3-} and ATP^{4-}) between the cytosol and the mitochondrial matrix, located in the inner mitochondrial membrane.

ACTIVE TRANSPORT

In active transport, the transport protein moves a specific molecule against the concentration gradient,

i.e. from a lower concentration to the higher concentration. It is a process that requires energy which, in most cases, is coupled to the hydrolysis of ATP (Fig. 3.10). The active transport can be grouped as:

- Primary active transport, and
- Secondary active transport.

Primary Active Transport

This transport system has the same characteristics as the passive transport system but it is an **endergonic process**. Examples of such transporters include membrane-bound ATPases that translocate cations. They are further classified as:

- *P type transporters:* The transporter protein is phosphorylated and dephosphorylated during the transport activity.
- *V type transporters:* These are present in the membrane of the lysosomes, the Golgi vesicles and the secretory vesicles. These are responsible for acidification of the interior of these vesicles.
- *F type transporters:* These are present in mitochondria and are involved in ATP synthesis.

Some of the Primary Active Transport Systems

Primary active transport systems are important in the maintenance of electrochemical gradient in biological systems and consume nearly one-third of the total energy expenditure of a cell. Examples of primary active transport system include Na^+/K^+-ATPase, Ca^{2+}-ATPase, H^+/K^+-ATPase and neurotransmitter transporters:

1. *Na^+/K^+-ATPase:* The Na^+/K^+-ATPase (Na^+-K^+ pump) is an antiport that moves three Na^+ out of the cell and two K^+ into the cell, with the concomitant hydrolysis of intracellular ATP (Fig. 3.13). The pump is an integral part of the membrane and has binding sites for both ATP and Na^+ on the cytoplasmic side of the membrane, and K^+ binding site on the extracellular side of the membrane. Drugs that inhibit the Na^+-K^+ pump are of clinical importance (Chemistry to Clinics 3.4).

2. *Ca^{2+}-ATPase:* Ca^{2+} is an important intracellular messenger referred to as a second messenger. It regulates various cellular processes such as muscle contraction, release of neurotransmitters and glycogen breakdown. It is also an important activator of oxidative metabolism. In order to maintain low cytosolic Ca^{2+} concentration, it is actively transported out of the cell across the plasma membrane, the endoplasmic reticulum or the sarcoplasmic reticulum. The Ca^{2+}-ATPase (Ca^{2+} pump) actively pumps two Ca^{2+} out of the cytosol at the expense of ATP hydrolysis. The mechanism of Ca^{2+}-ATPase resembles that of the Na^+/K^+-ATPase. In eukaryotes, the Ca^{2+} transporter is regulated by the cytosolic Ca^{2+} level through a calcium binding protein termed calmodulin.

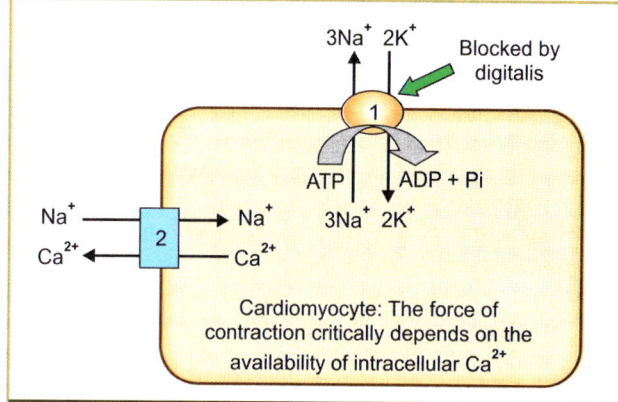

Fig. 3.14: Role of digitalis in heart failure: Normally, the Na^+-K^+-ATPase (1) in the cardiomyocyte membrane moves Na^+ out of the cell in exchange for K^+. The low cytosolic Na^+ maintains the Na^+ gradient for the functioning of the Na^+-Ca^{2+} exchanger (2) so that low cytosolic Ca^{2+} levels are maintained. In a failing heart, the aim of treatment is to make the myocardium contract with greater force. This is achieved with digitalis, which, by inhibiting Na^+-K^+-ATPase, abolishes the Na^+-gradient. Consequently, Ca^{2+} cannot exit the cell and attains sufficiently high intracellular levels to mediate excitation-contraction coupling and generate **greater contractile force**. As more blood is pumped out, the symptoms of heart failure are alleviated.

3. *H^+/K^+-ATPase:* Parietal cells in the gastric mucosa secrete HCl. Intracellular hydration of CO_2 by carbonic anhydrase forms carbonic acid (H_2CO_3) which splits into H^+ and HCO_3^-. The secretion of H^+ involves the H^+/K^+-ATPase, also called the proton pump, in the luminal membrane. This is an antiport and as H^+ is pumped out, the K^+ which enters the cell is subsequently externalized to the lumen. The chloride channels secrete Cl^- into the lumen so that the overall secreted product is HCl. Inhibition of H^+/K^+-ATPase is of clinical importance (Chemistry to Clinics 3.5).

4. *Neurotransmitter transporters:* Regulating the temporal availability of synaptically released neurotransmitter is critical to normal neuronal function. The removal of neurotransmitter from the synaptic cleft by active transport back into the presynaptic terminal or perisynaptic astrocytes (in the central nervous system) is the major way in which synaptic signaling is terminated at most of the synapses. Many disease processes in the central and peripheral nervous systems are due to disorders of synaptic signaling, and may involve altered function of neurotransmitter transporters (Chemistry to Clinics 3.6).

Chemistry to Clinics 3.4: Heart Failure

The cell membrane of cardiomyocytes (cells of the myocardium) contain many transport pumps. Two of them are, Na^+/K^+-ATPase and Na^+/Ca^{2+} exchanger. The Na^+/K^+-ATPase serves its usual function of maintaining low intracellular Na^+ concentrations. The Na^+/Ca^{2+} exchanger relies on this Na^+ gradient to extrude Ca^{2+} out of the cells. Cardiac glycosides (digitalis) such as digoxin and ouabain abolish this gradient by inhibiting the Na^+/K^+-ATPase. High intracellular Na^+ concentration slows the extrusion of Ca^{2+} by the Na^+/Ca^{2+} exchanger. Increased availability of Ca^{2+} results in increased force of contraction that is clinically useful in the management of cardiac failure (Fig. 3.14).

3

Chemistry to Clinics 3.5: Peptic Ulcer

Excess production of HCl along with a failure of mucosal defense mechanisms, can damage the gastric mucosa and may lead to peptic ulcer. The H^+/K^+-ATPase of the gastric mucosa is activated by histamine stimulation of the cell surface receptor (type 2 histamine receptors). Compounds, such as cimetidine and its analogs (type 2 antihistamine drugs) block the process by competing with histamine for its binding to the receptor and, in turn, reduce HCl production. These drugs are therefore widely used to alleviate the painful and otherwise fatal symptoms of peptic ulcer. However, proton pump inhibitors such as omeprazole are better because they are selective inhibitors of H^+/K^+-ATPase and are therefore more powerful than the antihistamines. It is now recognized that many ulcers are caused by infection with the bacteria *Helicobacter pylori* and can better be cured by the use of antibiotics besides a reduction in acidity.

Chemistry to Clinics 3.6: Neurotransmitter Transport Disorders

Dopamine, serotonin, glutamate, norepinephrine, etc. are some of the well-known neurotransmitters. Each has its own reuptake mechanism mediated by specific membrane transporters which may be affected in several diseases:

- *Defect in the dopamine transporter:* Alzheimer's disease, attention deficit hyperactivity disorder, obesity, Parkinson's disease, schizophrenia and substance abuse.
- *Defect in the serotonin transporter:* Autism, gastric motility disorders, mood disorders and obsessive-compulsive disorder.
- *Defect in the glutamate transporter:* Amyotrophic lateral sclerosis, epilepsy, schizophrenia, and stroke.
- *Defect in the norepinephrine transporter:* Mood disorders, severe orthostatic hypotension and substance abuse.

Knowing the tertiary and quaternary structure of the transporters is important for developing selective drugs to target them.

Secondary Active Transport

Secondary active transport is also called as **ion gradient-driven active transport**. In this process, free energy of the electrochemical gradient, generated by an ion-pumping ATPase, drives the transport of another substance, such as a sugar or an amino acid, against its concentration gradient. Na^+ glucose transport system and the amino acid transport system are the examples of secondary active transport system.

1. *Na^+ glucose transport system:* An example is the absorption of glucose in the proximal renal tubules and the small intestine (Fig. 3.13). Glucose enters the intestinal epithelial cells by active transport using the electrogenic Na^+ glucose transporter-1 (**SGLT1**) in the apical membrane. This increases the intracellular glucose concentration above the blood glucose concentration, and the glucose molecules move passively out of the cell and into the blood via an equilibrating carrier mechanism (**GLUT2**) in the basolateral membrane. The intestinal GLUT2, like the erythrocyte GLUT1, is a sodium-independent transporter that moves glucose down its concentration gradient. However, unlike GLUT1, the GLUT2 transporter can accept other sugars, such as galactose and fructose for absorption. The **Na^+/K^+-ATPase** that is located in the basolateral membrane pumps out the Na^+ (that enter the cell with glucose via SGLT1). In short, the successful uptake of glucose and sodium (symport) is '*secondarily*' dependent on the Na^+ gradient maintained by the primary active Na^+/K^+-ATPase. The **polarized** organization of the epithelial cells and the integrated functions of the plasma membrane transporters form the basis by which cells accomplish transcellular movement of both glucose and sodium ions, and is also exploited clinically (Chemistry to Clinics 3.7).

A comparison between passive mediated transport (facilitated diffusion) and active transport is shown in Table 3.2.

2. *Amino acid transport systems:* Amino acids are transported by luminal epithelial cells of the intestine by the Na^+-dependent pathway, similar to the Na^+-dependent glucose transport system.

Chemistry to Clinics 3.7: Oral Rehydration Solution

The administration of oral rehydration solution (ORS) has dramatically reduced the mortality resulting from cholera and other diseases that involve extreme losses of water/solutes from the gastrointestinal tract. The main ingredients of ORS are glucose, NaCl or $NaHCO_3$, KCl and water. The glucose and Na^+ are reabsorbed by the sodium-glucose transporter-1 (SGLT1) in the apical membrane of enterocytes, i.e. epithelial cells lining the lumen of the small intestine. Transfer of solutes on the basolateral aspect of the enterocytes increases the osmolarity compared with the luminal osmolarity thereby favoring the osmotic absorption of water. In this manner, the absorption of glucose accompanied by the obligatory increase in absorption of NaCl and water, help to compensate for the diarrhoeal losses of water/solutes, and treat dehydration.

Table 3.2: Comparison between facilitated diffusion and active transport

Parameter	Facilitated diffusion	Active transport
Specific binding site	Present	Present
Saturation kinetics	Yes	Yes
Inhibition by structural analogs	Yes	Yes
Direction of operation	Uni- or bidirectional	Unidirectional
Mode of operation	Along electrical/chemical gradient	Against electrical/ chemical gradient
Energy dependent	No	Yes

At least seven different brush-border specific transport systems have been identified for the uptake of different classes of L-amino acids and the dipeptides in the luminal membrane. These include the amino acid transporter for:

1. Neutral amino acids with short or polar side chain such as serine, threonine and alanine.
2. Neutral amino acids with aromatic or hydrophobic side chain, e.g. phenylalanine, tyrosine, tryptophan, methionine, valine, leucine and isoleucine.
3. Imino acids, e.g. proline and hydroxyproline.
4. β-amino acids, such as β-alanine and taurine.
5. Basic amino acids, e.g. lysine and arginine as well as cystine.
6. Acidic amino acids, such as aspartate and glutamate, and
7. Dipeptides.

Each one of these transport systems is specific for a group of closely related amino acids and operates as Na^+ symport system. Several pathological conditions due to a defect in the membrane transport system for specific amino acids are known (Chemistry to Clinics 3.8).

VESICULAR TRANSLOCATION

Cells translocate certain macromolecules across the plasma membrane by mechanisms which involve vesicle formation with or from the plasma membrane

Chemistry to Clinics 3.8: Amino Acid Transport Disorders

- *Hartnup's disease* is due to a decrease in the transport of neutral amino acids including tryptophan in the epithelial cells of the intestine and in the renal tubules. It is characterized by pellagra-like features due to niacin deficiency consequent to tryptophan deficiency.
- In *cystinuria*, renal reabsorption of cystine and basic amino acids (arginine and lysine) is abnormal. This in turn may result in the formation of cystine stones in the kidney.

and are referred to as **endocytosis** and **exocytosis** (Fig. 3.9). All these processes require energy (ATP), Ca^{2+} and the cytoskeletal system for proper functioning.

Endocytosis

Endocytosis is a mechanism for the uptake of large molecules such as polysaccharides, proteins or polynucleotides into the cytoplasm. In this process, a region of the plasma membrane invaginates, enclosing a small volume of the extracellular fluid and its contents within a bud, and generates endocytotic vesicles. The vesicle then pinches-off, as fusion of the plasma membrane seals the neck of the vesicle at the original site of invagination. The resulting small vesicle is called an **endosome**. It moves into the interior of the cell and delivers its contents to some other organelle, bound by a single membrane, e.g. a lysosome, by fusion of the two membranes. This 'hybrid vesicle' is called a **secondary lysosome**. Due to the presence of hydrolytic enzymes, the macromolecular contents are digested to their monomers, such as amino acids, simple sugars or nucleotides, which then diffuse out of the vesicle in the cytoplasm.

There are two general types of processes referred to as endocytosis, i.e. phagocytosis and pinocytosis.

- *Phagocytosis (or cell eating):* It occurs only in specialized cells like macrophages and granulocytes for the ingestion of large particles, such as bacteria, viruses, etc.
- *Pinocytosis:*
  - *Simple pinocytosis* (or *cell drinking*) leads to cellular uptake of fluid and its contents as a result of invagination of the plasma membrane (Fig. 3.15).
  - *Absorptive pinocytosis* or *receptor mediated pinocytosis* is a very selective type of

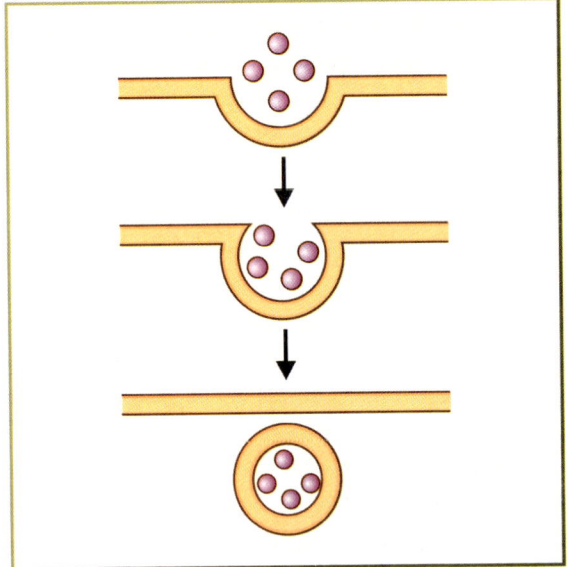

Fig. 3.15: Endocytosis.

pinocytosis that occurs in coated pits, lined with the protein **clathrin**, resulting in the formation of the clathrin-coated vesicles. The high affinity receptors permit selective concentration of the ligand from the medium, e.g. low density lipoproteins (LDL), transferrin, etc. and the receptors are subsequently internalized by means of the coated-pits containing the receptors. The coated vesicle may fuse with lysosomes, the contents are digested and clathrin is recycled back to the membrane (Fig. 3.16).

– Sometimes, in case of some hormones, clathrin is not required for receptor-mediated pinocytosis. The internalized vesicle fuses with another organelle such as Golgi complex, i.e. no secondary lysosomes are formed. The process is known as *adsorptive pinocytosis*.

Exocytosis

Exocytosis is the reverse of endocytosis. It involves contact of two inside surface monolayers from the cytosolic side and release of macromolecules to the exterior of a cell. A secretory vesicle in the cytoplasm, originating in the Golgi complex or the endoplasmic reticulum, moves to the inner surface of the plasma membrane and fuses with it, releasing the vesicular contents outside the membrane (Fig. 3.17).

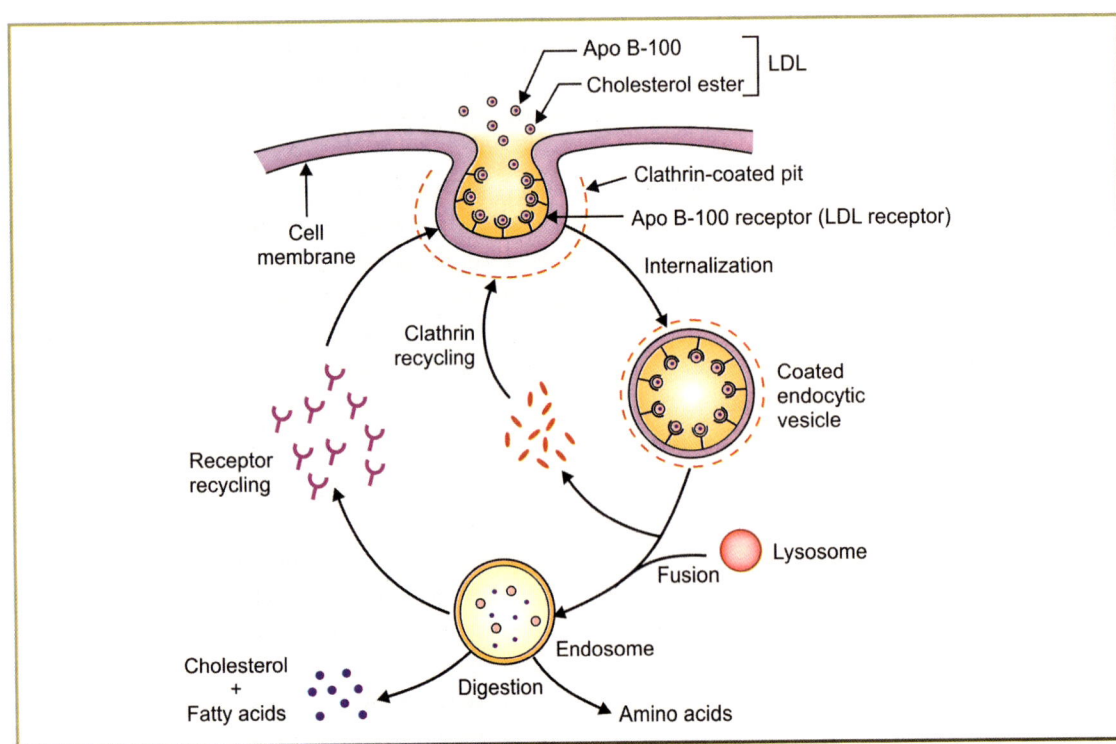

Fig. 3.16: Receptor-mediated endocytosis of LDL.

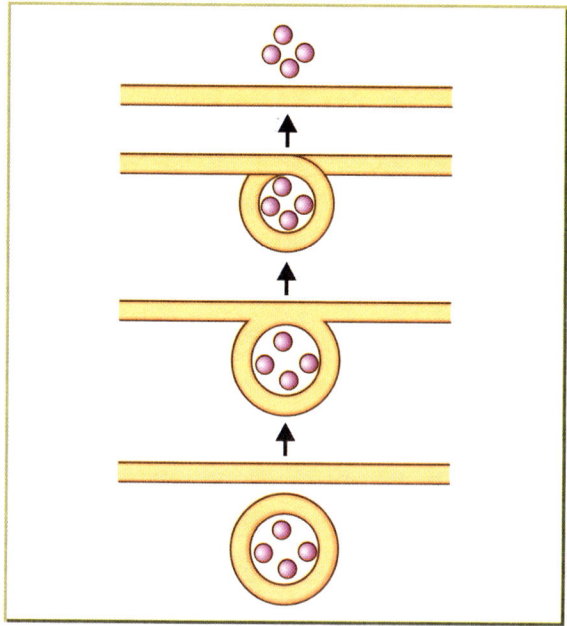

Fig. 3.17: Exocytosis.

All cells contain the machinery for the targeted destruction of intracellular macromolecules when they are no longer needed. For example, 'proteasomes' are meant for targeted destruction of proteins and 'exosomes' are meant for targeted degradation of RNA. Exosomes contain RNase PH activity for RNA cleavage and all the RNA as substrates, marked for degradation. In cells undergoing rapid division, exosomes may be thrown out into the surrounding. Hence, the term 'exosomes' also refers to small microvesicles surrounded by lipid bilayer, shed by tumors into the blood. The exosomes contain the complete set of messenger RNAs (mRNAs) and micro-RNAs (miRNAs), collectively known as the transcriptome. The exosomes can be isolated from the blood and the transcriptome subjected to reverse transcription polymerase chain reaction for detecting DNA mutations. Such blood-based detection of mutations is very valuable in diagnosing tumors where there may be constraints in obtaining a tissue biopsy, as in case of cancers of lungs, pancreas and ovaries.

The secreted/exocytosed molecules may have either of three possible fates:

1. They become a part of the cell membrane surface, e.g. antigens.
2. They become a part of the extracellular matrix, e.g. collagens.
3. They enter the blood and carried to distant sites, e.g. hormones like insulin.

In some diseases characterized by uncontrolled cell division, vesicles may be thrown out to the cell exterior, and contain molecules actually meant for intracellular use only. The process is not a true exocytosis and such vesicles are not true secretory vesicles. They are called **exosomes** (Chemistry to Clinics 3.9).

MEMBRANE ASSOCIATED PHENOMENON: GIBBS DONNAN EQUILIBRIUM

Consider two solutions separated by a semi-permeable membrane as shown in Fig. 3.18. Both the solutions I and II contain diffusible ions such as Na^+ and Cl^-; in addition, solution I contains impermeable/non-diffusible anions designated as ND^-. According to Gibbs and Donnan, the ND^- create an osmotic gradient and influence the distribution of the permeable ions across the membrane so that **at equilibrium**:

1. The product of diffusible ions in solutions I and II are equal ($36 \times 16 = 24 \times 24 = 576$).
2. Both the solutions remain electrically neutral.
3. The total number of every ion remains the same as that before equilibrium; however, the total ion concentration is higher on the side containing the non-diffusible ions (ND^-).

Gibbs Donnan equilibrium has **important biological applications**:

- Responsible for the **differential solute** (glucose, urea, electrolytes, etc.) distribution between plasma and other biological fluids such as intracellular fluid, interstitial fluid, gastric juice, cerebrospinal fluid, etc.

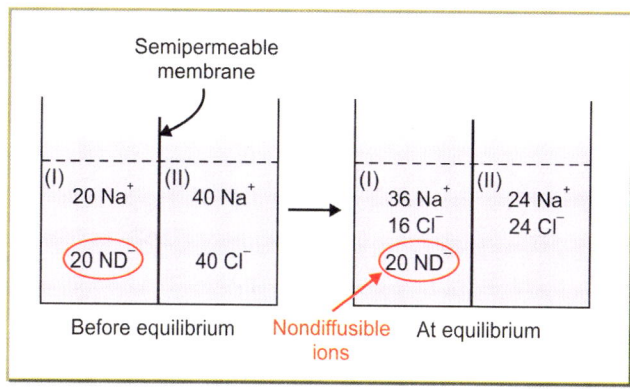

Fig. 3.18: Gibbs Donnan membrane equilibrium.

3

- Explains the **osmotic gradient and pH gradient** between plasma and other biological fluids.
- Explains the **'chloride-shift'** in RBC.

- Finds its clinical application in **dialysis** (Chemistry to Clinics 3.10).

Chemistry to Clinics 3.10: Dialysis

Dialysis (Greek 'dialusis' = 'dissolution'; 'dia' = 'through'; 'lysis' = 'loosening'), an artificial means to purify blood, works on the principle of Gibbs Donnan membrane equilibrium. It is a useful maneuver to partly compensate for the loss of renal function in patients of renal failure. The blood (in case of **hemodialysis**) from a peripheral artery of the patient is allowed to flow on one side of a semipermeable membrane while an artificially prepared fluid of known solute concentration, called the **dialysate**, flows by the other side but in opposite direction (Fig. 3.19). Proteins present in the blood are the large non-diffusible ions. The solute concentration in the dialysate is so designed as to maximize diffusion of water and solutes across the membrane. The net effect is the reduction of toxic molecules to low levels in the blood while improving the levels of the essential ones. The 'purified' blood is returned through a peripheral vein.

The basic procedure is the same in case of **peritoneal dialysis**. Here, the dialysate is run through a tube into the peritoneal cavity and the peritoneal membrane itself serves as the semipermeable membrane. The dialysate is retained for sometime and eventually drained out through the tube, removing excess water and waste products.

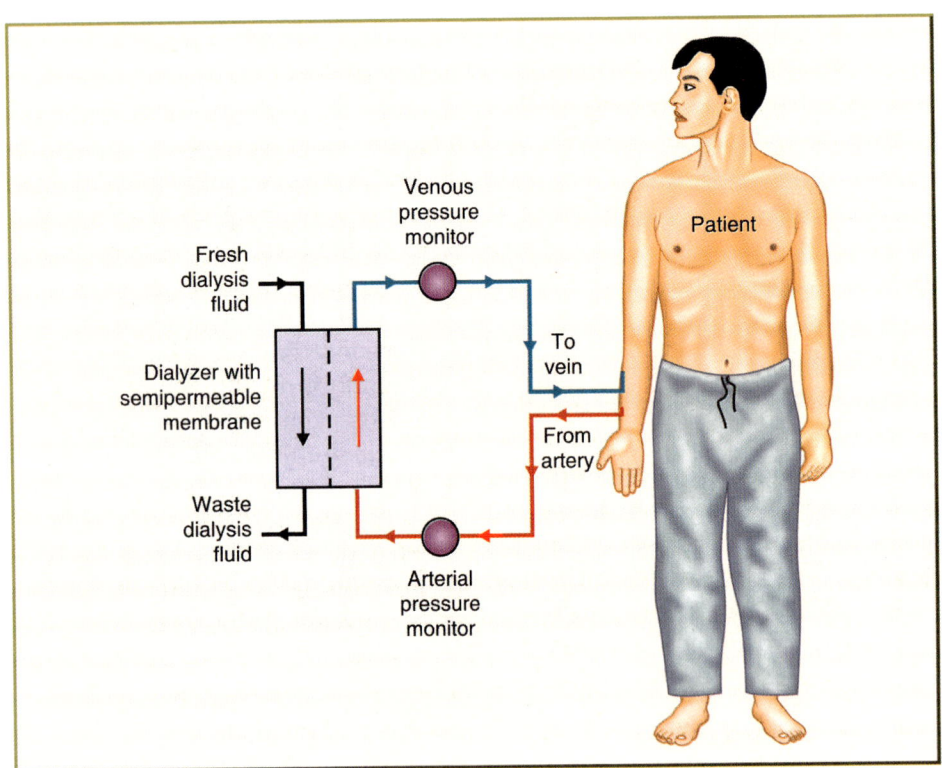

Fig. 3.19: Application of Gibbs Donnan membrane equilibrium in hemodialysis.

SOME IMPORTANT QUESTIONS

1. Discuss composition of a biological membrane.
2. Describe:
    i. Fluid-mosaic model of cell membrane
    ii. Important functions of a biological membrane

iii. Ion channels
iv. Carrier-mediated transport
v. Amino acid transport systems
vi. Transport disorders

3. Write notes on:
i. Micelles
ii. Lipid bilayer
iii. Liposomes
iv. Integral membrane proteins
v. Peripheral proteins
vi. Non-mediated transport
vii. Channelopathies

viii. Ionophores
ix. Facilitated diffusion
x. Group translocation
xi. Endocytosis
xii. Exocytosis
xiii. Pinocytosis
xiv. Gibbs Donnan equilibrium

MULTIPLE CHOICE QUESTIONS

1. **Liposomes can be used to deliver:**
   A. DNA
   B. Enzymes
   C. Amphotericin B
   D. All of the above

2. **In the myelin sheath, lipid:protein ratio is nearly:**
   A. 4:1
   B. 1:4
   C. 1:1
   D. 3:2

3. **Membrane fluidity depends on:**
   A. Its cholesterol content
   B. Its unsaturated fatty acid content
   C. Degree of unsaturation of unsaturated fatty acids
   D. All of the above

4. **In myasthenia gravis, autoantibodies are directed against the following membrane receptor:**
   A. Dopamine
   B. Epinephrine
   C. Acetylcholine
   D. Serotonin

5. **Cystic fibrosis transmembrane conductance regulator (CFTR) is a:**
   A. cGMP-dependent Ca^{2+} channel
   B. cGMP-dependent Cl^- channel
   C. cAMP-dependent Ca^{2+} channel
   D. cAMP-dependent Cl^- channel

6. **In the renal collecting tubules, expression of aquaporin-2 (AQP2) is increased by:**
   A. ADH
   B. ANP
   C. Aldosterone
   D. Angiotensin II

7. **Valinomycin and nigericin translocate:**
   A. K^+
   B. Na^+
   C. Ca^{2+}
   D. Cl^-

8. **Cardiac glycosides act by:**
   A. Increasing intracellular Ca^{2+}
   B. Decreasing intracellular Ca^{2+}
   C. Decreasing intracellular Na^+
   D. Increasing intracellular K^+

9. **Gastric proton pump is:**
   A. A uniport
   B. A symport
   C. An electrogenic antiport
   D. A neutral antiport

10. **Oral rehydration solution (ORS) therapy exploits the following transport system in the small intestine:**
    A. GLUT
    B. SGLT-1
    C. AQP
    D. Neutral amino acid transporter

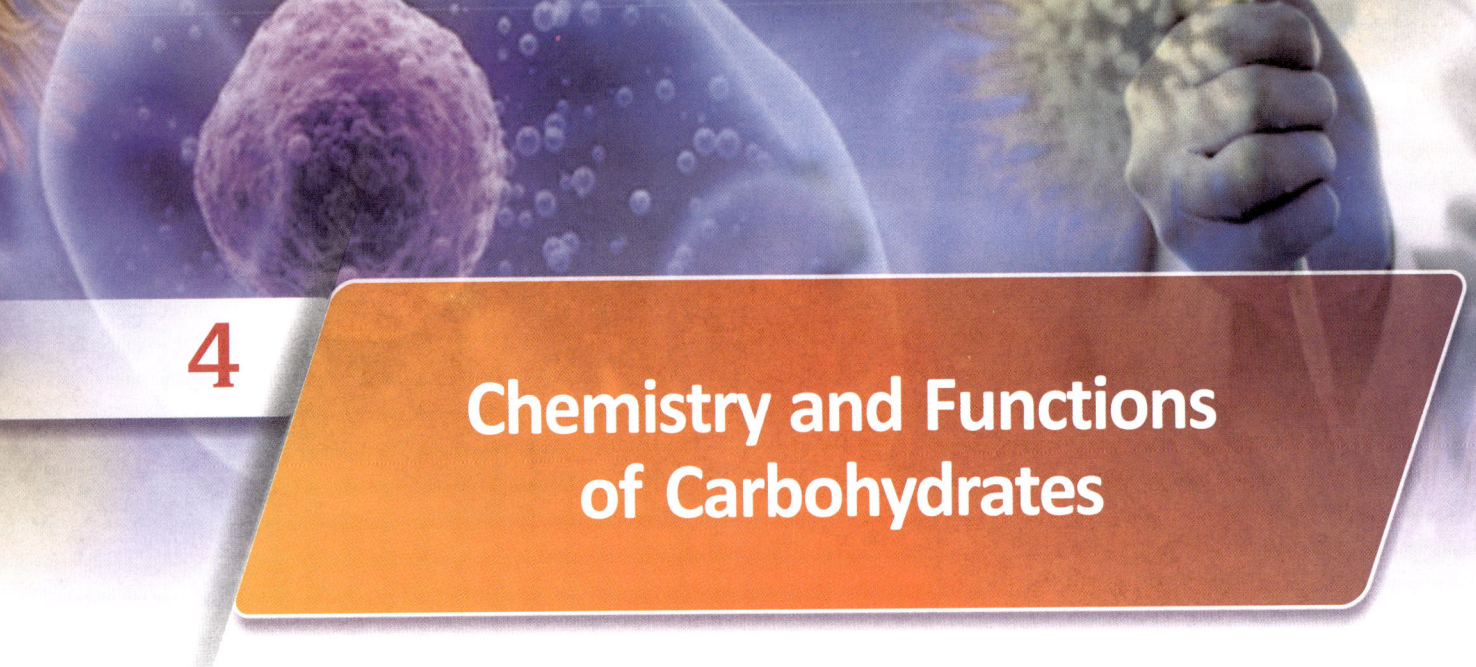

4

Chemistry and Functions of Carbohydrates

Carbohydrates, also called saccharides (Greek-Sakcharon: Sugar), are aldehyde or ketone derivatives of polyhydroxy alcohols. They are the most abundant biological molecules containing just three elements, i.e. C, H and O which are combined as $(CH_2O)n$, where $n \geq 3$.

CLASSIFICATION OF CARBOHYDRATES

Depending upon the number of monomeric units present in the molecule, carbohydrates are classified as monosaccharides, disaccharides and polysaccharides (Fig. 4.1).

MONOSACCHARIDES

Simple sugars are called monosaccharides. They join together in various ways to form di- and poly-saccharides. These are the aldehyde or ketone derivatives of straight chain polyhydroxy alcohols which contain 3 or more carbon atoms.

Different monosaccharides can be separated from a mixture by the technique known as chromatography.

Classification of Monosaccharides

Monosaccharides are divided into different groups according to the chemical nature of their carbonyl group, or the number of carbon atoms in a chain (Table 4.1).

According to the chemical nature of the carbonyl group, monosaccharides are divided into two groups, as aldoses and ketoses:

Aldoses: A sugar is an aldose when it contains an aldehyde (–CHO) group on Cl, e.g. glucose.

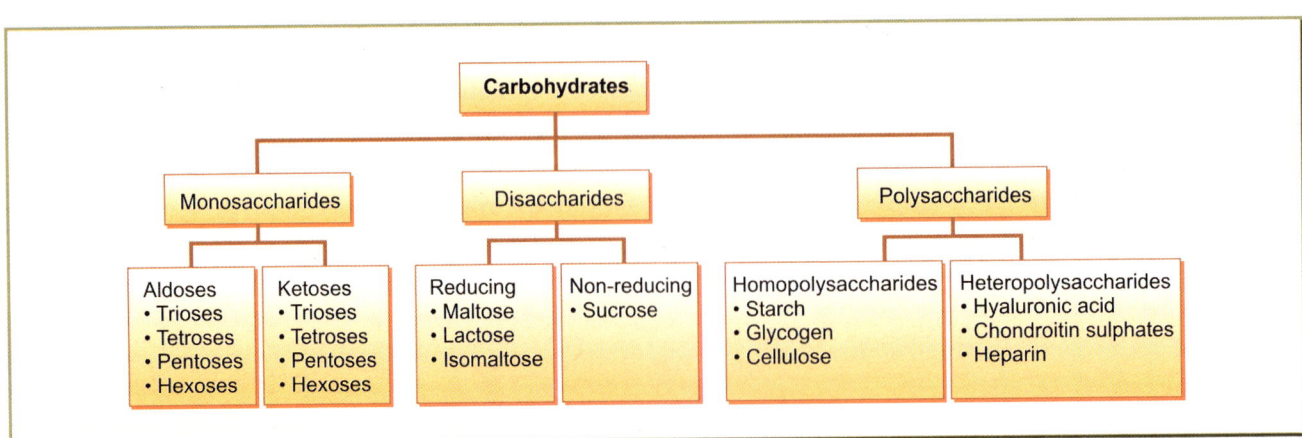

Fig. 4.1: Classification of carbohydrates.

Table 4.1: Classification of monosaccharides

Monosaccharides	Number of C-atoms	Aldoses	Ketoses
Trioses	3	Glyceraldehyde	Dihydroxy-acetone
Tetroses	4	Erythrose	Erythrulose
Pentoses	5	Ribose	Ribulose
Hexoses	6	Glucose	Fructose

Ketoses: The sugar is a ketose when it has a ketone (–CO) group at C_2, e.g. fructose.

Some of the ketoses are named by inserting '-ul-' before the suffix '-ose' in the name of the corresponding aldose, e.g. erythrulose, from erythrose (an aldose).

According to the number of carbon atoms, monosaccharides are designated as trioses, tetroses, pentoses, etc.:

Trioses: The smallest monosaccharides with three carbon atoms, include glyceraldehyde (an aldotriose) and dihydroxyacetone (a ketotriose). Both of these molecules are of physiological significance since the phosphate esters of these sugars, i.e. glyceraldehyde-3-phosphate and dihydroxyacetone phosphate, are important intermediates in glycolysis.

Tetroses: These are compounds with four carbon atoms, e.g. erythrose (an aldotetrose) and erythrulose (a keto-tetrose). Erythrose, as erythrose-4-phosphate, is an intermediate in hexose monophosphate (HMP) shunt.

Pentoses: These are sugars containing five carbon atoms such as ribose (an aldopentose) and xylulose (a ketopentose), both of which are intermediates in the HMP shunt.

Ribose is also an important constituent of nucleotides present in RNA.

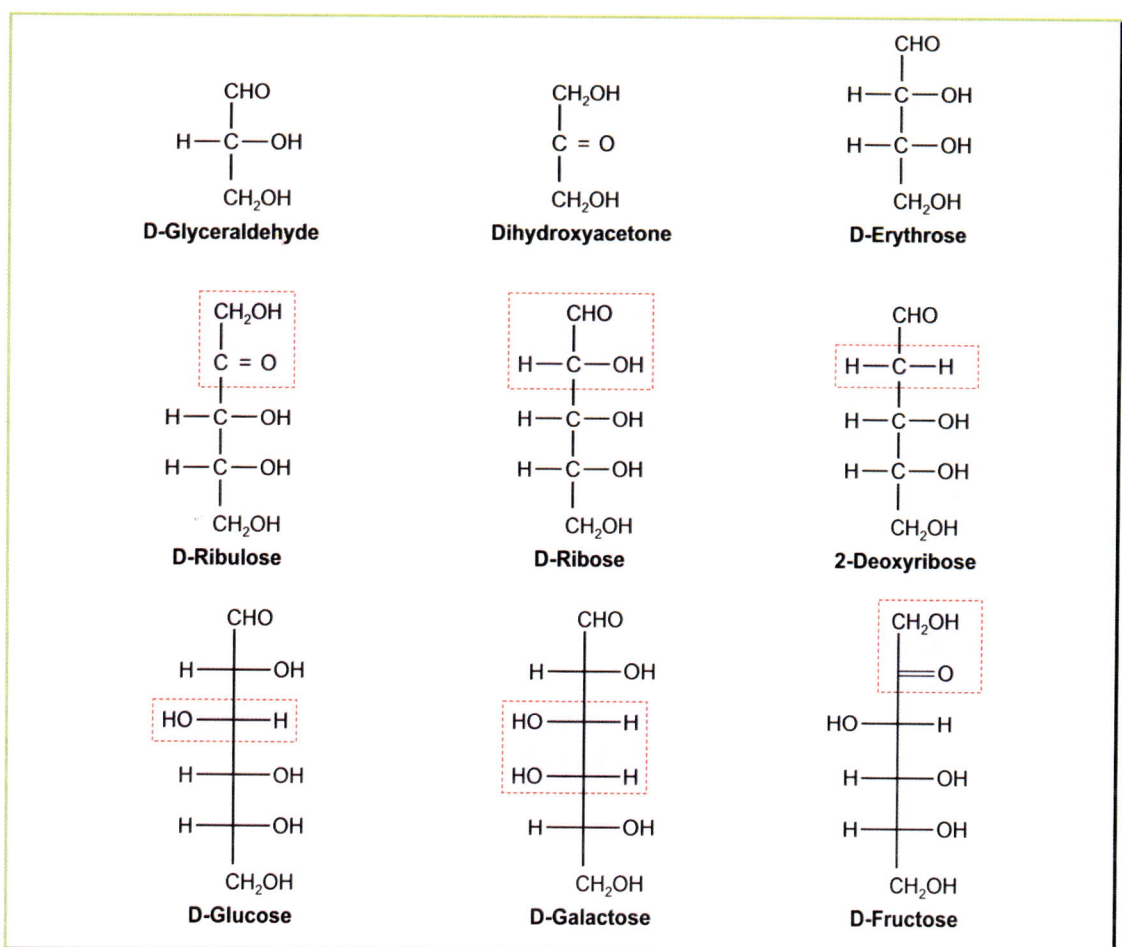

Fig. 4.2: Some monosaccharides of biological significance.

4

Hexoses: They contain six carbon atoms, e.g. glucose (an aldohexose) and fructose (a ketohexose). Glucose, commonly known as dextrose, is an important source of energy in the body. Fructose is an important constituent of the common sugar, sucrose.

Some of the monosaccharides of biological significance are given in Fig. 4.2.

Structural Configuration: General Concepts

Chiral centre: Monosaccharides are optically active compounds and can rotate the plane of polarized light either to right or to left (Fig. 4.3).

Such a property is characteristic of substances having tetrahedral carbon that has four different substituents, i.e. the carbon atom having four different atoms or groups attached to it. The central carbon atom in such a molecule is called as the asymmetric carbon atom (asymmetric center or chiral center) (Fig. 4.4).

Simple sugars contain centers of asymmetry and are thus chiral molecules.

Stereoisomers/enantiomers: A compound having one asymmetric carbon atom may occur in two forms, both of which are the non-superimposable mirror images of each other. These two molecules are spatial isomers or stereoisomers (also called enantiomers)

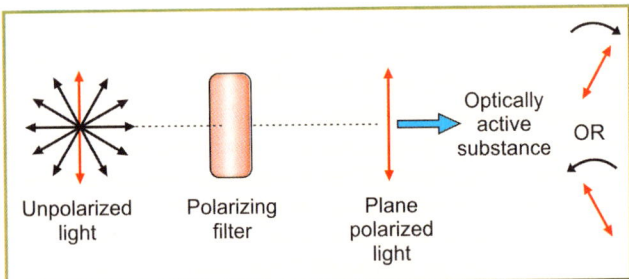

Fig. 4.3: Light is characterized by electric and magnetic fields that oscillate in planes that are perpendicular to one another. In 'normal', unpolarized light, these oscillations are randomly oriented in all planes. Light passed through a polarizing filter oscillates in only one direction, and is called plane polarized light. An optically active (chiral) substance is one which can rotate the plane of polarization of plane polarized light, either clockwise (to the right) or anti-clockwise (to the left). A polarimeter is an instrument used to measure the angle of rotation. Although geometric isomers (e.g. *cis-* and *trans*-isomers) have completely different physical and chemical properties, optical isomers (enantiomers) differ in only one characteristic—the direction of rotation of plane polarized light (the degree of rotation being the same). In every other way, such as boiling point, density, refractive index, viscosity, etc., two optical isomers are identical.

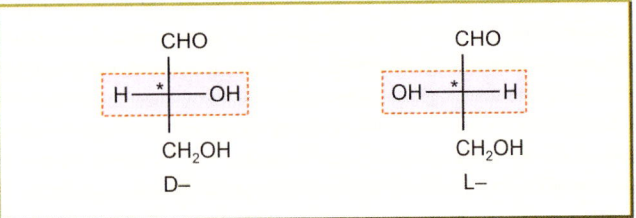

Fig. 4.4: D- and L-isomers (*asymmetric carbon atom) of glyceraldehyde.

of one another. Both the enantiomers can rotate the plane of polarized light to the same degree but in opposite directions.

'D' and 'L' forms: According to Fischer, two isomers of the parent compound of carbohydrate family, i.e. glyceraldehyde, are designated as D-glyceraldehyde and L-glyceraldehyde. The D or L form of a monosaccharide is determined with respect to its spatial relationship with the glyceraldehyde.

In Fischer projection, glyceraldehyde molecule with an –OH group around the asymmetric center (i.e. the α-carbon atom or the carbon atom adjacent to the carbon atom with the terminal primary alcoholic group) present on the right hand side when –CHO group is at the top, is designated as D-glyceraldehyde. Its non-superimposable mirror image, which has an –OH group around the asymmetric center on the left, is designated as L-glyceraldehyde (Fig. 4.4).

Number of possible isomers: Any successive addition of carbon atom in the form of –CHOH (secondary alcoholic group) to the parent compound D-glyceraldehyde, gives rise to the family of D-sugars. Thus, D-sugars give the same absolute configuration at the asymmetric center farthest from their carbonyl group as does D-glyceraldehyde (e.g., the -OH at C5 of D-glucose is on the right similar to -OH at C_2 of D-glyceraldehyde). Since each new carbon atom (as a secondary alcoholic group) is added as an asymmetric center, the number of possible isomers increases with the increasing number of carbon atoms as the asymmetric centers. The number of isomers so formed thus depends upon the number of the asymmetric centers (n) in a molecule. It is represented by the formula n^2. Since the number of asymmetric carbon atoms in a glucose molecule is four (n = 4), glucose therefore has 4^2 = 16 stereoisomers.

Every sugar thus exists in a D- or L- form, each being a mirror image of the other. The D-forms of monosaccharides though are present in abundance than the L-sugars in mammalian carbohydrates, L-isomers of monosaccharides, e.g. L-xylulose are also found in the human body.

Dihydroxyacetone (a ketotriose) is a monosaccharide which does not occur as a D or L isomer.

'd' and 'l' forms: An isomer which rotates the plane of polarized light to the right is designated as dextrorotatory (*d* or +) while the other isomer which rotates polarized light to the left is designated as levorotatory (*l* or –).

A chiral molecule with D-configuration thus can either be dextrorotatory [D(+)] or levorotatory [D(–)] indicating its structural relationship to the D or L glyceraldehyde but exhibiting different optical rotations.

Racemic mixture: A mixture containing equal amounts of each of the two isomers, i.e. the mixture of a dextrorotatory and the levorotatory isomers of a chiral molecule is called a racemic mixture (*dl*-mixture).

Configuration versus Conformation

The term 'configuration' refers to the geometric possibilities for a given set of atoms, e.g. D- and L-forms as discussed above. Different configurations of a molecule are achieved by breaking and rearranging covalent bonds. On the other hand, the term 'conformation' refers to the overall 3-dimensional architecture of a molecule. Different conformations of a molecule are achieved without breaking any covalent bond.

Formation of the Ring Structure: Pyran and Furan

Monosaccharides normally adopt a ring conformation. When D-glucose adopts a six-membered ring structure, a hemiacetal bond is formed between the aldehyde carbonyl group of carbon 1 and the hydroxyl group on carbon 5. Cyclization of glucose thus results in the formation of ring structure, which is analogous with the structure of pyran, a six-membered ring containing five carbon and one oxygen atoms (Fig. 4.5).

Sugars with a six-membered pyran ring are designated as pyranoses. Cyclization of D-glucose

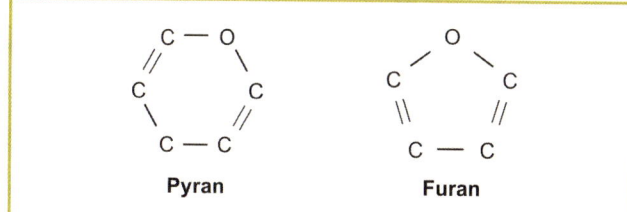

Fig. 4.5: Pyran and furan rings.

thus yields a cyclic hemiacetal, i.e. glucopyranose. Fructose, on the other hand, forms a five-membered ring with four carbon and one oxygen atom called as a furan ring. The linear form of D-fructose thus cyclizes between the carbonyl group of the second carbon (C2) and the alcoholic group of the fifth carbon (C5), and yields a hemiketal, i.e. fructofuranose. The smallest monosaccharide having furanose ring structure is ribose. These ring structures of the sugars were proposed by Haworth and are called Haworth structures.

Anomers

When a monosaccharide cyclizes, its carbonyl carbon (called anomeric carbon) also becomes asymmetric with two possible configurations, i.e. α and β forms. Such stereoisomers that differ in configuration at the anomeric carbon, i.e. at C1 in an aldose (e.g. glucopyranose) or at C2 in a ketose (e.g. fructofuranose) are called anomers. In an α-anomer, the –OH substituent of the anomeric carbon is on the opposite side from the –CH$_2$OH group at the chiral center, such as C5 in hexoses. The other anomeric form is designated as the β-form (Fig. 4.6).

The two anomers of D-glucose (α-D-glucopyranose and β-D-glucopyranose) have different physical and chemical properties including optical rotation.

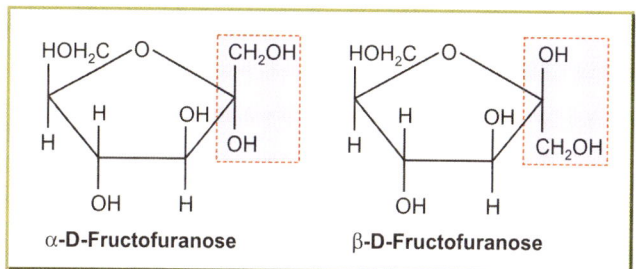

Fig. 4.6: Anomers.

4

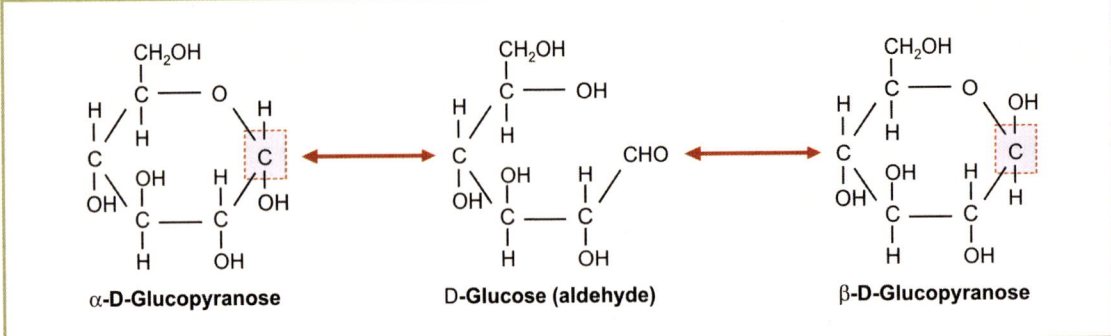

Fig. 4.7: Mutarotation.

Mutarotation

Two anomers of glucose are freely interconvertible in an aqueous solution. At equilibrium, D-glucose is a mixture of β-anomer (63.6%) and α-anomer (36.4%) in a ratio of nearly 2:1. Interconversion of the two anomers also results in a change in optical rotation of glucose. During equilibration, optical rotation of D-glucose slowly changes with time and reaches a constant value of 52.5°. This phenomenon of change in optical rotation of D(+) glucose in an aqueous solution, reaching a constant value due to interconversion of the two anomers at equilibrium is called mutarotation (Fig. 4.7) (Chemistry to Clinics 4.1).

Epimers

Sugars that differ by configuration of its –H and –OH groups around only one of the optically active carbon atoms are known as epimers. D-Mannose differs in configuration around the second carbon atom (C2) with respect to D-glucose. Similarly, D-galactose has a different configuration than

Chemistry to Clinics 4.1: Mutarotation and Mutarotases
Although the phenomenon of mutarotation is spontaneous, it may be catalyzed by enzymes called mutarotases as observed in the tissues of some animals and birds. Mutarotase activity can be measured with a precision polarimeter. It can be used in ELISA and Western blot along with anti-mutarotase (antibody against mutarotase, an example of an abzyme, i.e. antibody against enzyme).

D-glucose around fourth carbon atom (C4). D-Mannose and D-galactose therefore are the two epimers of D-glucose (Fig. 4.8).

Monosaccharide Derivatives

Derivatives of sugars include sugar acids, sugar alcohols, amino sugars and methylglycosides.

Sugar Acids

Oxidation of C1 of an aldose converts its aldehyde group to a carboxylic acid group and forms an acid called aldonic acid, such as D-gluconic acid. Similarly, oxidation of the primary alcoholic group of C6 of

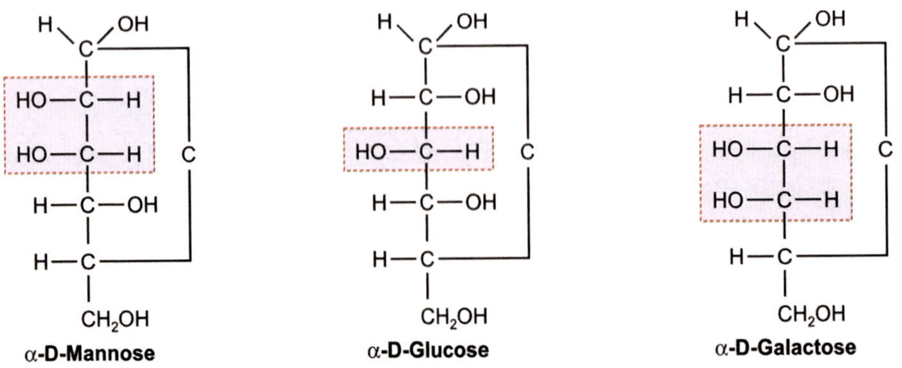

Fig. 4.8: Epimers.

aldose produces uronic acid, such as D-glucuronic acid (Fig. 4.9).

Sugar Alcohols

Sugars get reduced under mild reducing conditions and produce cyclic polyhydroxy alcohols called alditols, e.g. ribitol (a component of FMN and FAD) and xylitol (a sweetener used in gums and candies).

Amino Sugars

Amino sugars, such as glucosamine and galactosamine, are formed by the replacement of one of the –OH group by the –NH$_2$ group on C2 (Fig. 4.10).

Amino sugars are often present as their N-acetyl derivatives in various compounds called as glycosaminoglycans, such as hyaluronic acid, chondroitin sulfates, erythromycin, etc. N-acetylneuraminic acid and its derivatives are called sialic acids.

Glycoproteins and glycolipids: Glycosaminoglycans and sialic acids are important constituents of glycoproteins (complexes of sugars with proteins). Complexes of sugars with lipids are called glycolipids. The glycoproteins and glycolipids of infectious organisms play an important role in human disease (Chemistry to Clinics 4.2 and 4.3).

Methylglycosides

Carbon atom number 1 of a sugar may react with an alcohol, such as methanol and yields methylglycosides. These are also found in glycosaminoglycans.

DISACCHARIDES

Disaccharides consist of two similar or dissimilar units of monosaccharides linked by a glycosidic bond. Maltose, lactose and sucrose are the disaccharides of biological significance.

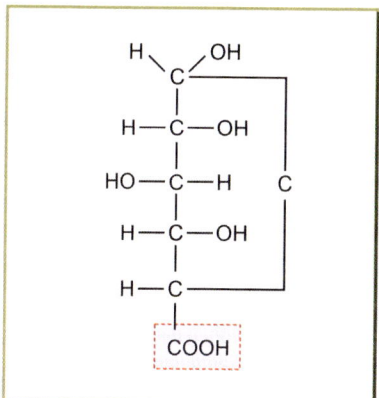

Fig. 4.9: D-glucuronic acid.

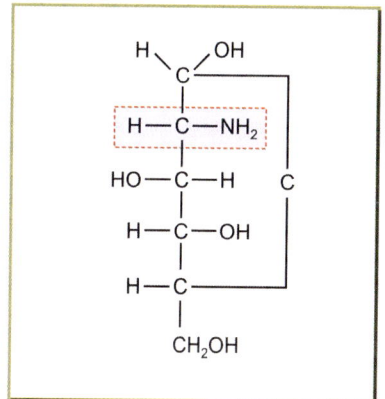

Fig. 4.10: D-glucosamine.

Chemistry to Clinics 4.2: Influenza Virus Glycoproteins

The surfaces of influenza viruses include two glycoproteins named hemagglutinin (H) and neuraminidase (N), **coded by the viral RNA genome**. Each of these molecules is required for successful infection and spread in a host animal. The hemagglutinin attaches influenza viruses to sialic acid on the surfaces of cells, enabling them to enter and infect cells. Following replication, neuraminidase (also called sialidase) removes sialic acid from the cell membrane, enabling the newly assembled viruses to be released in order to spread and infect other cells. Based on the primary structures of H and N, the influenza A viruses are classified into various serotypes or subtypes, such as H1N1, H2N2, H3N2 and so forth. The viral neuraminidase can be inhibited by the drugs oseltamivir (brand name Tamiflu, the first orally active neuraminidase inhibitor commercially developed) and zanamivir (brand name Relenza), that bind to the active site of the enzyme by induced-fit and behave as transition state analogs. The drugs are indicated both for prophylaxis and for treatment within two days of the onset of symptoms. Unlike Tamiflu, which is given orally, Relenza is usually administered by inhalation, or can be injected. The influenza pandemic of 2010–2011 was caused by H1N1 virus which is a type of swine influenza derived originally from a strain that lived in pigs and this origin gave rise to the common name of 'swine flu'. However, despite its origin in pigs, this strain is transmitted between people and not from swine to people unless one is in very close association with infected swine. Further, there is no risk of contracting flu from eating cooked pork products.

4

Chemistry to Clinics 4.3: Sugar-based Vaccine

Out of the various malaria parasites known, *Plasmodium falciparum* is particularly notorious to cause life-threatening complications. The membrane surface of *P. falciparum* contains glycosylphosphatidyl inositols (GPIs), a type of glycolipid which behaves like antigen. The GPIs are implicated in several pathologic processes in severe falciparum malaria. Reactive antibodies are commonly found in the sera of people residing in endemic zones whereas they are absent in non-endemic areas. It has been observed that the antibodies may offer partial protection against serious outcomes of falciparum malaria. Hence, sugar (GPIs)-based malaria vaccines are currently being developed.

Maltose

Maltose [α-D-glucopyranosyl-(1→4)-α-D-glucopyranose] consists of **two glucose** (α-D-glucopyranose) units which are linked together by α-1,4-glycosidic linkage. The symbol (1→4) indicates that the glycosidic bond links C1 of a glucose molecule to C4 of the other molecule of glucose. Accordingly, in maltose –OH group at C4 of a glucose molecule is linked to the –OH group at C1 (the anomeric carbon) of another glucose molecule. This leaves a free –OH group at the anomeric carbon (C1) of the first glucose molecule, which can form a reducing aldehyde group if the ring opens. Thus, maltose is a reducing disaccharide (Fig. 4.11).

Maltose is usually obtained as a hydrolyzed product of polysaccharides such as starch, glycogen and dextrins. It can be hydrolyzed to its component monosaccharides, i.e. the two glucose units, by the enzyme maltase in the intestinal lumen.

Partial hydrolysis of glycogen and starch produces **isomaltose**. This is also a **reducing** sugar which contains **two glucose** units linked through **α-1,6 linkage**.

Lactose (Milk Sugar)

Lactose [β-D-galactopyranosyl-(1→4)-β-D-glucopyranose] consists of galactose (β-D-galactopyranose) and glucose (β-D-glucopyranose) which are linked together by the β-1,4-glycosidic linkage. The glycoside bond links C1 of galactose to C4 of glucose residue. There is a free –OH group at the anomeric carbon (C1) of β-D-glucose, which can form a reducing aldehyde group if the ring opens. Thus, lactose is a reducing disaccharide (Fig. 4.12).

Lactose occurs naturally in milk hence it is also called as milk sugar. In females, lactose is synthesized during lactation and is secreted in milk. During late pregnancy and lactation, lactose may be excreted in the urine of these females (physiological lactosuria). Lactose is hydrolyzed by the intestinal enzyme lactase (β-D-galactosidase) to its component monosaccharides, i.e. glucose and galactose.

Sucrose (Table Sugar, Cane Sugar or Invert Sugar)

Sucrose [α-D-glucopyranosyl-(1→2)-β-D-fructofuranose] consists of glucose (α-D-glucopyranose) and fructose (β-D-fructofuranose) which are linked by β-1, 2-glycosidic linkage (Fig. 4.13). Since the carbonyl groups of both the monosaccharides, i.e. the C1 in glucose and C2 in fructose participate in the glycosidic bond, there is no free carbonyl carbon on any of its monosaccharides. Thus, sucrose is a non-reducing sugar.

Sucrose, commonly known as invert sugar, is the most abundant disaccharide found in plants and is familiar to human beings as the common table sugar or cane sugar. It is hydrolysed to its monosaccharide components, i.e. glucose and fructose by the intestinal sucrase (also called invertase). Sucrose is a notorious cariogenic substance (Chemistry to Clinics 4.4).

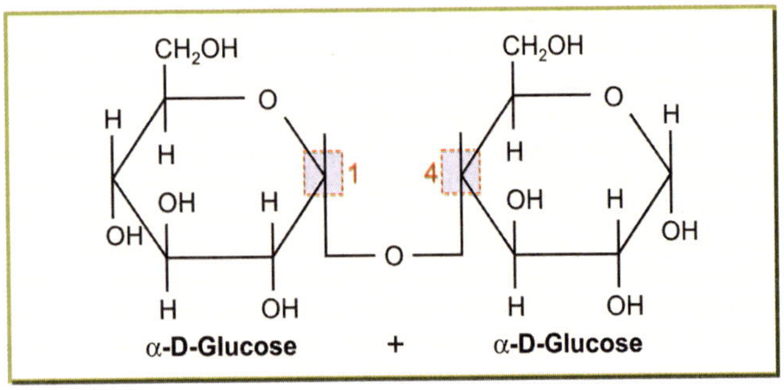

Fig. 4.11: Maltose.

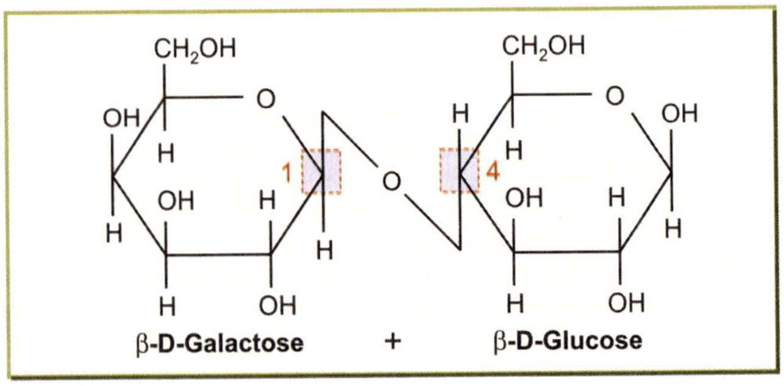

Fig. 4.12: Lactose.

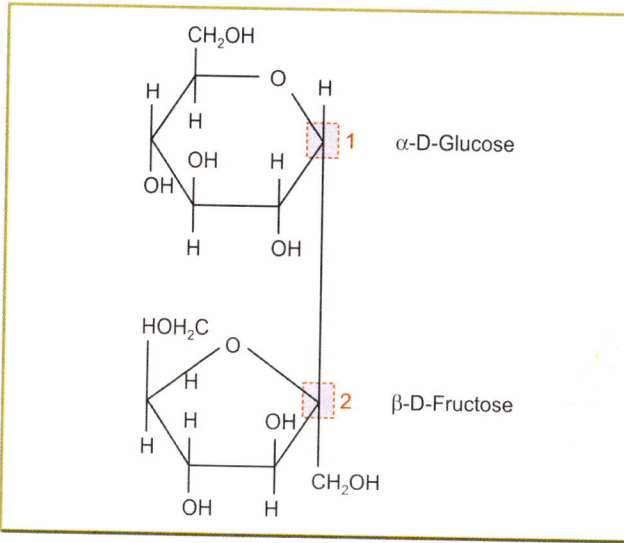

Fig. 4.13: Sucrose.

Lactulose: It is a semisynthetic disaccharide of fructose and galactose (Chemistry to Clinics 4.5).

POLYSACCHARIDES

Polysaccharides are also called glycans. These are polymers of large number of monosaccharides which are linked together by the glycosidic bonds. Where the number of monosaccharide units is <10, these are termed as oligosaccharides. Polysaccharides are

sparingly soluble in cold water but form a colloidal solution in hot water. These are neither sweet in taste nor have reducing properties. These exist as linear and/or branched polymers, and are classified as homopolysaccharides and heteropolysaccharides.

Homopolysaccharides

Homopolysaccharides (homoglycans) are the polymers of identical monosaccharide units. Common homopolysaccharides of biological significance are starch, glycogen and cellulose (the homopolymers of glucose, also called glucosans), and inulin (the homopolymer of fructose, also called fructosan).

Starch

Starch is stored as a reservoir of food in cereals and tubers of plants. Starch consists of two polysaccharides, i.e. α-amylose and amylopectin.

The α-amylose is a linear polymer of glucose residues linked by α-(1→4) glycosidic bonds. Amylopectin is a branched molecule with both α-1, 4 straight chain and α-(1→6) branch points which occur after every 24 to 30 glucose residues (Fig. 4.14).

Starch is a main source of carbohydrate in the human diet. Amylase present in the saliva and in the pancreatic juice randomly hydrolyses α-(1→4) glycosidic bonds of starch and degrades it to a mixture of maltose, maltotriose and dextrins.

Glycogen

Glycogen is the storage polysaccharide of animals and is therefore also called as animal starch. It is present in all cells but is most prevalent in the skeletal muscle and the liver. Structure of glycogen is similar to amylopectin with a linear chain of α-(1→4) glycosidic bonds and α-(1→6) branch points, but branching occurs more frequently, i.e. after every 10–12 glucose residues. Glycogen is thus highly branched with a tree like structure (Fig. 4.15).

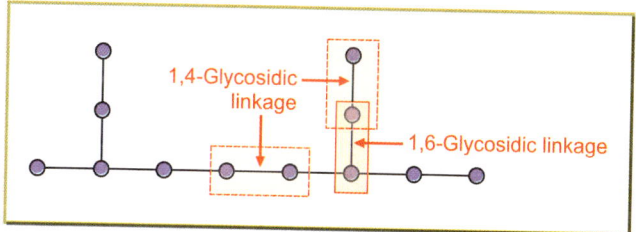

Fig. 4.14: Starch (–O– represents a glucose unit).

4

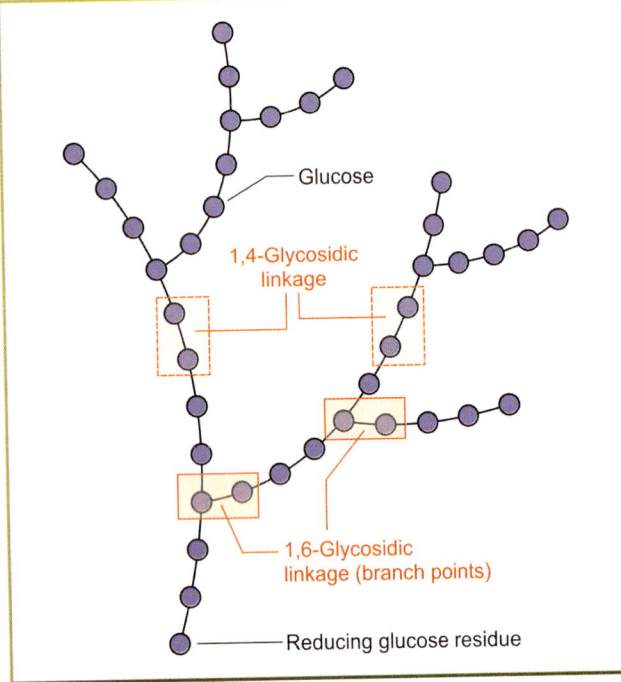

Fig. 4.15: Glycogen.

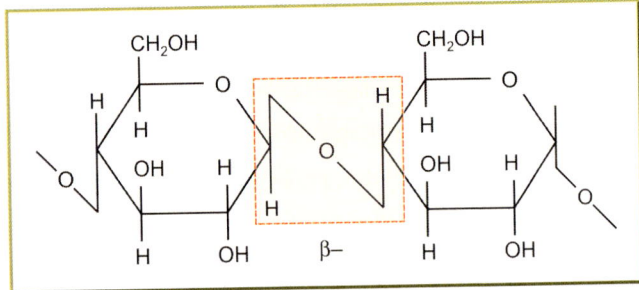

Fig. 4.16: Cellulose.

In the liver, glycogen is degraded by phosphorylase and serves as a readily available source of glucose especially during the initial 18–24 hours of fasting.

Table 4.2 lists various differences between starch and glycogen.

Cellulose

Cellulose is the primary structural component of the plant cell wall. It is a linear polymer of [-β-D-glucosyl-(1→4)-α-D-glucosyl-] repeating units. Cellulose thus has β-(1→4) glycosidic bonds (Fig. 4.16).

Cellulose cannot be digested by human beings because of lack of cellulases, the enzymes which are capable of hydrolyzing β-(1→4) linkages present in cellulose. Cellulose though cannot be utilized by the human body, it still forms a considerable part of the vegetable food and adds to the bulk of the feces.

Inulin

Inulin is a linear polymer of β-D-fructose. It occurs in bulbs of dahlia, onion and garlic. Though inulin is not utilized by human beings, it is of biological significance as it is used for determining the glomerular filtration rate (GFR).

Dextrans

Dextrans are highly branched homopolymers of glucose units with 1–6, 1–4 and 1–3 linkages. They are produced by various microorganisms growing in sucrose media. They have high molecular weight. They are used in:
1. Intravenous infusion as plasma volume expanders in the treatment of hypovolemic shock.
2. Food additives and as cryopreservatives.

'Dextran' is different from 'dextrose' (glucose solution, so called because of its dextrorotatory nature) and 'dextrin' (also called limit-dextrins. They are partially hydrolyzed products of starch containing α1→4 linkages with one or more α1→6 linkages. Iodine gives blue-purple color with starch whereas amylodextrin gives violet, erythrodextrin red, and acrodextrin no color).

Table 4.2: Differences between starch and glycogen

Starch	Glycogen
• Plant reserve food stored in seeds	• Animal reserve food stored in liver and muscles
• Less branched, branching after every 24–30 glucose units	• Highly branched, branching after every 10–12 glucose units
• Consists of amylose and amylopectin	• No such structure present
• Sparingly soluble in cold water, forms paste in hot water	• Readily soluble in water forming opalescent solution
• Gives violet color with iodine solution	• Gives brown to reddish color with iodine solution

Chitin

Chitin is present in the exoskeleton of insects and is composed of units of N-acetyl-glucosamine joined by β-1,4-glycosidic linkages.

Heteropolysaccharides

Heteropolysaccharides (heteroglycans) are the polymers of non-identical monosaccharide units, also referred to as glycosaminoglycans (GAGs). The GAGs (originally designated as mucopolysaccharides) are large complexes of negatively charged heteropolysaccharides associated with a small amount of protein, forming proteoglycans which are the gel forming components of the extracellular matrices. The GAGs are unbranched polysaccharides and consist of alternating uronic acid and hexosamines residues. Solutions of GAGs have slimy, mucus like consistency due to their high viscosity and elasticity. Most important glycosaminoglycans are hyaluronic acid, chondroitin sulfates, heparin, etc. (Fig. 4.17).

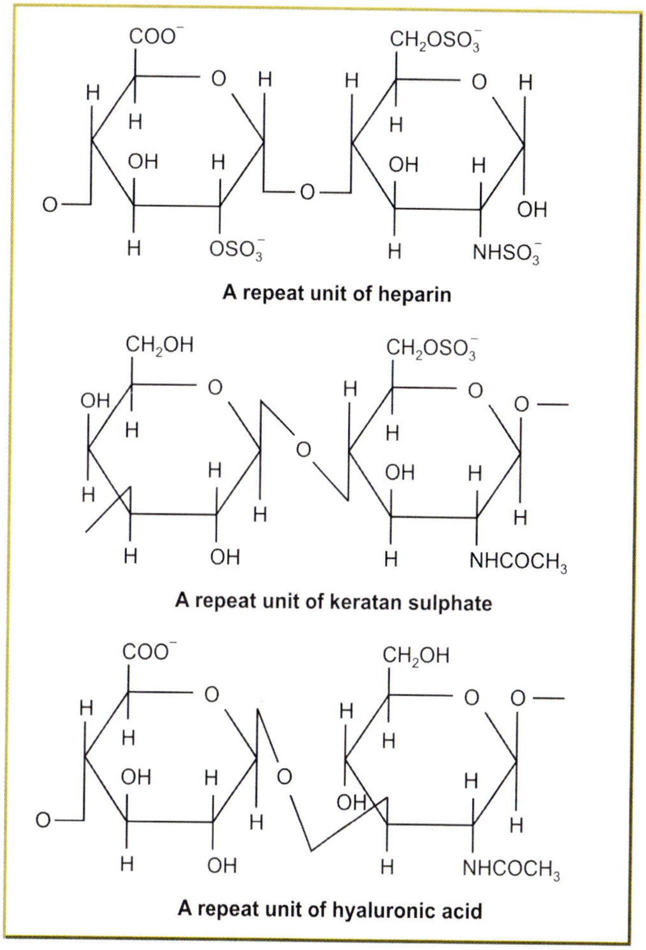

Functions of Glycosaminoglycans

1. Provide structural support to tissues, especially cartilage and connective tissue.
2. Enable the tissues to withstand torsion and shock.
3. Provide a balance between integrity and flexibility.
4. Perform specific functions in certain organs such as liver, kidney, cornea, etc.

Structure and Classification of Glycosaminoglycans

Each glycosaminoglycan chain is composed of a repeating disaccharide unit which comprises of an acidic sugar and an amino sugar, i.e. it has the structure as:

$$[\text{Acidic sugar – Amino sugar}]_n$$

The acidic sugar is either D-glucuronic acid or its carbon 5 epimer called L-iduronic acid. The amino sugar is either D-glucosamine or D-galactosamine in which the amino group is usually acetylated. It may also be sulfated on carbon 4 or 6, or on non-acetylated nitrogen.

The GAGs are divided into six major classes according to monomeric composition, type of

Fig. 4.17: Some of the heteropolysaccharides.

glycosidic linkage and degree and location of sulfate units.

Composition of GAGs and their distribution are shown in Table 4.3.

Hyaluronic Acid

Hyaluronic acid is composed of repeating units of D-glucuronic acid and N-acetyl-D-glucosamine. This polysaccharide chain is the longest of the GAGs and is the only one which is non-sulfated. It is not covalently attached to protein and is not limited to animal tissues but also found in bacteria. It is an important component of synovial fluid and the vitreous humor. The viscoelastic behavior of hyaluronate solution makes them excellent biological shock absorbers and lubricants. Its concentration is decreased in osteoarthritis (Chemistry to Clinics 4.6).

4

Table 4.3: Composition and functions of glycosaminoglycans

Glycosaminoglycan	Repeating disaccharide unit	Tissue location	Major functions
Hyaluronic acid	[GlcUA-GlcNAc]	Joint and ocular fluids	Serves as excellent biological shock absorber and lubricant
Chondroitin sulfates	[GlcUA-GalNAc]	Cartilage, tendons, bone	Bind collagen and give it strength
Dermatan sulfate	[IdUA-GalNAc]	Skin, valves, blood vessels	Valve integrity
Heparan sulfate	[IdUA-GlcNAc]	Cell surfaces	Initiation of signaling processes
Heparin	[IdUA-GlcNAc]	Mast cells, liver	Serves as an anticoagulant
Keratan sulfates	[Gal-GlcNAc]	Cartilage, cornea	Corneal transparency

Chemistry to Clinics 4.6: Osteoarthritis

Degenerative disorders of large weight-bearing joints, e.g. knee joints, are common in old age. However, obesity may result in premature osteoarthritis. The condition is characterized by reduced joint space, damage to articular cartilage and limitation of movement associated with reduced content of hyaluronic acid in synovial fluid. Commercially available hyaluronic acid is sometimes required to be injected intra-articularly.

Chondroitin Sulfates

Chondroitin sulfates contain glucuronic acid and N-acetylgalactosamine with sulfate on the hydroxyl group of either carbon 4 (chondroitin-4-sulfate) or carbon 6 (chondroitin-6-sulfate). They are the major components of cartilage where they bind collagens and hold fibers in a tight, strong network. They are also found in aorta, tendons and ligaments.

Dermatan Sulfate

Dermatan sulfate is derived from chondroitin by enzymatic epimerization of carbon 5 of glucuronate residues to form iduronate residues. Thus, dermatan sulfate contains L-iduronic acid (with variable amounts of glucuronic acid) and N-acetylgalacto-samine. It is found in skin, blood vessels, tendons and heart valves.

Heparan Sulfate

Heparan sulphates are not constructed of identical disaccharides but exhibit structural diversity. They consist of glucuronic or iduronic acid and glucosamine. Some glucosamines are acetylated and may have N- and O-sulfate groups. It is a ubiquitous cell-surface component as well as extracellular substance in blood vessel walls and brain. Heparan sulfates

which function directly at the cell surface interact with a variety of proteins including growth factors and their receptors (such as fibroblast growth factors and their receptors) to initiate signaling processes.

Heparin

Heparin consists of glucuronic or iduronic acid and glucosamine. Most of its glucosamine units are N-sulfated. Sulfate is also bound to the hydroxyl group on carbon 2 of the uronic acid residues and the carbon 3 or 6 of glucosamine. It is a highly charged polymer found in the intracellular granules of the mast cells that occur in arterial walls, especially in liver, lungs and skin. Heparin is clinically important (Chemistry to Clinics 4.7).

Keratan Sulfates

Keratin sulfate is the most heterogeneous group of GAGs as its sulfate content is variable and it contains small amounts of fucose, mannose, N-acetyl-glucos-amine and sialic acid. The repeating disaccharide generally is N-acetyl-glucosamine and galactose. Keratan sulfates are linked to protein either by an N-linked (keratan sulfate I) or O-linked (keratan sulfate II) oligosaccharide. Keratan sulfate I is found in cornea while keratan sulfate II occurs in loose connective tissue proteoglycan aggregates with chondriotin sulfate. Corneal clouding in macular

Chemistry to Clinics 4.7: Clinical Applications of Heparin

Heparin inhibits clotting of blood and is thus widely used to inhibit blood clotting after sample collection from a patient. It is also used to periodically flush intravenous lines/cannulas to keep them clot-free. Suitably modified low-molecular weight heparin is used in the prophylaxis and treatment of deep vein thrombosis (Fig. 4.18).

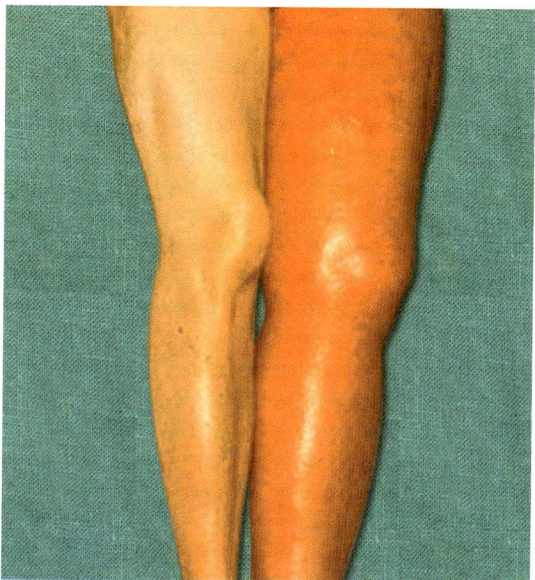

Fig. 4.18: Deep vein thrombosis caused by a thrombus in the deep veins (ileofemoral veins) in the left groin. The affected limb has all the cardinal signs of acute inflammation—swelling, heat, redness, pain and loss of function. The condition mandates **urgent treatment with intravenous heparin**.

corneal dystrophy is associated with undersulfation of keratan sulfate I.

Please refer to Chapter 37 for details about degradation of glycosaminoglycans.

CARBOHYDRATES AS MEDICINE

Some of the important carbohydrates available as medicine and their clinical use are summarized in Table 4.4.

Table 4.4: Carbohydrates as medicine

Carbohydrate	Type	Clinical application
Glucose/dextrose	Monosaccharide	Hypoglycemia
Lactulose	Synthetic disaccharide	Ammonia intoxication
Cellulose	Homopolysaccharide	Insoluble fibre for weight reduction in obesity
Dextran	Branched homopolysaccharide	Plasma expander for hypovolemic shock
Hyaluronic acid	Glycosaminoglycan	Osteoarthritis
Heparin	Glycosaminoglycan	Anticoagulation, deep vein thrombosis

SOME IMPORTANT QUESTIONS

1. Define carbohydrate. Give their classification. Explain stereoisomerism of carbohydrates.

2. What are polysaccharides? Classify them.

4

3. Write notes on:

i. Cellulose
ii. Anomers
iii. Epimers
iv. Mutarotation
v. Inulin
vi. Homopolysaccharides

vii. Heteropolysaccharides
viii. Hyaluronic acid
ix. Chondroitin sulfates
x. Heparin
xi. Carbohydrates as medicine

MULTIPLE CHOICE QUESTIONS

1. **Two enantiomers rotate the plane of polarized light:**
   A. To the same degree in the same direction
   B. To the same degree but in opposite directions
   C. To different degrees in the same direction
   D. To different degrees in opposite directions

2. **Parent compound of the carbohydrate family is:**
   A. Glucose
   B. Glycogen
   C. Galactose
   D. Glyceraldehyde

3. **In a glucose solution at equilibrium, mutarotation results in a fixed optical rotation of:**
   A. 55.2°
   B. 5.52°
   C. 5.25°
   D. 52.5°

4. **With respect to D-glucose, D-mannose and D-galactose are epimers at:**
   A. C2 and C4 respectively
   B. C4 and C2 respectively
   C. C2 and C1 respectively
   D. C1 and C2 respectively

5. **An example of a non-reducing disaccharide is:**
   A. Maltose
   B. Isomaltose
   C. Lactose
   D. Sucrose

6. **The most notorious cariogenic sugar is:**
   A. Sucrose
   B. Glucose
   C. Fructose
   D. Lactose

7. **Inulin is a:**
   A. Glucosan
   B. Lactosan
   C. Fructosan
   D. Galactosan

8. **In the prophylaxis and treatment of deep vein thrombosis, low molecular weight derivatives of the following heteropolysaccharides are used:**
   A. Hyaluronic acid
   B. Chondroitin sulphate
   C. Heparan
   D. Heparin

9. **The following heteropolysaccharide is commercially available for injecting into synovial joints in patients suffering from advanced osteoarthritis:**
   A. Hyaluronic acid
   B. Chondroitin sulphate
   C. Heparan
   D. Heparin

10. **Cornea and heart valves are rich in the following heteropolysaccharide(s):**
    A. Keratan sulphate
    B. Chondroitin-4-sulphate and chondroitin-6-sulphate
    C. Dermatan sulphate
    D. Keratan sulphate and dermatan sulphate

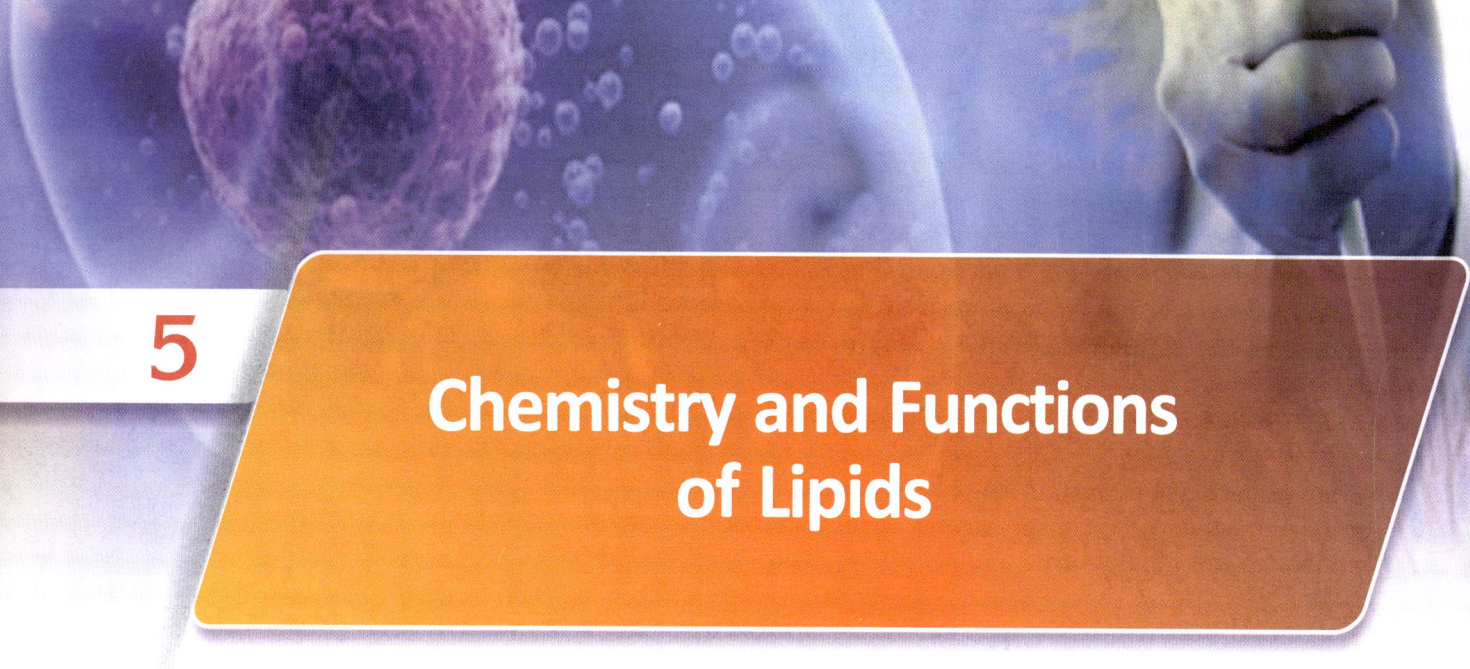

5 Chemistry and Functions of Lipids

ipids (Greek *lipos*: Fat) are the heterogeneous group of largely hydrophobic organic molecules found in all cells. They are sparingly soluble in water but are soluble in organic solvents, such as acetone, ether, alcohol or chloroform. Lipids therefore, can be easily separated from other biological materials by their extraction into organic solvents.

CLASSIFICATION OF LIPIDS

Lipids are classified into three groups, i.e. simple lipids, compound lipids and derived lipids (Fig. 5.1).

Simple Lipids

Simple lipids are the esters of fatty acids with various types of alcohol, e.g. fats, oils and waxes.

Fats and oils are complex mixtures of triacylglycerols (triglycerides) whose fatty acid composition may vary with the source. Thus, 'lipids' and 'fats' are not synonymous; fats are just a type of simple lipids.

Fats and oils differ only in that **fats are solid while oils are liquid at room temperature**.

Fats are obtained from animal sources, have more saturated fatty acids and thus higher melting points. Oils are abundant in plant seeds. These are usually rich in unsaturated fatty acids.

The esters of long chain fatty acids with high molecular weight monohydroxy aliphatic alcohols are called **waxes**. These are used in the manufacturing of various types of wax polish.

Compound Lipids

In addition to fatty acids and alcohol, certain lipids also contain some amphipathic group. These are thus called as compounds lipids, e.g. lipids conjugated with phosphate to form phospholipids.

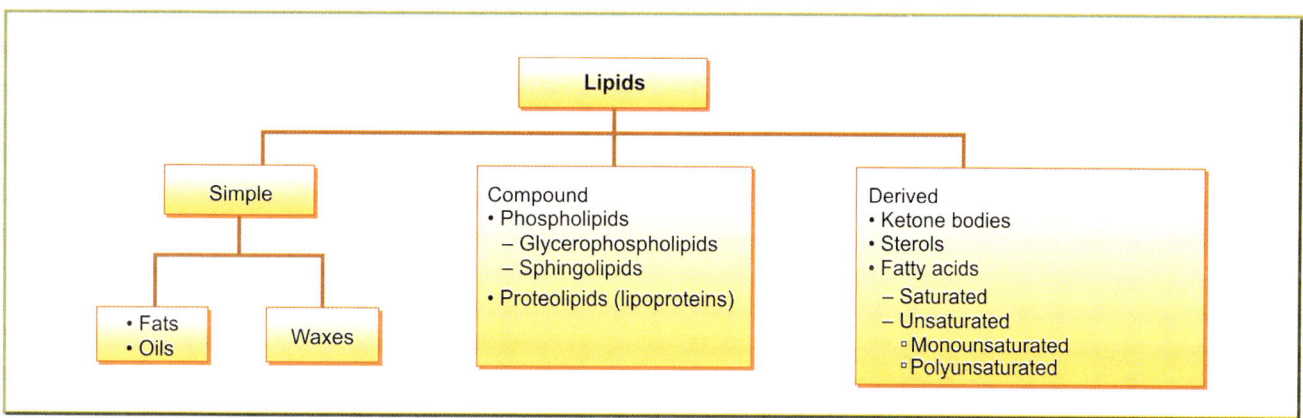

Fig. 5.1: Classification of lipids.

5

Derived Lipids

These are derived from the hydrolysis of the simple lipids and the compound lipids, e.g. fatty acids, glycerol, etc.

Biological Significance of Lipids

1. Important dietary constituents of food; have high calorific value.
2. Enhance the palatability of food (Chemistry to Clinics 5.1).
3. Dietary lipids are the source of lipid soluble vitamins and essential fatty acids.
4. Serve as energy stores.
5. Subcutaneous and peri-visceral fat acts as a thermo-insulating material.
6. Lipids around the nerves, such as myelin sheath, act as electrical insulators.
7. Lipid bilayers together with proteins are important components of biological membranes.
8. Involved in various intra and intercellular signaling events.

FATTY ACIDS

Fatty acids are the carboxylic acids with a long hydrocarbon chain. The hydrocarbon chain in turn may be **saturated** (no double bond) or **unsaturated** with one or more double bonds.

Chemistry to Clinics 5.1: Artificial Fat

Sucrose polyester, i.e. a sucrose molecule attached to 6–8 fatty acid molecules is called artificial fat or synthetic fat replacer, commercially available as Olestra. It is prescribed to patients who need to markedly cut down their dietary fat intake for medical or cosmetic reasons. It is undigested and unabsorbed in the gastrointestinal tract, hence, it is devoid of any energy value. However, it tastes like fat and is used in potato chips, tortilla chips, corn chips, crackers, etc. It is fortified with fat-soluble vitamins.

Most fatty acids in the body are esterified in triacylglycerols or phospholipids which act as storage or structural forms, or transport vehicles for fatty acids. The major source of circulating free fatty acids is the adipose tissue which releases fatty acids after hydrolysis of its storage triacylglycerols. Although the plasma concentration of free fatty acids is low, they have a very rapid turnover and are an important source of energy for many tissues of the body. They have a limited solubility in water and are mainly bound to plasma albumin which has specific binding sites for free fatty acids.

Nomenclature of Fatty Acids

The nomenclature of a fatty acid depends upon the name of the hydrocarbon chain with the same number of carbon atoms where the suffix '-oic' is substituted for the final 'e' in the name of the hydrocarbon. There are two systems of nomenclature:

Delta system: Various carbon atoms in a fatty acid are numbered, beginning with the **carboxyl carbon** (–COOH) as carbon atom number 1. The next carbon atom, to which the carboxyl carbon group is attached, is designated as α-carbon. Accordingly, carbon-3 (C3) is the β-carbon and C4 is the γ-carbon. This system of numbering of the carbon atoms of a fatty acid is called as delta (Δ) system of nomenclature of fatty acids.

Omega system: The carbon atoms in a fatty acid are counted beginning at the **methyl terminal** (CH$_3$-) end of the chain and the position where a double bond is first encountered. This carbon atom at the terminal CH$_3$-group is called omega (ω) carbon. Hence, this system of nomenclature of a fatty acid is called omega (ω) system (Fig. 5.2). However, replacement of the symbol ω by the letter 'n' has been recommended as an n-numbering system.

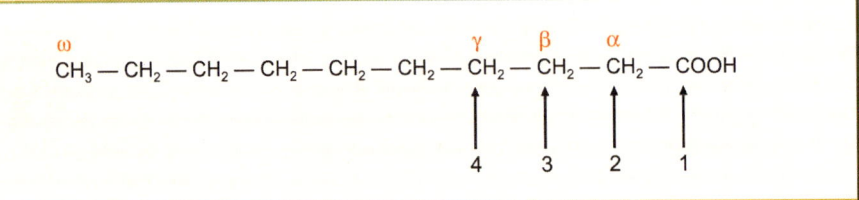

Fig. 5.2: Nomenclature of a fatty acid.

Table 5.1: Saturated fatty acids.

Fatty acids	No. of C-atoms	Formula	Sources
Acetic acid	2	CH_3-COOH	Carbohydrate fermentation
Butyric acid	4	$CH_3-(CH_2)_2-COOH$	Butter
Caproic acid	6	$CH_3-(CH_2)_4-COOH$	Butter and some plant fats
Caprylic acid	8	$CH_3-(CH_2)_6-COOH$	- do -
Capric acid	10	$CH_3-(CH_2)_8-COOH$	- do -
Lauric acid	12	$CH_3-(CH_2)_{10}-COOH$	Coconut oil
Myristic acid	14	$CH_3-(CH_2)_{12}-COOH$	- do -
Palmitic acid	16	$CH_3-(CH_2)_{14}-COOH$	Animal and plant fats
Stearic acid	18	$CH_3-(CH_2)_{16}-COOH$	- do -
Arachidic acid	20	$CH_3-(CH_2)_{18}-COOH$	Peanut oil

Saturated/Unsaturated Fatty Acids

The hydrocarbon side chain in a fatty acid may be saturated or unsaturated. Accordingly, fatty acids may be divided into two groups, i.e. saturated fatty acids and unsaturated fatty acids.

Most of the naturally occurring fatty acids have even number of carbon atoms because they are synthesized from acetyl CoA, i.e. by the combination of 2C units. They are divided into three groups, i.e. short chain (4–8C), medium chain (9–14C) and long chain fatty acids (15C or more). They have different physicochemical properties and are handled differently in the body. In higher plants and animals, the predominant fatty acids are those containing 16 or 18 carbon atoms, such as palmitic acid, oleic acid, linoleic acid and stearic acid.

Saturated fatty acids end in '-anoic', e.g. octadecanoic acid (stearic acid) is a fatty acid with 18 carbon atoms. Saturated fatty acids are highly flexible molecules and can assume a wide range of conformations because there is relatively free rotation around each of their C–C bonds. These are obtained from animal fats, e.g. butter fat. Saturated

fatty acids of common biological significance are listed in Table 5.1.

Unsaturated fatty acids, i.e. those with one or more double bonds, end with '-enoic', e.g. octadecenoic acid (oleic acid), a fatty acid with 18 carbon atoms and a double bond. Widely used convention to name an unsaturated fatty acid is to indicate the number of carbon atoms, followed by the number of double bonds with their positions in the carbon chain, such as octadecenoic acid may be written as 18:1; 9, i.e. a fatty acid with 18 carbon atoms and one double bond present on C9, i.e. between C9 and C10 (Fig. 5.3).

The location of the double bond can also be indicated by the symbol Δ, followed by a superscript

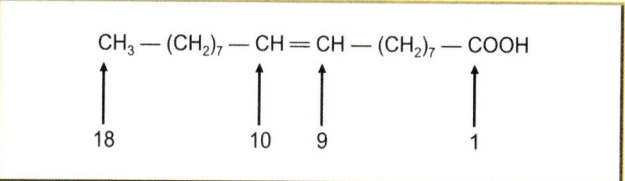

Fig. 5.3: Oleic acid or octadecenoic acid (18:1; 9).

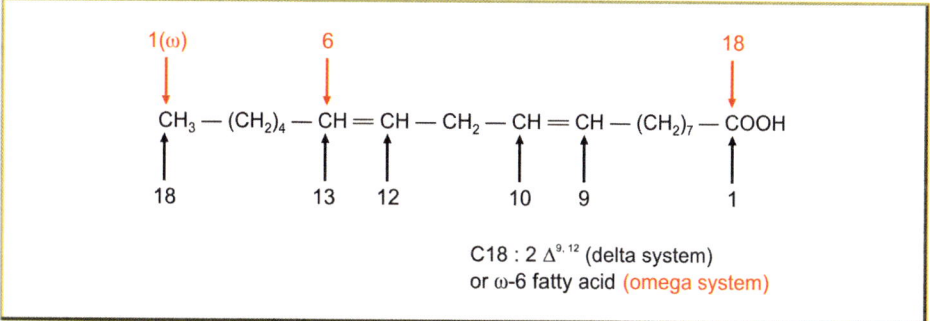

Fig. 5.4: Linoleic acid.

indicating the number of carbon atoms. Thus, linoleic acid, which has 18 carbons and two double bonds at C9 and C12, is written as $18:2\ \Delta^{9,12}$. According to the ω system, linoleic acid is designated as ω-6 fatty acid because the double bond (closest to the ω-end) is located six carbon atoms away from the ω-end (Fig. 5.4).

Over half of the fatty acid residues of plant and animal lipids are unsaturated, i.e. they contain double bonds. The double bond of a monounsaturated fatty acid commonly occurs between C9 and C10, and is called as a Δ^9 double bond, e.g. oleic acid (Fig. 5.3). The double bonds may be *cis-* or *trans-* in their orientation. Naturally occurring fatty acids have predominantly *cis-* double bonds (Chemistry to Clinics 5.2).

Chemistry to Clinics 5.2: *Trans*-Fatty Acids

Majority of the unsaturated fatty acids occurring in nature are *cis*-fatty acids, i.e. the H-atoms next to the double bonds lie on the same side of the hydrocarbon chain. Only a few are *trans*-fatty acids, i.e. the H-atoms next to the double bonds lie on opposite sides of the hydrocarbon chain (Fig. 5.5). Milk fat and butter contain traces of *trans*-fatty acids. In the body, *trans*-fatty acids behave more like saturated fatty acids than like unsaturated fatty acids and are associated with cardiovascular disease.

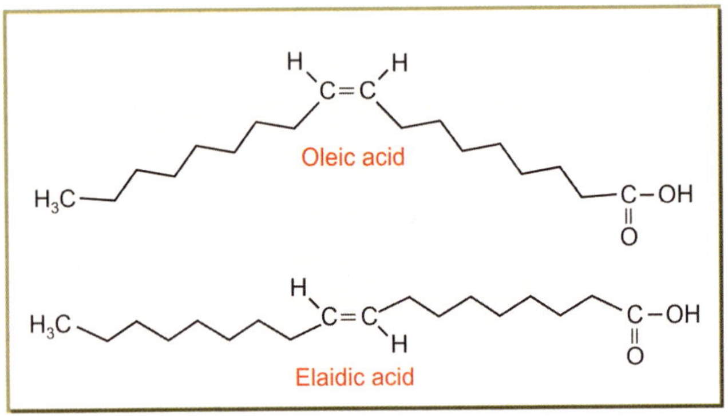

Fig. 5.5 *Cis-trans* isomerism in fatty acids: The steric geometry of unsaturated fatty acids can vary so that the acyl groups can be oriented on the same side or on opposite sides of the double bond. When both the acyl groups are on the same side of the double bond it is referred to as a *cis* bond, e.g. oleic acid (18:1). When the acyl groups are on opposite sides the bond is termed *trans* such as in elaidic acid, the *trans* isomer of oleic acid. The majority of naturally occurring unsaturated fatty acids exist in the *cis*-conformation. *Trans*-fatty acids occur in some foods and as byproducts of the process of hydrogenating saturated fatty acids to make them solids at room temperature, such as in partially hydrogenated vegetable oils.

Unsaturated fatty acids are chemically more reactive than the saturated fatty acids and are prone to alterations by processes such as lipid peroxidation. Unsaturated fatty acids pack together less efficiently than the saturated fatty acids. Unsaturated fatty acids also have reduced van der Waals interactions and low melting points; the melting point decreases with the degree of unsaturation. On the other hand, the fluidity of lipid increases with the degree of unsaturation.

Physical and Chemical Properties of Fatty Acids

- Generally, short chain fatty acids, i.e. those between 4C and 8C, are liquid while long chain fatty acids, i.e. those with >15 carbon atoms are solid at room temperature.
- Fatty acids present in various oils react with alkali and form salts. Salts of the various acids are used as soaps and emulsifying agents.
- Unsaturated fatty acids undergo reduction and are converted to saturated fats, such as hydrogenation of a vegetable oil results in the formation of ghee.
- Unsaturated fatty acids exhibit *cis-trans* isomerism, due to the presence of a double bond.
- Various fatty acids can be separated from a mixture by gas-liquid chromatography.

Polyunsaturated Fatty Acids

Fatty acids obtained from plant seeds usually contain two or more double bonds. These fatty acids are called polyunsaturated fatty acids (**PUFA**). In PUFA, double bonds generally occur after every three carbon atoms and always have a *cis*-configuration. The PUFA are obtained mainly from plant oils, e.g. soya bean oil, sunflower oil, groundnut oil, etc. The PUFA, such as linoleic acid, linolenic acid and arachidonic acid are designated as essential fatty acids (Figs 5.4 to 5.7).

Essential Fatty Acids

Though the body can introduce a double bond and prolong an aliphatic chain, polyunsaturated fatty acids (PUFA) cannot be synthesized in the body and thus are to be essentially included in the diet; hence these are called essential fatty acids, e.g. linoleic acid, linolenic acid and arachidonic acid

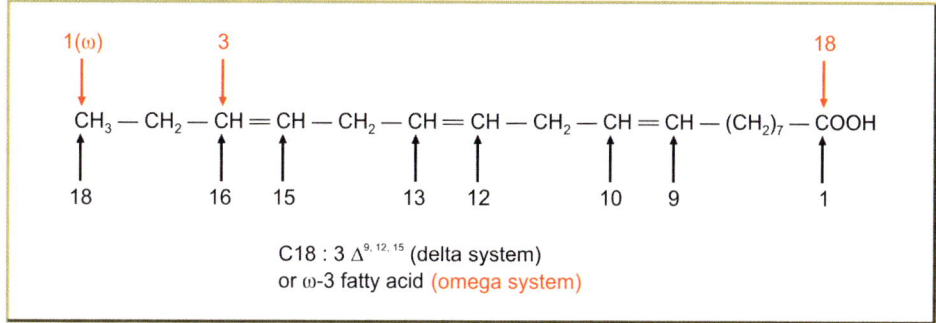

C18 : 3 $\Delta^{9, 12, 15}$ (delta system)
or ω-3 fatty acid (omega system)

Fig. 5.6: Linolenic acid.

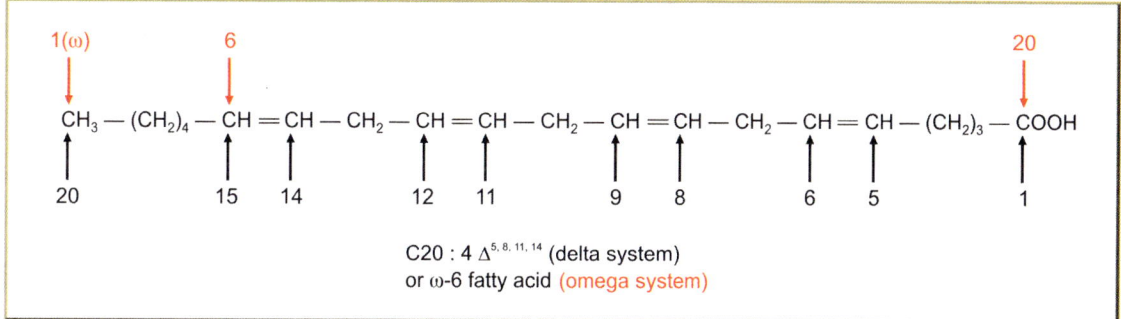

C20 : 4 $\Delta^{5, 8, 11, 14}$ (delta system)
or ω-6 fatty acid (omega system)

Fig. 5.7: Arachidonic acid.

(Figs 5.4 to 5.7). Since linoleic acid can be converted to arachidonic acid in the body, only **linoleic acid** and **linolenic acid** are truly essential in a human diet. Arachidonic acid however, becomes essential only if there is insufficient amount of linoleic acid in the diet.

Deficiencies of these three PUFA leads to the development of a condition characterized by retarded growth, hair loss, dermatitis ('toad-skin' or phrenoderma, Fig. 5.8) and poor wound healing. These are essential for the body since:

• They form an important constituent of the phospholipids.
• Essential fatty acids also help in lowering blood cholesterol level and help in its esterification in the liver.
• Arachidonic acid is also a precursor of eicosanoids such as prostaglandins, thromboxanes and leukotrienes.

Essential fatty acids are sometimes also classified by the position of the first double bond, numbered from the methyl (or ω) end of the fatty acid chain. Thus, linoleic acid is an example of an ω-6 and α-linolenic acid of an ω-3 fatty acid. Both types are

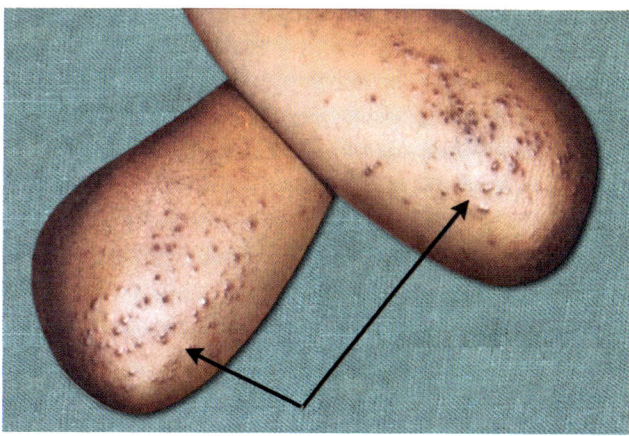

Fig. 5.8: Phrenoderma (or phrynoderma): A child with hard papules on the extensor surfaces (arrows) due to deficiency of essential fatty acids, resembling **'toad skin'**. However, sometimes, similar findings may be seen in vitamin A deficiency.

essential and can be converted into many biologically important compounds (Fig. 5.9).

Arachidonic acid (20C : 4 $\Delta^{5,8,11,14}$), an ω-6 fatty acid can be synthesized from linoleic acid. It is a precursor of the 2-series of prostaglandins and thromboxanes, and the 4-series of leukotrienes. The α-linolenic acid is converted in the body to eicosapentaenoic acid

5

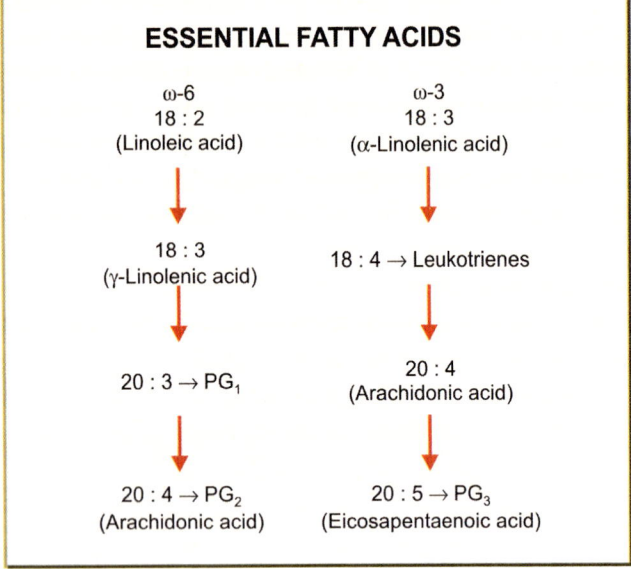

Fig. 5.9: Biological significance of essential fatty acids.

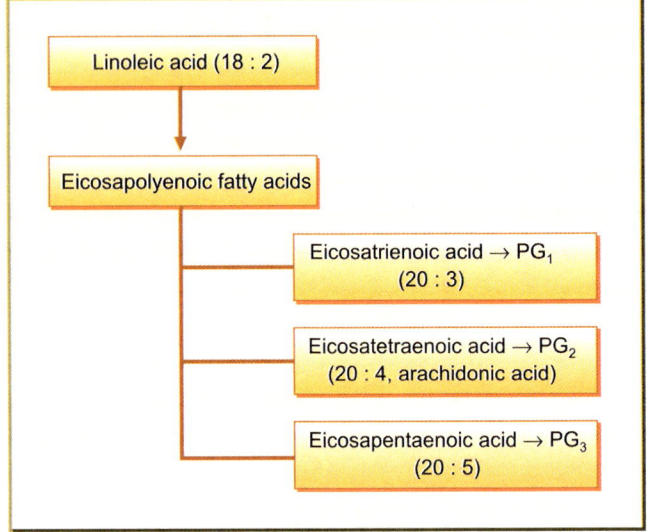

Fig. 5.10: Eicosapolyenoic acids.

(20:5 ω-3), a precursor of the 3-series of prostaglandins and thromboxanes.

Biological Significance of PUFA

1. Necessary for normal growth and health.
2. Important constituents of all biological membranes.
3. Required for the esterification of cholesterol and thus help in its transport and metabolism.
4. Diet rich in ω-6 PUFA (principally linoleic acid) promotes a reduction in cholesterol level.
5. Diet rich in ω-3 PUFA promotes a reduction in plasma triacylglycerols.
6. Arachidonic acid is a precursor of eicosanoids.

Eicosanoids

Eicosanoids (Greek *eicosa*: Twenty) are physiologically and pharmacologically active compounds such as prostanoids (prostaglandins, prostacyclins and thromboxanes), and the leukotrienes. Eicosanoids are derived from 20C containing polyunsaturated fatty acids (20C PUFA), also called as eicosapolyenoic fatty acids, such as arachidonic acid. Three different eicosapolyenoic fatty acids, i.e. eicosatrienoic acid (20C:3), eicosatetraenoic acid (20C:4 or arachidonic acid), and eicosapentaenoic acid (20C:5) with three, four and five-double bonds respectively, can be synthesized in the body from

other essential fatty acids, i.e. linoleic acid and α-linolenic acid (Fig. 5.10).

Three different eicosapolyenoic acids act as precursors of three separate series of eicosanoids designated as 1, 2 and 3 (i.e. the compounds containing 3, 4 and 5 double bonds respectively, such as PG_1, PG_2 and PG_3 series of prostaglandins). Variations in the substituent groups attached to the cyclic ring present in the eicosanoids further give rise to different types of compounds in each series. For example, the E type of prostaglandin (such as PGE_2) has a keto group in position 9 while the F type (such as PGF_1) has a hydroxyl group.

The Cyclooxygenase and Lipoxygenase Pathways

Eicosapolyenoic acids such as arachidonic acid follow one of the two metabolic pathways—the cyclooxygenase (COX) pathway or the lipoxygenase (LOX) pathway, producing different series of products. Cyclooxygenase pathway of eicosapolyenoic acid metabolism results in cyclization at the center of the 20 carbon chain. This results in the formation of a cyclopentane ring containing endoperoxides called PGG_2 which acts as precursors for the synthesis of prostaglandins, prostacyclins and thromboxanes. On the other hand, lipoxygenase pathway leads to the formation of leukotrienes (Fig. 5.11).

The specific products, so formed, are tissue dependent. For example, the endothelial cells predominantly synthesize prostacyclins whereas platelets produce thromboxanes. Eicosanoids act at very low concentrations and are important for the regulation of blood pressure, blood coagulation, vascular tone, inflammatory response, immune response, reproduction, gastric HCl secretion, maintaining the patency of fetal ductus arteriosus, smooth muscle contraction, etc. (Fig. 5.11).

Isoenzymes of cyclooxygenase (COX): Prostaglandin endoperoxide synthase (PGH_2 synthase) or cyclooxygenase (COX) catalyzes two steps in succession, i.e. oxidation of arachidonate to PGG_2 and the latter to PGH_2. The enzyme has two isoforms. COX-1 is responsible for the normal production of prosta-

glandins. COX-2 is induced by cytokines, mitogens and endotoxins during inflammation (Chemistry to Clinics 5.3).

Prostaglandins

Prostaglandins are 20 carbon containing fatty acid derivatives having one or more unsaturated bonds, several hydroxyl groups, sometimes a keto group and a cyclopentane ring. Prostaglandins are so named because of their initial isolation from the prostate gland secretion. They are now known to be produced and released by nearly all mammalian cells except red blood cells. Prostaglandins act as local hormones and have a very short half-life. Soon after their

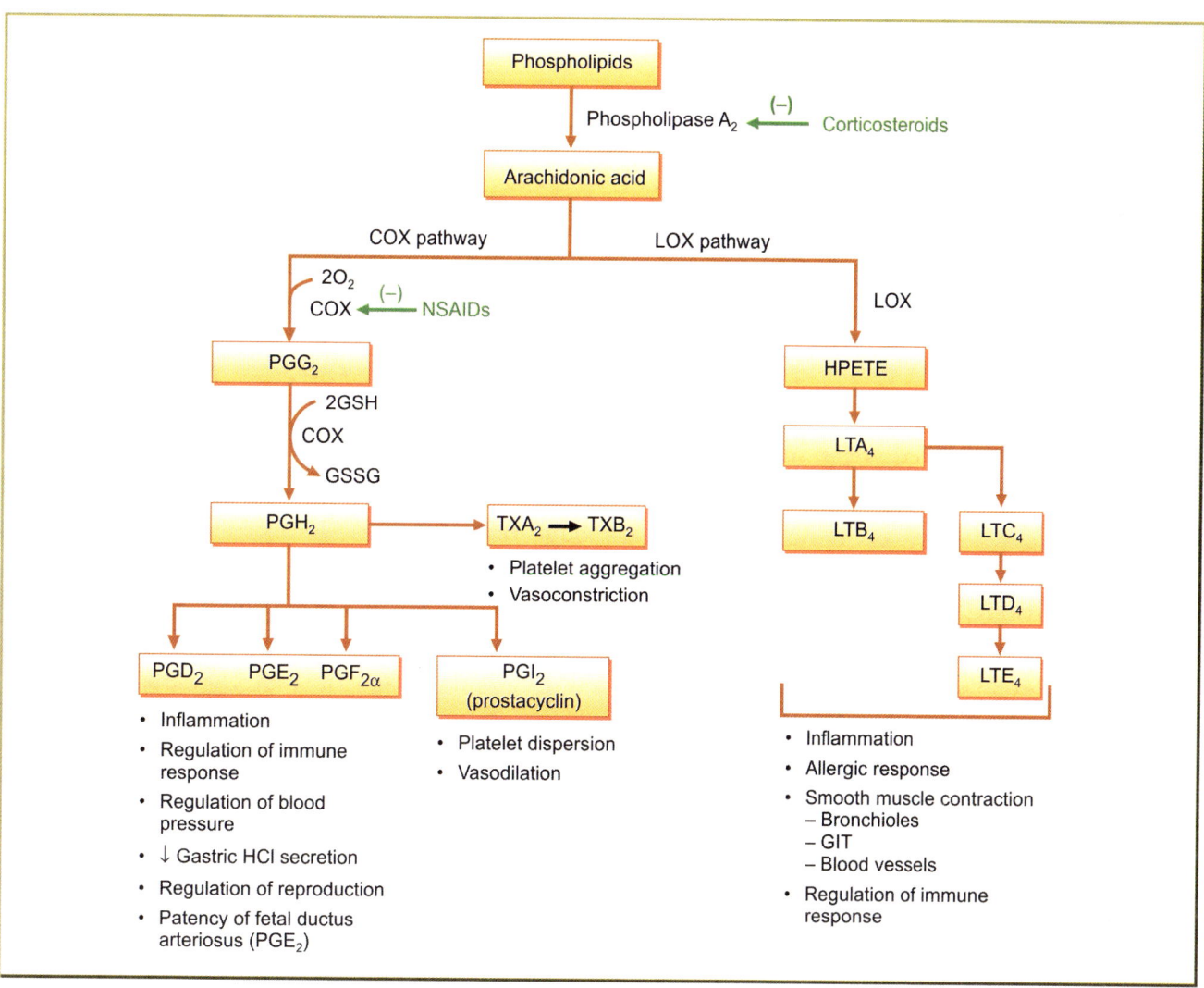

Fig. 5.11: Synthesis and functions of eicosanoids.

Chemistry to Clinics 5.3: Anti-inflammatory Drugs and Prostaglandin Synthesis

There are two broad categories of anti-inflammatory drugs:

- The **non-steroidal anti-inflammatory drugs** (NSAIDs) such as aspirin irreversibly acetylate Ser[530] of both COX-1 and COX-2. Others, such as indomethacin and ibuprofen, inhibit COX-1/COX-2 by other mechanisms and thus block the conversion of eicosanoic acids, e.g. arachidonic acid to cyclic endoperoxides thereby inhibiting the bio-synthesis of various prostaglandins. These drugs are non-specific COX inhibitors. Recently, specific COX-2 inhibitors have been developed that selectively suppress the role of eicosanoids during inflammation only. Such inhibitors, called 'coxibs' (e.g. celecoxib and etoricoxib), also produce less gastric and renal side effects.

- The **steroidal anti-inflammatory drugs** like hydrocortisone, prednisone and betamethasone, on the other hand, block the entire eicosanoid biosynthetic pathway by inhibiting phospholipase A_2 activity so as to interfere with the mobilization of arachidonic acid, an essential substrate for the subsequent reactions. Thus, steroids are more potent anti-inflammatory drugs than NSAIDs.

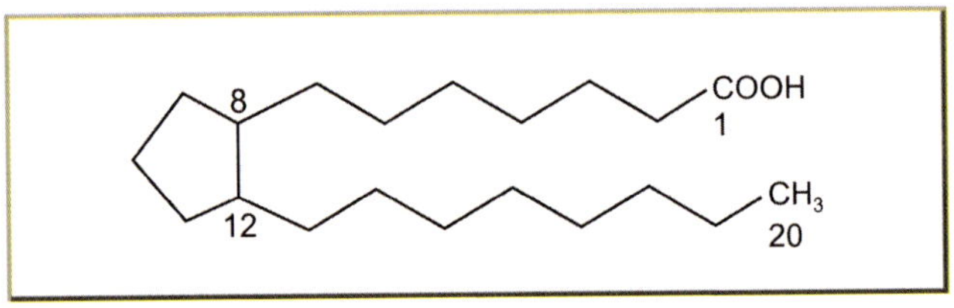

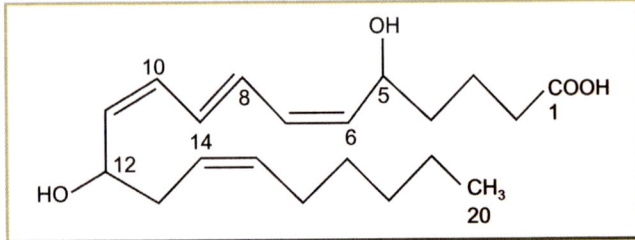

Fig. 5.12: Prostanoic acid.

release, they are rapidly taken up by the cells where they exert very short-lived effects and are rapidly catabolized.

There are three major classes of primary prostaglandins, i.e. the A, E and F series. All are related to the hypothetical parent compound, prostanoic acid (Fig. 5.12). They are distinguished on the basis of functional groups around the cyclopentane ring, i.e. the E series contains a β-hydroxy-ketone, the F series are 1,3-diols, and those in the A series are α, β-unsaturated ketones. The subscript numerals 1, 2 and 3 refer to the number of double bonds in the side chain.

Prostacyclins

Prostacyclins (PGI_2) are derived from eicosapolyenoic acids such as arachidonic acid in the vascular endothelium. These have a powerful vasodilatory action especially on the coronary arteries. These are also responsible for inhibiting platelet aggregation.

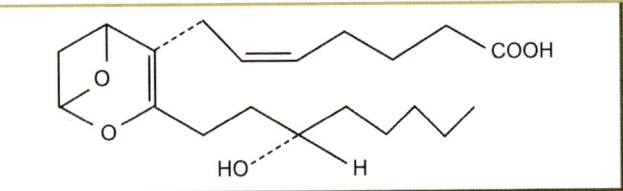

Fig. 5.13: Thromboxane A_2 (TXA_2).

Thromboxanes

The term 'thromboxane' is derived from the fact that these compounds have thrombus-forming potential. They are highly active metabolites of PGG_2 and PGH_2 type prostaglandin endoperoxides whose cyclo-pentane ring is replaced by a six-membered oxygen containing ring called as oxane ring (Fig. 5.13). The substituent groups attached to different positions of the ring give rise to different types in each series of thromboxanes, i.e. A, B, etc.

The thromboxane TXA_2 is the main prostaglandin endoperoxide formed in platelets. It causes release of serotonin and Ca^{2+} from platelet granules. It produces vasoconstriction and increase blood pressure besides contraction of arterial smooth muscle and platelet aggregation.

Leukotrienes

Leukotrienes are a family of conjugated trienes formed from eicosapolyenoic fatty acids by the lipoxygenase pathway. Twenty carbon polyunsaturated fatty acids, such as arachidonic acid, are first converted to their hydroperoxy-eicosatetraenoic acids (HPETE) and serve as precursors of different types of leukotrienes. Leukotrienes do not have a ring in their structure but have three conjugated double bonds (Fig. 5.14).

Leukotrienes are synthesized in leukocytes, mast cells and macrophages in response to immunologic and non-inflammatory stimuli. They stimulate mucus secretion and cause constriction of the bronchial smooth muscles (Chemistry to Clinics 5.4).

Fig. 5.14: Leukotriene B_4 (LTB_4).

Chemistry to Clinics 5.4: Leukotrienes and Bronchial Asthma

Elevated levels of leukotrienes (LT) are associated with various inflammatory and hypersensitivity disorders, such as bronchial asthma. Specifically, a combination of LTC4, D4 and E4, previously known as the 'slow reacting substance of anaphylaxis or SRSA', is notorious to produce bronchospasm. Drugs blocking the leukotriene receptors are currently being used in the treatment of bronchial asthma. Further, it is useful to bear in mind that aspirin and other NSAIDs suppress the cyclooxygenase pathway and thereby divert the eicosanoid pathway towards the synthesis of leukotrienes. This can precipitate an asthmatic attack in aspirin-sensitive individuals.

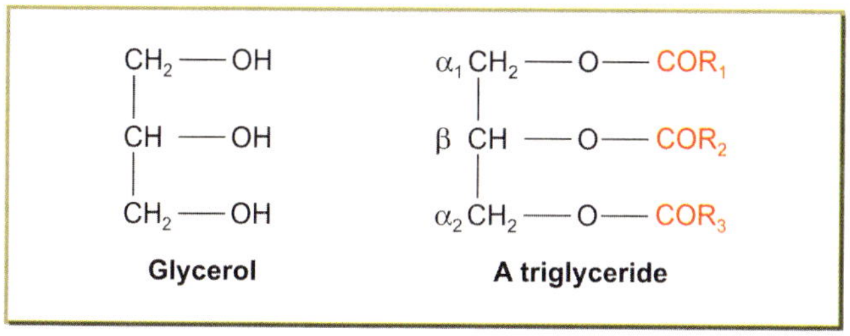

Fig. 5.15: Structure of glycerol and a triglyceride (triacylglycerol or neutral fat).

TRIACYLGLYCEROLS

Triacylglycerols or neutral fats (also called triglycerides) are fatty acid tri-esters of glycerol (glycerin, a trihydric alcohol) and are simple lipids. Glycerol with one molecule of a fatty acid is called **monoacylglycerol**, with two molecules of fatty acids is called a **diacylglycerol** while with three fatty acid residues it is known as **triacylglycerol** (Fig. 5.15).

A molecule of triacylglycerol may contain three similar or dissimilar fatty acid residues which may be saturated and/or unsaturated. Triglycerides are named according to the presence of the fatty acid residues on the glycerol moiety, e.g. 1-palmitoyl-2-arachidonoyl-3-stearoylglycerol has palmitic acid at C1, arachidonic acid at C2 and stearic acid at C3 of glycerol. All natural fats and oils invariably are complex mixtures of triacylglycerols whose fatty acid composition varies with the source. Plant oils are usually rich in unsaturated fatty acids compared to animal fats. Generally, with the primary alcoholic groups, i.e. at the α positions (C1 and C3 of glycerol), there are saturated fatty acids while at C2 there is an unsaturated fatty acid.

Dietary fat, which is an important source of energy for the body, mainly contains triacylglycerols. In the body also triacylglycerols are the store of energy. Fat is stored in the body in the form of triacylglycerols, mainly in the adipose tissue. Triacylglycerols are transported in the plasma either as chylomicrons (which are produced by the intestine for the transport of exogenous fat) or as very low density lipoprotein particles (which are produced in the liver for the transport of endogenous triglycerides).

Physical and Chemical Properties of Triacylglycerols

1. *Energy reserve:* Triacylglycerols are the major storage form of energy in the body. In animals, fat cells (adipocytes) are specialized for the synthesis and storage of triacylglycerols. The average fat content of normal human being is about 21% for man and 26% for woman. This allows them to survive for 2–3 months.
2. *Hydrolysis:* Triacylglycerols are hydrolysed by lipases to release free fatty acids and glycerol (Fig. 5.16).
3. *Rancidity:* Naturally occurring fats, particularly from animal sources, develop unpleasant odour and taste, if stored under moist conditions. This is called rancidity. It is due to partial hydrolysis of triacylglycerols and the subsequent oxidation of the released fatty acids to aldehydes and ketones. Antioxidants, e.g. vitamin E can prevent atmospheric oxidation of fats and thus rancidity.
4. *Iodine number:* Unsaturated fatty acids, present in triacylglycerols can accept halogens, such as iodine at the double bond. This process is termed as **halogenation**. It is a measure of the degree of unsaturation of a fat. Number of grams of iodine used for the iodination of 100 g of fat is referred to as iodine number. High iodine number indicates that more unsaturated fatty acids are present in a particular fat, thus suggestive of high degree of unsaturation.

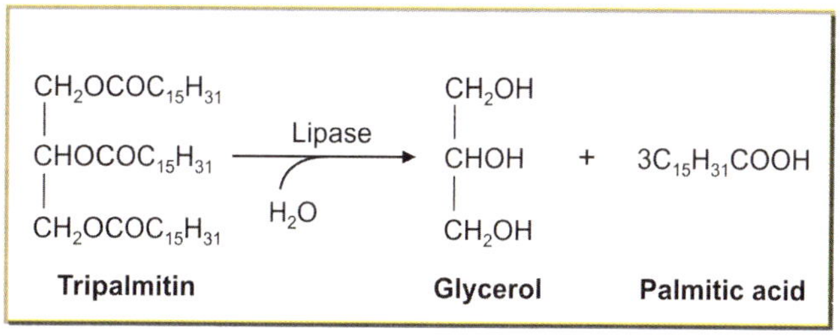

Fig. 5.16: Hydrolysis of tripalmitin, a triglyceride.

5

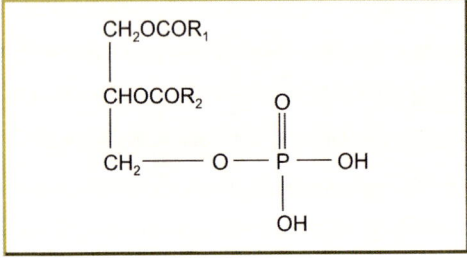

Fig. 5.17: Phosphatidic acid.

PHOSPHOLIPIDS

Phospholipids are a heterogeneous group of compound lipids which contain one or more phosphoric acid and a polar group, which may be a nitrogenous base, an amino acid or a polyalcohol. In addition, they also contain long chain fatty acid residues. With cholesterol, phospholipids are the important constituents of the cell membrane. Classification of phospholipids is given in Table 5.2.

Glycerophospholipids

Phospholipids which are derivatives of glycerol are called glycerophospholipids or phosphoglycerides. Glycerophospholipids are the major lipid components of the biological membrane. A glycerophospholipid consists of glycerol, two residues of fatty acids and a molecule of phosphoric acid. Phosphoric acid is attached at C3 of glycerol, forming glycerol-3-phosphate. The C1 and C2 positions of glycerol-3-phosphate are esterified with two fatty acids. A saturated fatty acid usually occurs at C1 (α1-carbon) while a polyunsaturated fatty acid is commonly attached at C2 (β-carbon) of glycerol. Glycero-phospholipids are thus amphiphilic molecules with nonpolar tails and polar heads.

1, 2-Diacylglycerol

Some of the hydrolyzed products of glycero-phospholipids, such as 1,2-diacylglycerol, serve as intra- and extracellular signaling molecules. 1,2-diacylglycerol is derived from membrane lipids by the action of phospholipase C. It is an intracellular signal molecule that activates protein kinase.

Phosphatidic Acid

The simplest glycerophospholipid is phosphatidic acid (Fig. 5.17). It is produced by hydrolysis of the membrane lipids in blood platelets and injured cells, and stimulates cell growth as a part of the wound repair process. The phosphoryl group of phosphatidic acid may be linked to a nitrogenous compound such as ethanolamine, choline or serine, or to some other group like inositol thereby forming various glycerophospholipids, e.g. phosphatidylcholine (lecithin), phosphatidylethanolamine (cephalin), phosphatidylinositol, etc.

Lecithins

Lecithins contain choline (a nitrogenous base) at C3 in a phosphatidic acid (Fig. 5.18). Lecithins are surface active agents and help in emulsification of fat. These are widely distributed in brain, lungs, nerve cells, sperm and egg yolk.

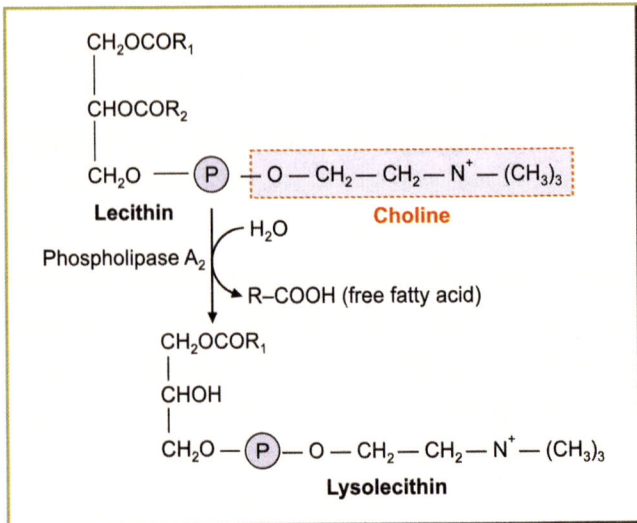

Fig. 5.18: Lecithins.

Chemistry to Clinics 5.5: Snake Venom

The venom of Indian cobra (*Naja naja*) is rich in phospho-lipase A_2. Entry of the venom into the circulation of a victim of cobra-bite results in extensive hydrolysis of fatty acids at position C2 of membrane glycerophospholipids. This alters the membrane integrity especially of RBC. Further, the released lysolecithin acts as detergent and disrupts the membrane leading to hemolysis. The liberation of hemoglobin into the circulation may be sufficiently high (exceeding the capacity of haptoglobin and hemopexin, the hemoglobin-binding plasma proteins) to block the renal tubules and cause acute renal failue.

Various hydrolytic enzymes, known as phospho-lipases, act at different sites in glycerophospholipids and hydrolyze them. This leads to the formation of various products, e.g. phospholipase A_2 hydrolytically excises a fatty acid residue from C2, leaving a lysophospholipid (Chemistry to Clinics 5.5).

Lung Surfactant

Chemical nature: Pulmonary surfactant is a lipo-protein rich in phospholipid. The principal agent responsible for its surface tension-reducing properties is dipalmitoyl phosphatidylcholine (DPPC), also called dipalmitoyl lecithin.

Biosynthesis: The alveolar epithelium consists of two cell types: Alveolar type I and type II cells. Alveolar type II cells, often referred to as type II pneumocytes, synthesize surfactant. Compared with type I cells, they are rich in mitochondria and are metabolically more active. Electron-dense lamellar inclusion bodies are a distinguishing feature of the type II cell and are the storage sites for surfactant (Fig. 5.19).

Principle of action
- The alveolar lining is coated with pulmonary surfactant which not only lowers surface tension at the gas-liquid interface but also changes surface tension with changes in alveolar diameter (Fig. 5.20). Therefore, pulmonary surfactant makes it possible for alveoli of different diameters that are connected in parallel to coexist and be stable at low lung volumes, by lowering surface tension proportionately more in the smaller alveoli.
- When the water and gas molecules are compressed during lung deflation, surfactant causes a decrease in surface tension. At low lung volume, when the molecules are tightly compressed, some surfactant

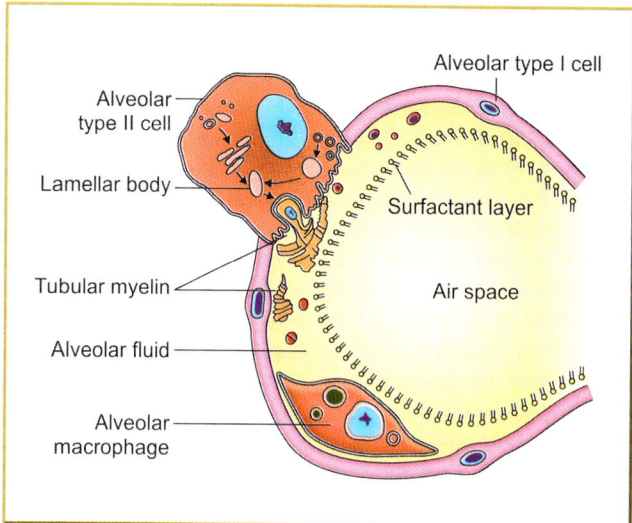

Fig. 5.19: Surfactant layer inside an alveolus. Alveolar type II cells synthesize surfactant and store it as lamellar bodies which are later exocytosed and complexed with proteins to form tubular myelin. Subsequently, the surfactant layer is formed.

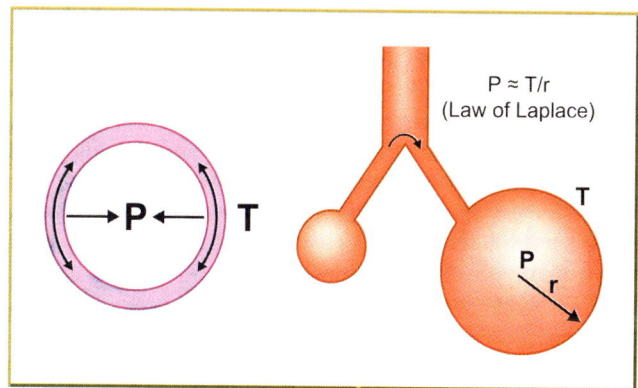

Fig. 5.20: The Law of Laplace states that the pressure (P) inside a sphere is inversely proportional to the radius (r) at constant surface tension (T). Thus, if surface tensions are equal, during deflation (expiration), a small alveolus will experience a greater inward force than a large alveolus. If both alveoli are connected to the same airway, the small alveolus will be more likely to collapse, expelling its contents into the large alveolus. This is prevented by the **action of surfactant which lowers surface tension more in** the small alveolus.

is squeezed out of the surface. On expansion (reinflation), new surfactant is required to form a new film that is spread on the alveolar surface lining.

- In addition to lowering alveolar surface tension and promoting alveolar stability, surfactant helps to prevent edema in the lungs. The inwardly contracting force that tends to collapse alveoli also

5

tends to lower interstitial pressure, which 'pulls' fluid from the capillaries. Pulmonary surfactant reduces this tendency by lowering surface forces.

Lung maturity: Because the lungs are among the last organs to develop, the synthesis of surfactant appears rather late in gestation. In humans, surfactant appears at about week 34 (a full-term pregnancy is 40 weeks). Failure of proper lung maturation during the perinatal period is still a major cause of death in newborns (Chemistry to Clinics 5.6). On the other hand, surfactant deficiency in a mature lung may result in adult respiratory distress syndrome (Chemistry to Clinics 5.7).

Chemistry to Clinics 5.6: Infant Respiratory Distress Syndrome

Premature birth and certain hormonal disturbances (such as those seen in diabetic pregnancies) interfere with the normal control and timing of lung maturation. These infants have structurally intact but functionally immature lungs at birth which often leads to infant respiratory distress syndrome (IRDS), also called **hyaline membrane disease**. Breathing is extremely labored because surface tension is high, making it difficult to inflate the lungs. These infants develop pulmonary edema and atelectasis (alveolar collapse, Fig. 5.21). They are at high risk until the lungs become mature enough to secrete surfactant. The syndrome can be diagnosed by obtaining amniotic fluid (amnio-centesis, Fig. 5.22) and calculating the lecithin: Sphingo-myelin ratio (**L/S ratio**). The condition can be treated with exogenous surfactants and hydrocortisone injection during antenatal period.

Cephalins

Cephalins are glycerophospholipids where instead of choline present in lecithins, either ethanolamine or serine is attached as a nitrogenous base with the

Chemistry to Clinics 5.7: Adult Respiratory Distress Syndrome (ARDS)

It is the name given to diffuse lung injury of various causes which include trauma from chest injury (e.g., car accidents), long bone injury, and pelvic injury. Two other major causes include sepsis (presence of pathogen or toxin in the blood) and aspiration of gastric contents. The latter occurs with gastric reflux and usually occurs at night during sleep. Other causes include cardiopulmonary bypass, high altitude, smoke inhalation and exposure to irritant gases. Exposure to irritant gases was the cause of the widespread ARDS cases that occurred at the disaster in Bhopal, India. ARDS is characterized by decreased lung compliance, pulmonary edema, focal atelectasis and hypoxemia (low partial pressure of O_2 in the arterial blood), with an inflammatory reaction that leads to an infiltration of neutrophils into the lung.

Neutrophil aggregation is a key underlying mechanism of ARDS, causing capillary endothelial damage by releasing a number of toxic products. These include oxygen free radicals, proteolytic enzymes, arachidonic acid metabolites (leukotrienes, thromboxanes, prostaglandins), and platelet-activating factor. Collectively, these factors lead to a loss of surfactant and an increase in lung stiffness (i.e., decreased compliance). The condition warrants the use of mechanical ventilation and drugs to reduce neutrophil chemoattraction and aggregation in the pulmonary capillaries.

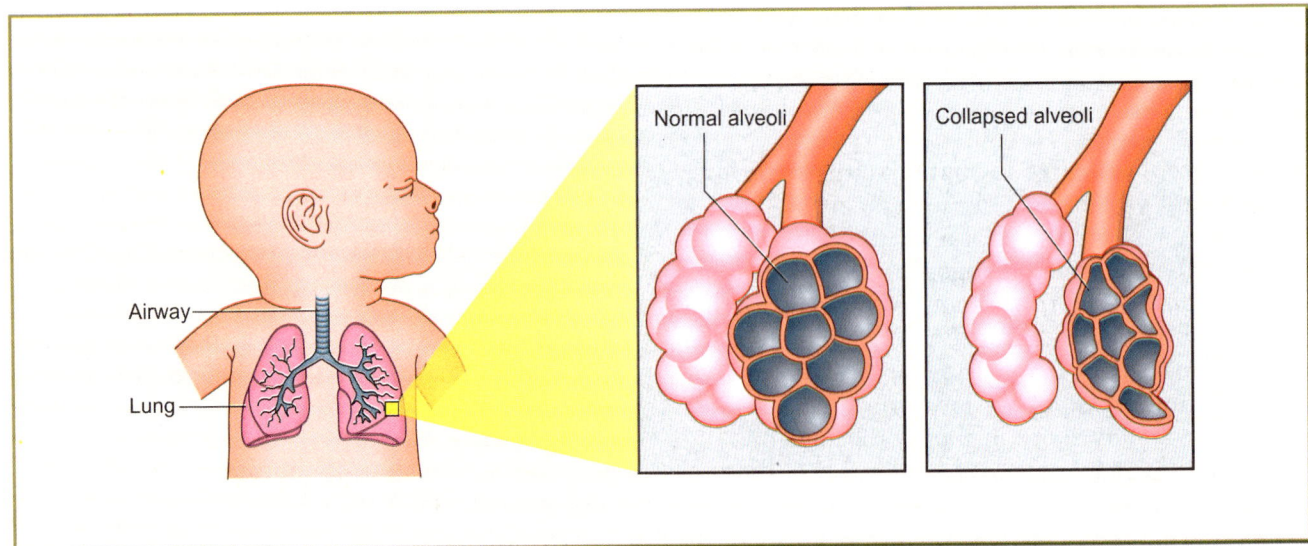

Fig. 5.21: Collapsed alveoli in infantile respiratory distress syndrome.

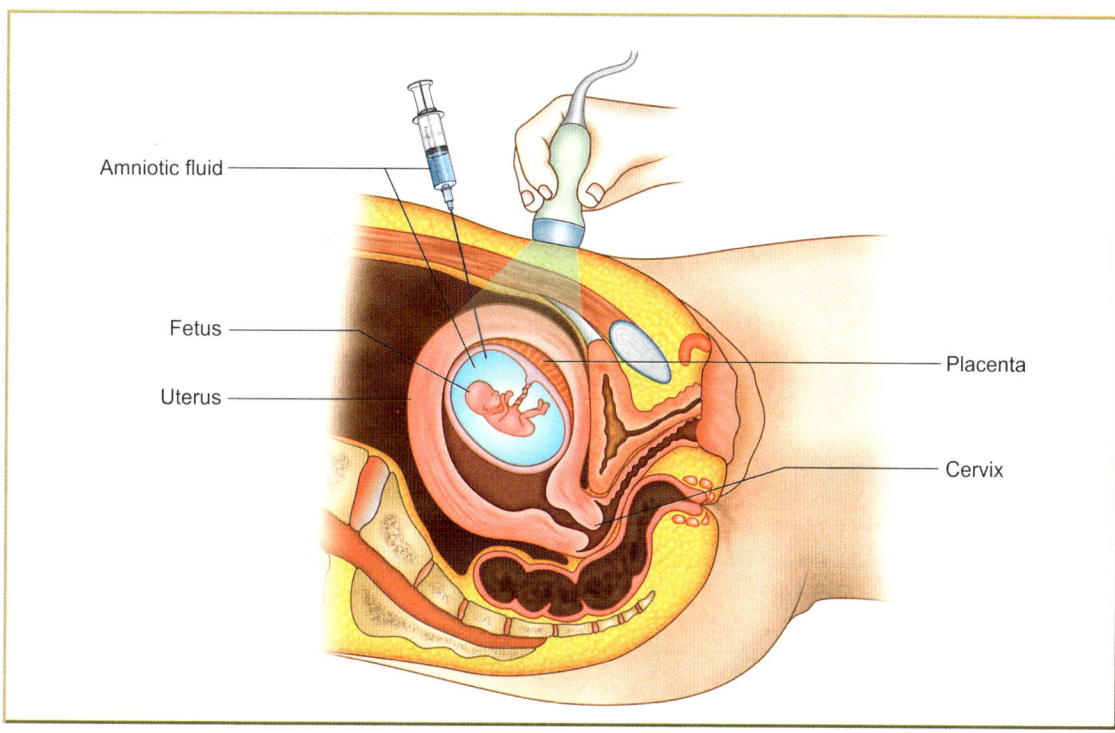

Fig. 5.22: Amniocentesis: The aspiration of amniotic fluid under ultrasound guidance. Lecithin: Sphingomyelin ratio (L/S ratio) in the amniotic fluid is used for the evaluation of fetal lung maturity. Before 33–35 weeks of gestation, the ratio is nearly 1.0. At term, there is a marked increase in lecithin concentration and thus the L/S ratio increases to more than 5.0. In a premature low birth weight fetus, the ratio is <2.0. Such infants are likely to develop respiratory distress syndrome.

phosphoric acid residue. Cephalins are present in erythrocyte membrane, brain, etc.

Phosphatidylinositols

Phosphatidylinositols are glycerophospholipids containing phosphatidic acid bound to inositol instead of a nitrogenous base. These are found mainly in the brain.

Plasmalogens

Plasmalogens are glycerophospholipids in which C1 of glycerol is linked to an α, β-unsaturated fatty acid by an ether linkage in the *cis*-configuration, rather than to a saturated fatty acid through an ester linkage. Plasmalogens are present in cardiac and skeletal muscles, and in semen. Because of their large concentration in cardiac muscles these are also called cardiolipins.

Sphingolipids

Sphingolipids do not contain glycerol but are derivatives of an unsaturated amino alcohol sphingosine which has 18 carbon atoms and a double bond with a *trans*-configuration. Most sphingolipids are sphingoglycolipids, i.e. their polar head groups consist of carbohydrate units.

N-Acyl derivatives of sphingosine (N-acyl sphingosines) are known as **ceramides**. The ceramides are parent compounds of most sphingolipids, e.g. sphingomyelins, cerebrosides and gangliosides.

Sphingomyelins

Sphingomyelins are ceramides with either phosphocholine or phosphoethanolamine. These are the most common sphingolipids and are also called sphingophospholipids. The membranous myelin sheath that surrounds and electrically insulates many nerve cell axons is particularly rich in sphingomyelins.

Sphingolipids, like glycerophospholipids, are a source of smaller lipids that have discrete signaling activity. Sphingomyelin as well as ceramide portions of the more complex sphingolipids, modulate activities of protein kinases and protein phosphatases that are involved in the regulation of cell growth and differentiation.

The lecithin:sphingomyelin ratio (**L/S ratio**) in amniotic fluid is an index of fetal lung maturity (Fig. 5.22).

Cerebrosides

Cerebrosides are glycosphingolipids and contain a ceramide with a sugar residue (such as galactose or glucose), i.e. cerebrosides are ceramide monosaccharides. Most prevalent cerebrosides are galactocerebrosides and glucocerebrosides. In contrast to phospholipids, cerebrosides lack phosphate groups and hence are nonionic.

A number of cerebrosides are found in white matter of the brain and in myelin sheath of nerves. These are named with respect to the fatty acid they contain, e.g. a galactosylceramide called cerebran contains cerebronic acid. Similarly, nervon has an unsaturated derivative of lignoceric acid called nervonic acid.

Gangliosides

Structure: Gangliosides are the most complex glycosphingolipids. They are ceramides with attached oligosaccharides that include hexosamines (glucosamine or galactosamine) and at least one molecule of N-acetyl-neuraminic-acid (sialic acid). In other words, gangliosides are sialic acid containing ceramide oligosaccharides.

Nomenclature: Numerous gangliosides are known and each one of them has different oligosaccharide head groups. These are designated as G_{M1}, G_{M2}, G_{M3} etc. (G refers to a ganglioside; M, D or T indicate mono-, di- or tri-sialic acid residues; the number with each subscript denotes the carbohydrate sequence that is attached to the ceramide).

Distribution: Gangliosides are primarily components of cell membrane surface and constitute a significant fraction of brain lipids. They are present in large amount in the ganglion cells of the central nervous system, particularly in the nerve endings.

Importance
1. Their complex carbohydrate head-groups act as specific receptors for certain pituitary glycoprotein hormones that regulate a number of important physiological functions.

2. Gangliosides are receptors for certain bacterial protein toxins such as cholera toxin (Fig. 5.23), tetanus toxin and certain viruses.
3. Gangliosides are specific determinants of cell-recognition and thus have a role in growth and differentiation of tissues as well as in carcinogenesis.

STEROIDS

Steroids are the derivatives of **cyclopentanoperhydrophenanthrene ring**, also called as **steroid nucleus**, a component that consists of four fused, nonpolar rings labeled as A, B, C and D (Fig. 5.24).

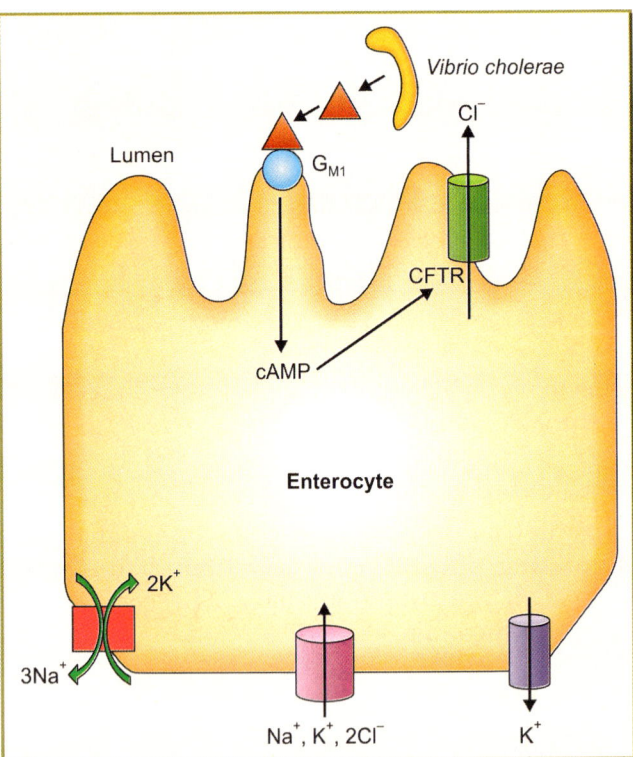

Fig. 5.23: Cholera toxin induced diarrhea: The bacterium *Vibrio cholerae* secretes a toxin (red triangle) which binds to the ganglioside receptor G_{M1} (blue sphere) on the enterocyte luminal brush border membrane. Activation of adenylate cyclase forms cAMP which stimulates secretion of Cl^- through cystic fibrosis transmembrane regulator (**CFTR channels**), with associated sodium and water secretion. Cl^- and Na^+ reabsorption are also inhibited. The abundance of water and mucus in the stool gives the name 'rice water' diarrhea, causing severe dehydration. The various ion channels in the contraluminal membrane fail to compensate for the deficiency. The condition requires treatment with oral rehydration solution or, in an emergency, with intravenous fluids/electrolytes.

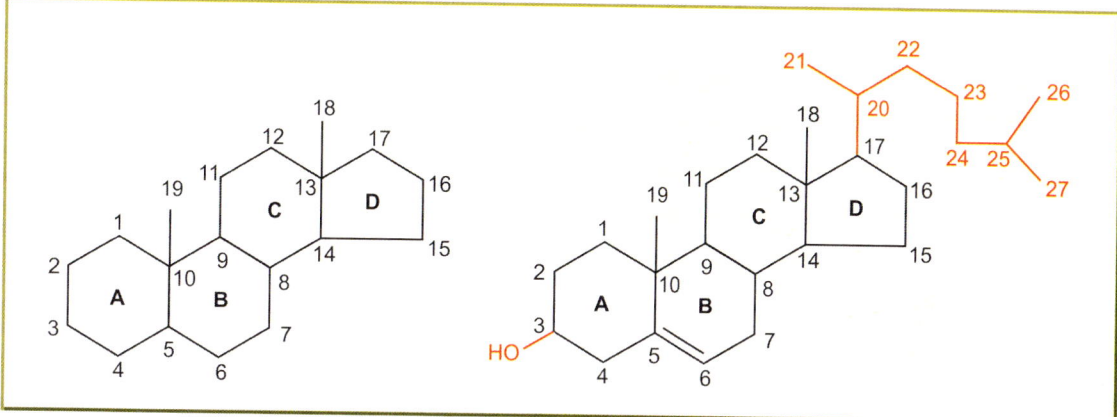

Fig. 5.24: Steroid nucleus (cyclopentanoperhydrophenanthrene ring) and cholesterol.

Cholesterol

Structure: Cholesterol is the most abundant steroid in animals. It has 27 carbon atoms, a hydroxyl group at C3, a double bond between C5 and C6, two methyl groups at C18 and C19, and a side chain at C17 (Fig. 5.24). Because of the OH group (at C3), cholesterol is a steroid alcohol (sterol) and can be esterified to long-chain fatty acids to form cholesteryl esters.

Functions

1. The body of an adult contains about 1 g cholesterol/kg body weight. About 25% of it is in the membranes of the nervous system where it is a major component of the myelin sheath.

2. Cholesterol is a major component of all biological membranes where it exists as free/unesterified cholesterol.

3. It is a precursor of steroid hormones (gluco-corticoids, mineralocorticoids, androgens and estrogens), vitamin D and bile acids.

Normal serum cholesterol level is 150–250 mg/dl although the desirable level in adults is <220 mg/dl. Eggs, meat and milk are the main dietary sources of cholesterol. It is also synthesized in the body by nearly all cells and the process is controlled by the intracellular cholesterol content. The amount synthesized each day is at least twice of that ingested in the average diet which is nearly 250–750 mg/day.

LIPOPROTEINS

Lipids such as triacylglycerols, cholesterol and phospholipids are sparingly soluble in aqueous solution (plasma). Hence, these are transported in blood in complex with proteins (called apolipoproteins or simply apoproteins), as hydrophilic complexes known as lipoproteins. These are globular micelle-like particles that consist of nonpolar core of triacylglycerols and cholesteryl esters surrounded by an amphiphilic coating of proteins, phospholipids and cholesterol.

Separation of lipoproteins: According to their densities, various lipoproteins can be separated by ultracentrifugation (Fig. 5.25). These can also be separated according to their protein contents, by electrophoresis (Fig. 5.26).

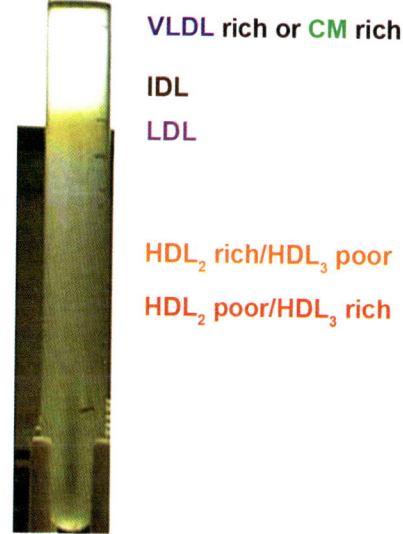

VLDL rich or **CM** rich

IDL

LDL

HDL$_2$ rich/**HDL$_3$** poor

HDL$_2$ poor/**HDL$_3$** rich

Fig. 5.25: Separation of serum lipoproteins by ultracentrifugation. HDL subfractions, i.e. HDL$_2$ and HDL$_3$ are discussed in Chapter 12.

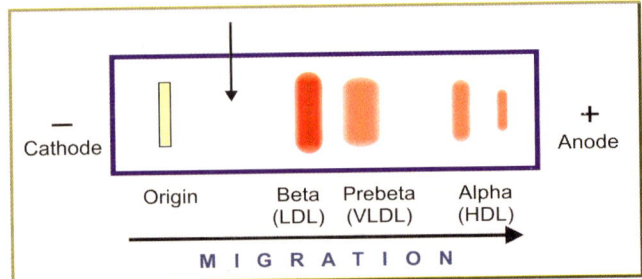

Fig. 5.26: Electrophoretogram of serum lipoproteins after 12 hours of fasting. For approximately 2–8 hours following a meal, there is an additional lipoprotein class (position indicated by blue arrow), called chylomicrons, representing the transport of dietary lipids absorbed in the intestine. The small band to the right of HDL represents free fatty acid-albumin complex.

Classification of lipoproteins: Lipoproteins are classified into different classes (Table 5.3).

Table 5.3: Salient characteristics of plasma lipoproteins

Lipoprotein class	Density on ultra-centrifugation	Diameter (nm)	Protein/lipid (%)	Major apoproteins	Major lipids	Source	Functions
Chylomicrons (cm)	<0.95	100–1000	2/98	B-48, A, C, E	TG	Small intestine	Transport dietary TG from intestine to extrahepatic tissues
Very low density lipoproteins (VLDL)	0.95–1.006	30–80	10/90	B-100, C, E	TG	Liver	Transport hepatic TG to extrahepatic tissues
Intermediate density lipoproteins (IDL)	1.006–1.019	25–50	18/82	B-100, E	TG, CHOL	Circulating VLDL	Transport hepatic TG and CHOL
Low density lipoproteins (LDL)	1.019–1.063	18–28	25/75	B-100	CHOL	Circulating VLDL and IDL	Transport CHOL to various tissues
High density lipoproteins (HDL)	1.063–1.21	5–15	33/67	A, C, D, E	CHOL, PL	Liver	Reverse CHOL transport from periphery to liver complex
Free fatty acid-albumin	1.21–1.3	–	99/1	Albumin	FFA	FFA: Adipose tissue, albumin: Liver	Transport FFA to liver and muscles

TG: Triacylglycerol; CHOL: Cholesterol; PL: Phospholipids; FFA: Free fatty acids

SOME IMPORTANT QUESTIONS

1. What are lipids? Classify them. Give biological significance of lipids.

2. What are phospholipids? Describe various types of phospholipids with example.

3. What are fatty acids? Classify them. Write biological significance of polyunsaturated fatty acids.

4. Describe briefly:

i. Lipoproteins
ii. Chemistry and functions of prostaglandins.
iii. Classification of lipids with suitable examples
iv. Leukotrienes
v. Lipoproteins and their functions
vi. Lung surfactants
vii. Plasmalogens
viii. Sphingolipids
ix. Chemistry and functions of cholesterol
x. Cerebrosides
xi. Lipoproteins
xii. Apolipoproteins

5. Write notes on:

i. Triacylglycerols
ii. Iodine Number
iii. PUFA
iv. Thromboxanes
v. Essential Fatty acids
vi. Eicosanoids
vii. Lecithins
viii. Respiratory distress syndrome
ix. L/S ratio
x. Cardiolipins

MULTIPLE CHOICE QUESTIONS

1. The omega system of nomenclature of a fatty acid begins with the:
   A. Methyl-carbon atom
   B. Carboxyl-carbon atom
   C. Carbon atom next to the methyl-carbon atom
   D. Carbon atom next to the carboxyl-carbon atom

2. The following are associated with an increased risk of cardiovascular disease:
   A. Diet rich in saturated fatty acids
   B. Diet rich in *trans*-fatty acids
   C. Increased plasma oxidized LDL
   D. All of the above

3. Phrenoderma results from a dietary deficiency of:
   A. Essential amino acids
   B. Essential fatty acids
   C. Phytanic acid
   D. Propionic acid

4. In polyunsaturated fatty acids (PUFA), double bonds generally occur after every:
   A. Two carbon atoms
   B. Three carbon atoms
   C. Four carbon atoms
   D. Six carbon atoms

5. In general, in triacylglycerols present in the body, an unsaturated fatty acid is esterified to glycerol at:
   A. C1
   B. C2
   C. C3
   D. Any of the above

6. An ether linkage between glycerol and fatty acid is characteristic of:
   A. Lecithin
   B. Cephalin
   C. Phosphatidylinositol
   D. Plasmalogen

7. N-acyl sphingosine is:
   A. Ceramide
   B. Choline
   C. Cephalin
   D. Cardiolipin

8. Infantile respiratory distress syndrome is most likely with an amniotic fluid L/S ratio:
   A. <2
   B. 3
   C. 4
   D. >5

9. Cholesterol is a precursor of:
   A. Glucocorticoids
   B. Mineralocorticoids
   C. Androgens
   D. All of the above

10. Phosphate groups are absent in:
    A. Cerebrosides
    B. Lecithin
    C. Cephalin
    D. Plasmalogen

Chemistry and Functions of Amino Acids and Proteins

PROTEINS

Proteins (Greek *proteios*, primary) are polymers of amino acids linked through peptide bonds in a specific sequence dictated by the corresponding DNA sequence. They are a class of macromolecules containing nitrogen. All proteins are composed of 20 different amino acids.

AMINO ACIDS

Amino acids are the hydrolyzed products of proteins and are also called as the monomeric building blocks of proteins. The commonly occurring amino acids are α-amino acids because they have a primary amino group (–NH$_2$) and a carboxylic group (–COOH) as substituents on the α-carbon atom. The general structure of an amino acid is represented in Fig. 6.1.

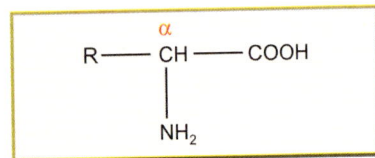

Fig. 6.1: General structure of an amino acid.

Classification of Amino Acids

Amino acids may be classified either based on their side chains or according to their nutritional requirements.

Depending upon the presence of their side chain (the R group attached to the α-carbon atom), amino acids may be classified into two groups:

1. According to the type of the reaction of the R group.
2. According to the polarity of the side chain.

A side chain thus defines the chemical nature and structure of an amino acid.

According to the type of reaction, i.e. based on the ionic charge, amino acids are classified into different groups as follows:

Neutral Amino Acids

These amino acids are neutral in reaction and have one amino (–NH$_2$) and one carboxylic (–COOH) group. These are also called as mono-amino mono-carboxylic acids. According to the presence of the R group, neutral amino acids are further subdivided into two categories, i.e. the aliphatic amino acids and the aromatic amino acids.

Aliphatic Amino Acids

i. **Simple aliphatic amino acids:** Such as glycine and alanine (Fig. 6.2). Glycine has the smallest possible side chain, i.e. a hydrogen atom (–H) as the R group. Alanine has a methyl group (–CH$_3$) in its side chain.

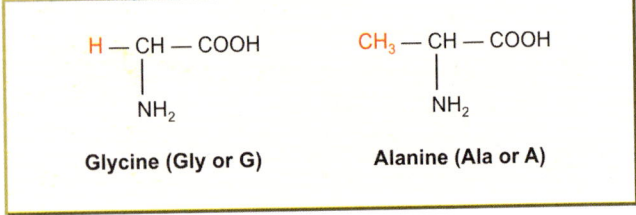

Fig. 6.2: Simple aliphatic amino acids.

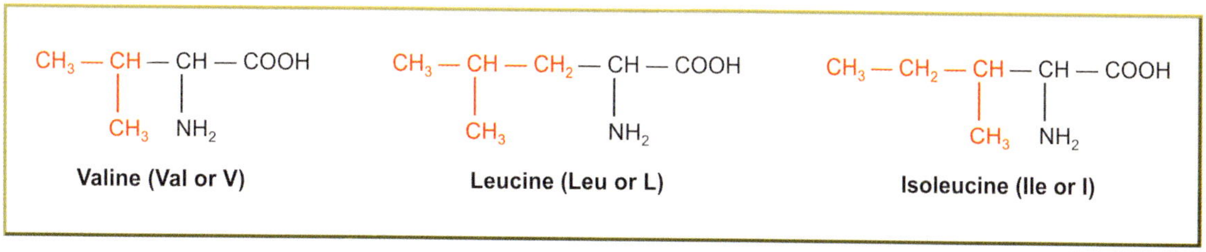

$$CH_3 - CH - CH - COOH$$
$$| \quad |$$
$$CH_3 \quad NH_2$$

Valine (Val or V)

$$CH_3 - CH - CH_2 - CH - COOH$$
$$| \qquad\qquad |$$
$$CH_3 \qquad\qquad NH_2$$

Leucine (Leu or L)

$$CH_3 - CH_2 - CH - CH - COOH$$
$$| \quad |$$
$$CH_3 \quad NH_2$$

Isoleucine (Ile or I)

Fig. 6.3: Branched chain amino acids.

ii. **Branched chain amino acids:** These amino acids have an aliphatic hydrocarbon side chain which has a branch in its structure, i.e. some group is attached to one of the carbon atoms of the aliphatic side chain. There are 3 amino acids which are labeled as branched chain amino acids. These are valine, leucine and isoleucine (Fig. 6.3).

iii. **Hydroxy amino acids:** There are 2 amino acids which have a hydroxyl (–OH) group in their aliphatic side chain. These are serine and threonine (Fig. 6.4).

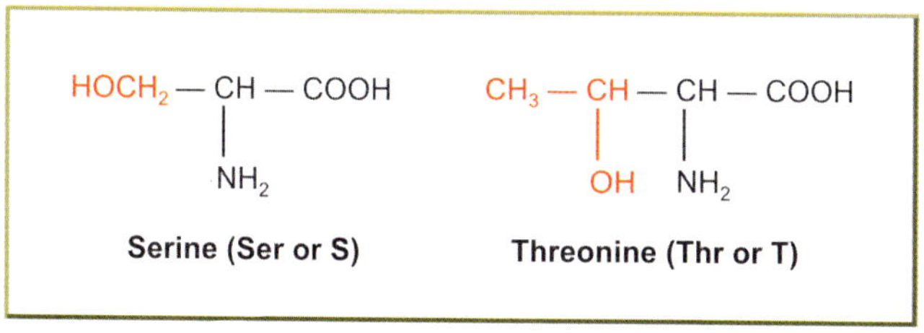

$$HOCH_2 - CH - COOH$$
$$|$$
$$NH_2$$

Serine (Ser or S)

$$CH_3 - CH - CH - COOH$$
$$| \quad |$$
$$OH \quad NH_2$$

Threonine (Thr or T)

Fig. 6.4: Hydroxy amino acids.

iv. **Sulfur** (also spelt 'sulphur') **containing amino acids:** Some amino acids, in addition to C, H, O and N, also contain sulfur (S) as a part of its aliphatic side chain. These are cysteine and methionine.

Cysteine has a free thiol group (–SH) which can form a disulfide bond (–S–S–) with another cysteine residue. Through the oxidation of the two thiol groups, it can form another amino acid called cystine or dicysteine. Certain oxidative processes can convert two molecules of cysteine to cystine, in a protein, in the body.

Methionine does not contain a free –SH group. Instead, it has a thiol linkage as CH_3—S– in its side chain (Fig. 6.5).

Aromatic Amino Acids

These amino acids have an aromatic ring which is neutral in reaction. There are three amino acids which are grouped as aromatic amino acids. These are phenylalanine (alanine with a phenyl group), tyrosine (4-hydroxy-phenylalanine) and tryptophan (alanine attached to an indole ring), as shown in Fig. 6.6.

Acidic Amino Acids and their Amides

These amino acids are acidic in reaction since they have one amino group but more than one (generally two) carboxylate groups. These amino acids are also called as mono-amino dicarboxylic acids. There are two amino acids which are acidic in nature. These are aspartic acid and glutamic acid. Besides, there are two other amino acids which are not actually acidic in nature but are derived from the acidic amino acids.

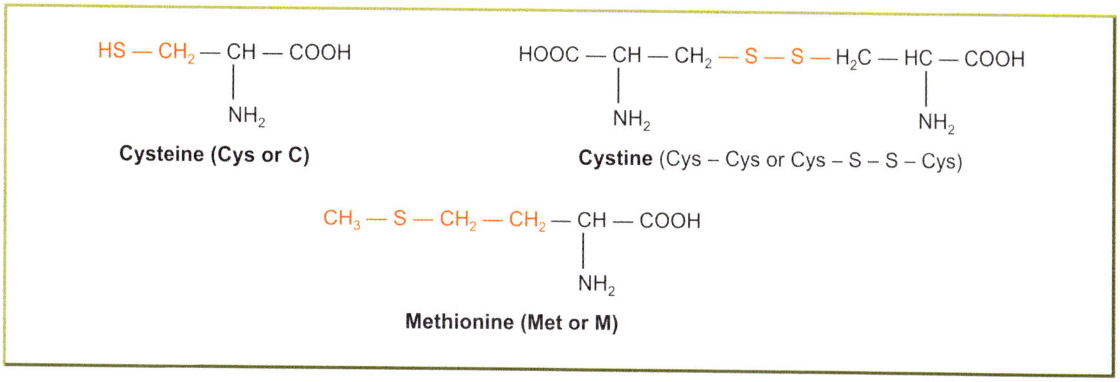

$$HS - CH_2 - CH - COOH$$
$$|$$
$$NH_2$$

Cysteine (Cys or C)

$$HOOC - CH - CH_2 - S - S - H_2C - HC - COOH$$
$$| \qquad\qquad\qquad\qquad\qquad |$$
$$NH_2 \qquad\qquad\qquad\qquad\qquad NH_2$$

Cystine (Cys – Cys or Cys – S – S – Cys)

$$CH_3 - S - CH_2 - CH_2 - CH - COOH$$
$$|$$
$$NH_2$$

Methionine (Met or M)

Fig. 6.5: Sulfur containing amino acids.

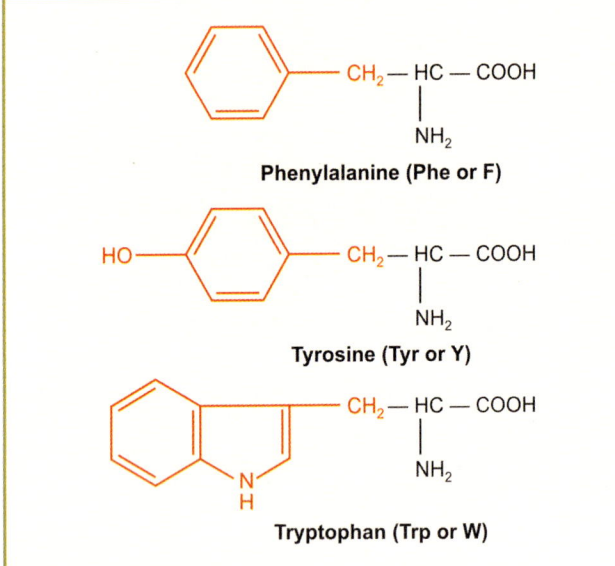

Fig. 6.6: Aromatic amino acids.

These are thus the amides of the acidic amino acids (Fig. 6.7).

The amide of aspartic acid is called as asparagine. It is required in cell multiplication. The amide of glutamic acid is called glutamine. Its formation within the body helps to remove ammonia from the brain.

Glutamine is also needed in many biosynthetic reactions.

Basic Amino Acids

These amino acids are basic in reaction and have one carboxylic group but either >1 amino group in the aliphatic side chain or a heterocyclic ring which is basic in reaction. These are lysine, arginine and histidine:

- Lysine has two –NH_2 groups.
- Arginine has a guanidine group in the aliphatic chain.
- Histidine has a heterocyclic imidazole ring (Fig. 6.8).

Imino Acids

In addition to the above amino acids which are found in most proteins, collagen is rich in proline, which is an imino acid. Proline does not contain a primary α-amino group (–NH_2) but has a secondary imino group (–NH–) in a heterocyclic ring (pyrrolidine ring). In collagen, proline is converted to its 4-hydroxy derivative called 4-hydroxyproline. Though proline has a secondary imino group, for the uniformity of classification, it is also referred as an α-amino acid (Fig. 6.9).

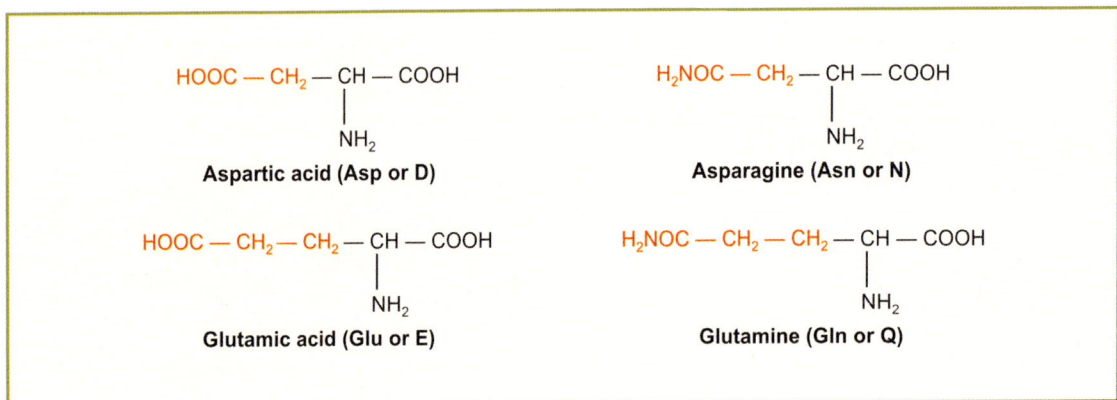

Fig. 6.7: Acidic amino acids and their amides.

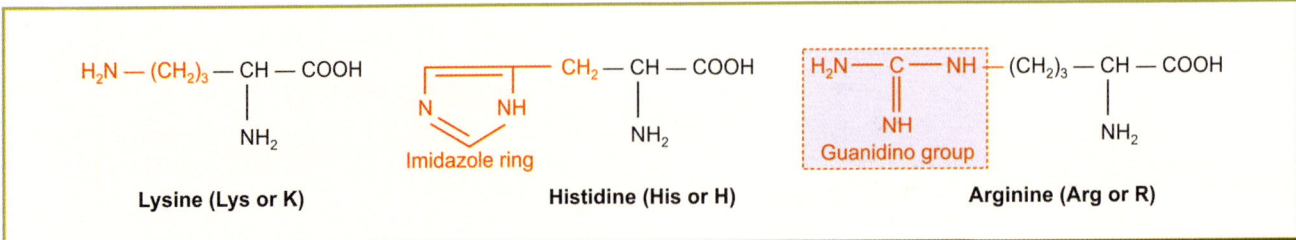

Fig. 6.8: Basic amino acids.

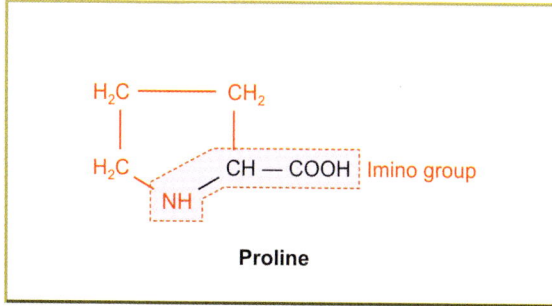

Fig. 6.9: Proline (Pro or P), an imino acid.

Table 6.1: Classification of amino acids according to polarity of their side chains

Non-polar side chain	Polar side chain	
	Uncharged	*Charged*
• Glycine	• Serine	• Lysine
• Alanine	• Threonine	• Arginine
• Valine	• Asparagine	• Histidine
• Leucine	• Glutamine	• Aspartate
• Isoleucine	• Tyrosine	• Glutamate
• Methionine	• Cysteine	
• Phenylalanine		
• Tryptophan		
• Proline		

According to the polarity of the side chain, amino acids may be classified as nonpolar (hydrophobic) or polar (hydrophilic).

Nonpolar Amino Acids

As listed in Table 6.1, there are nine amino acids which have a nonpolar side chain. These amino acids contribute hydrophobic properties to a protein and tend to stabilize its tertiary structure.

Polar Amino Acids

Amino acids contributing hydrophilic properties to a protein are further subdivided into two groups, i.e. those with uncharged side chains (neutral polar amino acids) and those with a charged side chain (charged polar amino acids).

There are six amino acids which have an **uncharged polar side chain** (R group). These amino acids carry no charge on the R group but have a hydroxyl (–OH), sulfhydryl (–SH) or amide (–CONH$_2$) group. These groups frequently participate in hydrogen bonding and, in turn, stabilize protein conformation.

Charged polar amino acid residues in a protein chain are the dicarboxylic (acidic) amino acids which have anionic groups as well as the basic amino acids which have the cationic groups. Depending upon the pH of the surrounding medium, the anionic or cationic group can exist in charged or uncharged state. Thus, at low pH, the protein will have a positive charge because acidic amino acid residues (aspartic acid and glutamic acid) will be uncharged whereas the basic amino acid residues (lysine, arginine and histidine) will be protonated. In a medium of high pH, the protein will have a negative charge since the basic amino acids will be uncharged while the acidic amino acids will have a negative charge. Thus, the net charge of a protein at physiological pH depends upon the relative amounts of acidic and basic amino acids. There are five amino acids which have a charged polar side chain (Table 6.1).

Depending upon the nutritional requirement, amino acids are divided into three groups, as essential amino acids, semi-essential amino acids and non-essential amino acids (Table 6.2).

Among the various amino acids found in proteins, all cannot be synthesized in the body. Those which cannot be synthesized are essentially required in the diet and are called indispensible or **essential amino acids**. There are eight amino acids which are essential for an adult human being. These are methionine, threonine, tryptophan, valine, isoleucine, leucine, phenylalanine and lysine.

Arginine and histidine, though are not essential for normal adult human beings but their synthesis is not sufficient during growth, pregnancy and lactation or during high-grade fever and chronic infections

Table 6.2: Classification of amino acids according to their dietary requirement

Essential	Semi-essential	Non-essential
• Methionine	• Arginine	• Glycine
• Threonine	• Histidine	• Alanine
• Tryptophan		• Serine
• Valine		• Cysteine
• Isoleucine		• Tyrosine
• Leucine		• Aspartate
• Phenylalanine		• Glutamate
• Lysine		• Asparagine
		• Glutamine
		• Proline

when their requirements are increased. Under these conditions arginine and histidine also become essential. These two amino acids are thus called as **semi-essential amino acids** or conditionally essential amino acids.

The remaining amino acids are **non-essential** and can be synthesized in the human body.

BIOLOGICAL VALUE OF A PROTEIN

A protein which has the right quantity of each essential amino acid required for growth and maintenance has high biological value (nutritionally superior), e.g. milk proteins and egg albumin. On the other hand, a protein with poor biological value (nutritionally inferior) has a limited supply of one or more essential amino acids, e.g. proteins from cereals and pulses. Besides the contents of essential amino acids, biological value of a protein is also influenced by digestibility of the protein.

NON-PROTEIN AMINO ACIDS

Besides the 20 amino acids commonly found in proteins, there are some amino acids which do not occur in proteins but are synthesized in the body. They are called non-protein amino acids (Table 6.3).

Table 6.3: Non-protein amino acids

Amino acid	Importance
Ornithine	Intermediate in urea cycle; precursor of polyamines
γ-Aminobutyric acid (GABA)	Neurotransmitter
Dopamine	Neurotransmitter
Histamine	Local mediator of allergic reactions
Thyroxine	Iodine containing thyroid hormone
β-Alanine	Constituent of pantothenic acid and hence of coenzyme A

BIOLOGICAL SIGNIFICANCE OF AMINO ACIDS

1. *Source of nitrogen*: Amino acids are important dietary sources of nitrogen.
2. *Protein synthesis*: Amino acids are used in protein biosynthesis.
3. *Gluconeogenesis*: Some amino acids can be converted to glucose and serve as an important source of energy for the body. Such amino acids are called glucogenic amino acids, e.g. alanine.

4. *Synthesis of specialized products*: Several amino acids are used in the synthesis of various specialized products in the body:
   i. Glycine is an important constituent of creatine, glutathione (a tripeptide, important in oxidation-reduction processes), heme, bile acids and the purine ring.
   ii. Sulfur containing amino acids are also the source of sulfur for the body. Besides, cysteine is also used in the biosynthesis of glutathione while methionine (as S-adenosylmethionine or SAM or active methionine) is an important component of one carbon metabolism.
   iii. Aromatic amino acids are essential for the biosynthesis of thyroid hormones, catecholamines (hormones of the adrenal medulla, i.e. dopamine, norepinephrine and epinephrine) and melanin (a brown-black pigment present in the skin).
   iv. Acidic amino acids are important for transamination reactions.
   v. Aspartate and glutamine are required in the biosynthesis of purines and pyrimidines.

GENERAL PROPERTIES OF AMINO ACIDS

All the naturally occurring amino acids except glycine have at least one asymmetric carbon atom (α-carbon atom) and are optically active. Two spatial isomers of an amino acid, i.e. D and L forms are therefore possible (Fig. 6.10).

All the amino acids derived from proteins, though have L-configuration, some of the D-amino acids (common constituents of the bacterial cell wall) may also be found in the body as components of some oligopeptides.

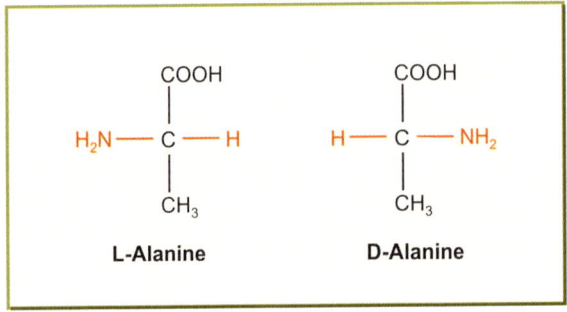

Fig. 6.10: Optical isomers of alanine.

Amino Acids have Acid–Base Properties

At physiological pH of 7.4, an amino acid never exists in an uncharged form as shown in Fig. 6.1, but its carboxyl group is dissociated (R–COO⁻) while the amino group in protonated (R–NH_3^+). Due to the presence of these two ionizable groups, amino acids exhibit acid–base properties.

These properties of amino acids also depend upon the presence of the acidic (–COOH) or basic (NH_2) functional groups present in the side chain (R). Amino acids thus may have a net positive, negative or zero charge and are weak acids.

Relative strength of a weak acid may be expressed by its acid dissociation constant (K_a).

The pK_a is expressed as the negative log of the dissociation constant, i.e. $pK_a = -\log K_a$.

This kind of ionized molecule, having co-existent negative and positive charges, is called a **dipolar ion** or an **ampholyte**.

Zwitterions and Isoelectric pH

Generation of zwitterions: At low pH, an amino acid is in the cationic form, i.e. both the amino group and the carboxyl group are protonated as NH_3^+ and –COOH. As the pH rises, the carboxyl group loses its proton and the **ampholyte** form appears. With a further increase in pH, the amino group (–NH_3^+) is also de-protonated and the anionic form of the molecule is formed. Ampholytes when contain equal number of ionizable groups of opposite charges (i.e. the number of cations are equal to the number of anions) and bear no net charge, become **iso-ionic** species and are called as **zwitterions**.

Isoelectric pH: The pH of the medium/solution at which molecules exist as zwitterions with net charge equal to zero, is called the isoelectric pH (**pI**) The pI is thus the pH at the midpoint between the pK_a values on either side of the iso-ionic species. At a pH greater than its pI, an amino acid is negatively charged and at a pH less than its pI, it is positively charged (Fig. 6.11). This rule also holds true for proteins. The pI of some proteins is as follows: Casein: 4.6; Albumin: 4.7; Globulins: 3.5–4.5; Hemoglobin: 6.7.

Properties of zwitterions

- The molecule (amino acid or protein) being electrically neutral, does not migrate in an electric field.
- The molecule has minimum solubility, hence maximum precipitation.
- The molecule has minimum buffering capacity.

Application: During gel electrophoresis with a pH gradient, various proteins get precipitated at their respective pI. This is called isoelectric focusing (Fig. 6.12). and is employed to:
- Separate proteins in a mixture.
- Identify proteins by suitable staining.
- Purify proteins.

Amino Acids form Peptide Bonds

- The most important property of amino acids is the formation of a peptide bond (–CO–NH) where an

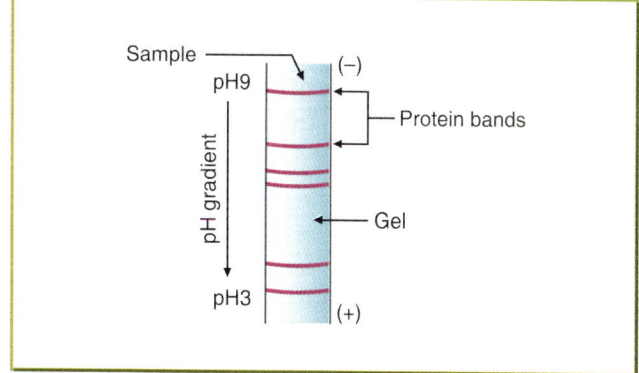

Fig. 6.12: Isoelectric focusing during vertical tube gel electrophoresis.

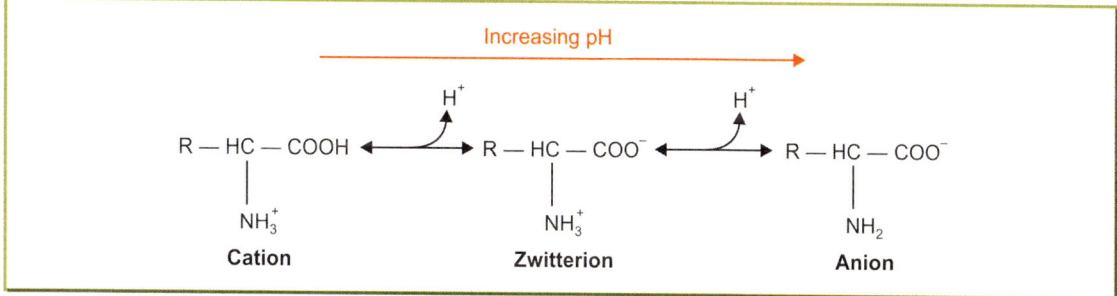

Fig. 6.11: Ionic forms of an amino acid.

6

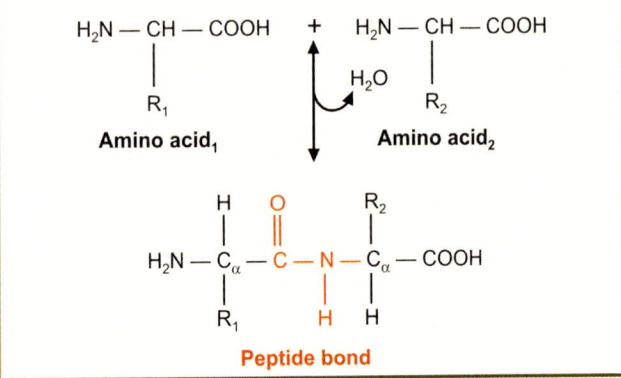

Fig. 6.13: Formation of a peptide bond (red) between two amino acids to form a dipeptide.

α-carboxylic group from one amino acid reacts with the α-amino group of the other amino acid.

- It is a condensation reaction resulting in a covalent (amide) linkage with the elimination of a molecule of water (Fig. 6.13).
- It is planar, rigid with partial double bond character and no freedom of rotation.
- The –C=O and –NH groups are *trans*, polar and participate in H-bonding.
- It is the backbone of a polypeptide which is formed when several amino acids are linked together through peptide linkages (Fig. 6.14).
- The C_α–C and N–C_α bonds are single bonds allowing adequate rotational freedom and hence the folding of the polypeptide.

$$H_2N — AA_1 — AA_2 — AA_3 \ldots\ldots\ldots AA_{n-1} — AA_n — COOH$$

N-terminal end   C-terminal end

Fig. 6.14: A polypeptide.

PROTEINS, POLYPEPTIDES, OLIGOPEPTIDES AND PEPTIDES

Each protein has a free α-amino group (from the first amino acid) represented on the left hand side of the protein chain. It is called an **amino terminal or N-terminal end**. A protein also has free α-carboxylic group (from the last amino acid), which is present on the right hand side of the chain and is called the **carboxy terminal or C-terminal end**.

The term '**polypeptide**' is used when the number of amino acids is 51–100, e.g. insulin (51 amino acids). **Peptides** contain ≤50 amino acids and those which contain ≤20 amino acids are called **oligopeptides**. A **dipeptide** and a **tripeptide** contain two and three amino acids respectively. Some physiologically important peptides are listed in Table 6.4.

STRUCTURAL ORGANIZATION OF PROTEINS

Variations in the number and order of different amino acids or the manner in which these amino acids are arranged in a polypeptide chain, reflects the type of protein structure. There are 4 levels of structural organization of proteins:

Primary Structure of a Protein

Primary structure of a protein refers to the order and sequence of covalently linked amino acid residues in a polypeptide chain (Fig. 6.15).

Some proteins are synthesized as single polypeptides that are later cleaved into two or more chains, such as insulin. Such molecules may also have intrachain as well as inter-chain disulfide linkages.

Secondary Structure of a Protein

Secondary level of protein structure includes folding or twisting patterns of the polypeptide chains in a

Table 6.4: Physiologically important peptides

Peptide	Source	Importance
Glutathione (tripeptide = 3 amino acids; γ-glutamylcysteinylglycine)	All cells especially RBC	Detoxification of peroxides
Thyrotropin releasing hormone (TRH; tripeptide = 3 amino acids)	Hypothalamus	Release of thyrotropin (thyroid stimulating hormone—TSH) from anterior pituitary
Angiotensin II (octapeptide = 8 amino acids)	Plasma angiotensin I	Vasoconstrictor, maintains blood pressure
Oxytocin (nonapeptide = 9 amino acids)	Posterior pituitary	Parturition; milk ejection
Antidiuretic hormone (ADH, nonapeptide = 9 amino acids)	Posterior pituitary	Water reabsorption from distal nephrons
Substance P (undecapeptide = 11 amino acids)	Sensory nerve terminals	Pain perception

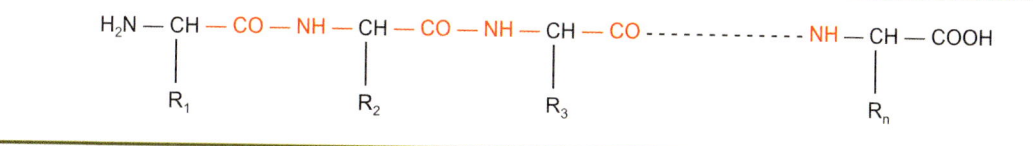

$$H_2N - CH - CO - NH - CH - CO - NH - CH - CO ----------- NH - CH - COOH$$

R_1 R_2 R_3 R_n

Fig. 6.15: Primary structure of a protein.

protein. Secondary structure is thus the local spatial arrangement of a polypeptide's backbone atoms without taking into account the conformations of its side chains. Various forces which stabilize protein conformation include hydrogen bonds, hydrophobic interactions, electrostatic interactions and van der Waals forces. Secondary structures include α-helix and β-pleated sheets.

α-Helix

- A coil or helix is formed by twisting the backbone of a polypeptide chain. As a result of its folding, hydrogen bonds may be formed between –CO (of residue 'n') and –NH (of residue 'n + 4') groups within the same polypeptide chain (Fig. 6.16). These are called intra-chain linkages. The side chains of amino acids extend outward.
- A polypeptide helix may be either right-handed (α-helix) or left-handed (β-helix, rare). The α-helix has the lowest-energy and is the most stable conformation for a polypeptide chain formed spontaneously.
- There are 3.6 amino acid residues in one complete turn.
- Pitch (the distance the helix rises along its axis per turn) is 0.54 nm.
- Proline interferes with the formation of α-helix.
- Hemoglobin, myoglobin, myosin, tropomyosin, fibrin and α-keratin are rich in α-helices.

β-Sheet

- The second regular structure present in most of the proteins is the β-structure ('β' denotes that it was the second regular structure described after α-helix).
- It is stretched-out with a rippled or pleated appearance when viewed from edge/side, hence called pleated sheet-like structures; the amino acid side chains and C_α are alternately above and below the plane of the sheet.

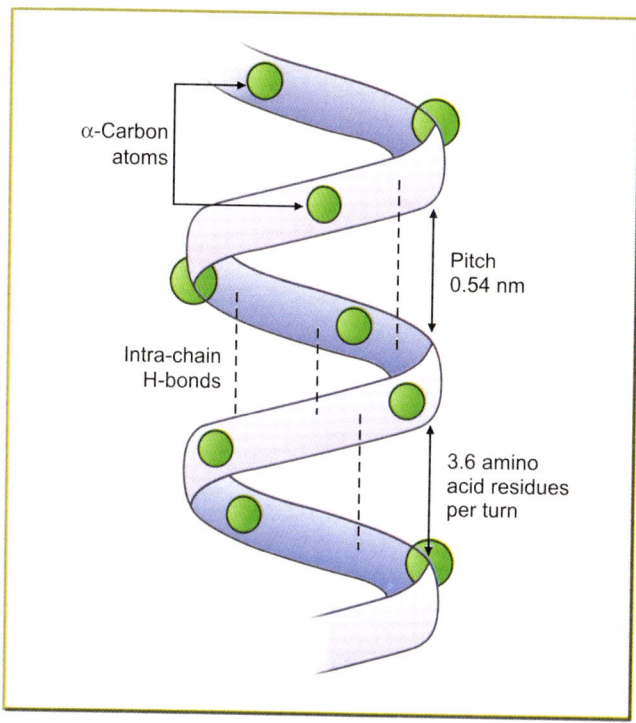

Fig. 6.16: A right-handed α-helix.

- β-sheet orientation is formed due to stretching of the helices of the polypeptide chains, as a result of formation of hydrogen bonds between –CO and –NH groups of the neighboring strands of the polypeptide rather than within one strand (as in an α-helix). Therefore, it has inter-chain linkages (Fig. 6.17).
- Ribonuclease A, carbonic anhydrase, flavodoxin, silk fibroin and wool are rich in β-sheets.
- **Antiparallel β-sheet:** The neighboring hydrogen-bonded polypeptide chains run in opposite directions (Fig. 6.18). Thus, the N-terminus of one strand is adjacent to the C-terminus of the next, e.g. fibroin.
- **Parallel β-sheet:** The hydrogen bonded chains extend in the same direction (Fig. 6.19). Thus, the N-termini of successive strands are oriented in

6

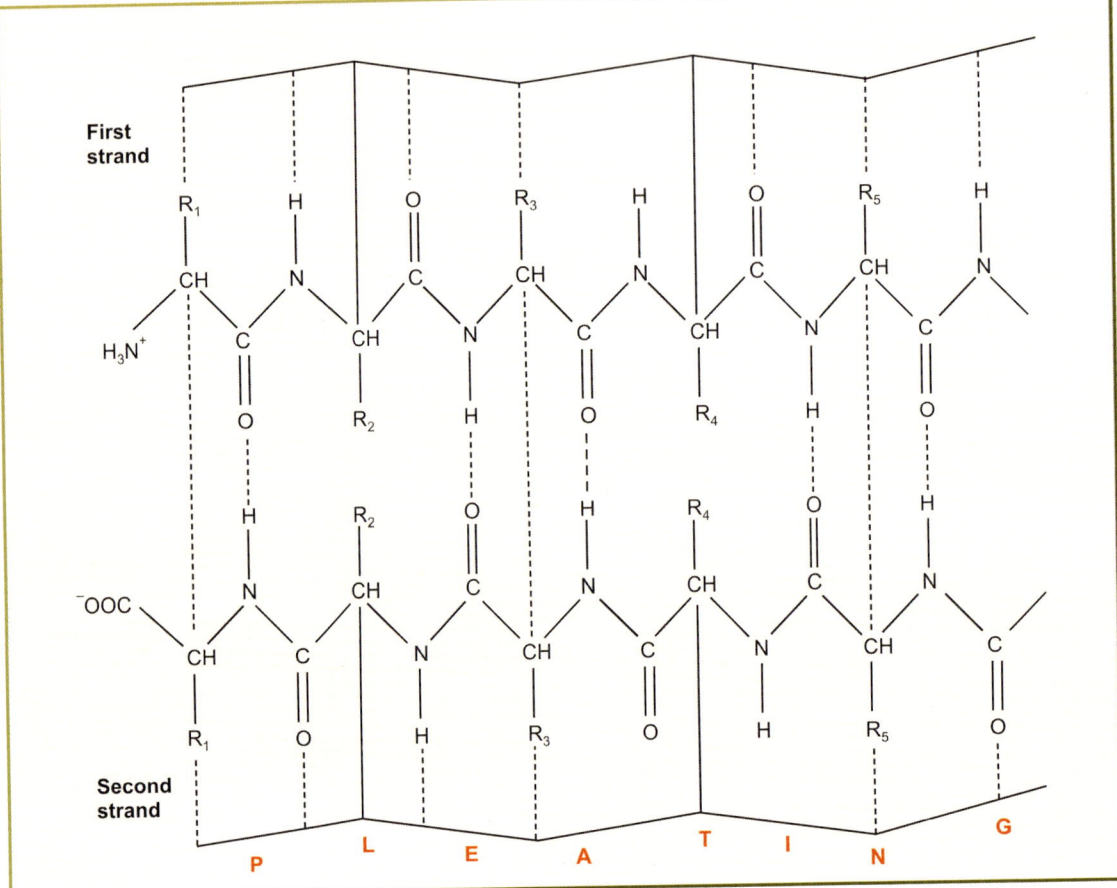

First strand

R₁   H   O   R₃   H   O   R₅   H

Second strand

P   L   E   A   T   I   N   G

Fig. 6.17: β-pleated sheet.

the same direction, e.g. flavodoxin (a prokaryotic electron-transfer protein).

- **Mixed β-sheet:** The protein has a mixture of the two types, e.g. carbonic anhydrase.

Supersecondary structures: Certain combinations of secondary structure are also observed in different folded protein structures. They are referred to as **structural motifs**. These longer pattern lengths of secondary structure may include multiple structural motifs and when commonly observed in more than one protein are referred to as **supersecondary structures**. These include helix-turn-helix, leucine-zipper, zinc-finger (found in DNA binding proteins). etc.

Tertiary Structure of a Protein

Tertiary structure involves the intra-molecular folding of the polypeptide chain into a compact three-dimensional structure with a specific shape. Thus, the

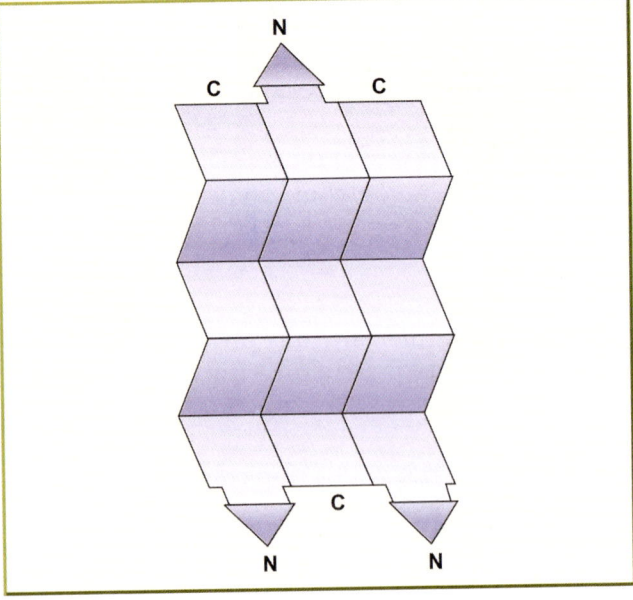

Fig. 6.18: Antiparallel β-sheets.

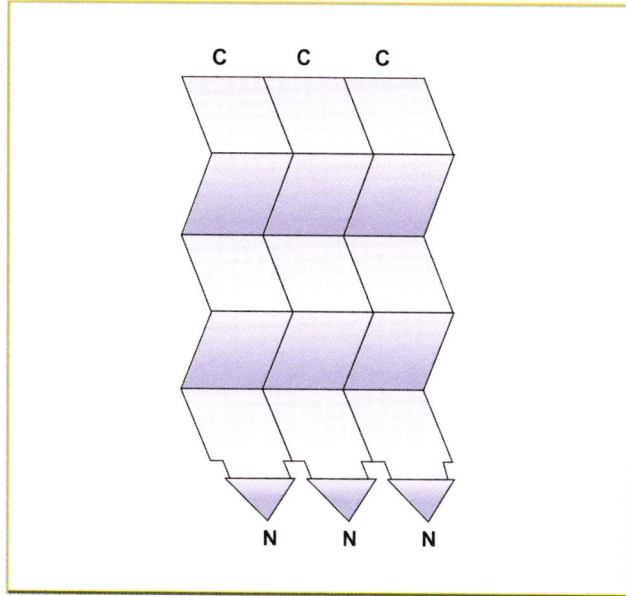

Fig. 6.19: Parallel β-sheets.

difference between the secondary and tertiary structures is rather arbitrary (Fig. 6.20).

Localized regions of specific three-dimensional arrangements (α-helix, β-sheet, etc.) are the secondary structures whereas all the secondary structures along with the intervening regions give the protein its final three-dimensional shape, i.e. the tertiary structure. The latter is also called the **conformation** of a protein. Tertiary structure is maintained by electrostatic linkages, hydrogen bonds, disulfide bridges, van der Waals forces and hydrophobic interactions. Hydrophobic interactions are the major forces in maintaining the unique tertiary structure of a protein.

Configuration versus Conformation

The term **'configuration'** refers to the geometric possibilities for a given set of atoms, e.g. D- and L-amino acids as discussed above. Different configurations of a molecule are achieved by breaking and rearranging covalent bonds. On the other hand, the term **'conformation'** refers to the overall 3-dimensional architecture of a molecule, generally a protein. Different conformations of a molecule are achieved without breaking any covalent bond.

FOLDING OF A PROTEIN

Correct and timely folding is an important phenomenon critical to the biological function of a protein. Its salient features are:

- **Formation of secondary structure:** Initially, the secondary structures (α-helices and/or β-sheets) are formed which associate and pack close together.

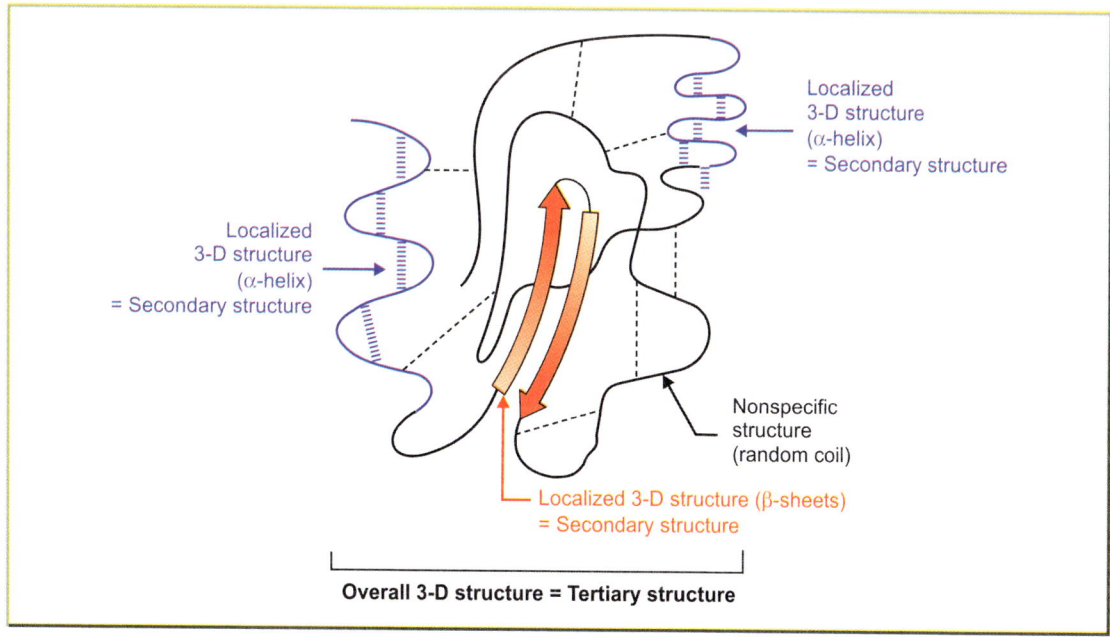

Fig. 6.20: Secondary and tertiary levels of protein structure. Various non-covalent stabilizing forces are shown as dotted lines.

6

The peptide segments between the secondary structures are short and direct, without any complicated twist or turn.

- *Stabilization*: The most stable structure is preferred which is characterized by:
    i. Large number of intra-molecular H-bonds.
    ii. Reduced exposed surface area accessible to solvents.
    iii. Buried hydrophobic core and hydrophilic surface, driven by hydrophobic interactions.
- *Chaperones*: The folding process may be assisted by other proteins called molecular chaperones, e.g. hsp60 (known as chaperonins), hsp70 and hsp90. The 'hsp' refers to 'heat-shock proteins' (originally observed in cells given brief exposure to high temperature, nearly 42°C) and the numbers are their M_r in kD. The chaperones help in:
    i. Appropriate burial of hydrophobic core, otherwise adjacent proteins may aggregate.
    ii. Moving proteins to their cellular destinations.
    iii. Rescuing and refolding of mature proteins that become partly unfolded.
- *Abnormal or delayed folding*: It is associated with diseases such as Alzheimer's disease, Creutzfeldt-

Chemistry to Clinics 6.1: Disorders of Protein Folding

It has been observed that many diseases result from an abnormal or delayed folding of a protein. Interestingly, the primary structure of the protein may be normal or altered, i.e. mutated. Important examples include:

- **Alzheimer's disease:** Misfolded β-amyloid peptide accumulates as plaques in the brain (Fig. 6.21).
- **Creutzfeldt-Jakob disease:** Normal cellular prion protein (PrP^C) is replaced by protease-resistant prion protein (PrP^{SC}) in the brain. Prion refers to 'proteinaceous infectious particles'.
- **Hereditary emphysema (called Z-variant):** Correct but slow folding of mutated α_1-antitrypsin in the lungs. Unopposed action of neutrophil elastase degrades the lung elastin.
- **Cystic fibrosis:** Mutant CFTR (**C**ystic **F**ibrosis **T**ransmembrane **R**egulator, a membrane Cl^- channel protein in the exocrine glands) fails to dissociate from chaperones and thus cannot reach its destination, i.e. cell membrane.

Jakob disease, hereditary emphysema and cystic fibrosis (Chemistry to Clinics 6.1).

Quaternary Structure of a Protein

Multisubunit or multimeric proteins contain several identical and/or different chains where each of the polypeptide chain is called a subunit. These polypeptide subunits associate with a specific geometry.

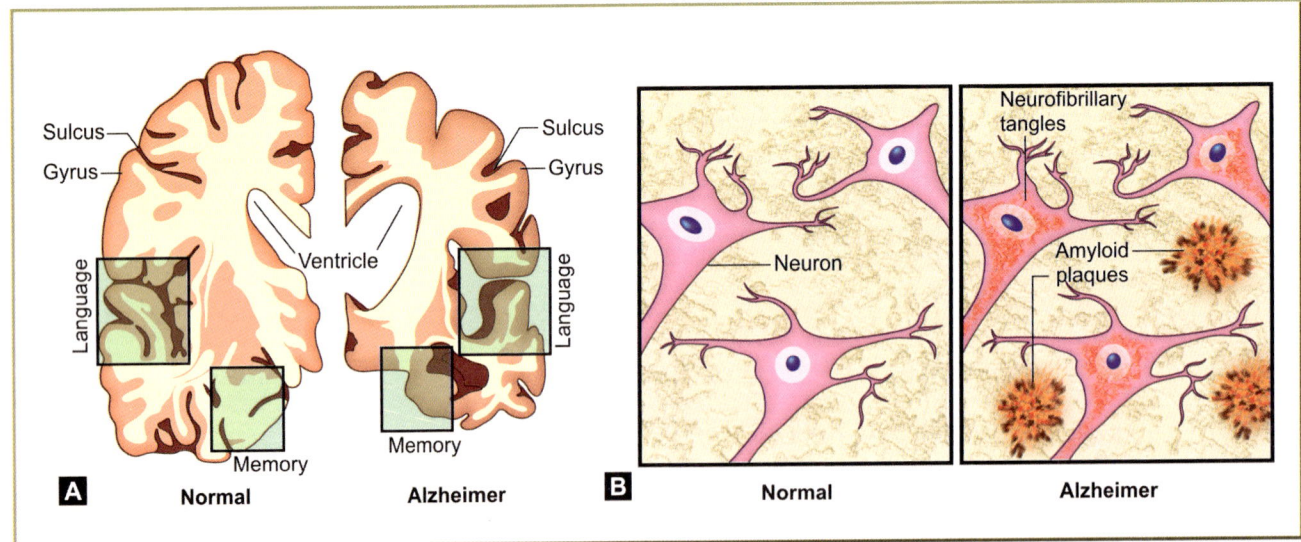

Fig. 6.21: Alzheimer's disease (AD). (A) Cut section of brain showing shrinkage of gyri and widening of sulci, particularly involving the memory and language areas of the brain, explaining the symptoms of AD. (B) **Hallmarks of AD:** β-amyloid plaques and neurofibrillary tangles. β-amyloid is a protein fragment cleaved from an amyloid precursor protein. In a healthy brain, these protein fragments are broken down and eliminated. In AD, the fragments accumulate to form insoluble plaques between the neurons. Neurofibrillary tangles are insoluble twisted fibers found inside the neurons, consisting primarily of a protein called tau (normal components of microtubules). The microtubule helps transport nutrients and other important substances from one part of the neuron to another. In AD, the tau protein is abnormal and the microtubule structures collapse. Both β-amyloid plaques and neurofibrillary tangles contribute to the neuronal loss in AD.

The spatial arrangement of these subunits refers to the quaternary structure of a protein.

Proteins with more than one subunit are also called **oligomers** while their individual units are called **protomers** which may or may not be identical (Figs 6.22 and 6.23). For example, hemoglobin is an oligomer which has four subunits. It has a subunit composition as $\alpha_2\beta_2$. In other words, it is a dimer of $\alpha\beta$ protomers.

Disintegration of the monomeric subunits results in a loss of biological activity of the protein.

Advantages of Quaternary Structure

1. **Enhanced protein stability:** Due to reduced surface area : volume ratio (increasing the radius increases the volume).
2. **Genetic economy:** Less DNA is required to code for a monomer that assembles into a multimer, than for a large protein of the same M_r.
3. **Enhanced catalytic efficiency:** By bringing catalytic sites close together in multisubunit enzymes.
4. **Cooperativity:** Binding of a ligand at one subunit changes the affinity of binding at successive subunits. If the affinity is enhanced it is called positive cooperativity; if reduced, it is called negative cooperativity.

CLASSIFICATION OF PROTEINS

Several criteria are used to classify proteins (Fig. 6.24).
1. *Depending upon the physical and chemical properties,* proteins are divided into three categories, i.e. simple proteins, conjugated proteins and derived proteins.

Simple Proteins

Based on their solubility, simple proteins are further subdivided into different groups, as follows:
- **Albumins:** Present in serum, milk and eggs. These are soluble in water as well as in a neutral salt solution.
- **Globulins:** Also present in serum, milk and eggs. These are, however, sparingly soluble in water but are soluble in dilute neutral salt solutions.
- **Prolamines:** Gliadin of wheat and zein of maize are the examples. These are insoluble in water but are soluble in 60–80% alcohol.
- **Glutelins:** Soluble in dilute acids and alkalis, e.g. gluten in wheat and oryzenin in rice.
- **Scleroproteins:** Highly insoluble proteins present in supporting tissues, such as bones and cartilages. These are also present in the protective tissues like skin, hair, nail and horn.
- **Histones:** Rich in basic amino acids and are soluble in water, e.g. nucleohistones.

Conjugated Proteins

These are simple proteins which are conjugated with a nonprotein molecule called **prosthetic group. Nucleoproteins** (histones conjugated with nucleic acids), **glycoproteins** (proteins in combination with carbohydrates), **phosphoproteins** (phosphoric acid

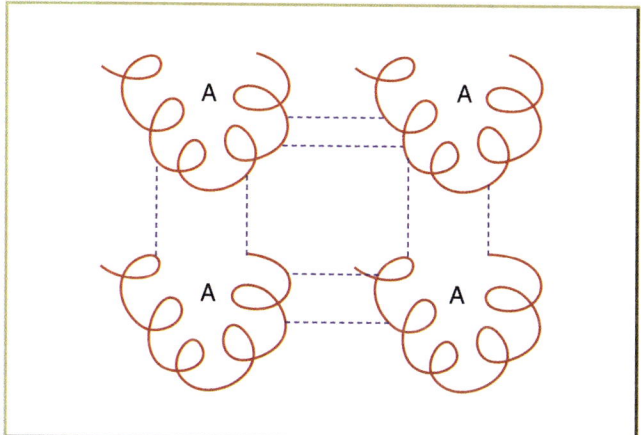

Fig. 6.22: Quaternary level of protein structure with four identical protomers = A_4.

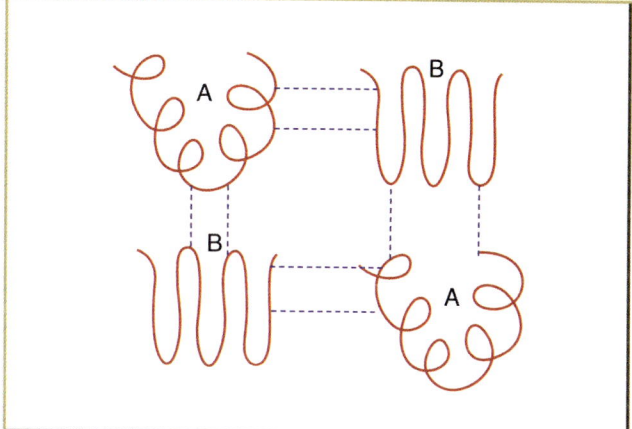

Fig. 6.23: Quaternary level of protein structure with two pairs of different protomers = A_2B_2.

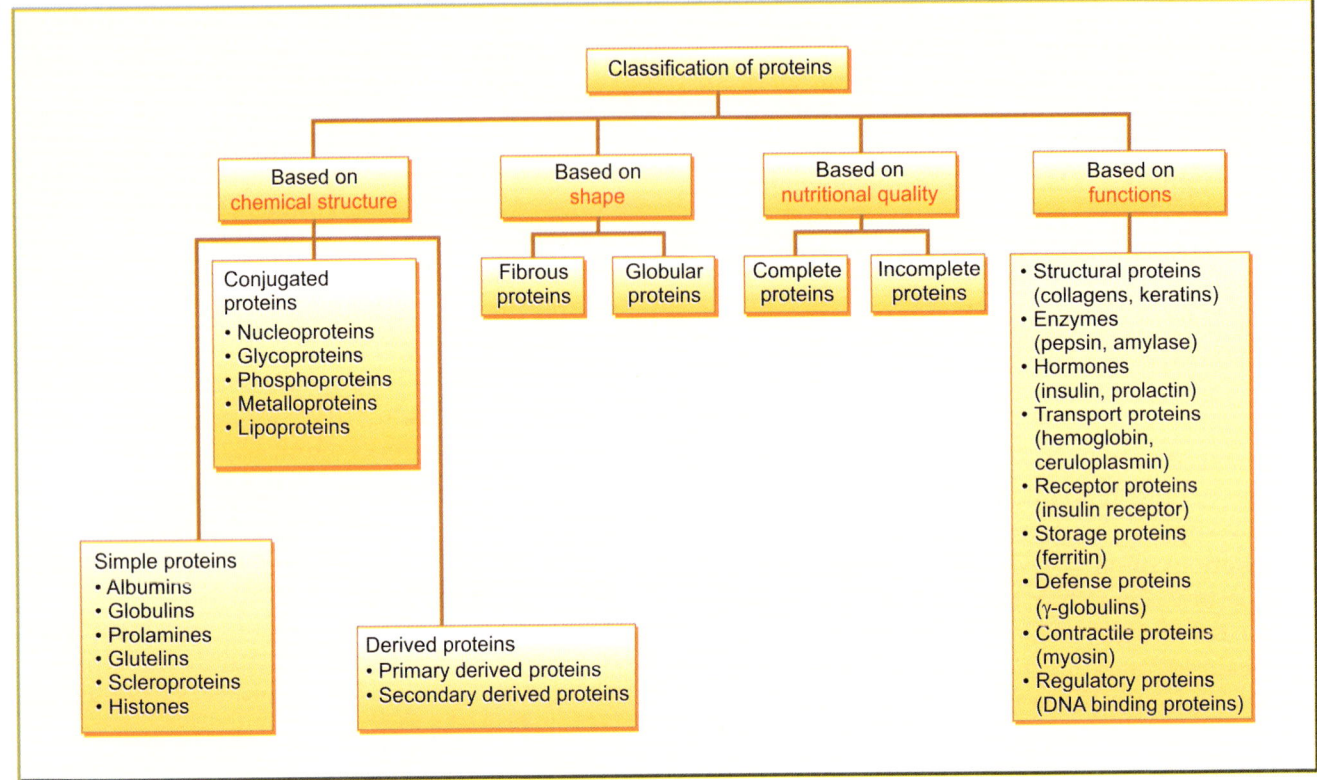

Fig. 6.24: Classification of proteins based on several criteria.

attached to a serine moiety of the protein, like casein of milk), **metalloproteins** (metal containing proteins, such as ceruloplasmin—a cuproprotein), and **lipoproteins** (lipid associated proteins) are the examples of conjugated proteins.

Derived Proteins

These are the derivatives of simple proteins, such as the denatured and the coagulated proteins called as **primary derived proteins**, or those which are produced due to the cleavage of the peptide bonds and are called as **secondary derived proteins**, such as proteoses and peptones.

2. *Depending on their overall morphology/shape,* proteins are classified as either fibrous or globular proteins based on their axial ratio, i.e. length/width ratio (Table 6.5).

3. *From the nutritional perspective,* proteins are categorized into complete and incomplete proteins. **Complete proteins** such as milk casein and egg albumin contain all the essential amino acids.

Table 6.5: Fibrous versus globular proteins

Parameter	Fibrous proteins	Globular proteins
Axial ratio	>10	<10, usually <5
Shape	Rod-like, elongated and cylindrical	Nearly spheroidal
Water solubility	Lower	Higher
Regular secondary structures	Predominant	Variable
Biological role	Structural: Protective, connective, supportive	Functional: Catalysts, transporters, metabolic regulators
Examples	Collagen, α-keratin, tropomyosin	Hemoglobin, myoglobin, triose phosphate isomerase

Cereal proteins, collagens and gelatin (obtained by denaturation of collagens) lack one or more essential amino acids and are therefore called **incomplete proteins**.

4. *With respect to their biological functions,* proteins are divided into different groups (Fig. 6.24, functional classification).

PROTEIN DENATURATION, COAGULATION, PRECIPITATION AND FLOCCULATION

Denaturation refers to the loss of the native protein structure and hence its biological function, on exposure to some physical/chemical agents. The primary structure is, however, preserved. If denaturation becomes irreversible, it results in **coagulation**. Reversal of denaturation is renaturation, e.g. ribonuclease in concentrated urea solution may be reversibly denatured by controlling the molarity of the solution. **Precipitation** of proteins requires neutralizing their surface charge or surface dehydration. Precipitation at isoelectric pH is called **flocculation** (Fig. 6.25).

SEPARATION TECHNIQUES

Various physicochemical properties of proteins are used to separate a protein of interest from a mixture.

Most commonly used separation techniques include chromatography and electrophoresis.

Chromatography

Chromatography is a physical method of separation in which the components to be separated are distributed between two phases, one of which is stationary while the other moves in a definite direction. It is a powerful tool for the separation and quantification of various clinically useful compounds.

Mobile phase and stationary phase: In most modern chromatographic procedures a mixture of substances to be separated is introduced into a flowing stream of liquid or gas, called the **mobile phase**. It then passes through a bed, layer or column, containing a porous solid matrix, called the **stationary phase**. As the mobile phase carries a sample, the solute with lesser affinity for the stationary phase remains in the mobile phase and travels faster, thereby getting separated from the one with a greater affinity for the stationary phase.

Paper Chromatography

It is one of the earliest chromatographic techniques in which a strip of filter paper is used. Cellulose of the filter paper absorbs water and acts as a stationary

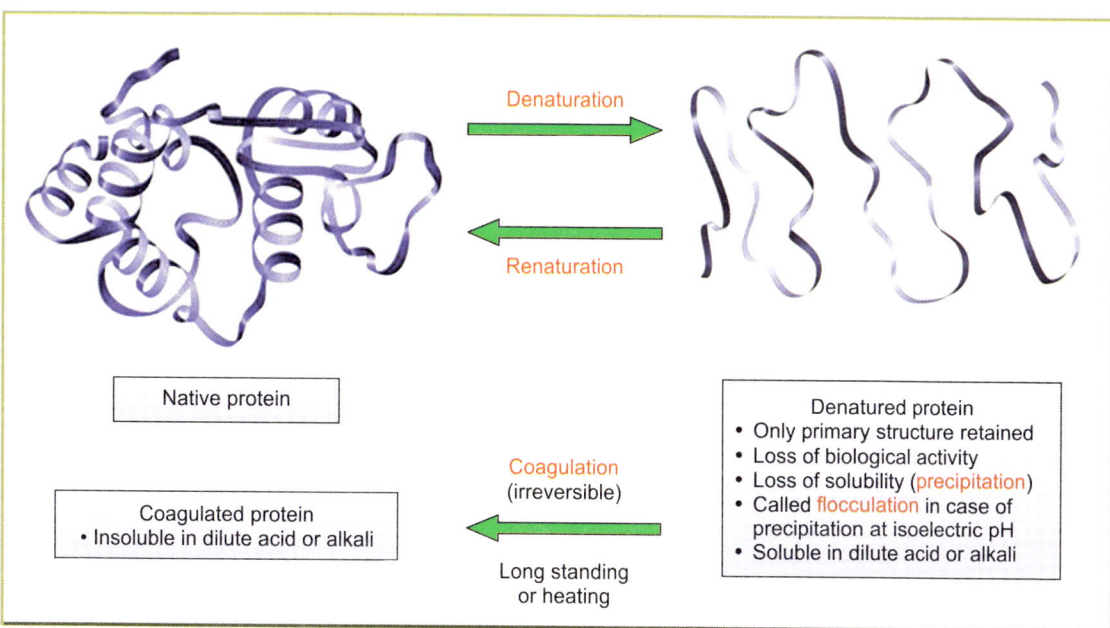

Fig. 6.25: A native protein may undergo reversible or irreversible denaturation. The key processes are highlighted in red.

phase. The mobile phase is a nonpolar solvent, such as n-butanol, which migrates up (ascending chromatography, Fig. 6.26) or down (descending chromatography).

Thin Layer Chromatography

In thin layer chromatography (TLC, Fig. 6.27), a thin layer of polar material, such as silica gel, is spread uniformly on a glass plate or a plastic sheet. This is mainly used for the separation of lipids.

Column Chromatography

In column chromatography, support particles and the stationary phase are contained within a tube called column.

Gas Chromatography

If the mobile phase is a gas, the technique is known as gas chromatography.

Ion Exchange Chromatography

In ion exchange chromatography, charged molecules bind to the oppositely charged groups that have been

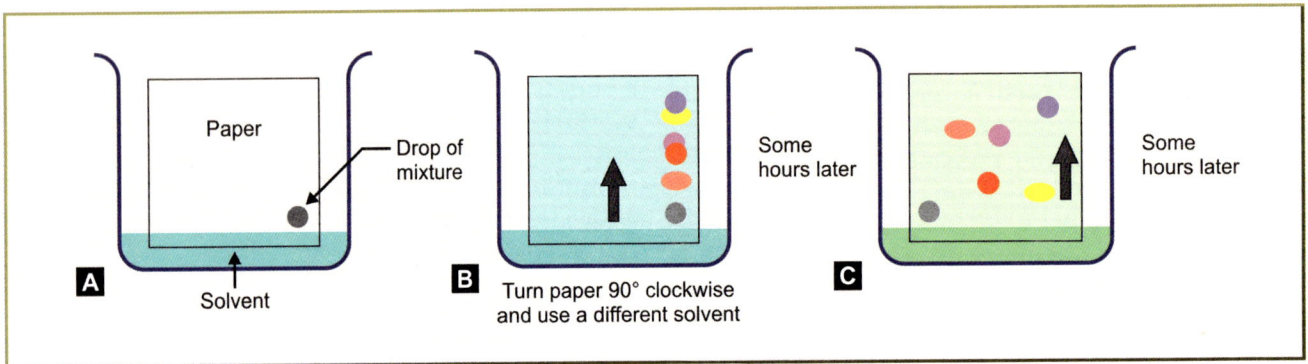

Fig. 6.26: Ascending paper chromatography. (A) A drop of protein mixture is placed in one corner of filter paper. One edge of the paper is immersed in a solvent. (B) The solvent migrates up the sheet by capillary attraction. As it does so, each protein in the drop migrates at a rate that reflects its size and its solubility in the solvent. (C) After a second run at right angles to the first (often using a different solvent), the various proteins are spread out at distinct spots across the sheet, forming a chromatogram. The identity of each spot can be determined by comparing its position with the positions occupied by known proteins under the same conditions. The spots may also be identified by chemical methods.

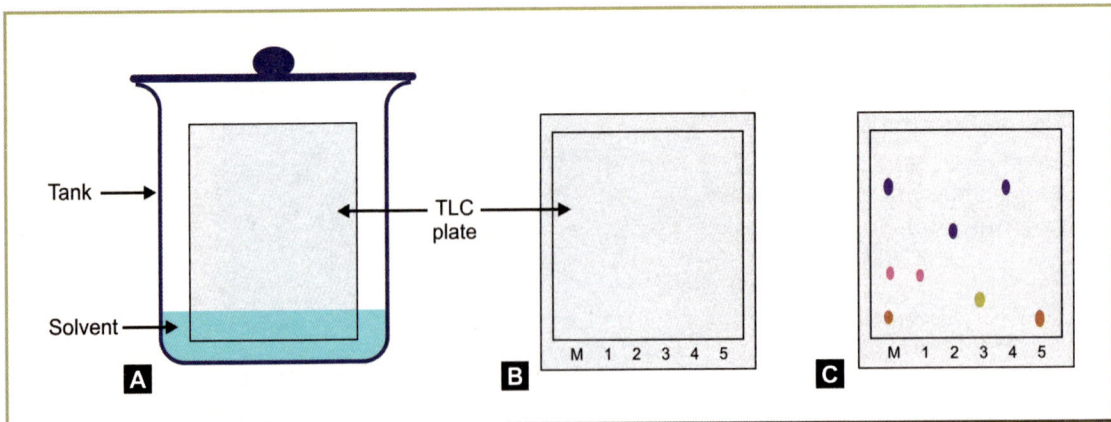

Fig. 6.27: Thin layer chromatography (TLC). (A) TLC apparatus. (B) A small drop of a mixture of amino acids (M) is placed on the baseline of the thin layer plate, and similar small spots of the known amino acids (labeled 1 to 5) are placed alongside. The plate is then placed in a suitable solvent and left for a few hours in the tank. The spots are separated but invisible. (C) After spraying with ninhydrin, compare the spots in the mixture with those of the known amino acids, with respect to their positions and colors. In this example, the mixture contains the amino acids labeled as 1, 4 and 5. α-amino acids give blue-purple color (called Ruhemann's purple) while proline gives yellow-brown color with ninhydrin.

immobilized on the matrix. The anions bind to the cationic groups on anion exchangers while the cations bind to the anionic groups on cation exchangers.

The most frequently used anion exchanger is a matrix with attached diethylaminoethyl (DEAE) group, e.g. DEAE-cellulose (Fig. 6.28). A frequently used cation exchanger is a matrix bearing carboxymethyl (CM) group, such as CM-cellulose.

Gel Filtration Chromatography

In gel filtration chromatography (also called size exclusion or molecular sieve chromatography), molecules are separated according to their size and shape. The stationary phase consists of gel-beads containing pores that span a relatively narrow size range. If an aqueous solution of molecules of various sizes is passed through a column containing such molecular sieves, the molecules that are too large to pass through the pores are excluded from the gel beads. These large molecules therefore traverse the column more rapidly than small molecules that pass through the pores (Fig. 6.29).

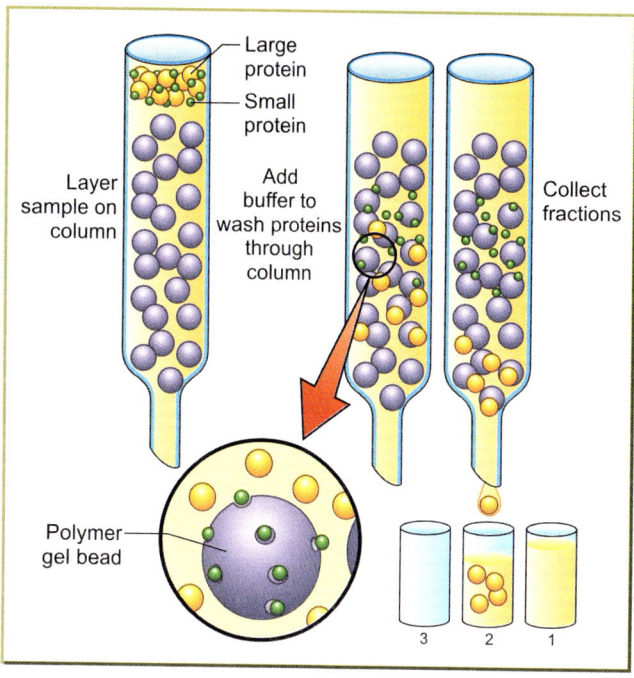

Fig. 6.29: Gel filtration or size exclusion or molecular sieve chromatography.

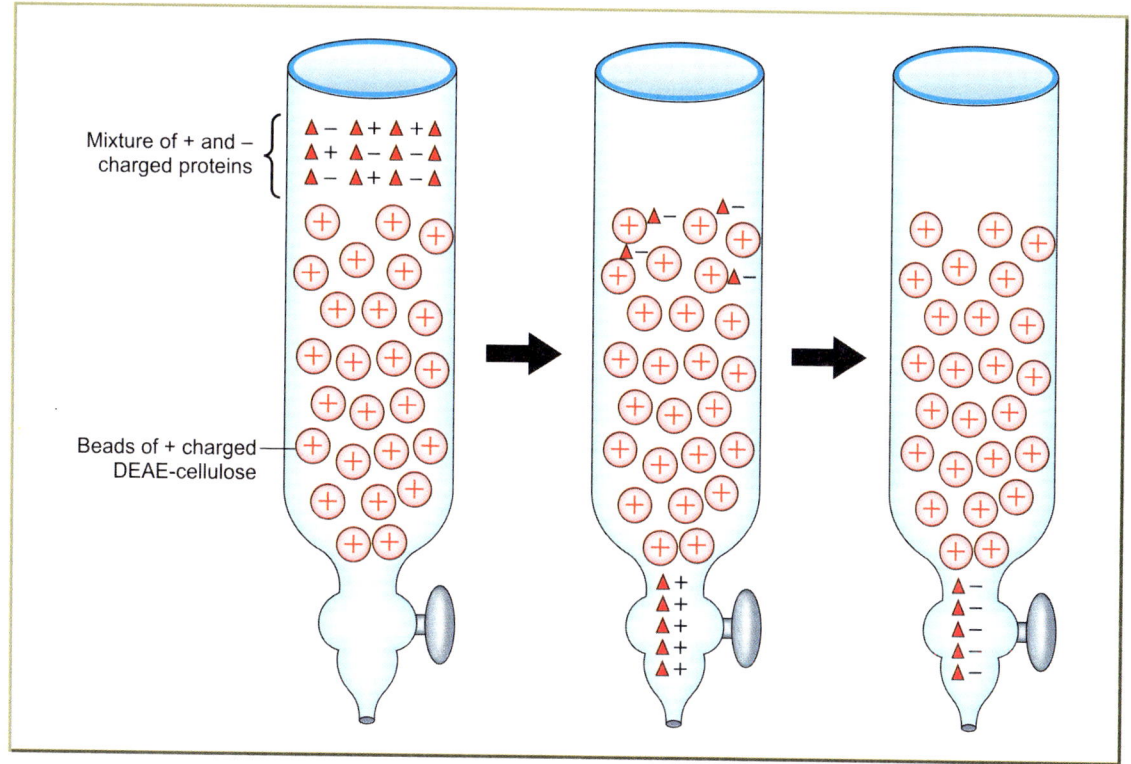

Fig. 6.28: Ion exchange chromatography.

Affinity Chromatography

In affinity chromatography, a molecule (a ligand, such as an enzyme, antibody or antigen, lectin or nucleic acid) that specifically binds to the protein of interest is covalently attached to an inert (column) matrix. When a protein solution is passed through this chromatographic material, the desired protein binds to the immobilized ligand whereas other substances are washed through the column with the buffer. The desired protein can then be recovered in highly purified form by changing the elution conditions, to release the protein from the matrix (Fig. 6.30).

High Performance Liquid Chromatography (HPLC)

The HPLC technique employs an automated system with precisely applied samples with controlled flow rates at high pressure (up to 5000 psi) and a chromatographic matrix of specially fabricated glass or plastic beads (3–300 mm diameter) which is coated with a uniform layer of chromatographic material. The technique depends on the use of microfine column mixtures to give high resolution, rapidly (Fig. 6.31).

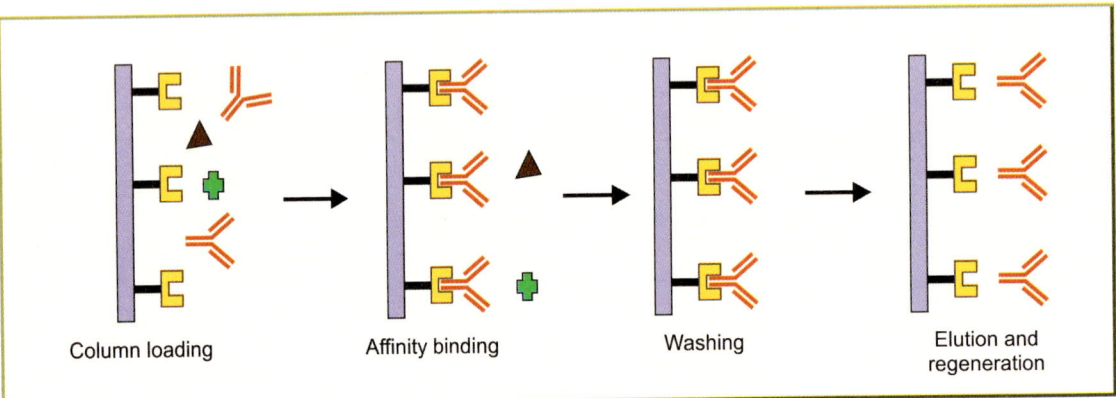

Fig. 6.30: Affinity chromatography. The antibody (red) to be separated from a mixture is made to bind with the respective antigen (yellow) already attached to the column support. Undesirable substances (brown, green) are washed out, followed by regeneration of antibodies in pure form.

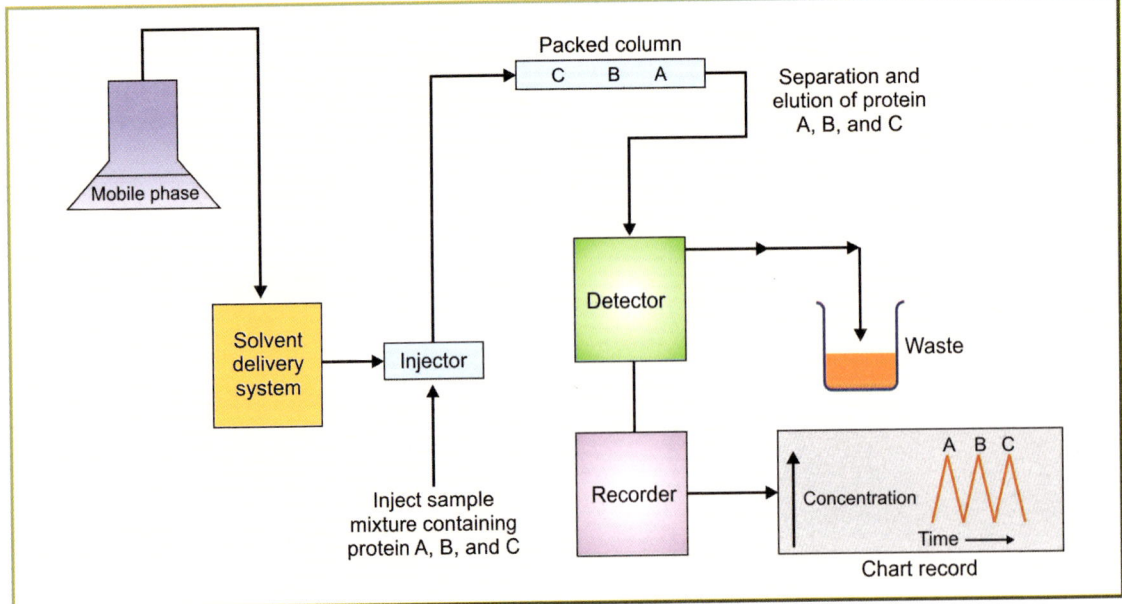

Fig. 6.31: High performance liquid chromatography **(HPLC).**

Electrophoresis

Electrophoresis is a technique for the separation of the charged particles by means of an electric current. A charged particle, when placed in an electric field, migrates towards the anode or the cathode, depending upon the net charge carried by the particle. Different molecules migrate at different speeds depending upon their charge, molecular weight, particle size and shape. Movement occurs in a buffer solution supported on an inert material like filter paper, cellulose acetate strip, agar gel, starch gel or polyacrylamide gel.

Paper Electrophoresis

In paper electrophoresis, a strip of filter paper is dipped in a buffer solution (commonly barbitone buffer, pH 8.6) and is laid on a plastic platform. The ends of the paper strip are dipped in buffer chambers. The entire apparatus is covered to minimize evaporation. Voltage is applied through the two electrodes dipped in the buffer compartments. The electric current is supplied through a power supply which may supply either constant current or constant voltage, or both. The electric current is carried by the charged ions of the buffer solution and depending upon the charge, a protein or amino acid molecule migrates either towards the anode (positive electrode) or the cathode (negative electrode) (Fig. 6.32).

Polyacrylamide Gel Electrophoresis (PAGE)

Principle: In this technique, proteins are separated on the basis of their charge and molecular size. The phenomenon is also referred to as molecular sieving.

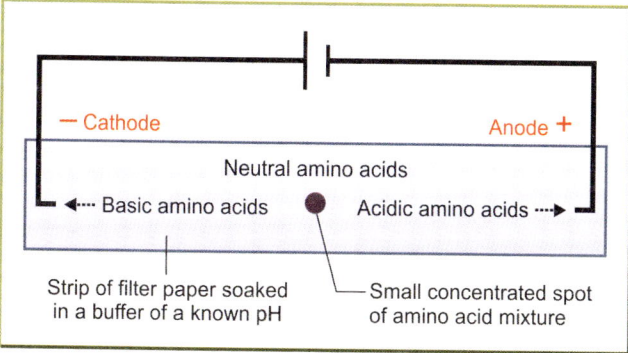

Fig. 6.32: Paper electrophoresis.

Polyacrylamide gel: PAGE is carried out in polyacrylamide gel with a characteristic pore size.

Individual gels are prepared *in situ* in glass tubes (0.5×4.0 cm) by polymerizing a gel monomer and a cross-linking agent with the aid of an appropriate catalyst. A serum sample is applied at the top, and proteins, following electrophoresis, are stained with amido black. It may yield 20 or more fractions and is widely used to study individual proteins in serum, especially genetic variants and isoenzymes.

SDS-PAGE: PAGE can also be carried out in the presence of sodium dodecyl sulphate (SDS), called as SDS-PAGE. By this technique, oligoproteins can be separated into their subunits.

Proteins are suspended in 1% solution of SDS. This detergent disrupts most protein-protein and protein-lipid interactions. The solution is layered on an acrylamide gel containing SDS and subjected to electrophoresis. A pattern of bands appears when the gel is stained with Coomassie Blue.

SDS molecules are negatively charged and, in turn, coat the proteins. The negative charge on each protein varies with the number of peptide bonds in a protein. Since the number of peptide bonds is proportional to the molecular weight of a protein, the rate of migration on electrophoresis is therefore an index of molecular weight of the protein.

Isoelectric focusing: This was discussed earlier (Fig. 6.12).

High Voltage Electrophoresis

It is mainly used for the separation of amino acids. Amino acids can be separated by the process of electrophoresis but in this case instead of low voltage (100 V) as used in paper electrophoresis for serum proteins, very high voltage (800–1000 V) is used. Different amino acids migrate at different positions which can be observed as bands after the separated amino acids are stained with a solution of ninhydrin.

PLASMA PROTEINS

Plasma contains over 300 proteins. Albumin, globulins and fibrinogen are the major plasma proteins, all of which are synthesized in the liver (except γ-globulins). Others include apolipoproteins (present in lipoproteins), protein hormones (such as insulin, prolactin etc.), enzymes and coagulation proteins.

Total plasma protein concentration varies from 6.3–8.0 g/dl out of which albumin constitutes 3.7–5.3 g/dl while globulins constitute 1.8–3.7 g/dl. The range for the various globulin fractions are—α_1 plus $\alpha_2 = 0.4$–1.4 g/dl, $\beta = 0.5$–1.3 g/dl and $\gamma = 0.6$–1.5 g/dl.

A/G RATIO

A/G ratio refers to plasma albumin:globulin ratio. The normal plasma A/G ratio is 1.2–2.0:1 which may be altered in a number of conditions (Chemistry to Clinics 6.2).

ACUTE-PHASE PROTEINS

The liver has the capacity to enhance or reduce the synthesis of various proteins in response to diseases.

Chemistry to Clinics 6.2: A/G Ratio

- An increase in total plasma proteins occurs in dehydration due to prolonged diarrhea, vomiting and diabetes insipidus. Because of hemoconcentration, both albumin and globulins are increased proportionately so that A/G ratio remains unaltered.
- A decrease in total plasma proteins is generally due to hypoalbuminemia as seen in liver cirrhosis, nephrotic syndrome, kwashiorkor, etc. It may be accompanied by either no increase in globulins or an increase in globulins that is proportionately less than the fall in albumin, resulting in a reversal of A/G ratio. It is clinically manifested as edema involving the feet, pre-tibial area (Fig. 6.33), pre-sacral area, periorbital area, etc. If not timely diagnosed and treated, it leads to generalized edema known as anasarca.
- Reversal of A/G ratio due to increased γ-globulins is observed in gammopathies such as multiple myeloma.

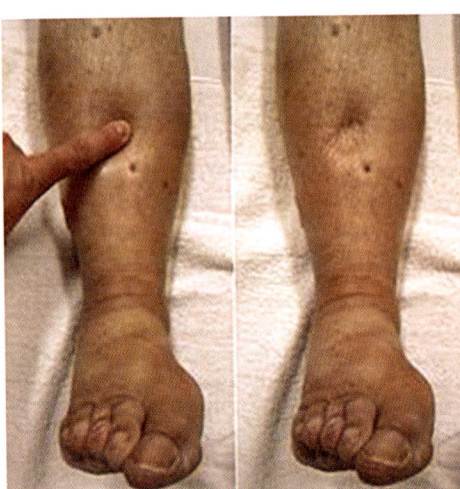

Fig. 6.33: Pitting edema of the lower extremity: The depression persists for sometime after the finger is removed.

Chemistry to Clinics 6.3: Acute-Phase Proteins

The liver responds to inflammation by increasing the synthesis of some plasma proteins and decreasing the synthesis of others. These proteins are called 'positive acute-phase proteins' or 'negative acute-phase proteins' respectively and the overall response is called the acute-phase response. Common examples include:

Positive acute-phase proteins: C-reactive protein (so named because it was first identified as a substance in the serum of patients with acute inflammation that reacted with the C-polysaccharide of Pneumococcus), fibrinogen, α_1-antitrypsin, α_2-macroglobulin, ferritin, ceruloplasmin, etc.

Negative acute-phase proteins: Albumin, transferrin, transthyretin, transcortin, retinol-binding protein, etc.

These are called acute-phase proteins or acute-phase reactants (Chemistry to Clinics 6.3).

Functions of Plasma Albumin

Albumin performs several functions:
- Maintenance of **plasma colloidal osmotic pressure** and hence the regulation of blood volume.
- **Transport** of various molecules such as long chain fatty acids, unconjugated bilirubin, steroids, Cu^{2+} and drugs like salicylates, barbiturates, penicillin, sulfonamides and warfarin.
- As plasma **antioxidant** because of the presence of sulfhydryl (–SH) groups.
- **As protein reserve** in case of nutritional depletion.

Functions of Plasma Globulins

The α and β globulins transport various molecules such as hormones, copper, iron, etc. (Table 6.6). γ-globulins constitute the defense proteins that combat antigenic challenge.

Table 6.6: Transport proteins and their ligands

Protein	Ligand
Albumin	Cu^{2+}, Fe^{3+}, bilirubin, free fatty acids, steroids, heme
Ceruloplasmin	Copper
Transferrin, ferritin, hemosiderin	Iron
Haptoglobin, hemopexin	Free hemoglobin
Thyroid binding globulin	Thyroid hormones
Cortisol binding globulin	Cortisol
Sex hormone binding globulin	Androgens, estrogens

Clinical Uses of Plasma Proteins

- **Treatment of hypoalbuminemia:** A 20–40% colloidal solution of human albumin is administered by intravenous infusion to treat patients suffering from gross hypoalbuminemia and massive edema.
- **Diagnosis of pulmonary embolism:** Radiolabeled albumin is used in the screening of pulmonary embolism (the movement of a blood clot or other plug from the systemic veins through the right heart and into the pulmonary circulation, where it lodges in one or more branches of the pulmonary artery). It involves the injection of aggregates of human serum albumin labeled with a radionuclide into a peripheral vein. These albumin aggregates travel through the right side of the heart, enter the pulmonary vasculature and lodge in small pulmonary vessels. Only those lung areas receiving blood flow will manifest an uptake of the tracer; the nonperfused region will not show any uptake of the tagged albumin. The aggregates fragment and are removed from the lungs in about a day.
- **Passive immunization:** Sera rich in γ-globulins (hyperimmune sera) are used to confer artificial passive immunity in certain cases, e.g. administration of anti-tetanus serum (ATS) in tetanus.

Separation of Plasma Proteins by Electrophoresis

The separation of plasma proteins is performed on paper or cellulose acetate in 0.1 M barbitone buffer (pH 8.6). About 10 µl of plasma is applied along a thin line near the cathode. At pH 8.6, all plasma proteins carry a net negative charge and migrate towards the anode. At a constant current of 1–2 mA, different proteins migrate at different rates depending on their mass and surface charge. At the end, their positions are revealed by some dye such as bromophenol blue which stains the proteins to produce separate bands, called an **electrophoretogram**. In case of normal plasma, five bands are formed (Fig. 6.34A). Albumin is the lightest and carries the largest negative charge, hence it moves fastest. γ-globulin possess the opposite properties and move the least. Starting from the anode, the bands are designated as albumin, α_1-globulin, α_2-globulin, β-globulin and γ-globulin.

Concentrations of individual proteins may be determined by an instrument called a **densitometer** which scans and **quantifies** the proteins (Fig. 6.34B).

Electrophoretograms are useful in the diagnosis of diseases (Fig. 6.34C to J).

Plasma Protein Disorders

Hypoalbuminemia

It refers to low plasma albumin and may arise due to a number of reasons such as:
- Protein malnutrition, e.g. kwashiorkor and marasmus.
- Malabsorption, e.g. inflammatory bowel disease and following bowel-resection.
- Impaired synthesis in chronic liver disease, e.g. cirrhosis.
- Excessive losses in urine (nephrotic syndrome, Fig. 6.35) or stool (protein-losing enteropathy) or through skin (severe burns).
- Leakage and trapping in extravascular sites known as 'third space fluid losses, e.g. ascitis (accumulation in peritoneal cavity, Fig. 6.36) and pleural effusion (accumulation in pleural cavity).
- Increased catabolism (major surgery or trauma, sepsis, malignancy and following repeated radiation therapy).
- Overhydration (artifact causes), e.g. pregnancy or dilution of sample due to taking a blood sample from a site close to an intravenous infusion.

Analbuminemia

Analbuminemia refers to a condition in which plasma albumin is almost completely absent (<100 mg/dl). There may be compensatory increase in plasma globulins concentrations.

Hyperglobulinemia

Increase in globulins occurs most commonly in:
- Advanced liver disease, e.g. cirrhosis.
- Chronic diseases which may be infectious (tuberculosis, viral hepatitis) or non-infectious (rheumatoid arthritis).
- Multiple myeloma.

Liver disease, chronic infection or an autoimmune disease such as rheumatoid arthritis give rise to sustained stimulation of B lymphocytes and hence an increased production of γ-globulins, which is revealed as a broad/diffuse band on serum protein electrophoresis (Fig. 6.34C and H).

6

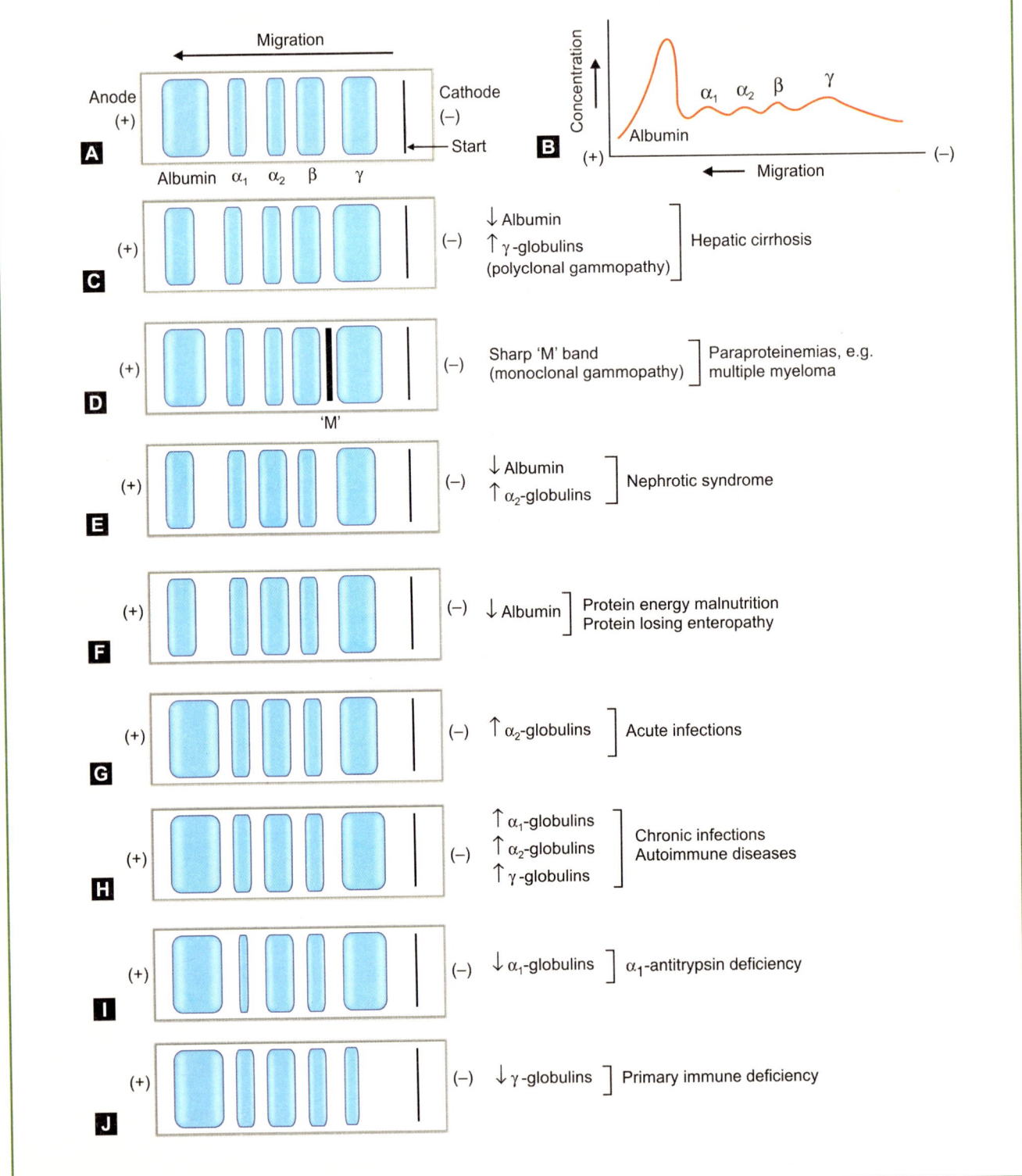

Fig. 6.34: Normal electrophoresis (A), and densitometric (B) patterns of plasma proteins. Various abnormal electrophoresis patterns are shown from (C to J).

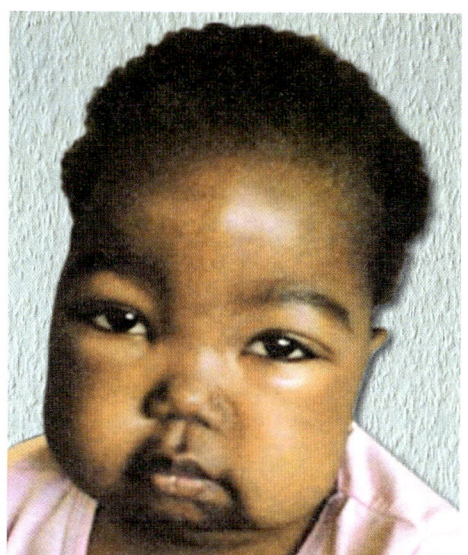

Fig. 6.35: Facial and periorbital edema in a child with **nephrotic syndrome**.

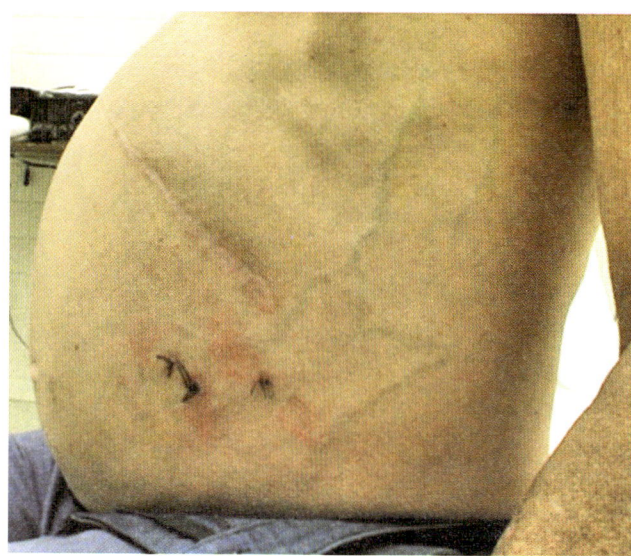

Fig. 6.36: Ascites: Note the prominent superficial veins in the lateral abdominal wall. An operative scar and sites of fluid drainage are also seen.

Paraproteinemia

Discrete immunoglobulin bands visible on serum protein electrophoresis are known as **paraproteins** or monoclonal components. They are observed in multiple myeloma and lymphoid tumors. They are due to overproduction of a single immunoglobulin class or immunoglobulin fragment by a single class (clone) of B cells (Chemistry to Clinics 6.4).

Chemistry to Clinics 6.4: Multiple Myeloma and Bence Jones Proteins

Normally, B lymphocytes mature into plasma cells which are responsible for the production of immunoglobulins/antibodies. **Multiple myeloma** is a disease characterized by malignant proliferation of B lymphocyte precursors generating excessive plasma cells, which overproduce complete IgG or IgA immunoglobulins and the amount is proportional to the tumor mass. Plasma protein electrophoresis reveals a characteristic, intense and narrow **'M' band** with the γ-globulin (Fig. 6.34D).

In some patients, dimers of immunoglobulin light chains (either κ or λ) are found in the urine. These are called **Bence Jones proteins** and they show a characteristic differential heat solubility—gradual heating of the urine sample kept in a water bath results in precipitates between 40° and 50°C, disappearing at nearly 90°C. On cooling, the precipitates reappear at nearly 70°C.

SOME IMPORTANT QUESTIONS

1. **What are amino acids? Based on the ionic charge classify various amino acids.**

2. **What are proteins? Based on their solubility classify various proteins.**

3. **Describe:**

   i. Biological value of a protein
   ii. Structural organization of proteins
   iii. Chromatography
   iv. Electrophoresis

4. **Discuss briefly:**

   i. α-Helix
   ii. β-Sheets
   iii. Quaternary structure of proteins
   iv. Separation of serum proteins
   v. SDS-PAGE
   vi. Protein folding
   vii. Protein denaturation

5. Write notes on:

i. Neutral amino acids
ii. Branched chain amino acids
iii. Aromatic amino acids
iv. Acidic amino acids
v. Basic amino acids
vi. Essential amino acids
vii. Isoelectric point
viii. Zwitterion
ix. Functions of plasma albumin
x. Functions of plasma globulins
xi. A/G ratio
xii. Hypoalbuminemia
xiii. Hyperglobulinemia
xiv. Bence Jones protein
xv. Edema
xvi. Acute phase proteins

MULTIPLE CHOICE QUESTIONS

1. **The bond between γ-COOH group of glutamate and α-NH$_2$ group of cysteine in glutathione is:**
   A. A true peptide bond
   B. An isopeptide bond
   C. Not a peptide bond
   D. An unstable bond

2. **In an insulin molecule, the disulphide bonds are:**
   A. 2 interchain, 1 intrachain
   B. 1 interchain, 2 intrachain
   C. 3 interchain
   D. 3 intrachain

3. **A compact, globular functional unit of a protein is called a:**
   A. Secondary structure   B. Motif
   C. Domain   D. Catalytic site

4. **Isoelectric pH of casein is:**
   A. 7.0   B. 7.4
   C. 4.6   D. 6.7

5. **The following is a prolamine:**
   A. Gliadin   B. Insulin
   C. Albumin   D. Collagen

6. **The following is a structural protein:**
   A. Collagen   B. Phaseolin
   C. Zein   D. Hemoglobin

7. **The following can result in protein denaturation:**
   A. Heat   B. UV rays
   C. Urea   D. All of the above

8. **The following proteins are known to be associated with abnormal folding resulting in disease:**
   A. CFTR   B. α$_1$-AT
   C. β-Amyloid   D. All of the above

9. **The normal plasma albumin/globulin (A/G) ratio is:**
   A. 1.2 : 1   B. 2.2 : 1
   C. 1 : 1.2   D. 1 : 2.2

10. **Hyperglobulinemia may occur in:**
   A. Tuberculosis
   B. Rheumatoid arthritis
   C. Hepatic cirrhosis
   D. All of the above

7

Chemistry and Functions of Nucleotides and Nucleic Acids

Nucleic acids are the macromolecules constituted by the repeated monomeric units called nucleotides, i.e. nucleotides are the building blocks for nucleic acids, as amino acids to proteins or monosaccharides to polysaccharides. Nucleic acids occur in association with basic proteins, such as histones and protamines. Nucleic acids store information and make it available to the cell. These are strongly acidic in nature and thus are negatively charged at physiological pH.

A **nucleotide has 3 components**, i.e. a pentose sugar, a nitrogenous base and phosphoric acid.

PENTOSE SUGARS

The presence of a pentose sugar defines the type of a nucleic acid. There are two classes of nucleic acids, viz. deoxyribonucleic acid (DNA) and ribonucleic acid (RNA). As the name suggests, deoxyribonucleic acid contains deoxyribose sugar while ribonucleic acid contains ribose.

Ribose has three –OH groups at carbon numbers 1, 2 and 3 of the pentose molecule. **Deoxyribose**, on the other hand, does not contain an oxygen atom at the second carbon and thus has only two –OH groups, i.e. at carbon atoms, 1 and 3. Deoxyribose, thus, is also called as 2-deoxyribose (Fig. 7.1).

The sugar molecule is linked to a nitrogenous base on one side (through carbon atom one, i.e. C1) and to phosphoric acid on the other side (through carbon atom five, i.e. C5).

To differentiate between the carbon atom of a sugar molecule from the carbon atom of a nitrogenous base,

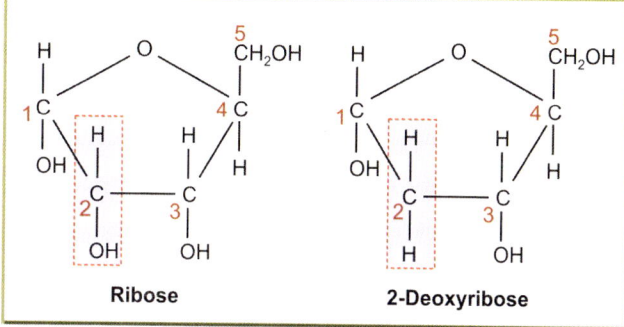

Fig. 7.1: Sugars present in nucleic acids.

in the nomenclature of a nucleotide, the position of a carbon atom of the sugar moiety is represented by a sign called **prime (′)**. These are thus written as C1′ or C5′, etc. On the other hand, the carbon and the nitrogen atom of the nitrogenous bases are written without the prime sign, such as N1 or C2, etc.

NITROGENOUS BASES

Nitrogenous bases found in various nucleotides are either the derivatives of a purine ring or of a pyrimidine ring. Purine ring is a nine-membered ring containing 5 carbon and 4 nitrogen atoms while pyrimidine is a six-membered ring which has 4 carbon and 2 nitrogen atoms (Fig. 7.2).

Various nitrogenous bases are formed with the appropriate substitutions on the parent heterocyclic ring, and are accordingly called the derivatives of purines and pyrimidines.

There are two types of **purine bases** present in nucleic acids, viz. adenine (6-aminopurine) and

7

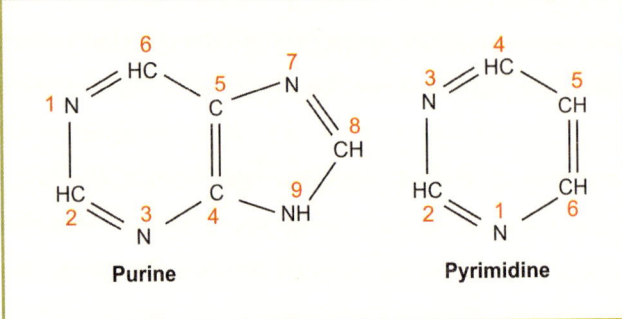

Fig. 7.2: Purine and pyrimidine rings.

guanine (2-amino-6-oxypurine). The **pyrimidine bases**, found in nucleic acids, are designated as cytosine (2-oxy-4-aminopyrimidine), uracil (2,4-dioxypyrimidine) and thymine (2,4-dioxy-5-methylpyrimidine, also called as 5-methyluracil) (Fig. 7.3). Out of these three pyrimidines, only two are repeatedly found in a nucleic acid. Usually cytosine and uracil are found in RNA while cytosine and thymine are found in DNA.

Lactam-Lactim Tautomerism

Due to the presence of an oxy group, purine and pyrimidine bases of nucleic acids can assume different tautomeric forms, called as keto (lactam) and enol (lactim) forms. Tautomers are easily convertible isomers that differ only in hydrogen positions (Fig. 7.4).

Under physiological conditions, guanine and thymine occur predominantly in the lactam (keto) form.

Unusual Nitrogenous Bases

Besides the four nitrogenous bases (2 purines and 2 pyrimidines), which are commonly found in nucleic acids, there also occur some unusual nitrogenous bases in nucleic acids of certain bacteria and viruses. These are called as minor bases, e.g. 5-methylcytosine, 5-hydroxymethylcytosine, pseudouracil (where structural positions of N1 and C5 in the uracil molecule are interchanged), N6-methyladenine, N7-methylguanine, etc. (Fig. 7.5).

Besides, there are some other purine derivatives which are of biological significance. These are either found as intermediates in purine biosynthesis, e.g. hypoxanthine and xanthine, or as the end product of their catabolism, such as uric acid (Fig. 7.6).

NUCLEOSIDES

A nucleoside has two components, i.e. it consists of a **nitrogenous base** and a molecule of **sugar**. In a nucleoside, a pentose sugar (ribose or deoxyribose) is linked to a nitrogenous base by an N-glycosidic linkage. The first carbon atom of the sugar moiety (C1) is linked either with the N1 of a pyrimidine or with N9 of a purine.

Base – N – 1' – Sugar

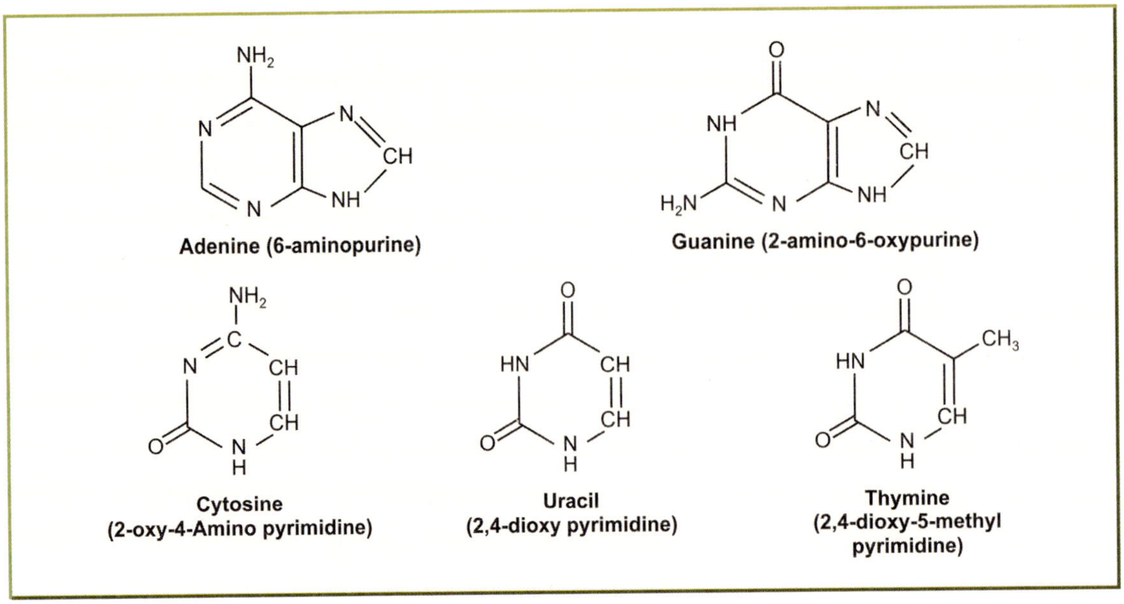

Adenine (6-aminopurine)

Guanine (2-amino-6-oxypurine)

Cytosine (2-oxy-4-Amino pyrimidine)

Uracil (2,4-dioxy pyrimidine)

Thymine (2,4-dioxy-5-methyl pyrimidine)

Fig. 7.3: Nitrogenous bases found in nucleic acids.

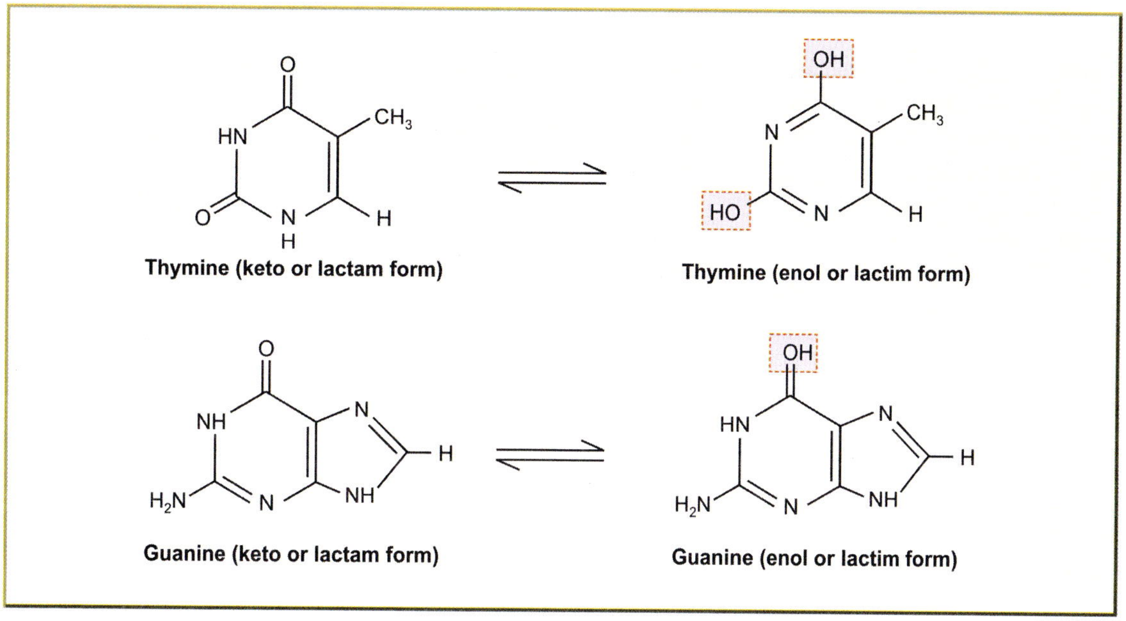

O
HN
CH3
O
N
H
H
Thymine (keto or lactam form)
OH
N
CH3
HO
N
H
Thymine (enol or lactim form)
O
NH
N
H
H2N
N
NH
Guanine (keto or lactam form)
OH
HN
N
H
H2N
N
NH
Guanine (enol or lactim form)

Fig. 7.4: Keto-enol or lactam-lactim tautomerism.

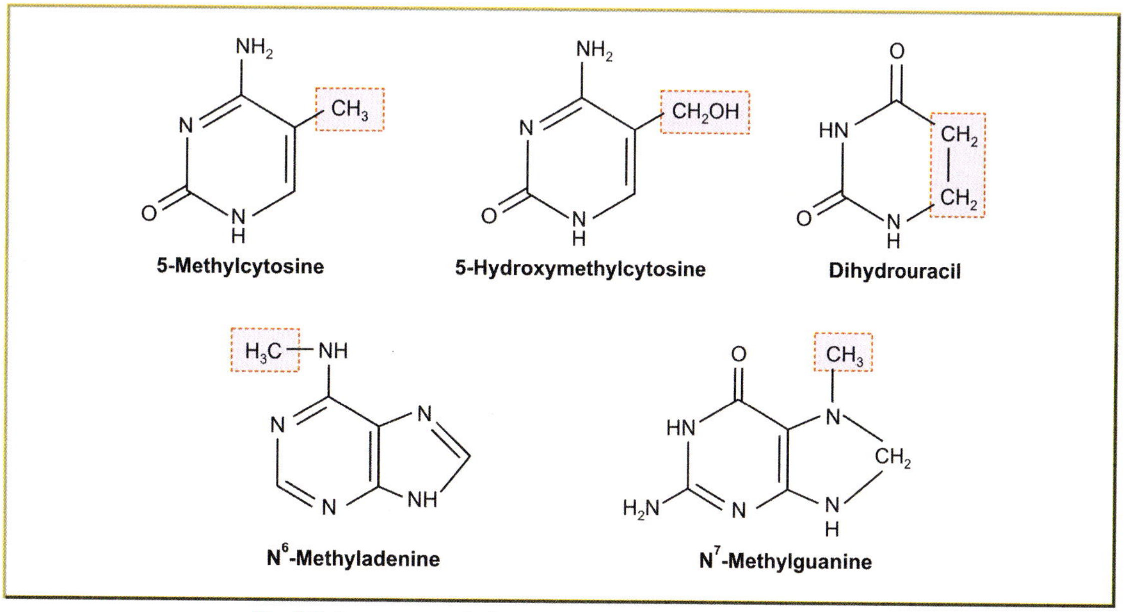

NH2
CH3
N
O
N
H
5-Methylcytosine
NH2
CH2OH
N
O
N
H
5-Hydroxymethylcytosine
O
HN
CH2
CH2
O
N
H
Dihydrouracil
H3C—NH
N
N
N
NH
N6-Methyladenine
O
CH3
HN
N
CH2
H2N
N
N
H
N7-Methylguanine

Fig. 7.5: Some unusual nitrogenous bases found in nucleic acids.

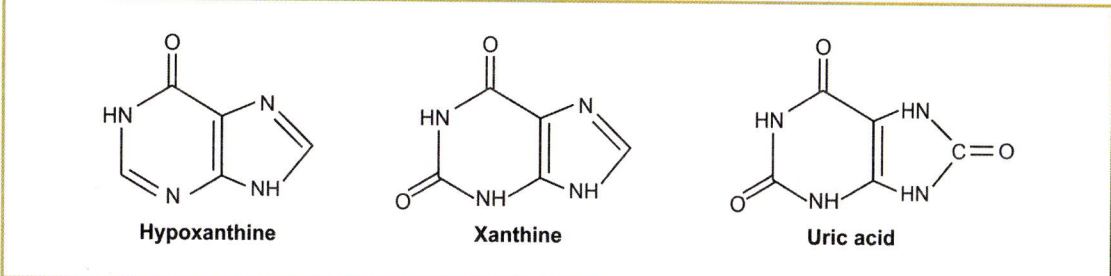

O
HN
N
N
NH
Hypoxanthine
O
HN
N
O
NH
NH
Xanthine
O
HN
HN
C=O
O
NH
HN
Uric acid

Fig. 7.6: Some purine bases of metabolic significance.

7

Ribonucleosides

The nucleosides of ribose are called ribonucleosides. Ribonucleosides of adenine, guanine, cytosine and uracil are designated as adenosine, guanosine, cytidine and uridine respectively (Fig. 7.7). Adenosine has attained considerable clinical importance (Chemistry to Clinics 7.1).

Chemistry to Clinicis 7.1: Significance of Adenosine

- Adenosine is a local hormone, known as an **autacoid**. During exercise, contracting muscles release adenosine which causes local vasodilation thereby enhancing the supply of nutrients including oxygen to the muscles.
- Adenosine participates in sleep regulation. Prolonged wakefulness increases the extracellular adenosine levels in the brain which induce sleepiness by binding to specific adenosine receptors. Interestingly, this interaction is blocked by caffeine, explaining the tendency of coffee to promote wakefulness.
- Intravenous administration of adenosine is employed in the emergency treatment of supraventricular tachycardia characterized by uncontrolled rapid heart beats (Fig. 7.8).

Deoxyribonucleosides

Nucleosides of deoxyribose are designated as deoxyribonucleosides. Various deoxyribonucleosides are written with a prefix d- (deoxy). Thus, deoxyadenosine, deoxyguanosine, deoxycytidine and deoxythymidine are the nucleosides of deoxyribose with adenine, guanine, cytosine, and thymine respectively. Since thymine is usually found in DNA where it is linked to a deoxyribose only, its nucleoside is commonly designated as thymidine and not deoxythymidine (Fig. 7.9).

NUCLEOTIDES

A nucleotide, as mentioned earlier, consists of a **nitrogenous base**, a **pentose sugar** and **phosphoric acid**. The sugar molecule (ribose or deoxyribose) is linked both to a nitrogenous base on one side and to phosphoric acid on the other side. As in a nucleoside, C1 of the sugar molecule is linked to a nitrogenous

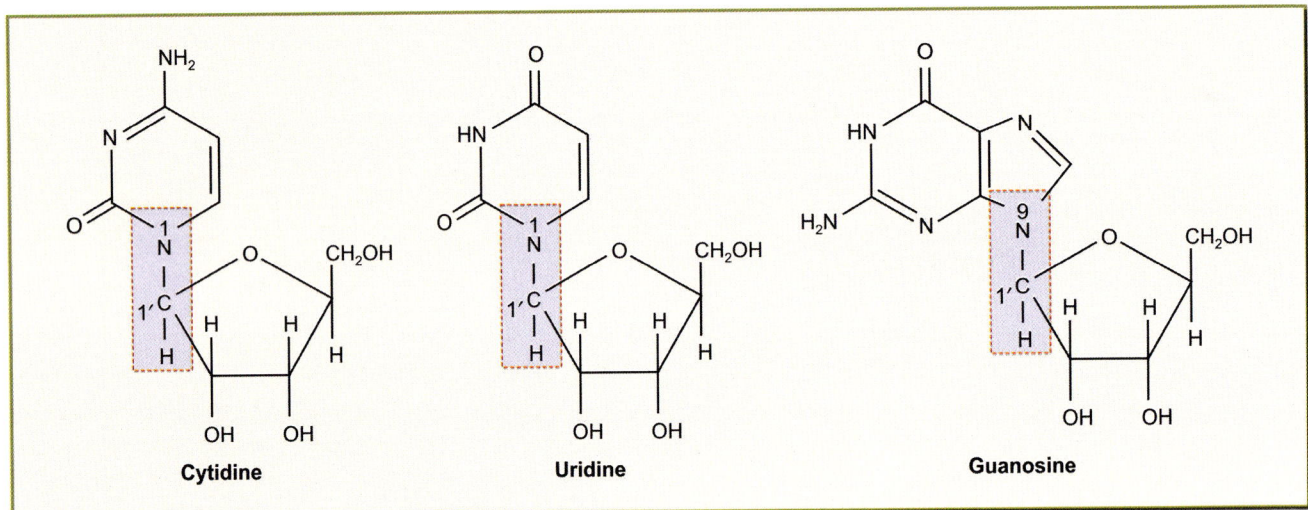

Fig. 7.7: Ribonucleosides.

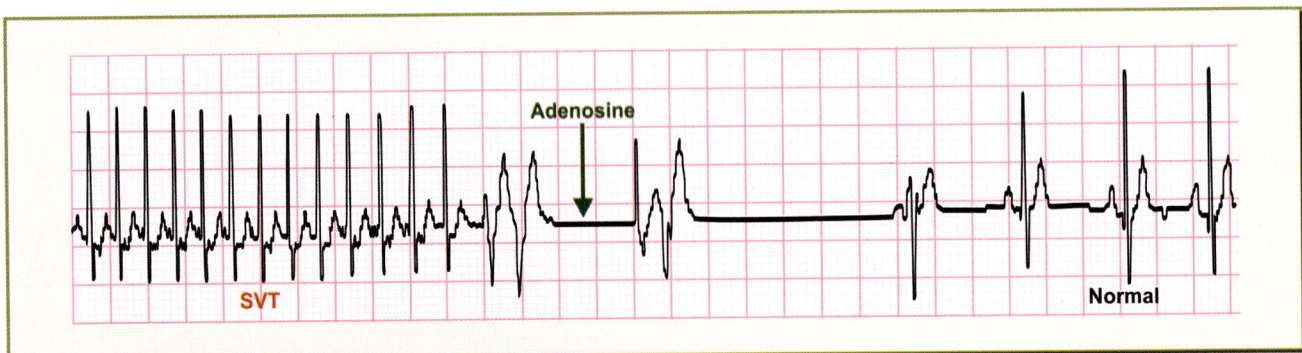

Fig. 7.8: ECG showing supraventricular tachycardia (SVT: Abnormally rapid heart rate which may be life-threatening) being normalized by intravenous **adenosine**.

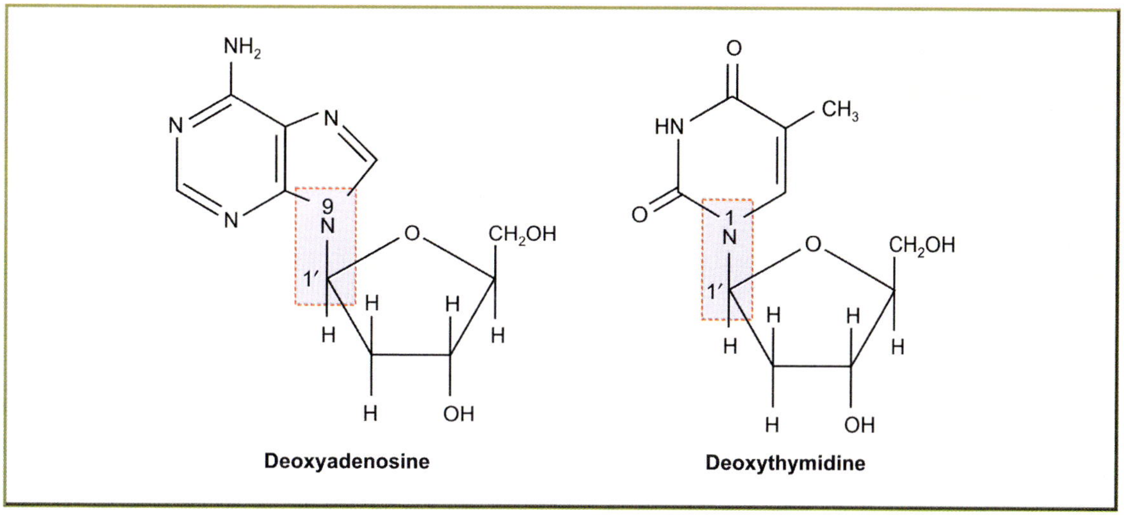

Fig. 7.9: Deoxyribonucleosides.

base either through N1 of a pyrimidine or N9 of a purine. The sugar is also linked to phosphoric acid. Although any hydroxyl group (–OH) of the sugar can get esterified with phosphoric acid, more commonly C5 of the sugar is linked to a phosphate moiety.

Base – N – 1′ – Sugar – 5′ – Phosphate

Ribonucleotides

A nucleotide containing a ribose sugar is called ribonucleotide. Four ribonucleotides obtained on hydrolysis of RNA are designated as adenosine monophosphate or adenylate (AMP), guanylate (GMP), cytidylate (CMP) and uridylate (UMP) (Fig. 7.10).

Deoxyribonucleotides

The corresponding deoxyribonucleotides obtained on hydrolysis of a DNA molecule are designated as dAMP, dGMP, dCMP and TMP respectively. Some of the deoxyribonucleotides are shown in (Fig. 7.11).

Various nitrogenous bases, nucleosides and nucleotides found in nucleic acids are shown in Table 7.1.

Attachment of a phosphate in a nucleotide during hydrolysis of a nucleic acid

As discussed above, though C5′ of the sugar moiety is usually linked with the phosphate in a nucleotide, during hydrolysis of a nucleic acid, the phosphate

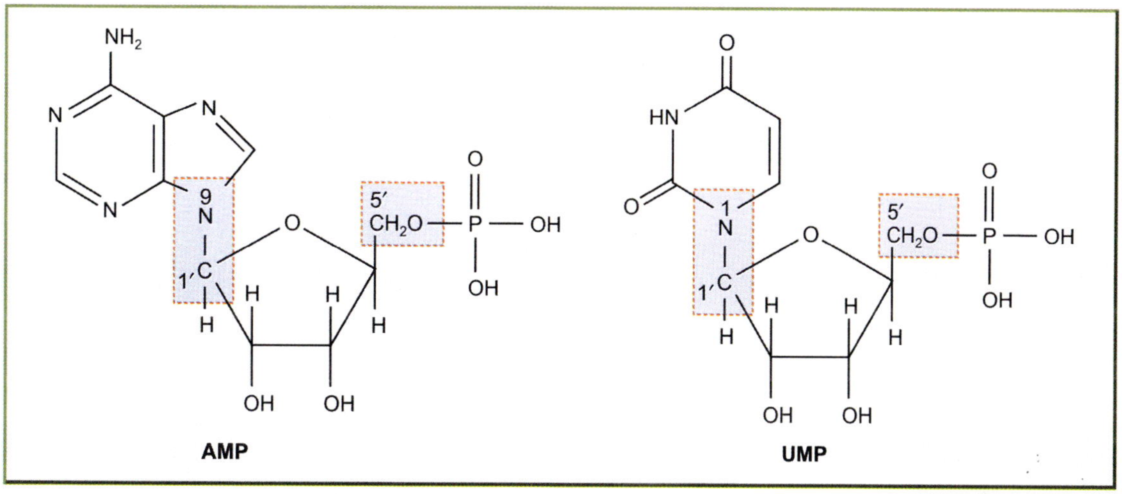

Fig. 7.10: Ribonucleotides.

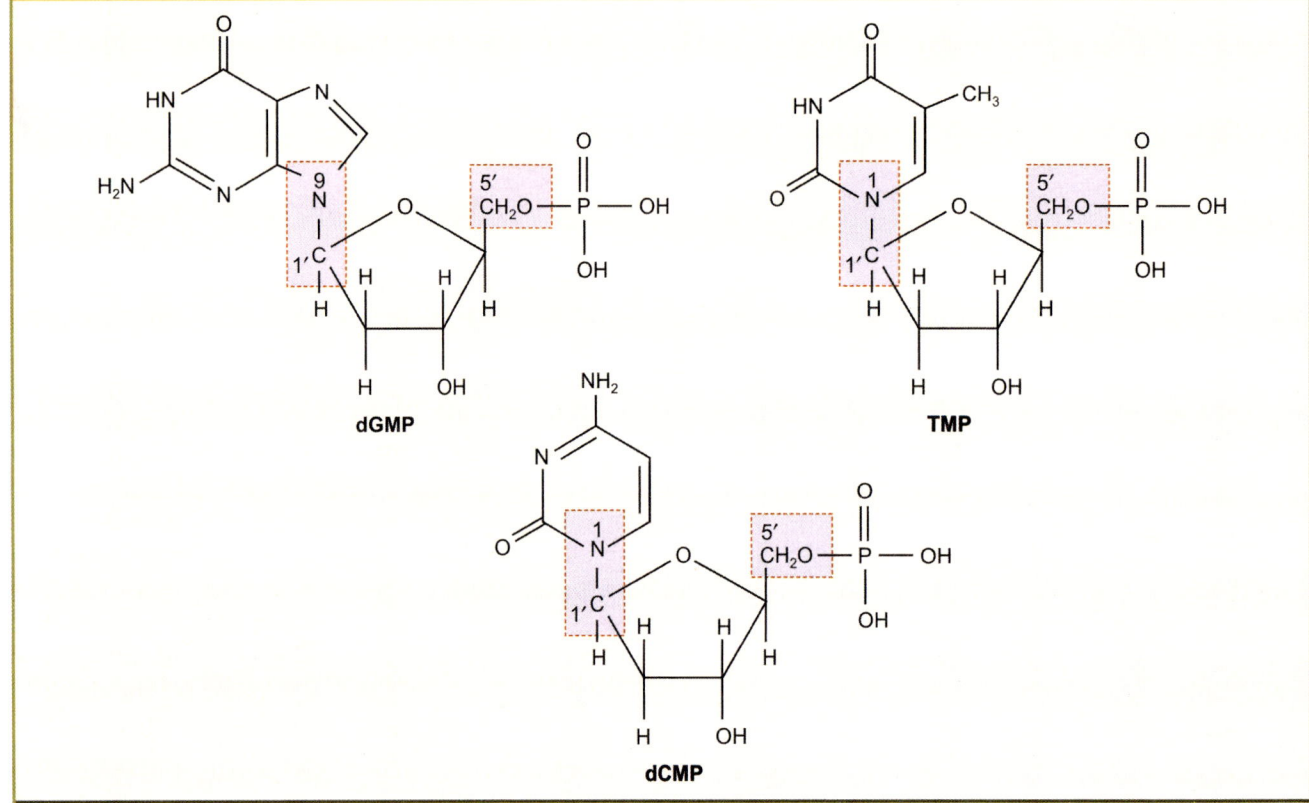

Fig. 7.11: Deoxyribonucleotides.

Table 7.1: Different nitrogenous bases, nucleosides and nucleotides found in nucleic acids

Nitrogenous base	Nucleoside (base + sugar)	Nucleotide (base + sugar + P)
RNA		
Adenine	Adenosine	AMP
Guanine	Guanosine	GMP
Cytosine	Cytidine	CMP
Uracil	Uridine	UMP
DNA		
Adenine	Deoxyadenosine	dAMP
Guanine	Deoxyguanosine	dGMP
Cytosine	Deoxycytidine	dCMP
Thymine	Thymidine	TMP

moiety may get attached even on to other –OH groups of sugar molecule. Thus, a deoxyribonucleotide may have a phosphoric acid attached to the –OH group of its deoxyribose either at C3′ or C5′, forming deoxyribonucleoside-3′-monophosphate (dN-3′-MP) or dN-5′-M-P (N refers to a nucleoside of any nitrogenous base).

In a ribose, since the –OH group is also present at C2′, in addition to N-3′-MP (nucleoside-3′-monophosphate) and N-5′-MP, N-2′-MP is also obtained during hydrolysis of an RNA molecule.

Different nucleoside monophosphates are shown in Fig. 7.12.

Nucleotide Derivatives of Biological Significance

Besides the nucleotides of adenine, guanine, cytosine, uracil or thymine which are the hydrolyzed products of nucleic acids, there also occur di- and triphosphate derivatives of various nucleosides, e.g. ADP, ATP, GTP, CTP, UTP, etc. (Fig. 7.13).

Important biological functions of nucleotides include

• Energy metabolism, e.g. ATP is the cellular energy currency.
• Monomeric units of nucleic acids.

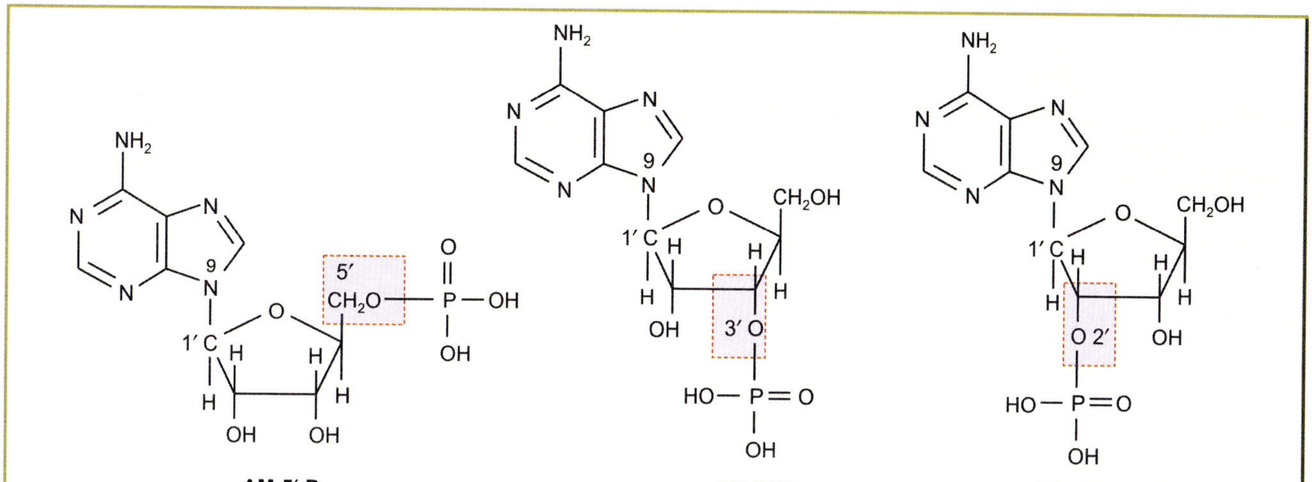

Fig. 7.12: Attachment of a phosphate at different positions in a nucleotide to produce various nucleoside monophosphates.

- Physiological mediators, e.g. cAMP is the second messenger for epinephrine.
- Metabolic precursors, e.g. GTP for tetrahydro-biopterin synthesis.
- Components of coenzymes, e.g. NAD, FAD, etc.
- Activated metabolic intermediates, e.g. S-adenosyl methionine (SAM).
- Allosteric effectors, e.g. hexokinase is allosterically activated by ADP whereas it is allosterically inhibited by ATP.
- Interconversion of monosaccharides by UDP-glucose and UDP-galactose.
- Conjugation reactions, e.g. UDP-glucuronic acid is used for the conjugation of bilirubin.

Synthetic Analogs

An alteration either in the heterocyclic ring or in the sugar moiety may produce pharmacologically active compounds. When this analog gets incorporated into the nucleic acid, it shows toxic effects. Some of them may be inhibitory to various enzymes and may thus inhibit DNA synthesis (Chemistry to Clinics 7.2).

POLYNUCLEOTIDES

- Polymerization of the monomeric units, i.e. nucleotides results in the formation of a polynucleotide. Various nucleotide units are linked

Chemistry to Clinics 7.2: Purine/Pyrimidine Analogs as Drugs

Some of the synthetic analogs, such as 5-fluorouracil (a derivative of pyrimidine with the analogous heterocyclic ring), 6-thioguanine and 6-mercaptopurine (sulfur substituted analogs of purine) are used as anticancer drugs. Allopurinol (4-hydroxy-pyrazolo-pyrimidine, an analog of purine) is an inhibitor of xanthine oxidase and is used in the treatment of hyperuricemia.

Some analogs of sugar moiety, such as arabinosylcytosine (cytosine with arabinose instead of cytidine which contains cytosine and ribose) are also used in cancer chemotherapy (Fig. 7.14).

together by a 3', 5' phosphodiester linkage where a hydroxyl group of the sugar molecule of one nucleotide is linked to the hydroxyl group of the sugar moiety of the other nucleotide, between C3' and C5', forming a polynucleotide.

- One end of the polynucleotide is a hydroxyl or 5'-phosphate terminus while the other end is a 3'-phosphate or 3'-hydroxyl terminus. They are called as the 5'-end and 3'-end respectively.
- Conventionally, nucleotides are represented by the first letter of the base, e.g. AGCT, etc. Since each nucleotide is linked through the phosphate moiety (p), thus pApGpT specifies that the polynucleotide sequence starts with AMP which has phosphate moiety at the 5' terminus and ends at TMP having a hydroxyl group at the 3' terminus (Fig. 7.15).
- Polymers of nucleotides are known as deoxy-ribonucleic acid (DNA) and ribonucleic acid (RNA). These are the primary players in the storage and decoding of genetic information.

7

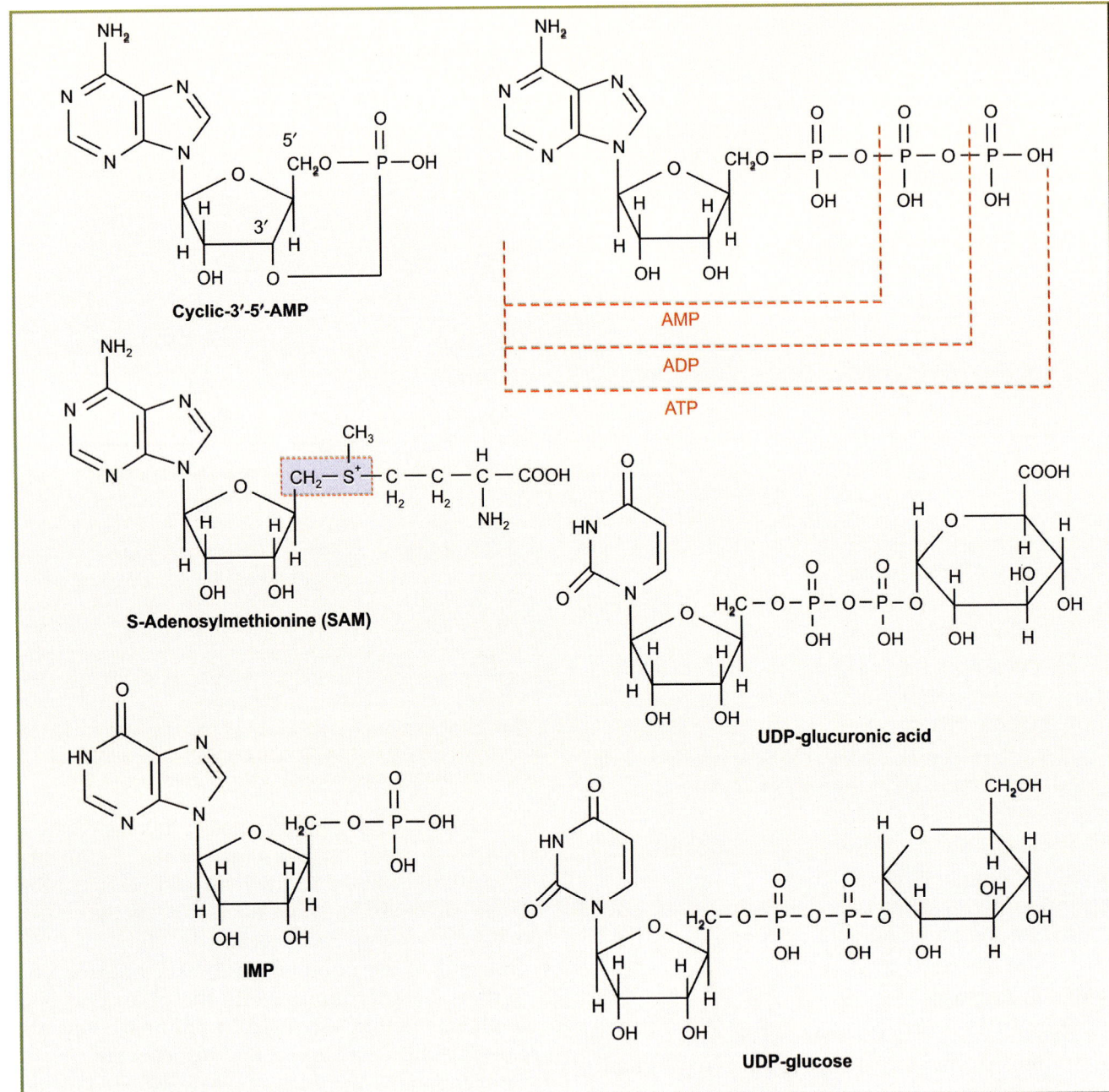

Fig. 7.13: Some nucleotide derivatives of biological significance.

DEOXYRIBONUCLEIC ACID (DNA)

Structure of DNA: Watson-Crick Model

Deoxyribonucleic acid (DNA) stores genetic information and is called as the chemical basis of heredity. DNA is a double-stranded polymer of deoxyribonucleotides which are linked by phosphodiester bonds. Various features of DNA structure were first described by Watson and Crick, therefore it is called as the Watson-Crick model or Watson-Crick structure of DNA. They described that:

• DNA is a **polynucleotide** of deoxyadenylate (dAMP), deoxyguanylate (dGMP), deoxycytidylate (dCMP) and thymidylate (TMP).

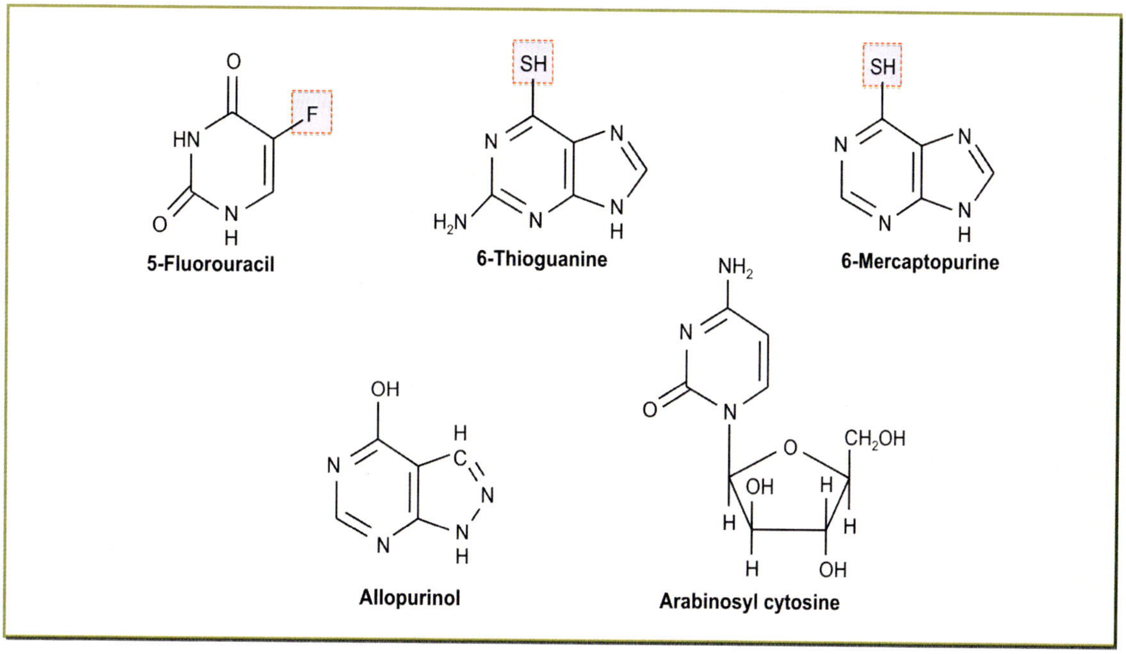

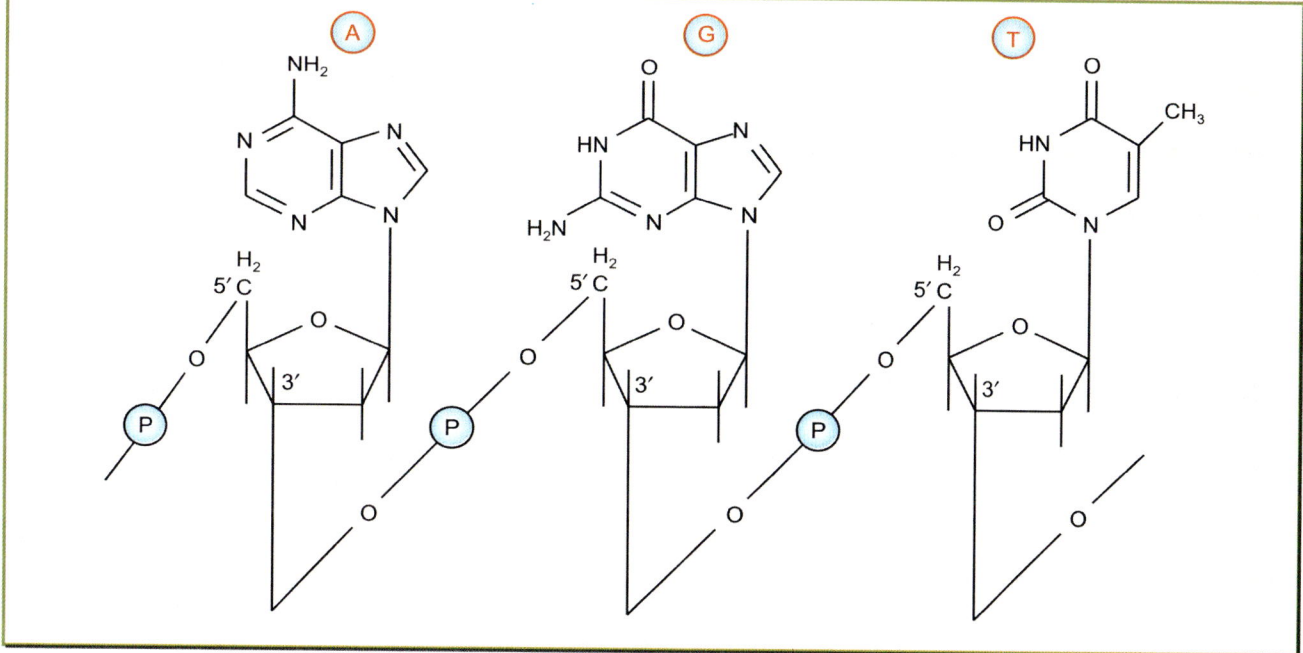

Fig. 7.14: Some synthetic nucleotide analogs.

5-Fluorouracil

6-Thioguanine

6-Mercaptopurine

Allopurinol

Arabinosyl cytosine

Fig. 7.15: A polynucleotide.

• The information content of a DNA molecule resides in the **sequence** in which these monomers (purine and pyrimidine deoxyribonucleotides) are ordered.

• The polymer possesses a **polarity** where one of its end has a 5′-hydroxyl or phosphate terminus while the other end has a 3′-phosphate moiety or a hydroxyl group.

7

```
5' ── A ── G ── C ── C ── C ── T ── T ── A ── A ── A ── G ── C ── G ── T ── A ──────── 3'
       │    │    │    │    │    │    │    │    │    │    │    │    │    │    │
3' ── T ── C ── G ── G ── G ── A ── A ── T ── T ── T ── C ── G ── C ── A ── T ──────── 5'
```

Fig. 7.16: A double-stranded nucleic acid molecule.

- DNA molecule is **double-stranded**.
- The two chains run **antiparallel** to each other, i.e. one strand runs in the $5' \rightarrow 3'$ direction while the other in the $3' \rightarrow 5'$ direction (Fig. 7.16).
- Both the polynucleotide chains are wound around a common axis so as to form a **right-handed helix**. The double helix so formed is nearly 2 nm in diameter.
- A base occupies the core of the helix while sugar-phosphate chains run along the periphery and form two grooves of unequal width. These are called as the **major groove** and the **minor groove** (Fig. 7.17).
- The helix has a **pitch** (rise/turn) of 3.4 nm and has 10 base pairs within each turn.
- The two strands of the double-stranded molecule are held together by **hydrogen bonds** between a purine base and a pyrimidine base of the respective polynucleotide chain.
- **Chargaff's rule:** The base-pairing is very specific, as A is linked to T with two hydrogen bonds and G is linked to C with three hydrogen bonds (Fig. 7.18).

DNA molecule, thus has equal number of adenine and thymine residues (A = T) as well as guanine and cytosine residues (G = C). This relationship is known as Chargaff's rule.

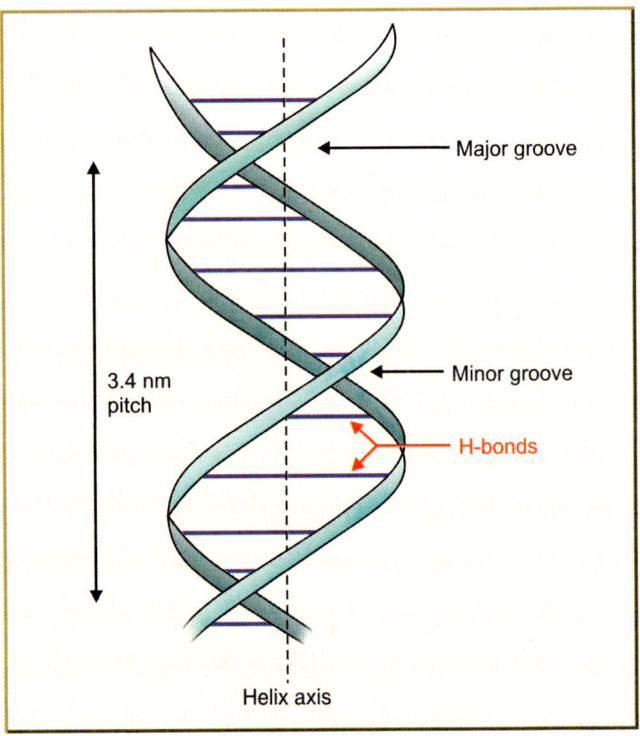

Fig. 7.17: DNA double-helix.

The hydrogen-binding interaction, a phenomenon known as **complementary base pairing**, results in

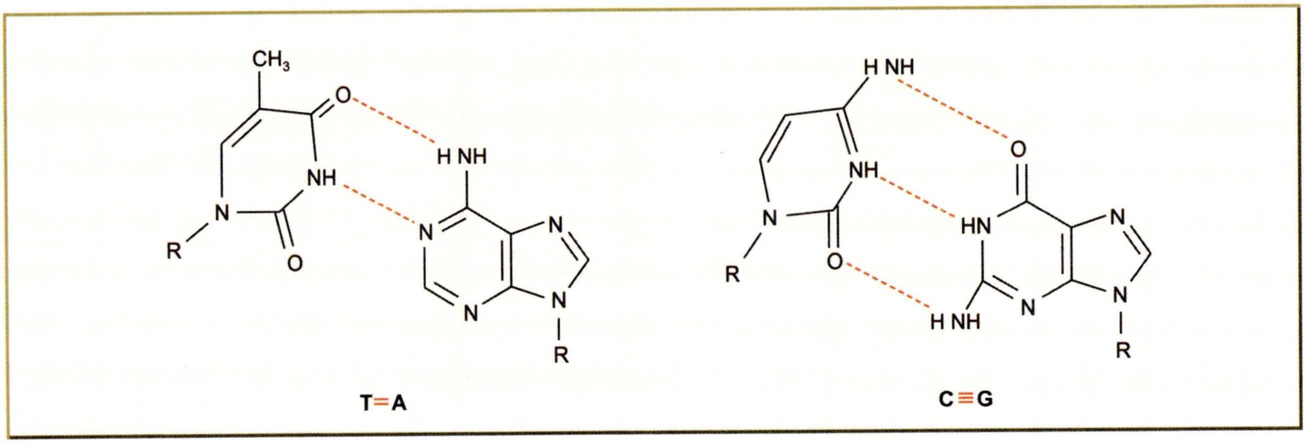

Fig. 7.18: Hydrogen bonding in DNA.

specific association of the two chains of a double helix. It finds application in DNA denaturation/renaturation.

Denaturation and Renaturation (Melting and Annealing) of DNA

Two strands of the DNA double helix get separated (**melted**) when a solution of duplex DNA is heated above a certain temperature. This process of complete separation or unwinding of the two strands *in vitro* is called as **denaturation**. It results in breakage of the hydrogen bonds between bases and the separation of the base pairs. Denaturation of DNA also results in qualitative changes in physical properties of the DNA, such as a decrease in viscosity or increase in ultraviolet absorbance of DNA (called **hyperchromicity**, observed at 260 nm).

The temperature at which DNA is half denatured is called as **melting temperature** or **Tm** of DNA. At Tm, absorbance of UV light is 50% between the maximum and minimum. The Tm depends on nature of the solvent, concentration of the ions in solution, its pH and base composition of the DNA.

When the melted sample of DNA is slowly cooled at temperature below Tm, it results in reformation of the complementary base pairs as per Chargaff's rule, and formation of the DNA double helix, i.e. **renaturation**. This process of renaturation of DNA is called **annealing** (Fig. 7.19).

The denaturation/renaturation cycle is used in the polymerase chain reaction. The formation of the RNA-DNA hybrid double helix from the complementary strands of RNA and DNA is called **hybridization**.

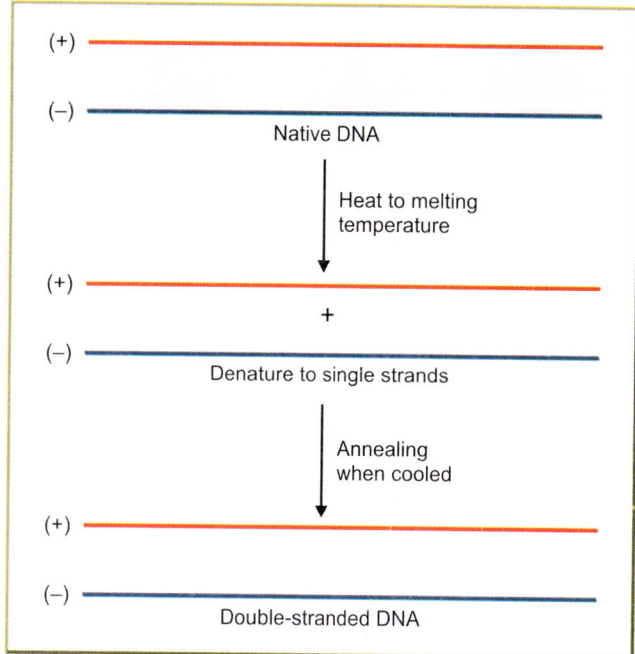

Fig. 7.19: Denaturation and annealing of DNA.

Short stretches of RNA-DNA hybrids occur during the initiation of DNA replication by small fragments of RNA.

Structural Forms of Double Helix DNA

A double helix DNA can assume various distinct structures, depending upon the base sequence as well as composition of the solvent. There are 3 major structural forms of DNA, i.e. the B form originally described by Watson and Crick, the A form and the Z form (Table 7.2).

Table 7.2: Comparison of different types of DNA

Parameter	B-DNA	A-DNA	Z-DNA
Formation	Commonest form	Formed from B-DNA under dehydrating conditions	Transiently formed from B-DNA during transcription; may relieve torsional strain
Overall proportions	Long, thin	Short, broad	Elongated, slim, zig-zag [due to complementary poly-nucleotides with alternating purines and pyrimidines, such as poly d(CG) • poly d(GC) or poly d(AC) • poly d(TG)]
Helix rotation sense	Right-handed	Right-handed	Left-handed
Base pairs per turn	10	11	12
Pitch	3.4 nm	2.8 nm	4.5 nm
Helix axis location	Through base pairs	Major groove	Minor groove
Major groove	Wide, intermediate depth	Very narrow and deep	Flattened out
Minor groove	Narrow, intermediate depth	Very broad and shallow	Very narrow and deep

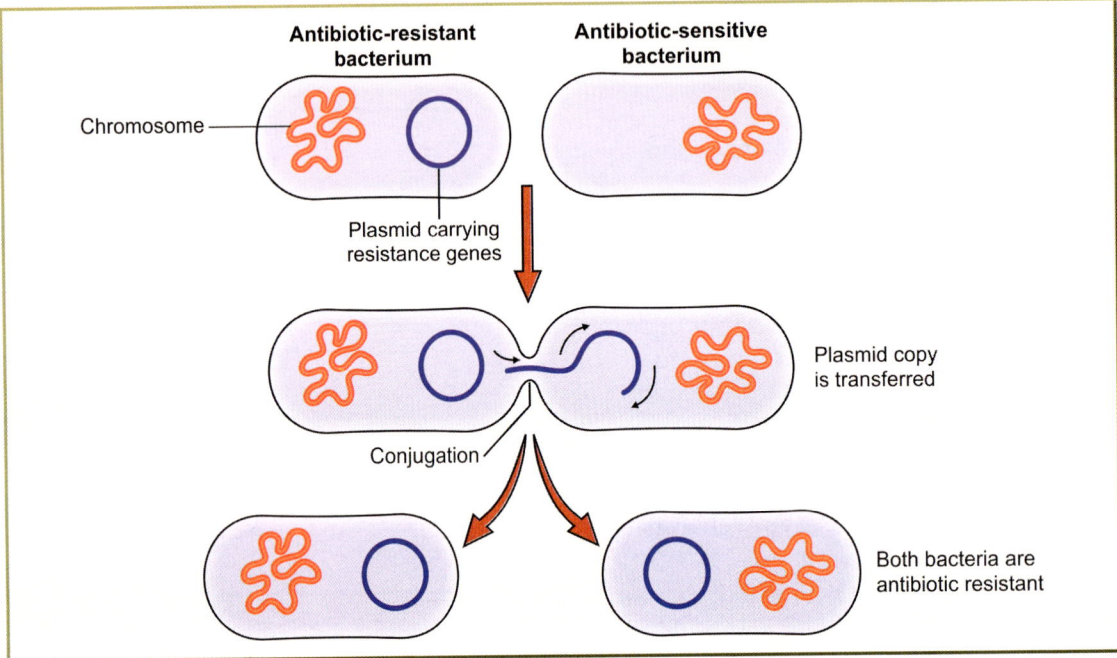

Fig. 7.20: Plasmid-mediated transfer of antibiotic resistance.

Plasmids

Plasmids are small, circular, **extrachromosomal DNA** molecules, of 1–200 Kb, found in most species of bacteria. Plasmid DNA carries genetic information and undergoes replication. Plasmids facilitate the transfer of genetic information from one bacterium to another and are used as vectors in recombinant DNA technology, e.g. *E. coli* plasmid pBR322. The small circular DNA molecule automatically replicates in a bacteria or yeast cell and provides resistance to antibiotics (Fig. 7.20).

Plasmids that contain DNA sequences, called cos sites, required for packaging λ DNA into the phage particle are designated as **cosmids**. Cosmids can accept very large DNA fragments (35–40 Kb).

Mitochondrial DNA

Mitochondria contain circular molecules of DNA (mtDNA) each one of which codes for various polypeptides required for the process of oxidative phosphorylation. The mtDNA is maternally inherited and has a high rate of mutation (please refer to Chapter 2 for details).

Cellular Functions of DNA

DNA controls every aspect of cellular function, i.e.
• It makes copies of itself as a cell divides and thus transfers genetic information from one generation to the next. This process is known as replication.
• DNA also determines the properties of a living cell and regulates biological information by controlling protein synthesis.
• The biological information passes from one class of nucleic acid to another, i.e. from DNA to RNA. This is known as transcription.
• The sequence of bases in RNA is then translated into the sequence of amino acids and forms a protein. This is called translation.
DNA molecule thus serves as a template, both for the transcription of information into RNA as well as for the replication of information into daughter DNA (Fig. 7.21).

RIBONUCLEIC ACIDS (RNAs)

Like DNA, RNA (ribonucleic acids) also have purine and pyrimidine bases, and 3′,5′-phosphodiester linkages but RNAs have several specific structural differences from DNA.

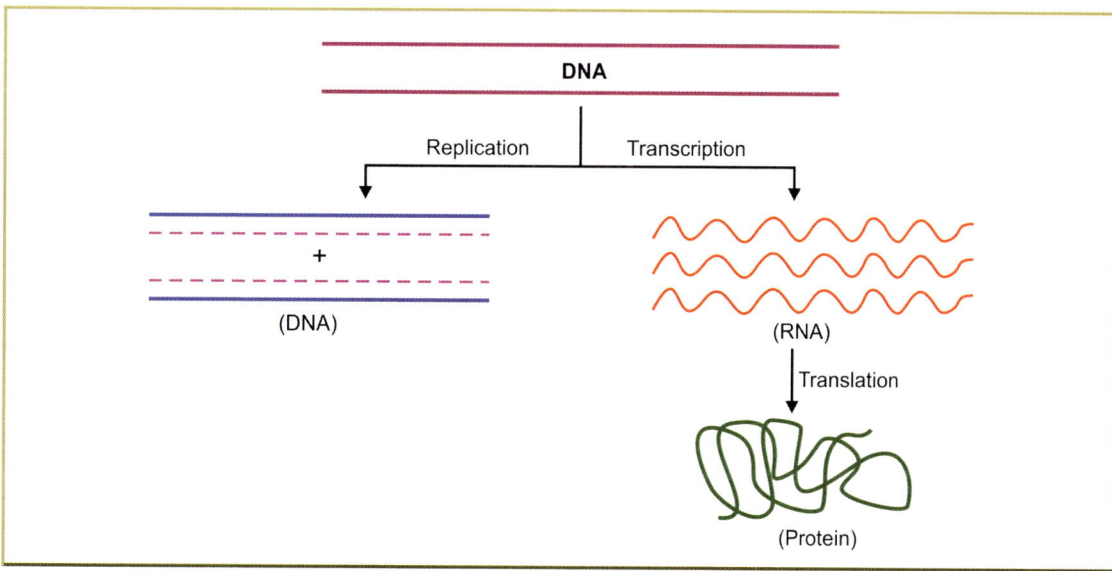

Fig. 7.21: Cellular functions of DNA.

Differences between DNA and RNA

1. As the name suggests, the sugar moiety in RNA is ribose instead of deoxyribose in DNA.
2. RNA does not contain thymine (which is present in DNA); instead, it has uracil.

   RNA is a polymer of ribonucleotides of adenine, guanine, cytosine and uracil.
3. Unlike DNA, RNA is generally a single-stranded molecule. Therefore, in RNA, guanine content may not necessarily be equal to its cytosine content. Similarly, the adenine content need not to be equal to the uracil content.
4. RNA is alkali labile because of the presence of 2'-hydroxyl groups.

Types of RNA

Three main classes of RNA, i.e. messenger RNA, ribosomal RNA and transfer RNA are found in all eukaryotic as well as prokaryotic cells. Although all three types of RNA are involved in protein bio-synthesis, they differ from each other with respect to their size, composition, location within the cell, and functions.

Messenger RNA

Messenger RNAs (mRNA) are most heterogeneous, highly elongated and short-lived molecules. These are synthesized within the nucleus as a result of the transcription of a DNA molecule. Their features include:

- The mRNA transcript has $5' \rightarrow 3'$ polarity which is complementary to the coding strand of its gene (DNA molecule) but there occurs a difference in the pyrimidine base, as mRNA contains uracil in place of thymine present in the DNA strand (Fig. 7.22).
- The mRNA conveys message (information) from the gene to the protein synthesizing machinery. This information is present in the mRNA molecule in the form of codons (the sequence of nucleotides as triplets). Each mRNA serves as a template on which specific sequence of amino acids is polymerized to form a specific protein, the ultimate product of a gene.
- The mRNA are generally stable in eukaryotes but quite unstable in prokaryotes.
- In mammalian cells, the primary transcription product of DNA is a larger molecule called hetero-geneous nuclear RNA (**hnRNA**). The hnRNA molecules undergo post-transcriptional changes and form mRNA which are released into the cytoplasm where they serve as templates for protein biosynthesis.

Transfer RNA

Transfer RNAs (tRNA) are much smaller in size, and consist of nearly 75 to 90 ribonucleotides.

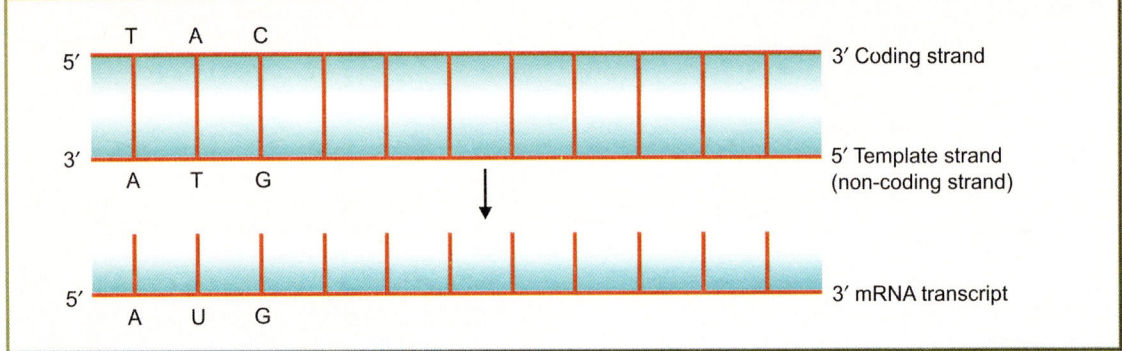

Fig. 7.22: mRNA transcript from a DNA molecule.

tRNA molecules comprise about 15% of the total cellular RNA. tRNA is also known as soluble RNA (sRNA) because it is found in the soluble fraction of the cell.

There are about 40 different tRNA, each one of which fulfills the role of an adaptor molecule and has a sequence called anticodon. Thus, each tRNA, bearing an amino acid, has a unique property of locating itself at the correct codon for translation of information (present in the sequence of nucleotides of mRNA) into specific amino acids in the protein chain.

Specific tRNA although differ from each other in their nucleotide sequence, as a class they have many common features:

• The nucleotide sequence (the primary structure) allows extensive folding and intra-molecular base-pairing to form a secondary structure, giving the clover-leaf like appearance (Fig. 7.23).

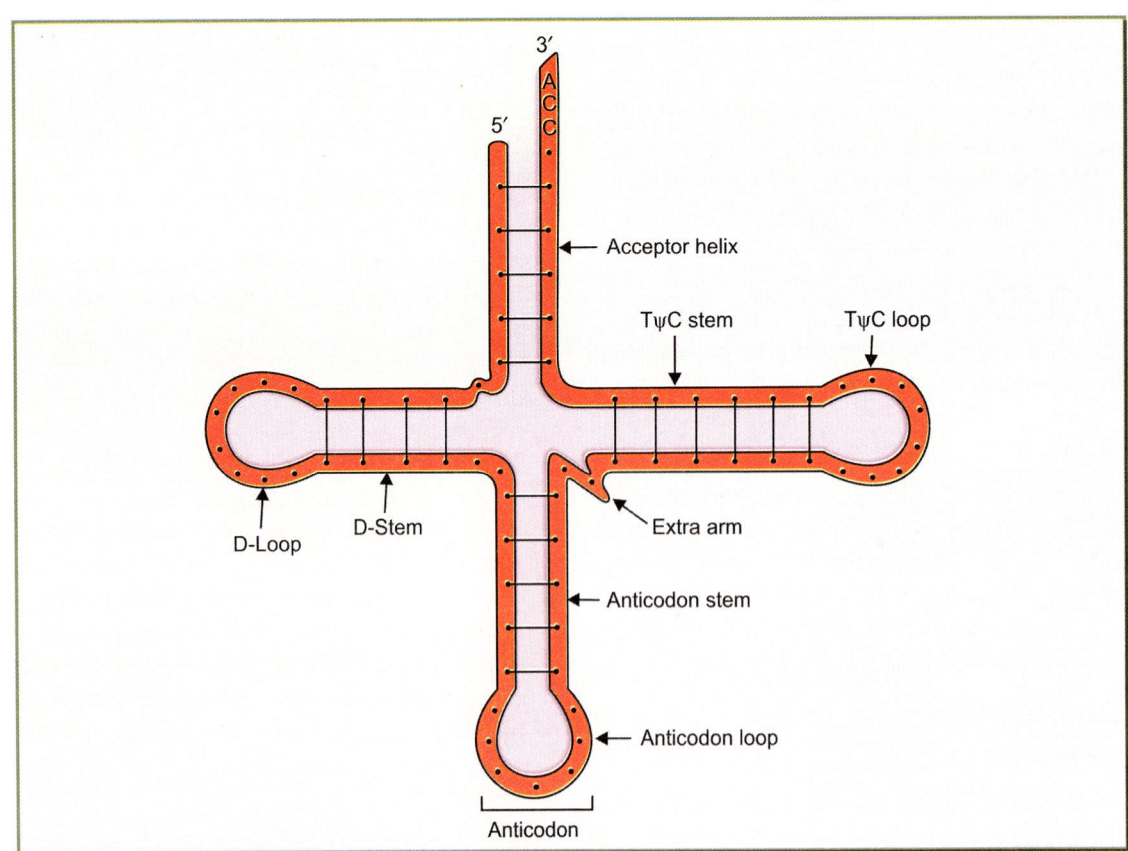

Fig. 7.23: Clover-leaf model of tRNA.

- All tRNAs, in addition to the 4 usual bases (A, G, C and U), have several unusual (modified) bases, e.g. 7-methylguanine, thymine, dihydrouracil, pseudouracil, hypoxanthine, etc.
- All tRNA molecules have 4 main arms, i.e. the amino acid acceptor arm, the anticodon arm, DHU arm and TΨC arm. In addition, there is also an extra arm as a small loop.

Amino acid acceptor arm: The amino acid acceptor arm has a 7 base-paired stem which terminates in CCA (5′ → 3′ sequence) whose A (the adenosyl moiety) accepts an amino acid. The carboxyl group of the amino acid forms an ester linkage with 3′-hydroxyl group of the adenosyl moiety.

Anticodon arm: The anticodon arm has 5 base pairs and a loop which has a triplet nucleotide sequence (the anticodon), complementary to the codon. This anticodon is responsible for the specificity of a tRNA molecule.

The other two arms have unusual bases and are named accordingly as the DHU arm and the TΨC arm.

DHU arm: The DHU arm has dihydrouracil (DHU) in its loop and 3 or 4 base-paired stem.

TΨC arm: The TΨC arm has a sequence of thymine (T), pseudouracil (Ψ) and cytosine (C) in the loop, and a stem having 5 base pairs.

Extra arm: An extra arm may have 3–5 base pairs.

RIBOSOMAL RNA

Ribosomal RNAs (rRNA) are present in the ribosomes, in association with a number of polypeptides. Ribosomes are found in the cytoplasm and contain nearly 80% of the total cellular RNA. Ribosomes combine to form polyribosomes which are the active units in protein biosynthesis.

Both mRNA and tRNA interact on ribosomes to translate the information transcribed from the gene into the specific protein molecule. Mammalian ribosomes are very complex with a sedimentation velocity of 80S. Each ribosome has 2 subunits—a larger subunit (60S) and a smaller subunit (40S). The larger subunit contains 3 different rRNAs, i.e. 5S, 5.8S and 28S along with more than 50 specific polypeptides. The smaller subunit has an 18S rRNA and nearly 30 polypeptides (Fig. 7.24).

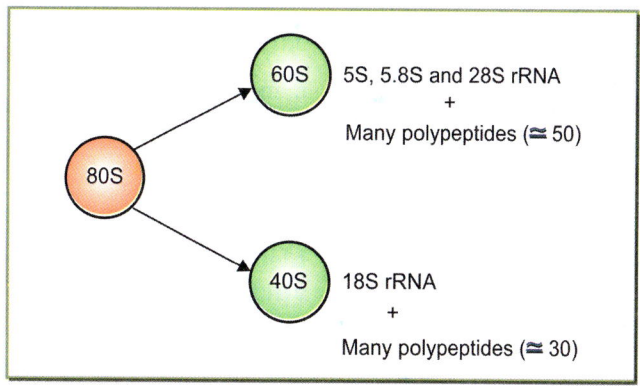

Fig. 7.24: Mammalian ribosomes.

SOME IMPORTANT QUESTIONS

1. Describe various special features of the Watson-Crick model of DNA.

2. What are various type of RNAs? Describe their functions.

3. Explain:
   i. Structure and function of tRNA
   ii. Differences between DNA and RNA
   iii. Various nitrogenous bases found in nucleic acids
   iv. Unusual nitrogenous bases

7

4. Write notes on:

i. Ribosomes
ii. B-DNA
iii. A-DNA
iv. Z-DNA
v. Unusual nitrogenous bases
vi. Nucleosides

vii. Nucleotides
viii. Plasmid
ix. Mitochondrial DNA
x. hnRNA
xi. Importance of adenosine
xii. Purine/pyrimidine analogs

MULTIPLE CHOICE QUESTIONS

1. At physiological pH, nucleic acids are:
   A. Negatively charged
   B. Positively charged
   C. Uncharged
   D. Uncharged zwitterions

2. The following are vasodilators *except*:
   A. Prostacyclin
   B. Adenosine
   C. Nitric oxide
   D. Endothelin

3. In the Watson-Crick DNA model, the number of H-bond(s) between G and C is/are:
   A. 1   B. 2
   C. 3   D. 4

4. During DNA denaturation, the following bond(s) is/are broken:
   A. Phosphodiester   B. Hydrogen
   C. Glycosidic   D. All of the above

5. The Watson-Crick model originally described the following:
   A. Z-DNA
   B. B-DNA
   C. A-DNA
   D. Denatured DNA

6. The biologically commonest form of DNA is:
   A. B-DNA
   B. A-DNA
   C. Z-DNA
   D. None of the above

7. The diameter of Watson-Crick B-DNA double helix is:
   A. 0.2 nm   B. 2.0 nm
   C. 0.34 nm   D. 3.4 nm

8. hnRNA is found in the:
   A. Nucleus
   B. Cytoplasm
   C. Ribosomes
   D. Smooth endoplasmic reticulum

9. The specificity of a tRNA molecule lies in the:
   A. Amino acid acceptor arm
   B. Anticodon arm
   C. TψC arm
   D. DHU arm

10. 80% of total cellular RNA is present in the:
    A. Cytosol
    B. Ribosomes
    C. Nucleoplasm
    D. Nucleolus

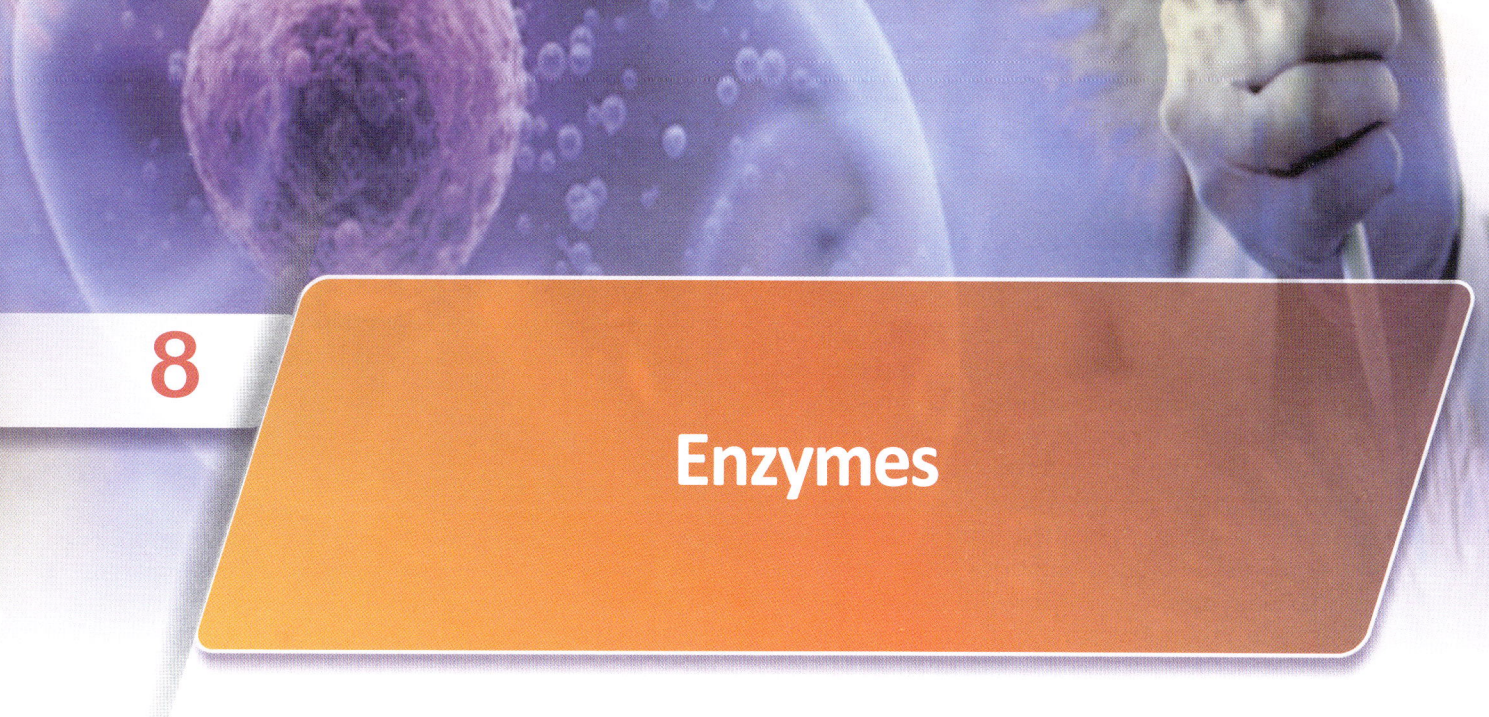

Enzymes

Enzymes are biological catalysts, nondialyzable, colloidal, organic macromolecules which are produced in the living organisms and catalyze biochemical reactions without being utilized in the process. They are so-called since they were discovered as the substances found in yeast (Greek *en* = in, and zyme = yeast) and were capable of catalyzing the reactions of fermentation. Most of them are proteins (except ribozymes), thermolabile, and accelerate the rate at which a reaction proceeds towards equilibrium, by lowering the free energy barrier that separates the substrates (reactants) from the products.

Differences between an Enzyme and a Chemical Catalyst

An enzyme differs from a chemical catalyst in several ways:
1. An enzyme catalyzed reaction has higher reaction rate than that of the corresponding chemically catalyzed reaction.
2. An enzymatic reaction occurs under relatively milder conditions, such as at temperature near 37°C, pH near neutrality and at atmospheric pressure.
3. Enzymes have a greater degree of specificity for their substrates as well as products.
4. Several enzyme catalyzed reactions are under regulatory control.

CHEMICAL NATURE OF AN ENZYME

Most of the enzymes are protein in nature with large molecular weight though certain RNAs, called ribozymes, also show highly substrate specific catalytic activity.

MULTIMERIC PROTEINS

Most of the enzymes though are simple proteins having a single polypeptide chain, there are several enzymes which have more than one polypeptide chain. These are called as multimeric proteins which may be found as either oligomeric enzymes or as multienzyme complexes.

Oligomeric Enzymes

Enzymes with two or more subunits are called oligomeric enzymes, e.g. phosphorylase, hexokinase, lactate dehydrogenase, etc. These occur as tetramers, i.e. each enzyme has four protein subunits. Others like phosphofructokinase, fructose-1,6-bisphosphatase and creatine phosphokinase are dimers, i.e. each has two protein subunits.

Multienzyme Complexes

Several enzymes occur in the form of a multienzyme complex, i.e. they have more than one enzyme activities. Such a complex catalyzes the conversion of a substrate, in a sequential series of reactions, to different products, e.g. pyruvate dehydrogenase complex, α-ketoglutarate dehydrogenase complex, etc. Each of these complexes contains three enzymes. Fatty acid synthase is a multienzyme complex with six different enzyme activities.

INTRACELLULAR LOCALIZATION

Most of the enzymes are produced by the cells of a particular tissue and function within the cell. Such enzymes are called **intracellular enzymes**, e.g. the enzymes of glycolysis, TCA cycle and fatty acid synthesis. On the other hand, there are certain enzymes which are produced by the cells of a particular tissue and liberated from there for use in the other tissues. Such enzymes are called **extra-cellular enzymes**, e.g. various proteolytic enzymes like trypsin, chymotrypsin, etc. These are secreted by the pancreas for their action in the small intestine.

Zymogens

Most of the intracellular enzymes are secreted in their active forms called **'zymases'**. Proteolytic enzymes, on the other hand, are usually synthesized as somewhat larger inactive precursors, known as **'zymogens'** (Chemistry to Clinics 8.1). These molecules are stored in the storage vesicles known as zymogen granules, secreted as zymogens and undergo modifications in structure, after coming in contact with certain activating agents (Table 8.1).

An activating agent can be H^+, another enzyme or an active form of the zymogen itself. For example, gastric juice contains pepsin which is secreted as pepsinogen (a zymogen). Pepsinogen is transformed to its active form pepsin by the H^+ of the gastric juice.

Once formed, pepsin itself also acts on pepsinogen and catalyzes its own conversion into pepsin. This process is called **autocatalysis** (Fig. 8.1).

NOMENCLATURE AND CLASSIFICATION OF ENZYMES

Nomenclature of Enzymes

Enzymes are commonly named by putting the suffix '-ase' to the name of the substrate or with the catalytic action of the enzyme, e.g. a lipase is an enzyme which catalyzes the hydrolysis of a lipid, a fatty acid synthase is an enzyme that catalyzes the synthesis of a fatty acid. These names of the enzymes are called as the trivial names for which no systematic rules are followed.

Classification of Enzymes

For the rational naming of each enzyme, International Union of Biochemistry and Molecular Biology (IUBMB) adopted a scheme and suggested functional classification of enzymes. As per IUBMB, enzymes are named with the suffix '-ase' with the name of the substrate and/or the type of the reaction it catalyzes. Each enzyme is assigned a name and a systematic four digit enzyme code, commonly known as **Enzyme Commission number** (EC number):

Chemistry to Clinics 8.1: Acute Pancreatitis

The inactivity of zymogens is crucial because if these enzymes were synthesized in their active forms within the cell, this situation would be potentially self-destructing. Acute pancreatitis, a painful and sometimes fatal condition is characterized by the premature activation of the digestive enzymes synthesized by this organ. The enzymes damage the pancreas and spill over into the circulation. Pancreatic amylase and lipase are significantly raised in the serum of these patients and help to establish the diagnosis.

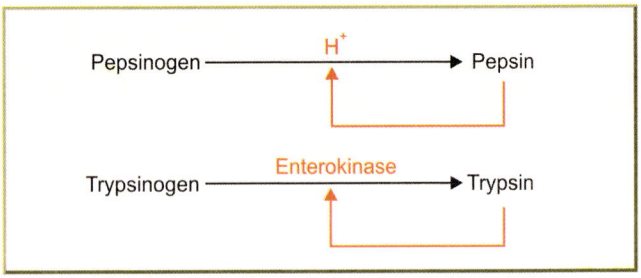

Fig. 8.1: Activation of zymogens.

Table 8.1: Gastric and pancreatic proenzymes/zymogens

Proenzyme/zymogen	Site of synthesis	Activator	Active enzyme
Pepsinogen	Chief cells of stomach	H^+, pepsin	Pepsin
Trypsinogen	Pancreatic acinar cells	Trypsin	Trypsin
Chymotrypsinogen	Pancreatic acinar cells	Trypsin	π- or α-chymotrypsin
Procarboxypeptidase A	Pancreatic acinar cells	Trypsin	Carboxypeptidase A
Procarboxypeptidase B	Pancreatic acinar cells	Trypsin	Carboxypeptidase B
Proelastase	Pancreatic acinar cells	Trypsin	Elastase

- Its first digit denotes the main class which is according to the general type of a chemical reaction that an enzyme catalyzes.
- The second digit characterizes the subclass, based on the nature of a chemical group removed or transferred, or any bond split or formed.
- The third digit indicates the sub-subclass and is used for more detailed subdivision of the subclass.
- The last digit of the EC number indicates an arbitrarily assigned serial number to each enzyme in a sub-subclass.
- For example, 1.1.1.1 is the enzyme code for alcohol dehydrogenase that catalyzes the oxidation of an alcohol to yield an aldehyde. It removes $2e^-$ and $2H^+$, and in turn reduces NAD^+. It is the first enzyme of the sub-subclass 1 (NAD^+ utilizing), of the subclass 1 (dehydrogenases) and belongs to class 1 (oxidoreductase).

Enzymes are thus classified according to the nature of a chemical reaction they catalyze. Accordingly, there are six major classes of enzymatic reactions (Table 8.2).

1. **Oxidoreductases**: These are enzymes involved in the oxidation and reduction of their substrates, i.e. they catalyze addition of oxygen or removal of hydrogen or electrons. Accordingly, several sub-classes include dehydrogenases, oxidases, oxygenases, etc. Examples of oxidoreductases are alcohol dehydrogenase, xanthine oxidase, glutathione reductase, etc.

2. **Transferases**: These are enzymes which catalyze the transfer of a functional group from one substrate (donor) to another (acceptor). On the basis of the transferring group, transferases are further subclassified as aminotransferases, phosphotransferases, etc. Glutamate oxaloacetate transaminase, hexokinase, glucose-1-phosphate uridyltransferase are some of the examples of the class transferase.

3. **Hydrolases**: These enzymes bring about cleavage of a substrate by the addition of a molecule of water, termed as hydrolysis. According to the nature of the group or the bond being hydrolyzed, hydrolases are subclassified as peptidases, glycosidases, etc.

Table 8.2: Enzyme classification according to the type of reaction catalyzed

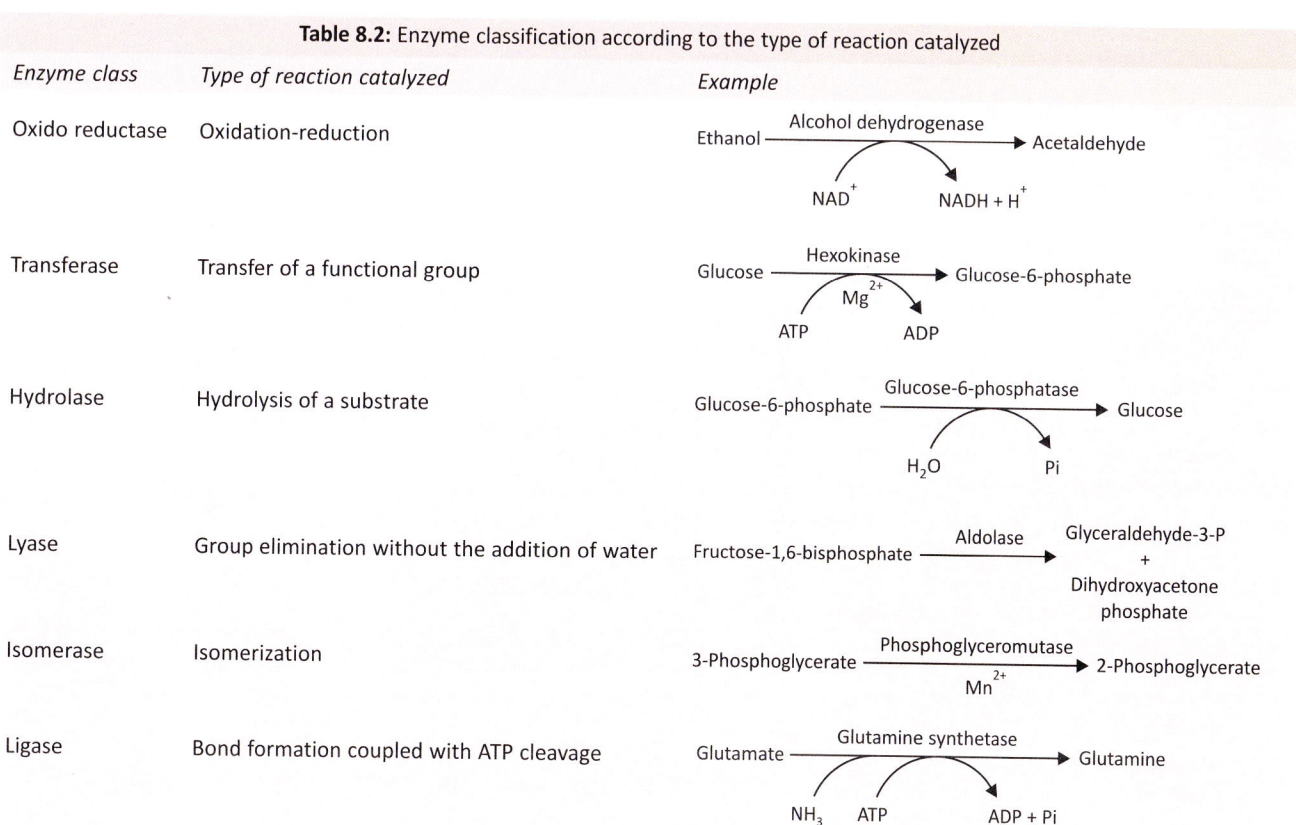

Enzyme class	Type of reaction catalyzed	Example
Oxido reductase	Oxidation-reduction	Ethanol $\xrightarrow{\text{Alcohol dehydrogenase}}$ Acetaldehyde (NAD^+ → $NADH + H^+$)
Transferase	Transfer of a functional group	Glucose $\xrightarrow{\text{Hexokinase}}$ Glucose-6-phosphate (Mg^{2+}, ATP → ADP)
Hydrolase	Hydrolysis of a substrate	Glucose-6-phosphate $\xrightarrow{\text{Glucose-6-phosphatase}}$ Glucose (H_2O → Pi)
Lyase	Group elimination without the addition of water	Fructose-1,6-bisphosphate $\xrightarrow{\text{Aldolase}}$ Glyceraldehyde-3-P + Dihydroxyacetone phosphate
Isomerase	Isomerization	3-Phosphoglycerate $\xrightarrow{\text{Phosphoglyceromutase}}$ 2-Phosphoglycerate (Mn^{2+})
Ligase	Bond formation coupled with ATP cleavage	Glutamate $\xrightarrow{\text{Glutamine synthetase}}$ Glutamine (NH_3, ATP → ADP + Pi)

Examples include glucose-6-phosphatase, amylase, pepsin, etc.

4. *Lyases*: These enzymes catalyze the removal of a small molecule such as water, ammonia or CO_2, from a large substrate, i.e. they bring about the cleavage without the addition of water. These enzymes are further subclassified on the basis of the linkage they attack. Examples include aldolase, argininosuccinase, histidase, etc.

5. *Isomerases*: These are involved in the isomerization of a substrate and catalyze the interconversion of one isomeric form to the other. Racemases, epimerases and mutases are some of the subclasses of this class. Examples of isomerases include phosphohexose isomerase, phosphoglucomutase, alanine racemase, etc.

6. *Ligases*: These are also called as synthetases (ligate means to bind), as they are involved in the synthesis of a molecule, by joining two different compounds together, at the expense of a high energy phosphate bond of ATP. Various subclasses include the ligases forming a C–C, C–N or C–S bond. Examples of ligases are glutamine synthetase, glutathione synthetase, etc.

COFACTORS AND COENZYMES

Cofactors

Some of the enzymes require the presence of certain small nonprotein factors, such as a metal ion or an organic molecule for their activity. The inorganic ions, such as Mg^{2+}, Zn^{2+} or Cl^- required for the catalytic activity of an enzyme are called **'inorganic cofactors'**. Sometimes, a metal ion is loosely associated with the enzyme and forms a metal-enzyme complex. Such enzymes are called **metal-activated enzymes** (Table 8.3). On the other hand, a metal ion may form an integral part of the enzyme. Such enzymes are called **metalloenzymes**. Transition metal ions, such as Fe, Cu, Zn or Mn may form an integral part of several metalloenzymes (Table 8.4).

Table 8.3: Metal-activated enzymes

Metal-activated enzymes	Cofactor
Lipase, ATPase, succinate dehydrogenase	Ca^{2+}
Phosphorylase, enolase, DNA polymerase	Mg^{2+}
Arginase, phosphoglucomutase, cholinesterase	Mn^{2+}
Salivary amylase	Cl^-
Pyruvate kinase	K^+

Table 8.4: Metalloenzymes

Metalloenzymes	Cofactor
Peroxidases, catalase	Fe
Cytochrome oxidase, tyrosinase	Cu
Xanthine oxidase	Mo
Carbonic anhydrase	Zn
Glutathione peroxidase	Se

Coenzymes

'Organic cofactors' which are dialyzable, thermostable and of low molecular weight are called coenzymes. Some of them are only transiently associated with the enzyme and function as cosubstrates. Others, known as **prosthetic groups**, are permanently associated with their proteins, often by covalent bonds. For example, heme, the prosthetic group of cytochromes. It is tightly bound to the protein through extensive hydrophobic and hydrogen bonding interactions, together with the covalent bonds.

The catalytically active form of an enzyme is the **enzyme cofactor complex**, called as the **holoenzyme**. The inactive enzyme resulting from the removal of a cofactor from the holoenzyme is referred as **apoenzyme** while the nonprotein component of the holoenzyme is called as **coenzyme**.

$$\text{Holoenzyme} = \text{Apoenzyme} + \text{Coenzyme}$$
$$\text{(active)} \qquad \text{(inactive)}$$

Vitamins as coenzymes: Coenzymes are the derivatives of the B complex group of vitamins (see Chapter 28 for details). These are chemically changed by the enzymatic reaction in which they participate but regenerated to their original state after the completion of the catalytic cycle. For example, NAD^+ is reduced to NADH in alcohol dehydrogenase reaction, but is oxidized back, may be by a different enzyme. Table 8.5 lists various coenzymes, their precursor vitamins, along with the type of reaction in which the coenzyme participates.

ENZYME SPECIFICITY

An enzyme binds to a substrate and forms an **enzyme-substrate complex** which is subsequently transformed into a product and releases the enzyme.

$$E + S \rightarrow ES \rightarrow P + E$$

Enzymes are highly specific catalysts—both with regard to their substrates as well as to the type of

Table 8.5: Coenzymes, their precursor vitamins and corresponding reactions

Coenzyme	Parent vitamin	Enzyme	Reaction
TPP	Thiamin	Pyruvate dehydrogenase complex, α-ketoglutarate dehydrogenase complex	Pyruvate ⟶ Acetyl CoA α-Ketoglutarate ⟶ Succinyl CoA
FMN	Riboflavin	L-Amino acid oxidase	L-Amino acids ⟶ α-Keto acids
FAD	Riboflavin	D-Amino acid oxidase	D-Amino acids ⟶ α-Keto acids
		Succinate dehydrogenase	Succinate ⟶ Fumarate
NAD⁺	Niacin	Lactate dehydrogenase	Lactate ⟶ Pyruvate
NADP⁺	Niacin	Glucose-6-P-dehydrogenase	Glucose-6-Phosphate ⟶ 6-P-Gluconolactone
PLP	Pyridoxine	Glutamate pyruvate transaminase	Alanine + α-Ketoglutarate ⟶ Pyruvate + Glutamate
CoA	Panthothenic acid	Pyruvate dehydrogenase complex, Fatty acyl CoA synthetase	Pyruvate ⟶ Acetyl CoA Fatty acid ⟶ Fatty acyl CoA
Carboxybiocytin	Biotin	Acetyl CoA carboxylase	Acetyl CoA ⟶ Malonyl CoA
		Pyruvate carboxylase	Pyruvate ⟶ Oxaloacetate
Tetrahydrofolic acid	Folic acid	Serine hydroxymethyl transferase	Glycine ⟶ Serine
Cobamides	B₁₂	Methyl malonyl CoA isomerase	Methyl malonyl CoA ⟶ Succinyl CoA

reaction. Some enzymes show **absolute specificity for substrate**, e.g. L-amino acid oxidase. The enzyme binds only to L-amino acids and not to D-amino acids (Fig. 8.2). Others have **broader specificity**. Such an enzyme can accept several analogs of the specific substrate. For example, hexokinase can catalyze phosphorylation of glucose, fructose or mannose (Fig. 8.3). Hexokinase thus has a broader specificity and is **reaction specific**. On the other hand, glucokinase is specific for its substrate, i.e. glucose only.

The specificity of an enzyme is located in a particular region on the enzyme surface that is designated as the active site/center.

Active Site/Center

The specificity of an enzyme is located in a particular region called the active site/center whose salient features are:

1. A small cleft in the tertiary structure (Fig. 8.4) of an enzyme molecule made up of:
   (i) **Substrate binding site**: A substrate binds to the enzyme through various noncovalent forces, such as van der Waals forces, electrostatic forces, hydrogen bonds and hydrophobic interactions.
   (ii) **Catalytic site**
      • Lined by specific amino acids called catalytic residues, most commonly serine (others

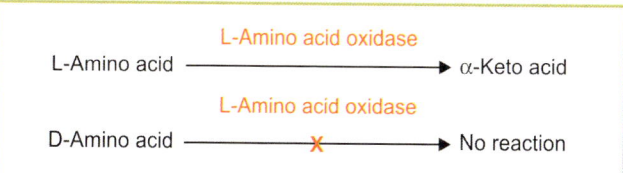

Fig. 8.2: Absolute specificity of an enzyme.

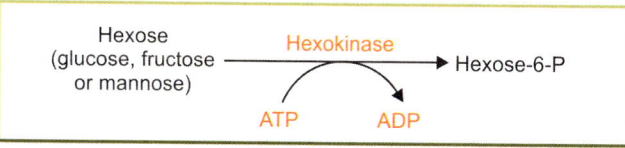

Fig. 8.3: Reaction specificity of an enzyme.

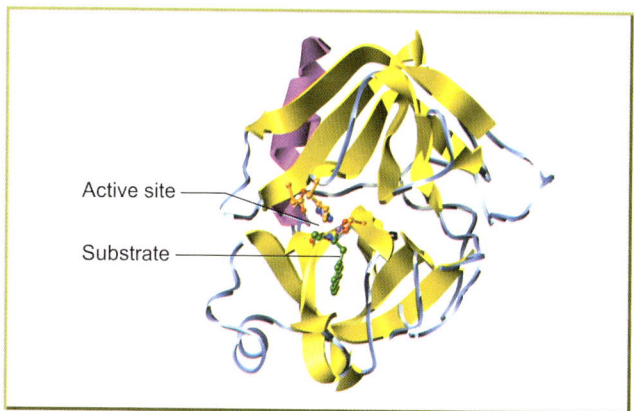

Fig. 8.4: Active site/center of an enzyme is a small cleft in the tertiary structure

include cysteine, aspartate, histidine, tyrosine, arginine, lysine, etc.).

- Catalytic residues are spatially close but actually distant from each other in the primary structure.
- Cofactors are a part of the catalytic site.
- Specific nucleotides are present in ribozymes.

2. Binding of substrate with the active site is explained by **'lock-and-key' model** (assumes a rigid character of active site) or **'induced-fit' model** (assumes a flexible character of active site).

3. May be inactivated by alterations in temperature and pH.

4. May be blocked by various compounds resembling the substrate (reversible competitive enzyme inhibition) or by unrelated substances (irreversible enzyme poisoning).

5. Identification and analysis of active site is crucial in the process of drug discovery (Chemistry to Clinics 8.2).

6. A software-based technology called comparison of protein active site structures (CPASS) helps to compare active sites and hence in new drug designing.

Chemistry to Clinics 8.2: HIV Protease Inhibitors
Proteases play an important role in the pathogenesis of diseases caused by retroviruses such as HIV. The 3-dimensional characterization of HIV protease and identification of its active site helped to develop a popular antiretroviral drug called ritonavir. It is a tetrapeptide resembling the protein that is the substrate of HIV protease. Thus, it inhibits protease through competitive inhibition.

Interaction of the Enzyme with the Substrate: Formation of the Enzyme-Substrate Complex

Lock-and-Key Model

- The first proposal, by Emil Fischer, to explain the interaction of substrate with the active site of an enzyme and the formation of enzyme-substrate complex.
- Also called the **rigid** template model.
- Based on the complementarity between the enzyme and its substrate. In other words, a pocket or cleft on the surface of the enzyme contains a 'negative impression' of the molecular features of the substrate, thus allowing specificity of the enzyme for a particular substrate (Fig. 8.5).

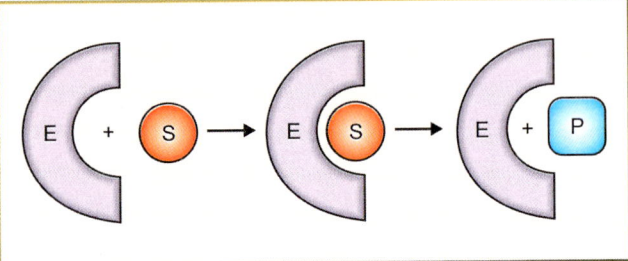

Fig. 8.5: Lock-and-key theory.

- The amino acid residues that form the binding site are so arranged that they interact specifically with the substrate. During the process of formation of an enzyme-substrate complex, the substrate attaches itself onto the specific amino acid residues in the active site on the enzyme molecule like a key fits into its lock.

- The model implies rigidity of the enzyme's active site; explains enzyme specificity but fails to explain alteration in the structure of active site in the presence of allosteric modulators.

Induced-Fit Model

- A **flexible** model, proposed by Koshland, to explain the interaction of substrate with the active site of an enzyme and the formation of enzyme-substrate complex.

- The substrate binding site of enzyme undergoes some conformational change on its binding with the substrate. That is to say, during its binding with the enzyme, a substrate induces conformational changes in the enzyme's active site, so as to attain a desired shape, in such a way that the substrate can fit the active site conveniently (Fig. 8.6).

- The model implies flexibility of the enzyme's active site; explains enzyme specificity plus alteration in

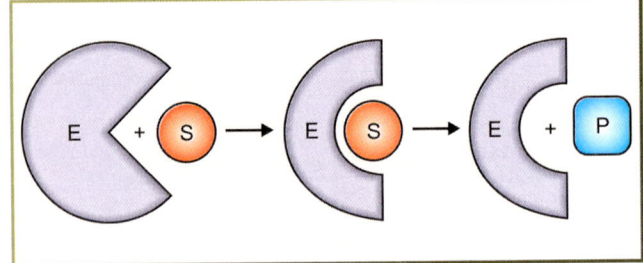

Fig. 8.6: Induced-fit theory.

the structure of active site in the presence of allosteric modulators.

- Explains competitive inhibition and enzyme inactivation.

MULTISUBSTRATE REACTIONS

If an enzyme utilizes more than one substrate or acts upon a substrate and a coenzyme together to generate one or more products, such a reaction is called as a multisubstrate reaction which may proceed by any of the following two mechanisms, i.e. the ping-pong mechanism or the sequential mechanism.

Ping-Pong Mechanism

A substrate (S1) reacts with an enzyme (E) forming an enzyme-substrate complex (ES1) to produce a product (P1). The release of product (P1) in turn results in some modification in the enzyme structure, e.g. E to

E1. The second substrate (S2) thereafter binds to the modified enzyme (E1) and is converted to the second product (P2). After the release of P2, the enzyme (E1) is regenerated in its original form (E) (Fig. 8.7).

For example, in a transaminase catalyzed reaction, the enzyme-bound pyridoxal phosphate accepts α-amino group from an amino acid and releases the amino acid as α-keto acid. Another α-keto acid then binds to the modified enzyme from where the amino group is transferred on to the α-keto acid resulting in the formation of a new amino acid. With the release of this amino acid, the enzyme is regenerated in its original form (Fig. 8.8).

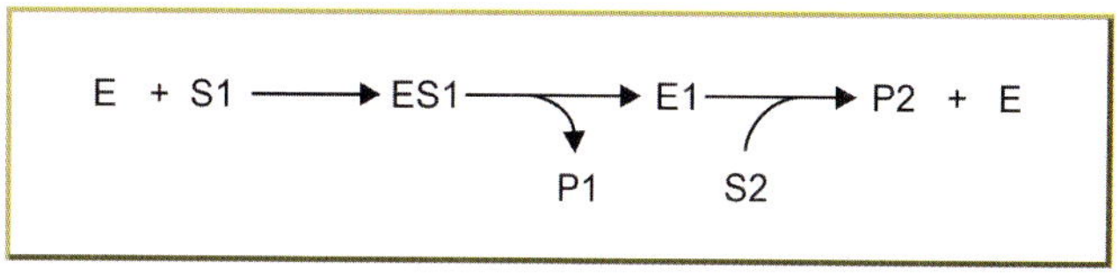

E + S1 ⟶ ES1 ⟶ E1 ⟶ P2 + E

P1   S2

Fig. 8.7: Ping-pong mechanism of enzyme catalyzed reaction.

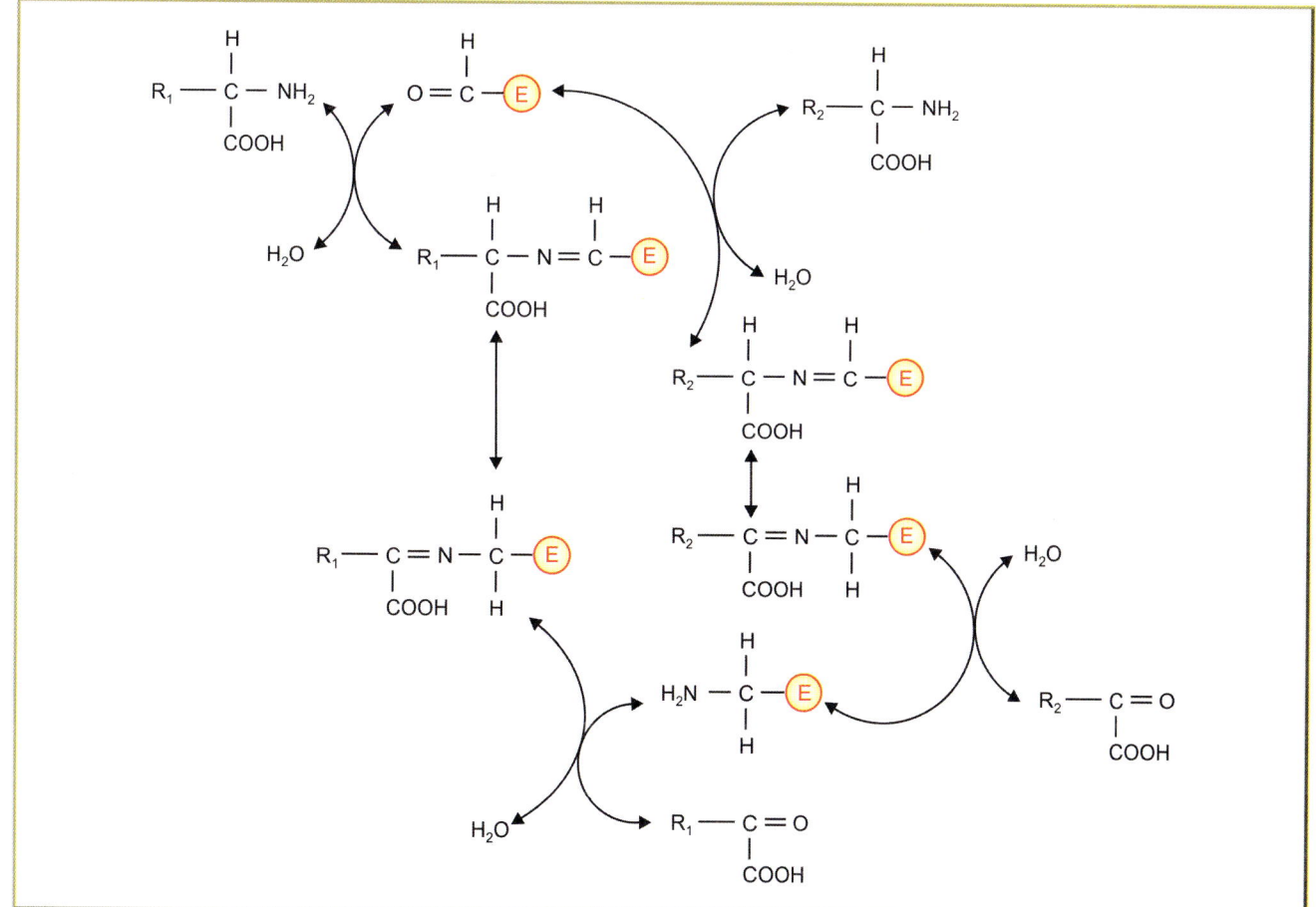

Fig. 8.8: Enzyme catalyzed reaction: Ping-pong mechanism of transamination.

8

Sequential Mechanism

In sequential mechanism, the reaction is bimolecular, i.e. if there are two substrates (S1 and S2) both of them bind with the enzyme before the reaction occurs and the product is released. An example is a dehydrogenase catalyzed reaction where the second substrate is a coenzyme (NAD^+ or FAD). These reactions are also designated as single displacement reactions because the group undergoing transfer is directly passed from the donor (the first substrate) to the acceptor (the second substrate).

MECHANISMS OF ENZYME CATALYSIS

It shown in Fig. 8.9, the reactants and the products are in states of minimum free energy whereas the transition state corresponds to the point of highest free energy. The difference in free energy between the reactants and the transition state is known as the **free energy of activation** ($\Delta G°$). A catalyst such as an enzyme acts by lowering the transition state free energy for the reaction it catalyzes. The enzyme-substrate complex, in the transition state, can break down to products or go back to reactants. Since the overall energy difference between the reactants and

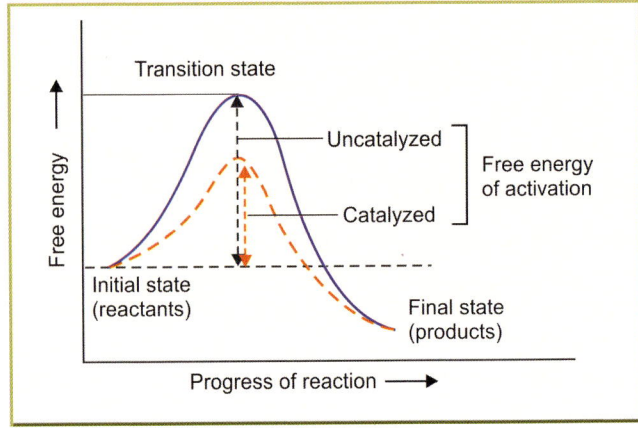

Fig. 8.9: Energy state for a catalyzed versus a noncatalyzed reaction.

the products is the same, the enzyme equally accelerates the forward and the backward reaction.

Enzymatic catalysis may take place by several processes (Table 8.6).

FACTORS AFFECTING ENZYME ACTIVITY

Enzymes exhibit maximum activity under optimal conditions. The activity of an enzyme is markedly affected by several factors as discussed below.

Table 8.6: Mechanisms of enzyme catalysis

Mechanism	Example
Acid–Base Catalysis: The catalytic activity of an enzyme may be sensitive to pH, since pH can influence the state of protonation of the side chain at the active site. At physiological pH, the protonated form of histidine is the most important general acid while its conjugate base is an important general base. Besides, the imidazole group of histidine, the −SH group of cysteine, the −OH group of tyrosine, and the ε-amino group of lysine can also act as acids. The general bases are carboxylic acid anions and the conjugate bases of the general acids.	Ribonuclease A (RNase A, a digestive enzyme secreted by the pancreas into the small intestine) hydrolyzes RNA to its component nucleotides with the formation of 2′,3′-cyclic nucleotides as the intermediates. The enzyme has two His residues, His 12 and His 119, which act in a concerted manner as a general base and general acid, respectively.
Covalent Catalysis: It accelerates the reaction rate through the transient formation of a catalyst-substrate covalent bond, by the reaction of a nucleophilic group (negatively charged) on the catalyst with an electrophilic group (positively charged) on the substrate. Hence, this form of catalysis is also called nucleophilic catalysis.	Functional groups in proteins, such as the ε-amino group of Lys, the imidazole group of His, the −SH group of Cys, the −COOH group of Asp and the −OH group of Ser, which have high polarity, are good covalent catalysts. In addition, several coenzymes, such as TPP and pyridoxal phosphate, also function in association with their apoenzymes, as covalent catalysts. Serine proteases, such as trypsin, chymotrypsin and thrombin are some other examples.
Metal Ion Catalysis: Metalloenzymes require the presence of a metal ion (Fe^{2+}, Fe^{3+}, Cu^{2+}, Zn^{2+} etc.) for their catalytic activity. Metal ions facilitate substrate binding and thus catalysis, by forming several kinds of bridge complexes of the enzyme, the metal and the substrate.	Carbonic anhydrase contains Zn^{2+} which is implicated in the catalytic mechanism of the enzyme.
Transition State Stabilization: In an enzyme catalyzed reaction, the point of highest free energy is called as the transition state of the system. An enzyme binds in the transition state of the reaction it catalyzes with greater affinity than either of its substrate or the product.	By taking the enzyme-substrate complex in the transition state as an antigen, antibodies can be synthesized artificially. These antibodies have catalytic activity and are called as abzymes. The potential applications of catalytic antibodies are discussed later.

1. Temperature

Rate of an enzyme-catalyzed reaction increases with the increase in temperature of the reaction mixture, because a rise in temperature increases the energy of activation of the system which in turn increases reaction velocity. But it is possible only up to an **'optimum temperature'** which is defined as the temperature at which enzyme activity is maximum. For most of the enzymes, optimum temperature is near the body temperature, i.e. 37°C. With further rise in the temperature, the enzyme (protein) is denatured and results in a loss of its activity. The relationship of the enzyme activity to a change in temperature is usually represented by a bell-shaped curve, the peak of which denotes optimum temperature (Fig. 8.10).

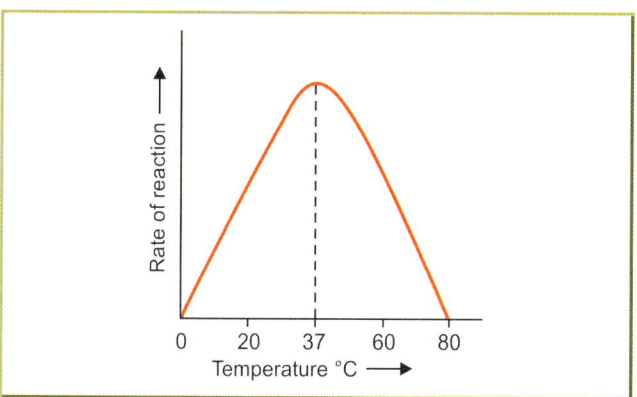

Fig. 8.10: Effect of temperature on enzyme activity.

2. pH

The relationship between enzyme activity and pH of the reaction medium is also represented by a bell-shaped curve which has its peak at the **optimum pH**. This pH is characteristic for each enzyme (Fig. 8.11).

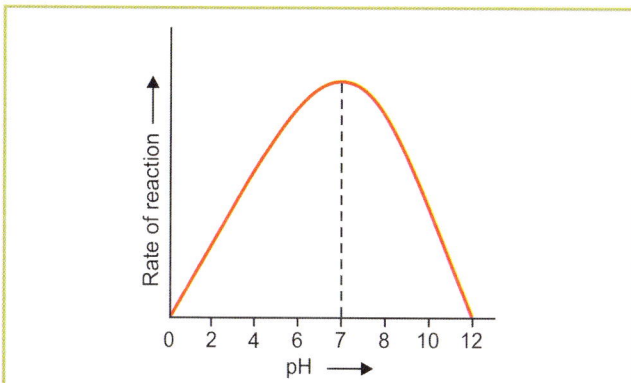

Fig. 8.11: Effect of pH on enzyme activity.

Optimum pH for most of the intracellular enzymes is in the neutral range, i.e. around 7.0. The optimum pH for pepsin, however, is about 2.0 while for the enzymes of the pancreatic juice, optimum pH is nearly 8.0. The optimum pH of an enzyme depends upon the ionization of the enzyme as well as of the substrate. A change in pH affects ionization of the protein molecule thereby decreasing the number of active sites. At an extremely low or high pH, enzyme (protein) gets denatured.

3. Substrate Concentration

For an enzyme catalyzed reaction (with a single substrate and a single product), the reaction rate is directly proportional to substrate concentration. If the concentration of a substrate (S) is increased while all other conditions are kept constant, the measured initial velocity (V_o), i.e. the reaction velocity at zero time, increases as the substrate concentration increases, up to a point where the enzyme is said to be saturated with the substrate. The measured initial velocity reaches a maximal value and is unaffected by a further increase in the substrate concentration. This, however, is true only up to a certain point, i.e. the point at which the enzyme will be working at its maximum velocity (V_{max}). Any further increase in substrate concentration thereafter, does not increase the reaction rate (Fig. 8.12).

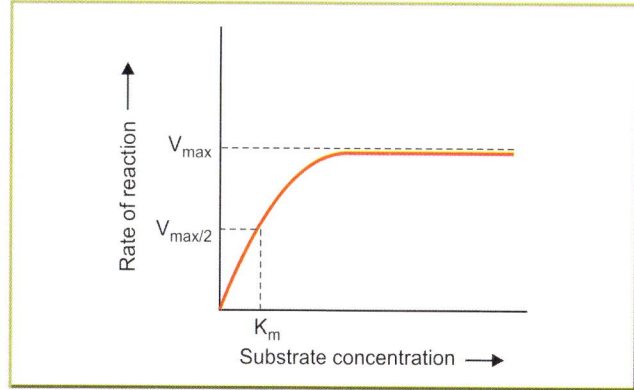

Fig. 8.12: Effect of substrate concentration on enzyme activity.

Reaction Order

- For a simple one-substrate/one-product reaction such as S → P, the reaction velocity is proportional to the substrate concentration, i.e. V = k[S] where k is a constant. This is a **first order reaction**.

- For reactions involving multiple substrates/products such as S1 + S2 → P1 + P2, V = k[S1][S2]. This is an overall **second order reaction** although it is first order with respect to S1 as well as first order with respect to S2.
- If V_{max} (maximum velocity) is independent of substrate concentration, it indicates a saturation effect and the reaction is **zero order**.

Michaelis-Menten Equation

The relationship between substrate concentration and reaction velocity can be derived by Michaelis-Menten equation. Michaelis and Menten proposed that an enzyme (E) forms enzyme-substrate complex (ES), with a single substrate (S). The complex (ES) is broken down, relatively slowly, into free enzyme (E) and the product (P). Accordingly, Michaelis and Menten derived an equation called **Michaelis-Menten equation** (Fig. 8.13), where V_o is the initial reaction velocity, V_{max} is the maximum velocity of a reaction, [S] is concentration of the substrate and K_m is a constant, called **Michaelis constant**.

Michaelis constant (K_m): It is defined as the concentration of the substrate at which the reaction velocity is half of the maximum velocity ($V_{max/2}$) (Fig. 8.12). The K_m is independent of the enzyme concentration. Therefore, if an enzyme has a small value of K_m, it achieves maximal catalytic efficiency at low substrate concentration.

For convenience, a linear form of the Michaelis-Menten equation is used to determine K_m and V_{max} obtained from a plot of the reciprocal of the reaction rate (1/V) against the reciprocal of the substrate concentration, 1/[S]. The Michaelis-Menten equation, when inverted, can be written as shown in Fig. 8.13.

When $1/V_o$ (the reciprocal of V_o) is plotted against 1/[S] (the reciprocal of [S]), such a plot is called as a double reciprocal plot or Lineweaver-Burk plot.

The intercept at the Y axis is given by $1/V_{max}$. On the other hand, the extrapolation at the X-axis (the negative X intercept) denotes $-1/K_m$. The slope of the plot represents $-K_m/V_{max}$. Thus, K_m can be calculated by using either the slope and the Y intercept, or the negative X intercept. Its extrapolation intercepts the 1/[S] line and gives the value of $-1/K_m$, from which K_m can be calculated (Fig. 8.14).

Significance of K_m

- **Physiological significance:** Glucose can be phosphorylated to glucose-6-phosphate by glucokinase (the enzyme, present in the liver, is specific for glucose) or hexokinase (nonspecific for hexoses except galactose, present in all tissues). Glucokinase has a high K_m (i.e. low affinity for glucose), hence it is important during the fed state when glucose is in excess and needs to be stored as glycogen. On the other hand, under post-absorptive/fasting conditions, hexokinase having a low K_m (i.e. high affinity for glucose) is important so that glycolysis continues to provide energy to the vital organs even at comparatively lower blood glucose levels.

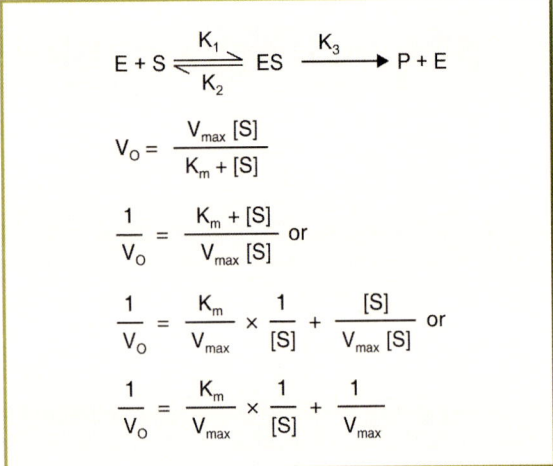

Fig. 8.13: Michaelis-Menten equation (linear and reciprocal forms).

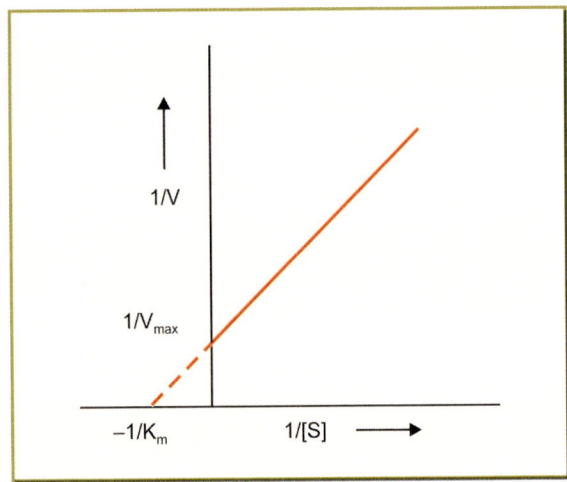

Fig. 8.14: Lineweaver-Burk plot (double-reciprocal plot).

Chemistry to Clinics 8.3: Aldehyde Dehydrogenase
This enzyme oxidizes acetaldehyde (formed from alcohol) into acetic acid. People having a low K_m (i.e. high affinity) variant of the enzyme metabolize acetaldehyde rapidly and are less susceptible to its adverse effects such as headache and flushing. On the other hand, people having the high K_m variant are more prone to these side effects of alcohol.

- **Laboratory significance:** During enzyme assays in the laboratory, the substrate concentration is kept at saturating amounts (at least 10 times the K_m) so that the reaction proceeds to completion.
- **Clinical significance:** The K_m value for a given enzyme may differ from person to person and explains the varied response to drugs/chemicals (Chemistry to Clinics 8.3).

4. Enzyme Concentration

The rate of an enzyme catalyzed reaction is proportional to the concentration of the enzyme present in a reaction mixture. When concentration of the enzyme is doubled, it combines with twice the amount of substrate and the amount of product formed will also be two-fold. This relationship holds good for low concentration of enzyme but with adequate substrate concentration (Fig. 8.15).

5. Enzyme Inhibition

Chemical substances which inhibit enzyme activity and reduce the velocity of an enzyme catalyzed reaction are called inhibitors, and the phenomenon is called enzyme inhibition. There are several classes of inhibitors:

Competitive Inhibitors

A substance that competes directly with a normal substrate for an enzyme's substrate-binding site is known as a competitive inhibitor. Competitive inhibition thus occurs when both substrate and inhibitor can fit into the active site and compete with each other to occupy the same. Chemical structure of the competitive inhibitor closely resembles with that of the substrate. It is called a **structural analog**. For example, in a reaction catalyzed by the enzyme succinate dehydrogenase, that converts succinate to fumarate, malonate, a structural analog of succinate, acts as a competitive inhibitor for the enzyme (Fig. 8.16).

The inhibitor forms a complex with the enzyme called **enzyme-inhibitor** (EI) **complex**, instead of the enzyme substrate (ES) complex, and inhibits the enzyme from acting on the substrate (Fig. 8.17). A competitive inhibitor thus reduces concentration of free enzyme available for the substrate binding. The binding of the enzyme with the inhibitor or with the substrate depends upon the relative concentrations of the substrate as well as the inhibitor. It is, therefore, usually a reversible process, as the degree of inhibition can be reduced by increasing the concentration of the substrate. The presence of a competitive inhibitor therefore increases the apparent K_m for the substrate, without any change in V_{max} (Fig. 8.18). Some of the competitive inhibitors are shown in Fig. 8.19.

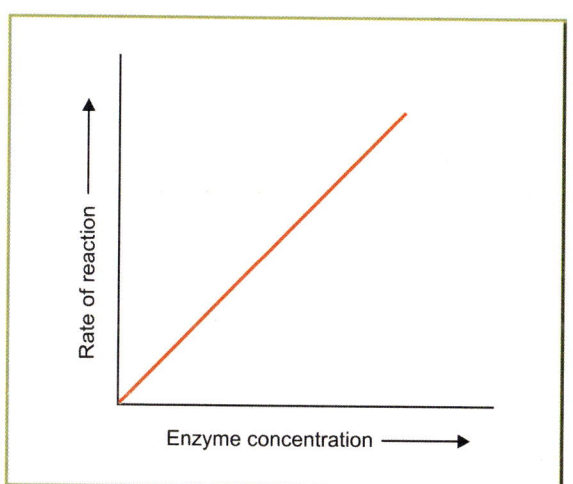

Fig. 8.15: Effect of enzyme concentration on enzyme activity.

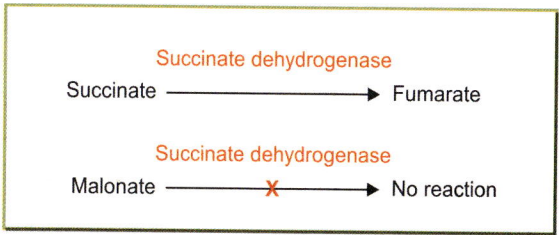

Fig. 8.16: Inhibition of succinate dehydrogenase by malonate.

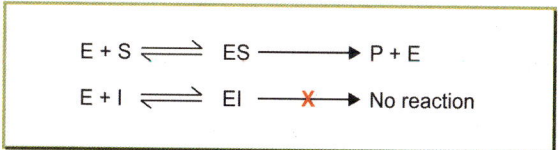

Fig. 8.17: Competitive inhibition.

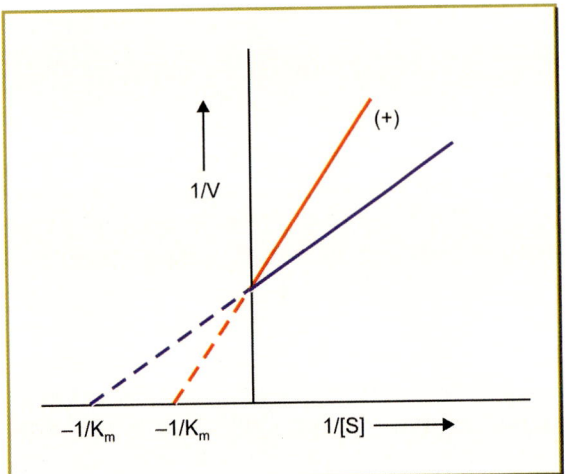

Fig. 8.18: Lineweaver-Burk plot for a competitive inhibitor (+); V_{max} unaltered, apparent K_m increased.

Competitive inhibitors are clinically very useful (Table 8.7) (Chemistry to Clinics 8.4).

Chemistry to Clinics 8.4: Ethanol in the Treatment of Methanol Poisoning

Methanol as such is only mildly toxic, in the liver. However, when acted upon by the enzyme alcohol dehydrogenase, methanol is converted into a highly toxic compound, i.e. formaldehyde.

The toxicity of methanol can be overcome by giving ethanol. Since ethanol competes with methanol for binding to the active site of the enzyme and slows down the conversion of methanol to formaldehyde, this in turn facilitates the excretion of methanol from the body in the urine, without being converted into formaldehyde. Ethanol thus is used in the treatment of methanol poisoning due to its competitive inhibition of the enzyme alcohol dehydrogenase.

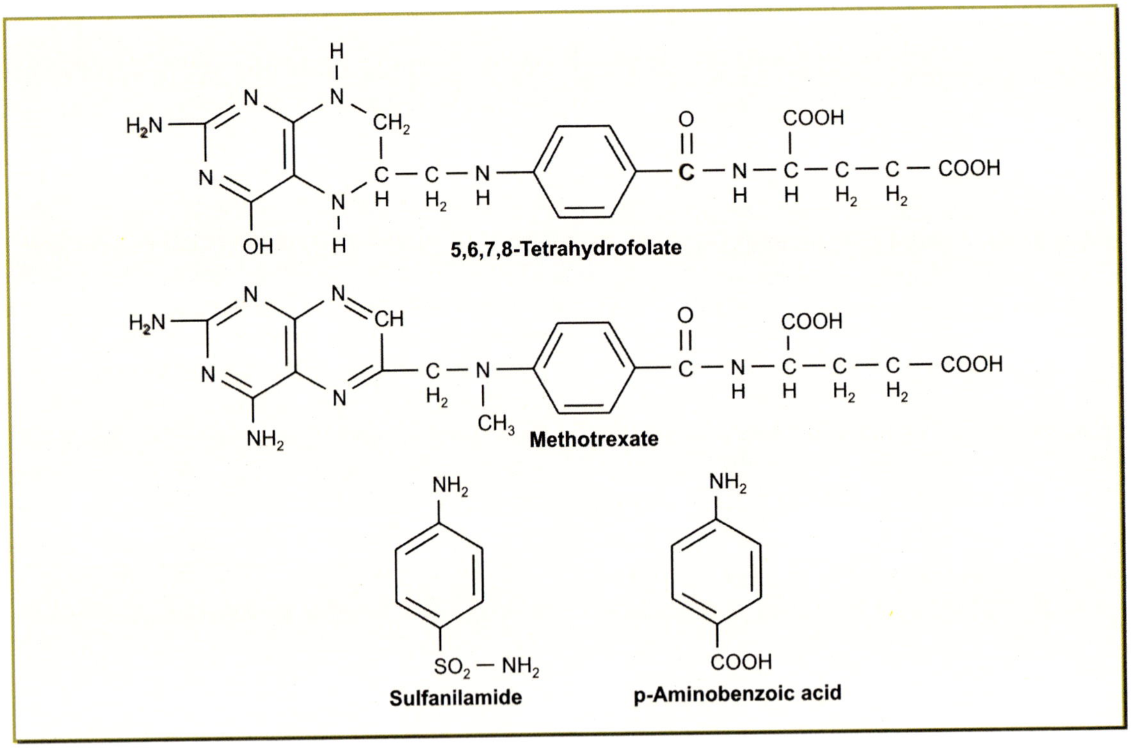

Fig. 8.19: Competitive inhibitors.

Table 8.7: Clinical applications of competitive enzyme inhibition			
Drug	*Enzyme*	*True substrate*	*Clinical application*
Allopurinol	Xanthine oxidase	Hypoxanthine	Gout
Sulfonamides	Bacterial dihydropteroate synthase	Para-amino benzoic acid (PABA)	Bacterial infections
Methotrexate	Dihydrofolate reductase	Dihydrofolate	Cancer
Dicumarol	Epoxide reductase	Vitamin K epoxide	Thrombosis
Ethanol (alcohol)	Alcohol dehydrogenase	Ethanol (alcohol)	Methanol poisoning
Succinyl choline	Acetyl cholinesterase	Acetyl choline	Muscle relaxant

Non-competitive Inhibitors

The inhibitor (I) usually bears no structural similarity to the substrate (S) and thus there occurs no competition between I and S. A noncompetitive inhibitor binds at a site other than the substrate binding site, hence, the enzyme as well as the enzyme-substrate complex can bind to inhibitor. Therefore, both binary (EI) and ternary (ESI) complexes can be formed. Since, ESI may break down to form a product but at a slower rate, a reversible noncompetitive inhibitor decreases V_{max} but does not change K_m (Fig. 8.20). Many antimetabolites act by this mechanism (Chemistry to Clinics 8.5).

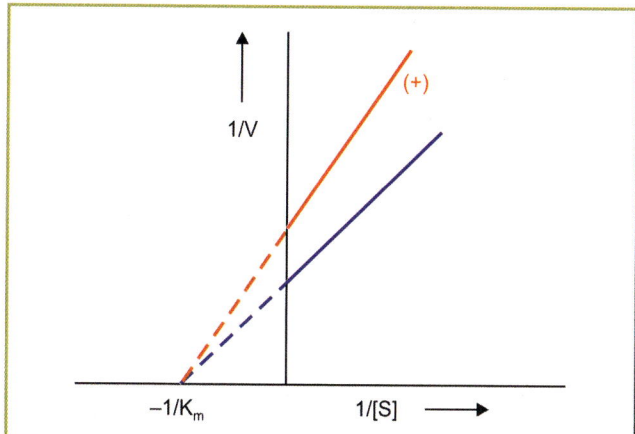

Fig. 8.20: Lineweaver-Burk plot for a non-competitive inhibitor (+); V_{max} reduced, K_m unaltered.

Chemistry to Clinics 8.5: Antimetabolites

Certain analogs of purines and pyrimidines (called antimetabolites) are noncompetitive inhibitors of some of the enzymes of purine/pyrimidine biosynthetic pathways. This blocks DNA synthesis, hence these antimetabolites are used as anticancer drugs. For example, 5-fluorouracil, an analog of thymine (Fig. 8.21), inhibits thymidylate synthetase, noncompetitively.

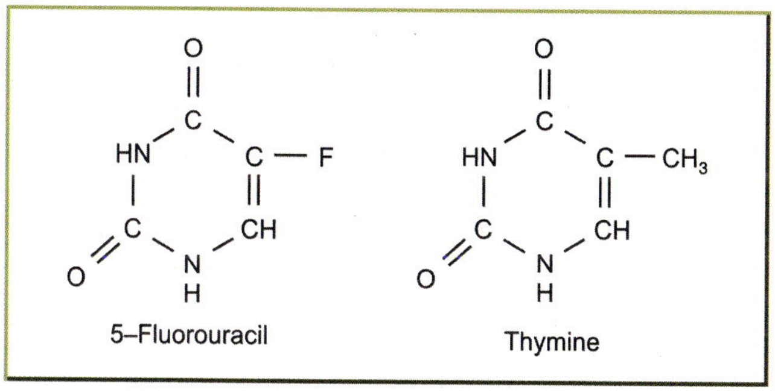

Fig. 8.21: Non-competitive inhibitors.

Uncompetitive Inhibitors

Uncompetitive inhibition occurs when the inhibitor binds after the substrate has bound to the enzyme, and then stops the reaction. The uncompetitive inhibitor thus binds directly to the enzyme substrate complex and not to free enzyme. Such an inhibitor may not resemble the substrate (Chemistry to Clinics 8.6).

The uncompetitive inhibitor affects catalytic function of the enzyme but not the substrate binding. Both K_m and V_{max} are decreased (Fig. 8.22).

Chemistry to Clinics 8.6: Lithium

Lithium (as lithium carbonate) is commonly used in the treatment of a psychiatric disorder called manic depressive psychosis (MDP), characterized by alternating periods of mania and depression. Normally, inositol monophosphatase (IMPase) catalyzes the hydrolysis of myoinositol monophosphate to myoinositol, which is important in stabilizing mood and behaviour through a complex mechanism. In MDP, there is altered metabolism of phosphatidylinositol in the brain. Lithium prevents inositol recycling through uncompetitive inhibition of IMPase.

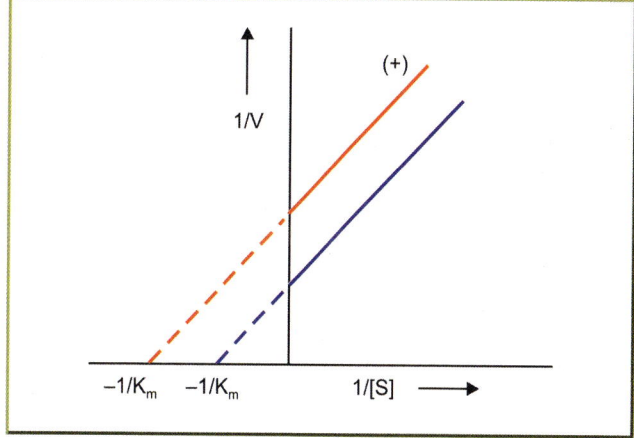

Fig. 8.22: Lineweaver-Burk plot for an uncompetitive inhibitor (+); both V_{max} and apparent K_m are reduced.

Irreversible Inhibitors

Several oxidizing agents, enzyme poisons and heavy metals cause irreversible inhibition of enzyme activity. As these inhibitors bear no structural similarity to the substrate, the inhibition cannot be reversed by increasing substrate concentration. These inhibitors result in chemical modification of the enzyme molecule and inactivate it (Chemistry to Clinics 8.7).

Reagents that chemically modify specific amino acid residues can act as inactivators, e.g. di-isopropyl-

Chemistry to Clinics 8.7: Aspirin

Eicosanoids are an important group of compounds synthesized in the body from unsaturated fatty acids. Their concentration increases during acute inflammation. Aspirin (acetylsalicylic acid) is a very popular non-steroidal anti-inflammatory drug (NSAID). It irreversibly acetylates and inactivates cyclooxygenase, an important enzyme required for eicosanoid biosynthesis.

phosphofluoridate, used for the detection of active site Ser of serine protease, irreversibly inactivates the enzyme. These inactivators reduce V_{max} at all levels of [S], without changing K_m.

Table 8.8 summarizes the effect of various types of inhibitors on K_m and V_{max} of an enzyme catalyzed reaction.

Table 8.8: Effect of various types of inhibitors on V_{max} and K_m of an enzyme catalyzed reaction

Type of inhibition	Effect of inhibition on	
	V_{max}	K_m (Apparent change)
Reversible		
Competitive	Unaltered	↑
Noncompetitive	↓	Unaltered
Uncompetitive	↓	↓
Irreversible	↓	Unaltered

Suicide Inhibition

A special class of irreversible enzyme inhibition is suicide inhibition in which an inhibitor binds to the active center of the enzyme and, through the catalytic action of the enzyme, is converted to a reactive compound that binds tightly with a functional group at the active center thereby irreversibly inactivating the enzyme. This type of inhibition is also known as **mechanism-based enzyme inactivation** (the inhibitor is called a **suicide substrate** or **Trojan horse substrate**). It also depends upon both the structural similarity of the inhibitor to the substrate and the mechanism of action of the target enzyme (Chemistry to Clinics 8.8).

Chemistry to Clinics 8.8: Allopurinol and Hyperuricemia

Allopurinol, a structural analog of hypoxanthine, is a competitive inhibitor as well as a substrate for xanthine oxidase. By itself it is not capable of inhibiting the enzyme; however, when transformed to alloxanthine (oxypurinol) by the host enzyme (xanthine oxidase), it becomes a competitive inhibitor. Allopurinol, which affects both the penultimate and ultimate steps in the formation of uric acid, is used to lower plasma uric acid levels in clinical conditions associated with excessive uric acid production and hyperuricemia (e.g. gout, hematological disorders and antineoplastic therapy).

REGULATION OF ENZYME ACTIVITY

The regulation of a metabolic pathway occurs through modification of the activity of one or more key enzymes of the pathway, in the following manner:

1. **Change in enzyme quantity:** The absolute quantity of an enzyme is determined by a balance between the rate of synthesis of the enzyme and its rate of degradation. Cells can synthesize a specific enzyme in response to a substance called **inducer**; such enzymes are called **inducible enzymes**. Tryptophan pyrrolase, tyrosine transaminase and HMG CoA reductase are some of the inducible enzymes. On the other hand, enzymes whose concentrations are always maintained at a particular level, independent of the inducer, are **constitutive enzymes**.

Sometimes, accumulation of a metabolite may inhibit its own synthesis. This is called as repression and such a metabolite is called as a repressor. A repressor thus inhibits synthesis of the enzyme. The exhaustion of the repressor overcomes the inhibition of synthesis of the enzyme and the biosynthesis of the enzyme can again occur. This is called derepression.

2. **Change in catalytic efficiency of the enzyme:** Catalytic activity of an enzyme is modulated by allosteric regulation, feedback inhibition or covalent modification:

   (i) **Allosteric regulation:** The catalytic activity of some of the **regulatory enzymes** called **allosteric enzymes** is modulated by certain low-molecular weight substances. These substances bind at a site which is different than the catalytic site, i.e. they occupy another space, hence they are called **allosteric effectors** (**allosteric modulators**, Table 8.9). The catalytic site where the substrate binds, and the allosteric site where the effector molecule binds, is physically distinct and often located far away from each other.

   The effector may activate an enzymatic reaction (**allosteric activation**) and is called as a **positive effector** or **allosteric activator**. The converse is **allosteric inhibition** and such an effector molecule is called a **negative effector** or **allosteric inhibitor**. Reversal of such an inhibition can be brought about by increasing the amount of the substrate, relative to the amount of the inhibitor.

Table 8.9: Allosteric modulation of some enzymes

Enzyme	Allosteric activator	Allosteric inhibitor
Hexokinase	ADP	Glucose-6-P, ATP
Isocitrate dehydrogenase	ADP	Glucose-6-P, ATP
Glutamate dehydrogenase	ADP	ATP, NADH
Pyruvate carboxylase	Acetyl CoA	ADP

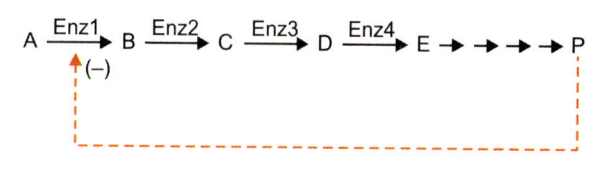

Fig. 8.24: Feed-back inhibition (–).

If the effector substance is the substrate itself, the phenomenon is called a **homotropic** effect; if it is a substance other than the substrate, the effect is **heterotropic**.

Based on the effect of an allosteric effector on the K_m or the V_{max}, allosteric enzymes are divided into two classes, i.e. the K class and the V class. In the **K class**, the effector alters the K_m but not the V_{max} whereas in the **V class** the effector alters the V_{max} but not the K_m.

When reaction velocity is plotted against substrate concentration, a characteristic **sigmoidal curve** (S-shaped curve) is obtained. The presence of an allosteric activator (a positive modulator or '+') shifts the entire curve to the right whereas an allosteric inhibitor (a negative modulator or '–') shifts the curve to the left (Fig. 8.23).

(ii) **Feedback inhibition:** It refers to the inhibition of an enzyme by the end product of a reaction. When a substrate (A) is converted to an end product (P) through various intermediates, such as B, C, D, etc., the end product of the reaction inhibits the first enzyme of the pathway (Fig. 8.24). Accumulation of the end product slows down the whole reaction

sequence. As the end product is consumed, the synthesis continues.

(iii) **Covalent modification:** Activity of many enzymes is regulated by covalent modification. There are two well-known processes leading to covalent modification, i.e. phosphorylation and partial proteolysis.

Phosphorylation-dephosphorylation: The activity of many enzymes is regulated by ATP-dependent phosphorylation with subsequent hydrolysis of the phosphate group as inorganic phosphate. The phosphorylation of Ser, Thr and Tyr residues is catalyzed by protein kinases. Subsequent removal of the inorganic phosphate (dephosphorylation) is catalyzed by another set of enzymes called as protein phosphatases, the activities of which are also regulated.

Phosphorylation-dephosphorylation is a reversible process of a regulatory cascade, in response to the signal triggered by a hormone or a secondary messenger, e.g. Ca^{2+} or cAMP. Catalytic activities of pyruvate dehydrogenase and glycogen synthase are altered by covalent phosphorylation-dephosphorylation.

Partial proteolysis: Some enzymes are synthesized in the form of their inactive precursors called **proenzymes** or **zymogens** (Table 8.1). Conversion of an inactive proenzyme to an active enzyme occurs by selective proteolysis at one or more sites, irreversibly. Digestive enzymes, e.g. pepsin A, trypsin, etc. are secreted as inactive zymogens (as pepsinogen A or trypsinogen) and are converted to active enzymes by partial proteolysis.

ENZYME UNITS

The amount of an enzyme in the sample of a biological fluid, such as serum or in a tissue extract is measured in terms of the rate of reaction catalyzed by the enzyme. Under appropriate conditions, the measured

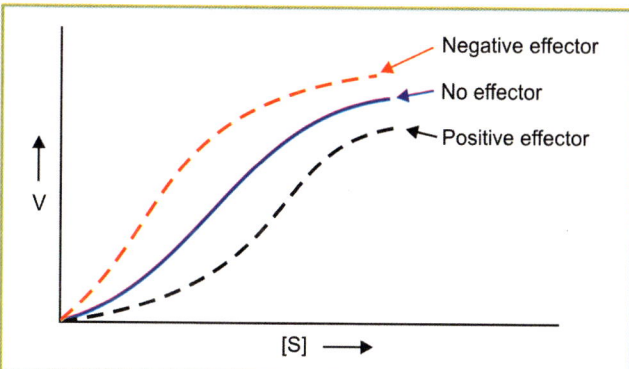

Fig. 8.23: Effect of positive/negative effector on reaction velocity for an allosteric enzyme.

rate of a reaction is directly proportional to the quantity of the enzyme present in the sample. Since it is difficult to determine the number of molecules or mass of enzyme present, results are expressed in terms of enzyme units.

Older units: Historically, a multiplicity of units for expressing enzyme activity were introduced by different workers which are still in use, e.g. King-Armstrong units (KA units) or Bodansky units for alkaline and acid phosphatases, or Somogyi units for amylase, etc.

International Unit: As per Enzyme Commission of the International Union of Biochemistry (IUB), a unit of enzyme activity is designated as the International Unit (IU), which is defined as the quantity of enzyme that catalyzes the reaction of 1 μmol of substrate reacting or product transformed per minute (1 μmol/min). This catalytic concentration is expressed in terms of some convenient numerical value e.g. IU/L.

SI unit: To overcome the problem of different units being reported by different laboratories, the SI (Systeme Internationale, i.e. International System) scheme of units has been suggested by the IUB. According to SI units, mole should be a measure of the substrate transformed and the second should be the unit of time. The enzyme activity should be expressed in terms of **Katals** which is defined as moles/second and the enzyme concentration should be expressed in terms of Katals per liter (Kat/L).

ISOENZYMES

Isoenzymes (isozymes) are the physically distinct forms of an enzyme which have the same specificity but may be present in different tissues of the same organism, in different cell types or sub-cellular compartments. Besides the source, they also differ from each other with respect to their structure, electrophoretic mobility and immunological properties. The most common mechanism for the formation of isoenzymes involves the arrangement of subunits, arising from different genetic loci, in different combinations to form the active polymeric enzyme.

Isozymes that have wide clinical applications include lactate dehydrogenase, creatine kinase and alkaline phosphatase (Table 8.10).

Lactate Dehydrogenase

Lactate dehydrogenase (LD or LDH) is a tetramer, i.e. it has four polypeptide subunits. Each subunit may be one of the two types, known as the H type (**heart type**) and the M type (**muscle type**). LD exists in serum in five distinct forms (isoenzymes) which have different proportions of the H and the M subunits. LD-1 has 4H type of polypeptide chains (H_4) and is predominantly found in myocardium while LD-5 has 4M subunits (M_4) and is the predominant form in the hepatic tissue (Chemistry to Clinics 8.9). The other forms are LD-2 (H_3M), LD-3 (H_2M_2) and LD-4 (HM_3). LD-6 and LD-7 have also been reported.

Table 8.10: Diagnostic importance of some isoenzymes

Enzyme	Isoenzymes	Predominant location	Diagnostic significance ($\uparrow$ serum levels)
Creatine kinase (CK, a dimer with 2 polypeptide chains B [brain] and M [muscle])	CK-1 (BB)	Brain	Cerebrovascular accidents
	CK-2 (MB)	Myocardium	Myocardial infarction
	CK-3 (MM)	Skeletal muscle	Muscular dystrophies
Lactate dehydrogenase (LD, a tetramer with 4 polypeptide chains, H [heart] and M [muscle])	LD-1 (H_4)	Myocardium	Myocardial infarction
	LD-2 (H_3M)	Erythrocytes	Hemolytic anemia
	LD-3 (H_2M_2)	Brain	Cerebrovascular accidents
	LD-4 (HM_3)	Liver	Hepatocellular damage
	LD-5 (M_4)	Skeletal muscle	Muscular dystrophies
Alkaline phosphatase (ALP, monomeric isoenzymes because of differences in carbohydrate contents [sialic acid residues])	α_1-ALP	Liver	Obstructive jaundice
	α_2-ALP-heat labile	Liver	Hepatitis
	-heat stable	Placenta	Pregnancy
	Pre β-ALP	Bones	Osteoblastic bone diseases
	γ-ALP	Colon	Ulcerative colitis
	Regan ALP	Some primary tumors	Bronchogenic carcinoma

Chemistry to Clinics: 8.9. Flipped Ratio

LD-1 and LD-2 predominate in myocardium and RBC, respectively. Normally, serum LD-1 concentration is less than that of LD-2 i.e. LD-1/LD-2 ratio is <1. However, serum LD-1 becomes greater than LD-2 (known as a flipped ratio) between 12 and 24 hours following myocardial infarction.

Creatine Kinase

Creatine kinase (CK) exists in three forms. Each isoenzyme is a dimer composed of two subunits, i.e. M (**muscle** type) and B (**brain** type). The three isoenzymes are CK-1 (BB) found in brain, CK-2 (MB) in myocardium, and CK-3 (MM) in skeletal muscle. Serum CK-1 activity may increase in patients with cerebrovascular disease and head injury. CK-2 isoenzyme is present in very small amount in serum. Its level rises within 4–6 hours of myocardial infarction and reaches to a maximum within 1 day of the infarction (Fig. 8.25). CK-3 activity is greatly elevated in all types of muscular dystrophies. However, in a neurogenic muscle disease, such as myasthenia gravis, serum enzyme activity is normal.

Alkaline Phosphatase

Different tissues contain different forms of alkaline phosphatase. A major portion of alkaline phosphatase in serum is derived from liver and its level rises in post-hepatic jaundice. In growing children, the major isoenzyme is from the bone which is related to its increased osteoblastic activity. During the last trimester of pregnancy, there is an increase in alkaline phosphatase which is of placental origin. This isoenzyme is heat-stable and is called **heat-stable alkaline phosphatase**.

DIAGNOSTIC SIGNIFICANCE OF ENZYMES

Principles of Diagnostic Enzymology

1. **Functional plasma enzymes:** These are normally present at all times in the circulation where each performs a physiological function. They generally are synthesized in the liver but are present in the blood in equivalent or higher concentrations than in tissues, e.g. lipoprotein lipase, pseudocholine esterase, and the enzymes of blood coagulation.

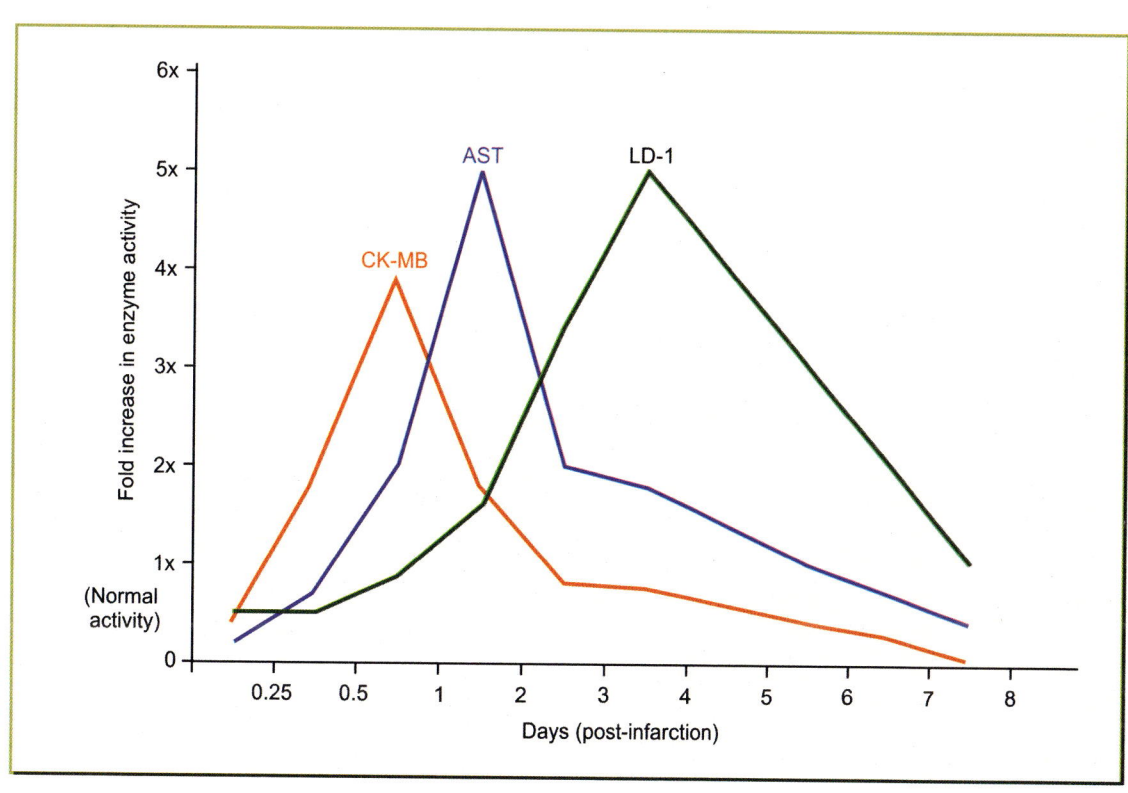

Fig. 8.25: Serum enzyme profile in **myocardial infarction.**

8

2. **Nonfunctional plasma enzymes:** These are present in very low concentrations in the blood where they perform no physiological function. Elevation in the levels of these enzymes suggests an increased rate of tissue destruction and thus provides valuable diagnostic information to the physician (Chemistry to Clinics 8.10 to 8.12).

3. **Isoenzymes:** Whenever possible, the specific isoenzyme relevant to the clinical condition should be estimated (Table 8.10).

4. **Enzyme clearance:** Besides the release of the enzyme from damaged or dying cells resulting in increased enzyme activity in the serum, clearance of enzyme from the circulation can also influence its concentration in the serum and other body fluids.

Chemistry to Clinics 8.10: Liver Enzyme Panel

Transaminases: Serum aspartate aminotransferase (**AST**) also called as serum glutamate oxaloacetate transaminase (**SGOT**), and alanine aminotransferase (**ALT**) also called as serum glutamate pyruvate transaminase (**SGPT**), have great clinical significance. Both serum AST and ALT levels are raised even before the clinical signs and symptoms of the disease appear. However, ALT is more liver specific. Levels may increase multiple folds. The duration of illness is variable and enzyme levels may be raised for sometime even after clinical recovery (Fig. 8.26).

Alkaline phosphatase (ALP): Intrahepatic obstruction of the bile flow raises serum ALP to a lesser extent, i.e. up to 2–3 times of the upper normal limit only. However, a marked rise (up to 10 times or more) occurs in **post-hepatic obstruction**.

γ-Glutamyl transpeptidase (γ-glutamyl transferase, γ-GT): Serum γ-GT primarily originates from the hepatobiliary system. Its activity is increased in all forms of liver disease. Elevated levels are of special significance in detecting **alcohol-induced liver disease**. Levels are increased not only in patients with alcoholic cirrhosis but also in majority of people who are heavy drinkers.

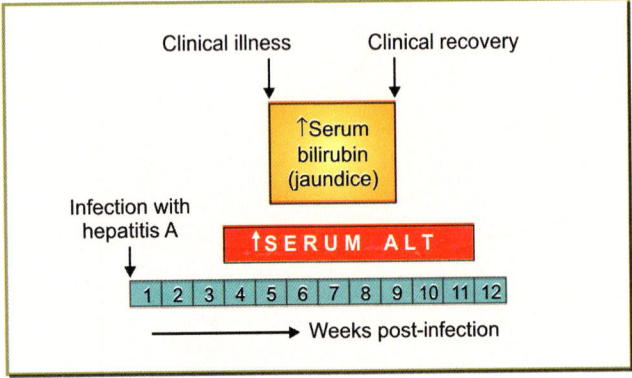

Fig. 8.26: Serum alanine transaminase (ALT) is raised prior to serum bilirubin in **viral hepatitis**. High levels persist for sometime even after clinical recovery and clearance of jaundice.

Chemistry to Clinics 8.11: Amylase and Lipase

Estimations of amylase activity in serum and urine are significant in the diagnosis of diseases of the pancreas (**P type amylase**) and the salivary glands (**S type amylase**). In acute pancreatitis, a transient rise (4–6 folds) in serum P type amylase activity occurs within 2 to 12 hours of the onset and levels return to normal by the 3rd to 5th day. Nowadays, estimation of serum lipase is preferred to strengthen the diagnosis; it rises within 4 to 8 hours and normalizes by the 7th to 14th day post-treatment. Diseases of salivary glands (e.g. mumps) result in increased serum S type amylase.

Chemistry to Clinics 8.12: Cardiac Enzyme Panel

- The measurement of serum CK-2 (CK-MB) is the most commonly used enzymatic test for the diagnosis of myocardial infarction. An initial rise occurs in 4 to 6 hours. Peak levels are found at approximately 24 hours while return to normal occurs within 48 to 72 hours (Fig. 8.25).

- Rise in LD starts 12 to 18 hours after the onset of myocardial infarction, with peak at 48 to 72 hours. The levels return to below the upper normal level after 6 to 10 days. Rise in total LD parallels LD-1 isozyme.

- Increased SGOT (AST) activity appears in serum as its concentration is highest in the cardiac muscle. Since SGPT (ALT) concentration is much less than SGOT in the cardiac muscle, it is only marginally increased. Peak level of SGOT is reached after 18 to 24 hours and falls to within normal limit by the fourth or fifth day.

For example, increased level of serum amylase after acute pancreatitis is also accompanied by its increased excretion in the urine.

5. **Serial analysis:** It is often useful to measure the level of enzyme activity on more than one occasion, as the time course over which the activity changes is characteristic of the condition. Further, it also helps to assess the response to treatment.

6. **Supporting parameters:** The results of enzyme analysis should always be assessed along with the results of other non-enzymatic parameters (such as bilirubin in acute hepatitis) and the clinical findings of the patient.

The main enzymes of established diagnostic significance together with their tissue of origin and clinical applications are listed in Table 8.11.

ENZYMES AS ANALYTICAL REAGENTS

Enzymes are widely used as analytical reagents in the measurement of activity of other analytes (enzymes/non-enzymes):

Table 8.11: Some serum enzymes of diagnostic significance

Enzyme	Principal sources	Conditions in which altered ($\uparrow$, increase; $\downarrow$, decrease)
Acid phosphatase	Prostate, RBC	$\uparrow$Carcinoma prostate
Alkaline phosphatase	Liver, bone, placenta, kidney	$\uparrow$Obstructive jaundice, rickets, Paget's disease, hyperparathyroidism, growing children
Aldolase	Skeletal muscle, heart	$\uparrow$Muscular dystrophies, acute hepatitis
Amylase	Salivary glands	$\uparrow$Acute parotitis
Amylase	Pancreas	$\uparrow$Acute pancreatitis, intestinal obstruction
Ceruloplasmin	Liver	$\uparrow$Cirrhosis, $\downarrow$Wilson's disease
Cholinesterase	Liver	$\uparrow$Nephrotic syndrome, organophosphorus poisoning
Creatine phosphokinase	Skeletal muscle, brain, heart	$\uparrow$Myocardial infarction, muscular dystrophies
Glutamate oxaloacetate transaminase (GOT)	Liver, skeletal muscle, heart, kidney, RBC	$\uparrow$Myocardial infarction, toxic liver cell necrosis, acute hepatitis, myositis
Glutamate pyruvate transaminase (GPT)	Liver, skeletal muscle, heart	$\uparrow$Viral hepatitis
γ-Glutamyl transferase	Liver, kidney	$\uparrow$Alcoholism, hepatobiliary disease
Glutamate dehydrogenase	Liver	$\uparrow$Hepatocellular damage
Lactate dehydrogenase	Heart, liver, skeletal muscle, RBC, platelets	$\uparrow$Myocardial infarction, acute hepatitis, myositis, hemolysis
Lipase	Pancreas	$\uparrow$Acute pancreatitis, pancreatic carcinoma
5'-Nucleotidase	Hepatobiliary tract	$\uparrow$Obstructive jaundice, hepatocellular carcinoma
Trypsin	Pancreas	$\uparrow$Acute pancreatitis

Immobilized enzymes: Glucose, cholesterol, uric acid, etc. are frequently quantitated by enzymatic reactions which measure the concentration of the analyte due to the specificity of the concerned enzyme. Immobilized enzymes are chemically bonded to a solid support, e.g. agarose. When a sample containing substrate (the analyte to be estimated) is passed through the preparation, the product is retrieved and analyzed whereas the enzyme (being a recoverable reagent) becomes free to react with more substrate. Immobilized enzymes are more stable than enzymes in solution and are suited for batch analysis.

Enzyme-linked immunosorbent assay (ELISA): Certain enzymes such as horseradish peroxidase, alkaline phosphatase, glucose-6-phosphate dehydrogenase, β-galactosidase, etc. are employed as reagents in immunoassays to measure HIV antibodies, therapeutic agents and tumor antigens.

ENZYMES AS THERAPEUTIC AGENTS

Enzymes are widely used as drugs in the therapy of specific medical problems:

Treatment of inherited disorders

1. **Adenosine deaminase (ADA):** It is used in severe combined immunodeficiency (SCID, due to lack of ADA); the first successful application of enzyme replacement therapy for an inherited disease.
2. **Glucocerebrosidase:** As enzyme replacement therapy for Gaucher's disease.

Treatment of acquired disorders

1. **Streptokinase**: It is obtained from streptococci and is used in blood clot-dissolution during myocardial infarction or in deep vein thrombosis. Tissue plasminogen activator (tPA) serves the same purpose.
2. **Asparaginase:** It is used for some types of leukemias based on the rationale that the tumor cells are asparagine-dependent for their multiplication and survival.
3. **Deoxyribonuclease (DNase):** It is administered by the respiratory route to clear up the viscid secretions in patients of cystic fibrosis.
4. **Serratiopeptidase**: It is used to minimize the edema that accompanies a physical trauma or an acute inflammation of the skin.

8

5. **Hyaluronidase:** It is used for hypodermoclysis, to facilitate the subcutaneous administration of water/electrolyte solutions in patients with hypovolemic shock where the collapsed veins are difficult to locate.

6. **Hemocoagulase**: It is used as a hemostat.

7. **Fungal diastase (amylase) and pepsin:** They are used in digestive preparations.

8. **Ribozymes and abzymes** (Chemistry to Clinics 8.13 and 8.14).

Chemistry to Clinics 8.13: Ribozymes

Structure and properties: These are certain ribonucleic acids (RNAs) which exhibit highly substrate specific catalytic activity. They catalyze hydrolysis of phosphodiester bonds within the RNA molecule and play a key role in the intron splicing events, which are essential in the conversion of pre-mRNAs to mature mRNAs. Many ribozymes have a hair-pin or hammer-head shaped active center and require divalent metal ions (e.g. Mg^{2+}) as cofactors. They obey simple Michaelis-Menten kinetics and some of them can be allosterically modulated.

Examples: RNAse P from *E. coli*, self-splicing RNA introns, telomerase and eukaryotic peptidyl transferase.

Applications: Synthetic ribozymes have been developed that possess better catalytic activity than the natural ones and their biomedical applications include:

1. Tools for RNA cleavage *in vitro.*
2. Designing of specific catalytic RNA molecules to cleave nucleic acids of infectious viruses (HIV, hepatitis C, herpes simplex, etc.) and malignant cells.
3. Study of gene expression, function and use in gene therapy.

Protein versus RNA catalysts: Compared with protein catalysts, ribozymes have the following drawbacks:

1. Ribozymes are not as efficient and versatile as protein catalysts since there are only four different nucleotide building blocks for RNA rather than the twenty amino acids available for proteins.
2. Ribozymes generally act only once in a chemical event whereas protein enzymes are reused after each round of catalysis.
3. Rate of catalysis is slower for ribozymes because for substrate binding, they rely mostly on H-bonding and less on hydrophobic plus electrostatic interactions exploited by protein catalysts.

Chemistry to Clinics 8.14: Abzymes

These are the artificially synthesized catalytic antibodies against the enzyme-substrate complex in the transition state of the reaction. They are also called 'catmab' (catalytic monoclonal antibody) since they are monoclonal antibodies possessing catalytic activity. However, sometimes natural abzymes may be found in the blood, e.g. anti-vasoactive intestinal peptide autoantibodies, DNA-hydrolyzing abzymes seen in systemic lupus erythematosus, etc. Abzymes exhibit the same kind of substrate specificity as do enzymes and yield products with defined stereochemistry. Abzymes can be useful in the treatment of various diseases, e.g. abzymes against the gp120 envelope protein of HIV may potentially prevent the virus entry into the host cell.

SOME IMPORTANT QUESTIONS

1. What are enzymes? Classify them. Discuss factors affecting enzyme activity.

2. Define enzyme, coenzyme and cofactor. Discuss the role of B-complex group of vitamins as coenzymes.

3. What are isoenzymes? Discuss the importance of enzymes in clinical diagnosis.

4. What are allosteric enzymes? How is their activity modulated? Give examples.

5. Give a brief account of factors affecting enzyme activity.

6. Discuss briefly:
   i. Mechanisms of enzyme action.
   ii. Various types of enzyme inhibition, giving examples.
   iii. Apoenzyme, holoenzyme and coenzyme.
   iv. Classification of enzymes with suitable examples.
   v. Michaelis-Menten equation
   vi. Regulation of enzyme activity.

7. Write notes on:

i. Diagnostic significance of enzymes.
ii. Noncompetitive inhibition of enzyme activity.
iii. K_m.
iv. Isoenzymes and their clinical importance.
v. Zymogens.
vi. Competitive inhibitors.
vii. Specificity of enzyme action.
viii. Coenzymes.
ix. Classification of enzymes.
x. Ribozymes.
xi. Abzymes.
xii. Allosteric regulation.
xiii. Feedback inhibition.
xiv. Enzyme units.

MULTIPLE CHOICE QUESTIONS

1. **The following is not a lyase:**
   A. Glucose-6-phosphatase
   B. Aldolase
   C. Argininosuccinase
   D. Histidase

2. **Hexokinase does not phosphorylate:**
   A. Glucose
   B. Fructose
   C. Mannose
   D. Galactose

3. **In enzyme catalysis, the following is reduced:**
   A. Free energy of substrate
   B. Free energy of transition state
   C. Free energy of product
   D. All of the above

4. **K_m is:**
   A. Directly proportional to enzyme concentration
   B. Inversely proportional to enzyme concentration
   C. Half of enzyme concentration
   D. Independent of enzyme concentration

5. **5-Fluorouracil inhibits thymidylate synthetase by:**
   A. Competitive inhibition
   B. Non-competitive inhibition
   C. Uncompetitive inhibition
   D. Allosteric inhibition

6. **Isoenzymes may be present in:**
   A. Different tissues
   B. Different cell types of a tissue
   C. Different subcellular compartments of a cell
   D. All of the above

7. **In myocardial infarction, the marker to rise earliest in serum is:**
   A. CPK-MM
   B. LDH-1
   C. CPK-MB
   D. ALT

8. **The following serum analyte is a good index of recent alcohol intake:**
   A. ALT
   B. γ-GT
   C. LDH-5
   D. Ceruloplasmin

9. **Ribozymes may function in/as:**
   A. Intron splicing
   B. Peptidyl transferase
   C. Both
   D. None of the above

10. **Abzymes are directed against:**
    A. Substrate
    B. Enzyme
    C. Enzyme-substrate complex in transition state
    D. Product

Digestion and Absorption of Carbohydrates, Lipids and Proteins

DIGESTION AND ABSORPTION OF CARBOHYDRATES

Digestion of Dietary Carbohydrates

- Digestion of a dietary carbohydrate starts **in the mouth** when food comes in contact with the saliva. Salivary amylase (**S type amylase**) hydrolyzes $1,4\alpha$-glycosidic linkages randomly, within the polysaccharide chain of starch or glycogen and produces maltose and various oligosaccharides. After food reaches the stomach, salivary amylase becomes inactive in the acidic environment.

- **In the duodenum**, pancreatic amylase (**P type amylase**), present in the pancreatic juice, helps in further hydrolysis of the remaining polysaccharide units. Pancreatic amylase is similar in action to salivary amylase and hydrolyzes the partially hydrolyzed products of starch and glycogen to maltose, isomaltose, maltotriose, limit dextrin and glucose (Table 9.1).

- Digestion continues **in the small intestine** as the intestinal juice also contains **oligosaccharidases** which hydrolyze the terminal $1,4\alpha$-glycosidic linkage from the oligosaccharides. At the same time, various **disaccharidases** (maltase, lactase and sucrase) hydrolyze disaccharides, i.e. maltose, lactose and sucrose respectively, to their constituent monosaccharide units (Table 9.1).

Lack of the enzyme lactase results in **lactose intolerance** (Chemistry to Clinics 9.1). Congenital sucrase deficiency results in symptoms similar to those of lactase deficiency.

Dietary Fibres

These refer to indigestible though nutritionally important carbohydrates and are discussed in Chapter 25.

Absorption of Monosaccharides

After digestion by the action of various enzymes, dietary carbohydrates are released as monosaccharides which are almost completely absorbed from the small intestine. Galactose and glucose are

Table 9.1: Digestion of dietary carbohydrates

Enzyme	Site of action	Catalytic action
Salivary amylase	Mouth	Starch/glycogen → Partially hydrolyzed dextrins, oligosaccharides, isomaltose and maltose
Pancreatic amylase	Small intestine	Partially hydrolyzed dextrins/oligosaccharides → Dextrins, maltose, isomaltose, maltotriose
α-Dextrinase	Small intestine	α-Limit dextrins → Maltotriose, glucose
Disaccharidases	Small intestine	
Sucrase		Sucrose → Glucose and fructose
Lactase		Lactose → Glucose and galactose
Maltase		Maltose/maltotriose → Glucose
Isomaltase		Isomaltose → Glucose

Chemistry to Clinics 9.1: Lactose Intolerance

It is a condition resulting from a deficiency of intestinal **lactase** so that the individual is unable to digest the milk sugar. It is different from milk allergy that is due to an immune reaction to milk protein. Lactase deficiency results in the accumulation of undigested lactose which is osmotically active. Lactose moves to the colon where its bacterial fermentation generates CO_2 and organic acids. The symptoms include abdominal cramps, diarrhea and flatulence.

It is very rare for an infant to be born with lactase deficiency. Lactase activity is highest immediately after birth and by adulthood only 5–10% of the initial activity remains. Only 30% of people retain enough lactase to digest lactose efficiently throughout adult life. Secondary lactase deficiency may result from damage to villi caused by drugs, prolonged diarrhea and malnutrition. Cheese is well tolerated since lactose gets removed with the whey during manufacturing.

The management strategy is to gradually decrease the intake of milk products, to take them with other foods and to spread their intake over the day. Further, medications containing lactose as filler must be avoided and adequate supplementation of riboflavin, calcium and vitamin D should be taken. **'Acidophilus milk'**, i.e. milk pre-treated with the bacteria *Lactobacillus acidophilus* is commercially available. The bacterial lactase cleaves lactose into glucose plus galactose, thus producing a sweet though lactose-free product.

Chemistry to Clinics 9.2: Hexose Malabsorption

Malabsorption of hexoses in the small intestine can be the indirect result of an increase in intestinal motility or defects in digestion because of pancreatic insufficiency. Although less common, malabsorption may be a direct result of a specific defect in hexose transport. Regardless of the cause, the symptoms are common and include diarrhea, abdominal pain and excessive gas formation. The challenge is to identify the cause so that the proper treatment can be applied. Some infants develop a copious watery diarrhea when fed milk that contains glucose or galactose or the disaccharides lactose and sucrose. The latter are degraded to glucose, galactose and fructose by enzymes in the intestine. The dehydration can begin during the first day of life and can lead to rapid death if not corrected. Fortunately, the symptoms disappear when a carbohydrate-free formula fortified with fructose is used instead of milk. This condition is a rare inherited disease known as **glucose-galactose malabsorption**. At least 10% of the general population has glucose or lactose intolerance, however, it is possible that these people may have milder forms of disease.

A specific defect in absorption of glucose and galactose can be demonstrated by tolerance tests in which oral administration of these monosaccharides produces little or no increase in plasma glucose or galactose. The primary defect lies in SGLT1 located in the apical plasma membrane of intestinal epithelial cells. Glucose and galactose have very similar structures, and both are substrates for transport by SGLT1. Fructose transport is much slower than glucose and galactose absorption and is not affected by a defect in SGLT1 because a specific fructose transporter named GLUT5 is present in the apical membrane.

absorbed from the small intestine very rapidly, by the active process which is linked to the transport of sodium and requires energy, in the form of hydrolysis of a high energy phosphate bond of ATP. **Sodium-glucose transporter-1 (SGLT1)** binds both glucose and sodium at separate sites and transports them through the plasma membrane of the intestinal cells (Fig. 3.13, Chapter 3). The process is inhibited by ouabain (a cardiac glycoside) and phlorhizin (an inhibitor of glucose reabsorption in the renal tubules). A defect in SGLT1 may reduce the absorption of glucose and galactose (Chemistry to Clinics 9.2).

There is also a **sodium-independent glucose transporter-2 (GLUT2)** which facilitates the transport of sugar out of the cell. Fructose and mannose are absorbed by facilitated transport which requires a carrier protein but not energy. Pentoses are absorbed passively by simple diffusion.

DIGESTION AND ABSORPTION OF LIPIDS

An adult human consumes nearly 50–100 g of lipids per day. Normally, triacylglycerols (triglycerides) constitute >90% of the dietary lipids with only a small amount of free fatty acids, phospholipids, cholesterol, vitamin A and their esters. Excess lipid consumption

may result in turbid urine in some individuals (Chemistry to Clinics 9.3).

Chemistry to Clinics 9.3: Lipuria

Ingestion of large amounts of lipids may lead to a condition called alimentary lipuria (**adiposuria**). The urine of such individuals becomes opalescent, turbid or sometimes even milky. In rare instances, when its lipid content is very high, a peculiar creamy layer is also seen. Lipuria may also be observed in lipemia of diabetes mellitus, lipoid nephrosis, fractures of the long bones with injury to the bone marrow and in phosphorus poisoning.

Digestion of Dietary Lipids

Lipids, as we know, are poorly soluble in water and thus cannot be easily accessible to digestive enzymes in the aqueous phase. To facilitate the same, dietary triacylglycerols form emulsion droplets which, in turn, increases the interfacial area between the aqueous and the lipid phase. Digestion of dietary lipids takes place with the participation of several enzymes (Table 9.2).

- The process is initiated **in the stomach** by an acid stable lipase which is present in the sublingual glands as well as in the stomach.

9

Table 9.2: Digestion of dietary lipids

Enzyme	Site of action	Action of the enzyme
Lingual lipase (important in neonates)	Mouth	Triglycerides ⟶ Fatty acids, monoglycerides, glycerol
Lipase/colipase	Pancreas	Triglycerides ⟶ Fatty acids, monoglycerides, glycerol
Phospholipase A/B	Pancreas	Lecithin ⟶ Fatty acid, lysolecithin
Cholesterol esterase	Pancreas	Cholesterol ester ⟶ Cholesterol, fatty acid
Retinyl ester hydrolase	Pancreas	Retinyl ester ⟶ Retinol, fatty acid
Monoglyceride lipase	Small intestine	Monoglyceride ⟶ Glycerol, fatty acid
Lecithinase	Small intestine	Lecithin ⟶ Fatty acids, glycerol, phosphoric acid, choline

- The main enzyme for the hydrolysis of triacylglycerol is the **pancreatic lipase (steapsin)** present in the pancreatic juice. Thus, the main site of lipid digestion is the **small intestine**.
- Pancreatic lipase is an α-lipase and prefers long chain fatty acids, i.e. fatty acids of more than 10 carbon atoms. It also requires a co-lipase. The enzyme specifically attacks ester linkages at 1- and 3-position of a triacylglycerol, leaving mono-acylglycerol with a fatty acid at C2 of glycerol, i.e. a β-monoacylglycerol. The free fatty acids and β-monoacylglycerol are released at the surface of the lipid emulsion droplet and are incorporated into **micelles**.

  Micelles provide a major vehicle for moving lipids from the intestinal lumen to the cell surface where absorption occurs. Micelles also serve as a transport vehicle for cholesterol and lipid soluble vitamins.
- In addition to lipase, pancreatic juice also contains a less specific lipid esterase which acts upon monoacylglycerols, cholesterol esters and esters of retinoic acid.
- Dietary phospholipids are hydrolyzed by specific phospholipases. Pancreatic juice is especially rich in proenzyme for phospholipase A_2 which is activated by trypsin. Phospholipase A_2 also requires bile acids for its activity.

Bile Acids

Bile acids are composed of 24 carbon atoms and are synthesized in the hepatocytes, directly from the cholesterol. **Primary bile acids**, i.e. cholic acid and chenodeoxycholic acid, are derivatives of cholanic acid. They contain two or three OH groups and have a side chain with a carboxyl group which is often conjugated via amide linkage either to glycine or to taurine and form glycocholic acid or taurocholic acid. Since the carboxyl group is ionized at pH 7.0, hence these are named as *bile salts*. They can bind to cations and commonly exist as sodium glycocholate, sodium taurocholate, potassium glycocholate and potassium taurocholate.

Bile acids are secreted into bile canaliculi and carried to the gallbladder for storage and ultimately to the small intestine for excretion. With the removal of one OH group by microorganisms in the gut, the **primary bile acids**, i.e. cholic acid and chenodeoxycholic acid are converted to deoxycholic acid and lithocholic acid, respectively. These are called as **secondary bile acids**. Enterohepatic circulation carries bile acids from the intestine back to the liver.

Functions of bile acids

1. Cholesterol is excreted in the bile as free cholesterol and as bile acids.
2. Bile acids and phospholipids function to solubilize cholesterol in the bile and act as emulsifying agents.
3. Bile acids are the biological detergents; they reversibly form aggregates called micelles (Fig. 9.1) without which dietary lipids cannot be digested and absorbed (Chemistry to Clinics 9.4).
4. Bile acids also play a role in the activation of pancreatic lipase.
5. They also facilitate the absorption of lipid soluble vitamins from the intestine.

Absorption of Lipids

- **Absorption of the products of lipid digestion**, primarily **free fatty acids** (≈70%) and **β-monoacylglycerols** (≈25%), occurs from micelles in the brush border of the enterocytes by passive diffusion. Within the enterocytes, the fate of the absorbed fatty acids depends on their chain-length.

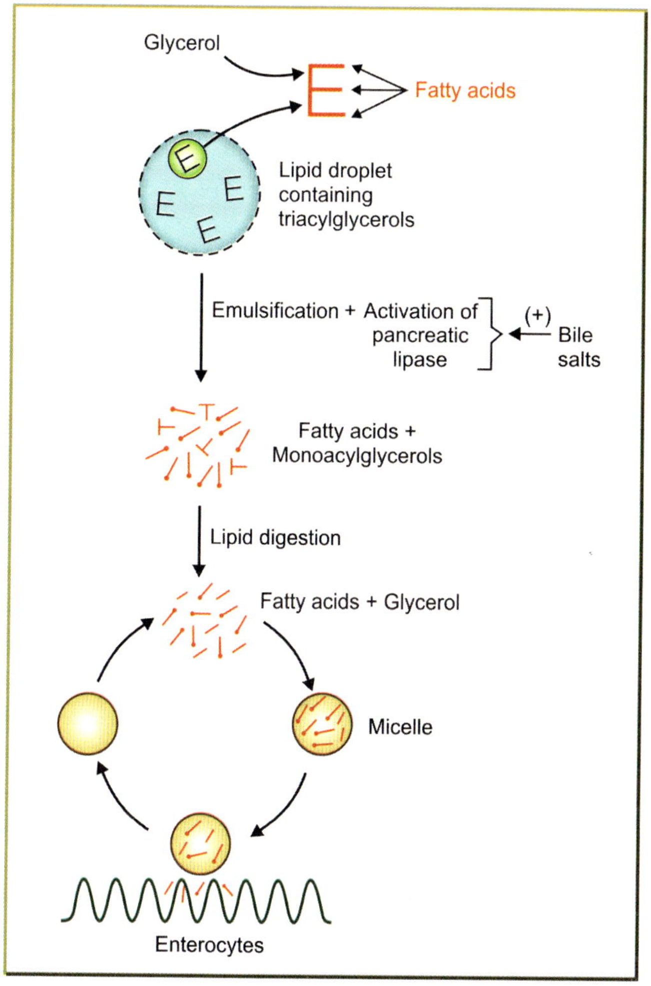

Fig. 9.1: Role of bile salts in emulsification, digestion and absorption of dietary lipids.

Chemistry to Clinics 9.4: Steatorrhea

Digestion and absorption of triacylglycerols is drastically reduced in the absence of bile acids. As a result, a bulk of the dietary lipids is excreted in the stool which becomes clay-colored. This condition is known as steatorrhea. Naturally, the absorption of lipid soluble vitamins is also compromised. The first vitamin whose deficiency becomes manifest clinically is that of vitamin K (increased bleeding tendency after minor cuts). Steatorrhea is commonly seen in obstructive jaundice (impaired flow of bile from the liver to the small intestine) and in advanced cases of hepatic jaundice (decreased hepatic synthesis of bile acids).

– **Short** to **medium chain fatty acids** (4–12 C-atoms) as well as unsaturated fatty acids are absorbed more readily and without any modification. These fatty acids thus reach the liver directly via portal blood, for their utilization in the hepatic tissue.

– On the other hand, **long chain fatty acids**, i.e. those with chain length of >12 C-atoms, bypass the liver. These fatty acids bind to a fatty acid binding protein in the cytoplasm and are transported to the endoplasmic reticulum where they are used for the resynthesis of triacylglycerols. Glycerol required for this purpose is obtained from the absorbed β-monoacylglycerols, and a small amount from glucose, via glycolysis.

- **Absorption of the hydrolyzed products of phospholipids**, i.e. fatty acids, glycerol, phosphoric acid and nitrogenous bases are absorbed along with the digestive products of triacylglycerols. Phospholipids are then resynthesized in the intestinal mucosa and form a part of the chylomicrons.

- **Cholesterol is absorbed** in the free form but is re-esterified in the intestinal mucosa. Cholesterol esters are also incorporated into the chylomicrons.

Formation of Chylomicrons

The resynthesized **triacylglycerols** form **fat globules** onto which phospholipids and some specific proteins, designated as apoproteins, are absorbed. Within the membrane bound vesicles, the complexes migrate through Golgi apparatus to the basolateral plasma membrane and released into the intercellular space. Since these fat globules are several microns in diameter and are released from the intestine as milky juice via lymph vessels called chyle, these fat globules are termed as chylomicrons. Apolipoprotein B is essential for the release of chylomicrons from enterocytes into the lymphatics.

Thus, *all dietary lipids*, i.e. triacylglycerols, phospholipids, free and esterified cholesterol along with the apoproteins (apolipoproteins) are incorporated into and released as chylomicrons (Fig. 9.2). Via the thoracic duct, intestinal lymph vessels drain into the large veins and thus (through blood), dietary triacylglycerols finally reach the peripheral tissues (Chemistry to Clinics 9.5).

Chemistry to Clinics 9.5: Chyluria

An obstruction to the thoracic duct may result in milky appearance of the urine. This is due to the reason that lymph vessels of the urinary tract become distended and burst thereby allowing lymph to pass directly into the urine. Hence, this condition, i.e. the presence of chylomicrons in the urine, is called as chyluria. It is common in endemic zones of lymphatic filariasis.

9

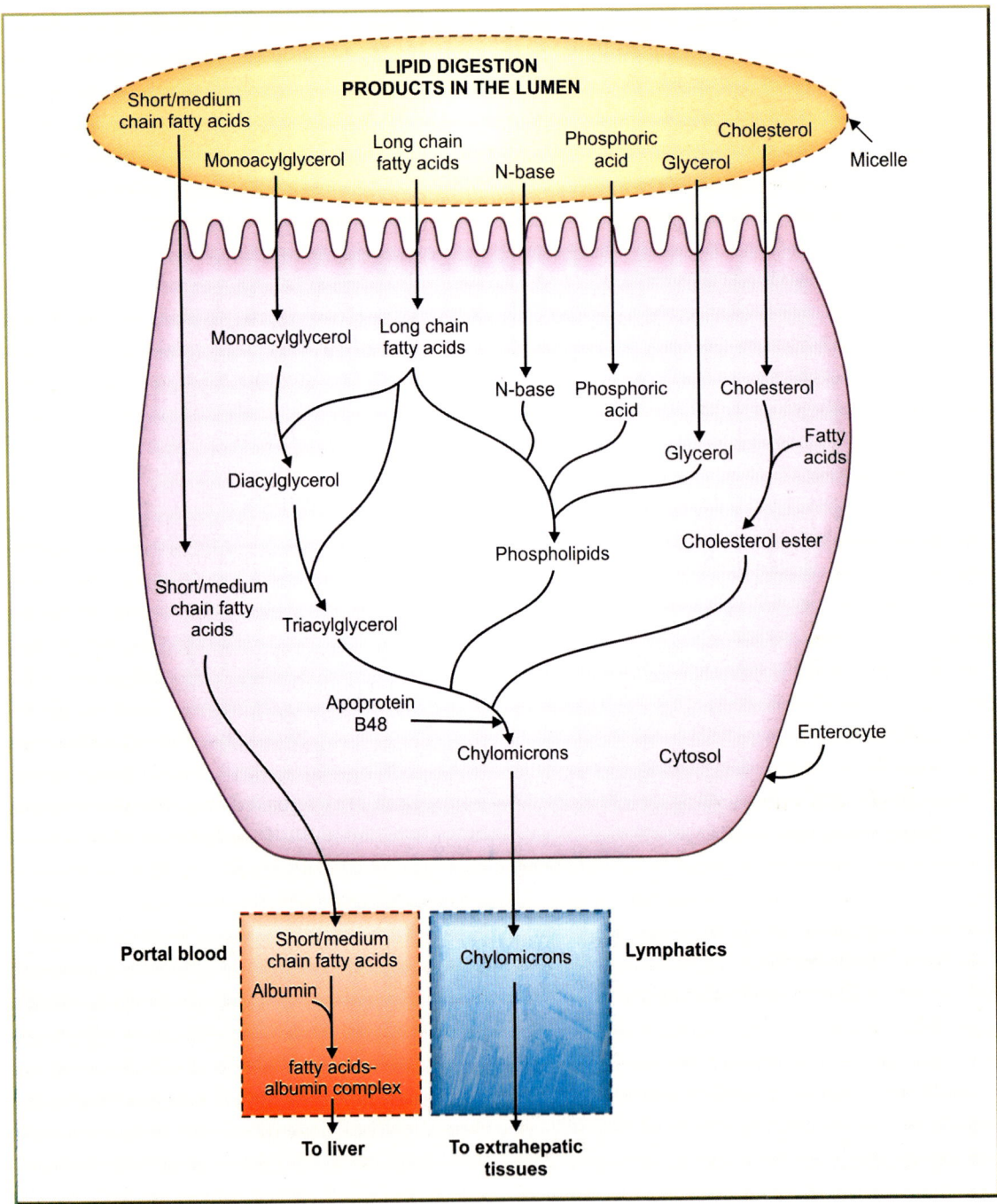

Fig. 9.2: Lipid absorption in the intestine.

Cells of the adipose tissues and the muscles take up large amounts of these dietary lipids for either storage or metabolism, and bypass the liver from a lipid overload after a meal. Intestinal lipid absorption is associated with a marked increase in lymph flow called the **lymphagogic effect of fat feeding**. This increase in lymph flow plays an important role in the transfer of lipoproteins from the intercellular spaces to the central lacteal. Apoprotein A–IV (apo A–IV) secreted by the small intestine, may be an important factor contributing to anorexia after fat feeding.

DIGESTION AND ABSORPTION OF PROTEINS

Digestion of Dietary Proteins

Digestion of proteins begins with the hydrolysis of peptide bonds which link successive amino acid residues together, in a polypeptide chain. The process is known as **proteolysis** and enzymes responsible for the hydrolysis of peptide linkages are called 'proteases' or 'peptidases'. Endo-acting proteases (acting on peptide linkages other than N- or C-terminal peptide bonds) are called '**endopeptidases**' or '**proteinases**' whereas exo-acting proteases (acting on N- or C-terminal peptide bonds) are called '**exopeptidases**'.

Proteolytic digestion of the dietary proteins takes place in the gastrointestinal tract and is carried out by proteases secreted by the stomach, the pancreas and the small intestine:

- Digestion of proteins starts *in the stomach* by the action of a proteolytic enzyme **pepsin**, at pH of the gastric juice (1.5–2.5). Pepsin is secreted by chief cells of the gastric mucosa in the form of a zymogen (proenzyme) called **pepsinogen A** which is activated by hydrogen ions of the gastric juice (HCl) and later on autocatalytically by the pepsin itself (Fig. 9.3).

  Pepsin preferentially hydrolyzes peptide linkages towards the amino group of either an aromatic

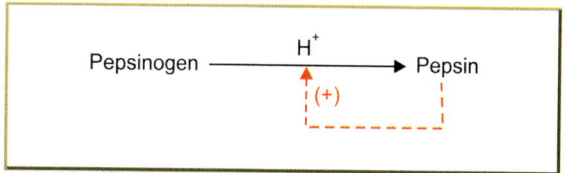

Fig. 9.3: Activation of pepsinogen.

amino acid, i.e. phenylalanine, tyrosine or tryptophan or a dicarboxylic acid, i.e. aspartate or glutamate (Fig. 9.4). In infants, another enzyme rennin hydrolyzes milk protein casein.

- Proteolytic products of pepsin pass on to the *small intestine* where they are attacked by proteases that are secreted by the pancreas, i.e. trypsin, chymotrypsin and carboxypeptidases.

  – **Trypsin** is secreted in the zymogen form as **trypsinogen** (Fig. 9.5) which is converted to trypsin by another enzyme called enterokinase (enteropeptidase) which acts as an activator of trypsinogen and is secreted by the intestinal mucosa. Once trypsin is formed, it acts on trypsinogen and converts it to trypsin, autocatalytically. Trypsin is most effective on a partially digested protein and hydrolyzes peptide linkages formed by carboxylate group contributed by a basic amino acid, i.e. arginine or lysine (Fig. 9.6).

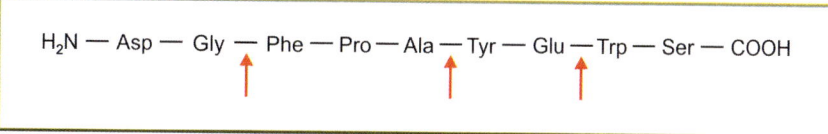

Fig. 9.4: Sites of action of pepsin.

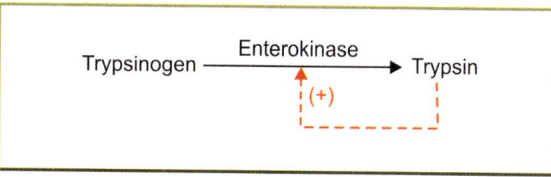

Fig. 9.5: Activation of trypsinogen.

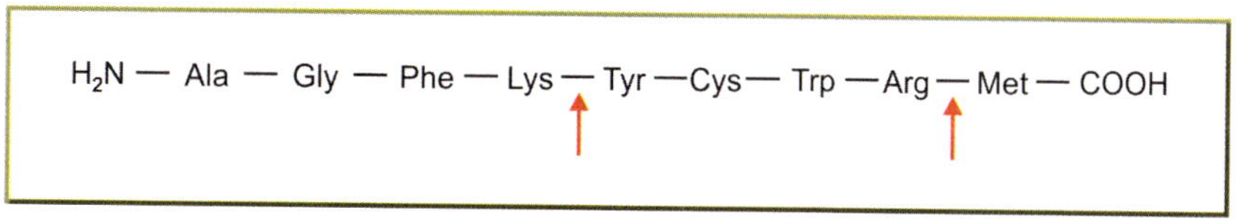

Fig. 9.6: Sites of action of trypsin.

9

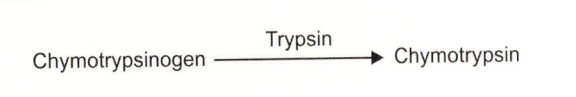

Fig. 9.7: Activation of chymotrypsinogen.

– **Chymotrypsin** is also synthesized and secreted as a zymogen designated as **chymotrypsinogen** (Fig. 9.7). It is activated by trypsin. It preferentially cleaves peptide bonds involving the carboxyl group contributed by the aromatic amino acids as well as those of leucine, methionine, asparagine and histidine (Fig. 9.8).

– Pancreatic juice also contains collagenase and elastase which specifically act on collagen and elastin, respectively.

– In addition to the above endopeptidases, two exopeptidases are also secreted by the pancreatic juice in the zymogen forms. These are pro-carboxypeptidase A and procarboxypeptidase B. These zymogens are also activated by trypsin (Fig. 9.9). These two enzymes attack peptide linkages specifically those having a free carboxyl group. **Carboxypeptidase A** hydrolyzes the C-terminal amino acid in peptides particularly of those where the terminal amino acid is an aromatic or aliphatic amino acid while **carboxypeptidase B** hydrolyzes the terminal peptide bond of the basic amino acids (arginine and lysine).

• The digestion of proteins thereafter is completed by the action of **aminopeptidases** and **dipeptidases** which are secreted by mucosa of the small intestine.

Absorption of Amino Acids

The end products of digestion of proteins are amino acids which are absorbed from the small intestine into the portal blood. Amino acid content of the portal blood rises only temporarily during digestion of proteins, indicating that absorption mechanisms are so efficient that amino acids are absorbed immediately after they are formed from digestion of proteins.

Absorption of L-amino acids is a Na^+-dependent active transport and requires ATP and specific transport proteins. Pyridoxal phosphate (vitamin B_6) is also required for the absorption of amino acids.

• Both an L-amino acid and the Na^+ attach to the carrier protein which is present on the mucosal surface of the microvillous membrane and form L-amino acid-carrier protein-Na^+ complex.

• The complex passes into the inner surface of the membrane and dissociates to liberate free amino acid and Na^+ (Fig. 3.13, Chapter 3).

• Carrier protein returns to the brush border while the amino acid, through portal blood, enters the liver. On the other hand, Na^+ is actively pumped out of the cell membrane by the Na^+/K^+ pump. At the same time, ATP is hydrolyzed by ATPase, to release energy required for this process.

At least seven different brush-border specific transport systems have been identified for the uptake of different classes of L-amino acids and the dipeptides in the luminal membrane. These include:

1. A carrier for neutral amino acids with short or polar side chains, such as for Ala, Ser and Thr;

2. A carrier for neutral amino acids with an aromatic or hydrophobic side chain, such as for Phe, Tyr, Met, Val, Leu and Ile;

3. A specific carrier for imino acids, i.e. for Pro and hydroxyproline (HO-Pro);

4. A separate carrier for Lys, Arg and Cystine (Cys-Cys);

5. A carrier for acidic amino acids, i.e. for Asp and Glu;

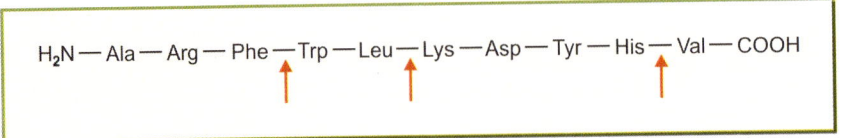

Fig. 9.8: Sites of action of chymotrypsin.

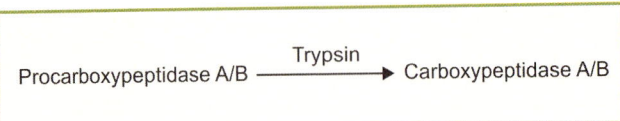

Fig. 9.9: Activation of procarboxypeptidase A and B.

6. A separate carrier for β-amino acids, e.g. for β-Ala and taurine; and

7. A separate carrier for dipeptides, e.g. peptide-1 (pep-1), glycylsarcosine, etc. The dipeptides are absorbed through the intestinal cells where they are hydrolyzed by dipeptidases to the constituent amino acids.

Besides, the small intestine of the fetus and the neonate can absorb intact proteins by endocytosis (pinocytosis).

Glutathione also participates in the active transport of L-amino acids in some of the tissues such as in the small intestine, kidneys and liver. The process is called group-translocation (Fig. 3.11, Chapter 3).

Absorption of amino acids may be affected in specific transport disorders or other diseases involving the small intestine or the immune system (Chemistry to Clinics 9.6 and 9.7).

Chemistry to Clinics 9.6: Genetic Disorders of Amino Acid Transport Carriers

• **Hartnup's disease:** It is a genetic lesion in epithelial amino acid transport named after the family in which the disease was first recognized. The transport and absorption of neutral amino acids including that of tryptophan is decreased in epithelial cells of the small intestine and proximal tubules of the kidney. The intestinal defect results in malabsorption of free amino acids from the diet. The inability to reabsorb amino acids by the kidney manifests in the excretion of neutral amino acids including that of tryptophan and other indole derivatives in the urine resulting in **neutral amino aciduria**. Symptoms of the disease are mainly those due to essential amino acid and nicotinamide deficiencies. Due to tryptophan deficiency there are **pellagra like features**, such as dermatitis, diarrhoea and dementia. Women are more susceptible to pellagra since kynurenine hydroxylase (an enzyme of the tryptophan-niacin pathway) is inhibited by estrogen.

• **Cystinuria:** It involves the carrier for sulfur-containing amino acids (e.g. cystine) and the basic amino acids (e.g. lysine and arginine). Because the apical membrane of enterocytes also possess a peptide transport system that is unaffected in these disorders, treatment with supplemental dipeptides containing the specific amino acids is possible. However, the treatment fails if the renal transporter is also involved as in the case of cystinuria.

Chemistry to Clinics 9.7: Celiac Disease

It is also called **celiac sprue** or **gluten-sensitive enteropathy**, a common disease caused by the sensitivity of the small intestine to gluten, the protein present in cereal grains such as wheat, barley, rye and oats. Wheat gluten proteins consist of two major fractions: the gliadins (monomeric) and the glutenins (polymeric). Tissue transglutaminase (tTG, an enzyme present in many tissues including small intestine) is the autoantigen in celiac disease since anti-tTG antibodies (IgA and IgG) are found in the sera of these patients. Besides, anti-gliadin antibodies are also found. Upon exposure to gliadins, tTG modifies the proteins which then bind to specific HLA molecules in the intestine to trigger an inflammatory reaction.

It is important to note that celiac disease is different from '**wheat allergy**' characterized by an exaggerated mast cell-mediated IgE response to wheat proteins.

The disorder can result in the malabsorption of all nutrients as a result of the shortening or total loss of intestinal villi, which reduces the mucosal enzymes for nutrient digestion and the mucosal surface for absorption. The elimination of dietary gluten is a standard treatment for these patients. Occasionally, the symptoms are improved with glucocorticoid therapy because of the immunosuppressive and anti-inflammatory actions of these hormones. tTG is a potential target for therapeutic intervention.

SOME IMPORTANT QUESTIONS

1. Briefly discuss the following:

i. Digestion of dietary carbohydrates
ii. Absorption of monosaccharides
iii. Digestion of dietary lipids
iv. Absorption of fatty acids
v. Digestion of dietary proteins
vi. Absorption of amino acids
vii. Malabsorption

2. Write notes on:

i. Lactose intolerance
ii. Hexose malabsorption
iii. Bile acids
iv. Micelles
v. Steatorrhea
vi. Hartnup's disease
vii. Cystinuria
viii. Celiac disease

9

MULTIPLE CHOICE QUESTIONS

1. **Salivary amylase acts on:**
   A. 1,4 α-glycosidic linkage, randomly
   B. 1,4 β-glycosidic linkage, randomly
   C. 1,4 α-glycosidic linkage, from terminal end only
   D. 1,4 β-glycosidic linkage, from terminal end only

2. **Generally, lactase activity is highest:**
   A. Immediately after birth
   B. In children
   C. In young adults
   D. In elderly

3. **The lowest intestinal absorption rate is of:**
   A. Fructose
   B. Glucose
   C. Galactose
   D. All are absorbed at equal rates

4. **Sodium glucose transporter-1 (SGLT-1) is:**
   A. Present in apical membrane of enterocytes
   B. Inhibited by ouabain
   C. Inhibited by phlorhizin
   D. All of the above

5. **Pancreatic lipase hydrolyzes triacylglycerol preferentially at:**
   A. C1, C2
   B. C2, C3
   C. C1, C3
   D. C1, C2, C3

6. **The following is most commonly observed in steatorrhea:**
   A. Increased bleeding tendency
   B. Night blindness
   C. Bone pain
   D. Painful micturition

7. **Pepsin cleaves peptide bonds where amino group is contributed by:**
   A. Aromatic amino acids
   B. Aspartate
   C. Glutamate
   D. Any of the above

8. **The intestinal absorption of amino acids requires:**
   A. Vitamin B_6
   B. Niacin
   C. Vitamin B_1
   D. Folic acid

9. **The following is not true for Hartnup's disease:**
   A. Neutral aminoaciduria
   B. Pellagra-like features
   C. Genetic defect in epithelial amino acid transport
   D. Inability to absorb basic amino acids and sulfur-containing amino acids

10. **The following is true for cystinuria:**
    A. Neutral aminoaciduria
    B. Pellagra-like features
    C. Acquired defect in epithelial amino acid transport
    D. Inability to absorb basic amino acids and sulfur-containing amino acids

Biological Oxidation and Oxidative Phosphorylation

Cells possess a complicated system of energy producing and energy utilizing chemical reactions. The reactions involved in energy generation result in the breakdown of complex macromolecules such as carbohydrates, lipids and proteins, to the smaller molecules like pyruvate and acetyl CoA, and ultimately to CO_2 and H_2O with the liberation of energy. These **catabolic pathways** require oxygen and thus the process of oxidation of nutrients in biological systems is designated as **biological oxidation**.

The metabolic pathways involved in the biosynthesis of complex macromolecules from smaller precursors are called as the **anabolic pathways** and require the expenditure of energy. Besides anabolic processes, requirement for energy is also for performing various tissue specific cellular functions, active transport systems by which compounds or ions can be moved across biological membranes against a concentration gradient, nerve impulse conduction, muscle contraction, thermogenesis, transfer of genetic information and growth (Fig. 10.1).

BIOENERGETICS

The potential energy is inherent in various macromolecules in the form of chemical bonds and reducing equivalents. This is released after these molecules undergo oxidation either through combustion or through controlled catabolic oxidation, as it happens

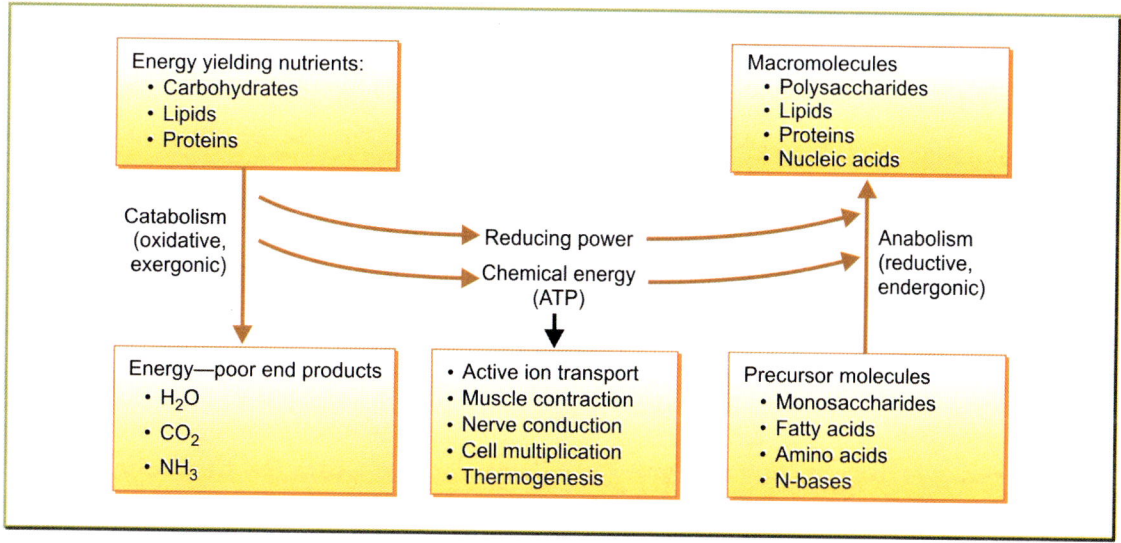

Fig. 10.1: Energy producing and energy utilizing processes.

10

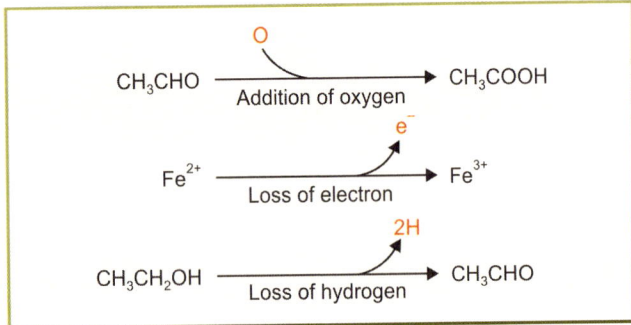

Fig. 10.2: Oxidation.

Table 10.1: Redox potentials of some redox systems

Redox system	E_0' (Volt)
NADH/NAD$^+$	−0.32
Succinate/fumarate	−0.03
FADH$_2$/FAD	0.0
Coenzyme Q.H$_2$/CoQ	0.10
Cytochrome b (Fe^{2+}/Fe^{3+})	0.12
Cytochrome c$_1$ (Fe^{2+}/Fe^{3+})	0.22
Cytochrome a (Fe^{2+}/Fe^{3+})	0.29
Cytochrome a$_3$ (Fe^{2+}/Fe^{3+})	0.39
H$_2$O/½O$_2$	0.82

within the cell. **Oxidation** thus refers to the state of addition of oxygen or loss of electrons or loss of hydrogen (Fig. 10.2).

Reversal of these states is termed as **reduction**. Since there is no free flow of electrons or atoms, a compound 'X' gets oxidized only when an equivalent amount of the other compound 'Y' is simultaneously reduced. In a chemical reaction, we therefore have two **oxidation-reduction systems**, e.g. X_{red}/X_{ox} and Y_{red}/Y_{ox}. In a biological system, X and Y refer to two compounds, one of which is a substrate while the other one is usually a cofactor.

Oxidation-Reduction Potential

Various substances or systems differ in their affinity for electrons. This affinity of an oxidation-reduction system for electrons is referred to as oxidation-reduction potential or **redox potential** (E_0). The redox potential of a system is usually compared against the potential of hydrogen electrode which at pH 0 is designated as 0.0 volt (0.0 V).

Standard Redox Potential

In a biological system, oxidation and reduction occur at physiological temperature and pressure, carried out by various enzymes, and the hydrogen and electron carrier systems. The redox potential at physiological pH is expressed as standard redox potential (E_0'). The value of standard redox potential of a hydrogen electrode is −0.42 V.

A biological system which has a strong tendency to donate electrons, i.e. to oxidize other systems, has a **negative redox potential**. On the other hand, the system which has a strong tendency to accept electrons, i.e. reduce other systems, has a **positive**

redox potential. The redox potentials of some of the redox systems are given in Table 10.1.

Free Energy (ΔG) and its Significance

When two oxidation-reduction systems, as mentioned above (i.e. a substrate and a cofactor), react with one another, the difference in redox potential between the two systems (designated as $\Delta E'_0$) is related to the changing free energy of the reaction, as per the following equation:

$$\Delta G^{o'} = -nF\Delta E_0'$$

The free energy released ($\Delta G^{o'}$) is directly proportional to the difference in the standard reduction potential (E'_0) between the parameters of the redox pair, where $\Delta G^{o'}$ is the standard free energy change in calories, n is the number of electrons transferred and F is a constant called Faraday (the electric charge carried by one gram equivalent and its value is 23,080 calories). The concept of ΔG is useful to understand:

1. *Exergonic/endergonic reactions*: Spontaneous processes, at constant temperature and pressure, are said to be **exergonic**, and have **negative ΔG$^{o'}$** values (−ΔG$^{o'}$). On the other hand, the processes that do not occur spontaneously have **positive ΔG$^{o'}$** values (+ΔG$^{o'}$). These are said to be **endergonic** and are driven by the input of free energy. In a reversible set of reactions, if a reaction is exergonic, it releases energy but when it proceeds in the reverse direction, it is driven by the input of free energy and is said to be endergonic. At equilibrium, when the forward and the back-ward reactions are exactly balanced, ΔG$^{o'}$ is zero (ΔG$^{o'}$ = 0).

2. *Energy homeostasis*: Catabolic degradation of macromolecules liberates energy which is required to drive various energy requiring processes. A part of this liberated energy is salvaged in high-energy

intermediates whose subsequent exergonic breakdown drives endergonic processes. These intermediates thus form a sort of 'free energy currency' through which energy-producing reactions pay for the energy-consuming processes occurring in biological systems (Fig. 10.1).

3. *High energy compounds*: This is discussed below.

HIGH-ENERGY COMPOUNDS

There are several compounds, esters and mixed anhydrides, which on hydrolysis of their high energy bonds yield nearly 10.0–15.0 kcal/mol, e.g. phosphoenolpyruvate, 1,3-bisphosphoglycerate, etc. These compounds are called as high-energy compounds or **phosphagens** including active phosphate carriers such as the various nucleoside triphosphates, e.g. ATP, GTP, CTP and UTP as well as the metabolites like 1,3-bisphosphoglycerate, phosphoenolpyruvate and creatine phosphate.

Besides, there are several relatively inert phosphate compounds called ester phosphates, like glucose-6-phosphate. These compounds yield relatively less energy, nearly 3.0 kcal/mol.

Adenosine-5'-Triphosphate

Adenosine triphosphate (**ATP**) is a nucleoside triphosphate in which adenine is attached in a glycosidic linkage to D-ribose. Three phosphoryl groups are sequentially linked to the fifth position of the ribose moiety via a phosphoester bond followed by two phosphoanhydride bonds. The two terminal phosphoryl groups (i.e. γ and β phosphoryl groups) are involved in phosphoric acid anhydride bondings and are designated as the **energy-rich bonds** or **high-energy bonds** which are symbolized by the squiggle (~). ATP can therefore be represented as A-R-P~P~P (Fig. 10.3).

ATP is a high-energy intermediate, which occurs in all forms of life and is a primary cellular energy currency. Synthesis of ATP as a result of the catabolic processes or utilization of ATP in an energy dependent cellular function thus involves formation and either hydrolysis or transfer of the terminal phosphate group of ATP. When the terminal (γ) phosphate group of ATP is removed by hydrolysis, the reaction is strongly exothermic, yielding 7.3 to 7.8 kcal/mol (Fig. 10.4). Energy release from an ATP molecule occurs by enzymatic hydrolysis of the anhydride bond

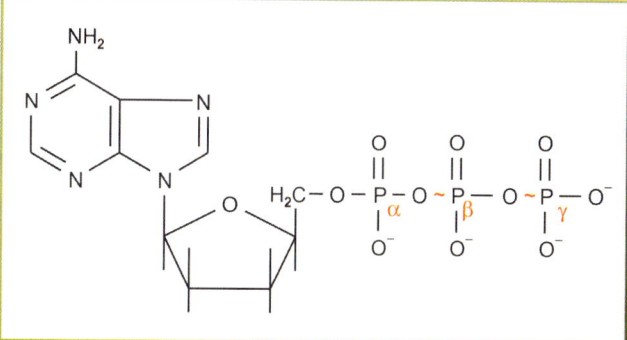

Fig. 10.3: ATP (~ = High energy bonds).

Fig. 10.4: Hydrolysis of ATP with release of energy.

connecting β- and γ-phosphates. Products of this hydrolysis are ADP and a free phosphate group (Pi).

Standard free energy of phosphate hydrolysis of some phosphorylated compounds of biological interest is listed in Table 10.2.

The universal cellular energy currency: As shown in Table 10.2, **ATP** occupies a middle rank with respect to the standard free energy of phosphate hydrolysis of various high energy phosphorylated compounds, since it is continually hydrolyzed as well as regenerated. After the phosphoanhydride hydrolysis of ATP, it can be regenerated by coupling its formation to a more exergonic metabolic process such as by the direct transfer of a phosphoryl group from another high-energy compound, like phosphoenolpyruvate

Table 10.2: Phosphorylated compounds of biological significance

Phosphorylated compound	Free energy of hydrolysis ($-\Delta G^{o}$/kcal/mol)
Phosphoenolpyruvate	14.8
1,3-Bisphosphoglycerate	11.8
Creatine phosphate	10.5
ATP	7.3*
Glucose-1-phosphate	5.0
Glucose-6-phosphate	3.3
AMP	2.2

*ATP occupies a central position, hence it is called the universal cellular energy currency.

10

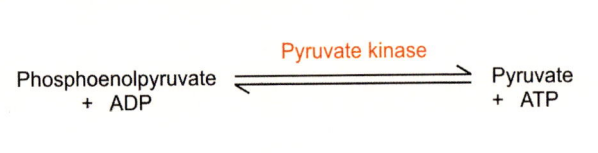

Fig. 10.5. Exergonic cleavage of phosphoenolpyruvate coupled with the regeneration of ATP.

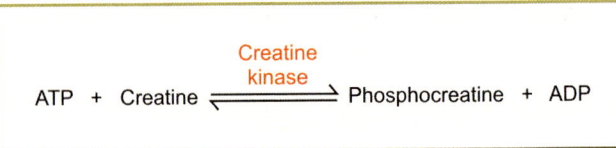

Fig. 10.6: Creatine kinase reaction.

(Fig. 10.5). Thus, there is a flow of energy from high energy phosphate compounds, such as 1,3-bis-phosphoglycerate to form ATP and from ATP to form low-energy compounds, such as glucose-6-phosphate and glycerol-3-phosphate whose free energy of hydrolysis is much below than the preceding high energy compound.

Coupled Reactions

Exergonic reactions of high energy compounds can be coupled to endergonic processes to drive them to completion and as long as the overall pathway is exergonic, these will operate in the forward direction. For example, the exergonic hydrolysis of ATP and release of ADP and Pi provides free energy for various processes in the body, such as for muscular contraction or transmembrane active transport.

Enol Phosphates

Several **phospho-anhydrides (enol-phosphates)** such as 1,3-bisphosphoglycerate and acyl-phosphates also have phosphoryl-group transfer potentials. ATP can therefore be regenerated from ADP by direct transfer of the phosphoryl-group from such a high-energy compound. This type of reaction is referred to as **'substrate level phosphorylation'**. Such compounds rank above ATP and are referred to as **high-energy phosphate donors**. On the other hand, there are other compounds such as glucose-6-phosphate and glycerol-3-phosphate, whose free-energy of hydrolysis is much less than the high-energy compounds mentioned above. Such compounds are referred to as the **low-energy phosphate acceptors** and rank below ATP in position.

Other Nucleoside Triphosphates

Various nucleoside triphosphates other than ATP such as CTP, GTP and UTP or the deoxynucleoside triphosphates, required for the synthesis of nucleic acids are also synthesized from ATP and the corresponding nucleoside diphosphates.

Phosphorylamidines

Phosphorylamidines or phosphoguanidines such as phosphocreatine and phosphoarginine, called phosphagens, have high phosphoryl-group transfer potentials. Phosphocreatine acts as an ATP buffer in cells that contain creatine kinase, such as muscle and nerve cells, which have a high ATP turnover (Fig. 10.6).

The intracellular concentrations of the reactants and the products however, operate close to equilibrium ($\Delta G^{\circ\prime} = 0$). Accordingly, when the cell is in a resting state and ATP concentration is relatively high, the reaction proceeds towards the synthesis of phospho-creatine. On the other hand, at the time of high metabolic activity when ATP concentration is low, the equilibrium shifts so as to yield ATP from phosphocreatine and ADP.

Pyrophosphate Cleavage

In some of the reactions such as attachment of amino acids to tRNA during protein synthesis, hydrolysis of ATP results in the pyrophosphate cleavage and yields AMP and PPi (pyrophosphate). Thereafter, PPi is rapidly hydrolyzed to 2 molecules of Pi. Thus, pyrophosphate cleavage of ATP ultimately consumes two high-energy phospho-anhydride bonds. These types of reactions are two step reactions where both the steps are readily reversible. The overall reaction is driven to completion by the irreversible hydrolysis of PPi (Fig. 10.7).

Thioesters

Thioesters, such as acetyl CoA (Fig. 10.8) and succinyl CoA, also act as high-energy compounds and a thioester bond is involved in substrate-level phosphorylation. Cleavage of succinyl CoA releases

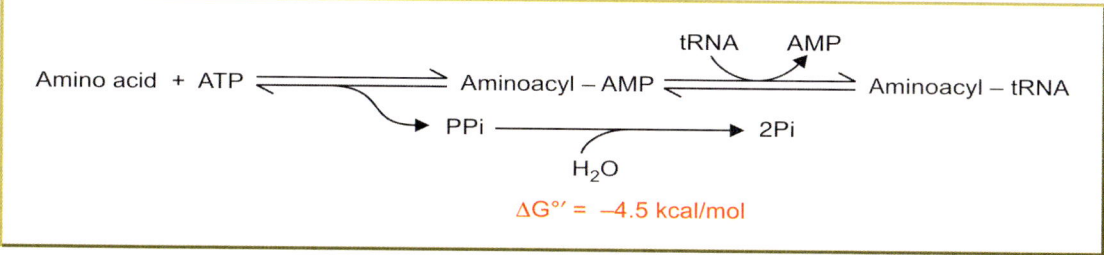

Fig. 10.7: Pyrophosphate cleavage.

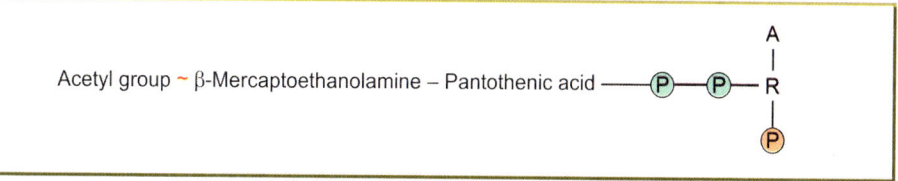

Fig. 10.8: Acetyl CoA.

sufficient free-energy to synthesize GTP from GDP and Pi, in the citric acid cycle.

Coenzyme A

Coenzyme A (HSCoA or CoA) consists of a β-mercaptoethanolamine group which is linked through an amide linkage to the vitamin pantothenic acid, which in turn is attached to the 3'- phosphoadenosine moiety via a pyrophosphate bridge (Fig. 10.9).

CoA functions as a carrier of the acetyl and other acyl groups. The formation of the thioester bond in a metabolic intermediate conserves a portion of the free energy of oxidation of a metabolic fuel and that free energy is used to drive the exergonic process.

The acetyl group in acetyl CoA is bound as a thio-ester to the sulfhydryl portion of the β-mercapto-ethanolamine (Fig. 10.8). Thus, acetyl CoA is also a high-energy compound. $\Delta G^{o'}$ for the hydrolysis of its thioester bond is –7.8 Kcal/mol which makes this reaction slightly more exergonic than the hydrolysis of ATP.

REDUCING EQUIVALENTS

As we know, lipids have greater caloric value (9 kcal/g) than carbohydrates and proteins (4 kcal/g). This is related to the oxidation state of the carbon atoms, which, in lipids are more reduced (or less oxidized) than those in carbohydrates or proteins which are comparatively more oxidized (or less reduced). Hence, during sequential breakdown of lipids, more reducing equivalents are extracted than from carbohydrates or proteins (Fig. 10.10).

A reducing equivalent thus may be defined as a proton plus electron ($H^+ + e^-$). These are utilized for ATP synthesis in the mitochondrial energy transduction sequence. To transduce this reducing power into utilizable energy, mitochondria have a system of electron carriers in the inner mitochondrial membrane. In the presence of O_2, this system of electron carriers converts reducing equivalents into utilizable energy by the process called **electron transport system**.

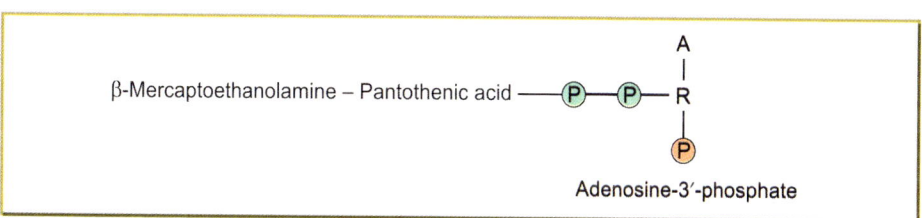

Fig. 10.9: Coenzyme A.

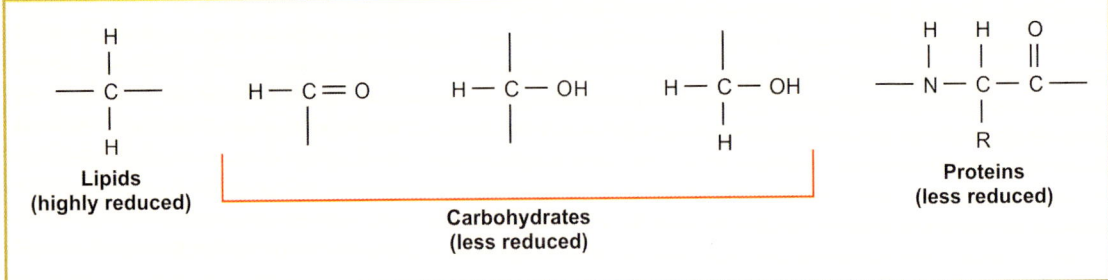

Fig. 10.10: State of different carbon atoms in a nutrient molecule.

ROLE OF ENZYMES IN BIOLOGICAL OXIDATION

Biological oxidation occurs either by the addition of oxygen or by the removal of hydrogen and/or electrons. These reactions are catalyzed by a class of enzymes termed as oxidoreductases and may be grouped as oxidases, oxygenases, hydroxylases or peroxidases (Table 10.3).

Oxidoreductases which remove hydrogen from a substrate and are involved in electron transfer may be grouped as **dehydrogenases**. Certain dehydrogenases which catalyze the removal of hydrogen atoms from a substrate and pass it directly to oxygen are called **aerobic dehydrogenases**, whereas **anaerobic dehydrogenases** catalyze the transfer of hydrogen from a substrate or some acceptor metabolite to another metabolite or some other acceptor molecule. The acceptor molecule may be a coenzyme, and may act as a cosubstrate (Table 10.4). As a result, the reduced substrate (e.g. AH_2) gets oxidized (AH_2 is converted to A) while the oxidized form of the cosubstrate such as NAD^+ or FAD, becomes reduced (NADH or $FADH_2$). Through the sequential transfer, the hydrogens and the electrons are ultimately transferred to molecular oxygen which is reduced to water.

Table 10.3: Oxidoreductases

Enzyme	Examples
Oxidases	Cytochrome oxidase
	Ascorbate oxidase
	Amino acid oxidase
Oxygenases	Tryptophan dioxygenase
	Homogentisate oxygenase
Hydroxylases	Phenylalanine hydroxylase
	Tyrosine hydroxylase
Peroxidases	Glutathione peroxidase
	Catalase

Table 10.4: Coenzyme-dependent dehydrogenases

Coenzyme	Examples
NAD	Alcohol dehydrogenase
	Lactate dehydrogenase
NADP	Glucose-6-phosphate dehydrogenase
	6-Phosphogluconate dehydrogenase
FAD	Succinate dehydrogenase

SHUTTLE SYSTEMS

The inner mitochondrial membrane is impermeable to various metabolites including NADH and $FADH_2$ which are produced in the cytosol during many biochemical reactions (e.g. glycolysis). There, however, exist several shuttle systems for the transport of reducing equivalents from the cytosol into the mitochondria. Two most common shuttles which transport these reducing equivalents include the malate-aspartate shuttle and the glycerophosphate shuttle.

Malate-Aspartate Shuttle

- In the cytosol, with the help of reducing equivalents (from the cytosolic NADH), oxaloacetate is reduced (by malate dehydrogenase) to malate and gets transported into mitochondria. In the matrix, after its reoxidation to oxaloacetate by the mitochondrial isoform of the same enzyme, malate releases its reducing equivalents.
- Oxaloacetate is impermeable through the mitochondrial membrane. Glutamate oxaloacetate transaminase, transaminates oxaloacetate to aspartate, and glutamate to α-ketoglutarate.
- Aspartate and α-ketoglutarate are transported through the mitochondrial membrane to the cytosol by the α-ketoglutarate transporter and the glutamate-aspartate transporter, respectively. Aspartate is reconverted back to oxaloacetate.

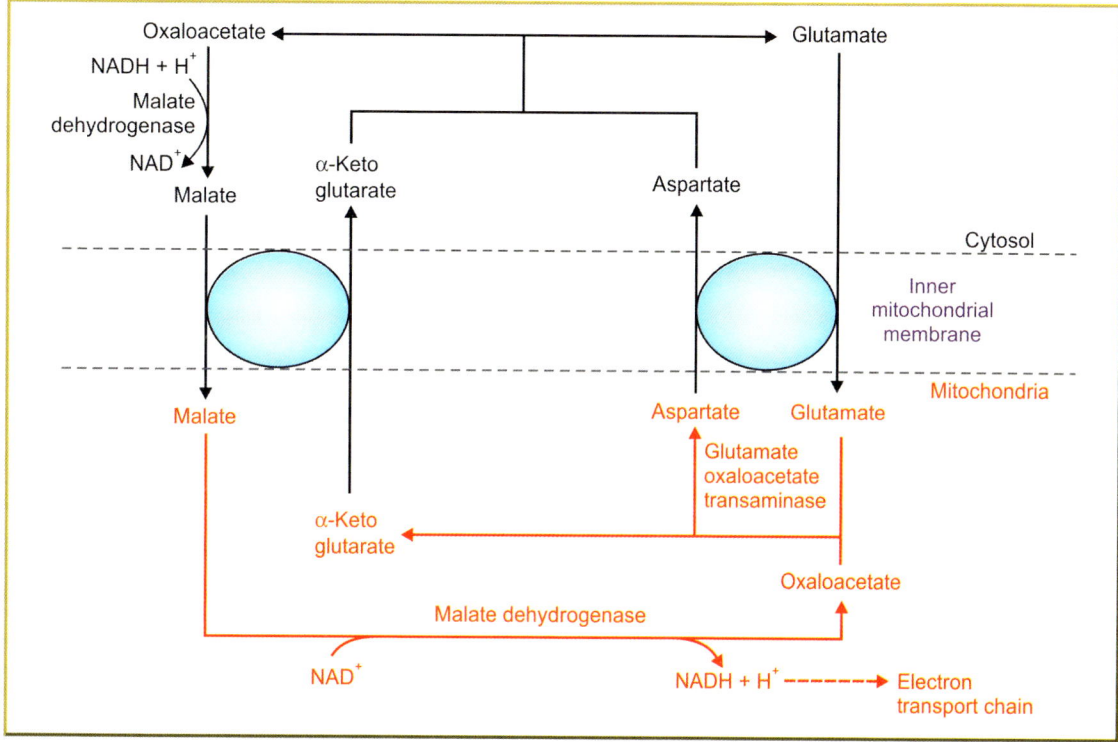

Fig. 10.11: Malate-aspartate shuttle.

- Thus, the cytosolic reducing equivalents are transported to the mitochondria for their entry into the electron transport chain (Fig. 10.11).
- This shuttle is more efficient compared with the glycerophosphate shuttle and is more widely distributed, e.g. in heart, kidney, liver, etc.

Glycerophosphate Shuttle

- Through the glycerophosphate shuttle, electrons are transported to the mitochondrial electron-transport chain via FAD.
- With the help of dihydroxyacetone phosphate, 3-phosphoglycerol dehydrogenase catalyzes the oxidation of cytosolic NADH to NAD^+ and reenters glycolysis.
- The electrons from 3-phosphoglycerol (glycerol phosphate) are transferred to a flavoprotein dehydrogenase. This oxidation of 3-phosphoglycerol results in the reduction of FAD to $FADH_2$.
- Since, flavoprotein dehydrogenase is situated on the outer surface of the inner mitochondrial membrane, it supplies electrons directly to the electron transport chain and results in the re-oxidation of $FADH_2$ to FAD.

- Thus, the cytosolic reducing equivalents are transported to the mitochondria for their entry into the electron transport chain (Fig. 10.12).
- This shuttle is limited to tissues like brain and white muscle.

ELECTRON TRANSPORT CHAIN

During catabolic reactions, there is generation of reducing equivalents in the TCA cycle, the β-oxidation sequence of fatty acids and various other dehydrogenase reactions. Although either of the two nicotinamide nucleotides, i.e. NAD^+ or $NADP^+$, may be involved in various metabolic reactions, reduced NADP, however, is not a substrate for the mitochondrial respiratory chain since it is used in reductive biosynthetic reactions, such as in the biosynthesis of fatty acids and cholesterol. Reducing equivalents from NADH enter the chain.

The electrons transferred from the cytosol to the mitochondria participate in the sequential oxidation-reduction of various redox centers in four enzyme complexes in the mitochondria. The sequence of electron carriers is called **electron transport chain**. It roughly reflects their relative reduction potentials so

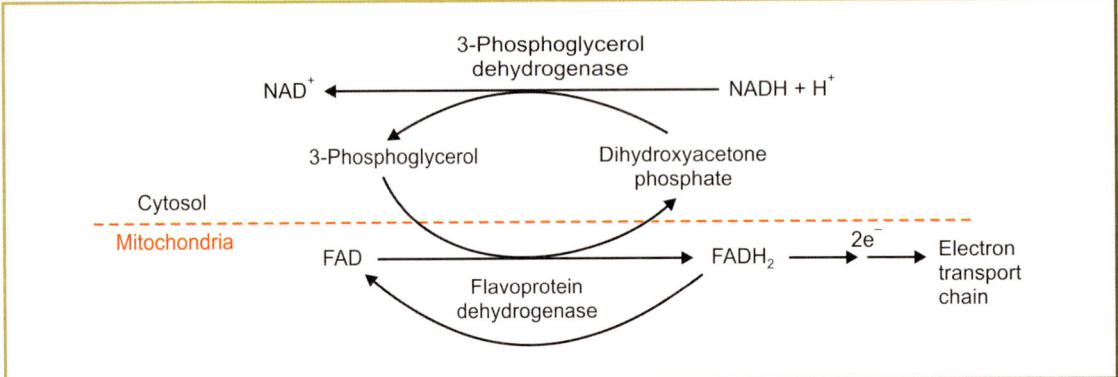

Fig. 10.12: Glycerol phosphate shuttle.

that the overall process of electron transport is exergonic.

Components of the Electron Transport Chain

Various enzymes and proteins required in the mitochondrial electron transfer system (electron transport chain) include an NAD^+-linked dehydrogenase, a flavin-linked dehydrogenase, iron-sulfur proteins, coenzyme Q and various cytochromes.

NAD-linked dehydrogenase: NAD-linked dehydrogenase reactions of the various pathways reduce NAD^+ to NADH while converting the reduced member of an oxidation-reduction reaction to the oxidized form, such as in the oxidation of malate (Fig.10.13).

In the dehydrogenation of a metabolite, two electrons and two protons are removed, out of which both the electrons and one of the protons are actually transferred to NAD^+. Since only one of the protons, as a hydride ion (i.e. H^-, a hydrogen atom containing an additional electron), is accepted by the nicotinamide moiety of the NAD^+, the second proton is released to the aqueous environment. Some of the **NAD-linked dehydrogenases** are malate dehydrogenase, lactate dehydrogenase, etc.

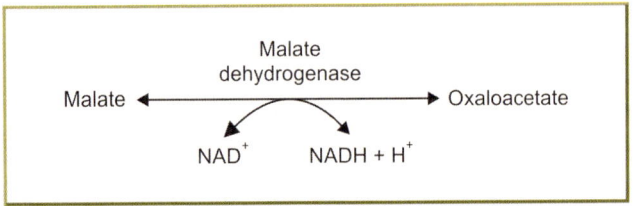

Fig. 10.13: Malate dehydrogenase, an NAD-linked dehydrogenase.

Flavin-linked dehydrogenase: The second type of the oxidation-reduction reaction, essential in the mitochondrial electron transport, employs a flavin as an electron acceptor, as a part of the flavin-linked dehydrogenases. The two flavin nucleotides commonly utilized in oxidation-reduction reactions are FMN and FAD. Both of these are derived from riboflavin.

NADH, produced as a result of NAD-linked dehydrogenase, is oxidized by **FMN-linked NADH dehydrogenase**. The isoalloxazine ring of the FMN molecule accepts two electrons and a proton from NADH plus one proton from the environment. NADH dehydrogenase is actually a **complex enzyme** having, in addition to a **flavoprotein**, at least four **iron-sulfur centers**. Various flavin-linked dehydrogenases are NADH dehydrogenase, succinate dehydrogenase, etc.

Iron-sulfur centers: As mentioned above, flavin-linked enzyme (e.g. NADH dehydrogenase) contains iron-sulfur centers (**iron-sulfur clusters**) which form prosthetic groups of the iron-sulfur proteins (**non-heme iron proteins**) involved in the catalytic mechanism. Iron component of the iron-sulfur center is bound in various arrangements, to the cysteine residues in a protein and to the acid-labile sulfur.

Iron-sulfur clusters undergo one-electron oxidation and reduction, i.e. the oxidized and the reduced states of the iron-sulfur clusters differ by one formal charge only. During the transfer of reducing equivalents, iron is converted from the oxidized form (Fe^{3+}) to the reduced form (Fe^{2+}).

Iron-sulfur centers function in the transfer of electrons from $FMNH_2$ to coenzyme Q and from cytochrome b to cytochrome c_1.

Coenzyme Q: The acceptor of electrons and protons from NADH dehydrogenase is coenzyme Q (**CoQ**) or **ubiquinone**. It is neither a protein nor a nucleotide but a **lipophilic electron carrier**. CoQ serves as a mobile electron transporter in the mitochondrial membrane which operates between a flavin-linked dehydrogenase and cytochrome b. By the addition of two reducing equivalents ($2H^+ + 2e$), the CoQ is alternatively oxidized and reduced ($CoQ \cdot H_2$). The hydrogen atoms collected by CoQ are released into the mitochondrial matrix and ultimately form water with the molecular oxygen.

Cytochromes: Their salient characteristics include:

- Cytochromes are a class of proteins called **hemoproteins** which are characterized by the presence of an iron containing heme bound to a protein. Unlike the heme group in hemoglobin or myoglobin in which the heme iron remains in the Fe^{2+} state, the iron in the heme of the cytochromes is alternatively reduced (Fe^{2+}) and oxidized (Fe^{3+}).

- Various cytochromes of the mammalian mitochondria are designated as **cytochrome a, cytochrome b, cytochrome c,** etc. on the basis of the α-band of their absorption spectrum and the type of the heme group.

- Cytochromes sequentially carry electrons from CoQ to molecular oxygen and act as carriers of electrons from $CoQ \cdot H_2$ on one hand to cytochrome oxidase on the other. Cytochromes thus act as *trans*-electronases. The electrons from a molecule of $CoQ \cdot H_2$ are accepted by two molecules of cytochrome b from where these are then passed on to the next member of the electron transport chain.

- Each cytochrome accepts a pair of electrons from its predecessor thereby converting the cytochrome into the ferrous form. Regeneration of the ferric form is accomplished by the transfer of electrons from one cytochrome to the next and eventually to the cytochrome oxidase. Cytochrome oxidase finally transfers its electrons to oxygen which, in its negatively charged state, combines with the hydrogen ions (released from $CoQ \cdot H_2$) to form water.

- The electron transfer from NADH through CoQ involves two e^- whereas reactions between CoQ and O_2, involving various cytochromes, are the one e^- transferring reactions.

- Cytochrome oxidase (cytochrome $a \cdot a_3$) is the terminal unit in the electron transport chain. Only the a_3 subunit of the cytochrome $a \cdot a_3$ is capable of reacting directly with oxygen. Copper ions are also involved in the transfer of electrons from cytochrome a to a_3.

- Various cytochromes thus form a link in the process by which the reduced CoQ is oxidized by molecular oxygen. No hydrogen transfer takes place within this segment of the electron transport chain.

Sequential Arrangement of the Various Components of the Electron Transport Chain

Various components, as mentioned above, are arranged in the inner mitochondrial membrane and participate in a sequential manner in the redox process known as **cellular/internal respiration**, which constitutes the electron transport chain (**respiratory chain**). The chain is constructed in such a way that the reduced member of the redox couple is oxidized by the oxidized member of the next component in the system (Fig. 10.14).

The components of the electron transport chain are located asymmetrically, thereby forming four different complexes (Fig. 10.15). These four complexes contain redox centres with progressively greater affinity for electrons, i.e. with the increasing standard reduction potentials. Electrons travel through this chain from a lower standard reduction potential to a higher one; from complex I or complex II to complex III by CoQ, and from complex III to complex IV by cytochrome c.

Complex I: The initial reaction is catalyzed by an **NADH dehydrogenase complex** [NADH dehydrogenase (FMN-Fe:S protein)] or NADH·CoQ oxidoreductase, designated as **Complex I**. It accepts protons and electrons from NADH + H^+ and transfers them to CoQ. Complex I thus catalyzes the oxidation of NADH by the reduction of CoQ. It is the largest protein complex found in the inner mitochondrial membrane. It contains one molecule of FMN and 6–7 iron-sulfur clusters.

FMN and CoQ can transfer either one or two electrons at a time. These, therefore provide an electron

10

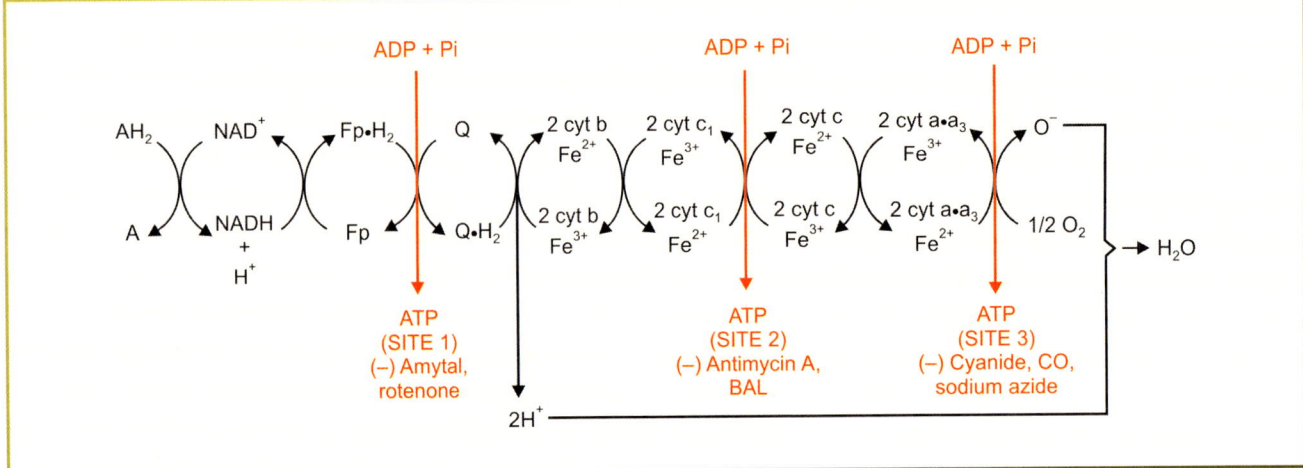

Fig. 10.14: Electron transport chain showing 3 sites of generation of ATP. Thus, if reducing equivalents enter through NAD, 3 ATP are synthesized. For the FAD-requiring reactions (not shown here), only 2 ATP can be synthesized because the first site is bypassed. However, based on **recent experimental evidence**, it is now suggested that instead of 3 (for NAD) and 2 (for FAD), the figures are actually **2.5** and **1.5**, respectively.

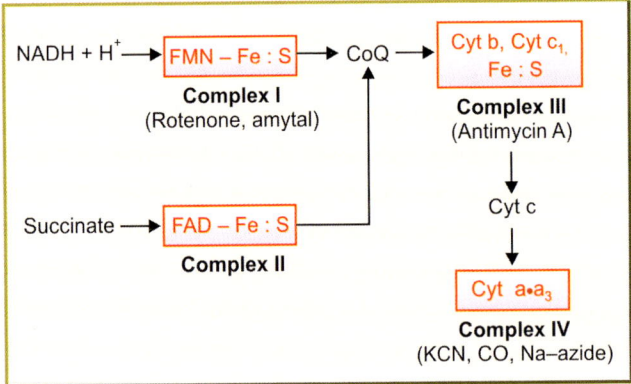

Fig. 10.15: Four complexes in the electron transport chain (inhibitors are shown in parentheses).

conduit between the two electron donors NADH and the one electron acceptors, the cytochromes. As electrons are transferred between the redox centers of complex I, four protons are translocated from the matrix to the intermembrane space.

$$NADH + 5H^+ + CoQ \longrightarrow NAD^+ + 4H^+ + CoQ \cdot H_2$$

Complex II: It consists of **succinate dehydrogenase-flavoprotein component** [succinate dehydrogenase (FAD-Fe:S protein)] which accepts reducing equivalents from succinate and in turn reduces FAD. Complex II thus catalyzes the oxidation of $FADH_2$ by CoQ. The metabolites which are directly oxidized

by flavin-containing dehydrogenases, e.g. succinate, bypass the NADH dehydrogenase step.

$$FADH_2 + CoQ \longrightarrow FAD + CoQ \cdot H_2$$

Complex III: The CoQ is a **mobile component** and facilitates the transfer of electrons from both the complexes, i.e. from complex I as well as complex II, on to complex III.

Complex III consists of cyt b, cyt c_1 and an Fe:S protein. It catalyzes the oxidation of the reduced CoQ by cytochrome c.

$$CoQ \cdot H_2 + \text{Oxidized cytochrome c} \longrightarrow CoQ + \text{Reduced cytochrome c}$$

Complex IV: Complex IV catalyzes the oxidation of the reduced cytochrome c by molecular oxygen ($\frac{1}{2} O_2$) which is the terminal electron acceptor of the sequence.

$$\text{Reduced cytochrome c} + \frac{1}{2}O_2 \longrightarrow \text{Oxidized cytochrome c} + H_2O$$

Inhibitors of the Electron Transport Chain

Inhibition of the electron transport chain is assessed by the effect of a compound on O_2 consumption. A variety of compounds specifically inhibit the electron transport chain at different points (Figs 10.14 and 10.15). These include rotenone (a plant toxin), amytal,

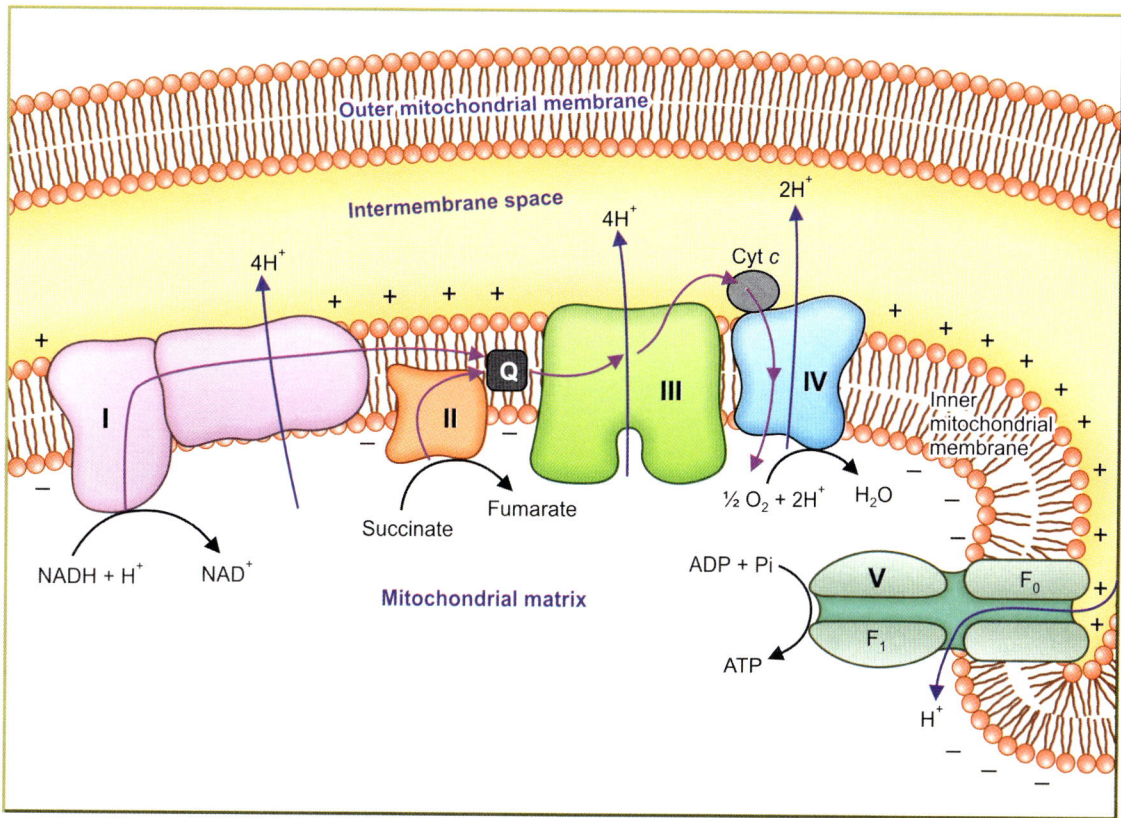

Fig. 10.16: Chemiosmotic theory of oxidative phosphorylation.

Inhibitors and Uncouplers of Oxidative Phosphorylation

Inhibitors and uncouplers of oxidative phosphory-lation stop ATP synthesis:

- *Inhibitors:* Oligomycin binds to the F_0 subunit of the mitochondrial F_1-F_0-ATPase, suppresses oxygen consumption and thus the phosphorylation of ADP to ATP.

- *Synthetic uncouplers:* 2,4-Dinitrophenol is a proton ionophore which uncouples phosphorylation from electron transport, resulting in the accumulation of ADP. The energy, normally conserved as ATP, is lost as heat. In this situation, electron transport may continue but without the generation of ATP.

- *Physiological uncouplers* (Table 10.6): They dissipate the chemical energy of ATP in the form of heat. They are one of the mechanisms for thermoregulation. One such protein called thermogenin or uncoupling protein-1 (UCP1, Chemistry to Clinics 10.2) is found in the mitochondria of brown adipose issue that is more

Table 10.6: Physiological uncouplers

- Uncoupling protein-1 (thermogenin)
- Unconjugated bilirubin
- Free fatty acids
- Thyroxine
- Estrogen

Chemistry to Clinics 10.2: Beige Fat

Adipose tissue containing cells resembling brown adipocytes (but genetically distinct, expressing low levels of UCP1 compared with brown adipocytes) have been discovered in the subcutaneous tissue near the clavicle and along the spine of adult humans. This is called 'beige fat' or 'brite fat' or 'inducible thermogenic adipose tissue'. A hormone called 'irisin' produced by exercising muscles, promotes the conversion of white fat into beige fat. Thus, with the help of novel drugs, it may be possible to further convert beige fat into brown fat with high expression of UCP1, with the potential to treat overweight/obesity and diabetes mellitus.

Table 10.7: Major uncoupling proteins

Type of uncoupling protein (UCP)	Major location	Major function
UCP1 (thermogenin)	Brown adipose tissue of human infants and hibernating mammals	Non-shivering thermogenesis to maintain body temperature
UCP2	Many tissues	Control of mitochondria-derived reactive oxygen species, immunity, regulation of glucose sensing in brain and pancreas
UCP3	Skeletal muscle, brown adipose tissue	Control of mitochondria-derived reactive oxygen species during exercise
UCP4	CNS	Energy homeostasis, protect against neurotoxins, regulate intracellular Ca^{2+} concentration, regulate gene expression
UCP5	CNS	Do

important in neonates. Many uncoupling proteins have been identified (Table 10.7).

SUBSTRATE LEVEL PHOSPHORYLATION

In addition to oxidative phosphorylation, i.e. the coupling of oxidation with phosphorylation of ADP to form ATP in the mitochondria, some ATP is also synthesized in the cytosol, within certain individual steps of a metabolic pathway. This process of transfer of a phosphate group from a very high-energy phosphate donor to ADP is called as substrate level phosphorylation, e.g. two reactions of glycolysis catalyzed by phosphoglycerokinase and pyruvate kinase (Fig. 10.17). Phosphorylation of ADP by creatine phosphate, catalyzed by creatine kinase, also

represents an important mode of ATP formation in the muscle. Besides, succinate thiokinase catalyzed reaction in Krebs cycle is also an example of substrate-level phosphorylation.

EXTRACTION OF ENERGY FROM FOOD

Energy is extracted from food in three stages (Fig. 10.18):
- Digestion of complex macromolecules into simpler ones and their absorption.
- Formation of acetyl CoA and its entry into the TCA cycle, and
- Transfer of reducing equivalents during the TCA cycle with harvesting of ATP, the final common

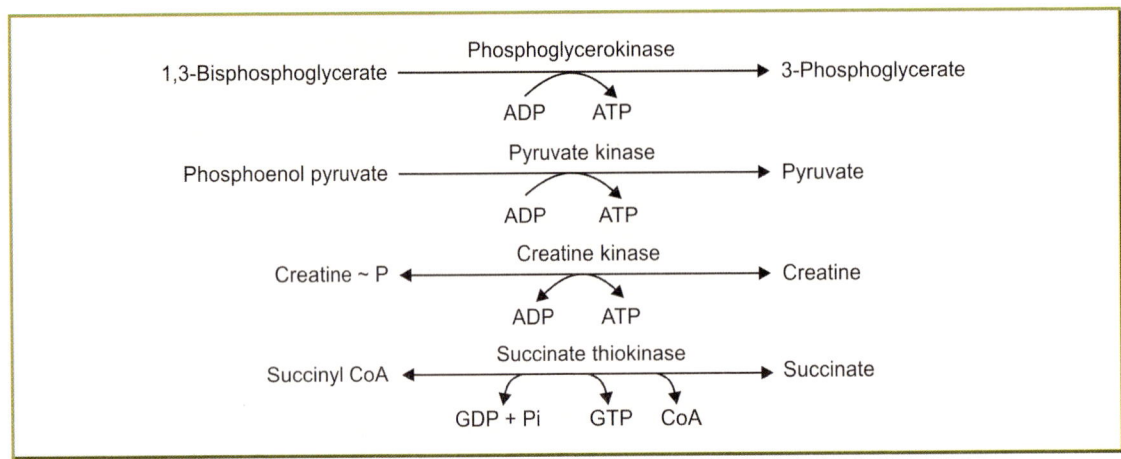

Fig. 10.17: Substrate level phosphorylation.

10

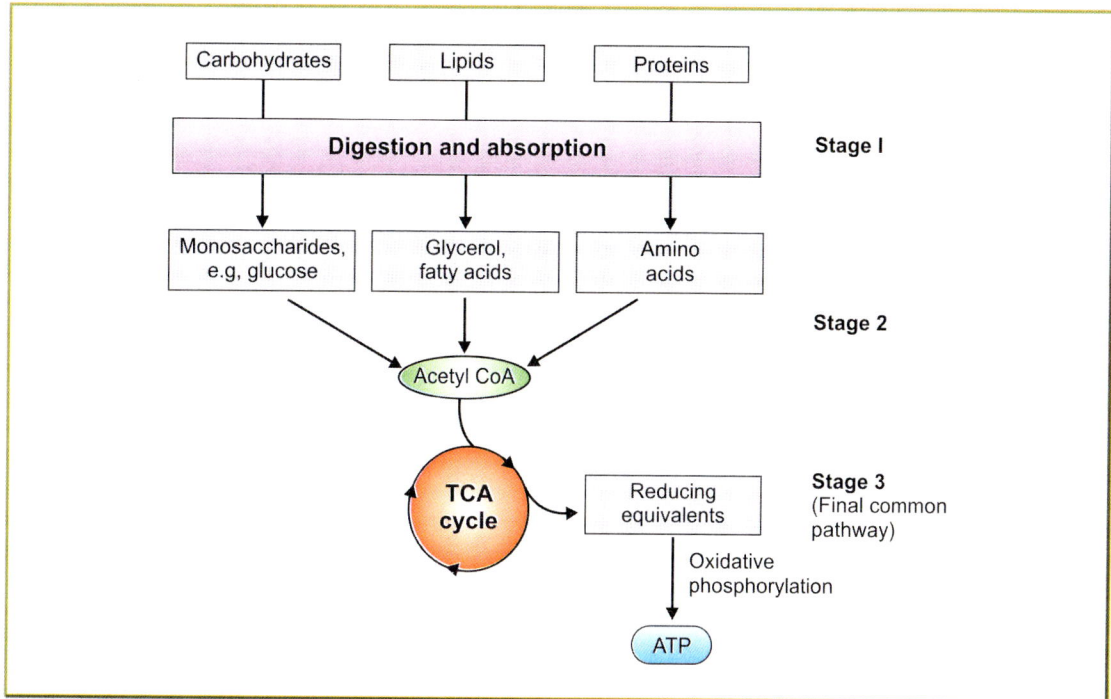

Fig. 10.18: Overview of metabolism.

pathway. ATP is used for various useful purposes (Fig. 10.1).

The three stages taken together represent the sum total of all the biochemical reactions in the living system, otherwise known as '**metabolism**'.

SOME IMPORTANT QUESTIONS

1. What is biological oxidation? Briefly discuss the role of enzymes in biological oxidation.

2. Discuss various high-energy compounds.

3. Write notes on:

   i. ATP
  ii. Phosphocreatine
 iii. Thioesters
 iv. Enol phosphates
  v. ATP as cellular currency of energy
 vi. Reducing equivalents
vii. Standard redox potential

 viii. Respiratory chain
  ix. Oxidative phosphorylation
   x. Substrate level phosphorylation
  xi. Iron-sulfur centers
 xii. Cytochromes
xiii. Cyanide poisoning
 xiv. P/O ratio

4. Explain oxidative phosphorylation and its inhibitors.

5. Discuss briefly:

  i. Respiratory chain and the sites of ATP production
 ii. Oxidative phosphorylation and uncouplers
iii. Diagrammatic representation of the electron transport chain

10

iv. Theory of oxidative phosphorylation
  v. Malate-aspartate shuttle
 vi. Glycerophosphate shuttle
vii. Inhibitors of oxidative phosphorylation
viii. Respiratory control
 ix. Beige fat

MULTIPLE CHOICE QUESTIONS

1. **The free energy of hydrolysis is maximum for:**
   A. Phosphoenolpyruvate
   B. ATP
   C. Creatine phosphate
   D. 1,3-BPG

2. **During catabolism, more reducing equivalents are extracted from:**
   A. Carbohydrates   B. Lipids
   C. Proteins   D. Same for all

3. **The inner mitochondrial membrane is impermeable to:**
   A. Glutamate   B. Oxaloacetate
   C. Malate   D. Aspartate

4. **Flavoprotein dehydrogenase is located in:**
   A. Outer surface of outer mitochondrial membrane
   B. Outer surface of inner mitochondrial membrane
   C. Inner surface of inner mitochondrial membrane
   D. Mitochondrial matrix

5. **In the electron transport chain (ETC), the following reacts directly with oxygen:**
   A. Coenzyme Q
   B. Cytochrome b
   C. Cytochrome c
   D. Cytochrome a_3

6. **Cytochrome a·a_3 requires:**
   A. Cu^{2+} B. Mg^{2+}
   C. Mn^{2+} D. Ca^{2+}

7. **Iron sulfur proteins are absent in:**
   A. Complex I
   B. Complex II
   C. Complex III
   D. Complex IV

8. **The following inhibit complex IV by binding to Fe^{3+}-heme *except*:**
   A. Carbon monoxide
   B. Sodium azide
   C. Potassium cyanide
   D. None of the above

9. **The following is not a physiological uncoupler:**
   A. Free fatty acid
   B. Thyroxine
   C. Insulin
   D. Unconjugated bilirubin

10. **The following is not an example of substrate level phosphorylation:**
    A. Phosphoglycerokinase and pyruvate kinase reactions of glycolysis
    B. Creatine kinase reaction
    C. Succinate thiokinase reaction of TCA cycle
    D. Oxidative phosphorylation

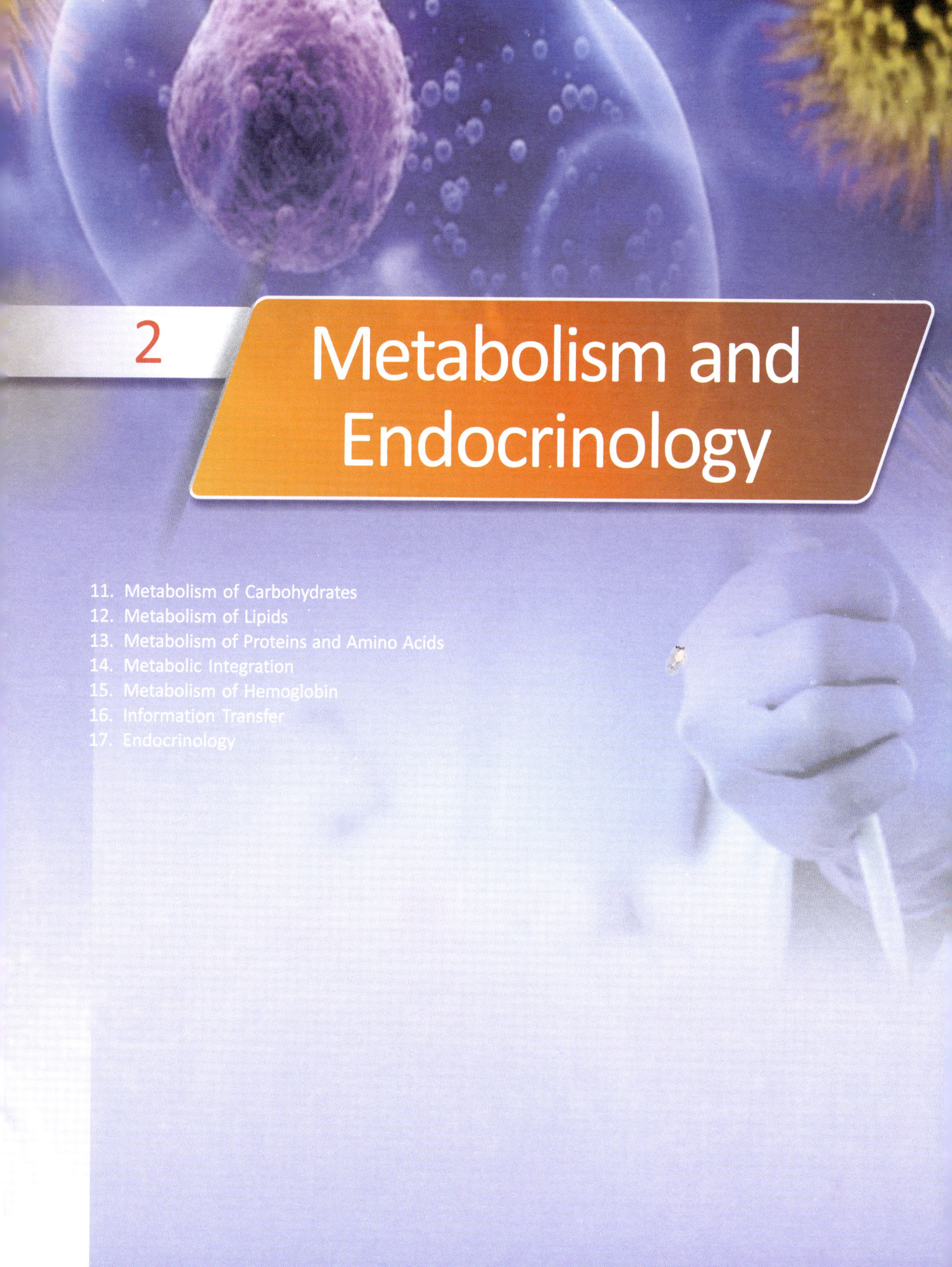

2

Metabolism and Endocrinology

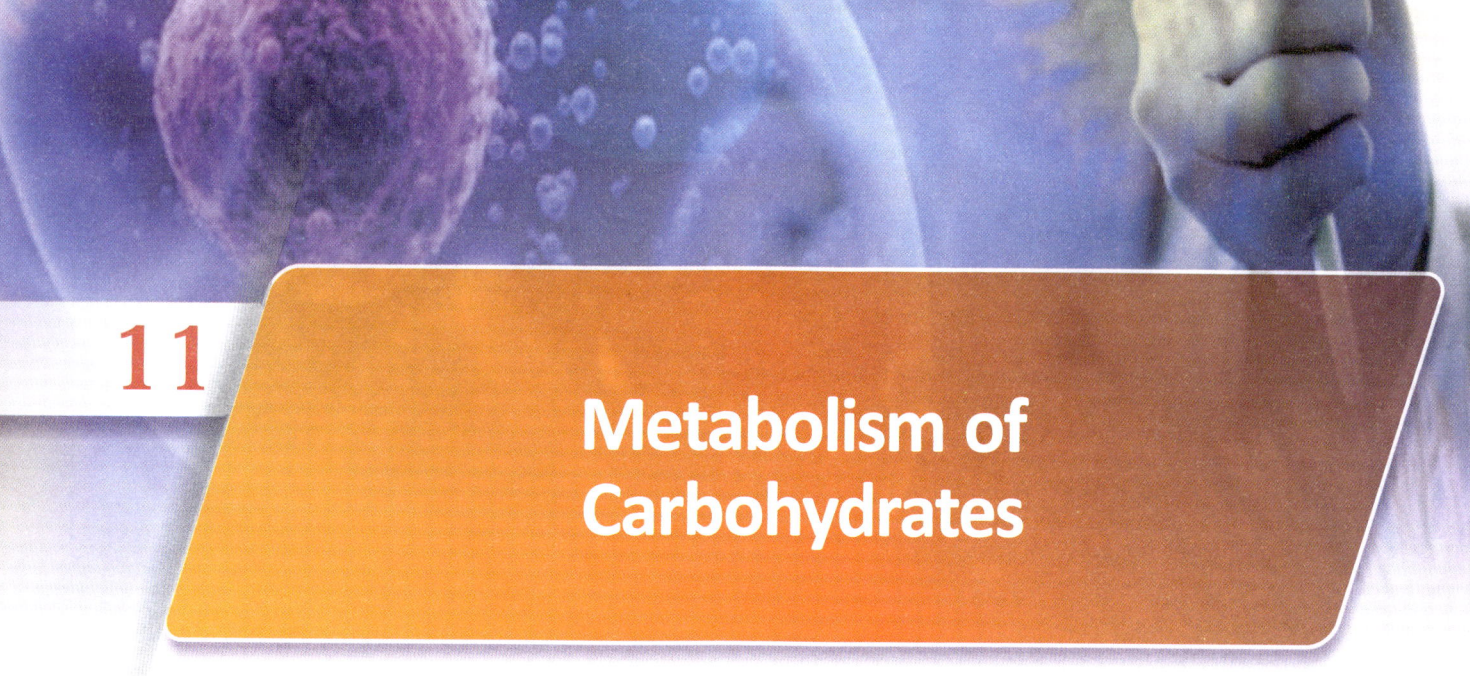

11

Metabolism of Carbohydrates

The digestion and absorption of dietary carbo-hydrates was discussed in Chapter 9.

Starch and glycogen are the main dietary carbo-hydrates which are hydrolyzed to their smaller units by the action of a number of digestive enzymes. After absorption from the intestine, the monosaccharides are transported to the liver. Glucose is the major monosaccharide which enters the liver. It is either converted to glycogen and stored in different tissues or is oxidized by different pathways in the liver and produces energy (Fig. 11.1). The liver also releases glucose to the systemic circulation for its utilization by the extrahepatic tissues.

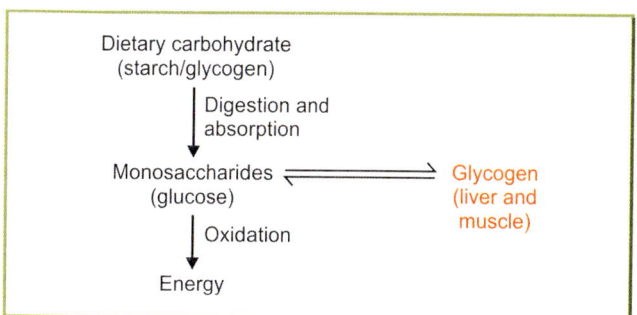

Fig. 11.1: Metabolic fates of dietary carbohydrate.

Glucose Transporters (GLUT): Salient Features

- At least 14 glucose transporters (GLUT) exist, some of which are listed in Table 11.1.
- They are membrane proteins.
- Not all GLUT are glucose-specific, e.g. GLUT5 transports fructose.

- A cell may contain >1 GLUT type so that hexose transport is unimpaired even if a particular GLUT is absent/non-functional, e.g. spermatozoa contain GLUT3, -5, -8 and -9.
- GLUT4 in muscles and adipose tissue are insulin-dependent.
- GLUT are important for the survival of tumor cells (Chemistry to Clinics 11.1).

Table 11.1: Examples of glucose transporters (GLUT)

GLUT type	Major location	Linked metabolic fate
GLUT1	RBC, brain, placenta	Glycolysis, HMP shunt
GLUT2	• Liver • Pancreas • Small intestine	• HMP shunt, glycogenesis, glucuronic acid pathway, glycolysis • Glycolysis • Exit of glucose through basal membrane into blood
GLUT3	Brain	Glycolysis, HMP shunt
GLUT4	• Skeletal/cardiac muscle • Adipose tissue	• Glycolysis, glycogenesis • Fatty acid synthesis, HMP shunt
GLUT5	Small intestine, skeletal muscle, testis	Fructose uptake

11

Tumor cells exhibit altered metabolic profiles, e.g. enhanced glucose uptake and glycolysis. Generally, the growth of solid tumors outpaces the growth of their blood supply so that the tumor cells are subjected to a relatively hypoxic condition. Hypoxia upregulates 'hypoxia-inducible transcription factor, HIF-1', which enhances the expression of glucose transporters along with many glycolytic enzymes. The HIF-1 also promotes vascularization. These metabolic adaptations allow tumor cells to survive hypoxia until vascularization (hence oxygenation) takes place.

METABOLISM OF GLUCOSE

Glucose utilizing and generating pathways: Various metabolic pathways which utilize glucose include glycolysis, hexose monophosphate shunt (HMP shunt) and glycogenesis. On the other hand, gluconeogenesis and glycogenolysis are the glucose generating pathways (Fig. 11.2).

GLYCOLYSIS

Glycolysis, also called **Embden-Meyerhof-Parnas pathway**, is the process of catabolism of glucose either in the presence of oxygen, such as in the liver, to pyruvic acid called **aerobic glycolysis** or in the lack of oxygen, such as during exercise in the skeletal muscle and in the erythrocytes to lactic acid by the process of **anaerobic glycolysis** (Fig. 11.3). Glycolytic enzymes are present in **cytosol**.

Various reactions of the glycolytic pathway are shown in Fig. 11.4 and discussed below:

1. **Activation of glucose:** Glucose is activated **irreversibly**, to glucose-6-phosphate by gluco-kinase or hexokinase, in the presence in ATP and

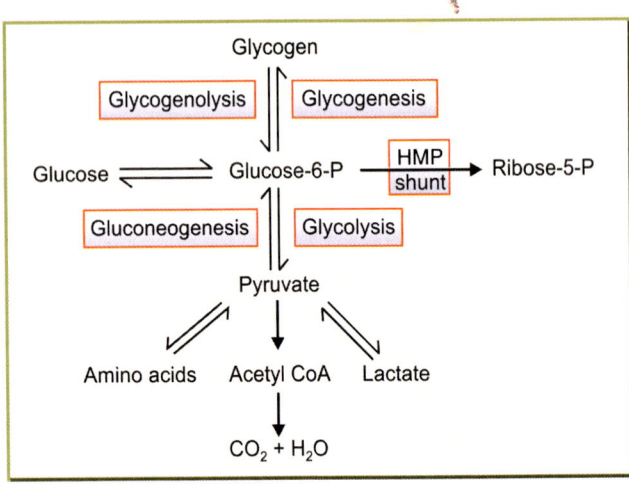

Fig. 11.2: Overview of glucose metabolism.

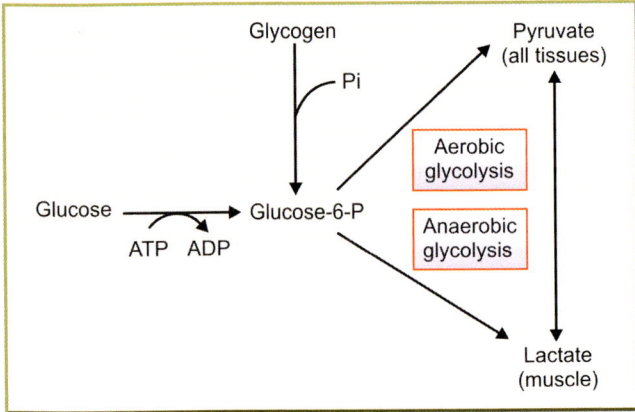

Fig. 11.3: Aerobic and anaerobic glycolysis.

Mg^{2+}. Hexokinase is allosterically inhibited by glucose-6-phosphate and has a high affinity (low K_m) for glucose. The enzyme is present in all extrahepatic tissues. In the liver, this reaction is also carried out by glucokinase, which is actually an isoenzyme of hexokinase. The catalytic activity of hexokinase is advantageously employed to detect tumors by **positron emission tomography** (**PET**, Chemistry to Clinics 11.2).

2. Glucose-6-phosphate is **isomerized**, in a freely reversible reaction, to fructose-6-phosphate by the enzyme phosphohexose isomerase.

3. Fructose-6-phosphate is **phosphorylated** by an allosteric enzyme phosphofructokinase (phospho-fructokinase-1) to form fructose-1, 6-bisphosphate. This is an **irreversible** reaction and requires ATP which acts as a cosubstrate as well as an allosteric inhibitor of the enzyme.

Another product, fructose-2,6-bisphosphate, formed by the action of phosphofructokinase-2, is an allosteric regulator of the enzyme phospho-fructokinase-1.

Bisphosphate and biphosphate: A bisphosphate is different from a biphosphate (diphosphate). In bisphosphate, two molecules of phosphoric acid

In this technique, 2-[^{18}F]fluoro-2-deoxy-glucose (FDG) is used as a molecular probe which is taken up by all cells and gets phosphorylated to FDG-6-phosphate by hexokinase. Cells accumulate FDG in direct proportion to the rate of glycolysis. Therefore, tumor cells accumulate more FDG since they have higher rate of glycolysis and are subsequently detected by PET scan which reveals abnormally high FDG accumulation (Fig. 11.5).

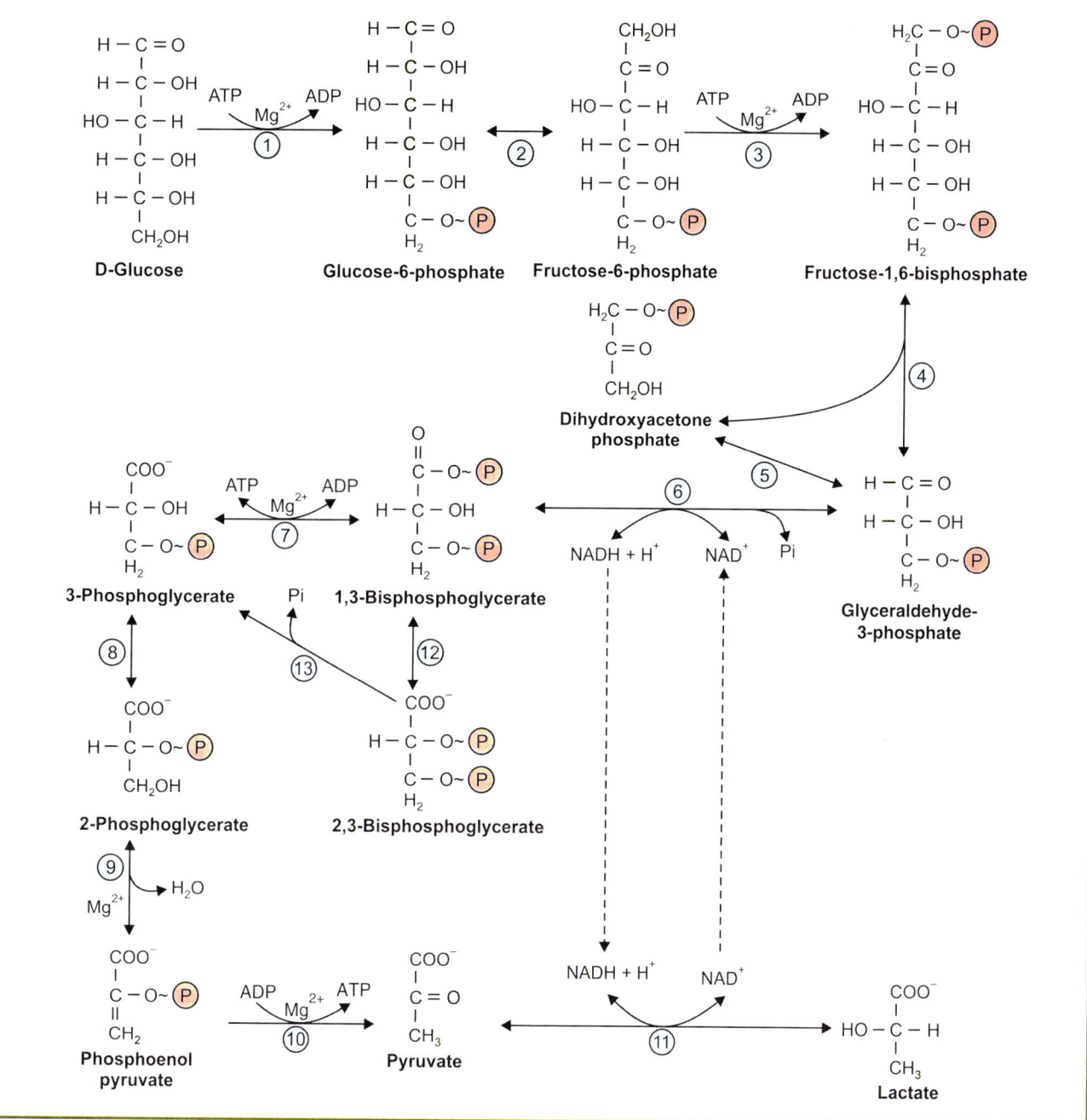

Fig. 11.4: Glycolysis. (1) Glucokinase/hexokinase, (2) Phosphohexose isomerase, (3) Phosphofructokinase, (4) Aldolase, (5) Phosphotriose isomerase, (6) Glyceraldehyde 3-phosphate dehydrogenase, (7) Phosphoglycerate kinase, (8) Phosphoglycerate mutase, (9) Enolase, (10) Pyruvate kinase, (11) Lactate dehydrogenase, (12) Bisphosphoglycerate mutase, (13) 2,3-Bisphosphoglycerate phosphatase. Reactions (12 and 13) are an off-shoot from glycolysis and constitute the Rapoport Luebering cycle in RBC, catalyzed by a single bifunctional enzyme.

are linked to two different carbon atoms while in a biphosphate these are attached through each other by the phosphodiester linkage, onto the same carbon.

Phosphofructokinase-1 plays a central role in the control of glycolysis because it catalyzes **one of the rate determining reactions** of the pathway. Citrate, ATP and hydrogen ions (low pH) are

11

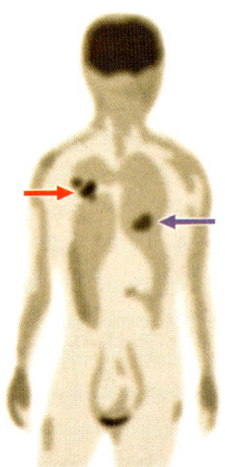

Fig. 11.5: PET scan showing the metabolic activity of different areas in the body using radio-labeled glucose. Areas of high glucose consumption are represented as dark spots. A tumor is revealed in the left lung (red arrow, viewing from behind the patient). The PET scan can also show whether the cancer has metastasized, or spread to other areas in the body (blue arrow). The brain and genitalia show physiologically high metabolic activity because the brain requires high amount of energy to function, and the genitalia are the site of spermatogenesis.

negative allosteric effectors whereas AMP and fructose-2,6-bisphosphate are positive allosteric effectors (activators) of the enzyme.

Congenital phosphofructokinase-1 deficiency causes severe muscular weakness.

4. Fructose-1,6-bisphosphate (the hexose molecule) is **cleaved** by an aldolase to 3-phosphoglyceral-dehyde (glyceraldehyde-3-phosphate) and dihydroxyacetone phosphate, i.e. the two trioses.

5. Since only 3-phosphoglyceraldehyde enters the pathway, dihydroxyacetone phosphate is also **isomerized** to 3-phosphoglyceraldehyde, catalyzed by phosphotriose isomerase. Glycerol can also enter glycolytic pathway through this reaction, i.e. via dihydroxyacetone phosphate.

6. In the presence of NAD^+ and inorganic phosphate, glyceraldehyde-3-phosphate dehydrogenase **oxidizes** 3-phosphoglyceraldehyde to 1,3-bisphos-phoglycerate.

7. 1,3-bisphosphoglycerate is converted to 3-phos-phoglycerate. This reaction is catalyzed by Mg^{2+}-dependent phosphoglycerokinase (phos-phoglycerate kinase) and generates one ATP. Since this reaction does not involve O_2, it is called **substrate-level production of ATP**.

Arsenic acid, if present, results in uncoupling of phosphorylation and inhibits ATP production.

Rapoport-Luebering cycle: In erythrocytes, conversion of 1,3-bisphosphoglycerate to 3-phos-phoglycerate by phosphoglycerate kinase is bypassed. Instead, 1,3-bisphosphoglycerate is converted to 2,3-bisphosphoglycerate **(2,3-BPG)** by bisphosphoglycerate mutase and is sub-sequently converted to 3-phosphoglycerate by 2,3-bisphosphoglycerate phosphatase. This results in a loss of high energy phosphate and thus there is no net production of ATP. This is called as Rapoport-Luebering cycle (Fig. 11.4).

Erythrocytes synthesize and degrade 2,3-BPG as an off-shoot from the main glycolytic pathway. The level of available 2,3-BPG regulates **oxygen-binding capacity of hemoglobin**. When 2,3-BPG levels are high, oxygen is loosely bound to hemoglobin and is released easily. On the other hand, when 2,3-BPG concentration is low, oxygen is bound more tightly and is released more slowly.

8. 3-phosphoglycerate is **isomerized** to 2-phospho-glycerate by phosphoglycerate mutase.

9. Enolase converts 2-phosphoglycerate to a **high energy compound** called phosphoenolpyruvate, in the presence of Mg^{2+} or Mn^{2+}. Enolase inhibition and its isoenzymes (Chemistry to Clinics 11.3 and 11.4) are of clinical importance.

10. Phosphoenolpyruvate is converted to pyruvate, **irreversibly**. The reaction is catalyzed by a Mg^{2+}-dependent allosteric enzyme pyruvate kinase which transfers a high energy phosphate from phosphoenolpyruvate to ADP and generates ATP.

The enzyme is inhibited by alanine. It is induced in the liver by insulin after a high carbohydrate

Chemistry to Clinics 11.3: Enolase Inhibition

Fluoride is a competitive inhibitor of enolase as it binds to the active site by competing with the physiological substrate 2-phosphoglycerate. This has two clinical implications:

Firstly, addition of fluoride to blood samples for the determination of blood glucose helps to maintain the true blood glucose. Otherwise, if RBC glycolysis continues, it would lead to false low blood glucose levels.

Secondly, fluoridated drinking water as well as fluoridated tooth-pastes should provide fluoride at concentrations which inhibit the enolase activity of oral bacteria without affecting mammalian cells. Blocking the bacterial glycolytic pathway prevents fermentation and hence dental caries.

Chemistry to Clinics 11.4: Enolase Isoenzymes

There are three subunits of enolase, α, β and γ, which can combine to form five different isoenzymes: $\alpha\alpha$, $\alpha\beta$, $\alpha\gamma$, $\beta\beta$ and $\gamma\gamma$. The more common isoenzymes in humans are—$\alpha\alpha$ or non-neuronal enolase (NNE or **enolase 1** found in many tissues), $\gamma\gamma$ or neuron-specific enolase (NSE, **enolase 2**) and $\beta\beta$ or muscle-specific enolase (MSE, **enolase 3**). Higher levels of NSE are found in the cerebrospinal fluid of patients suffering from stroke and some CNS cancers. Further, blood NSE determinations are likely to assume great importance as a biomarker in sports medicine. This is because higher blood levels are found up to two months after head injury in boxers. Thus, monitoring blood NSE levels would guide such athletes when they should abstain from training and competition.

intake. Deficiency of pyruvate kinase leads to **hemolytic anemia** (Chemistry to Clinics 11.5).

11. Pyruvate is either converted to acetyl CoA (aerobic glycolysis) or lactate (anaerobic glycolysis).

Under aerobic condition: Pyruvate is transported into the mitochondria via pyruvate transporter and is oxidatively decarboxylated to **acetyl CoA** by pyruvate dehydrogenase complex (Fig. 11.6). Acetyl CoA is coupled with oxaloacetate and is utilized in the **Krebs cycle**.

Pyruvate dehydrogenase complex: It is a **multi-enzyme complex** consisting of **three enzymes**, i.e. pyruvate dehydrogenase, dihydrolipoyl transacetylase and dihydrolipoyl dehydrogenase. In addition to Mg^{2+}, the complex requires **five coenzymes**, i.e. TPP, CoA, NAD^+, FAD and lipoic acid. It is regulated by phosphorylation-dephosphorylation involving an ATP-specific kinase. While **insulin stimulates** its activity, the enzyme is inhibited by:

Chemistry to Clinics 11.5: Pyruvate Kinase Deficiency

It results in reduced glycolytic activity, reduced ATP synthesis in RBC, failure to maintain membrane integrity and functions, leading to hemolysis. There is an accumulation of 2,3-BPG which partially compensates for the anemia, however, it also inhibits hexokinase and phosphofructokinase thereby further reducing the rate of glycolysis.

- Its products, i.e. acetyl CoA and NADH.
- Dietary deficiency of thiamin (as observed in nutritionally deprived alcoholics).
- Increased acetyl CoA/CoA, $NADH/NAD^+$ and ATP/ADP ratios.
- Arsenite and mercuric ions (which complex the –SH groups of lipoic acid).

Inhibition of the enzyme results in the accumulation of pyruvate and lactate and causes lactic acidosis. It also manifests as neurological disturbances.

Under anaerobic condition: Pyruvate is reduced to **lactate** (Fig. 11.4). The reaction is catalyzed by lactate dehydrogenase which also requires NADH + H$^+$. Tissues such as skeletal muscle, when function under hypoxic condition, produce large amounts of lactic acid. Pathological causes of sustained hypoxia lead to lactic acidosis (Chemistry to Clinics 11.6).

Energy Production during Glycolysis

Under anaerobic condition: Since each of the energy yielding steps, i.e. the conversion of 1,3-bisphosphoglycerate to 3-phoshoglycerate and phosphoenolpyruvate to pyruvate, produces one ATP, a total of 2 ATP are produced for each molecule of the triose oxidized, i.e. 4 ATP per hexose (Fig. 11.7).

Chemistry to Clinics 11.6: Lactic Acidosis

Elevated concentration of lactate in the blood is termed as lactic acidosis or lactacidosis. It occurs when there is reduced supply of oxygen to the tissues (hypoxia) such as in myocardial infarction, pulmonary embolism and hypovolemic shock. Hypoxia results in inadequate oxidative phosphorylation and decreased ATP synthesis, because oxygen is the terminal electron acceptor in the mitochondrial electron transport chain. To survive, cells rely on anaerobic glycolysis for generating ATP and thus produce lactic acid as the end product. The excess oxygen required to recover from a period of hypoxia is termed as the **'oxygen debt'**. It is related to the patient's morbidity or mortality. To assess the presence and severity of shock, measuring the blood levels of lactic acid helps in the rapid and early detection of oxygen debt.

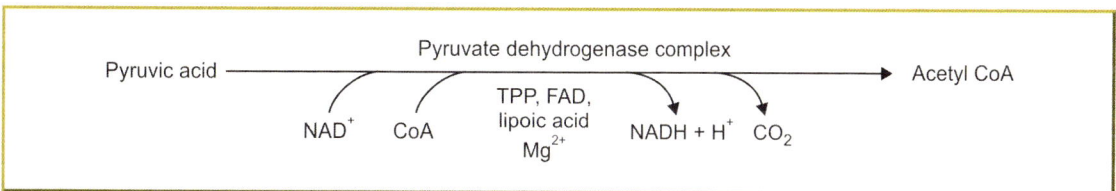

Fig. 11.6: Fate of pyruvate under aerobic condition.

11

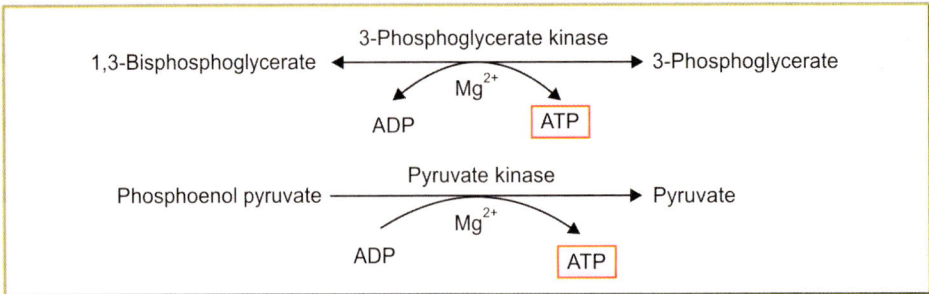

Fig. 11.7: Energy-yielding steps in glycolysis.

As 2 ATP are used in the initial reactions of the process, i.e. in the conversion of glucose to glucose-6-phosphate and fructose-6-phosphate to fructose-1,6-bisphosphate, the **net yield per molecule of glucose, is only 2 ATP**.

In the erythrocytes, when glycolysis occurs via 2,3-bisphosphoglycerate, the net energy yield is zero.

Under aerobic condition: In this process, since NADH produced during the conversion of 3-phosphoglycerate to 1,3-bisphosphoglycerate enters the electron transport chain and releases 2.5 ATP (by oxidative phosphorylation), additionally 5 ATP are produced per molecule of glucose. The total yield under these conditions is therefore 9 ATP. The **net yield thus becomes 7 ATP, per molecule of glucose.**

Regulation of Glycolysis

The **three irreversible steps** catalyzed by various kinases, i.e. hexokinase, phosphofructokinase-1 and pyruvate kinase are the sites of regulation of glycolysis. **Insulin stimulates** the activities of these enzymes, thereby increasing the utilization of glucose. On the other hand, **glucagon inhibits** the process.

TRICARBOXYLIC ACID CYCLE

Tricarboxylic acid cycle also called the **citric acid cycle or Krebs cycle**, is the process of oxidation of **acetyl CoA (active acetate)** to CO_2 and H_2O. During the process, **reducing equivalents** are produced which enter the respiratory chain and generate large amount of ATP during the process of **oxidative phosphorylation**. Enzymes of the Krebs cycle are located within the **mitochondria**. This, in turn, facilitates the transfer of reducing equivalents from the Krebs cycle to the respiratory chain, the enzymes of which are also located within the inner mitochondrial membrane.

Reactions of the Krebs cycle occur in a **cyclic manner** where two molecules of CO_2 are released and **oxaloacetate is regenerated** (Fig. 11.8).

1. In the first step, acetyl CoA (formed from pyruvate under aerobic condition) combines with oxaloacetate and forms citric acid (a tricarboxylic acid). The reaction is catalyzed by citrate synthase (condensing enzyme).
2. Citrate is then rearranged to form *cis*-aconitate.
3. *cis*-aconitate is subsequently changed to isocitrate. Both the steps are carried out by aconitase (the enzyme requires Fe^{2+}). The conversion of citrate to isocitrate is inhibited by fluoroacetate.
4. In the presence of isocitrate dehydrogenase, isocitrate is converted to oxalosuccinate.
5. Oxalosuccinate is later decarboxylated to form α-ketoglutarate.
6. α-ketoglutarate undergoes oxidative decarboxylation and is converted to succinyl CoA, catalyzed by α-ketoglutarate dehydrogenase complex. The reaction is similar to the conversion of pyruvate to acetyl CoA and also requires five coenzymes, i.e. TPP, NAD^+, FAD, coenzyme A and lipoic acid (Chemistry to Clinics 11.7).
7. Succinyl CoA is changed to succinate by succinate thiokinase (succinyl CoA synthase). During this reaction, a molecule of GTP is formed. This is known as **substrate level phosphorylation** since a high energy molecule is formed at the substrate level.

Chemistry to Clinics 11.7: Arsenic Poisoning

Both pyruvate dehydrogenase complex and α-ketoglutarate dehydrogenase complex require lipoic acid as a coenzyme. Arsenite forms a stable complex with the enzyme-bound lipoic acid and brings respiration to a halt. In arsenic poisoning, arsenic content in the hair is greatly increased which is an important observation in forensic science.

11

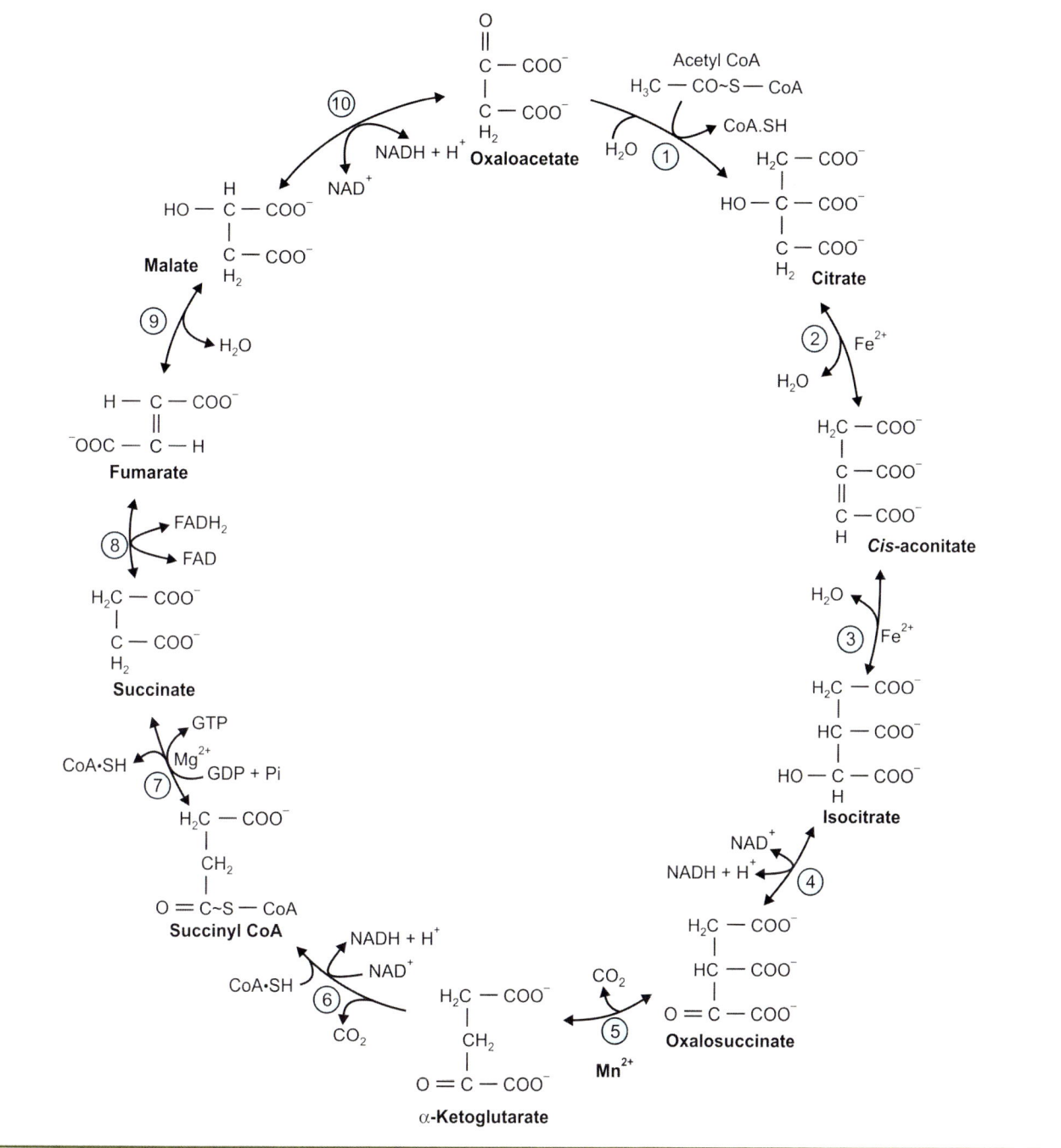

Fig. 11.8: TCA cycle. (1) Citrate synthase, (2 and 3) Aconitase, (4 and 5) Isocitrate dehydrogenase, (6) α-Ketoglutarate dehydrogenase complex, (7) Succinate thiokinase, (8) Succinate dehydrogenase, (9) Fumarase, (10) Malate dehydrogenase.

8. Succinate is converted to fumarate by an FAD containing enzyme succinate dehydrogenase. Due to the structural similarity between malonate and succinate, **malonate inhibits succinate dehydrogenase competitively**. The enzyme is also inhibited by oxaloacetate but is activated by ATP, Pi and succinate.

9. With the addition of a molecule of water by fumarase (fumarate hydratase, Chemistry to Clinics 11.8), fumarate is changed to L-malate.

11

Chemistry to Clinics 11.8: Fumarase Deficiency

The deficiency of an enzyme of TCA cycle is generally not compatible with intrauterine life. However, fumarase deficiency has been reported. Severe deficiency of fumarase, both in the mitochondria as well as in the cytosol of certain tissues, e.g. lymphocytes is characterized by severe neurological impairment and encephalopathy. Urine of such individuals contains abnormal amounts of fumarate and one or more of, succinate, α-keto-glutarate, citrate and malate.

10. Finally, malate dehydrogenase, in the presence of NAD^+, converts malate to oxaloacetate which can then re-enter the cycle.

Energy Production during Citric Acid Cycle

As a result of oxidation of one molecule of acetyl CoA in the Krebs cycle, three molecules of NAD^+ and one molecule of FAD are reduced. The reducing equivalents from one molecule of reduced NAD^+ ($NADH + H^+$) enter the respiratory chain and result in the production of 2.5 molecules of ATP. Similarly, reduced FAD ($FADH_2$) yields 1.5 ATP. Besides, there is a substrate level production of high energy phosphate bond as GTP. The **total energy yield, per molecule of acetyl CoA oxidized, is thus 10 ATP** (Table 11.2).

In addition, as mentioned earlier, conversion of pyruvate to acetyl CoA also generates one $NADH + H^+$, and gives 2.5 ATP. **Total number of ATP produced from the oxidation of pyruvate is therefore 12.5**.

Since 2 molecules of pyruvate are formed from one molecule of glucose, therefore in addition to the energy yield during aerobic glycolysis (i.e. 7 ATP), a molecule of glucose further produces 25 additional ATP via Krebs cycle. Thus, a **total of 32 ATP molecules are obtained when a molecule of glucose is completely oxidized to CO_2 and H_2O under aerobic condition**, i.e. via glycolysis and Krebs cycle.

Table 11.2: Energy yield in citric acid cycle		
Reaction	*Reducing equivalent*	*Number of ATP*
Isocitrate ⟶ α-Ketoglutarate	$NADH + H^+$	2.5
α-Ketoglutarate ⟶ Succinyl CoA	$NADH + H^+$	2.5
Succinyl CoA ⟶ Succinate	–	1.0
Succinate ⟶ Fumarate	$FADH_2$	1.5
Malate ⟶ Oxaloacetate	$NADH + H^+$	2.5
	Total	**10.0**

Role of Vitamins in Citric Acid Cycle

Four vitamins of the **B complex** group, i.e. **vitamin B_1** as thiamine pyrophosphate or TPP, **vitamin B_2** as FAD, **niacin** as NAD and **pantothenic acid**, a constituent of coenzyme A, play an important role in the citric acid cycle.

Biological Significance of Citric Acid Cycle: An Amphibolic Pathway

Citric acid cycle has a **dual role**, i.e. it is important both in the oxidation as well as synthetic processes. It is thus 'amphibolic' in nature. It is catabolic for the oxidation of carbohydrates, lipids and proteins as these substances are completely oxidized to CO_2 and H_2O, and release large amount of energy. It is also important for the anabolic reactions, as various intermediates of the cycle are used for the biosynthesis of nonessential amino acids. Various intermediates of the cycle are also potentially glucogenic and can give rise to glucose in the liver and the kidney (Fig. 11.9).

Reactions which replenish the intermediates of Krebs cycle are called 'anaplerotic reactions' (Greek Ana= 'up' and Plerotikos = 'to fill') whereas those which consume the intermediates are called 'cataplerotic reactions'.

Regulation of the Citric Acid Cycle

Citrate synthase, isocitrate dehydrogenase and α-ketoglutarate dehydrogenase are the **rate limiting enzymes** of the cycle. The most crucial regulators of the cycle are its substrates, i.e. acetyl CoA and oxaloacetate as well as NADH.

NADH, ATP and succinyl CoA function as inhibitors while ADP and Ca^{2+} are activators of the cycle.

GLUCONEOGENESIS

Gluconeogenesis (neoglucogenesis) is the process of **formation of glucose** from various **non-carbohydrate sources**:

- Glucogenic amino acids
- Lactate
- Glycerol
- Propionate

Importance of Gluconeogenesis

Gluconeogenesis occurs in the **fasting state or on a low carbohydrate diet**, particularly in the **liver** and

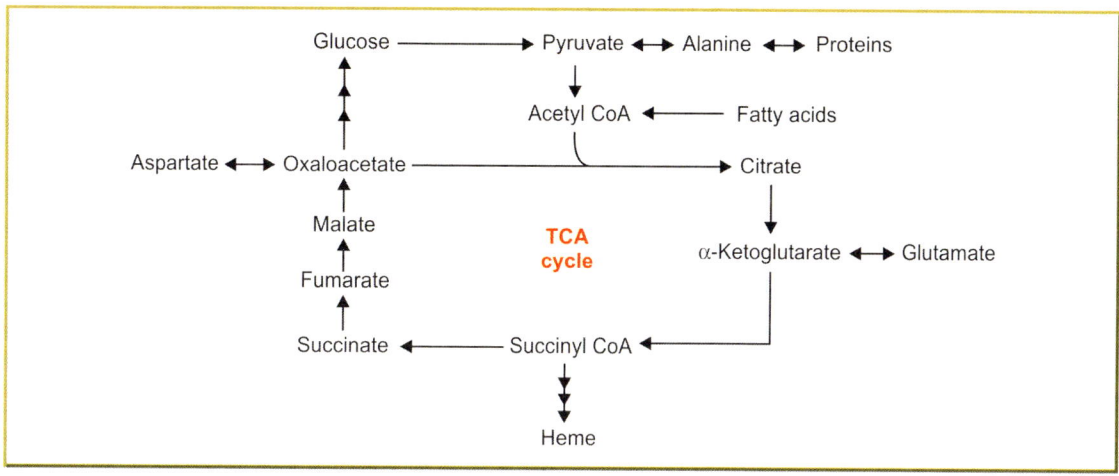

Fig. 11.9: Biological significance of Krebs cycle.

some other tissues which are solely dependent on glucose for their energy demand but not in the muscle. Gluconeogenesis thus enables the **maintenance of blood glucose** when all the dietary glucose has been absorbed and oxidized, and liver glycogen is nearly depleted. The process is essential since blood glucose level has to be maintained to support metabolism of the **tissues that use glucose as the primary substrate, such as the brain, the red blood cells and the lens**.

Formation of Glucose from Pyruvate

As discussed earlier, all the glycolytic reactions are reversible except the three steps of the pathway (Fig. 11.10). Gluconeogenesis is actually the reversal of these three irreversible reactions (Fig. 11.11).

1. **Reversal of pyruvate to phosphoenolpyruvate:** Firstly, pyruvate is changed to oxaloacetate by **pyruvate carboxylase** in the mitochondria. Active

biotin or biocytin is the coenzyme. The enzyme is regulated by induction, repression as well as allosteric regulation.

Oxaloacetate is then reduced to malate via citric acid cycle in the mitochondria from where it comes out to the cytoplasm and is re-oxidized to oxaloacetate. Oxaloacetate thus is formed from pyruvate by the reaction which occurs in the mitochondria whereas the enzymes which convert phosphoenolpyruvate to glucose are present in the cytoplasm. Oxaloacetate therefore has to be transported across the mitochondrial membrane. The enzyme malate dehydrogenase converts mitochondrial oxaloacetate to malate, which is readily transportable. In the cytosol, malate is reconverted back to oxaloacetate and in turn reduces NAD^+. The enzyme thus not only transports oxaloacetate (via malate) but also

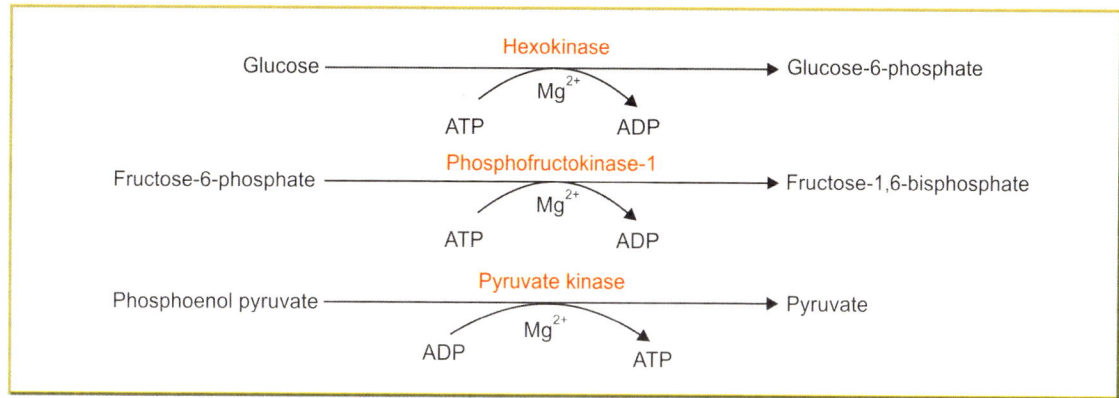

Fig. 11.10: Irreversible steps in glycolysis.

11

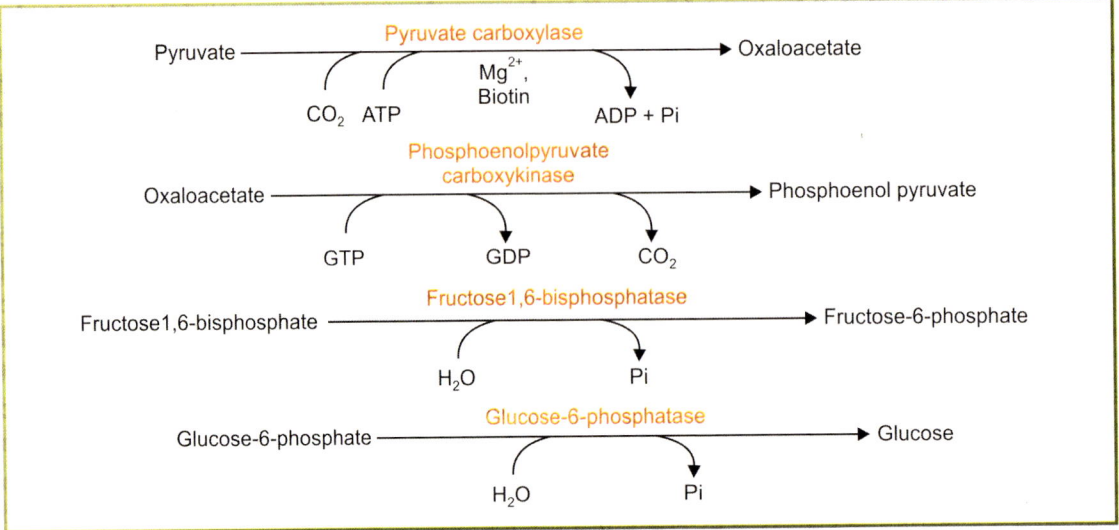

Fig. 11.11: Reactions of gluconeogenesis which bypass the irreversible steps of glycolysis.

transports reducing equivalents from mitochondria to the cytosol. Reactions of gluconeogenesis thus occur both in the cytosol as well as in the mitochondria.

In the cytoplasm, oxaloacetate is converted to phosphoenolpyruvate by **phosphoenolpyruvate carboxykinase** (PEP carboxykinase). The enzyme requires GTP as a coenzyme.

2. **Reversal of fructose-1,6-bisphosphate to fructose-6-phosphate:** The glycolytic reactions catalyzed by phosphofructokinase and hexokinase are endergonic in the gluconeogenesis direction and hence are bypassed by different enzymes.

   Fructose-1,6-bisphosphate is converted to fructose-6-phosphate by **fructose-1,6-bisphosphatase**. Deficiency or inhibition of fructose-1,6-bisphosphatase can impair synthesis of glucose from pyruvate.

   Fructose-6-phosphate is converted to glucose-6-phosphate.

3. **Reversal of glucose-6-phosphate to glucose:** Glucose-6-phosphate is converted to glucose by **glucose-6-phosphatase**. This enzyme is not found in the muscle and adipose tissue.

   PEP-carboxykinase and glucose-6-phosphatase are regulated by induction and repression.

   Energy expenditure during the synthesis of one molecule of glucose from two molecules of pyruvate is equivalent to 10 ATP [2(NADH + H$^+$) per molecule of pyruvate].

Table 11.3: Conversion of glucogenic amino acids to citric acid cycle intermediates

Amino acid	Citric acid cycle intermediate
Gly, Ala, Ser, Thr, Cys, Trp, HO-Pro	Pyruvate
Arg, His, Glu, Gln, Pro	α-Ketoglutarate
Phe, Tyr	Fumarate
Val, Ile, Met	Succinyl CoA

Formation of Glucose from Amino Acids

In the liver, various glucogenic amino acids transfer the α-amino group and release carbon skeletons which form certain intermediates of the citric acid cycle. These intermediates can enter gluconeogenic pathway and from glucose (Table 11.3).

Glucose-alanine cycle: During starvation, amongst the several amino acids which are transported from the muscle to the liver, alanine predominates. It is synthesized in the muscle by transamination of pyruvate (derived from glucose) and is transported via blood to the liver. In the liver, the carbon skeleton of alanine, i.e. pyruvate, is reconverted to glucose and released to the blood stream. It is then taken up by the muscle and used as a source of energy. The pyruvate so formed is again transaminated and is used to resynthesize alanine. This is called glucose-alanine cycle (Fig. 11.12).

Formation of Glucose from Lactate

Lactate produced during anaerobic glycolysis is also converted to glucose. To achieve this, lactate is first

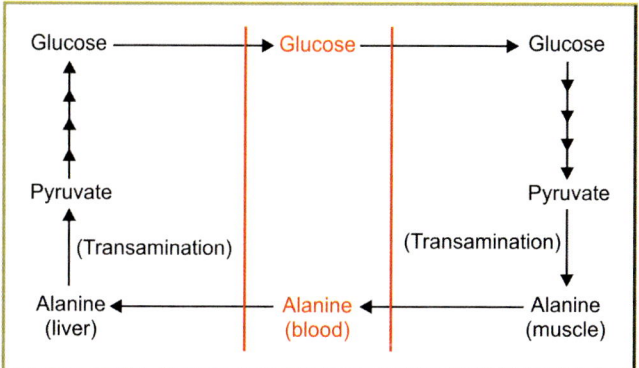

Fig. 11.12: Glucose-alanine cycle.

oxidized to pyruvate. The reaction is catalyzed by lactate dehydrogenase and requires NAD^+. Subsequently pyruvate is converted to glucose by the reversal of the glycolytic reactions.

Cori cycle: The end product of glycogen breakdown in the muscle is glucose-6-phosphate and not free glucose, due to the absence of glucose-6-phosphatase. Glucose-6-phosphate so produced is used for energy production, particularly during exercise (anaerobic glycolysis) and results in the production of lactic acid. Lactic acid is transported to the liver and reforms

glucose by the process of gluconeogenesis. Glucose via circulation again becomes available for its oxidation in the muscle and other tissues. This is called **lactic acid cycle** or Cori cycle (Fig. 11.13). It results in the net exchange of glycogen (via glucose-6-phosphate) and lactic acid in the two tissues, i.e. the muscle and the liver.

Formation of Glucose from Glycerol

Glycerol is produced as a result of lipolysis in the adipose tissue. Glycerol kinase converts it to α-glycerolphosphate in the liver which is later reduced by a dehydrogenase to dihydroxyacetone phosphate and enters glycolysis (Fig. 11.14). Due to the absence of glycerol kinase, adipose tissue cannot utilize glycerol.

Formation of Glucose from Propionate

Oxidation of **fatty acids containing odd number of carbon atoms**, in addition to acetyl CoA, also produces propionyl CoA. The latter is converted to D-methyl-malonyl CoA by propionyl CoA carboxylase. D-Methylmalonyl CoA is then changed to L-methyl-malonyl CoA and finally by an isomerase to succinyl

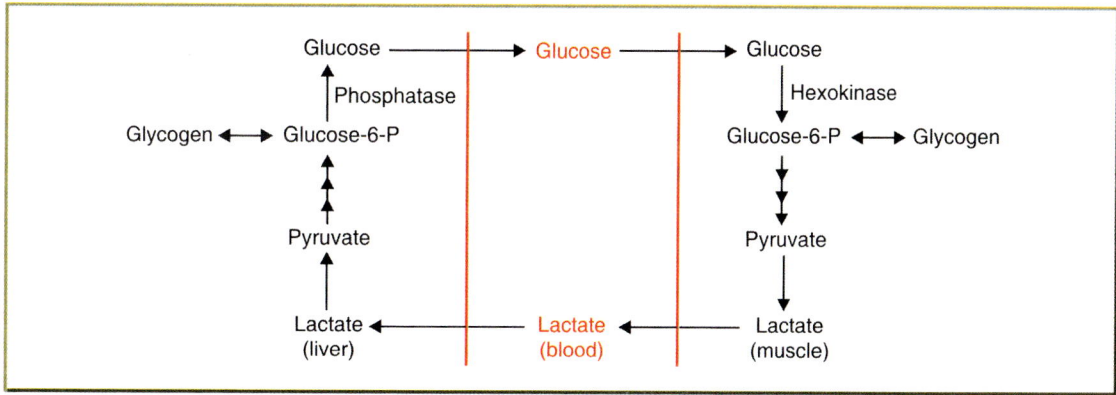

Fig. 11.13: Glucose-lactate cycle (Cori cycle).

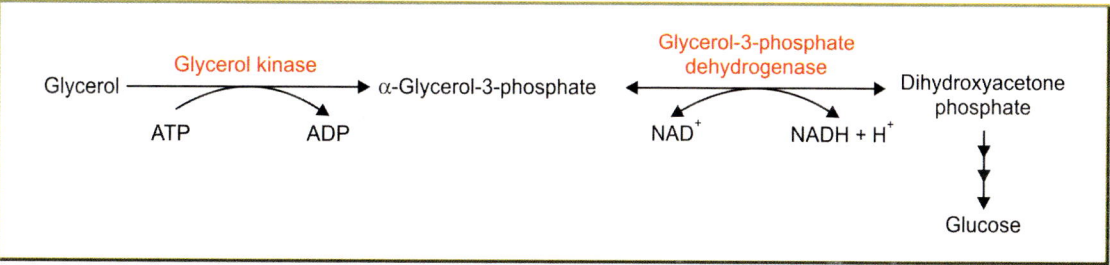

Fig. 11.14: Conversion of glycerol to glucose.

CoA (an intermediate of the citric acid cycle). Succinyl CoA enters the gluconeogenic pathway. **Vitamin B$_{12}$** is required as a coenzyme for the synthesis of glucose from propionyl CoA (Fig. 11.15). This mode of gluconeogenesis is more important in ruminants and less in humans.

Regulation of Gluconeogenesis

The two opposing pathways, i.e. **gluconeogenesis and glycolysis are 'reciprocally' regulated** to meet the glucose needs of the organism. Gluconeogenesis is regulated by the enzymes (pyruvate carboxylase, PEP carboxykinase, fructose-1,6-bisphosphatase and glucose-6-phosphatase) which catalyze to bypass the irreversible steps of glycolysis (hexokinase, phosphofructokinase-1 and pyruvate kinase). Turning-on gluconeogenesis is thus accomplished by shutting-off glycolysis (Fig. 11.16).

Glucagon and insulin also regulate gluconeogenesis by influencing the state of phosphorylation/dephosphorylation of the hepatic enzymes.

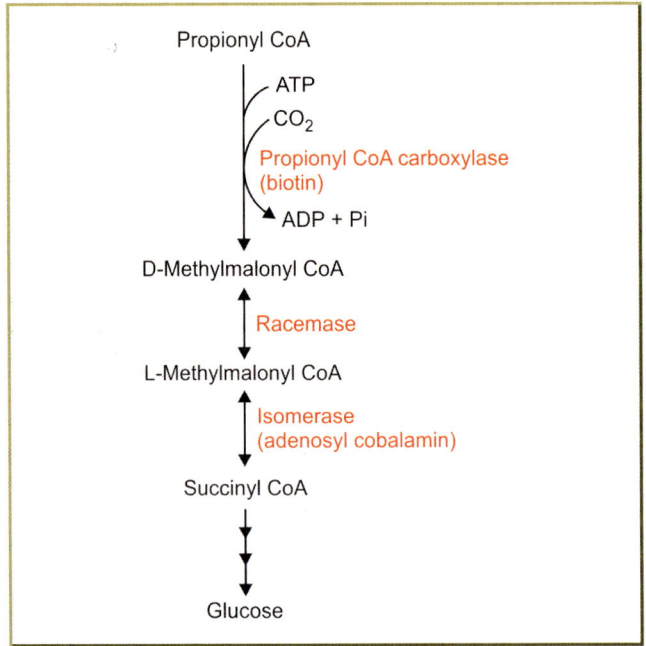

Fig. 11.15: Conversion of propionyl CoA to glucose.

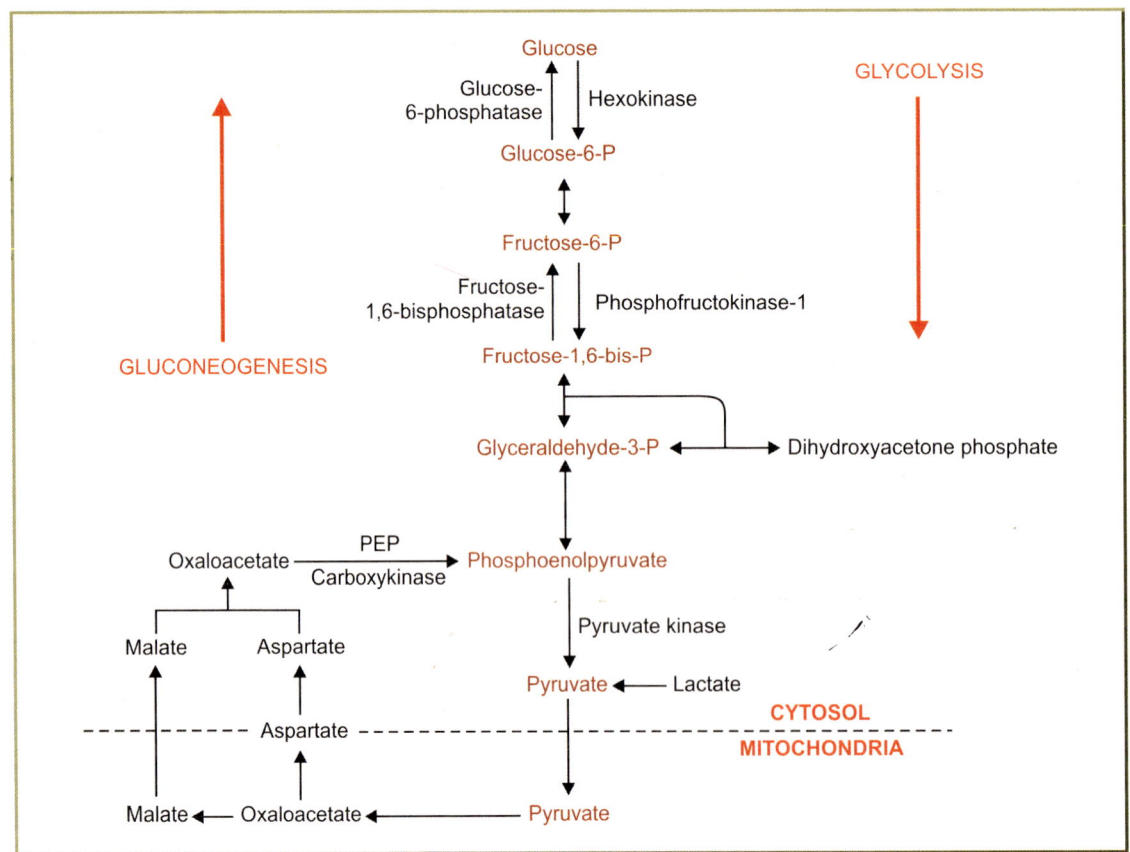

Fig. 11.16: Gluconeogenesis versus glycolysis: Reciprocal regulation.

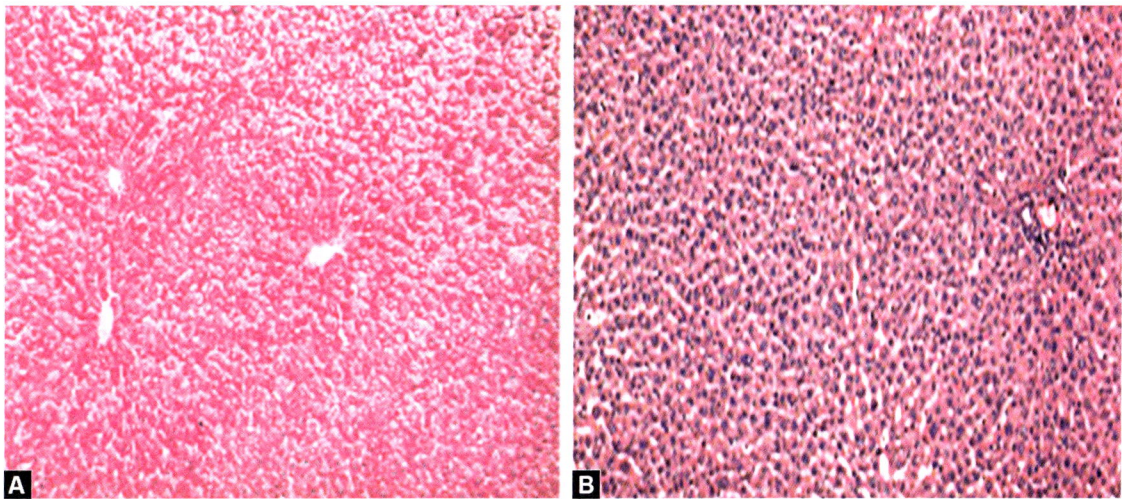

Fig. 11.17: Histological sections of liver. Pink color indicates the presence of hepatic glycogen. (A) **Fed state** with high glycogen content, (B) 24 hours **fasting state** with low glycogen content.

METABOLISM OF GLYCOGEN

Glycogen is the major form of carbohydrate present in the body. It corresponds to starch in plants but is comparatively more branched. It is stored in the body mainly in the **liver** (Fig. 11.17) and the **muscle**.

Importance of Glycogen

While glycogen stored in the liver is used for maintaining blood glucose level during the initial period of fasting and prevent hypoglycemia, the muscle glycogen is used for providing energy during exercise.

GLYCOGENESIS

Glycogenesis (**glycogen synthesis**) is the process of the conversion of **glucose to glycogen**. Although it is operative in several tissues, the liver and the muscle are the main organs for the synthesis of glycogen. Glycogenesis is **increased by insulin**. Glucose is converted to glycogen as follows (Fig. 11.18):

1. Glucose is first activated (phosphorylated) to form glucose-6-phosphate. The reaction is catalyzed by hexokinase in the extrahepatic tissues. The enzyme is allosterically inhibited by glucose-6-phosphate. In the liver, in the fed state, another enzyme, glucokinase converts most of the glucose into glucose-6-phosphate. This is an inducible enzyme and has greater specificity for its substrate.
2. Glucose-6-phosphate is epimerized to form glucose-1-phosphate by phosphoglucomutase.

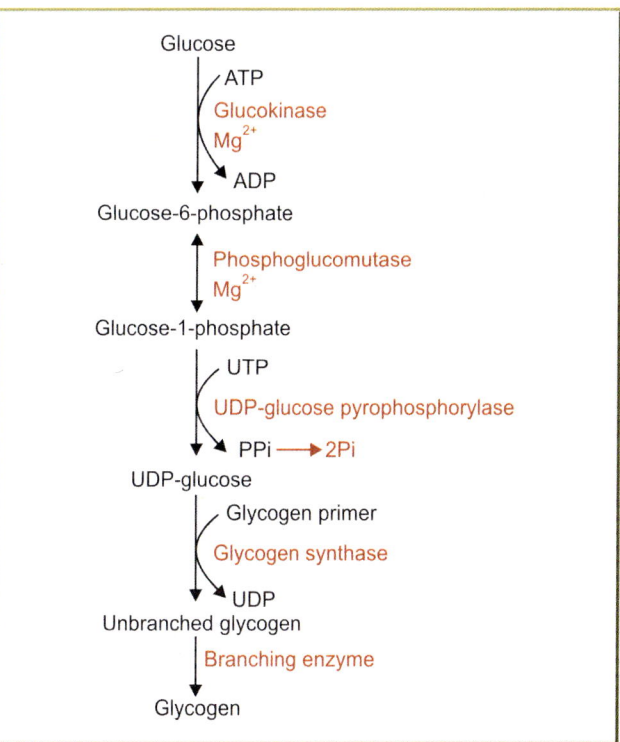

Fig. 11.18: Glycogenesis.

3. Glucose-1-phosphate reacts with UTP (a high energy compound) and is converted to uridine diphosphate glucose (UDP-glucose). The reaction is catalyzed by UDP-glucose pyrophosphorylase (glucose-1-phosphate uridyltransferase). The pyrophosphate so released is immediately

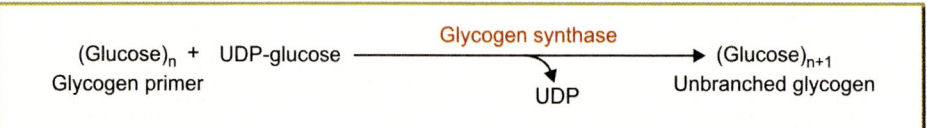

Fig. 11.19: Extension of glycogen primer.

hydrolyzed to two molecules of inorganic phosphate by the enzyme pyrophosphatase.

4. From UDP-glucose, the glucose moiety (a molecule of glucose) is transferred by the enzyme glycogen synthase to the pre-formed glycogen molecule, called **glycogen primer**. The glycogen primer is formed on a protein known as **glycogenin**.

   The incoming glucose is linked to the primer at the non-reducing end by 1,4-α-glycosidic linkage, resulting in elongation of the pre-existing branches. This results in the formation of an unbranched glycogen (Fig. 11.19).

   Both glycogen primer and UDP-glucose are the substrates for **glycogen synthase**. This is a **key enzyme** of glycogenesis. Muscle glycogen synthase is a homotetramer. The enzyme exists in two interconvertible forms, i.e. glycogen synthase a and glycogen synthase b. Glycogen synthase b is phosphorylated and is the inactive form. On the other hand, glycogen synthase a (dephosphorylated enzyme) is active (Fig. 11.20).

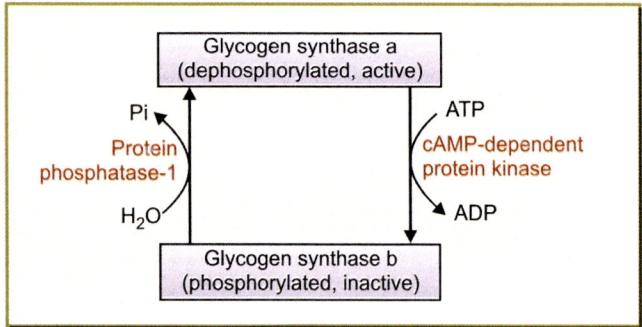

Fig. 11.20: Branching of glycogen.

   The enzyme is under allosteric control. It is strongly inhibited by physiological concentrations of ATP, ADP and Pi and is activated by glucose-6-phosphate.

5. Once a straight chain of about 11 residues has been formed, a branching enzyme (1,4-α-glucan branching enzyme) removes a block of about 7 glucosyl residues from a growing chain and transfers it to the neighbouring chain, to produce an α-1,6-linkage (Fig. 11.21). The branch again

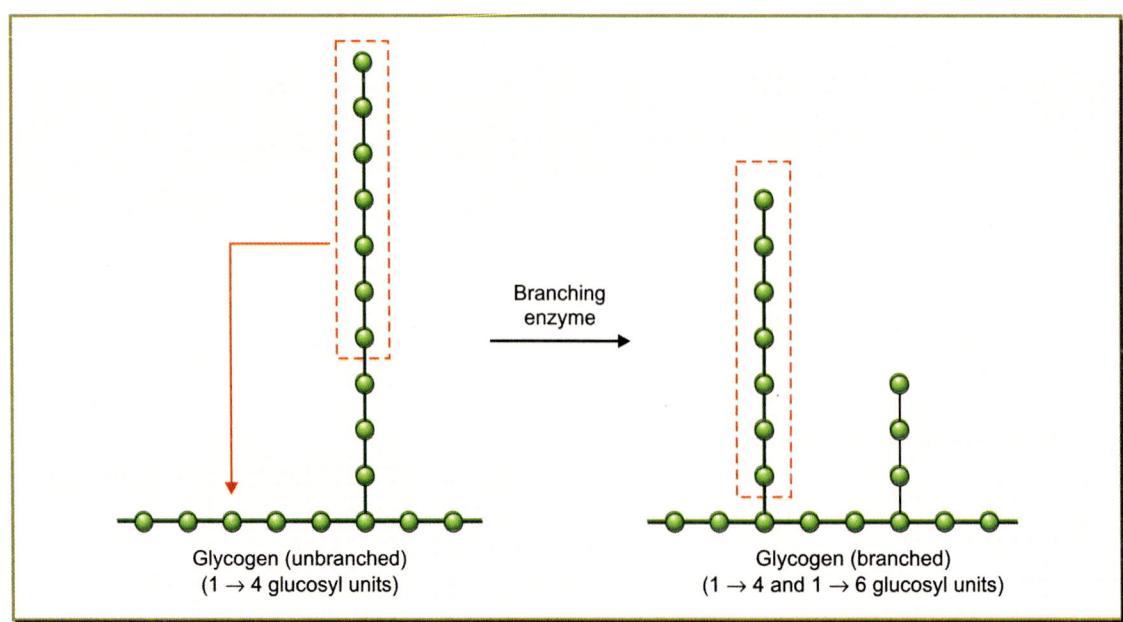

Fig. 11.21: Branching of glycogen

grows by addition of the glucose molecules at the $1\rightarrow4$ linkage and with further branching, it results in the formation of a highly branched polymer of glucose called as glycogen.

Since one ATP and one UTP molecule is used in the incorporation of each glucose unit in glycogen synthesis, the energy spent for the addition of each glucose unit on to the glycogen primer is equivalent to two ATP.

GLYCOGENOLYSIS

Glycogenolysis is the process of **breakdown of glycogen either to glucose-6-phosphate in the muscle or to free glucose in the liver and the kidney** (Fig. 11.22). In the liver, glycogenolysis is stimulated by glucagon. Glycogen is broken down to glucose as follows:

1. Glucose molecules are sequentially removed from glycogen as glucose-1-phosphate (Fig. 11.23). This is catalyzed by the enzyme **phosphorylase**, with **pyridoxal phosphate** as a **coenzyme**. The enzyme hydrolyzes α-1,4-glycosidic bonds until nearly four glucose residues are left on either side of the branch. After the action of phosphorylase, glycogen is partially hydrolyzed leaving a limit branch (**limit dextrin**).

Glycogen phosphorylase is subjected to allosteric activation by AMP and is allosterically inhibited by ATP, glucose-6-phosphate and glucose. The enzyme is a dimer and has two identical subunits. It is regulated both allosterically and by covalent modification (phosphorylation/dephosphorylation). The phosphorylated form of the enzyme is called phosphorylase a, the active form of the enzyme. The dephosphorylated form is called phosphorylase b, the inactive form.

The two forms of the enzyme are interconvertible by the actions of phosphorylase kinase and phosphoprotein phosphatase. Phosphorylase kinase is also subjected to regulation by a cyclic phosphorylation-dephosphorylation mechanism. Protein kinase A phosphorylates and activates phosphorylase kinase while phosphoprotein phosphatase in turn dephosphorylates and inactivates phosphorylase kinase (Fig. 11.24).

2. Debranching enzyme is a bifunctional enzyme that catalyzes two reactions necessary for the debranching of glycogen.

The **first unit of the enzyme** $1 \rightarrow 4$-α-D-glucan-transferase has glycosyltransferase activity in which a strand of three glucosyl residues is removed from a four glucosyl residue branch of the glycogen molecule to the non-reducing end of another branch. This reaction forms a new $\alpha(1 \rightarrow 4)$ linkage with three more units available for the phosphorylase reaction.

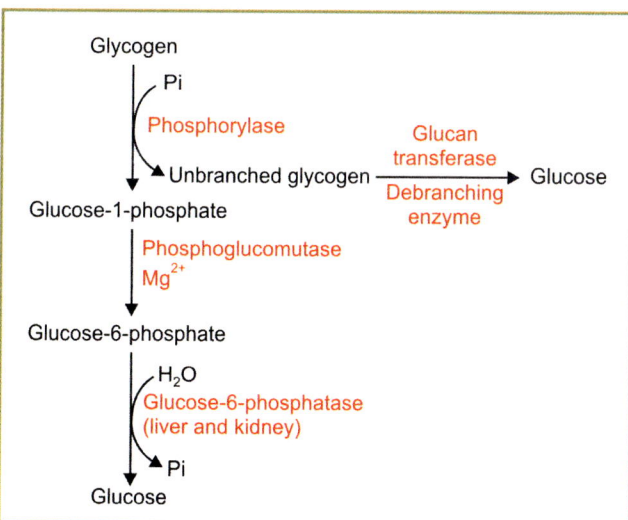

Fig. 11.22: Glycogenolysis.

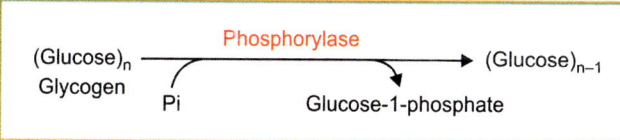

Fig. 11.23: Action of glycogen phosphorylase.

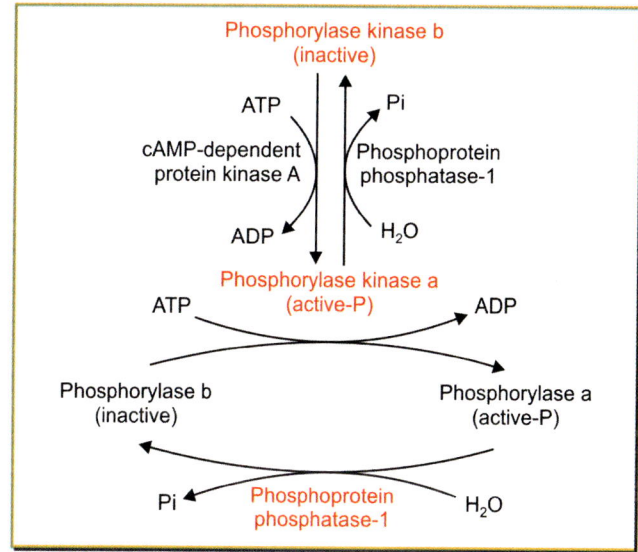

Fig. 11.24: Activation-inactivation of glycogen phosphorylase.

11

The $\alpha(1 \rightarrow 6)$ bond linking the remaining glucosyl residues in the branch to the main chain, is hydrolyzed by the **second enzyme activity** of the debranching enzyme, i.e. amylo-α-1,6-glucosidase. This glucosyl residue is released as glucose (rather than glucose-1-phosphate) leaving unbranched glycogen (Fig. 11.25).

The cooperative and repetitive actions of phosphorylase and debranching enzyme result in complete phosphorolysis of glycogen. During glycogenolysis, glucose-1-phosphate and glucose are liberated in the ratio of approximately 10:1.

3. Glucose-1-phosphate, produced as a result of the action of phosphorylase, is converted to glucose-6-phosphate by phosphoglucomutase.

In the **muscle**, this is the end product of glycogen breakdown and is used by the glycolytic pathway to give energy during exercise. Since glucose-6-phosphatase is absent in the muscle, glycogenolysis is immediately followed by glycolysis.

In the **liver and the kidneys**, glucose-6-phosphatase further hydrolyzes glucose-6-phosphate and produces glucose.

Thus, glycogen stored in the liver is used to maintain blood glucose during fasting so as to prevent a hypoglycemic state whereas glycogen stored in the muscle is used to provide energy during exercise.

Advantage of phosphorolysis over simple hydrolysis of glycogen: Phosphorolytic cleavage of glycogen is advantageous compared with hydrolytic cleavage because the released sugar (glucose-1-phosphate) is already phosphorylated; in case of hydrolysis, the released glucose would need to be phosphorylated in order to enter glycolysis. Further, glucose-1-phosphate is negatively charged and cannot come out of the cell.

Regulation of Glycogen Metabolism

Regulation of glycogen metabolism involves allosteric as well as hormonal control by covalent modification of the regulatory enzymes.

Allosteric Control

Both glycogen phosphorylase and glycogen synthase are under allosteric control by effectors that include ATP, glucose-6-phosphate and AMP.

As mentioned earlier, muscle glycogen phosphorylase is activated by AMP while inhibited by ATP and glucose-6-phosphate. On the other hand, glycogen synthase is activated by glucose-6-phosphate.

Hormonal Control

Glycogen metabolism in the liver is controlled by **glucagon** while in the muscles and various other tissues this control is exerted by **insulin and epinephrine/norepinephrine**. Hormones bind to the transmembrane receptors on surface of the cells and result in the release of second messengers, i.e. cAMP/Ca^{2+}.

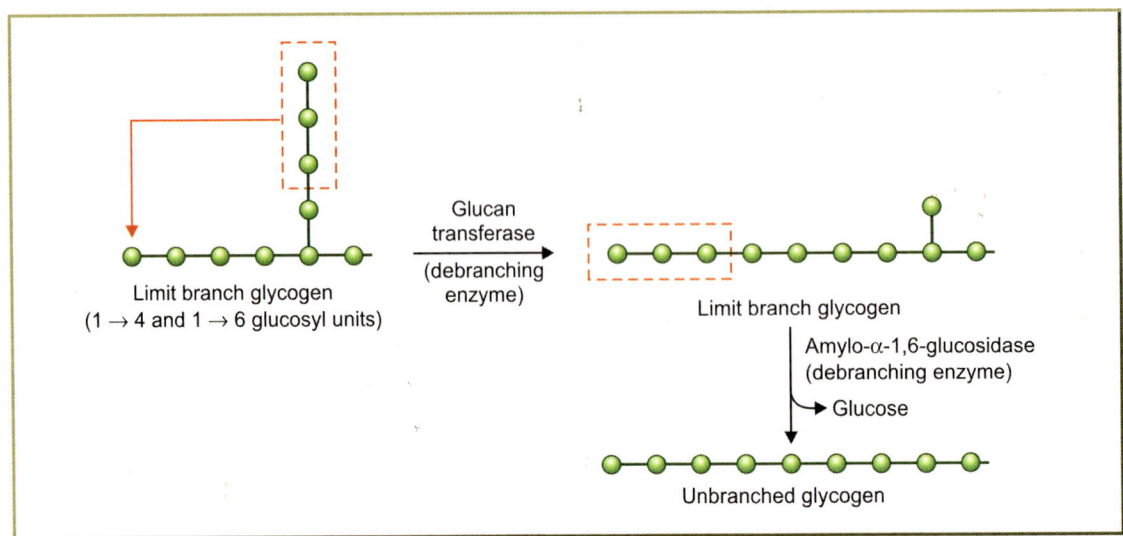

Fig. 11.25: Debranching of glycogen.

Glucagon binds to its receptors in the liver cells and increases intracellular cAMP concentration. This, in turn, promotes degradation of glycogen to glucose. Muscle cells, however, do not have receptors for glucagon.

There are two types of receptors for **epinephrine**:

- Epinephrine binds to α-adrenergic receptors on the **liver cells** and leads to increased cytosolic concentration of Ca^{2+} which promotes glycogenolysis and increases blood glucose concentration.

- Epinephrine binds to β-adrenergic receptors on the **liver and muscle cells**, and increases intracellular cAMP concentration. cAMP, in turn, promotes glycogen breakdown to glucose-6-phosphate for glycolysis in the muscle or to free glucose in the liver (Fig. 11.26).

When circulating glucose concentration is high, insulin increases the rate of glucose transport into many types of cells that have insulin receptors, such as the muscle cells and the fat cells (adipocytes). This, in turn, decreases cAMP concentration, promotes inactivation of glycogen phosphorylase and stimulates glycogen synthesis and thus stores excess of glucose as glycogen.

Covalent Modification of the Regulatory Enzymes

The key enzymes of glycogen metabolism, i.e. glycogen synthase and phosphorylase, as discussed earlier, exist in two different forms, designated as a and b. Interconversion of the a and b forms of these two enzymes is accomplished through enzyme-catalyzed phosphorylation and dephosphorylation under the control of various hormones, e.g. glucagon and epinephrine. **Glycogen phosphorylase is activated by phosphorylation whereas glycogen synthase is inactivated by phosphorylation**. On the other hand, dephosphorylation inactivates phosphorylase and activates glycogen synthase.

Phosphorylation of glycogen phosphorylase is under the control of three enzymes, i.e. phosphorylase kinase, cAMP-dependent protein kinase and phosphoprotein phosphatase-1.

cAMP dependent protein kinase: The intracellular concentration of cAMP is regulated between its rate of synthesis from ATP by adenylate cyclase as well as its breakdown by phosphodiesterase. The binding of the hormones (glucagon as well as epinephrine) to their cell-surface receptors stimulates adenylate cyclase which in turn catalyzes the synthesis of cAMP inside the cell. The cAMP is necessary for the activity of cAMP dependent protein kinase (cAMP-PK).

The enzyme consists of two regulatory subunits (R_2) and two catalytic subunits (C_2). In the absence of cAMP, the enzyme is an inactive tetramer (R_2C_2). The binding of cAMP to the regulatory subunits (R_2) causes dissociation of the active catalytic monomers (2C) (Fig. 11.27).

The intracellular concentration of cAMP thus activates cAMP-PK, which stimulates activation (phosphorylation) of phosphorylase kinase. The

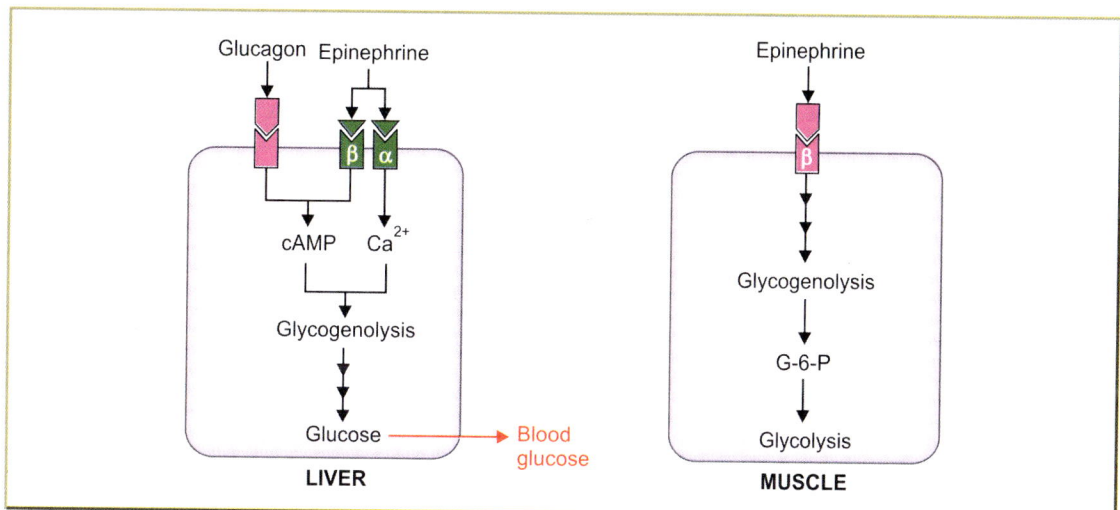

Fig. 11.26: Hormonal control of glycogen metabolism.

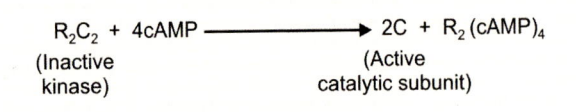

$$R_2C_2 + 4cAMP \longrightarrow 2C + R_2(cAMP)_4$$
(Inactive kinase)　　　　(Active catalytic subunit)

Fig. 11.27: Activation of cAMP-dependent protein kinase.

cAMP-PK also results in the phosphorylation of phosphorylase and glycogen synthase (Fig. 11.28).

The enzyme cAMP-PK also phosphorylates (activates) phosphoprotein phosphatase inhibitor-1 (Fig. 11.29).

Phosphorylase kinase: Phosphorylase kinase is a tetramer with four non-identical subunits, i.e. α, β, γ and δ. The γ subunit contains the catalytic site while the other three subunits have regulatory functions. The enzyme is activated by Ca^{2+} through its binding to the δ subunit which is also called **calmodulin**.

Phosphorylation of the α and β subunits of phosphorylase kinase also activates the enzyme.

Active phosphorylase kinase (phosphorylase kinase a) results in the activation (phosphorylation)

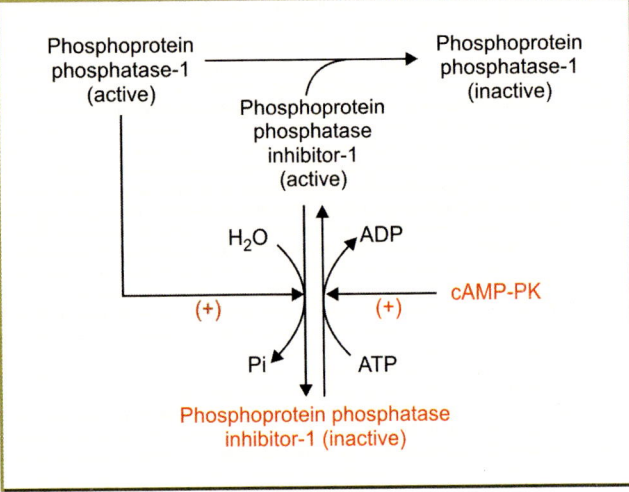

Fig. 11.29: Regulation of phosphoprotein phosphatase-1.

of glycogen phosphorylase and inactivation of glycogen synthase (Fig. 11.28).

Phosphoprotein phosphatase-1: Phosphoprotein phosphatase-1 removes phosphoryl groups from glycogen phosphorylase a, glycogen synthase b, and

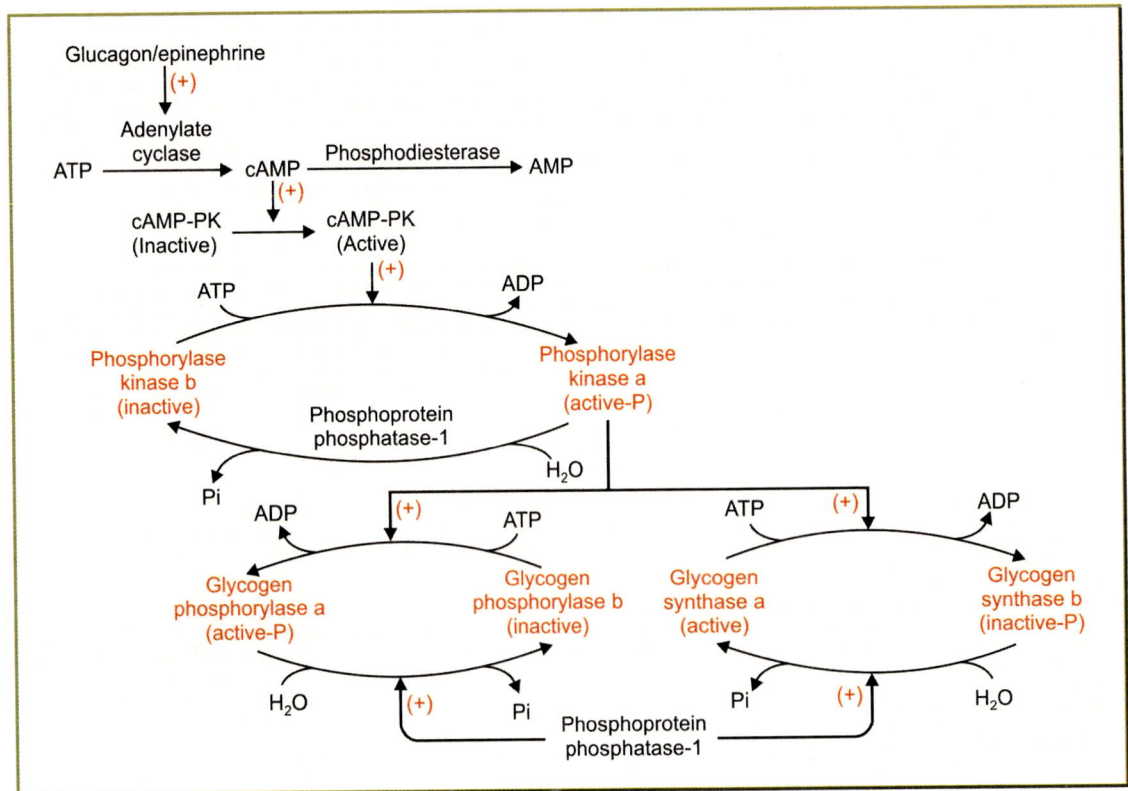

Fig. 11.28: Regulation of glycogen phosphorylase and glycogen synthase by covalent modification.

from the α and β subunits of phosphorylase kinase (Fig. 11.28).

Phosphoprotein phosphatase-1 itself is also inhibited by its binding to phosphoprotein phosphatase inhibitor 1. The Inhibitor 1, in turn, is activated by cAMP-PK but inactivated by the active phosphoprotein phosphatase-1 (Fig. 11.29).

The rates of phosphorylation and dephosphorylation of glycogen phosphorylase and glycogen synthase thus control glycogen synthesis as well as its breakdown.

Glycogen Metabolism in Liver versus Muscle

Table 11.4 shows glycogen metabolism differs in liver and skeletal muscle in several aspects.

Glycogen Storage Diseases

This is a group of inherited disorders associated with glycogen metabolism where an abnormal type or quantity of glycogen is deposited in different tissues. According to the deficiency of the enzyme involved, there are several types of glycogen storage diseases. All these are autosomal recessive disorders except Her's disease which is autosomal dominant (Table 11.5).

HEXOSE MONOPHOSPHATE SHUNT

Hexose monophosphate shunt (**HMP shunt**) or **pentose phosphate pathway** is the second major pathway for the metabolism of glucose. Enzymes for this pathway are localized in the **cytosol** and the reducing equivalents are accepted by **NADP$^+$ instead of NAD$^+$**. This pathway is operative in many tissues, such as the liver, erythrocytes, lactating mammary gland, testes and the adipose tissue. The rate of HMP shunt reactions is **increased by insulin**. Glucose is catabolized by HMP shunt as follows (Fig. 11.30):

Table 11.4: Comparison of glycogen metabolism in liver and skeletal muscle

Parameter	Liver	Skeletal muscle
Glycogen concentration	Higher: 10% w/w	Lower: 2% w/w
Absolute amount of glycogen in healthy adults in well-fed state	Lower: ~70 g	Higher: ~250 g because muscle mass (~35 kg) is much greater than liver mass (~1.8 kg)
Glucose-6-phosphatase	Present, hence free glucose is released after glycogenolysis	Absent, hence glucose-6-phosphate formed in glycogenolysis directly enters glycolysis in the muscle itself
Hormonal regulation of glycogenolysis	More responsive to glucagon	More responsive to epinephrine
Purpose of glycogenolysis	To regulate blood glucose levels in between meals, for use by brain, muscles, RBC	To provide glucose for its own use

Table 11.5: Glycogen storage diseases (glycogenoses)

Type	Glycogenoses	Deficient enzyme	Characteristics
0	Lewis disease	Hepatic glycogen synthase	Fasting ketotic hypoglycemia
I	von Gierke's disease	Glucose-6-phosphatase	Hypoglycemia, lactic acidosis, ketosis, hyperlipidemia, hyperuricemia. Liver, kidney and intestinal epithelial cells loaded with glycogen
II	Pompe's disease	Lysosomal acid maltase	Accumulation of glycogen in lysosomes, heart failure
III	Limit dextrinosis/Forbe's disease/ Cori's disease	Debranching enzyme	Accumulation of characteristic branched polysaccharide in liver, muscles, heart and WBC
IV	Amylopectinosis/Anderson's disease	Branching enzyme	Accumulation of polysaccharide with a few branch points, liver/cardiac failure leading to death in 1st year of life
V	McArdle's syndrome	Muscle phosphorylase	↓ exercise tolerance, muscles with very high glycogen content, little or no lactate in blood after exercise
VI	Her's disease	Liver phosphorylase	High liver glycogen content, tendency of hypoglycemia
VII	Tarui's disease	Phosphofructokinase	As per type V, possibility of hemolytic anaemia
VIII	–	Liver phosphorylase kinase	As per type VI

11

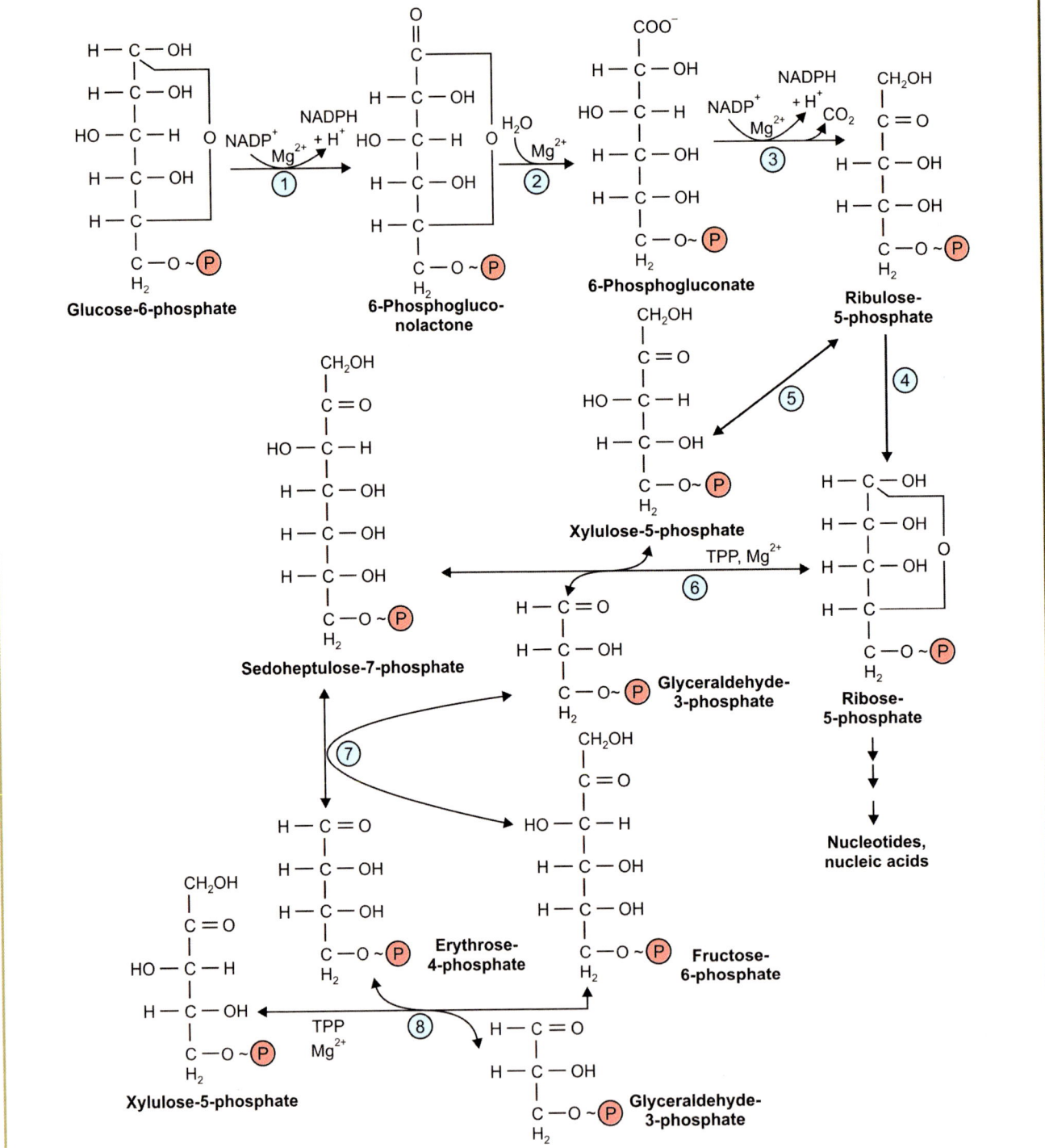

Fig. 11.30: Hexose monophosphate shunt or pentose phosphate pathway. 1. Glucose-6-phosphate dehydrogenase, 2. Gluconolactone hydrolase, 3. 6-Phosphogluconate dehydrogenase, 4. Ketoisomerase, 5. 3-Epimerase, 6. Transketolase, 7. Transaldolase, 8. Transketolase.

1. Firstly, glucose is activated to glucose-6-phosphate by hexokinase (Fig. 11.4). Thereafter, glucose-6-phosphate, by glucoses-6-phosphate dehydro-genase (**G6PD, induced by insulin**), is changed to 6-phosphogluconolactone. NADP+ is reduced to NADPH + H+. G6PD deficiency may be

associated with hemolytic anemia (Chemistry to Clinics 11.9).

2. 6-Phosphogluconolactone is converted to 6-phosphogluconate by gluconolactone hydrolase.

3. In the next reaction, **a hexose is converted to a pentose**. 6-Phosphogluconate is oxidized by 6-phosphogluconate dehydrogenase to form an intermediate 3-keto-6-phosphogluconate. This reaction also generates NADPH + H$^+$. Subsequently, by the enzyme 6-phosphogluconate decarboxylase, 3-keto-6-phosphogluconate is decarboxylated (the first carbon atom is removed as CO_2) to leave a pentose, ribulose-5-phosphate.

Chemistry to Clinics 11.9: Glucose-6-Phosphate Dehydrogenase (G6PD) Deficiency

It is an X-linked inherited disease characterized by hemolytic anemia due to an inability to detoxify oxidizing agents. The molecular defect is a point mutation in the *G6PD* gene and >300 variants are known. Highest prevalence is seen in the Middle East, tropical Africa and Asia, and parts of Mediterranean. Babies with G6PD deficiency suffer from neonatal jaundice appearing 1–4 days after birth due to increased bilirubin production resulting from hemolysis.

G6PD deficiency impairs the ability of RBC to form NADPH which is essential for the maintenance of reduced glutathione (GSH), a potent intracellular antioxidant (Fig. 11.31). This results in reduced detoxification of reactive oxygen species (free radicals such as superoxide anion as well as non-radicals like hydrogen peroxide) which damage the RBC membrane with consequent hemolysis. Further, there is oxidation of sulfhydryl groups in proteins including hemoglobin and leads to the formation of denatured proteins that form insoluble masses called **Heinz bodies**, which get attached to the cell membrane. **Extreme caution** should be taken when prescribing any drug to these patients since **oxidant-drugs readily trigger hemolysis**. Such drugs include antibiotics (sulfamethoxazole, chloramphenicol), anti-malarials (primaquine) and anti-pyretics (acetanilide).

Both glucose-6-phosphate dehydrogenase and 6-phosphogluconate dehydrogenase are **regulatory enzymes** of the shunt.

4. In the second stage of the shunt, ribulose-5-phosphate is utilized in a multicyclic process and is converted to other pentoses. Ribulose-5-phosphate is changed to ribose-5-phosphate by ribose-5-phosphate ketoisomerase.

5. Ribulose-5-phosphate is also converted to xylulose-5-phosphate by ribulose-5-phosphate epimerase.

6. The carbon skeletons of these pentoses are rearranged. A **transketolase** transfers a ketol group (the first 2 carbon atoms) from xylulose-5-phosphate onto ribose-5-phosphate forming sedoheptulose-7-phosphate and glyceraldehyde-3-phosphate. Transketolase requires **TPP as a coenzyme**.

7. An aldol group (3-carbon moiety) is transferred by transaldolase from sedoheptulose-7-phosphate onto glyceraldehyde-3-phosphate forming fructose-6-phosphate and erythrose-4-phosphate.

8. Transketolase also transfers a ketol group (2 carbon moiety) from xylulose-5-phosphate onto erythrose-4-phosphate, forming fructose-6-phosphate and glyceraldehyde-3-phosphate.

The Overall Process of HMP Shunt

Six molecules of hexoses (glucose) are utilized to give six molecules of CO_2 and six molecules of pentoses. These pentoses are rearranged to give four molecules of fructose-6-phosphate and two molecules of glyceraldehyde-3-phosphate which also forms a molecule of hexose by the reversal of glycolysis, thus regenerating five molecules of hexoses (Fig. 11.32).

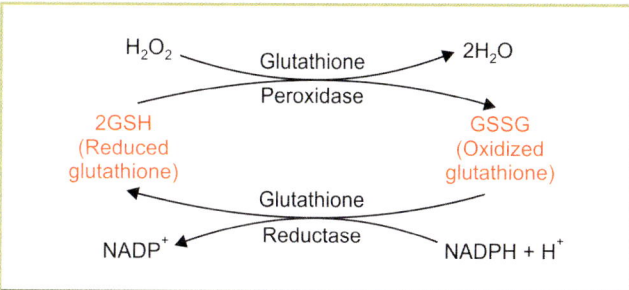

Fig. 11.31: Significance of HMP shunt in RBC.

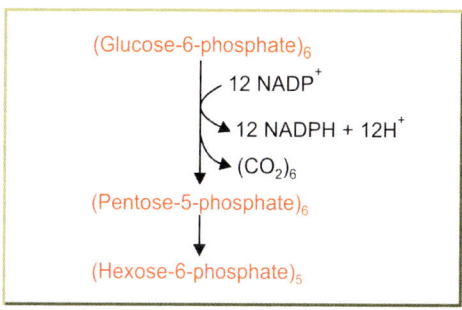

Fig. 11.32: HMP shunt—an overview.

11

Biological Importance of HMP Shunt

1. In the liver

- The NADPH produced in the HMP shunt is used for various **anabolic reactions**, such as for the synthesis of fatty acids and cholesterol.
- The liver is an important site for the **biotransformation of xenobiotics** which take place in the smooth endoplasmic reticulum and also require NADPH.
- HMP shunt is also important as a **source of pentoses** required for the biosynthesis of **nucleic acids** (Fig. 11.33).

2. In the erythrocytes

- NADPH is utilized by glutathione reductase to maintain the reduced state of glutathione, so as to **prevent RBC hemolysis**. This reaction is important for the detoxification of H_2O_2 produced in the erythrocytes since its accumulation decreases the lifespan of the erythrocytes (Fig. 11.31).
- NADPH is required for the activity of **methemoglobin reductase** that reduces the small amount of ferri-hemoglobin formed normally, back to ferrous-hemoglobin.

3. **Phagocytosis** by neutrophils and macrophages also requires NADPH.

Metabolic Partitioning of Glucose-6-Phosphate

Glucose-6-Phosphate is metabolized by glycolysis as well as by HMP shunt. It is carefully partitioned between these two metabolic routes depending on the cellular metabolic demand. Further, different tissues have varying requirements for NADPH or ribose so that the initial reactions (generating NADPH) or the

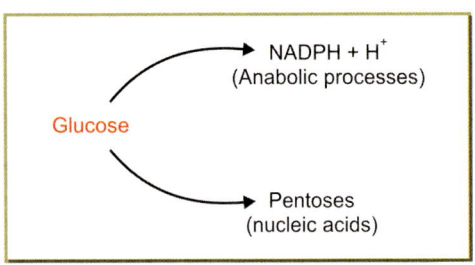

Fig. 11.33: Importance of HMP shunt in the liver.

later reactions (generating ribose) of HMP shunt become predominant (Table 11.6).

GLUCURONIC ACID PATHWAY

Glucuronic acid pathway or **uronic acid pathway** is also an alternative pathway for the oxidation of glucose but it **neither leads to the generation of ATP nor NADPH**. In this pathway, glucose may be converted to glucuronate, pentoses or ascorbate (but not in man, primates and Guinea pigs). This pathway mainly operates in the adipose tissue. Since uronic acid is an important intermediate, this pathway is also known as uronic acid pathway. The salient features of the pathway are as follows (Fig. 11.34):

1. Glucose is activated by hexokinase in the presence of ATP and Mg^{2+}, to form glucose-6-phosphate (Fig. 11.4).
2. Glucose-6-phosphate is converted to glucose-1-phosphate by the enzyme phosphoglucomutase.
3. Glucose-1-phosphate reacts with UTP in the presence of uridine diphosphate glucose pyrophosphorylase (UDP-glucose pyrophosphorylase) to form an active nucleotide, i.e. uridine diphosphate glucose (UDP-glucose).

Table 11.6: Metabolic partitioning of glucose-6-phosphate

Metabolic requirement	Metabolic location	Metabolic purpose
Ribose-5-phosphate >> NADPH	Rapidly dividing cells of bone marrow and small intestinal epithelium	Rapid synthesis of nucleic acids
Ribose-5-phosphate ~ NADPH	Hepatocytes	Repair/regeneration along with detoxification
Ribose-5-phosphate << NADPH	Adipocytes Liver Testis/ovary Mammary gland Adrenal gland	Fatty acid and cholesterol synthesis Fatty acid and cholesterol synthesis Steroidogenesis Fatty acid synthesis Steroidogenesis
NADPH (HMP shunt) and ATP (glycolysis)	RBC	To maintain reduced glutathione (GSH) along with proper membrane functions

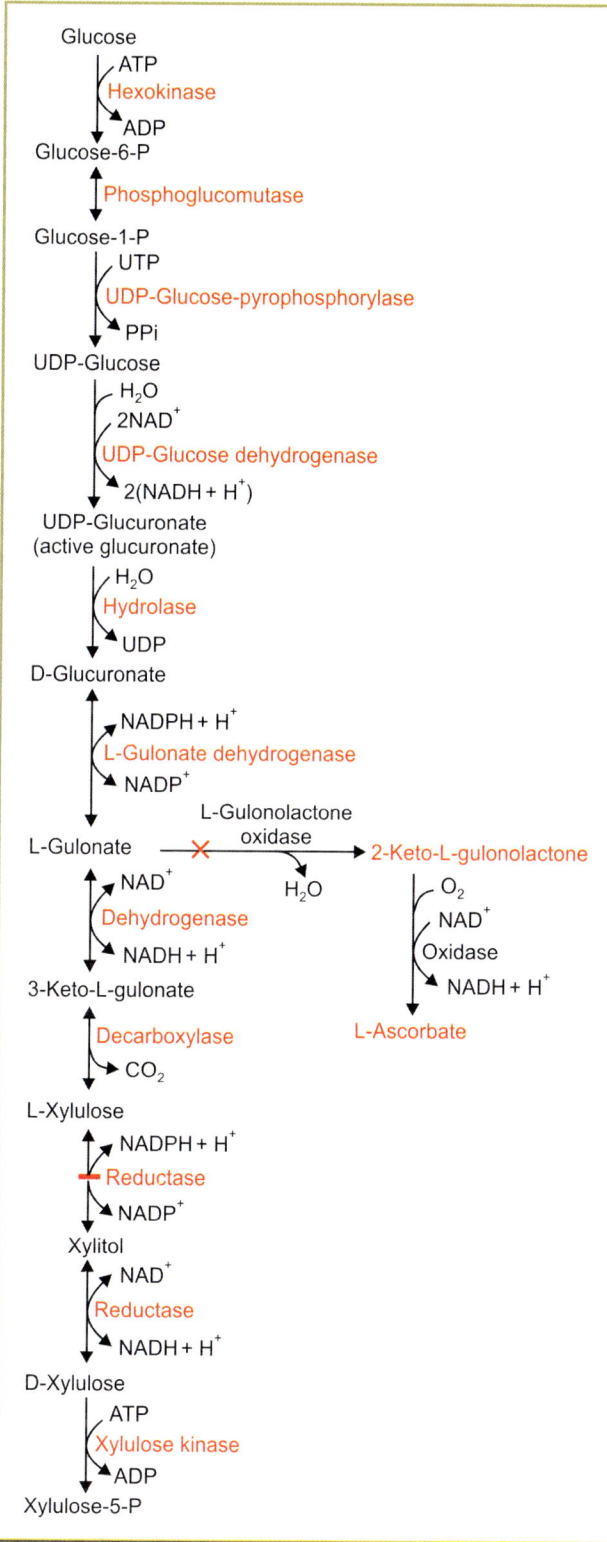

Fig. 11.34. Uronic acid pathway (X Blocked in humans), (▬ Blocked in essential pentosuria).

4. UDP-glucose is oxidized at C6 in the presence of NAD$^+$ dependent UDP-glucose dehydrogenase, to form **UDP-glucuronate**. This is the **active form of glucuronate** that is used in many conjugation reactions catalyzed by glucuronyl transferase, and is clinically important (Chemistry to Clinics 11.10).

5. UDP-glucuronate is hydrolyzed to form D-glucuronate.

6. D-glucuronate, in the presence of NADPH + H$^+$, is reduced to L-gulonate by L-gulonate dehydrogenase.

7. L-Gulonate is further metabolized differently, in different species. In **humans and other primates**, L-gulonate is oxidized to 3-keto-L-gulonate by dehydrogenase. The latter is subsequently decarboxylated to L-xylulose.

   In **plants and higher animals (except humans, other primates and guinea pigs)** which are capable of synthesizing **L-ascorbic acid (vitamin C)**, L-gulonate via L-gulonolactone, is converted to L-ascorbate. This reaction is catalyzed by L-gulonolactone oxidase. Human beings, other primates (e.g. monkeys) and Guinea pigs lack L-gulonolactone oxidase.

8. L-xylulose is reduced by NADPH-dependent L-xylulose reductase (xylitol dehydrogenase) to xylitol (Chemistry to Clinics 11.11).

9. Xylitol is then oxidized, in the presence of NAD$^+$ to D-xylulose.

Chemistry to Clinics 11.10: Neonatal Jaundice

With the help of the enzyme UDP-glucuronyl transferase, glucuronate gets conjugated with various compounds such as bilirubin, steroid hormones and several drugs. UDP-glucuronyl transferase converts these substances into their soluble glucuronides which can be easily excreted in the urine. Thus, bilirubin which is not soluble in water is also changed to **conjugated bilirubin (bilirubin glucuronides)** and becomes water soluble. However, development of the glucuronyl transferase conjugating mechanism occurs gradually and takes 10–12 days, after birth, to become fully active. The neonatal liver due to lack of glucuronyl transferase is thus unable to form bilirubin glucuronides at a rate comparable to that of bilirubin production. As a result, serum bilirubin (**unconjugated bilirubin**) level is higher in the newborns, in the first week of life. This condition is called **physiological jaundice of the newborn** or neonatal jaundice.

Glucuronyl transferase deficiency in adults is found in **Crigglar-Najjar syndrome**, a congenital familial non-hemolytic jaundice.

11

Reduced activity of NADP-linked L-xylulose reductase results in the excretion of large amounts of L-xylulose (a pentose) in the urine. This condition is called essential pentosuria.

10. D-xylulose, after phosphorylation with ATP by the kinase, is converted to D-xylulose-5-phosphate that can enter the HMP shunt.

SORBITOL PATHWAY

Glucose can also be converted to fructose by the cells of seminal vesicles (Fig. 11.35). These reactions are catalyzed by an NADPH-dependent reduction of glucose to sorbitol by aldose reductase and by an NAD^+-dependent oxidation of sorbitol to fructose by polyol dehydrogenase (sorbitol dehydrogenase).

Fructose is secreted from seminal vesicles in a fluid, forming part of the semen. Besides seminal vesicles, peripheral nerves, renal papillae, Schwann cells, glomerulus and retinal capillaries and lens (Chemistry to Clinics 11.12) also contain the two enzymes of the polyol pathway.

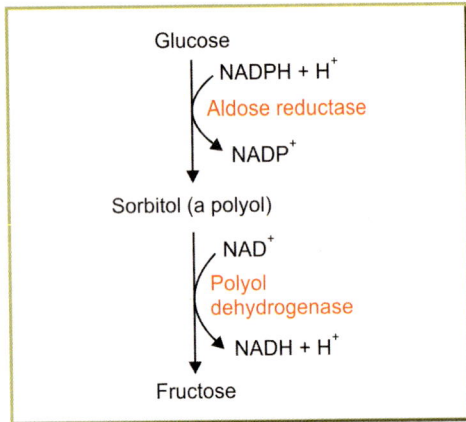

Fig. 11.35: Polyol pathway.

FRUCTOSE METABOLISM

Fructose is obtained by the body either directly from diet or as a result of hydrolysis of sucrose in the small intestine. **Highest concentration of fructose is found in the seminal fluid**. Fructose is converted to glucose for its utilization by the body by various routes (Fig. 11.37):

1. Fructose is changed to fructose-1-phosphate by a specific enzyme fructokinase present in the liver, muscle, intestine and kidneys. Fructose-1-phosphate is cleaved by the enzyme aldolase B. This enzyme is different from aldolase A which acts on fructose-1,6-bisphosphate. Aldolase B splits fructose-1-phosphate to dihydroxyacetone phosphate and D-glyceraldehyde (Chemistry to Clinics 11.13).

Subsequently, glyceraldehyde is phosphorylated by ATP in the presence of triose kinase and is changed to 3-phosphoglyceraldehyde that, in turn,

In diabetes mellitus, more glucose becomes available to enter the tissues which are not dependent on insulin for glucose uptake, such as the lens. Many proteins undergo non-enzymatic glycation to form **'advanced glycation end products' (AGE)** with partial loss of biological function. Such proteins include hemoglobin, albumin, and the lens protein crystallin. Further, the ratio of the activities of the two enzymes of the sorbitol pathway, favors sorbitol accumulation in the lens. This, in turn, increases osmolarity of the lens and affects structural organization of crystallin, thereby enhancing the rate of protein aggregation and denaturation leading to cataract (Fig. 11.36). Aldose reductase inhibitors such as tolrestat and epalrestat partly suppress cataractogenesis.

Fructokinase deficiency results in **essential fructosuria**, due to which fructose appears in the urine, after a high fructose or sucrose diet is ingested. On the other hand, individuals with **aldolase B deficiency** suffer from **hereditary fructose intolerance**.

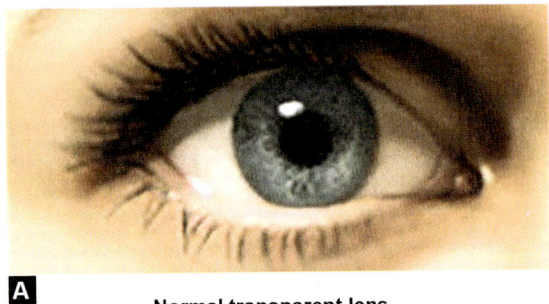
A   **Normal transparent lens**

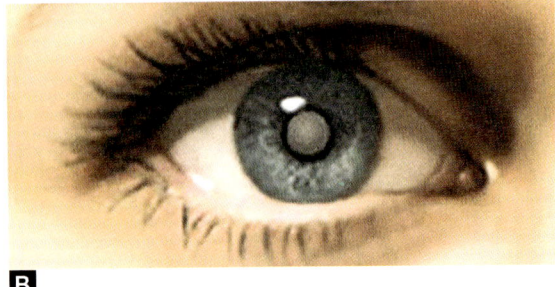
B   **Opaque lens (cataract)**

Fig. 11.36: Cataract: The normal transparent lens (A) becomes translucent or opaque (B), resulting in blurring or complete loss of vision.

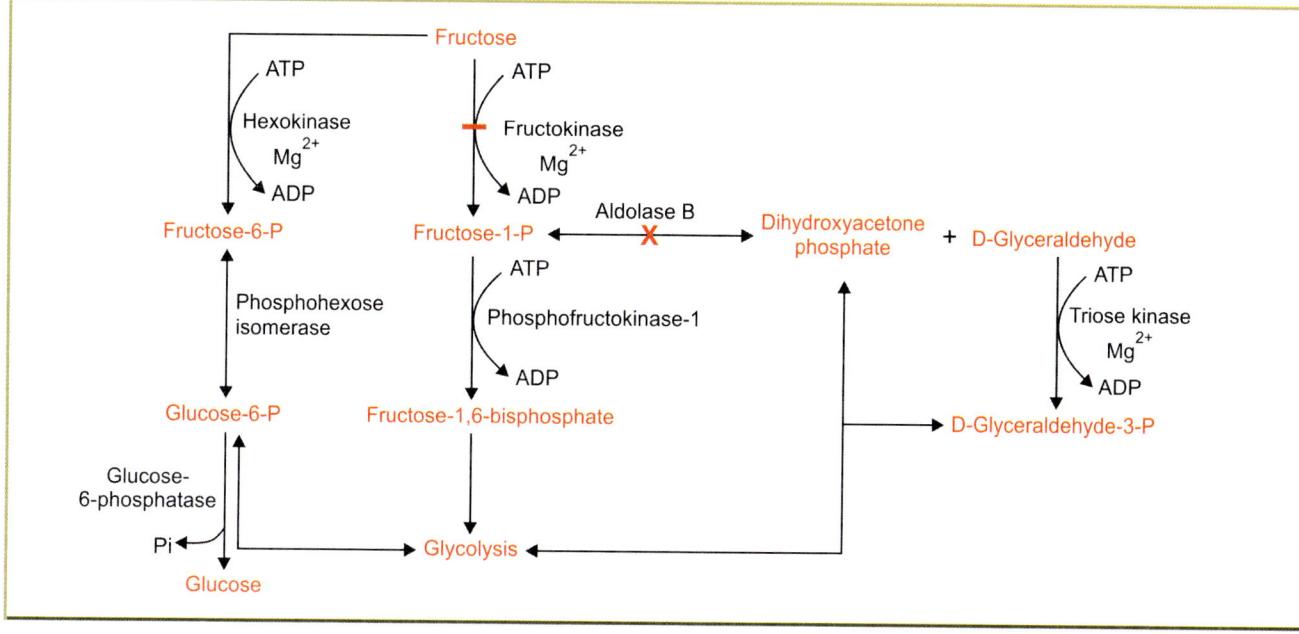

Fig. 11.37: Fructose metabolism (▬ Blocked in essential fructosuria) (**X** Blocked in hereditary fructose intolerance).

can get conjugated with dihydroxyacetone phosphate and form glucose-6-phosphate, by the reversal of the glycolytic reaction.

2. Alternatively, fructose-1-phosphate may be phosphorylated to form fructose-1,6-bisphosphate by the enzyme phosphofructokinase-1. The latter can then enter the glycolytic pathway.

3. Fructose may also be changed to fructose-6-phosphate by hexokinase. The latter is isomerized to glucose-6-phosphate and either enters glycolysis or hydrolyzed to produce glucose.

GALACTOSE METABOLISM

Galactose is released into blood stream by the **hydrolysis of lactose** due to the action of **lactase in the intestine**. Most of the dietary galactose is changed to glucose in the liver. This ability of the liver to utilize galactose is important in the assessment of the liver function test after a galactose load (**galactose tolerance test**).

Galactose is utilized in the liver, brain and lactating mammary gland by various routes (Fig. 11.38):

1. **In the liver**, galactose is phosphorylated by galactokinase and is converted to galactose-1-phosphate, more rapidly in children than in adults. Subsequently, galactose-1-phosphate reacts with uridine diphosphate glucose (UDP-glucose), in

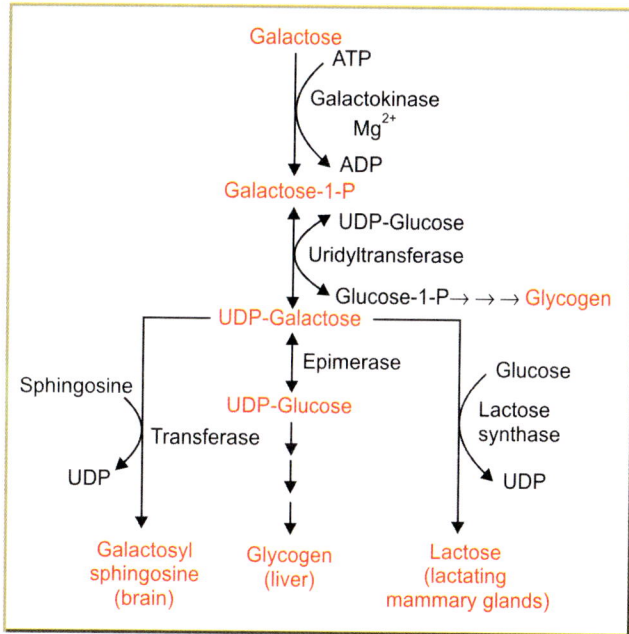

Fig. 11.38: Galactose metabolism.

the presence of galactose-1-phosphate uridyl-transferase and forms glucose-1-phosphate and UDP-galactose. The latter may be changed to UDP-glucose by the enzyme UDP-galactose-4-epimerase. Both glucose-1-phosphate and UDP-glucose can be used in glycogenesis. Several enzyme deficiencies in galactose metabolism can result in galactosemia (Chemistry to Clinics 11.14).

Chemistry to Clinics 11.14: Galactosemia

It refers to increased galactose levels in blood, and is of several types:

Type 1 (classical): Deficiency of galactose-1-phosphate uridyl-transferase.

Type 2: Deficiency of galactokinase.

Type 3: Deficiency of UDP-galactose-4-epimerase.

Features

1. Galactosemia, i.e. increased levels of galactose in the blood results in galactosuria (excretion of galactose in the urine).
2. Increased galactose concentration in the blood results in a higher galactose concentration in the lens of the eyes where this sugar is reduced to galactitol. This causes osmotic retention of water and damage to the lens protein (crystallin) with cataract formation.
3. In classical galactosemia, accumulation of galactose-1-phosphate inhibits glycogenolysis resulting in hypoglycemia and seizures. It also depletes the hepatic stores of inorganic phosphate (Pi) leading to liver damage and jaundice.
4. Deficiency of UDP-galactose impairs the synthesis of galactose-containing cerebral glycolipids, which, along with hypoglycemic episodes, hyperbilirubinemia and cerebral edema (due to accumulation of galactitol) may be responsible for mental retardation (Fig. 11.39).

Treatment: Galactose and lactose-free diet.

2. **In the brain**, UDP-galactose reacts with sphingosine, in the presence of the enzyme galactose-sphingosine transferase and is changed to galactosyl-sphingosine for use in the synthesis of gangliosides and cerebrosides.

3. **In the lactating mammary gland**, UDP-galactose combines with glucose in the presence of lactose synthase and forms lactose, for its secretion into the milk.

REGULATION OF BLOOD GLUCOSE

Blood glucose level is regulated by a balance between a number of factors that tend to reduce blood glucose, and others that tend to increase it. **Blood glucose homeostasis** requires tuning between:

1. Different metabolic pathways
2. Hormones
3. Kidneys.

Metabolic Pathways Regulating Blood Glucose Level

- Glycolysis, HMP shunt, and glycogenesis lower blood glucose concentration while glycogenolysis and gluconeogenesis increase blood glucose concentration.

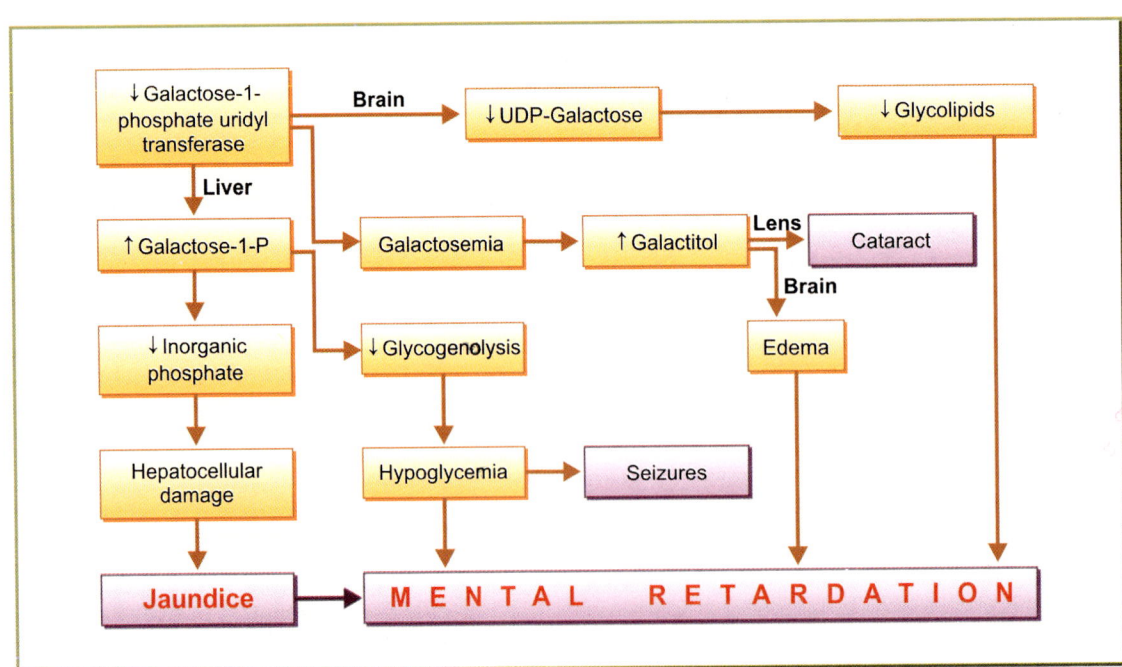

Fig. 11.39: Classical galactosemia: Biochemical-clinical correlations.

- In the **fasting state** or on a **low carbohydrate diet** when blood glucose level is reduced, glycogenolysis and gluconeogenesis are stimulated in the liver and add glucose to the blood. Lipolysis is also stimulated and lipids serve as a source of fuel for different tissues.
- In the **fed state**, when blood glucose concentration is increased, its cellular transport in the liver and its utilization by the glycolytic reactions is also increased. Glycogenesis is also stimulated in the liver and the muscle. At the same time, lipolysis is inhibited.

Hormonal Regulation of Blood Glucose

Several hormones regulate blood glucose concentration. While insulin is the only hormone which lowers blood glucose level, various other hormones increase blood glucose level (Fig. 11.40).

Hormone with Hypoglycemic Action: Insulin

Insulin is the only hormone with hypoglycemic action. It is released into the bloodstream under the direct influence of hyperglycemia. It is a polypeptide containing 2 chains and is produced by the **β-cells of the islets of Langerhans located in the tail of the pancreas**. Insulin **lowers blood glucose concentration** by:

- Increasing the GLUT-4-mediated uptake of glucose by the extrahepatic tissues, especially muscles and adipose tissue, for its oxidation.
- Promoting glycolysis and glycogenesis, both in the liver and the muscle.
- Suppressing glycogenolysis in the liver and the kidney.
- Suppressing gluconeogenesis.

These metabolic effects are achieved because the hormone stimulates the synthesis of various enzymes, such as glucose-6-phosphate dehydrogenase, 6-phosphogluconate dehydrogenase, ATP-citrate lyase, etc. while represses the synthesis of pyruvate

carboxylase, PEP carboxykinase and fructose-1,6-bisphosphatase.

The hormone also promotes the transport of amino acids across the cell membrane and thus **stimulates protein synthesis**. Insulin also **inhibits ketogenesis** and **promotes lipogenesis**.

Role of Amylin: Amylin is a 37-amino acid peptide that is expressed within **pancreatic β-cells**, where it is **co-packaged with insulin** in secretory granules. Consequently, amylin is **co-secreted with insulin** and the plasma concentrations of the two hormones display a similar pattern of low fasting levels and rapid increases in response to meals. **Amylin complements the actions of insulin in postprandial glucose homeostasis** via several mechanisms. These include a suppression of postprandial glucagon secretion and a slowing of the rate at which nutrients are delivered from the stomach to the small intestine for absorption. The net effect is to control the influx of glucose into the circulation and thus to support the rate of insulin-mediated glucose clearance from the circulation. Patients with type 1 diabetes mellitus have an absolute deficiency of both insulin and amylin whereas patients with type 2 diabetes have a relative deficiency of both hormones, including a significantly impaired amylin and insulin response to meals.

Mechanism of Insulin Secretion

- **Rising blood glucose is the most potent insulin secretagogue**. The glucose transporter GLUT2 mediates the uptake of glucose into the pancreatic β-cell. In addition to glucose, several other factors such as amino acids (arginine, lysine, leucine), incretin hormones and neural communication serve as important regulators of insulin secretion.
- In the cytosol, glycolysis converts glucose to pyruvate. The first rate-limiting step in this process is the phosphorylation of glucose to glucose-6-phosphate by the enzyme glucokinase. By determining the rate of glycolysis, **glucokinase functions as the glucose sensor of the β-cell** and this is the primary mechanism whereby the rate of insulin secretion adapts to changes in blood glucose.
- The increase in ATP synthesis from glycolysis and TCA cycle blocks the ATP-dependent K^+ channels (K_{ATP}) (Chemistry to Clinics 11.15) on the β-cell membrane. This induces membrane depolarization which activates voltage-gated Ca^{2+} channels, increasing the Ca^{2+} influx.

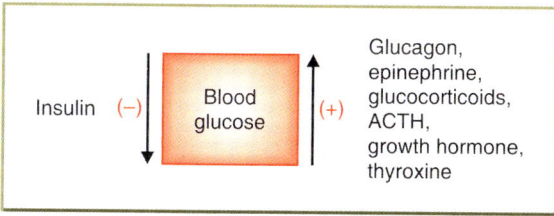

Insulin (−)   Blood glucose   (+)   Glucagon, epinephrine, glucocorticoids, ACTH, growth hormone, thyroxine

Fig. 11.40: Hormonal control of blood glucose.

11

Chemistry to Clinics 11.15: Sulfonylureas

The essential role of K_{ATP} channels in insulin secretion is the basis for sulfonylureas, a class of drugs used orally in the treatment of type 2 diabetes mellitus. The K_{ATP} channels comprise sulfonylurea receptors so that these drugs act as insulin secretagogues.

- The increase in cytosolic Ca^{2+} is the main spark for exocytosis, the process by which insulin-containing secretory granules fuse with the plasma membrane, leading to release of insulin into the circulation. The movement of insulin granules and exocytosis are also ATP-dependent processes.

Hormones with Hyperglycemic Action

Several hormones have been shown to have hyperglycemic action. These are called as 'insulin counter-regulatory hormones' or 'diabetogenic principles', which include glucagon, epinephrine, glucocorticoids, ACTH, growth hormone and thyroxine (Table 11.7).

Insulin/Glucagon Ratio: Critical Determinant of Metabolic Status

In most instances, insulin and glucagon produce opposing effects. Therefore, the relative levels of both hormones in the plasma, the insulin/glucagon ratio (**I/G ratio**), determine the net metabolic response. The I/G ratio varies considerably because the plasma concentration of each hormone changes rapidly in different nutritional states. In the fed state, the I/G ratio is approximately 30; after an overnight fast, it may fall to about 2 and with prolonged fasting it may fall to as low as 0.5.

A good example of the influence of I/G ratio on metabolic status is seen in type 1 diabetes mellitus. The insulin levels are low, so the insulin-stimulated metabolic pathways operate at a sub-optimum level. However, insulin is also necessary for the pancreatic α-cells to sense blood glucose appropriately; in the absence of insulin, the secretion of glucagon is inappropriately elevated. The result is an imbalance in the I/G ratio and an accentuation of glucagon effects well above what would be seen in normal states of low insulin, such as in fasting.

Role of Kidneys in the Regulation of Blood Glucose: Renal Glucose Threshold and Tubular Maximum

At normal blood glucose levels, all of the filtered glucose is reabsorbed by the proximal convoluted tubules and none is excreted in the urine. When the blood glucose exceeds a certain value (**≈180 mg/dl**),

Table 11.7: Major insulin counter-regulatory hormones

Hormone	Source	'Diabetogenic' action
Glucagon	α-cells of the islets of Langerhans of the pancreas	Hepatic glycogenolysis and gluconeogenesis
Epinephrine/Adrenaline (the first line of defense against hypoglycemia)	Adrenal medulla	• Glycogenolysis (both in liver and muscle) • Gluconeogenesis (liver) • Inhibits the release of insulin from the pancreas • Decreases the transport and utilization of glucose in different tissues • Stimulates glucagon secretion
Glucocorticoids (mainly cortisol)	Adrenal cortex	• Hepatic gluconeogenesis • Inhibit glycolysis • Facilitate other hyperglycemic hormones (permissive effects, see Chemistry to Clinics 11.16)
ACTH	Anterior pituitary	Effects are mediated through cortisol secreted from the adrenal cortex under its influence
Growth hormone	Anterior pituitary	• Decreases glucose uptake and utilization by muscle • Prolonged administration of growth hormone stimulates the secretion of insulin, exhaustion of β cells and diabetes mellitus-like situation.
Thyroxine	Thyroid gland	• Intestinal absorption of glucose • Hepatic glycogenolysis and gluconeogenesis • Destruction of insulin

Chemistry to Clinics 11.16: The Permissive Role of Glucocorticoids

The glucocorticoids are essential for the acceleration of gluconeogenesis during fasting. They play a permissive role in this process by maintaining gene expression and therefore the intracellular concentrations of many of the enzymes needed to carry out gluconeogenesis in the liver and kidneys. These include transaminases, pyruvate carboxylase, phosphoenolpyruvate carboxykinase, fructose-1,6-bisphosphatase, fructose-6-phosphatase and glucose-6-phosphatase. In an untreated, glucocorticoid-deficient person, the amounts of these enzymes in the liver are greatly reduced. As a consequence, the person cannot respond to fasting with accelerated gluconeogenesis and suffers from hypoglycemia. This is commonly seen in Addison's disease. In essence, the glucocorticoids maintain the liver and kidney in a state that enables them to carry out accelerated gluconeogenesis should the need arise.

Chemistry to Clinics 11.17: Renal Glucosuria (Renal Diabetes)

It results from an inherited defect in the proximal tubular Na^+-glucose cotransport (due to mutated SGLT2, the membrane protein responsible for majority of tubular glucose reabsorption). It is characterized by osmotic diuresis and glucosuria despite normal blood glucose levels. It is a benign condition not warranting any treatment.

significant quantities of glucose appear in the urine. This critical plasma concentration is called the **renal glucose threshold**. Any further increase in blood glucose lead to progressively more excreted glucose. Glucose appears in the urine because the filtered amount of glucose exceeds the capacity of the tubules to reabsorb it. At high filtered glucose loads, the rate of glucose reabsorption reaches a constant maximal value called the **tubular transport maximum** (Tm) for glucose (G), abbreviated as Tm_G. At Tm_G, the tubule glucose carriers are all saturated and transport glucose at the maximal rate.

Factors Affecting Renal Glucose Threshold

The glucose threshold is not a fixed value of blood glucose concentration. It **depends on three factors—glomerular filtration rate (GFR), Tm_G and splay:**

- A low GFR leads to an elevated threshold because the filtered glucose load is reduced and the tubules reabsorb all the filtered glucose despite elevated blood glucose.
- A reduced Tm_G lowers the threshold because the tubules have a diminished capacity lo reabsorb glucose.
- Splay refers to the phenomenon that the tubular glucose reabsorption does not abruptly attain Tm_G when blood glucose is progressively elevated. One reason for splay is that not all nephrons have the same filtering and reabsorbing capacities. Thus, nephrons with relatively high filtration rates and low glucose reabsorptive rates excrete glucose at a lower blood concentration than nephrons with relatively low filtration rates and high reabsorptive

rates. A second reason for splay is that the glucose carrier does not have an infinitely high affinity for glucose, so glucose escapes in the urine even before the carrier is fully saturated. An increase in splay causes a decrease in glucose threshold.

Osmotic Diuresis

In uncontrolled diabetes mellitus, the blood glucose levels are abnormally elevated, so more glucose is filtered at the glomerulus than can be reabsorbed by the tubules. The urinary excretion of glucose, called glucosuria, produces an osmotic diuresis. A diuresis is an increase in urine output. In osmotic diuresis, the increased urine flow results from the excretion of osmotically active solute. **Diabetes (from the Greek for 'syphon') gets its name from this increased urine output**. Interestingly, glucosuria may occur even without diabetes (Chemistry to Clinics 11.17).

DIABETES MELLITUS

Diabetes mellitus (DM) is the **commonest endocrine disease characterized by persistent hyperglycemia with or without glucosuria, caused by the deficiency in secretion or action of insulin**. Besides insulin, several other hormones (diabetogenic principles, as discussed above) also influence the metabolism of glucose. DM may be a result of genetic and/or environmental factors, classified into:

1. Type 1 diabetes mellitus, T1DM (formerly, insulin Dependent Diabetes Mellitus, IDDM).
2. Type 2 diabetes mellitus, T2DM (formerly, non-insulin dependent diabetes mellitus, NIDDM).
3. DM due to miscellaneous factors, e.g. due to prolonged use of corticosteroids, cystic fibrosis, hemochromatosis (bronze diabetes), etc.
4. Gestational DM.

Type 1 Diabetes Mellitus

T1DM is also called **juvenile-onset diabetes** because it usually appears in the childhood or in younger age

11

group (commonly <35 years of age). There is an **absolute deficiency of insulin** due to a gradual depletion of the β-cells of the pancreas which may get destroyed by an autoimmune process (Chemistry to Clinics 11.18).

T1DM is characterized by hyperglycemia, hyperlipoproteinemia (raised chylomicrons and VLDL) and severe **ketoacidosis**. This suggests that besides defects in carbohydrate metabolism, there are also abnormalities in lipid and protein metabolism in such patients.

Hyperglycemia in T1DM is a result of the inability of the insulin-dependent tissues to take up glucose as well as due to the accelerated hepatic gluconeogenesis from amino acids, derived from muscle protein. Increased lipolysis in the adipose tissue and accelerated fatty acid oxidation in the liver result in ketoacidosis. Insulin deficiency, in turn, also reduces lipoprotein lipase activity thereby resulting in hyperchylomicronemia.

Patients with T1DM can usually be recognized by an abrupt appearance of **polyuria** (frequent urination), **polydipsia** (excessive thirst), and **polyphagia** (excessive hunger), often triggered by stress or an illness. These symptoms are usually accompanied by fatigue, weight loss and weakness. The diagnosis can be confirmed by high fasting blood glucose commonly accompanied by ketoacidosis.

Patients with T1DM have virtually no functional β-cells and **rely on exogenous insulin**, injected subcutaneously, in order to control hyperglycemia and ketoacidosis. Insulin injections though do not cure the disease but promote glucose uptake by the tissues and inhibit gluconeogenesis, lipolysis and proteolysis.

Lifespan of the patient is reduced as a result of degenerative complications such as kidney malfunction, nerve impairment and cardiovascular disease. Hyperglycemia may also lead to blindness through retinal degeneration, and the accumulation of sorbitol along with the glycation of lens proteins causing cataract.

Type 2 Diabetes Mellitus

Majority of the diabetic patients suffer from T2DM. It is also called **maturity-onset diabetes** since this usually occurs in the middle-age group (usually ≥35 years of age), who are generally obese. The occurrence of the disease is almost completely determined by genetic factors. T2DM develops gradually without obvious symptoms. The metabolic alterations are milder than those for T1DM.

T2DM is characterized by hyperglycemia often with hypertriglyceridemia. Inspite of high levels of insulin, glucose levels are poorly controlled because of **lack of normal response to insulin** (Chemistry to Clinics 11.19). Insulin resistance in these patients may be due to receptor down-regulation caused by an increased expression of tumor necrosis factor-α in adipocytes of the obese individuals (receptor down-regulation refers to a decrease in the total number of receptors of a hormone and/or a decrease in the affinity of the receptors for the hormone and/or an impairment in the post-receptor events).

Hyperglycemia is mainly a result of poor peripheral utilization of glucose, especially in the muscle. Blood glucose concentrations are much higher than normal, particularly after a meal. **Ketoacidosis does not**

develop because the adipocytes remain sensitive to the effect of insulin on lipolysis. Rapid *de novo* synthesis of fatty acids and VLDL leads to hyper-triglyceridemia without hyperchylomicronemia.

Weight reduction and dietary modifications often correct the hyperglycemia of T2DM. Hypoglycemic agents such as sulfonylureas may be required to achieve a satisfactory fall in blood glucose level.

Salient features of the two types of diabetes mellitus are given in Table 11.8.

Complications of Diabetes Mellitus

1. **Acute complications:** Ketoacidosis and coma (T1DM), non-ketotic hyperosmolar coma (T2DM), or hypoglycemic coma (a consequence of insulin overdose or delaying/missing a meal after insulin injection).

2. **Chronic complications:** Myocardial infarction (diabetic patients often present with painless, i.e. silent myocardial infarction) due to accelerated atherosclerosis and coronary artery disease, cardiomyopathy, cerebrovascular disease, nephro-pathy, retinopathy, neuropathy, infections and delayed wound healing.

Biochemical Diagnosis of Diabetes Mellitus

It is based on the measurement of blood glucose or glycated hemoglobin (HbA_{1c}, discussed later) and interpreted according to standard protocol (Table 11.9).

Disease Monitoring

Once DM is diagnosed, short-term as well as long-term monitoring is essential to ensure the adequacy of glycemic control and to detect complications.

I. Short-term monitoring

A. Transcutaneous glucose measurement: It is predicted that by 2020, India may become the 'diabetic capital of the world'. Most methods of monitoring blood glucose require a blood sample, usually obtained by venepuncture or by using an automatic lancing device on a finger. Some glucometers use a blood sample from a less sensitive area such as the upper arm, forearm or thigh. Other devices use a beam of light instead of a lancet to pierce the skin.

Recent advances in insulin pump technology have created a demand for concurrent advances in the area of glucose sensing. A major reason for

Table 11.8: Type 1 versus type 2 diabetes mellitus

Features	Type 1 diabetes mellitus	Type 2 diabetes mellitus
Prevalence	≈ 15%	≈ 85%
Age of onset	<35 years (juvenile-onset)	≥35 years (maturity-onset)
Primary cause	↓ Insulin production due to β-cell destruction	Insulin resistance in target tissues
Body habitus	Underweight	Overweight/obese
Plasma insulin	↓/Absent	Normal/↑
Plasma glucagon	↑, suppressible	↑, resistant
Acute complications	Ketoacidosis	Non-ketotic hyperosmolar coma
Therapy	Insulin	Oral hypoglycemic agents

Table 11.9: Biochemical diagnosis of diabetes mellitus

	Fasting (12 h) plasma glucose (mg/dl)	Postprandial (2 h) plasma glucose (mg/dl)	Blood HbA_{1c}
Normal	<100	<140	<5.7%
Pre-diabetes	100–125 (impaired fasting tolerance)	140–199 (impaired glucose tolerance)	5.7–6.4%
Diabetes mellitus	≥126	≥200	≥6.5%

- Either fasting *OR* postprandial *OR* casual (random) plasma glucose *OR* blood HbA_{1c} may be estimated.
- In case of casual plasma glucose, value >200 mg/dl is required for a diagnosis in patients with classical diabetic presentation of polyuria, polydipsia and unexplained weight loss.

this is the desire to improve the quality of life of insulin pump users. When using a continuous insulin delivery system, the patients are required to check their blood glucose levels frequently throughout the day. As indicated above, many current devices rely on direct analysis of blood withdrawn from the tip of a finger. Many patients complain that these finger-sticks are painful and leave fingertips swollen and tender for many hours afterwards. The goal of many recent glucose-sensing devices is simply to minimize the pain associated with monitoring blood glucose levels.

Noninvasive blood glucose monitoring involves either radiation or fluid extraction. The most promising radiation technologies are: (1) mid-infrared radiation (Mid-IR) spectroscopy; (2) near-infrared radiation (Near-IR) spectroscopy; (3) radio wave impedance; and (4) optical rotation of polarized light. All of these technologies, except Mid-IR spectroscopy, involve application of an external energy source to the body. The interaction between the applied radiation (or thermal emissions, in the case of Mid-IR spectroscopy) and glucose in the blood is measured and converted into a blood glucose concentration.

B. **Urine glucose and ketone bodies:** This can be a bedside procedure using dipsticks.

II. Long-term monitoring

A. **Glycated hemoglobin:** Measurement of blood glucose though is a good index of diabetes mellitus, however, it changes quickly. This mandates the need to develop better parameters for the diagnosis as well as for the long-term monitoring of these patients. Such a parameter is glycated hemoglobin. The glycation reaction is **non-enzymatic and irreversible** with **covalent** attachment of carbohydrates to the globin chains of hemoglobin, known as 'Brownian reaction'. The important terms and facts in relation to hemoglobin glycation are outlined in Table 11.10. Various hemoglobin fractions may be separated and quantified by **chromatography** (Fig. 11.41) out of which HbA_{1c} is of special interest as far as DM is concerned.

Advantages of Glycated Hemoglobin (HbA$_{1c}$) Measurement over Blood Glucose Measurement

1. **Diagnostic value:** The amount of HbA_{1c} formed is proportional to the mean blood glucose levels.

Table 11.10: Important terms and facts about hemoglobin glycation in an adult

- **Total hemoglobin** = HbA (major adult Hb, $\alpha_2\beta_2$, 97%) + HbA_2 (minor adult Hb, $\alpha_2\delta_2$, 2.5%) + HbF (fetal Hb, $\alpha_2\gamma_2$, 0.5%)
- Some HbA is converted to various glycated forms, collectively called '**total glycated Hb**'
- Total glycated Hb = HbA_1 + HbA_0
- HbA_1: Glycation occurs at the N-terminal valine of the β-chain
- HbA_0: Glycation occurs at lysine residues of the β-chain or some amino acids in the α-chain
- HbA_1 = HbA_{1a} + HbA_{1b} + HbA_{1c}
- The annotations 'a', 'b' and 'c' depict the corresponding fraction of glycated hemoglobin eluted during chromatography
- HbA_{1a} has two subfractions: HbA_{1a} = HbA_{1a1} + HbA_{1a2}
- Carbohydrates attached during glycation: Fructose 1,6-bisphosphate in HbA_{1a1}, glucose-6-phosphate in HbA_{1a2}, pyruvic acid in HbA_{1b} and glucose in HbA_{1c}
- HbA_{1c} = 80% of HbA_1 but <5.7% of total Hb.

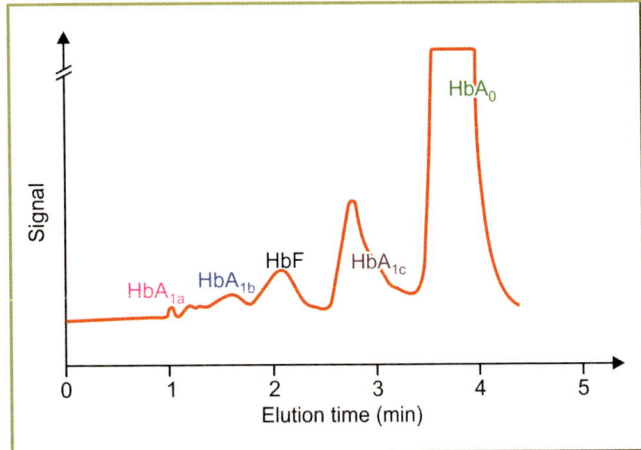

Fig. 11.41: Chromatogram showing the various hemoglobin fractions.

Thus, increased HbA_{1c} levels are observed in DM and may be used for its diagnosis (Table 11.9).

2. **Glycemic control:** It is an index of blood glucose control, whether by diet restriction and/or anti-diabetic drugs. Glycation being irreversible, it leaves a record of glycemia throughout the RBC lifespan of **90–120 days**. Thus, a unique advantage of HbA_{1c} measurement is that unlike simple blood glucose measurement, it reflects the time-average blood glucose over the preceding 2–4 months. A value >9% indicates poor glycemic control.

3. **Correlated with complications:** High HbA_{1c} levels indicate the ongoing glycation of other body

proteins forming advanced glycation end products (AGE). Loss of function of these proteins (e.g. LDL-receptors, lens proteins, etc.) is associated with complications like accelerated atherosclerosis, coronary heart disease, retinopathy, cataract, nephropathy, neuropathy.

4. **Prognostic value:** Persistently high HbA_{1c} levels indicate a poor prognosis.
5. **Low variability:** Values are fairly constant on a day-to-day basis.
6. **Convenient:** No special patient preparation is required, e.g. fasting or glucose load.

Disadvantages of Glycated Hemoglobin (HbA_{1c}) Measurement

1. Does not give an idea of daily blood glucose fluctuations, hence difficult to adjust insulin dosage on a day-to-day basis.
2. Results influenced by RBC turnover (Chemistry to Clinics 11.20).
3. Expensive.

B. **Plasma C-Peptide:** The β-cells of the pancreas secrete insulin. The product of the insulin gene is a peptide known as pre-proinsulin. As with other secretory peptides, the pre-peptide or signal peptide is cleaved off early in the biosynthetic process, yielding proinsulin, an 86-amino acid protein that is subsequently cleaved at two sites to yield insulin and a 31-amino acid peptide known as C-peptide. Insulin and C-peptide are therefore localized within the same secretory vesicle and are co-secreted into the blood stream. Measurement of plasma C-peptide is gaining clinical significance (Chemistry to Clinics 11.21).

C. **Others:** Plasma lipid profile, renal function tests, uric acid, urinalysis for microalbuminuria, etc. are useful long-term monitoring parameters.

Chemistry to Clinics 11.20: HbA_{1c} and RBC Turnover

All conditions that shorten the lifespan of RBC decrease HbA_{1c} as the average time during which erythrocytes are exposed to glucose is reduced. This is observed in hemolytic anemia. Conversely, following splenectomy, RBC survival time and hence HbA_{1c} is increased. Therefore, in patients with altered RBC turnover, it is recommended to use other tests for the determination of glycemic control, such as serum glycated albumin (turnover = 15–21 days, hence provides information on glycemic control over the past 2–4 weeks).

Chemistry to Clinics 11.21: C-Peptide

Measurements of circulating C-peptide levels can provide a valuable indirect assessment of β-cell insulin secretory capacity. In diabetic patients who are receiving exogenous insulin injections, the measurement of circulating insulin levels would not provide any useful information about their pancreatic function because it would primarily be the injected insulin that would be measured. However, an evaluation of C-peptide levels in such patients would provide an indirect measure of how well the β-cells were functioning with regard to insulin production and secretion.

Treatment Options for Diabetes Mellitus

Diet control, weight loss and exercise can be extremely effective in diabetes therapy and may be the only treatment necessary in the early stages. Patients are advised to switch over to foods having a low to moderate **glycemic index** (**GI**, a term that refers to the ability of a particular food to increase the blood glucose compared to 100% for an equal amount of pure glucose). Category of foods based on their GI:

• Low GI: Soybeans, apples, oranges, milk, yogurt.
• Moderate GI: Rye bread, bananas, pineapple, ice cream.
• High GI: White bread, corn flakes, potatoes, carrots, watermelon, soft drinks, honey.

For those patients who are reluctant to give up sucrose/glucose, artificial sweeteners are a good choice as a sugar substitute (Chemistry to Clinics 11.22).

Commonly, however, lifestyle intervention is supplemented by treatment with **insulin injections in case of T1DM** or one or more **oral agents in case of T2DM**. Multiple classes of drugs independently address different biochemical alterations that contribute to the development of type 2 diabetes. The available oral anti-diabetic agents can be divided by their mechanism of action into insulin sensitizers

Chemistry to Clinics 11.22: Artificial Sweeteners

Owing to the fact that diabetic patients and even those having impaired glucose tolerance are advised to avoid glucose or sucrose in their diet, 'artificial sweeteners' have become popular substitutes. The **non-nutritive sweeteners** do not yield energy, e.g. saccharin and sucralose. Their RDA is 5 mg/kg body weight. The **nutritive sweeteners**, e.g. aspartame, yield 4 kcal/g of energy that is insignificant owing to its RDA of 15 mg/kg body weight. However, aspartame also yields the amino acid phenylalanine, hence it should be avoided in patients suffering from phenylketonuria.

11

with primary action in the liver (e.g. biguanides), insulin sensitizers with primary action in peripheral tissues (e.g. glitazones), insulin secretagogues (e.g. sulfonylureas), agents that slow the absorption of carbohydrates (e.g. α-glucosidase inhibitors) and SGLT2 inhibitors (Chemistry to Clinics 11.23). In some cases, a patient with T2DM may be treated with insulin, just like the patient with T1DM.

Chemistry to Clinics: 11.23. Sodium-Glucose Linked Transporter-2 (SGLT2) and Diabetes Mellitus

In the kidneys, >90% of the filtered glucose is reabsorbed by SGLT2 in the proximal convoluted tubules and the rest by SGLT1 in the proximal straight tubules. Recently, a new drug called canagliflozin has been introduced in the market which inhibits SGLT2. Thus, majority of the filtered glucose fails to get reabsorbed and is eliminated in the urine. This helps to reduce blood glucose levels and is useful in the treatment of T2DM.

SOME IMPORTANT QUESTIONS

1. Outline the reactions of citric acid cycle. Give energetics of the cycle and explain the amphibolic role of this cycle.

2. Outline HMP shunt reactions. Discuss the significance of HMP pathway in different tissues.

3. Give outline of glycolytic reactions. What are the regulatory steps? What is the energy yield of this pathway?

4. Define glycogenolysis. Outline reactions of this pathway. How is it regulated?

5. What is glycogenesis? Give reactions of glycogenesis. How is it regulated?

6. Explain:
   i. Why aerobic glycolysis releases more energy than anaerobic glycolysis?
   ii. How glycolysis can be reversed?
   iii. TCA cycle and its energetics

7. Discuss briefly:
   i. Metabolism of galactose
   ii. Regulation of blood glucose
   iii. Glycogenolysis
   iv. Fructose metabolism

8. Write notes on:
   i. Diabetes mellitus
   ii. Galactosemia
   iii. Glycogenesis
   iv. Gluconeogenesis
   v. Glycogen storage diseases
   vi. Energetics of TCA cycle
   vii. Conversion of pyruvate to acetyl CoA
   viii. von Gierke's disease
   ix. Glycated hemoglobin
   x. GLUT
   xi. Artificial sweeteners

MULTIPLE CHOICE QUESTIONS

1. GLUT-1 is present in:
   A. Adipose tissue
   B. RBC
   C. Skeletal muscle
   D. Small intestine

2. Glycerol enters glycolysis via:
   A. Glucose-6-phosphate
   B. Fructose-6-phosphate
   C. Dihydroxyacetone phosphate
   D. Pyruvate

3. **Fluoroacetate inhibits:**
   A. Hexokinase
   B. Pyruvate dehydrogenase
   C. Aconitase
   D. Lactate dehydrogenase

4. **Gluconeogenesis occurs:**
   A. Mainly in liver, partly in kidneys, not in muscles
   B. Mainly in kidneys, partly in liver, not in muscles
   C. Mainly in muscles, partly in liver, not in kidneys
   D. Mainly in muscles, partly in kidneys, not in liver

5. **Cori cycle involves:**
   A. Glucose and alanine
   B. Malate and aspartate
   C. Glucose and lactate
   D. Q cycle

6. **Anderson's disease is due to deficiency of:**
   A. Lysosomal acid maltase
   B. Debranching enzyme
   C. Branching enzyme
   D. Muscle phosphorylase

7. **Physiological jaundice of the newborn is due to:**
   A. Decreased activity of glucuronyl transferase
   B. Increased activity of glucuronyl transferase
   C. G6PD deficiency
   D. Lack of β-glucuronidase

8. **Essential fructosuria is due to a deficiency of:**
   A. Aldolase 'A'
   B. Aldolase 'B'
   C. Fructokinase
   D. Phosphofructokinase-1

9. **The following is called a glucose sensor in pancreatic β-cells:**
   A. Glucokinase
   B. Insulin
   C. Amylin
   D. Glucose tolerance factor

10. **Glycated hemoglobin levels in blood are an index of blood glucose control over the past:**
    A. 3 hour
    B. 3 days
    C. 3 months
    D. 3 years

11

12

Metabolism of Lipids

The digestion and absorption of dietary lipids was discussed in Chapter 9.

OXIDATION OF FATTY ACIDS

Fatty acids that arrive at the surface of the tissues are taken up by the cells and are used (oxidized) for the production of **energy**. Oxidation takes place in the **mitochondria** where various enzymes for the oxidation of fatty acids are present, close to the enzymes of the electron transport chain.

β-Oxidation: The Most Important Mechanism for Fatty Acid Oxidation

The process of β-oxidation of fatty acids was proposed by Knoop and requires CoA, FAD and NAD. Oxidation of a fatty acid occurs at the β-carbon atom (carbon atom number 2) and results in the **elimination of two terminal carbon atoms as acetyl CoA**, leaving fatty acyl CoA which has two carbons less than the original fatty acid (Fig. 12.1).

1. **Activation of fatty acids:** The **first step** in the oxidation of a fatty acid is its **activation**. Fatty acid activation occurs in the cytoplasm, in the presence of ATP and is catalyzed by a thiokinase (acyl CoA synthetase). Thiokinases are fatty acid activating enzymes found, both, inside as well as outside the mitochondria. Several thiokinases are known, each one of which is specific for a group of fatty acids. These include:
   - **Acetyl CoA thiokinase:** This is found in the mitochondria and cause activation of acetic, propionic and butyric acids.
   - **Short-chain fatty acyl CoA thiokinases:** These are also found in the mitochondria and cause activation of fatty acids with 4–12 carbons.
   - **Long-chain fatty acyl CoA thiokinases:** These are found in the cytoplasm and cause activation of long-chain saturated as well as unsaturated fatty acids.

2. **Transport of a fatty acid through the inner mitochondrial membrane:** Short-chain fatty acids, as mentioned above, can cross the inner mitochondrial membrane as such and are activated to their CoA derivatives directly within the mitochondria. On the other hand, activation of long-chain fatty acids (>12C) occurs outside the mitochondria. Since the machinery for their oxidation is present within the mitochondria and the inner mitochondrial membrane is impermeable to CoA as well as to its derivatives, the long-chain fatty acids are thus to be transported from the cytoplasm to the mitochondria. This takes place with the help of **carnitine** which acts as a carrier of acyl group across the membrane. The enzymes that transfer a fatty acyl group between CoA and carnitine are found on both sides of the inner mitochondrial membrane.

Role of Carnitine in the Transport of a Long-chain Fatty Acid: Carnitine Shuttle

Carnitine (4-trimethylamino-3-hydroxybutyrate) is widely distributed in all the tissues especially the muscles. It is synthesized from **lysine and methionine** in the liver and the kidney and then redistributed to

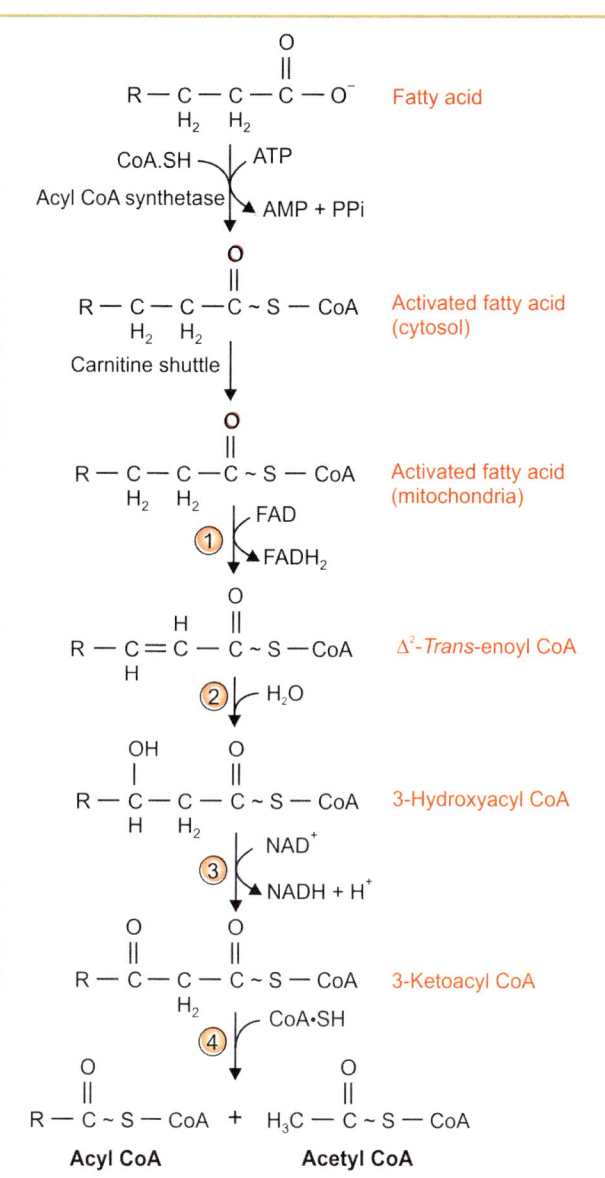

Fig. 12.1: β-Oxidation of fatty acids. 1. Acyl CoA dehydrogenase, 2. Δ²-Enoyl CoA hydratase, 3. 3-Hydroxyacyl CoA dehydrogenase, 4. Thiolase.

other tissues. It is used as a carrier of acyl group (chain length 12C–18C) across the mitochondrial membrane (Fig. 12.2).

The outer mitochondrial membrane contains an enzyme, carnitine palmitoyl transferase I (CPT-I). The enzyme converts long-chain fatty acyl CoA to acylcarnitine that exchanges across the inner mitochondrial membrane with free carnitine by a carnitine:acylcarnitine antiporter translocase. Finally,

the fatty acyl group is transferred back to CoA by carnitine palmitoyl transferase II (CPT-II), which is located on the matrix side of the inner membrane. The entire mechanism is also called carnitine shuttle and several disorders are associated with it (Chemistry to Clinics 12.1). Carnitine is emerging as an important health supplement (Chemistry to Clinics 12.2).

3. Reactions of β-oxidation

i. After activation and entry of the fatty acid into the mitochondria, flavoprotein containing acyl CoA dehydrogenase removes two hydrogen atoms from α- and β-positions of the fatty acyl CoA (Fig. 12.1). It forms enoyl CoA with a *trans*-double bond between C2 and C3, i.e. an α, β-unsaturated fatty acyl CoA.

Mitochondria contain several acyl CoA dehydrogenases with different chain length specificities. These are designated as short chain fatty acyl CoA dehydrogenase, medium

---

Chemistry to Clinics 12.1: Carnitine Deficiency Disorders

Primary carnitine deficiency: The entry of carnitine into the cell across the plasma membrane requires a sodium-dependent transporter encoded by the solute carrier family 22 member 5 (*SLC22A5*) gene. Mutations in *SLC22A5* result in autosomal recessive primary carnitine deficiency, which manifests with cardiac and skeletal symptoms because low levels of carnitine affect oxidation of long chain fatty acids. It requires lifelong oral L-carnitine supplementation.

Secondary carnitine deficiency: It is associated with inherited defects in β-oxidation pathway resulting in the accumulation of acyl CoA and acylcarnitine. Acylcarnitine is excreted in the urine and further lowers carnitine levels in the body.

Mutations in the Carnitine Palmitoyl Transferase II (*CPT II*) gene: These give rise to partial loss of CPT II activity. Patients generally experience muscle weakness during prolonged exercise. Myoglobinuria, due to breakdown of muscle tissue, is frequently observed. Severe deficiency of the enzyme may be precipitated by prolonged period of fasting and leads to hypoketotic hypoglycemia, hyperammonemia, cardiac malfunctions, etc.

Chemistry to Clinics 12.2: Carnitine Supplements

Intensive research on the role of carnitine supplements has shown partial benefit in the following conditions:

1. Heart failure
2. Peripheral vascular disease
3. Muscle wasting (as in cancer patients)
4. Hepatic encephalopathy
5. Type 2 diabetes mellitus

12

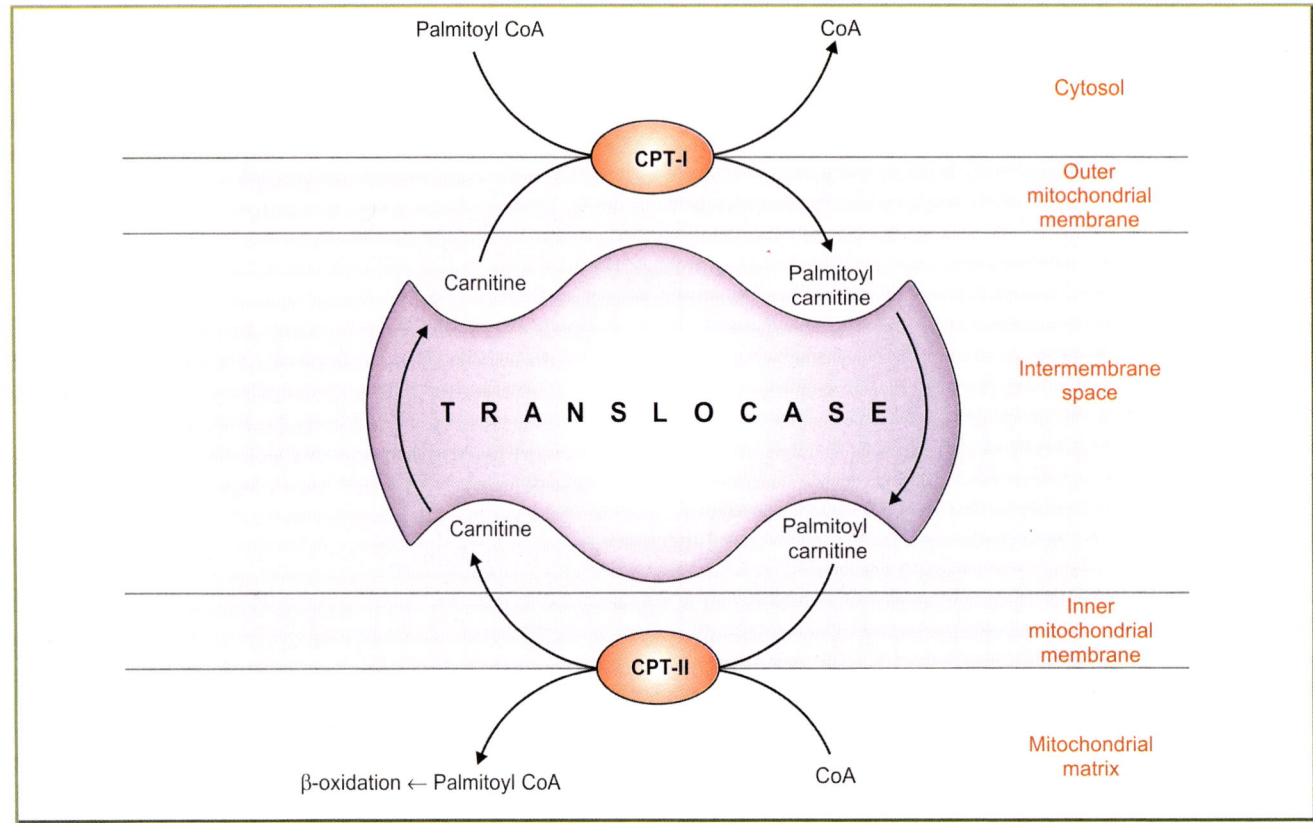

Fig. 12.2: Carnitine shuttle. Although translocase is located in the inner mitochondrial membrane, for simplicity of drawing it is shown here in the intermembrane space.

chain fatty acyl CoA dehydrogenase and long-chain fatty acyl CoA dehydrogenase. There may be a genetic deficiency of any of the three enzymes with several common clinical features. These are collectively called acyl CoA dehydrogenase deficiency diseases. Medium chain acyl CoA dehydrogenase deficiency disease is called sudden infant death syndrome (Chemistry to Clinics 12.3).

ii. Enoyl CoA hydratase adds a molecule of water at the double bond as a result of which α, β-unsaturated fattyacyl CoA is converted to β-hydroxyacyl CoA.

iii. In the presence of NAD⁺, β-hydroxyacyl CoA dehydrogenase oxidizes β-hydroxyacyl CoA to β-ketoacyl CoA.

iv. β-keto thiolase, in the presence of CoA, cleaves β-ketoacyl CoA and yields acetyl CoA and fatty acyl CoA having two carbons less than the original fatty acyl CoA. The enzyme is of clinical importance (Chemistry to Clinics 12.4).

Chemistry to Clinics 12.3: Sudden Infant Death Syndrome (Reye's Syndrome)

Acyl CoA dehydrogenase deficiency diseases are a group of inherited autosomal recessive defects resulting in impairment of the process of β-oxidation of fatty acids. The most common amongst them is the medium chain fatty acyl CoA dehydrogenase deficiency. This is also referred as sudden infant death syndrome (SIDS) or Reye's syndrome. Impairment in β-oxidation of medium chain fatty acids results in their accumulation in tissues, such as in the muscle. This, in turn, leads to their metabolism via ω-oxidation and transesterification to glycine and carnitine. Medium chain dicarboxylic acids as well as their glycine and carnitine esters may be detected in the urine of the affected individuals. Typical features include vomiting, lethargy and frequently coma, accompanied with hypoketotic hypoglycemia and dicarboxylic aciduria. Symptoms appear after more than 12 hours of fast and are more complicated on prolonged starvation, usually within first two years of life.

The newly formed fatty acyl CoA again undergoes a similar set of reactions, starting with acyl CoA dehydrogenase and is subsequently degraded to acetyl CoA.

Chemistry to Clinics 12.4: β-Ketothiolase

Heart muscles utilize free fatty acids as their primary fuel, via β-oxidation. In patients suffering from angina pectoris, parts of the heart muscles become ischemic. Under these conditions, one of the aims of treatment is to shift the metabolic fuel of heart muscles from fatty acids to glucose which also helps to reduce the accompanying acidosis. This is accomplished by administering trimetazidine, a drug which inhibits β-ketothiolase and thus stops β-oxidation, helping in a faster recovery from ischemia.

Regulation of β-oxidation: Availability of the substrates and the cofactors as well as the rate of removal of the product (acetyl CoA) regulates the process of β-oxidation.

Energy production during β-oxidation: When palmitic acid ($C_{15}H_{31}COOH$) undergoes β-oxidation, it releases 8 molecules of acetyl CoA in seven rounds of the oxidative process. In each round of β-oxidation, one molecule of $FADH_2$ and one molecule of NADH are produced. These, in turn, generate 1.5 and 2.5 ATP molecules, respectively. Thus, a total of 28 ATP are obtained during 7 rounds of the process. In addition, each molecule of acetyl CoA when oxidized in the citric acid cycle, gives 10 ATP. Therefore, additionally 80 ATP are produced from 8 molecules of acetyl CoA. A total of 108 ATP are hence generated from a molecule of palmitic acid.

As two high energy phosphate bonds are hydrolyzed from one molecule of ATP which is changed to AMP, a total of two ATP are used in the activation of a fatty acid. Therefore, there is a **net yield of 106 ATP when one molecule of palmitic acid (fatty acid with 16 carbons) is completely oxidized**.

Peroxisomal Oxidation of Fatty Acids

Besides β-oxidation, fatty acid oxidation also occurs in peroxisomes of the liver, kidney and other tissues. It differs from mitochondrial β-oxidation in two ways:

1. The initial dehydrogenation is carried out by a cyanide insensitive oxidase system. This results in the production of H_2O_2 which is detoxified by a catalase.

2. Specificity of the peroxisomal enzymes is for the long-chain fatty acids. This, in turn, results in chain shortening of the long-chain fatty acids to the stage of octanoyl CoA, i.e. up to 8C only.

Alternative Pathways of Fatty Acid Oxidation

α-Oxidation: Some of the fatty acids may be oxidized by the process of α-oxidation, in the **endoplasmic reticulum**, in the liver and the brain. α-oxidation occurs at carbon-2 (α-carbon) instead of the carbon-3 (β-carbon) in the process of β-oxidation.

In α-oxidation, there is a sequential removal of one carbon atom from the carboxyl end of a fatty acid which **neither forms CoA intermediates nor generates ATP** but is removed as CO_2. Reactions of α-oxidation are particularly important in the metabolism of methylated fatty acids, such as phytanic acid, a constituent of lipids in milk and other animal fats.

During the process of α-oxidation, a fatty acid is metabolized by α-hydroxylation (Chemistry to Clinics 12.5) followed by dehydrogenation and decarboxylation (Fig. 12.3).

ω-Oxidation: In another minor pathway, oxidation of medium and long-chain fatty acids may occur from **both the ends simultaneously**. Firstly, the end methyl group (–CH_3) of the acyl chain, called the ω-carbon, is

Chemistry to Clinics 12.5: Refsum's Disease

Genetic deficiency of the α-hydroxylating enzyme (a monooxygenase) of the α-oxidation system, results in the accumulation of large quantities of phytanic acid in tissues and serum. This leads to a neurological disorder called Refsum's disease.

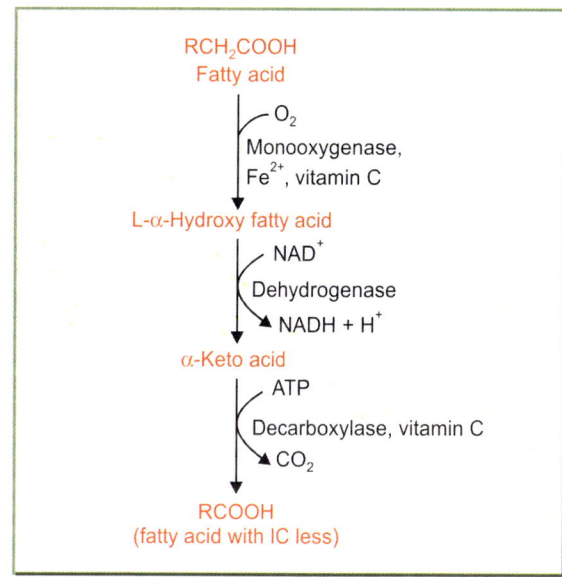

Fig. 12.3: α-Oxidation of fatty acid.

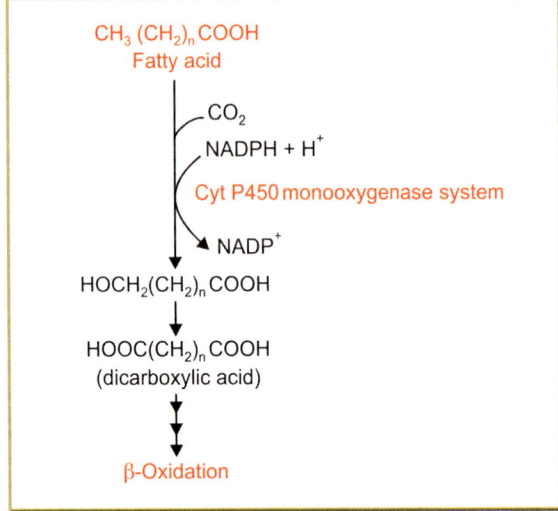

Fig. 12.4: ω-Oxidation of fatty acid.

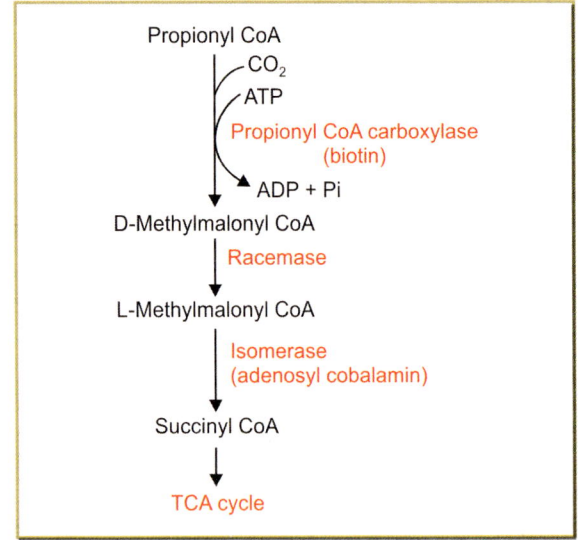

Fig. 12.6: Conversion of propionyl CoA to succinyl CoA.

oxidized to a carboxylic group (–COOH) and forms a dicarboxylic acid. The reaction is catalyzed by ω-hydroxylase in the presence of **cytochrome P450**. The dicarboxylic acid thereafter undergoes β-oxidation from both the ends, in a chain reaction (Fig. 12.4).

Oxidation of Fatty Acids with Odd Number of Carbon Atoms

Fatty acids with odd number of carbon atoms are also oxidized by the process of β-oxidation which in turn removes 2 carbon atoms as acetyl CoA in each round of the oxidative process. A molecule of **propionyl CoA**, containing 3 carbon atoms, is formed as the final product (Fig. 12.5). Propionyl CoA undergoes carboxylation, molecular rearrangement and is converted to succinyl CoA. This, in turn, forms an intermediate of the Krebs cycle (Fig. 12.6).

Oxidation of Unsaturated Fatty Acids

Unsaturated fatty acids are also activated, transported across the inner mitochondrial membrane and undergo β-oxidation, similar to that of saturated fatty

acids. But the double bonds of the naturally occurring unsaturated fatty acids are in the *cis*-configuration whereas those produced during β-oxidation have the *trans*-configuration. Hence, **three additional enzymes** are required for the oxidation of unsaturated fatty acids (Fig. 12.7):

1. An unsaturated fatty acid, such as linoleic acid, when undergoes the process of β-oxidation, after

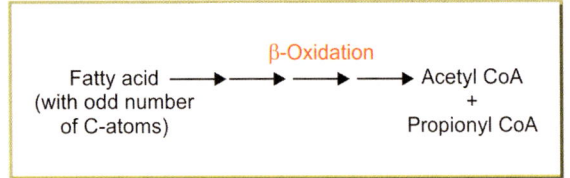

Fig. 12.5: Oxidation of fatty acid containing odd number of carbon atoms.

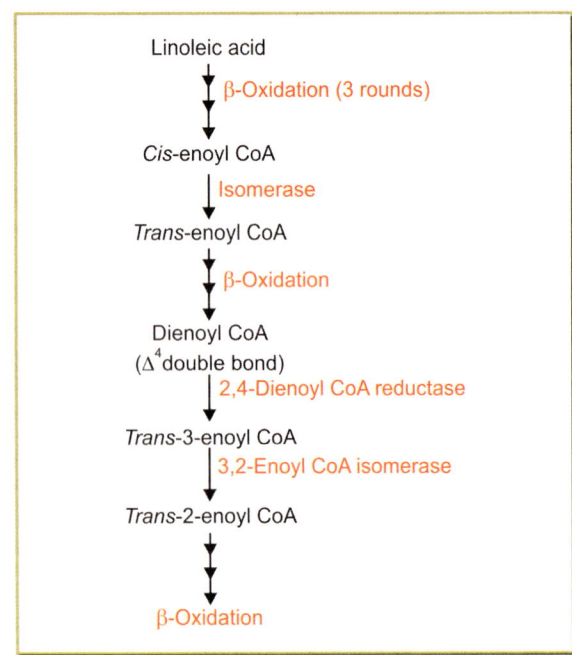

Fig. 12.7: Oxidation of an unsaturated fatty acid.

Metabolism of Lipids   191

12

three rounds, it results in the formation of enoyl CoA. This, however, has a *cis*-configuration and cannot be further oxidized by enoyl CoA hydratase since this enzyme acts only if the double bond has a *trans*-configuration. The shift of the double bond, from *cis*- to *trans*-configuration, is catalyzed by enoyl CoA isomerase. The process of β-oxidation thereafter again continues.

2. During the second round of β-oxidation, the product which is formed has a double bond at even numbered carbon atom, i.e. dienoyl CoA with Δ^4 double bond which is reduced by NADPH dependent dienoyl CoA reductase and the product is converted to *trans*-3-enoyl CoA.

3. *Trans*-3-enoyl CoA is subsequently isomerized to *trans*-2-enoyl CoA by 3,2-enoyl CoA isomerase.

Thereafter, the process of β-oxidation again continues resulting in complete oxidation of the unsaturated fatty acid.

Age Pigments/Lipofuscin: Auto-oxidation of lipids particularly that of PUFAs, result in the formation of hydroperoxides and dialdehydes, such as malondialdehyde (MDA) in the cell. These oxidized products of lipids and proteins accumulate in the cell in the form of a chemically heterogeneous pigmented substance called **lipofuscin** or **lipochrome** (Fig. 12.8).

Since lipofuscin, normally, accumulates in the cells of the older individuals and has been implicated in the ageing process, it is also called **age-pigments** or **'wear and tear' pigments**.

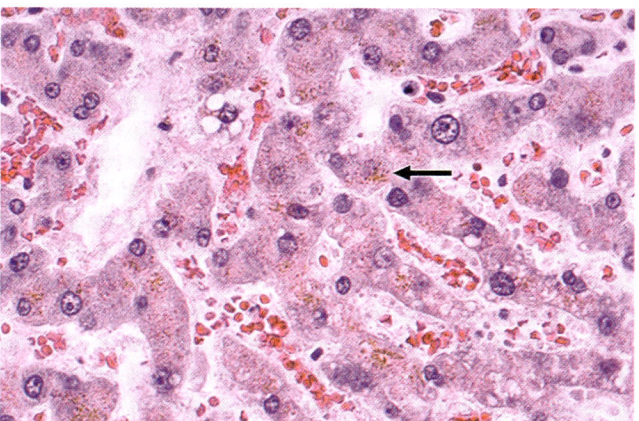

Fig. 12.8: Lipofuscin: The yellow-brown granular pigment (arrow), also called residual body or lipochrome or 'wear and tear' pigment, seen in the hepatocytes. It is the end result of autophagocytosis in which intracellular debris are sequestered and turned into lipofuscin in the cytoplasm.

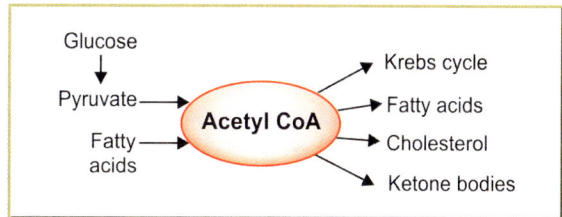

Fig. 12.9: Major sources and metabolic fates of acetyl CoA.

METABOLIC FATES OF ACETYL COA

In normal metabolic processes, as discussed above, oxidation of glucose (in glycolysis) as well as oxidation of fatty acids (via β-oxidation) produces acetyl CoA which is mainly used in the Krebs cycle. Besides, it is also used for the synthesis of fatty acids and cholesterol. A small quantity is converted to ketone bodies in the liver (Fig. 12.9).

BIOSYNTHESIS OF FATTY ACIDS

Other than the availability of fatty acids from dietary lipids, the second major source of fatty acids in the body is their biosynthesis from small molecules (intermediates) which are obtained as a result of the metabolism of sugars, some amino acids and fatty acids. Mammals can synthesize a major portion of the saturated as well as monounsaturated fatty acids. Saturated straight chain 16C fatty acid, i.e. **palmitic acid, is first synthesized** and all the other fatty acids are formed by modifications of the palmitic acid.

DE NOVO SYNTHESIS OF A FATTY ACID

Acetyl CoA is a direct source of all the carbon atoms for the biosynthesis of a fatty acid which mainly occurs in the liver, the mammary gland and the adipose tissue. Since the main enzymes for fatty acid synthesis, i.e. acetyl CoA carboxylase and fatty acid synthetase are found, primarily, in the cytosol, synthesis occurs in the **cytoplasm** by the sequential addition of the two-carbon units to the activated carboxyl end of a growing chain. This process of the biosynthesis of fatty acid is called *de novo* synthesis (*de novo* = 'a new', i.e. starting 'from scratch').

Acetyl CoA, as discussed earlier, is produced in the mitochondria from different sources, such as from pyruvate (obtained from carbohydrates via aerobic glycolysis) and glucogenic amino acids or directly from lipids (β-oxidation) and ketogenic amino acids. Since the mitochondrial membrane is impermeable to

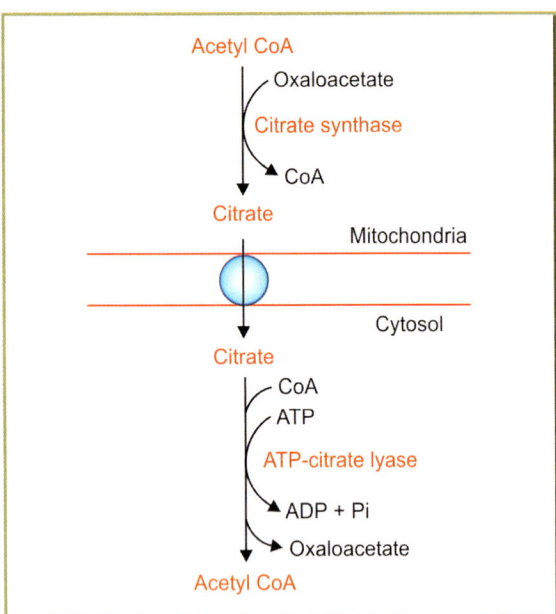

Fig. 12.10: Transport of acetyl CoA from the mitochondria to the cytosol.

acetyl CoA, a bypass mechanism moves it to the cytosol.

1. Transport of Acetyl CoA into Cytosol

For its entry into the cytosol, acetyl CoA first condenses with oxaloacetate and forms citrate. Citrate then enters the cytoplasm and is degraded to acetyl CoA and oxaloacetate by ATP citrate lyase (Fig. 12.10).

2. Synthesis of Malonyl CoA

In the cytoplasm, acetyl CoA is first converted to malonyl CoA by a biotin containing enzyme acetyl CoA carboxylase, irreversibly. The reaction occurs in the presence of ATP and CO_2 (HCO_3^-). Formation of malonyl CoA is a committed step in the synthesis of a fatty acid.

Acetyl CoA carboxylase regulates fatty acid synthesis by allosteric regulation, covalent modification, induction and repression. Acetyl CoA carboxylase is controlled by cAMP-mediated phosphorylation-dephosphorylation. Phosphorylation of the enzyme is promoted by glucagon and inactivates the enzyme. High carbohydrate or fat free diet increases the rate of synthesis of the enzyme while fasting or high fat diet decreases its rate of synthesis.

3. Synthesis of Palmitic Acid

Biosynthesis of palmitic acid requires NADPH besides biotin and pantothenic acid. Various reactions are catalyzed by fatty acid synthase which is a multi-enzyme complex.

Fatty acid synthase complex: It is composed of **two identical subunits, each one of which is a multienzyme complex** containing **6 enzymes** and an **acyl carrier protein (ACP)**. Six subunits of the multienzyme complex are designated as acetyl CoA-ACP transacylase, malonyl CoA-ACP transacylase, β-ketoacyl-ACP synthase (condensing enzyme), β-ketoacyl-ACP reductase, β-hydroxyacyl-ACP dehydratase, and enoyl-ACP reductase. The acyl carrier protein (ACP) contains pantothenic acid and has two –SH groups called the pantotheinyl-SH group and the cysteinyl-SH group.

The **reaction sequence for the synthesis of palmitic acid** is as follows (Fig. 12.11):

1. As discussed above, formation of malonyl CoA is a committed step in fatty acid biosynthesis.
2. Next, there is a transfer of an acetyl CoA to the cysteinyl-SH group of ACP. The reaction is catalyzed by acetyl CoA-ACP transacylase subunit of the fatty acid synthase complex and leads to formation of the acetyl-S-ACP.
3. At the same time, malonyl CoA-ACP transacylase transfers malonyl CoA on to the pantotheinyl-SH group of ACP and forms malonyl-S-ACP.
4. Next, the condensing enzyme (β-ketoacyl-ACP synthase) condenses acetyl-S-ACP with malonyl-S-ACP and forms acetoacetyl-S-ACP (β-ketoacyl-ACP).
5. β-Ketoacyl-ACP reductase with NADPH + H⁺ reduces acetoacetyl-S-ACP to form β-hydroxy-butyryl-S-ACP (-hydroxyacyl-S-ACP).
6. β-Hydroxyacyl-ACP dehydratase removes H_2O from β-hydroxyacyl-S-ACP and forms α-, β-transbutenoyl-ACP (crotonyl-S-ACP).
7. α, β-Transbutenoyl-ACP is reduced by enoyl-ACP reductase, utilizing NADPH + H⁺ and is converted to butyryl-S-ACP (acyl-ACP).
8. In the next cycle of reactions, butyryl-S-ACP again condenses with a molecule of malonyl CoA, chain elongation continues with the

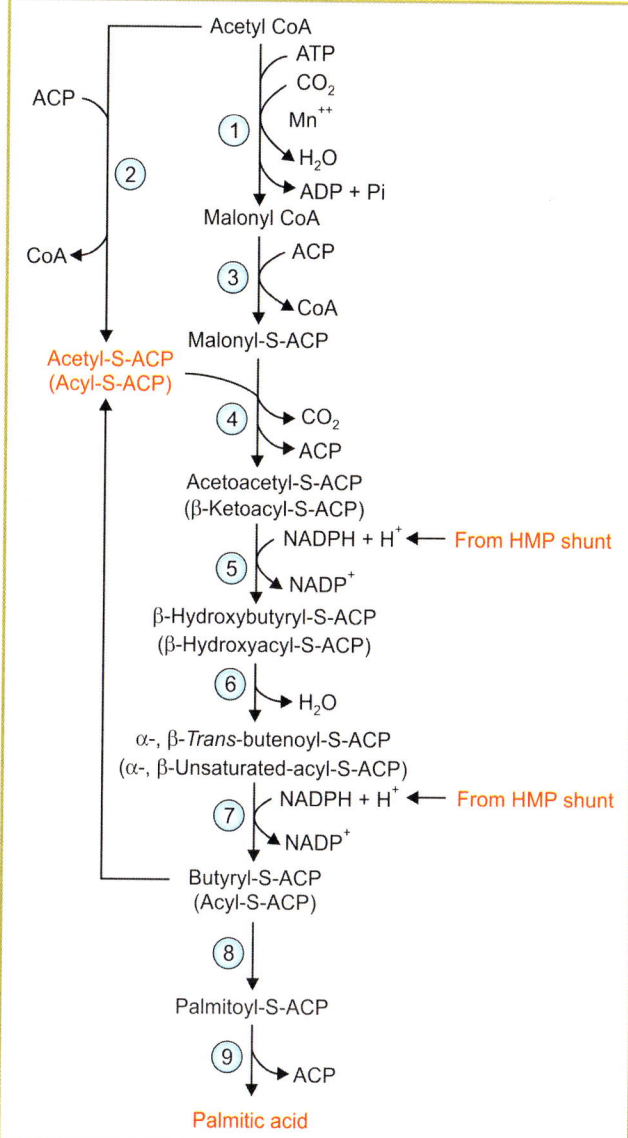

Fig. 12.11: *De novo* synthesis of palmitic acid. 1. Acetyl CoA carboxylase, 2. Acetyl CoA-ACP transacylase, 3. Malonyl CoA-ACP transacylase, 4. Condensing enzyme (β-ketoacyl ACP synthase), 5. Reductase, 6. Dehydratase, 7. Reductase, 8. Further condensation and chain elongation, 9. Thioesterase.

repeated rounds and finally palmitoyl-S-ACP is synthesized.

9. Thereafter, palmitoyl thioesterase removes ACP and yields palmitate. The reducing equivalents (NADPH + H$^+$) used in the biosynthesis of fatty acids are derived from pentose phosphate pathway.

Advantages of FAS existing as multienzyme complex: Multienzyme complexes are called 'metabolons' because they function as a discrete metabolic unit with distinct advantages:

i. The proximity of one enzyme to another minimizes the diffusion of the reaction intermediates thereby enhancing the overall reaction rate.

ii. The channeling of intermediates between successive enzymes reduces the opportunity for these intermediates to react with other molecules, thereby minimizing side reactions.

iii. The complex is more stable as compared to the constituent enzymes present in isolation.

iv. The individual enzymes are encoded by the same structural gene, hence all the enzyme constituents are coordinately expressed.

v. The multienzyme complexes are regulatory proteins so the reactions catalyzed by them are coordinately regulated.

4. Modifications of Palmitate to other Fatty Acids

The first fatty acid which is synthesized within the body is a saturated straight chain 16C fatty acid, called palmitic acid or palmitate (Fig. 12.12), which can be modified by three processes:

1. Chain elongation
2. Desaturation
3. Hydroxylation

Chain Elongation

Chain elongation of a fatty acid occurs either in the mitochondria or in the endoplasmic reticulum.

In mitochondria: Chain elongation in the mito-chondria takes place by the successive additions of acetyl CoA as two carbon units where both NADH as well as NADPH can serve as the reducing agent. The system operates by reversal of the pathway of β-oxidation with the exception that NADPH-linked enoyl CoA reductase replaces FAD-linked acyl CoA dehydrogenase. This process, primarily, results in the elongation of palmitate.

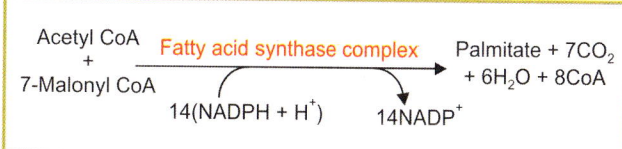

Fig. 12.12: Overall reaction of *de novo* synthesis of palmitate.

12

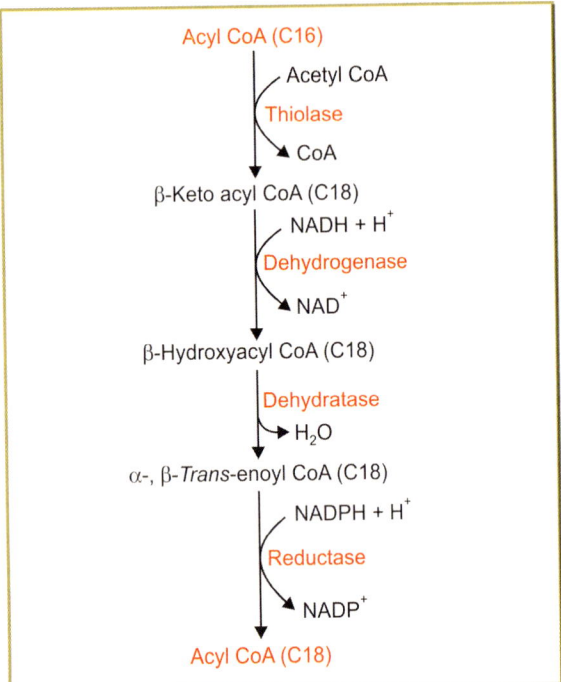

Fig. 12.13. Chain elongation of a fatty acid in the mitochondria.

- Firstly, acyl CoA condenses with acetyl CoA and forms β-ketoacyl CoA which utilizes NADH + H⁺ and is reduced to β-hydroxyacyl CoA.
- Removal of a molecule of water converts β-hydroxyacyl CoA to α, β-unsaturated fattyacyl CoA (enoyl CoA).
- The latter is reduced to a higher member of the series (Fig. 12.13).

In endoplasmic reticulum: The process of chain elongation in the endoplasmic reticulum is similar to fatty acid biosynthesis (*de novo* synthesis) in the cytoplasm. It utilizes malonyl CoA as the source of two carbon units but in the endoplasmic reticulum fatty acid is elongated as its CoA derivative rather than as ACP derivative as in fatty acid synthesis in the cytoplasm. In most of the tissues, chain elongation system in the endoplasmic reticulum converts palmitate to stearate. Brain, however, contains one or more additional elongation systems for the synthesis of long-chain fatty acids (up to 24C), which are needed for the synthesis of complex lipids within the brain.

Desaturation

Desaturation of a fatty acid occurs in higher animals in the endoplasmic reticulum, by desaturases (also

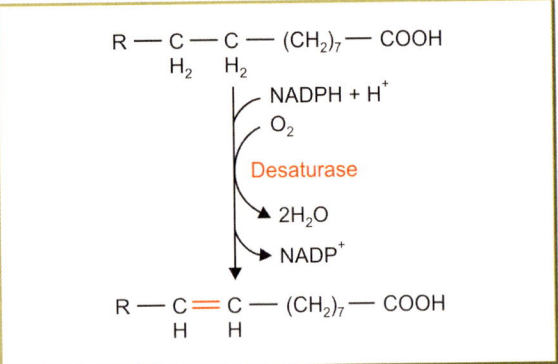

Fig. 12.14: Desaturation of a fatty acid in the endoplasmic reticulum.

termed as mixed function oxidases) (Fig. 12.14). The oxidizing system has 3 components, i.e. a desaturase, cytochrome b5 and NADPH-cytochrome b5-reductase.

A committed step in the formation of an unsaturated fatty acid from palmitic acid or stearic acid is the introduction of the first double bond between C-9 and C-10 by stearoyl CoA desaturase, to form palmitoleic acid or oleic acid, respectively. The activity of this enzyme and its synthesis are controlled by both dietary as well as hormonal mechanisms.

Increasing amounts of PUFA in the diet decreases the activity of this enzyme in the liver whereas insulin, triiodothyronine and hydrocortisone induce the enzyme.

Once the initial double bond has been introduced between carbons 9 and 10 by stearoyl CoA desaturase, additional double bonds can be introduced beyond C-4, C-5 or C-6.

Hydroxylation

Formation of α-hydroxy fatty acids in higher animals occurs in the mitochondria with the mixed function oxidase system which requires molecular oxygen and NADH or NADPH. Their synthesis is closely coordinated with the biosynthesis of sphingolipids that contain hydroxylated fatty acids in the nervous tissue.

Regulation of Fatty Acid Biosynthesis

- The conversion of acetyl CoA to malonyl CoA is a rate-limiting step in the biosynthesis of fatty acids. This reaction is catalyzed by **acetyl CoA carboxylase** which is stimulated by citrate, isocitrate and α-ketoglutarate. Citrate allosterically activates acetyl CoA carboxylase while long-chain fatty acyl CoA acts as an allosteric inhibitor for the same. Insulin also stimulates the activity of the enzyme whereas glucagon inhibits it.

- **High carbohydrate diet** increases the production of acetyl CoA which also increases the citrate pool. Citrate leaves the mitochondria and is cleaved by citrate lyase to produce acetyl CoA. Citrate also stimulates acetyl CoA carboxylase. Thus, high carbohydrate diet leads to increased synthesis of fatty acids.
- **Hormones** also regulate fatty acid biosynthesis. Insulin reduces cAMP levels, inhibits the activation of hormone sensitive lipase and favours lipogenesis. Glucagon, on the other hand, increases cAMP levels, activates hepatic lipase and inhibits fatty acid synthesis. Glucagon thus promotes the release of fatty acids from the adipose tissue (lipolysis) and opposes lipogenesis.
- **Fatty acid synthase** is the other key enzyme of palmitate biosynthesis. A high carbohydrate diet or a fat free diet stimulates fatty acid synthase activity by increasing enzyme synthesis. On the other hand, a high fat diet, fasting and glucagon decrease enzyme synthesis. Phosphorylated sugars, e.g. glucose-6-phosphate also cause allosteric activation of the enzyme.

METABOLISM OF FAT IN THE ADIPOSE TISSUE

After absorption, dietary fat is either oxidized in the liver and muscle or is stored in the body for use at the time of necessity. A major part of the dietary fat is stored in the fat depots called adipose tissue (**white adipose tissue**). Adipose tissue mainly possesses triacylglycerols which are utilized during prolonged starvation.

In a homeostatic situation, there is a continuous synthesis and breakdown of triacylglycerols in the adipose tissue. As the levels of triacylglycerols in the fat depots vary, these are called the **variable elements**. On the other hand, other lipids such as phospholipids form an essential component of the cell and the membrane structure. Their levels since do not alter during fasting, these are called **constant elements**.

Comparison of Glycogen and Neutral Fat (Triacylglycerol) as Energy Stores

As compared to glycogen, triacylglycerols/neutral fat are a more reduced as well as compact form of energy, highly calorigenic and more sustainable as energy stores (Table 12.1).

Brown adipose tissue: Besides white adipose tissue, newborns also have another type of adipose tissue called brown adipose tissue. It disappears during growth of the child. Brown adipose tissue has a **higher metabolic activity** and is capable of producing **large amount of heat**.

BIOSYNTHESIS OF TRIACYLGLYCEROLS

Triacylglycerols, as mentioned above, are the principle lipids of the fat depot in the body as well as the major dietary lipids. Excessive amounts of the dietary

Table 12.1: Comparison of glycogen and neutral fat (triacylglycerol) as energy stores

Parameter	Glycogen	Neutral fat
Form of energy	Less reduced	Highly reduced
Storage form	As granules (10–40 nm diameter) in the cytosol that do not coalesce; hence occupy a small volume of the cell	As droplets in the cytosol that coalesce; hence occupy most of the volume of the cell
Polarity and hydration	Relatively polar and hydrated	Highly nonpolar and anhydrous, hence more fat can be stored in a given volume compared with glycogen
Energy yield	Lower: 4 kcal/g	Higher: 9 kcal/g
Ability to sustain biological functions	18–24 h	4–8 weeks
Comparative advantage	Glycogenolysis yields glucose in between meals especially for brain and RBC. Further, glucose is a good source of energy during sudden, strenuous muscular activity. Glucose (not fatty acids) provides energy during anaerobic activity.	More suited as a long-term energy store that becomes useful during scarcity of carbohydrate as in starvation and diabetes mellitus.

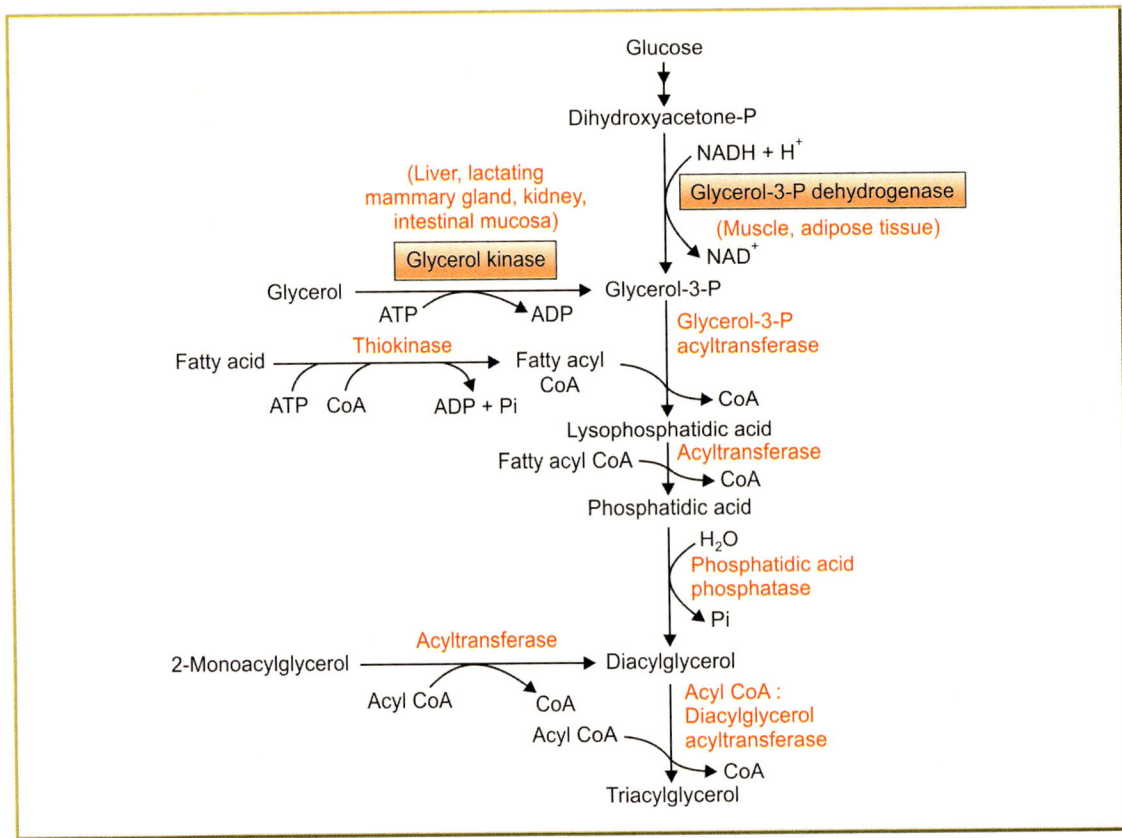

Fig. 12.15: Biosynthesis of a triacylglycerol.

proteins and carbohydrates are also readily converted to free fatty acids and are stored as triacylglycerols in the adipose tissue. Since their stores in the body continuously undergo synthesis as well as breakdown, the net result of the two processes determines the magnitude of **free fatty acid pool** in the adipose tissue. This, in turn, also determines free fatty acid levels in the blood.

Biosynthesis of triacylglycerols (**lipogenesis**), though mainly occurs in the liver and the adipose tissue, the lactating mammary glands, kidney and epithelial cells of the intestinal mucosa are also active in this respect. It requires activation of free fatty acids and α-glycerol phosphate (Fig. 12.15).

Synthesis of L-α-glycerol phosphate

L-α-glycerol phosphate, required for the esterification of fatty acids, can be synthesized in two ways:

1. In most of the tissues which contain glycerol kinase, glycerol is directly converted to L-α-glycerol phosphate.

2. Alternatively, in muscle and adipose tissue which lack glycerol kinase, L-α-glycerol phosphate is formed by the reduction of dihydroxyacetone phosphate, an intermediate of glycolysis. The reaction is catalyzed by glycerol-3-phosphate dehydrogenase.

Activation of Fatty Acid

Free fatty acids, in the presence of ATP and CoA, are activated to acyl CoA, by thiokinase (fatty acyl CoA synthetase).

Re-esterification of Glycerol Phosphate

After the synthesis of L-α-glycerolphosphate and the activation of fatty acids, triacylglycerols are synthesized by a process called re-esterification:

1. A molecule of acyl CoA combines with α-glycerol phosphate and forms l-acyl-glycerol-3-phosphate (lysophosphatidic acid). The reaction is catalyzed by glycerol-3-phosphate acyltransferase.

2. L-Acylglycerol-3-phosphate acyltransferase (lyso-phosphatidyl acyltransferase) converts l-acylgly-cerol-3-phosphate to 1,2-diacylglycerol phosphate (phosphatidic acid), a common intermediate for the biosynthesis of both triacylglycerols as well as phospholipids.

3. A phosphatase (phosphatidic acid phosphohydro-lase) hydrolyzes phosphatidic acid and forms 1,2-diacylglycerol. In many tissues, especially in the intestinal mucosa, 1,2-diacylglycerol is also formed from 2-monoacylglycerols since monoacylglycerols are directly absorbed in the intestinal mucosa. The reaction involves the transfer of an acyl group by the enzyme monoacylglycerol acyltransferase.

4. Diacylglycerol acyltransferase esterifies diacyl-glycerol and forms triacylglycerol.

Generally, palmitic acid is mainly present in position 1 while oleic acid at positions 2 and 3 of a triacylglycerol in the human adipose tissue.

CATABOLISM OF TRIACYLGLYCEROL

The process of breakdown of a triacylglycerol in the adipose tissue is called **lipolysis** and the key enzymes for the release of energy from these stores are called lipases. There are two types of lipases involved in the hydrolysis of triacylglycerols:

Lipoprotein lipase: This enzyme is located on the surface of the endothelial cells of capillaries and possibly of the adjoining tissues. Lipoprotein lipases remove fatty acids from 1 and/or 3 positions of triacylglycerols and/or diacylglycerols when they are present in lipoproteins (VLDL and chylomicrons). The enzyme requires apoprotein C-II for its activity. Insulin also activates the enzyme.

Fatty acids that are released are either bound to serum albumin or are taken up by the tissues. Monoglycerides, which are produced, may either pass into the cells or are further hydrolyzed by the serum monoacylglycerol hydrolase.

Hormone sensitive lipase: This is a distinct type of lipase which hydrolyzes fatty acids from triacyl-glycerols that are stored in the adipose tissue. It is regulated by lipolytic hormones such as epinephrine, glucagon and ACTH. These hormones stimulate cAMP mediated phosphorylation of the inactive enzyme. Insulin and prostaglandins inhibit the enzyme activity.

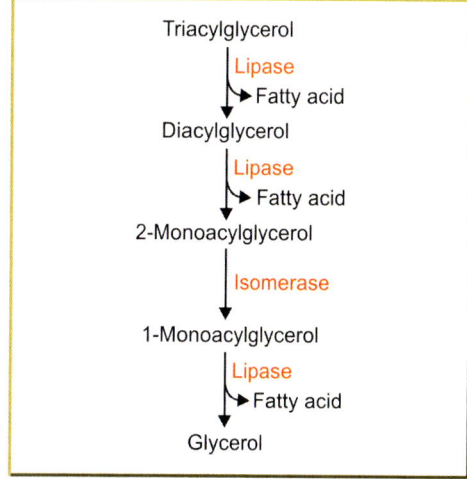

Fig. 12.16: Catabolism of triacylglycerol.

The sequence of hydrolysis of fatty acids from 3 positions of glycerol depends upon the specificities of the particular lipase (Fig. 12.16).

Fatty acids and glycerol so produced are released into the circulating blood. Fatty acids are bound to serum albumin, transported to different tissues and are oxidized to CO_2 and H_2O with the liberation of large amount of energy. Glycerol returns to the liver where it is converted to dihydroxyacetone phosphate and enters the glycolytic pathway or is converted to glucose via gluconeogenesis.

OBESITY

Obesity is the commonest form of malnutrition worldwide, characterized by a **body mass index (BMI, i.e. weight in kg/height in m^2) >30 kg/m^2**. A BMI of 20–25 is considered normal whereas 25–30 is considered overweight. It is multifactorial, involving a complex interplay between:

Genetic factors: Leptin, a protein product of *ob* gene, is secreted from adipose tissue and gastric mucosa (Chemistry to Clinics 12.6). High blood leptin levels are indicative of adequate stores of triacylglycerol (well-fed state) thereby abolishing the neural signals to eat more, and vice versa. It is thus a **lipostat** that acts through cerebral receptors and other local hormones in the CNS such as neuropeptide Y, to regulate the **feeding behavior** (Fig. 12.17). Mutations in *ob* gene result in suboptimal leptin levels with a persistent signal to eat more.

Chemistry to Clinics 12.6: Leptin and Peptic Ulcer Disease
Many cases of peptic ulcer disease have an infectious etiology attributed to the bacteria *Helicobacter pylori* (*H. pylori*). Infection-induced gastritis is associated with high gastric leptin expression resulting in reduced food intake and partly serves to explain the weight loss in these patients. Cure of infection restores the normal body weight.

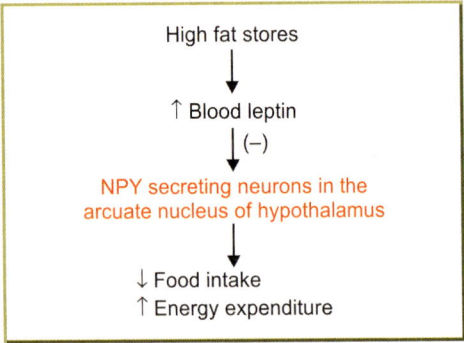

Fig. 12.17: Regulation of feeding behavior by leptin.

Environmental factors

i. *External environment:* High calorie intake versus reduced physical exercise.
ii. *Internal environment:* Low content of brown adipose tissue with or without specific endocrine disorders, e.g. diabetes mellitus, Cushing's syndrome, hypothyroidism, etc.

Biochemical Basis of Feeding Behavior

The regulation of eating behavior is part of a complex pathway that regulates food intake, energy expenditure and reproductive function in the face of changes in nutritional state. In general, the hypothalamus regulates calorie intake, use and storage in a manner that tends to maintain the body weight in adulthood. The 'set point' around which it attempts to stabilize body weight is remarkably constant but can be altered by changes in physical activity, composition of the diet, emotional states, stress, ageing, pregnancy and pharmacological agents.

Several **orexigenic** (stimulating appetite) and **anorexigenic** (causing loss of appetite) peptides and neurotransmitters contribute to the regulation of energy balance. Some, such as leptin and insulin, act on a longer time course to maintain body weight and blood glucose levels, while others such as cholecystokinin and ghrelin act on a shorter time course to

regulate initiation or cessation of a meal. Many of these signals are detected in the arcuate nucleus of the hypothalamus where two groups of neurons are critical. One group expresses **neuropeptide Y (NPY)**; activation of these neurons causes increased food intake and decreased energy expenditure. The other group expresses **pro-opiomelanocortin (POMC)**; activation of these neurons causes decreased food intake and increased energy expenditure.

Long-term regulation of feeding: A key player in the regulation of body weight is the hormone **leptin**, which is released by white adipocytes. As fat stores increase, plasma leptin levels increase and vice versa. On reaching the hypothalamus, leptin inhibits the NPY cells and stimulates the POMC cells. Physiological and biochemical responses to low leptin levels (starvation) are initiated by the hypothalamus to increase food intake, decrease energy expenditure, decrease reproductive function, decrease body temperature and increase parasympathetic activity. Likewise, the responses to high leptin levels (obesity) are initiated by the hypothalamus to decrease food intake, increase energy expenditure, and increase sympathetic activity (Fig. 12.17).

Short-term regulation of feeding: In addition to the long-term regulation of body weight, the hypothalamus also regulates eating behavior on a short term basis. Factors that limit the amount of food ingested during a single feeding episode originate in the gastrointestinal tract and influence the hypothalamic regulatory centers. These include the following:

- *Sensory signals* carried by the vagus nerve that signify stomach fullness.
- *Chemical signals* giving rise to the sensation of satiety, including absorbed nutrients (glucose, certain amino acids and fatty acids).
- *Gastrointestinal hormones* especially cholecystokinin, produced by endocrine cells in the gut wall, and ghrelin produced by the epithelia of the stomach and small intestine. Cholecystokinin is a satiety signal whereas ghrelin stimulates food intake by activating the NPY neurons in the arcuate nucleus. The success of gastric bypass surgery as a treatment for morbid obesity is thought to be a result of the decreased secretion of ghrelin.

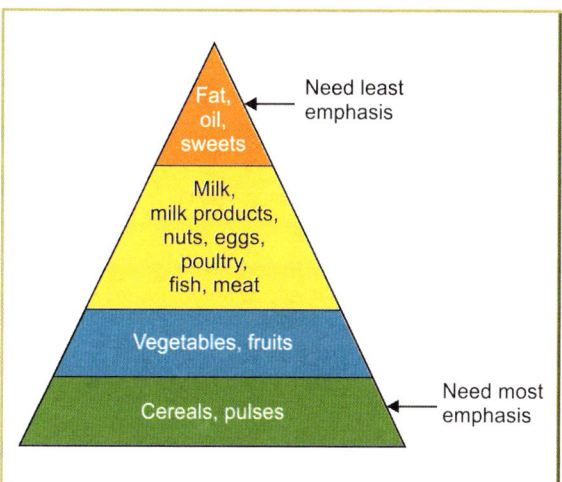

Fig. 12.18: Food guide pyramid.

Food Habits and Obesity

Foods that contain energy/calories (from carbohydrate and/or fat) but lack protein, vitamins and minerals are known as 'empty calorie foods'. A popular synonym is 'junk food'. Examples are potato chips, candies, colas, alcohol, etc. A preference for such foods during childhood and adolescence along with lack of adequate physical activity is a major factor contributing to premature obesity and other health problems. Therefore, the ABC of good health should be remembered and followed—Aim for fitness, Build a healthy base, Choose sensibly (food guide pyramid, Fig. 12.18).

Types of Obesity

- *Based on the time of onset and histological features:* It is of two types, i.e. **hyperplastic or juvenile-onset obesity** characterized by increase in adipocyte number, and **hypertrophic or adult-onset obesity** characterized by increase in adipocyte size mainly. Adipocyte number, once attained and largely fixed at puberty, cannot be reduced by weight-reduction programs, hence currently the attention is heavily directed towards early detection of hyperplastic obesity.
- *Based on the distribution of body fat:* It is again of two types, i.e. central obesity and pear-like obesity. **Central obesity** refers to excess intra-abdominal fat deposition around the organs. It is also called **apple-like obesity** and **android ('man-like') obesity**. It generally affects men and postmenopausal women.

The central body fat cells are larger and more insulin-resistant than the lower body fat cells. Hence, it is associated with diabetes mellitus and cardiovascular diseases, besides some cancers. On the other hand, lower body fat around the hips and thighs is called **pear-like obesity** and **gynoid ('woman-like') obesity**. It is common in women in their reproductive years and poses less of health problems.

Health Hazards of Obesity

Besides considered to be a social stigma, the adverse clinical outcomes of obesity include:
- Type 2 diabetes mellitus (Chemistry to Clinics 12.7)
- Hypertension and related cardiovascular disorders
- Osteoarthritis
- Gall stones
- Endometrial carcinoma
- Hypoventilation (Pickwickian syndrome).

Assessment of Obesity

Clinical assessment of obesity is made by skin-fold thickness or ideally by BMI. Striking biochemical features of obesity include marked elevation of serum free fatty acids, cholesterol and triacylglycerols irrespective of the dietary intake of fat. The other findings may include higher fasting blood glucose, decreased glucose tolerance and in some cases, other hormonal alterations.

Management of Obesity

Principles of management include diet control coupled with exercise (simply speaking, energy expenditure should exceed energy intake) which, it is again emphasized, reduces adipocyte size and not number. Resistant cases require anorexients, gastric bypass or liposuction surgery. Subcutaneous **recombinant**

Chemistry to Clinics 12.7: Metabolic Syndrome

Obesity is very often associated with an insulin-resistant state owing to down-regulation of insulin receptors (decrease in the number of insulin receptors or their affinity for insulin or both) resulting in various metabolic aberrations (Fig. 12.19). Further, obesity and insulin resistance may coexist with dyslipidemia and hypertension. Such combination is called 'metabolic syndrome' or 'syndrome X' and is associated with increased risk of cardiovascular disease.

12

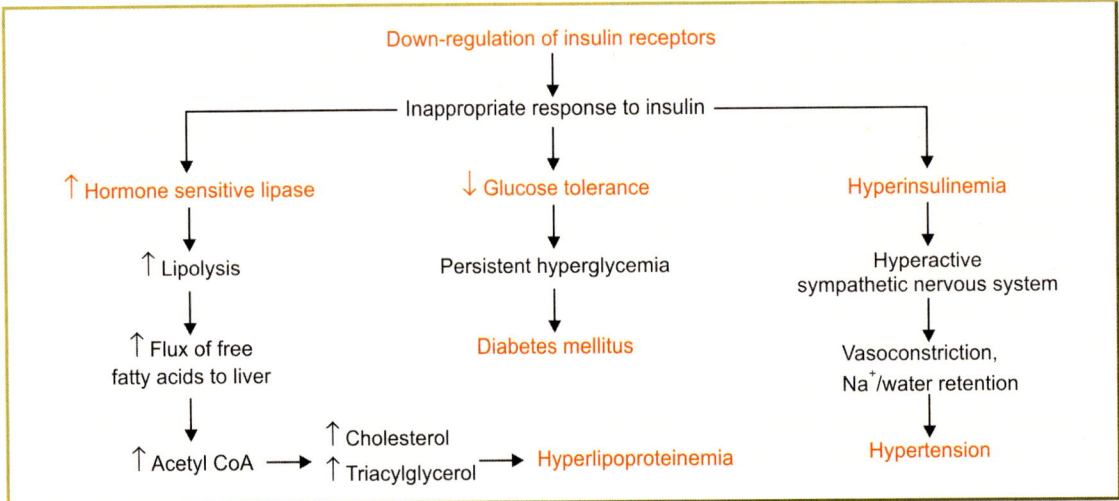

Fig. 12.19: Biochemical aberrations in obesity.

human leptin has shown encouraging results in preliminary studies.

METABOLISM OF CHOLESTEROL

Cholesterol is derived from the diet (**exogenous cholesterol**) as well as is synthesized in various tissues of the body (**endogenous cholesterol**).

Absorption: About 50% of the normal intake of dietary cholesterol is absorbed by small intestine and the rest is excreted in the feces. Nearly 300 mg of cholesterol is daily absorbed from the diet. Ingested cholesterol is absorbed with other lipids and is incorporated into chylomicrons and VLDL. More than 80% of it is esterified in the intestinal mucosa and is transported with lipoproteins.

Excretion: Cholesterol is excreted from the body either as fecal neutral sterols or as bile acids. About 600–750 mg of cholesterol is lost each day as bile acids, 500–600 mg as fecal neutral sterols, 75–100 mg is shed by skin and 35–50 mg is converted into steroid hormones.

Blood cholesterol: Cholesterol content in normal human blood varies from 150 to 250 mg/100 ml being equally distributed between the plasma and the erythrocytes. **Only about 30% of the circulating cholesterol occurs free while remaining exists in the form of cholesterol esters**. A long-chain fatty acid is attached, by an ester linkage, to the –OH group on carbon-3 of the A ring of cholesterol.

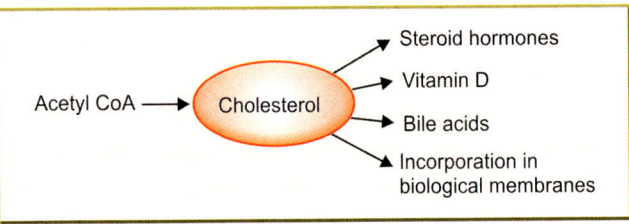

Fig. 12.20: Source and metabolic fates of cholesterol.

METABOLIC FATES OF CHOLESTEROL

Cholesterol occurs in the **free (unesterified) form in biological membranes**. Cholesterol is also a precursor of bile acids, steroid hormones and vitamin D (Fig. 12.20).

BIOSYNTHESIS OF CHOLESTEROL

A large quantity of cholesterol (about 1 g/day) is synthesized in the cytosol. Important sites for cholesterol biosynthesis include liver, skin, intestine, adrenal cortex and the reproductive tissues including ovaries, testes and placenta.

All the carbon atoms of cholesterol are derived from acetate (acetyl CoA) which is obtained from several sources, such as from the oxidation of long-chain fatty acids, ketogenic amino acids and glucose (via pyruvate). In addition, free acetate can also be activated by the enzyme acetokinase (acetothiokinase).

De novo **synthesis of cholesterol** takes place in the body as follows (Fig. 12.21):

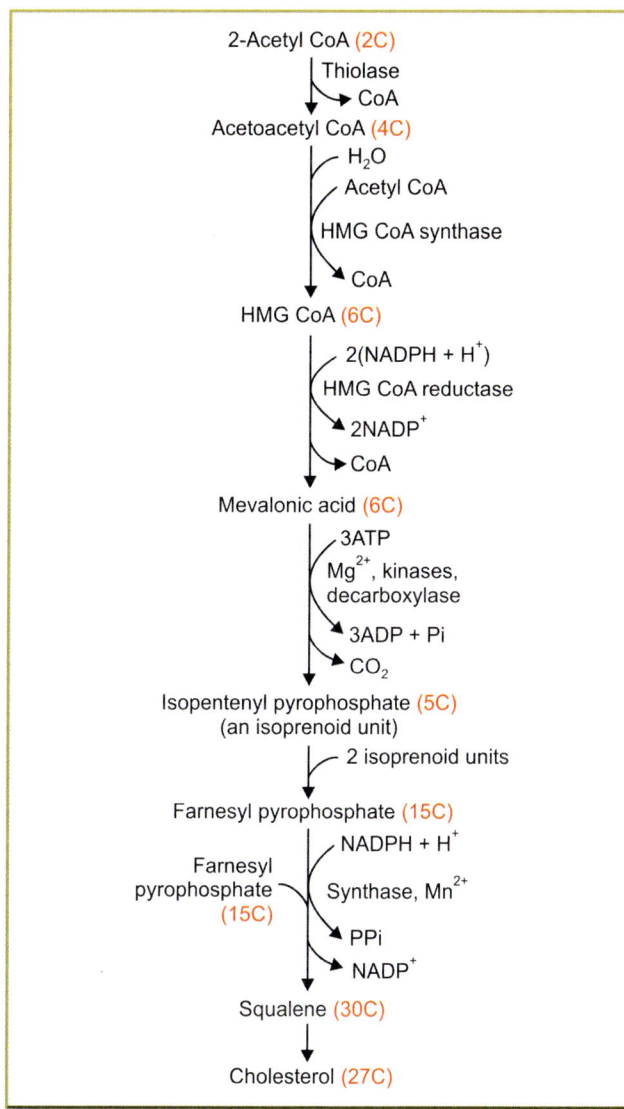

Fig. 12.21: Biosynthesis of cholesterol.

1. Firstly, two molecules of acetyl CoA condense to form acetoacetyl CoA. The reaction is catalyzed by acetoacetyl CoA thiolase.

2. In the presence of β-hydroxy-β-methylglutaryl CoA synthase (HMG CoA synthase), acetoacetyl CoA further condenses with another molecule of acetyl CoA and forms β-hydroxy-β-methylglutaryl CoA (HMG CoA).

   Liver parenchymal cells contain **two isoenzymes of HMG CoA synthase**. One is found in the cytosol and is involved in cholesterol biosynthesis while the other one is present in the mitochondria and is used for the synthesis of ketone bodies. HMG CoA

can also be obtained from oxidative degradation of leucine.

3. By an NADPH dependent enzyme **HMG CoA reductase**, HMG CoA is converted to mevalonic acid. This is a **regulatory step** in cholesterol biosynthesis.

4. Phosphorylation and decarboxylation of mevalonic acid forms an active isoprenoid unit, i.e. isopentenyl pyrophosphate.

   Stepwise transfer of two terminal phosphate groups from two molecules of ATP is catalyzed by two kinases called mevalonate kinase and phosphomevalonate kinase. Subsequent decarboxylation takes place by a decarboxylase (pyrophosphomevalonate decarboxylase).

5. In the next step, the isopentenyl pyrophosphate is isomerized to 3,3-dimethylallyl pyrophosphate, by isopentenyl pyrophosphate isomerase.

6. Stepwise condensation of the three isoprenoid (5C) units leads to the formation of farnesyl pyrophosphate (15C). Firstly, a molecule each of isopentenyl pyrophosphate and 3,3-dimethylallyl pyrophosphate condense to form geranyl pyrophosphate (10C units), which again condenses with another molecule of isopentenyl pyrophosphate and forms farnesyl pyrophosphate (15C). This reaction is catalyzed by geranyl transferase.

7. Fusion of two molecules of farnesyl pyrophosphate forms squalene (30C).

8. By ring closure and removal of three methyl groups, squalene is converted to cholesterol which has **27 carbon atoms**.

Regulation of Cholesterol Biosynthesis

Cholesterol biosynthesis is regulated by dietary cholesterol, feedback inhibition as well as by its disposal from the liver:

• **Dietary cholesterol:** The rate of *de novo* synthesis of cholesterol is inversely related to the amount of dietary cholesterol. When the amount of dietary cholesterol is reduced, cholesterol synthesis is increased in the liver and the intestine, to meet needs of the other tissues and organs. On the other hand, when the quantity of dietary cholesterol increases, endogenous cholesterol synthesis is suppressed.

• **Feedback inhibition:** Cholesterol inhibits its own synthesis by feed back inhibition. The primary site

12

for the control of cholesterol biosynthesis is the HMG CoA reductase step. Cholesterol inhibits the activity of HMG CoA reductase by suppressing synthesis as well as promoting rapid inactivation of the enzyme.

- **Disposal by the liver:** In a normal healthy adult on a low cholesterol diet, about 1300 mg of cholesterol is returned to the liver each day for disposal. The liver removes cholesterol by different processes:
    i. Esterification of cholesterol.
    ii. Excretion of cholesterol: Bile acids are the end products of cholesterol metabolism. Free cholesterol as well as bile acids/salts are excreted in the bile.
    iii. Incorporation of cholesterol into VLDL and secretion into the circulation.

METABOLISM OF KETONE BODIES

Acetoacetate, β-hydroxybutyrate and acetone are collectively known as **ketone bodies**. The process of the formation of ketone bodies is called **ketogenesis** (Chemistry to Clinics 12.8).

Chemistry to Clinics 12.8: Accelerated Ketogenesis

Ketosis: The concentration of ketone bodies in the blood is usually <3 mg/100 ml. In certain conditions such as during prolonged starvation or uncontrolled type 1 diabetes mellitus or a high-fat-low-carbohydrate diet, fat becomes the predominant source of energy and its degradation is greatly accelerated. It results in excessive production of acetyl CoA which cannot be fully utilized through Krebs cycle (due to the lack of oxaloacetate), and therefore, is converted to ketone bodies. Increased ketogenesis results in their raised concentration in the blood. This is called **ketonemia**. This, in turn, also results in increased excretion of ketone bodies in the urine, which is referred as **ketonuria**. A combination of ketonemia and ketonuria is called ketosis.

Ketoacidosis: Both acetoacetate and β-hydroxybutyrate are strong acids. These may slowly deplete alkali reserve of the body, causing metabolic acidosis. This condition is called ketoacidosis.

Diabetic ketoacidosis (DKA): It is an acute complication in patients with type 1 diabetes mellitus (insulin dependent diabetes mellitus) often triggered by an infection, trauma or surgery. Severe deficiency of insulin with excess glucagon and other hyperglycemic hormones, such as epinephrine, cortisol and growth hormone leads to marked hyperglycemia, ketoacidosis, and water and electrolyte imbalance. It should be noted that very often such patients are brought to the emergency in an unconscious state, however, the characteristic fruity odor of acetone (a volatile ketone body) in the expired breath of the patient helps an alert physician to clinch the diagnosis. The various features of this condition can be corrected by intravenous insulin administration only.

FORMATION OF KETONE BODIES

Formation of ketone bodies (**ketogenesis**, Fig. 12.22) occurs mainly in the **liver mitochondria** since liver has highly active system for the production of acetoacetate, the principle/parent ketone body:

1. In the liver, firstly, 2 molecules of acetyl CoA condense together and form acetoacetyl CoA which further reacts with one more molecule of acetyl CoA and forms HMG CoA.

   As already discussed under cholesterol biosynthesis, this step requires HMG CoA synthase. Thereafter, HMG CoA lyase, present in the mitochondria, splits HMG CoA to acetyl CoA and acetoacetate.

2. Acetoacetyl CoA can also be converted to acetoacetate by acetoacetyl CoA deacylase directly.

3. In some of the extrahepatic tissues such as the kidney and the muscle, acetoacetate may also be formed from acetoacetyl CoA by transacylation with succinate.

Acetoacetate is the parent ketone body. In the mitochondria, a portion of acetoacetate is subsequently reduced by NADH-dependent β-hydroxybutyrate dehydrogenase to β-hydroxybutyrate. Some of the acetoacetate is also spontaneously (non-enzymatically) decarboxylated to acetone (being **volatile**, it is lost through expiration).

UTILIZATION OF KETONE BODIES

Acetoacetate and β-hydroxybutyrate, produced by the liver, can be used as excellent sources of energy in the kidney and muscle. Although glucose is a major fuel for the brain in the well-nourished state but during starvation even the brain utilizes ketone bodies which are transported from the liver to the extrahepatic tissues.

The process of oxidation of ketone bodies is called **ketolysis** (Fig. 12.22):

1. **Oxidation of β-hydroxybutyrate:** Mitochondrial β-hydroxybutyrate dehydrogenase oxidizes β-hydroxybutyrate to acetoacetate.

2. **Oxidation of acetoacetate:** Acetoacetate is oxidized after its activation to acetoacetyl CoA either by transacylase or by thiokinase. Since liver does not contain these enzymes, ketone bodies therefore cannot be oxidized in the liver.

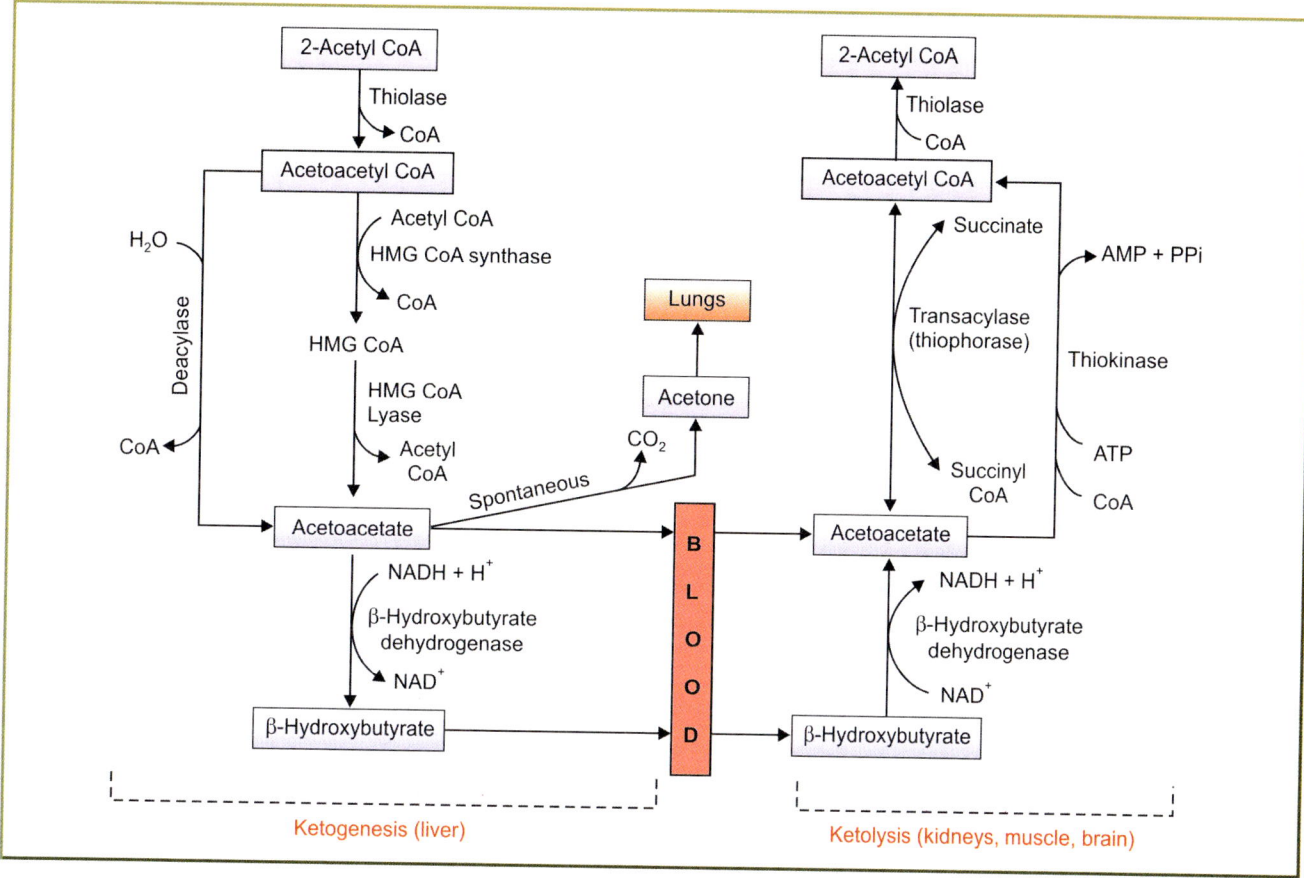

Fig. 12.22: Formation and utilization of ketone bodies.

- Acetoacetate reacts with succinyl CoA in the presence of transacylase (acetoacetate: Succinyl CoA transferase), also called as thiophorase, to form acetoacetyl CoA and succinate.
- Alternatively, acetoacetate thiokinase can also activate acetoacetate, directly. Thereafter, acetoacetyl CoA thiolase (β-ketothiolase) splits acetoacetyl CoA into two molecules of acetyl CoA.
3. **Oxidation of acetone:** Acetone is oxidized, though very slowly. It may be converted to acetoacetate by a reversal of decarboxylation. Some of it may also be converted to propionic acid via propanediol.

BIOSYNTHESIS OF PHOSPHOLIPIDS

All cells are capable of synthesizing phospholipids except the mature erythrocytes. Various phospholipids are synthesized in membranes, from where they are transported, in vesicles, to their final cellular destinations.

SYNTHESIS OF GLYCEROPHOSPHOLIPIDS

Glycerophospholipids are polar, ionic lipids composed of 1,2-diacylglycerol and a phosphodiester bridge that links the glycerol backbone to some base, usually a nitrogenous base. They comprise a molecule of glycerol with a saturated fatty acid at C1 and an unsaturated fatty acid at C2, i.e. 1,2-diacylglycerol. Various glycerophospholipids can be synthesized from 1,2-diacylglycerol and phosphatidic acid, the intermediates in the biosynthesis of triacylglycerols. A nitrogenous base (polar head group) is thereafter attached through a phosphodiester bond at C3 (Fig. 12.23).

Synthesis of Phosphatidylethanolamine/Phosphatidylcholine

1. For the synthesis of phosphatidylethanolamine or of phosphatidylcholine (also called **lecithin**) in the liver and brain, a nitrogenous group (ethanolamine or choline) is first activated. The reaction is

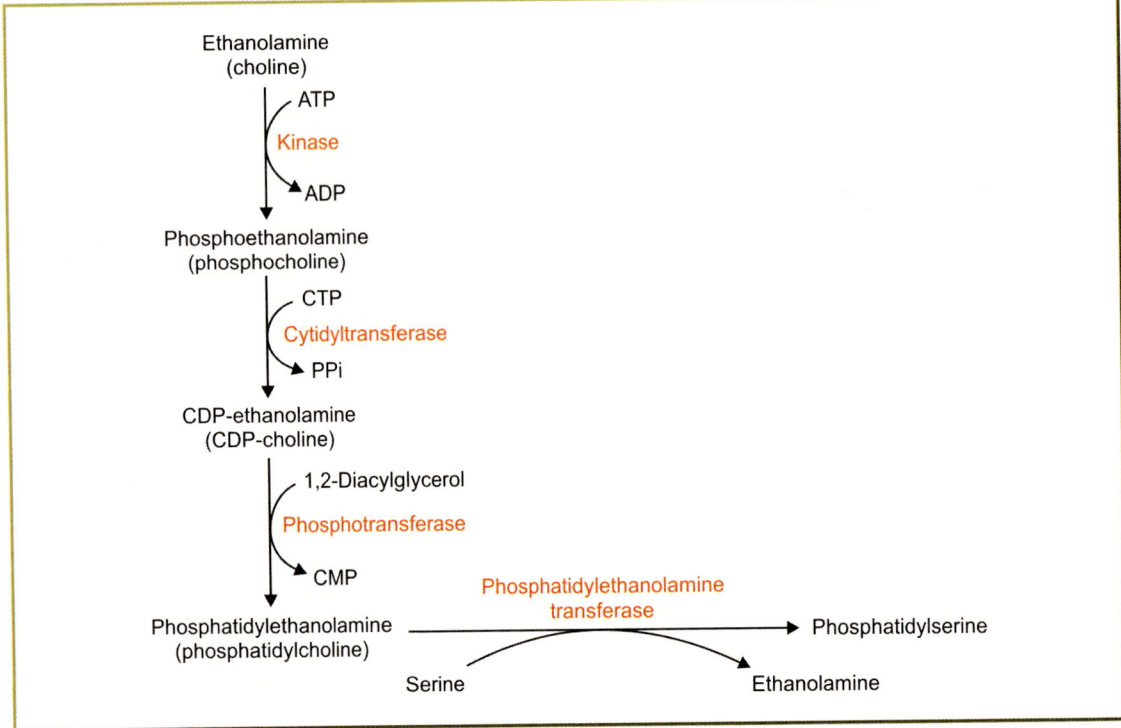

Fig. 12.23: Biosynthesis of phosphatidyl-X (X = ethanolamine/choline/serine).

catalyzed by a kinase (ethanolamine kinase or choline kinase) and requires ATP. Lecithin is of clinical importance (Chemistry to Clinics 12.9).

2. The phosphoryl group of phosphoethanolamine/ phosphocholine then reacts with CTP and leads to the formation of CDP-ethanolamine/CDP-choline. The reaction is catalyzed by phosphoethanolamine cytidylyltransferase/phosphocholine cytidylyl-transferase.

3. CDP-ethanolamine/CDP-choline then reacts with 1,2-diacylglycerol and gets converted to

Chemistry to Clinics 12.9: Lecithins as Lung surfactant

Dipalmitoyl lecithin (lecithin with two palmitic acid residues) also called surfactant is produced by type II epithelial cells in the alveoli. It comprises of >80% of the phospholipids in the extra-cellular liquid layer that lines alveoli of normal lungs and thus decreases surface tension of the aqueous surface layer. This, in turn, prevents atelectasis at the end of the expiration phase of breathing.

The maturity of the fetal lung can be predicted antenatally by measuring the **lecithin/sphingomyelin (L/S) ratio** in the **amniotic fluid**. The mean L/S ratio in normal pregnancy increases gradually with gestation. The ratio of 2.0 is achieved and is characteristic at the gestational age of about 34 weeks.

phosphatidylethanolamine/phosphatidylcholine. The reaction is catalyzed by ethanolamine phospho-transferase or choline phosphotransferase.

- Alternatively, phosphatidylcholine can also be formed by repeated methylation of phos-phatidylethanolamine in the liver. The reaction is catalyzed by phosphatidylethanolamine-N-methyl-transferase, an enzyme of the endo-plasmic reticulum.

    This enzyme catalyzes the transfer of three methyl groups from S-adenosylmethionine (SAM) onto phosphatidylethanolamine and forms phosphatidylcholine.

- Liver mitochondria can also generate phosphati-dylethanolamine by decarboxylation of phos-phatidylserine.

Synthesis of Phosphatidylserine

Phosphatidylserine is synthesized from phosphatidyl-ethanolamine by the transfer of serine with ethanolamine. The reaction is catalyzed by phos-phatidylethanolamine transferase (Fig. 12.23).

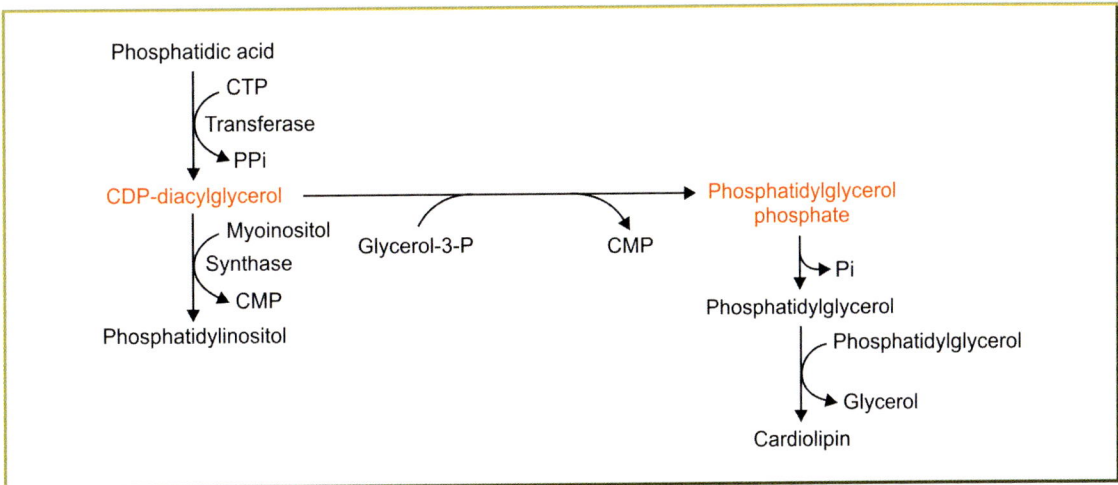

Fig. 12.24: Biosynthesis of phosphatidylinositol/glycerol and cardiolipin.

Synthesis of Phosphatidylinositols

Phosphatidic acid reacts with CTP and forms CDP-diacylglycerol which then reacts with free myoinositol and forms phosphatidylinositol. The reaction is catalyzed by phosphatidylinositol synthase (Fig. 12.24).

Phosphatidylinositols as signal transducers: Inositol containing phospholipids, called inosities, play several roles in the cell:

- Phosphatidylinositol is a structural component of membranes.
- It also serves as a source of arachidonic acid for the synthesis prostaglandins and leukotrienes.
- Phosphatidylinositol also serves to anchor glycoproteins to the plasma membrane.
- Phosphatidylinositol-4,5-bisphosphate (PIP_2) plays a central role in signal transduction system. After certain ligand binds to its receptor on the plasma membrane of a mammalian cell, receptor dependent phosphoinositidase hydrolyzes PIP_2, which is localized to the inner leaflet of the membrane. Hydrolysis of PIP_2, in turn, forms two intracellular signal molecules, i.e. inositol 1,4,5-triphosphate (IP_3), which triggers the release of Ca^{2+} from the endoplasmic reticulum, and 1,2-diacylglycerol which stimulates the activity of protein kinase C.

Synthesis of Cardiolipins

Cardiolipin (phosphatidylglycerol phosphoglyceride or diphosphatidylglycerol) is composed of two molecules of phosphatidic acid linked together covalently through a molecule of glycerol. It occurs primarily in the inner membrane of the mitochondria and in the bacterial membranes.

- Glycerol-3-phosphate reacts with CDP-diacylglycerol and forms phosphatidylglycerolphosphate (Fig. 12.24).
- Thereafter, with the removal of phosphoric acid, phosphatidylglycerol (phosphatidic acid) is synthesized.
- Two molecules of phosphatidylglycerol condense together and form a cardiolipin.

Synthesis of Plasmalogens

Plasmalogens may be designated as **ether glycerolipids**. These are synthesized from dihydroxyacetone phosphate, long-chain fatty acids and long-chain fatty alcohols (Fig. 12.25). About 20% of the mammalian glycerophospholipids are plasmalogens. They are present in membranes, nervous tissue and heart muscle. Large amounts of ethanolamine plasmalogen occur in myelin while choline plasmalogen is abundant in heart muscle. **Patients with Zellweger's disease lack peroxisomes and cannot synthesize adequate amounts of plasmalogens**.

SYNTHESIS OF SPHINGOLIPIDS

Sphingolipids are complex lipids which contain the long-chain amino alcohol sphingosine instead of glycerol. Their synthesis occurs as follows (Fig. 12.26):

12

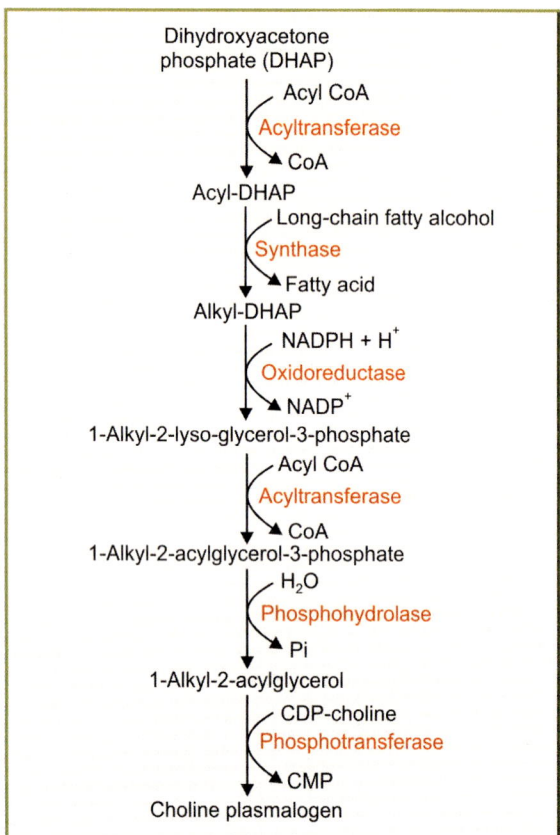

Fig. 12.25: Biosynthesis of a plasmalogen.

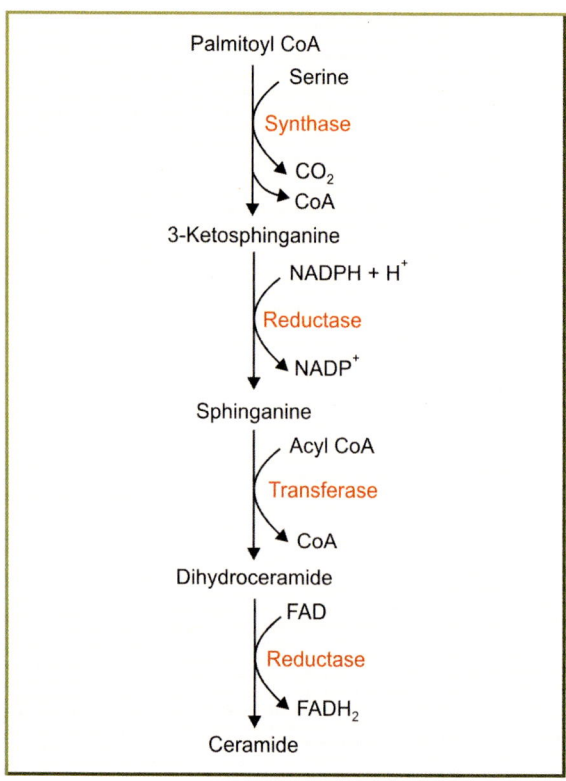

Fig. 12.26: Biosynthesis of a ceramide.

1. **Synthesis of sphingosine:** Sphingosine is synthesized by way of sphinganine from serine and palmitoyl CoA.
   - In the first reaction, palmitoyl CoA reacts with serine and forms 3-ketosphinganine. The reaction is catalyzed by 3-ketosphinganine synthase.
   - In the next reaction, 3-ketosphinganine is reduced to sphinganine (dihydrosphingosine) by 3-ketosphinganine reductase.
   - The conversion of sphinganine to sphingosine occurs not directly but at the level of a ceramide.
     Sphingosine does not occur naturally but forms an essential component of a ceramide, the core structure of the natural sphingolipids.
2. **Synthesis of a ceramide:** A ceramide is a long-chain fatty acid (mainly a saturated 22C fatty acid, i.e. behenic acid) amide derivative of sphingosine.
   - Dihydrosphingosine (sphinganine) condenses with a molecule of a long-chain fatty acyl CoA and forms dihydroceramide. The reaction is catalyzed by acyl CoA transferase.

- Dihydroceramide is reduced to form ceramide (N-acylsphingosine), catalyzed by dihydroceramide reductase.

Ceramide occurs as an intermediate in the biosynthesis and catabolism of sphingomyelin as well as glycosphingolipids.

3. **Synthesis of sphingomyelin:** Sphingomyelin is the **only sphingolipid which contains phosphorus**, i.e. a sphingophospholipid. It is the **major structural lipid of the membrane of the nervous tissue**. Sphingomyelin is synthesized with the transfer of phosphocholine from phosphatidylcholine on to a ceramide (Fig. 12.27). It is thus a **ceramide**

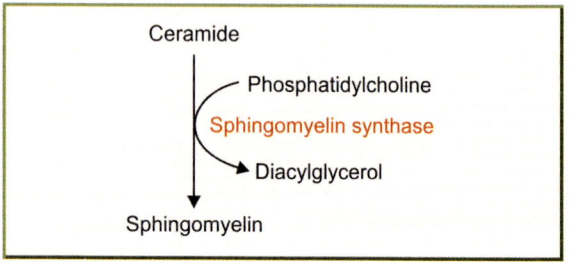

Fig. 12.27: Biosynthesis of sphingomyelin (ceramide phosphocholine).

phosphocholine. The sphingomyelins of the myelin contain long-chain fatty acids, such as lignoceric acid and nervonic acid while that of grey matter contain mainly stearic acid.

Synthesis of Glycosphingolipids

Glycosphingolipids usually have a glucose or galactose unit. The principal glycosphingolipid includes neutral sphingolipids such as cerebrosides or globosides, and acid sphingolipids which include sulfatides and gangliosides.

Cerebrosides: These are glycosylceramides, e.g. ceramide monohexosides. Two most common cerebrosides are glucocerebrosides and galacto-cerebrosides. Galactocerebrosides are more commonly found and are referred to as **galactolipids**. These are synthesized from a ceramide by the transfer of glucosyl units from the respective UDP-hexoses (Fig. 12.28). The reaction is catalyzed by glucosyl transferase or galactosyltransferase.

The **largest concentration of galactocerebrosides is found in the brain**.

Glucocerebroside is an intermediate in the metabolism of more complex glycosphingolipids and is not normally a component of the membrane.

Globosides: Globosides (ceramide oligosaccharides) are cerebrosides that contain two or more sugar residues, such as that of galactose, glucose or N-acetylgalactosamine. Some of the prominent globosides are lactosylceramide (a component of erythrocyte membrane) and ceramide trihexoside.

Sulfatide: Sulfatide (sulfogalactocerebroside) is a sulfuric acid ester of galactocerebroside. Galacto-cerebroside-3-sulfate is the major sulfolipid in the brain. It is synthesized from galactocerebroside and 3-phosphoadenosine-5-phosphosulfate (PAPS or active sulfate). The reaction is catalyzed by a sulfotransferase (Fig. 12.28).

Gangliosides: Gangliosides are sialic acid (N-acetyl-neuraminic acid or NANA) containing glycos-phingolipids. These are present in **high concentration in the ganglion cells** of the central nervous system, particularly in the nerve endings. The principle gangliosides in the brain are G_{M1}, G_{Dla}, G_{Dlb}, G_{Tlb}, where G refers to a ganglioside while M, D or T indicate mono, di or tri-sialic acid residues. The number with each subscript denotes the carbohydrate sequence that is attached to the ceramide.

A specific ganglioside on the intestinal mucosal cells mediates the action of **cholera toxin** (*see* Fig. 5.23). Some of the gangliosides may also act as receptors for other toxins, such as **tetanus toxin** and certain viruses.

CATABOLISM OF SPHINGOLIPIDS

Sphingolipids are normally degraded within the lysosomes of the phagocytic cells, particularly histiocytes or macrophages of the reticuloendothelial system which are primarily located in the liver, the spleen and the bone marrow. The overall pathway of sphingolipid catabolism is composed of several enzymes which cleave specific bonds, e.g. α- and β-galactosidases, glucosidase, neuraminidase, hexo-saminidase, sphingomyelinase, sulfatidase and ceramidase. These are lysosomal hydrolases with an optimum pH in the range of 3.5–5.5. Due to a genetic error when activity of any of the hydrolytic enzymes is markedly reduced, substrate for the defective enzyme accumulates and gets deposited within the lysosomes of the tissue responsible for the catabolism of that sphingolipid. These disorders are called **sphingolipid storage diseases** or sphingolipidoses (Chemistry to Clinics 12.10).

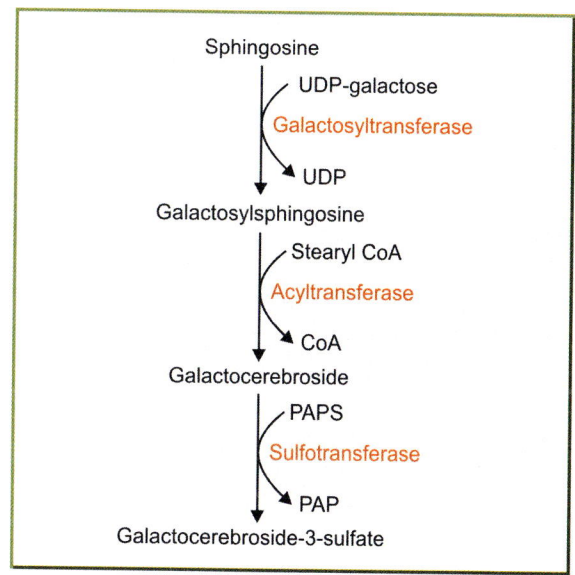

Fig. 12.28: Biosynthesis of a cerebroside and its sulfation.

12

Chemistry to Clinics 12.10: Sphingolipidoses

Common features of various sphingolipid storage diseases are that:

1. A catabolic enzyme is missing
2. The extent of deficiency is same in all the tissues
3. Usually, only a single sphingolipid accumulates in the affected organ while the rate of its biosynthesis is normal.
4. These are transmitted as recessive genetic abnormalities. Enzyme assay of serum or extracts of tissues, peripheral leukocytes and fibroblasts is useful in heterozygote detection.
5. Except for Gaucher's disease (treated with regular infusion of recombinant glucocerebrosidase for long-term), there is no therapy for these diseases.

    Various features of some of the sphingolipid storage diseases are given in Table 12.2.

METABOLISM OF LIPOPROTEINS

Lipoproteins are hydrophilic complexes comprising of lipids mainly triacylglycerols, phospholipids and free cholesterol as well as its esters in association with various **apoproteins (apolipoproteins)**. Four major classes of lipoproteins (as discussed in Chapter 5) are chylomicrons, very low density lipoproteins, low density lipoproteins and high density lipoproteins.

Apolipoproteins: Salient Features

- Protein components of lipoproteins are known as apolipoproteins or apoproteins.
- Functions:
    1. Transport lipids (water insoluble by nature) in plasma in a water-miscible form.
    2. Serve as structural components of lipoproteins
    3. Provide recognition sites for cell-surface receptors
    4. Serve as activators for enzymes involved in lipoprotein metabolism.

- Various apolipoproteins are divided into different classes from A to E, and at least nine are distributed in the lipoproteins, i.e. A-1, A-2, B-48, B-100, C-1, C-2, C-3, D and E.
- All apoproteins except B-100 are water soluble. Apolipoprotein B-100 (apo B-100) is one of the largest monomeric proteins known. It is synthesized by the liver and is present in LDL.

Metabolism of Chylomicrons

Chylomicrons are **triacylglycerol-rich particles** that are assembled in the **intestinal mucosal cells**. They carry **dietary/exogenous triacylglycerols** (the major lipids of chylomicrons), cholesterol and cholesteryl esters **to the peripheral (extrahepatic) tissues** where these lipids are subsequently metabolized (Fig. 12.29).

Intestinal mucosal cells release **nascent chylomicrons** which contain **apoB-48** that is synthesized in the intestine. These nascent chylomicron particles receive apoE and apoC from the circulating HDL. Apo C-2, in turn, activates lipoprotein lipase and hydrolyzes triacylglycerols to monoacylglycerols, free fatty acids and glycerol. As a result, chylomicron particles decrease in size and increase in density. Thereafter, ApoC is returned back to HDL and the leftover particles are called **chylomicron remnants**.

Chylomicron remnants bind to apoE receptors on the hepatocytes. These particles are then internalized and their lipids including cholesteryl esters can be either utilized or stored intracellularly. A small amount of the released fatty acids enters circulation and contributes directly to the plasma free fatty acid pool.

Table 12.2: Sphingolipid storage diseases (sphingolipidoses)			
Sphingolipidoses	*Defective enzyme*	*Accumulated substrate*	*Clinical features*
Tay-Sach's disease	Hexosaminidase A	Ganglioside G_{M2}	Mental retardation, blindness, cherry red spot on macula
Fabry's disease	α-Galactosidase A	Ceramide trihexosides	Lower limb pain, rashes, renal failure
Gaucher's disease	Glucocerebrosidase	Glucocerebrosides	Hepatosplenomegaly, erosion of long bones and pelvis
Krabbe's disease	Galactocerebrosidase	Galactocerebrosides	Absence of myelin leading to mental retardation
Niemann-Pick disease	Sphingomyelinase	Sphingomyelins	Hepatosplenomegaly, mental retardation
Metachromatic leukodystrophy	Sulphatidase	Sulphatides	Mental retardation
Generalized gangliosidosis	G_{M1} ganglioside: β-galactosidase	Ganglioside G_{M1}	Hepatomegaly, mental retardation

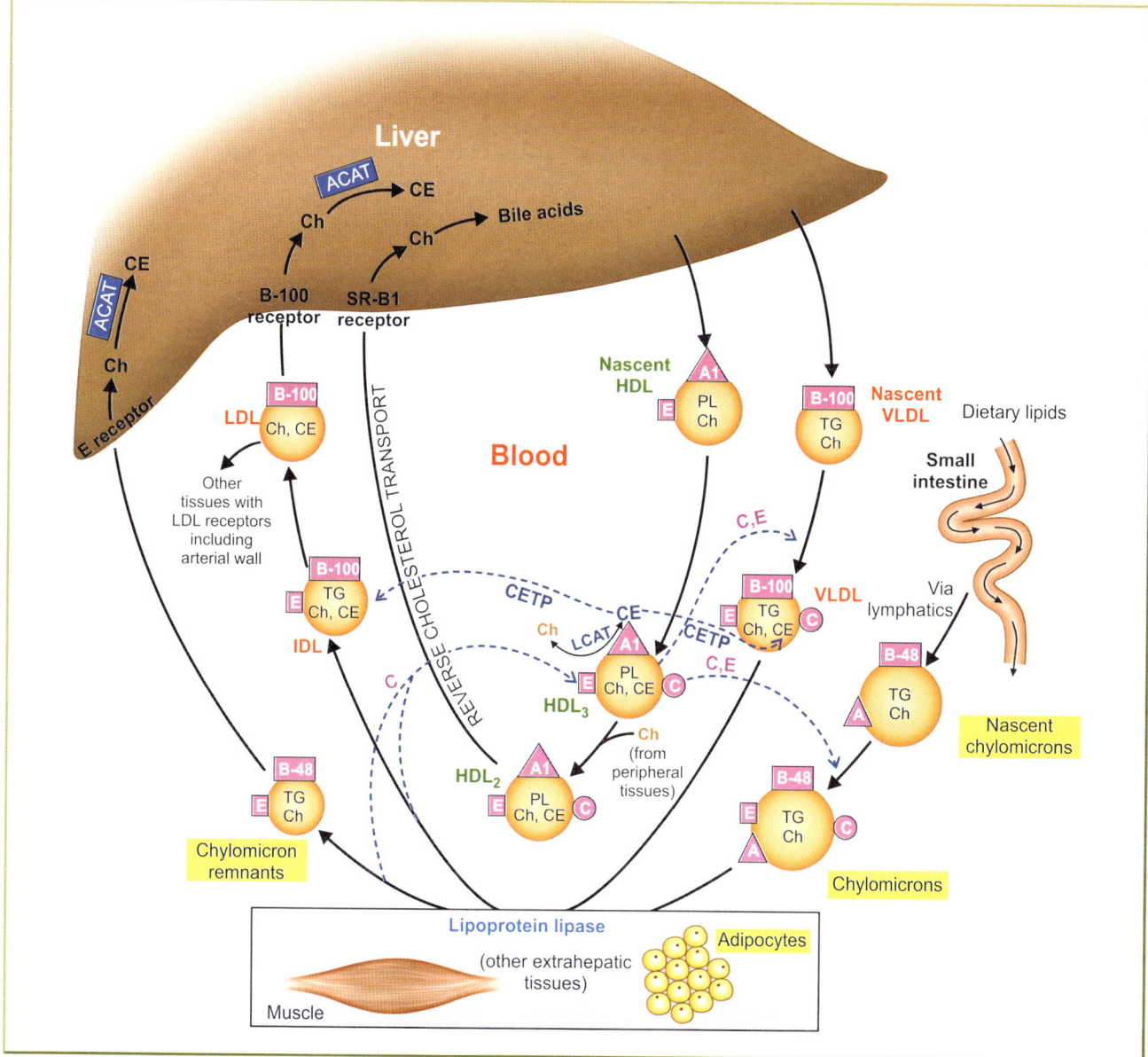

Fig. 12.29: Metabolism of lipoproteins. A=ApoA; A1=ApoA-1; ACAT=Acyl Cholesterol Acyl Transferase; B-48=ApoB-48; B-100=ApoB-100; C=ApoC; CE=Cholesterol Ester; CETP=Cholesterol Ester Transfer Protein; Ch=Cholesterol; E=ApoE; LCAT=Lecithin: Cholesterol Acyl Transferase; PL=Phospholipid; TG=Triglyceride.

Metabolism of Very Low Density Lipoproteins

Very low density lipoproteins (VLDL), also called **pre-β-lipoproteins**, are composed of triacylglycerols like chylomicrons but their function is to transport these lipids (**endogenous triacylglycerol**) from the **liver to the peripheral tissues (extrahepatic tissues)**. VLDL are released from the liver as **nascent VLDL** particles, similar to the release of nascent chylomicrons from the intestinal mucosa. Nascent VLDL particles contain **apoB-100** and apoA-1. They, subsequently, acquire apoC-2 and apoE from the circulating HDL and are converted to VLDL (Fig. 12.29).

During circulation, lipoprotein lipase hydrolyzes triacylglycerols and releases free fatty acids which are taken up by the peripheral tissues. Subsequently, apoC and apoE are transferred to HDL. In addition, cholesteryl esters are transferred from HDL to VLDL in exchange with the transfer of triacylglycerols and phospholipids from VLDL to HDL. As a result, their particle size is reduced and density is increased. VLDL particles are hence converted into **VLDL remnants** which are also designated as **intermediate density lipoproteins (IDL)**.

The **IDL particles are either removed by the liver or are further converted into circulating LDL particles**. During the process of this conversion (of IDL) to LDL, surface lipids and apoproteins, other than the molecule of apoB-100, are removed. Cholesteryl esters, which are synthesized in plasma as a result of the action of lecithin cholesterol acyltransferase (LCAT, discussed later) on HDL particles, are transferred from HDL to VLDL and IDL via cholesteryl ester transfer protein (CETP).

Metabolism of Low Density Lipoproteins

Low density lipoproteins (LDL) contain **high concentration of cholesterol and its esters**. They retain **apoB-100** and lose other apoproteins to HDL. The primary function of the LDL is to transport **cholesterol (initially released from the liver in VLDL) to the extrahepatic tissues** (Fig. 12.29). For their metabolism, LDL particles bind to their receptors on the cell membrane.

LDL receptors are negatively charged glycoproteins that are clustered in pits on the cell membrane and recognize apoB-100 of the LDL. The intracellular side of the pit is coated with a protein called **clathrin**, which stabilizes the shape of the pit. The number of these receptors is regulated by the cholesterol content of the cell. The ability of a tissue to take up LDL depends upon the rate of transcapillary transport as well as the number of receptors. The liver and the adrenals which have a fenestrated epithelium as well as large number of receptors, may take up LDL rapidly while the muscle and the adipose tissue which lack such an epithelium and have a few LDL receptors, take up LDL slowly.

After binding, LDL particles are **internalized** by endocytosis, in the form of vesicles. These LDL vesicles rapidly lose the clathrin coat, fuse with other similar vesicles and form endosomes (large vesicles). The receptors are recycled whereas LDL remnants, in the vesicles, are degraded and release cholesterol, fatty acids, phospholipids and amino acids (*see* Fig. 3.16).

Free cholesterol can be used for membrane biosynthesis or for its conversion to steroid hormones and bile acids. Excess of the cholesterol is re-esterified by acylcholesterol acyltransferase (**ACAT**) and is stored as cholesteryl esters.

Nearly 70–80% of the LDL particles are removed via LDL receptors while the rest of them are removed by nonspecific endocytosis, via the scavenger pathway. The latter is also a receptor mediated process involving phagocytic cells, in the reticuloendothelial system.

There are two LDL-subtypes that are clinically important (Chemistry to Clinics 12.11).

Lecithin–Cholesterol Acyltransferase (LCAT) and Reverse Cholesterol Transport (RCT)

HDL and the enzyme lecithin–cholesterol acyltransferase (LCAT) are important for the removal of cholesterol from the body. LCAT is a plasma enzyme produced mainly by the liver. The enzyme transfers a fatty acid from C2 position of lecithin to the 3-hydroxyl of cholesterol. The reaction (Fig. 12.30) is freely reversible and utilizes cholesterol which is present in HDL. Cholesterol esters so formed, diffuse into the core of the HDL particles where these are transported from tissues via plasma to the liver, the only organ capable of metabolizing and excreting cholesterol as bile acids. This mechanism, i.e. the action of LCAT on

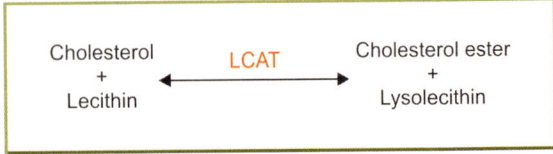

Fig. 12.30: Reaction catalyzed by lecithin–cholesterol acyltransferase (LCAT).

Table 12.3: Difference between LCAT and ACAT

Parameter	LCAT	ACAT
Site of esterification	Intravascular, extracellular	Extravascular, intracellular (hepatocytes)
Esterifying unit	Polyunsaturated fatty acids	Monounsaturated fatty acids
Activator	ApoA-1 in HDL	Unesterified cholesterol
Metabolic purpose	To esterify free cholesterol derived from peripheral tissues and transport it to the liver via HDL.	To store excess cholesterol as esters so as to maintain low intracellular free cholesterol levels.

HDL is referred to as **reverse cholesterol transport (RCT)**. HDL thus provides a vehicle for the transport of cholesterol from peripheral tissues to the liver and **protects from atherosclerosis**.

LCAT versus ACAT: Although both the enzymes are involved in acyl group transfer, they differ with respect to their location, the esterifying unit, activator and function (Table 12.3).

Metabolism of High Density Lipoproteins

High density lipoprotein (HDL) particles are synthesized in the **liver** and secreted into the bloodstream by exocytosis, as **nascent HDL** particles. They are discoidal in shape and are composed of apoA, apoE, phospholipids and free cholesterol. Among the various lipoproteins, they contain **highest concentration of phospholipids**.

As discussed above, there also occur the transfer of apoC to the nascent HDL from chylomicrons and VLDL (Fig. 12.29). Nascent HDL particles are thus converted to **mature HDL** called **HDL$_3$**. From HDL$_3$, cholesteryl esters (produced by the action of LCAT) are shifted to VLDL and IDL. At the same time, HDL$_3$ also acquires free cholesterol from the cell membrane. These HDL$_3$ particles are thus converted to **HDL$_2$**. (Note: HDL$_1$ is a very minor HDL fraction with higher phospholipid and lower apoA-1 content, detected in some patients of primary hyperlipoproteinemia or cholestasis). This is an important mechanism for the removal of excess cholesterol from the peripheral tissues and is called reverse cholesterol transport (RCT).

HDL thus **performs several important functions**

1. It is a circulating reservoir of apoC-2 which is transferred to chylomicrons and VLDL for the activation of lipoprotein lipase.
2. It removes free cholesterol from the extrahepatic tissues and esterifies it with the help of LCAT.

HDL thus transports cholesterol from the extra-hepatic tissues to the liver.

3. It transfers cholesteryl esters to VLDL and LDL in exchange for triacylglycerols and phospholipids from these particles.
4. It also carries cholesteryl esters to the liver.

In the liver, HDL is taken-up via SR-B1 (scavenger receptor class B, type 1) receptors, degraded and releases cholesterol. Cholesterol, in turn, is either repacked within the lipoproteins or is converted into bile acids and secreted into the bile for its removal from the body. Thus, HDL protects an individual against atherosclerosis (Chemistry to Clinics 12.12).

Good versus bad cholesterol: The risk of developing atherosclerosis is directly related to the plasma concentration of LDL cholesterol but inversely related to HDL cholesterol. Therefore, **LDL cholesterol** is called the **'bad cholesterol'** while **HDL cholesterol** is referred to as the **'good cholesterol'**, although chemically there is only one cholesterol.

DISORDERS OF LIPOPROTEIN METABOLISM

Hyperlipoproteinemias

Increased rate of synthesis or reduced clearance of lipoproteins from the bloodstream may result in a group of disorders referred to as hyperlipidemias or hyperlipoproteinemias (Table 12.4). Usually, they are detected by measuring plasma triacylglycerols and cholesterol, and are classified accordingly as follows:

Type I hyperlipoproteinemia: This condition is also called **hyperchylomicronemia or familial fat-induced hyperlipemia**. This is due to the accumulation of chylomicrons. These patients have very high levels of triacylglycerols in their plasma (over 1000 mg/dl) with a proportionally smaller increase in cholesterol. On electrophoresis, chylomicrons remain at the origin.

12

Chemistry to Clinics 12.12: Atherosclerosis (Arteriosclerosis)

Formation of atheroma: Atherosclerosis is a pathological process involving the arterial wall. It starts with repeated subtle injuries to the endothelium followed by migration of blood monocytes into the tunica media and accumulation as modified macrophages, accumulation of cholesterol and its esters in the macrophages (known as lipid-laden foam cells), smooth muscle cell proliferation, plaque formation and luminal narrowing (Fig. 12.31). Collectively, it results in thickening of the arterial wall, the atheroma.

Risk factors: *Major risk factors* include hypercholesterolemia, diabetes mellitus, hypertension, tobacco smoking, high plasma lipoprotein(a) and hyperhomocysteinemia, while the *accessory risk factors* are high calorie diet, sedentary lifestyle, obesity, alcohol, stress, estrogen supplements etc.

Complications: The most feared complications of atherosclerosis result from stenosis (narrowing) of arteries or the formation of thrombus on the plaque or dislodging of the thrombus as an embolus or rupture of the plaque itself, leading to myocardial infarction, stroke, peripheral vascular disease and accelerated hypertension with organ damage.

Management: The approach to management includes:

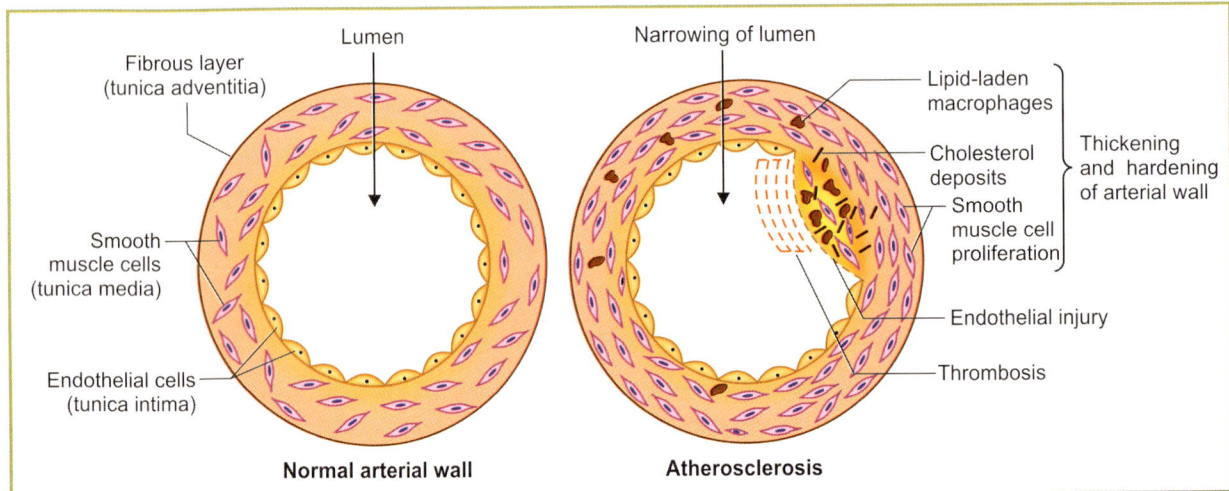

Fig. 12.31: Atherosclerosis.

1. Identification and management of risk factors.
2. Lifestyle interventions:
   - Increased physical activity (e.g. at least 30 minutes of brisk walking daily, at least 5 days/week), limit sedentary activity and stress, maintain close to ideal body mass index, reduce salt, quit smoking and alcohol.
   - Modify quantity and quality of lipid intake: <30% energy from fat (out of which <10% from saturated fat and the rest from unsaturated fat with <1% *trans*-fatty acids), cholesterol <300 mg/day, increase omega-3 fatty acids.
   - Liberal intake of fruits and vegetables: Excellent sources of micronutrients, antioxidants and dietary fibers.
3. Drugs (along with the above measures when these alone prove unsatisfactory):
   - Statins (such as lovastatin, simvastatin, atorvastatin and rosuvastatin) inhibit HMG CoA reductase, decrease endogenous cholesterol synthesis and stimulate LDL uptake (via LDL receptors) by the tissues.
   - Ezetimibe inhibits the intestinal absorption of cholesterol.
   - Cholestyramine binds bile salts and promotes its fecal excretion. This increases the rate of bile salt synthesis and LDL uptake by the liver.
   - Fibrates (such as clofibrate and gemfibrozil) decrease plasma triglyceride and VLDL by increasing lipoprotein lipase activity.
   - Nicotinic acid (high doses) suppresses hepatic VLDL production, and decreases plasma triglyceride and VLDL by increasing lipoprotein lipase activity.

Type I hyperlipoproteinemia may be due to **three different types** of genetic abnormalities:

- **Familial lipoprotein lipase deficiency:** It is usually present in infancy or childhood. There are recurrent episodes of abdominal pain due to attacks of acute pancreatitis which are triggered by very high plasma levels of triacylglycerols (Chemistry to Clinics 12.13). Patients may have skin lesions called

Table 12.4: Classification of hyperlipoproteinemias

Type	↑ Lipoproteins
Primary	
I Exogenous hypertriglyceridemia	Chylomicrons
IIa Hypercholesterolemia	LDL
IIb Combined hyperlipidemia	LDL + VLDL
III Remnant hyperlipidemia	Remnant VLDL
IV Endogenous hyperlipidemia	VLDL
V Mixed hyperlipidemia	VLDL + Chylomicrons
Secondary	
Type IV pattern: Diabetes mellitus, alcoholism, von Gierke's disease, lipodystrophies, acromegaly, oral contraceptives, uremia, hypothyroidism, high carbohydrate diet	VLDL

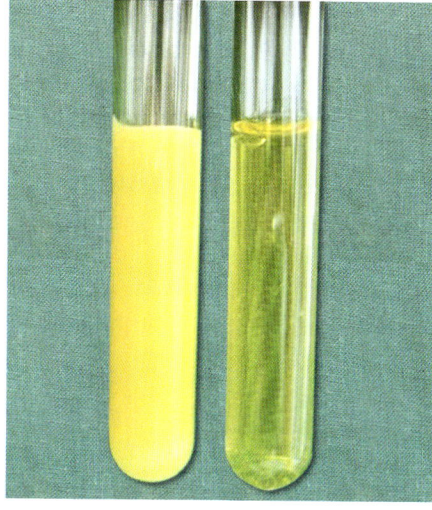

Fig. 12.32: Serum of a patient with triglyceride-related acute pancreatitis. **Left:** Lipemic serum before treatment with insulin and heparin. **Right:** Clear serum after 5 days of therapy.

eruptive xanthomata which appear on buttocks, back, knees and elbows. These lesions contain a lot of triacylglycerols due to the deposition of chylomicrons. Serum has a lipemic appearance (Fig. 12.32), and after an overnight refrigeration at 4°C, chylomicrons rise to the surface. Diagnosis is confirmed by measuring lipoprotein lipase activity in the plasma after a bolus injection of heparin.

- **Familial apoC-2 deficiency:** It is a rare condition, which is inherited as an autosomal recessive disorder. It is due to the deficiency of apoC-2 which is essential for the activation of lipoprotein lipase. Hence, there is impaired removal of both chylomicrons and VLDL from the plasma. This, in turn, results in the lipoprotein pattern which may be of type I or type V.
- **Familial lipoprotein lipase inhibitor:** It is an autosomal dominant condition of the type I

hyperlipoproteinemia. The patient has low post-heparin plasma lipolytic activity but high levels of lipoprotein lipase in the adipose tissue. Plasma of the affected individuals contains a nondialyzable, heat stable inhibitor of lipoprotein lipase. Occasionally, subjects with type I phenotype may also show a type V pattern, due to the accumulation of VLDL in their plasma. This is common if they ingest a high carbohydrate diet.

Type II hyperlipoproteinemia: It may be further sub-classified as:

- **Type IIa hyperlipoproteinemia:** It is also called **familial hypercholesterolemia or familial hyperbetalipoproteinemia.** There is high cholesterol in fasting plasma without increase in triacylglycerols. Electrophoretic pattern also shows an increase in β-lipoproteins. It may be a primary disorder due to some genetic abnormality or a secondary lipoprotein disorder.

  Primary type IIa hyperlipoproteinemia also called familial type IIa hyperlipoproteinemia may be seen in heterozygotes or homozygotes. Heterozygous familial type IIa hyperlipoproteinemia is an autosomal dominant inherited disease, usually from many different genetic mutations, affecting the gene for LDL, for apoB and apoE receptors. Mutations for LDL receptor gene can cause four different types of disorders:

Chemistry to Clinics 12.13: Hypertriglyceridemia and Acute Pancreatitis

Chylomicrons are usually formed 1–3 hours postprandially and cleared within 8 hours. However, in hypertriglyceridemia, chylomicrons are almost always present thereby increasing the viscosity of blood. Further, these particles are very large and may obstruct pancreatic capillaries leading to local ischemia and acidemia followed by cell necrosis and apoptosis. This local damage exposes triglycerides to pancreatic lipases. Triglycerides are hydrolyzed to free fatty acids which form self-aggregating micelles with detergent properties, damaging capillaries, platelets and pancreatic tissue. Cytotoxic injury, release of inflammatory mediators and free radicals, eventually manifests as acute pancreatitis.

12

– The most common type is mutant allele where no receptors are synthesized.
– The second common type of disorder is the one where receptors are synthesized but are transported slowly from the endoplasmic reticulum to the Golgi apparatus.
– Receptors are processed and reach the cell surface but fail to bind LDL.
– Receptors reach the surface and bind LDL but fail to cluster in the coated-pits, and cannot be internalized.

The heterozygotes have very high levels of plasma cholesterol and LDL.

Homozygous familial type IIa hyperlipoproteinemia is generally seen in children who present with planar or tuberous xanthomata since birth. Yellowish plaques or lumps occur on buttocks, knees, elbows and hands. Cardiovascular disease may develop before the age of 10 years.

Plasma LDL is several times higher than normal. Some of these patients may also show moderate elevation of triacylglycerols.

Secondary type IIa hyperlipoproteinemia results in hypercholesterolemia which can be caused by several common disorders unrelated to familial conditions, such as Cushing's syndrome, hypothyroidism, anorexia nervosa, nephrotic syndrome, primary liver cell carcinoma or diabetes mellitus.

• **Type IIb hyperlipoproteinemia:** It is called **familial combined hyperlipidemia or multiple lipoprotein-type hyperlipidemia**. There is an increase in total plasma cholesterol and triacylglycerols. On electrophoresis, there is an increase in the intensity of both β and pre β-bands, due to increased production of VLDL and LDL. Composition of the individual lipoproteins is normal. Obesity, high serum uric acid levels and glucose intolerance are common in patients with this pattern.

Type III hyperlipoproteinemia: It is also called **dysbetalipoproteinemia or remnant hyperlipoproteinemia or broad, floating beta disease or familial type III hyperlipoproteinemia**. There is a moderate hypercholesterolemia while hypertriacylglyceridemia is relatively uncommon. This is associated with the presence of chylomicron remnants and IDL in plasma. The disease rarely manifests itself before early adult life in males or before the menopause in females. Fasting serum or plasma is often turbid. The charac-

teristic finding on electrophoresis is a broad β-band but on ultracentrifugation these particles are isolated in the VLDL region.

Type IV hyperlipoproteinemia: This condition is also called **hyper-prebeta-hyperlipoproteinemia or endogenous hyperlipidemia or diet-induced hypertriglyceridemia or familial Type IV hyperlipoproteinemia**. These patients have a marked elevation of plasma triacylglycerols in VLDL. In some families, there is excessive VLDL secretion while in others the removal rate of VLDL from plasma is reduced. Fasting serum or plasma is turbid. On electrophoresis, there is a marked pre β-band with normal β and a normal or reduced α-band.

A **secondary type IV pattern** is quite common (Table 12.5).

Type V hyperlipoproteinemia: It is also called **mixed hyperlipidemia** since large amounts of both chylomicrons and VLDL are seen in the fasting plasma. It is occasionally seen in patients whose characteristic pattern is like type I (due to lipoprotein lipase deficiency) but rarely of type IV. Whole blood may be lipemic. Plasma is white and turbid. The electrophoretic pattern is characterized by raised chylomicrons and VLDL levels.

Hypolipoproteinemias

• *Abetalipoproteinemia:* Fat malabsorption is present from birth. In neonates, there is poor appetite, vomiting, diarrhea and failure to thrive. All plasma lipids, particularly triacylglycerols, are reduced to less then 50% of the normal levels. This is mainly due to the total absence of apoB, and thus of VLDL and LDL.

• *Familial hypobetalipoproteinemia:* There is a moderate reduction of plasma lipids. Both VLDL

Table 12.5: Causes of secondary type IV hyperlipoproteinemia

• Diabetes mellitus
• Alcoholism
• Hypothyroidism
• von Gierke's disease
• Lipodystrophies
• Acromegaly
• ↑use of oral contraceptives
• Uremia
• High carbohydrate diet

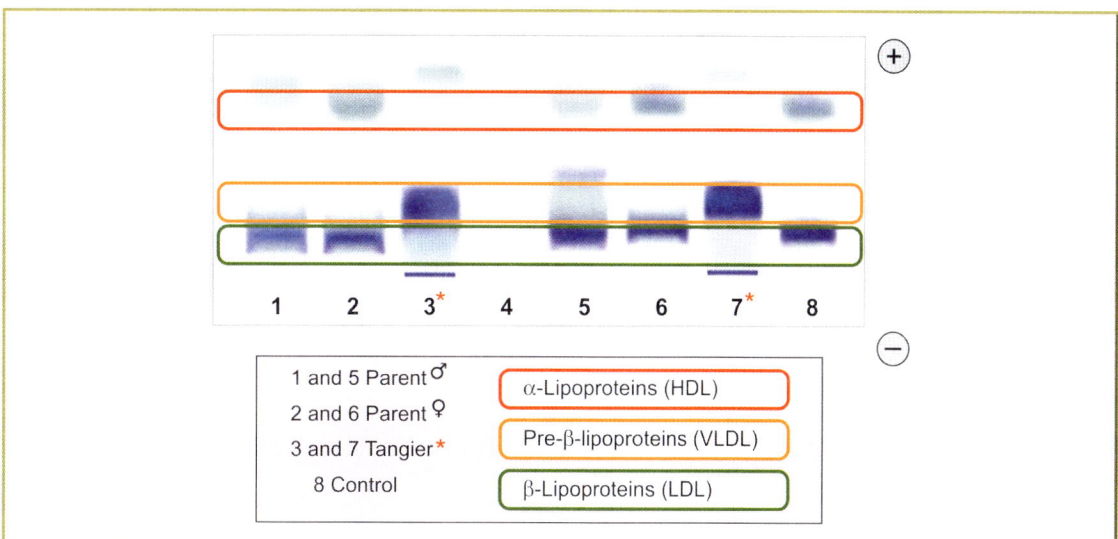

Fig. 12.33: Tangier disease. Two-dimensional lipoprotein electrophoresis: Patient sample (*columns 3 and 7) shows the **absence of α-band (red zone) indicating the absence of HDL**. Columns 1 and 5 show the father's sample; columns 2 and 6 show the mother's sample; and column 8, the control sample. The orange zone shows pre-β-lipoproteins; green zone, β-lipoproteins.

and LDL are low while HDL concentrations are variable. Low levels of apoB are also seen.

- *Tangier disease*: It is the HDL deficiency state (Fig. 12.33) where plasma triacylglycerol and VLDL levels are normal or moderately increased. LDL is rich in triacylglycerols. Total plasma cholesterol and LDL cholesterol are reduced by about two-third while HDL cholesterol is extremely low. ApoA-1 is around 1% of the concentration normally found in plasma and apoA-2 about 5–8% of the normal. Besides apoA-1 and apoA-2, there is also a moderate reduction in all the other apoproteins.

SERUM LIPID PROFILE (LIPIDOGRAM)

Serum lipids and lipoproteins should be measured after 12 hours of fasting to allow complete clearing of chylomicrons. Serum may appear hazy when serum triglycerides exceed 200 mg/dl. Chylomicrons can be easily detected because they form a white supernatant after refrigeration. The following parameters are included under a serum lipid profile or lipidogram:

- **Total cholesterol** (which is a sum of cholesterol distributed in LDL, VLDL and HDL): 150–250 mg/dl (desirable 140–220 mg/dl)
- **LDL-cholesterol**: 60–160 mg/dl
- **VLDL-cholesterol**: <32 mg/dl
- **HDL-cholesterol**: 30–60 mg/dl
- **Triglycerides**: 50–160 mg/dl

Chemistry to Clinics 12.14: Lipoprotein(a)

Lipoprotein(a) [**Lp(a)**] consists of an LDL-like particle and the specific apolipoprotein(a) [apo(a), synthesized by hepatocytes]. The apo(a) gene derives from a duplication of the plasminogen gene. Due to similarity between apo(a) and plasminogen, Lp(a) interferes with tissue plasminogen activator (tPA)-mediated plasminogen activation in fibrinolysis, thereby generating a hypercoagulable state. This predisposes to atherosclerosis and thrombosis.

According to **Friedwald's formula**, VLDL-cholesterol is given by triglycerides/5, provided triglycerides are <400 mg/dl. Thus, LDL-cholesterol can be calculated as follows:

LDL-cholesterol = Total cholesterol – [HDL-cholesterol + Triglycerides/5]

- **Cardiac risk ratio** = Total-cholesterol : HDL-cholesterol. A ratio >5 indicates an increased cardiovascular risk.

Special investigations may be performed in some cases and include plasma troponin, myoglobin, homocysteine, lipoprotein(a) (Chemistry to Clinics 12.14), C-reactive protein, etc.

ROLE OF THE LIVER IN LIPID METABOLISM

Lipids though are mainly stored in the adipose tissue, the liver has a central role in their metabolism:

- Synthesis of fatty acids from acetyl CoA, which is obtained from the oxidation of glucose.

- Synthesis of cholesterol from acetyl CoA.
- Synthesis of various plasma lipoproteins and phospholipids as well as their removal.
- Synthesis of ketone bodies.
- Fatty acid chain elongation and for the removal as well as introduction of a double bond in a fatty acid.
- Synthesis of bile acids from cholesterol.
- β-oxidation of fatty acids.

Abnormal deposition of fat in the liver is called fatty liver (Chemistry to Clinics 12.15).

Chemistry to Clinics 12.15: Fatty Liver and Lipotropic Factors

It refers to accumulation of >5% w/w of fat (triacylglycerol) in the liver. Normally, the input of free fatty acids to the liver from the adipose tissue is matched by its esterification into triacylglycerol, which is minimally retained by the liver and mainly exported as VLDL. However, fatty liver results when the flux of free fatty acids increases with or without a reduction in the capacity of the liver to synthesize lipoproteins. The latter can be due to reduced availability of certain dietary factors called lipotropic factors, which normally help to prevent fatty liver (Fig. 12.34). In some cases, especially in case of alcoholic liver disease, fatty liver progresses to cirrhosis (Fig. 12.35).

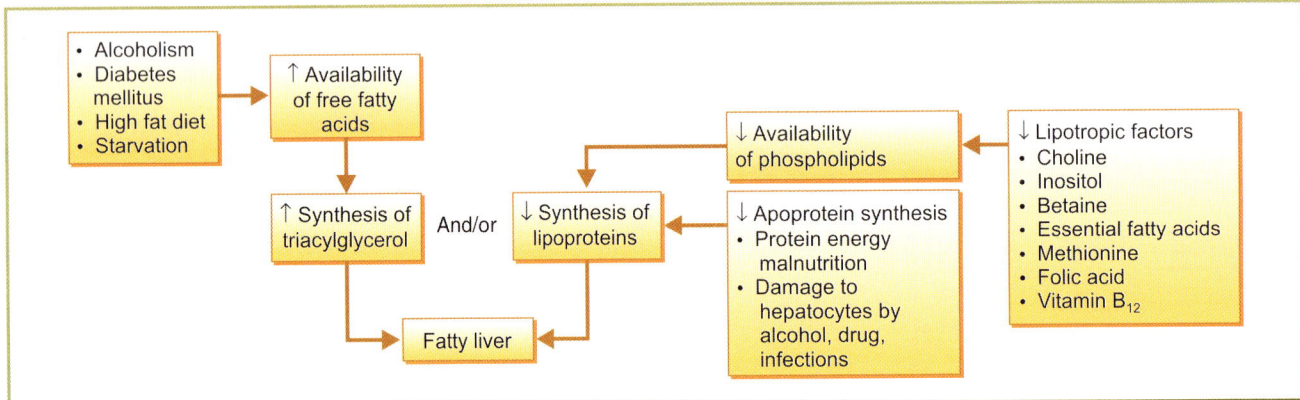

Fig. 12.34: Causes of fatty liver.

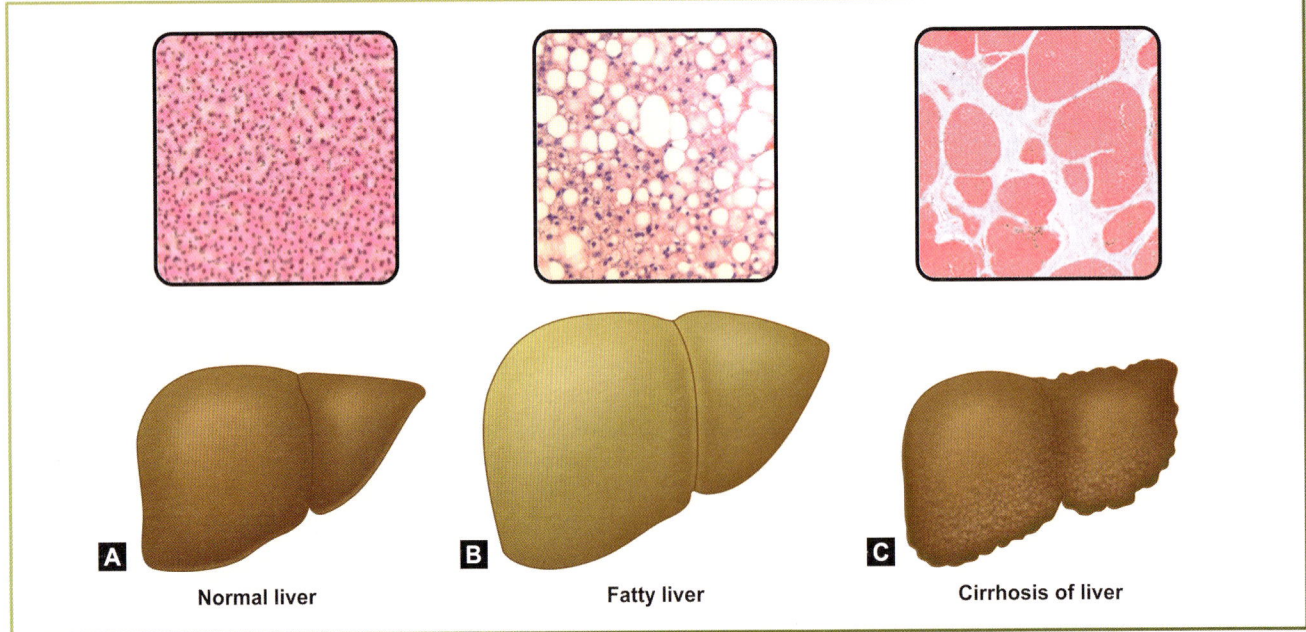

Fig. 12.35: Liver: Gross appearance and histology: A. **Normal liver**. B. **Fatty liver** is enlarged and discolored, with abundant lipid (triacylglycerol >5% w/w) droplets in the cytosol of hepatocytes. C. **Cirrhotic liver** is shrunken and scarred, with loss of hepatocytes and abundant fibrous tissue.

INFLUENCE OF HORMONES ON LIPID METABOLISM

Mobilization of fat from the adipose tissue releases fatty acids which serve as an important source of energy for the body. The key enzyme for lipolysis is the hormone sensitive triacylglyceral lipase which exists in two forms, the active (phosphorylated) form and the inactive (dephosphorylated) form. The two forms of the enzyme are regulated by a protein kinase and a phosphatase which are also stimulated or inhibited by cAMP. The concentration of cAMP is regulated by its own synthesis (from ATP by adenylate cyclase) as well as degradation (by phosphodiesterase). Various hormones are known to mediate the catalytic action of cAMP and thus control lipolysis:

- **Insulin:** It has anti-lipolytic effect and thus inhibits the release of fatty acids from the adipose tissue. It exerts its action by decreasing cAMP concentration either by inhibiting adenylate cyclase or by activating cyclic-3',5'-nucleotide phosphodiesterase. Reduced levels of cAMP inhibit the stimulation of cAMP dependent protein kinase and thus affect hormone sensitive lipase activity. Insulin also increases glucose transport into the adipose tissue. This, in turn, promotes the oxidation of glucose via HMP shunt and leads to increased production of NADPH which is essential for the synthesis of long-chain fatty acids and cholesterol.

  Insulin thus increases the synthesis of triacyl-glycerols in the liver as well as in the adipose tissue. Increased glucose catabolism (under the influence of insulin) also yields acetyl CoA and dihydroxy-acetone phosphate both of which further promote lipogenesis.

- **Other hormones:** Catecholamines, glucagon, growth hormone, ACTH, MSH, TSH and glucocorticoids promote lipolysis and thereby accelerate the release of free fatty acids from the adipose tissue. This, in turn, leads to ketogenesis and increases cholesterol biosynthesis. Administration of thyroid hormones reduces plasma lipoproteins, cholesterol and phospholipids but in insulin deficiency thyroid hormones increase release of fatty acids from the adipose tissue and promote ketogenesis.

SOME IMPORTANT QUESTIONS

1. Outline β-oxidation of fatty acids. How much energy is produced when one molecule of palmitic acid is completely metabolized to acetyl CoA?

2. Outline *de novo* synthesis of fatty acids. What is the source of reducing equivalents? How does *de novo* fatty acid synthesis differs from microsomal and mitochondrial fatty acid synthesis?

3. Describe briefly:
   i. Role of carnitine in fatty acid metabolism
   ii. Functions and fates of cholesterol
   iii. Regulation of cholesterol biosynthesis
   iv. Oxidation of fatty acids with odd number of carbon atoms

4. Write notes on:
   i. Ketone bodies
   ii. PUFA
   iii. ω-Oxidation
   iv. Sphingolipid storage diseases
   v. Atherosclerosis

5. What are triacylglycerols? How triacylglycerols are synthesized in the adipose tissue?

6. Write notes on:

i. Lipuria
ii. Digestion and absorption of dietary lipids
iii. Steatorrhea
iv. Chyluria
v. Sudden infant death syndrome
vi. Carnitine deficiency disorders
vii. α-Oxidation of a fatty acid
viii. Refsum's disease
ix. Lipofuscin
x. Metabolic fates of acetyl CoA

7. Write notes on:

i. Obesity
ii. Catabolism of triacylglycerols
iii. Hormone sensitive lipase
iv. Lipoproteins
v. Bile acids
vi. LCAT
vii. Diabetic ketoacidosis
viii. Lung surfactant
ix. Tay-Sach's disease
x. Gaucher's disease

8. Discuss:

i. Hyperlipoproteinemias
ii. Tangier disease
iii. Role of liver in lipid metabolism
iv. Abetalipoproteinemia
v. Fatty liver and lipotropic factors

MULTIPLE CHOICE QUESTIONS

1. **The commonest deficiency in Reye's syndrome is of:**
   A. Short-chain acyl CoA dehydrogenase
   B. Medium chain acyl CoA dehydrogenase
   C. Long-chain acyl CoA dehydrogenase
   D. None of the above

2. **Hormone sensitive lipase is stimulated by the following *except*:**
   A. ACTH
   B. Insulin
   C. Glucagon
   D. Epinephrine

3. **Increased circulating free fatty acids are observed in:**
   A. Diabetic ketoacidosis
   B. Starvation
   C. High-fat low-carbohydrate diet
   D. All of the above

4. **The following cannot use ketone bodies as a source of energy:**
   A. Liver
   B. Kidneys
   C. Muscles
   D. Brain

5. **The enzyme deficient in Gaucher's disease is:**
   A. Sphingomyelinase
   B. Galactocerebrosidase
   C. Glucocerebrosidase
   D. α-Galactosidase

6. **Very low density lipoproteins (VLDL) transport triacylglycerol from:**
   A. Liver to small intestine only
   B. Small intestine to liver
   C. Small intestine to extrahepatic tissues
   D. Liver to extrahepatic tissues

7. **The major lipid in chylomicrons is:**
   A. Dietary triglycerides
   B. Hepatic triglycerides
   C. Cholesterol
   D. Cholesterol esters

8. **The following is not a risk factor for atherosclerosis:**
   A. Increased plasma homocysteine
   B. Increased plasma lipoprotein(a)
   C. Increased plasma LDL-cholesterol
   D. Increased plasma HDL-cholesterol

9. **Tangier's disease is characterized by deficiency of circulating:**
   A. LDL
   B. VLDL
   C. Chylomicrons
   D. HDL

10. **Fatty liver may occur in:**
   A. Kwashiorkor
   B. Chronic alcoholism
   C. Diabetes mellitus
   D. All of the above

Metabolism of Proteins and Amino Acids

The digestion and absorption of dietary proteins was discussed in Chapter 9.

DEGRADATION OF MUSCLE PROTEIN

Protein degradation though occurs throughout the body but **muscle is the greatest source of free amino acids** in conditions such as starvation, trauma, burns and septicemia.

- Branched chain amino acids (Val, Leu and Ile) are released and used as the important source of fuel.
- Other amino acids undergo the process of transamination whereby their amino group is transferred to form alanine and glutamine. These amino acids are then transported to the liver and the kidney for the production of urea (from amino group of the amino acids) in the liver and ammonia (from glutamine) in the kidney, respectively. After the transfer of the amino group, their carbon skeletons are used either for energy or transported to the liver for gluconeogenesis (Fig. 13.1).

DEGRADATION OF AMINO ACIDS

Amino acids obtained from the diet or those synthesized in the body via transamination, undergo deamination to release ammonia and the carbon-skeleton of amino acids. Deamination may be oxidative or non-oxidative. Ammonia being a toxic molecule is detoxified and eliminated as urea whereas the carbon-skeletons, via amphibolic intermediates, form glucose and/or lipids (Fig. 13.2).

Transamination of alanine, glutamate and valine forms pyruvate, α-ketoglutarate and succinyl CoA,

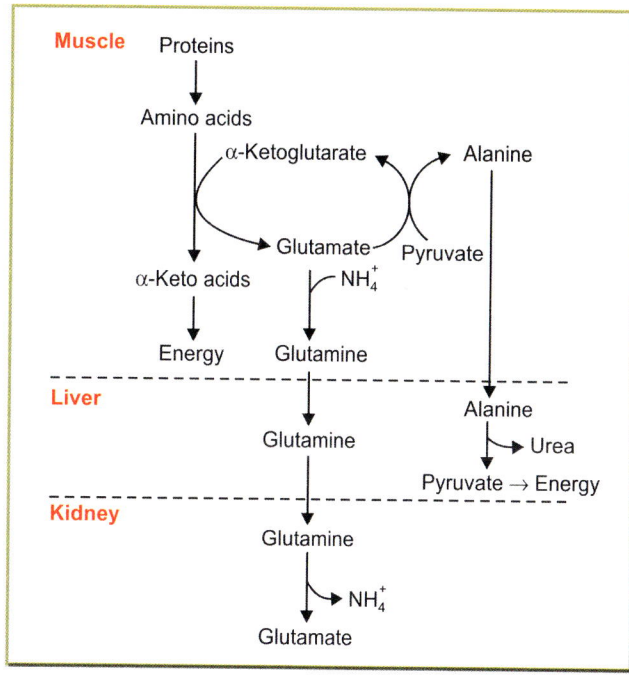

Fig. 13.1: Metabolic fate of muscle proteins.

respectively. These are the intermediates of the citric acid cycle and can be converted to glucose by the process of gluconeogenesis. Such amino acids are called **glycogenic or glucogenic** amino acids.

In addition to an intermediate of the Krebs cycle, catabolism of some of the amino acids, like phenylalanine, also form acetyl CoA or acetoacetyl CoA which are the precursors of ketone bodies. These amino acids are therefore, **both glycogenic as well as ketogenic**.

13

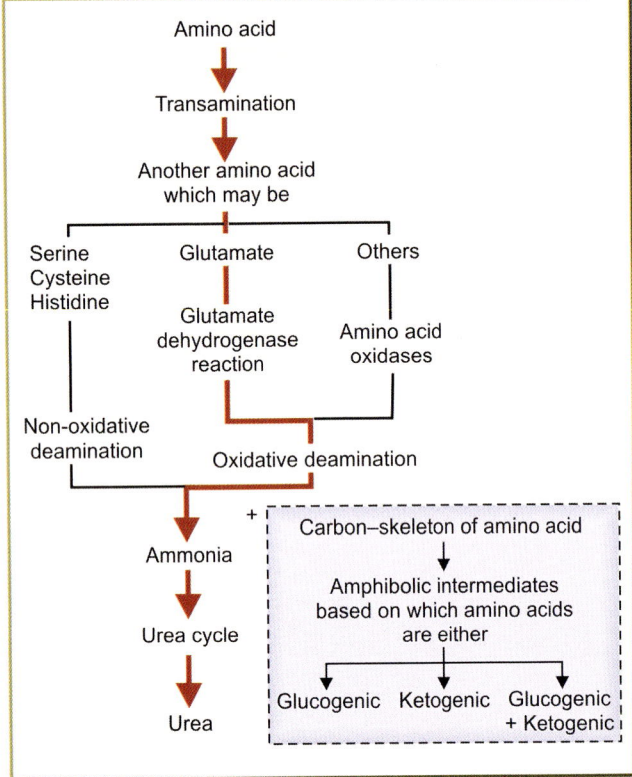

Fig. 13.2: Overview of amino acid metabolism. The scheme outside the dotted box indicates the overall flow of nitrogen and the major route is shown in bold lines.

Table 13.1: Classification of amino acids based on their catabolic fate

Amino acid	End product of catabolism
Glucogenic	
• Gly, Ala, Ser, Cys, Pro-OH	Pyruvate
• Glu, Gln, Pro, Arg, His	α-Ketoglutarate
• Val, Met	Succinyl CoA
• Asp, Asn	Oxaloacetate
Glucogenic and Ketogenic	
• Ile	Succinyl CoA and Acetyl CoA
• Phe, Tyr	Fumarate and Acetoacetyl CoA
• Trp	Pyruvate and Acetoacetyl CoA
• Thr	Pyruvate and Acetyl CoA
Ketogenic	
• Leu	Acetyl CoA and Acetoacetyl CoA
• Lys	Acetoacetyl CoA

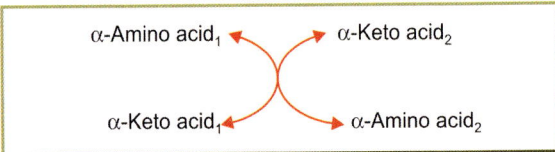

Fig. 13.3: The process of transamination of an amino acid.

Leucine is the amino acid whose catabolic end products are acetyl CoA and acetoacetyl CoA. Similarly, lysine is also a ketogenic amino acid, as the end product of its catabolism is acetoacetyl CoA. Hence, both leucine and lysine are **ketogenic** amino acids.

End products of catabolism of different amino acids as well as their metabolic fates are given in Table 13.1.

REMOVAL OF AMINO GROUP

Although it may occur in several tissues, liver is the major site for the removal of the α-amino group from an amino acid. There are two major routes for the removal of α-amino group, i.e. **transamination** and **deamination**.

Transamination

• Transamination is a process of transfer of the α-amino group from an amino acid to a keto acid, forming **a new amino acid and a keto acid**

(Fig. 13.3). Enzymes which catalyze this reversible set of reactions are called **transaminases or aminotransferases**.

• It is the **commonest reaction** involving free amino acids. **Threonine** and **lysine** (and **proline**, an imino acid), however, **do not participate** in this reaction.

• An obligate amino acid and α-keto acid pair in all these reactions is that of glutamate and α-ketoglutarate. Although liver contains several transaminases (except for threonine, lysine and proline), most important of these are glutamate pyruvate transaminase (**GPT**) also called alanine aminotransferase (**ALT**), and glutamate oxaloacetate transaminase (**GOT**) which is also known as aspartate aminotransferase (**AST**).

• Transaminases require **vitamin B$_6$ (pyridoxal-5-phosphate)** as a **coenzyme** (Fig. 13.4). An amino acid first reacts with the coenzyme pyridoxal-5-phosphate (PLP) and forms a Schiff base. The coenzyme is protonated and is subsequently hydrolyzed to release α-keto acid of the corresponding amino acid while retaining the α-amino group (–NH$_2$). The coenzyme thus gets aminated and is converted to pyridoxamine-5-phosphate.

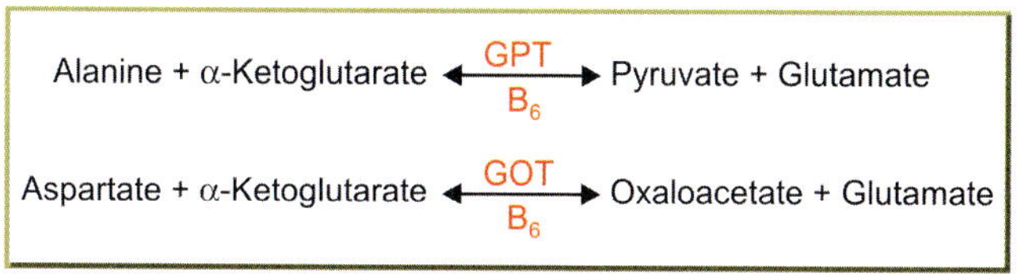

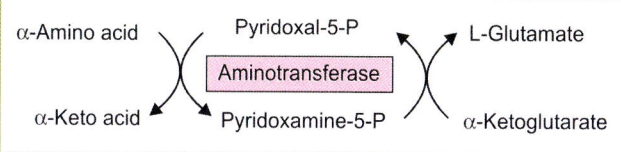

Fig. 13.4: Reactions catalyzed by two important transaminases, GPT (ALT) and GOT (AST).

α-Amino acid   Pyridoxal-5-P   L-Glutamate

Aminotransferase

α-Keto acid   Pyridoxamine-5-P   α-Ketoglutarate

Fig. 13.5: Role of pyridoxal-5-phosphate in transamination.

Thereafter, another α-keto acid (generally α-ketoglutarate) combines with the coenzyme bound amino group. This, in turn, releases the amino acid (mostly as glutamate) and regenerates the coenzyme (Fig. 13.5).

- **Importance**
  1. **Nonessential amino acids can be synthesized** from α-keto acid precursors via transfer of an amino group from another amino acid by various transaminases.
  2. Transamination followed by oxidative deamination (= **transdeamination**) ultimately releases the amino acid nitrogen as ammonia, to be detoxified in the urea cycle.
  3. Transaminases have clinical importance (Chemistry to Clinics 13.1).

Chemistry to Clinics 13.1: Diagnostic Significance of Transaminases

Both the enzymes, i.e. GOT and GPT are of diagnostic significance. They are present in large amounts in the cardiac muscle and the liver, respectively. Although serum levels of both the enzymes are raised in heart as well as liver diseases, serum levels of GOT (**SGOT** levels) are markedly raised in myocardial infarction while **SGPT** levels are more increased in liver disorders, such as in viral hepatitis and toxic liver necrosis (Table 13.2).

Table 13.2: Diagnostic significance of transaminases

Enzyme	Increased serum levels in
SGOT (AST)	Cardiac disorders, e.g. myocardial infarction
SGPT (ALT)	Liver disorders, e.g. viral hepatitis

Deamination

Since transamination involves only the transfer of α-amino group from an amino acid to α-keto acid and as such there is no net loss of the amino group, deamination is the actual process resulting in the removal of the α-amino group from an amino acid which is released in the form of ammonia. Though the process of deamination takes place in several tissues, the **liver** and the **kidney** are the main organs responsible for deamination of amino acids.

Deamination may take place as a result of removal of electrons which requires oxygen (**oxidative deamination**) or without the transfer of electrons (**non-oxidative deamination**).

Oxidative Deamination

The liver and the kidney contain several enzymes which catalyze deamination of amino acids, such as L-amino acid oxidases, D-amino acid oxidases and glutamate dehydrogenase, etc.

- **Amino acid oxidases**
  - **L-amino acid oxidases** catalyze oxidation of L-amino acids. An α-keto acid and ammonia are released as the final products. The enzyme has FMN as a prosthetic group (Fig. 13.6).
  - Tissues also contain FAD-linked **D-amino acid oxidase** which catalyzes the oxidation of D-amino acids, derived from the intestinal bacteria, and of glycine (Fig. 13.7).
- **Glutamate dehydrogenase:** Glutamate mostly acts as a common intermediate between free ammonia and amino group of majority of the amino acids. Glutamate is produced via α-ketoglutarate by

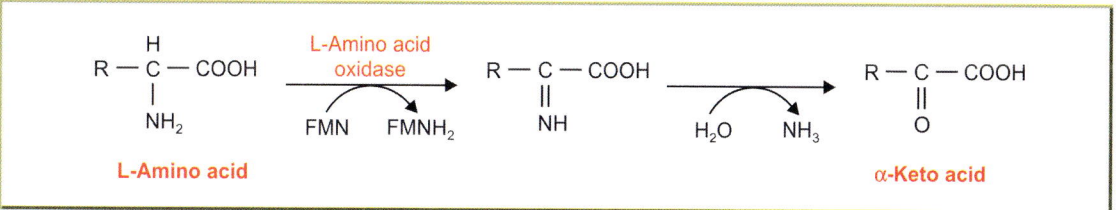

Fig. 13.6: Reaction catalyzed by L-amino acid oxidase.

13

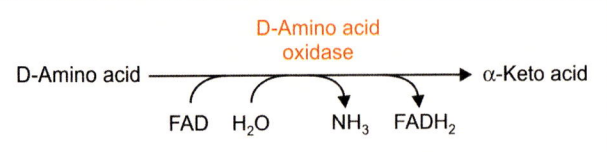

Fig. 13.7: Reaction catalyzed by D-amino acid oxidase.

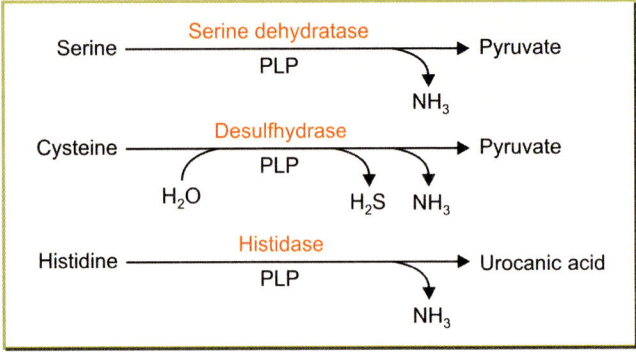

Fig. 13.9: Non-oxidative deamination of amino acids.

incorporating ammonia, as the amino group of nitrogen by the enzyme glutamate dehydrogenase. At the same time, this enzyme is also important in the production of ammonia from amino acids when these are catabolized for energy or are used as substrate for gluconeogenesis.

Glutamate dehydrogenase thus catalyzes a reversible set of reactions where NADPH is used as a coenzyme in the synthetic reaction while NAD^+ is used in the liberation of ammonia, in the degradative reaction.

Glutamate dehydrogenase is allosterically regulated by purine nucleotides. Its activity is increased by ADP and GDP in the direction of glutamate degradation when there is a need for the oxidation of amino acids for energy. On the other hand, ATP and GTP are allosteric activators in the direction of glutamate synthesis (Fig. 13.8).

Non-oxidative Deamination

Deamination of some of the amino acids such as **serine, cysteine and histidine** is catalyzed by dehydratase, desulfhydrase and histidase, respectively. These enzymes require pyridoxal-5-phosphate as a coenzyme and cause dehydration of the amino acid, spontaneously, followed by (non-oxidative) deamination ultimately resulting in the removal of NH_3 (Fig. 13.9).

Detoxification and Disposal of Ammonia

Ammonia, a highly toxic molecule, is detoxified and disposed by two processes:

First line of defense: Ammonia, a highly toxic molecule, is trapped by glutamate to form glutamine, especially in the brain. This is catalyzed by **glutamine synthetase** (Fig. 13.10). Further, glutamine is an important form for the transport of ammonia to the kidney where glutaminase hydrolyzes amide group of glutamine to glutamic acid and ammonia. The amide group of glutamine is also important as a nitrogen donor for purine bases, amino group of cytosine and amide group of asparagine.

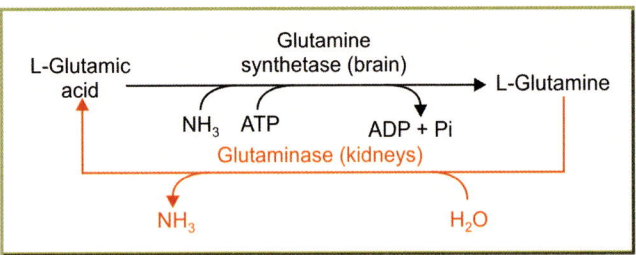

Fig. 13.10: Formation and disposal of glutamine.

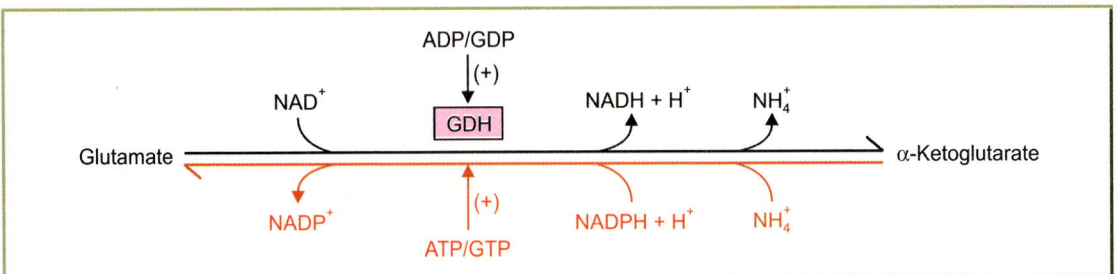

Fig. 13.8: Glutamate dehydrogenase (GDH) reaction.

Second line of defense: The **urea cycle** is a process by which ammonia is converted to urea, a less toxic and a soluble excretory waste product, in the liver as follows (Fig. 13.11):

Urea Cycle

1. In the first step, ammonia is activated by ATP and combines with carbon dioxide to from carbamoyl phosphate, in the mitochondria. The reaction is catalyzed by carbamoyl phosphate synthetase-I (CPS-I) and requires N-acetyl glutamate as a coenzyme.

Carbamoyl phosphate synthetases: There are two different enzymes called carbamoyl phosphate synthetase I (CPS-I) and II (CPS-II). The enzyme **CPS-I** is present in the mitochondria. It utilizes NH_3, and is absolutely dependent on N-acetyl glutamate for its activity. The enzyme produces carbamoyl phosphate for its entry into the urea cycle. On the other hand, **CPS-II** is found in the cytosol. It forms carbamoyl phosphate, by utilizing the amide group of glutamine (Fig. 13.12). Its activity is not affected by N-acetyl glutamate. The product carbamoyl phosphate so formed is used for the synthesis of pyrimidines.

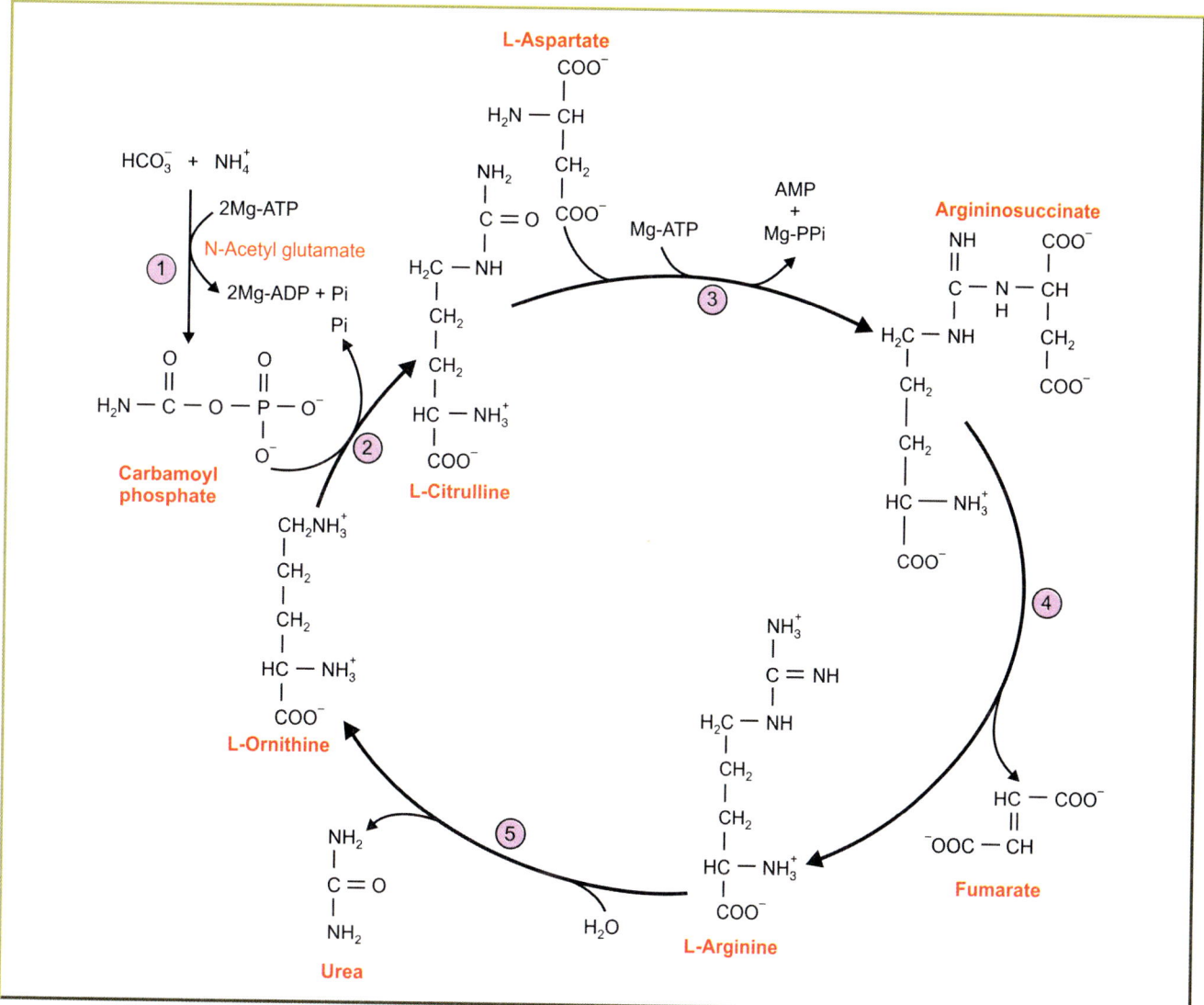

Fig. 13.11: Urea cycle. 1. Carbamoyl phosphate synthetase I (CPS-I), 2. Ornithine transcarbamoylase, 3. Argininosuccinate synthetase, 4. Argininosuccinase, 5. Arginase.

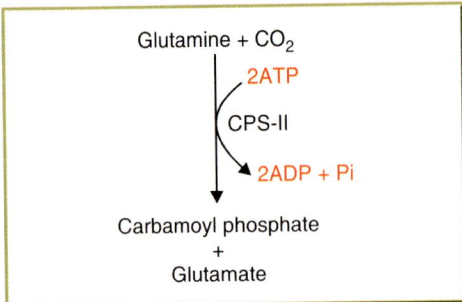

Fig. 13.12: Reaction catalyzed by CPS-II.

2. Ornithine transcarbamoylase transfers the carbamoyl group from carbamoyl phosphate to ornithine and produces citrulline, in the mitochondrial matrix. Citrulline is transported from the mitochondria to the cytosol where other reactions of the urea cycle occur.

3. In the presence of argininosuccinic acid synthetase and ATP, citrulline combines with L-aspartate and forms argininosuccinic acid (argininosuccinate).

4. Subsequently, argininosuccinase hydrolyzes argininosuccinic acid to liberate arginine and fumaric acid. Carbons from aspartate are released as fumarate and enter the mitochondria where it is metabolized to oxaloacetate, by the tricarboxylic acid cycle. Hence, urea cycle is coupled with the Krebs cycle, as **Krebs bicycle**, both of which were discovered by Krebs and coworkers.

5. In the last step, arginine is hydrolyzed by arginase to regenerate ornithine and forms urea.
   Ornithine is transported to the mitochondria and re-enters the cycle.

Importance of Urea Cycle

1. Urea cycle is the mechanism for **nitrogen excretion** in humans and other primates. The two nitrogen atoms in each urea molecule are derived from two different sources, i.e. one from free NH_3 and the other from the amino group of aspartate. As human beings cannot metabolize urea, it is transported to the kidney for filtration and excretion.

2. A small amount of urea may enter the **small intestine** where it is cleaved by bacteria. The NH_3 so formed is diffused into the circulation and used by the liver.

3. It is linked with Krebs cycle (**Krebs bicycle**, discussed above).

4. Synthesis of **arginine**, a semiessential amino acid.

5. Disorders of urea cycle result in hyperammonemias (discussed below).

Regulation of Urea Synthesis

- Carbamoyl phosphate synthetase is absolutely dependent on N-acetyl glutamate which acts as an allosteric activator for the enzyme. N-acetylglutamate is synthesized when acetyl CoA combines with glutamate. The reaction is catalyzed by N-acetylglutamate synthase and requires arginine.
- Induction of the urea cycle enzymes occurs when delivery of ammonia or amino acids to the liver increases. Thus, a high protein diet or starvation results in the induction of the enzymes of urea cycle.
- Compartmentalization of the cycle between the mitochondria and the cytosol.
- Presence of an ornithine-citrulline antiporter in the mitochondrial membrane ensures adequate exchange of the two compounds.

Metabolic Disorders of Urea Synthesis

As urea cycle is the major pathway for the elimination of **ammonia** from the body, which is a very **toxic** substance, metabolic disorders that may arise from abnormal function of the enzymes of urea synthesis are therefore potentially fatal and may cause coma when ammonia concentration becomes very high (Chemistry to Clinics 13.2). Inborn errors of all the enzymes of urea cycle have been reported and are shown in Table 13.3.

METABOLISM OF INDIVIDUAL AMINO ACIDS

As mentioned above, catabolism of various amino acids form the end products which are either

Chemistry to Clinics 13.2: Hyperammonemias and Ammonia Toxicity

Increased NH_3 in the brain is toxic for two reasons:
- First, the glutamate dehydrogenase reaction (Fig. 13.8) is favored in the direction of glutamate synthesis thereby depleting α-ketoglutarate, an intermediate of Krebs cycle. This results in slowing of the Krebs cycle and reduced ATP synthesis. Lack of ATP not only compromises neuronal functions but also slows the glutamine synthetase reaction (Fig. 13.10) that converts glutamate to glutamine by trapping NH_3.
- Second, increased glutamate synthesis promotes the synthesis of γ-aminobutyric acid (GABA), an inhibitory neurotransmitter that can cause CNS depression. It should be noted that a similar clinical picture is observed in acquired liver diseases where the liver fails to detoxify ammonia, e.g. liver cirrhosis.

Table 13.3: Inborn errors of urea cycle

Deficient enzyme	Metabolic disorder
Carbamoyl phosphate synthetase	Hyperammonemia type I
Ornithine transcarbamoylase	Hyperammonemia type II
Argininosuccinic acid synthetase	Citrullinemia
Argininosuccinase	Argininosuccinic aciduria
Arginase	Hyperargininemia

Table 13.4: Various products formed from some of the amino acids

Amino acid	Products formed
Glycine	Serine, purines, heme, bile acids, glutathione, creatine
Glutamic acid	Glutamine, ornithine, proline, γ-aminobutyric acid, folic acid, glutathione, N-acetyl glutamate
Phenylalanine and tyrosine	Catecholamines (dopamine, norepinephrine epinephrine), thyroxine, melanin, tyramine
Tryptophan	NAD^+, serotonin, melatonin, kynuramine
Arginine	Nitric oxide

glucogenic or ketogenic, or both. Besides, some of the amino acids are also used in the biosynthesis of several specialized products (Table 13.4).

GLYCINE

Glycine is the **simplest** amino acid found in proteins. It is a nonessential amino acid and is glucogenic in nature. Metabolic fates of glycine are:

1. Glycine, by a glycine cleavage complex, is degraded to CO_2 and ammonia (Fig. 13.13) (Chemistry to Clinics 13.3).
2. Glycine is also oxidatively deaminated by glycine oxidase to glyoxylate, which can be transaminated

Chemistry to Clinics 13.3: Hyperglycinemia

Deficiency of glycine cleavage complex results in nonketotic hyperglycinemia which is characterized by severe mental retardation. Neurological complications of the disease are due to hyperglycinemia since glycine is a major inhibitory neurotransmitter. Many patients do not survive infancy.

Chemistry to Clinics 13.4: Primary Hyperoxaluria

Excessive production of oxalate due to glycine transaminase deficiency results in primary hyperoxaluria. Oxalate forms calcium oxalate, high urinary excretion of which may lead to **renal calculi** (Fig. 13.15).

back to glycine or oxidized to oxalate (Fig. 13.14) (Chemistry to Clinics 13.4).

Besides, glycine performs most of the biochemical functions assigned to any amino acid.

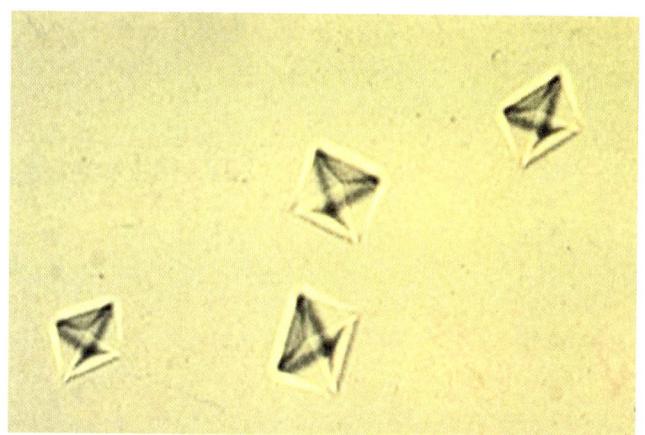

Fig. 13.15: Calcium oxalate crystals: Square shape with a characteristic 'X' mark. Calcium oxalate stones are the **most prevalent** renal stones.

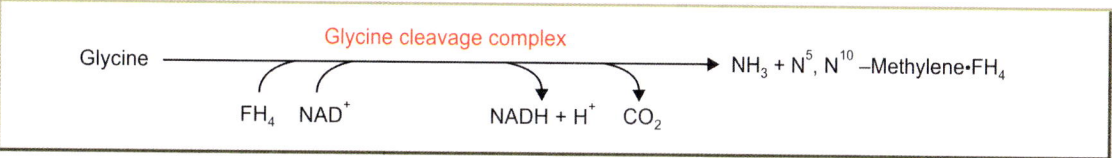

Fig. 13.13: Degradation of glycine.

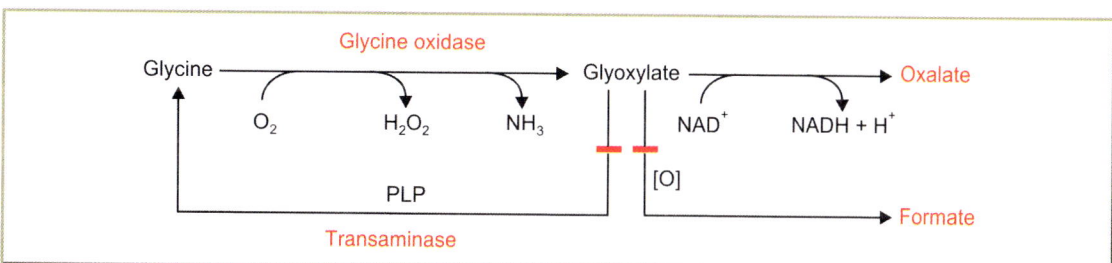

Fig. 13.14: Oxidation of glycine to oxalate. Sites of block (—) which can lead to primary hyperoxaluria and renal **oxalate stones**.

13

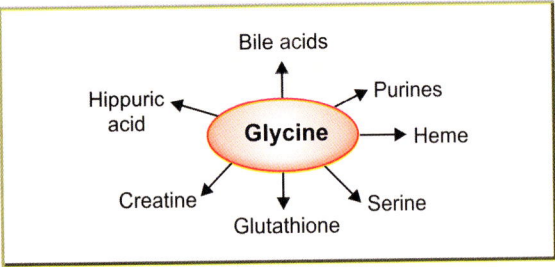

Fig. 13.16: Metabolic fates of glycine.

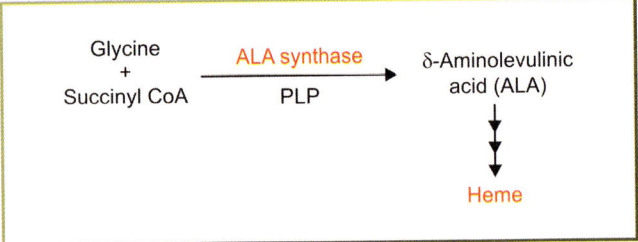

Fig. 13.19: First reaction in heme synthesis requires glycine.

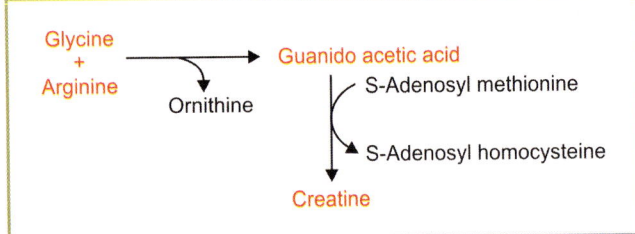

Fig. 13.20: First reaction in creatine synthesis requires glycine.

Glycine is a precursor for various compounds (Fig. 13.16).

1. Formation of **serine** from glycine is a reversible reaction catalyzed by serine hydroxymethyl-transferase, which requires pyridoxal-5-phosphate and N^5, N^{10}-methylene-tetrahydrofolate (N^5, N^{10}-methylene·FH_4) (Fig. 13.17). The demand for glycine or serine and the availability of N^5, N^{10}-methylene·FH_4 determine the direction of this reaction.

2. Glycine is an important contributor in the bio-synthesis of a **purine ring**. It contributes its nitrogen and both the carbons as N7, C4 and C5 in a purine ring (Fig. 13.18).

3. Glycine with succinyl CoA synthesizes δ-amino-levulinic acid, a precursor of **heme**. This reaction is catalyzed by aminolevulinic acid (ALA) synthase (Fig. 13.19).

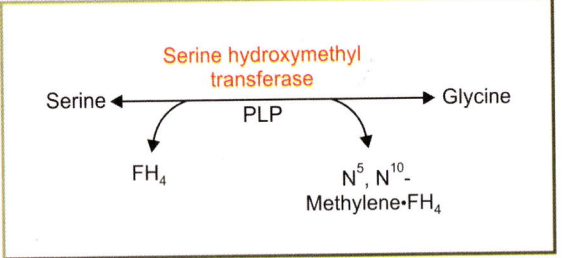

Fig. 13.17: Interconversion of glycine and serine.

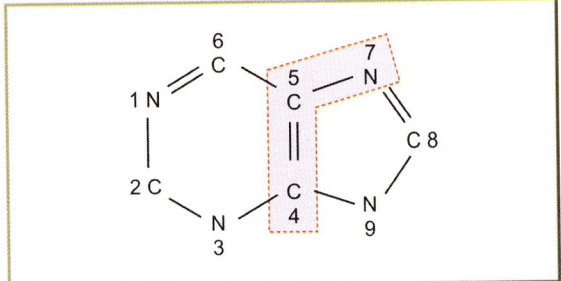

Fig. 13.18: Incorporation of glycine in a purine ring.

4. Glycine also contributes in the biosynthesis of **creatine**, a reservoir of energy in the muscle (Fig. 13.20). Creatine is stored in the muscle as creatine phosphate. After the phosphorylation of ADP by the high energy phosphate of creatine phosphate, the latter is converted to a waste product, creatinine.

5. Glycine is also a constituent of the tripeptide **glutathione**.

6. With cholic acid, glycine is used for the synthesis of **glycocholic acid** (a **bile acid**).

7. Glycine is also used in the **detoxification of benzoic acid,** which is excreted in the urine as hippuric acid.

ALANINE

Alanine (L-α-alanine) together with glycine makes up a considerable fraction of the amino acid nitrogen in human plasma. It is a nonessential amino acid and can be synthesized in the body by transamination of pyruvate with glutamate. The only known functions for alanine are its incorporation into protein and that it acts as a donor of the α-amino group for parti-cipation in a transamination reaction.

Reversible transamination of alanine yields pyru-vate, which is converted to glucose by the process of gluconeogenesis. Hence, alanine is a glucogenic amino acid.

L-Alanine is a main source for the removal of ammonia from the muscle and other peripheral tissues to the liver. This physiological process uses pyruvate, which is formed in the muscle during glycolysis. Pyruvate accepts ammonia by transamination from other amino acids and is converted to alanine which is transported to the liver via blood. In the liver, by reversible transamination, alanine is converted back to pyruvate and ammonia is removed. Ammonia is used in the synthesis of urea while pyruvate participates in gluconeogenesis and is converted to glucose which re-enters muscle and other tissues by circulation. Pyruvate and alanine thus constitute a shuttle mechanism for the transport of ammonia and its excretion as urea by the process known as **glucose-alanine cycle** (*see* Fig. 11.12).

Though L-alanine is mainly found in the body, small amount of D-alanine may also be found as a constituent of the bacterial cell wall.

Besides α-alanine, β-alanine is also present in mammalian tissues, which is formed from the catabolism of uracil. It is an important constituent of pantothenic acid as well as the dipeptides carnosine and anserine, found in the muscle.

SERINE

Serine is a hydroxyl group containing amino acid. It is a nonessential amino acid and is readily synthesized *de novo*.

Chemistry to Clinics 13.5: Serine Deficiency Syndrome

It has been reported in infants and may result from a deficiency of 3-phosphoglycerate dehydrogenase or phosphoserine phosphatase. Serine deficiency leads to partial glycine deficiency, which may explain the neurological manifestations since glycine (and possibly serine also) is an inhibitory neurotransmitter.

Synthesis of serine starts with 3-phosphoglycerate, which is obtained from the glycolytic pathway:

- 3-Phosphoglycerate undergoes oxidation, and is converted to 3-phosphopyruvate. The reaction is catalyzed by phosphoglycerate dehydrogenase and requires NAD^+.
- An aminotransferase transfers an amino group from glutamate and converts 3-phosphopyruvate to 3-phosphoserine, which is ultimately converted to serine by a phosphatase (Fig. 13.21) (Chemistry to Clinics 13.5).

Metabolic Fates of Serine

Serine has several metabolic fates and acts as a precursor of various compounds in the body (Fig. 13.22):

1. Serine, as discussed above, is converted reversibly to **glycine** in a reaction catalyzed by serine hydroxymethyltransferase that requires pyridoxal phosphate and tetrahydrofolate (FH_4). As shown in Fig. 13.17, tetrahydrofolate, in turn, is converted to N^5, N^{10}-methylene tetrahydrofolate (N^5, N^{10}-methylene·FH_4).

2. Serine is degraded to 3-phosphoglycerate, which can enter **glycolysis**. By an aminotransferase, serine is first converted to 3-hydroxypyruvate, which is then reduced to D-glycerate by D-glycerate dehydrogenase. Thereafter, a phosphate group is added and glycerate is converted to 3-phos-

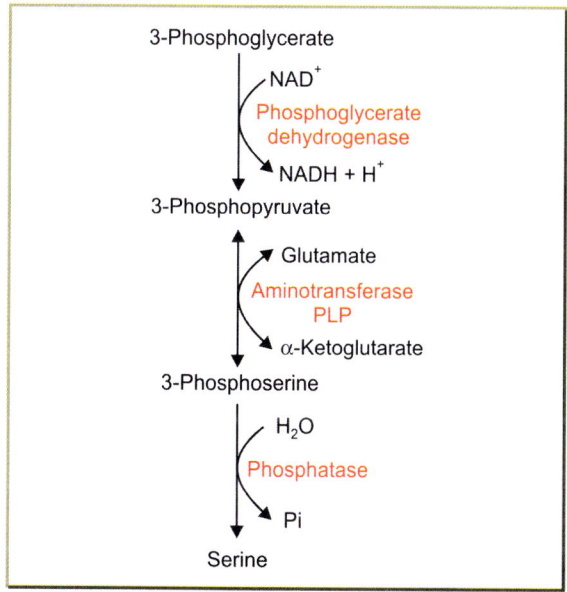

Fig. 13.21: Synthesis of serine.

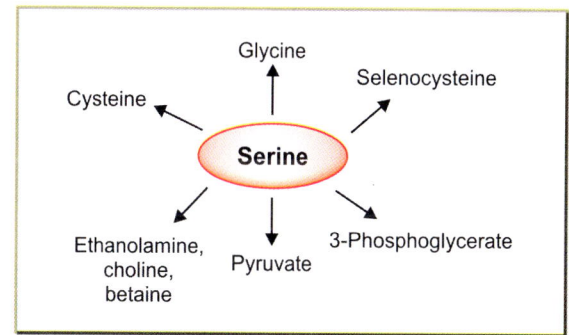

Fig. 13.22: Metabolic fates of serine.

13

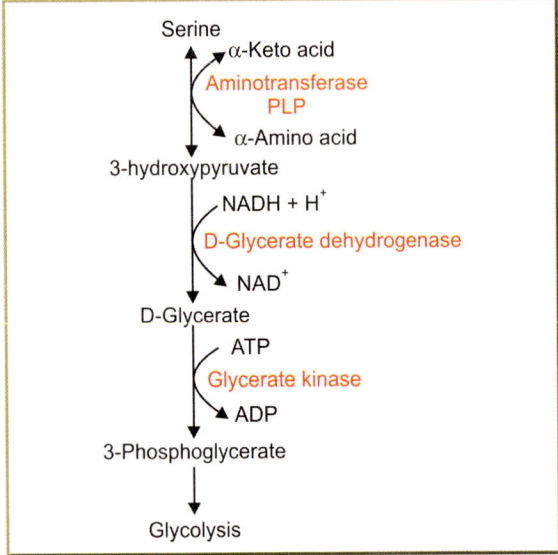

Fig. 13.23: Conversion of serine to 3-phosphoglycerate.

phoglycerate. This reaction is catalyzed by glycerate kinase and requires ATP (Fig. 13.23).

3. With the loss of the amino group, as ammonia, serine can form **pyruvate** by the process of

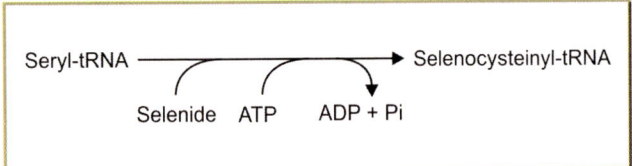

Fig. 13.24: Role of serine in the formation of selenocysteinyl-tRNA.

non-oxidative deamination. This reaction is catalyzed by serine dehydratase (Fig. 13.9).

4. Serine is a precursor of an unusual amino acid called **selenocysteine** (SeC) (Fig. 13.24). During translation, serine-tRNA complex (seryl-tRNA) is changed to selenocysteinyl-tRNA and thus incorporates selenocysteine in a growing polypeptide chain in certain proteins such as glutathione peroxidase.

5. Serine is a precursor for **ethanolamine**, **choline** and **betaine**. Ethanolamine and choline are components of phospholipids while betaine is a methyl donor.

6. Serine is also a precursor of **cysteine**. Serine accepts a sulfhydryl group from homocysteine and is converted to cysteine via cystathionine (Fig. 13.25).

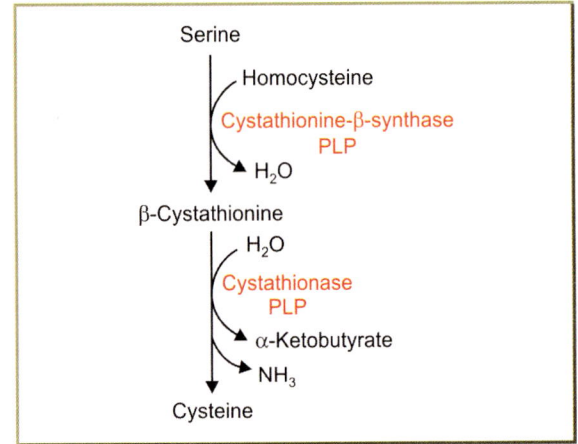

Fig. 13.25: Synthesis of cysteine from serine.

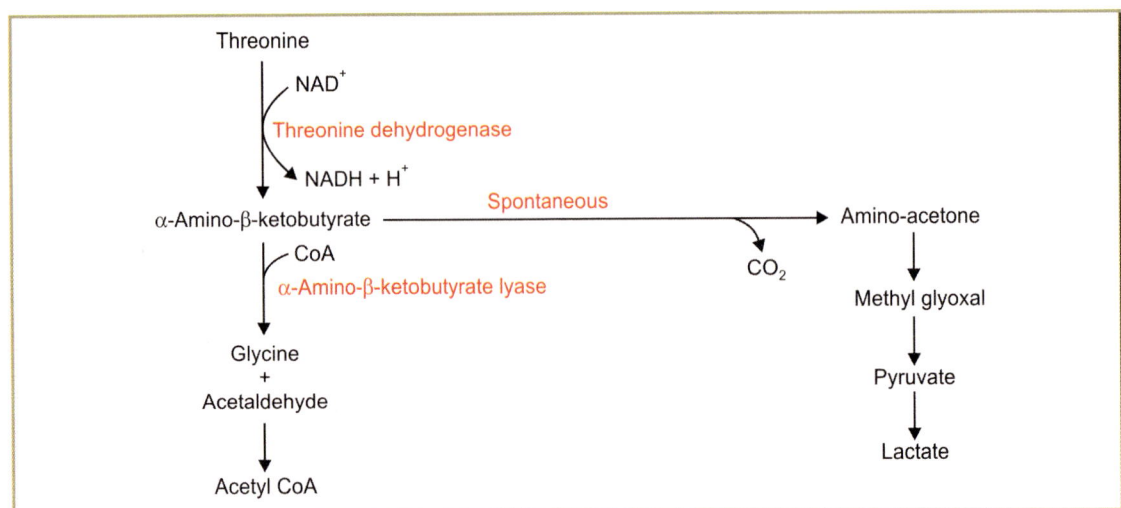

Fig. 13.26: Degradation of threonine.

THREONINE

Threonine, an essential amino acid, is both glucogenic and ketogenic since it generates both pyruvate as well as acetyl CoA:

1. Threonine is degraded through threonine dehydrogenase, producing α-amino-β-ketobutyrate. The latter undergoes thiolysis with CoA by α-amino-β-ketobutyrate lyase to form glycine and acetyl CoA. Glycine can be converted to serine and the α-carbon atom of threonine thus can contribute to one carbon pool (Fig. 13.26). α-Amino-β-ketobutyrate can also be converted to lactate via pyruvate.

2. Threonine can also be converted to α-ketobutyrate. The reaction is catalyzed by threonine dehydratase. α-Ketobutyrate can be subsequently converted to propionyl CoA by α-keto acid dehydrogenase (Fig. 13.27).

ACIDIC AMINO ACIDS AND THEIR AMIDES

Aspartic acid and glutamic acid are the two dicarboxylic monoamino acids called acidic amino acids. Both are nonessential and form key amino acids for the transamination of various keto acids. These amino acids can be readily synthesized from and converted to glucose via oxaloacetate and α-ketoglutarate by transamination or oxidative deamination.

The corresponding amides of these two acidic amino acids are called asparagine and glutamine respectively. They can be interconverted to aspartate and glutamate, reversibly.

GLUTAMIC ACID

Glutamic acid is one of the nonessential amino acids. By the reversible reaction catalyzed by glutamate dehydrogenase, glutamic acid is formed in the liver from α-ketoglutaric acid and ammonia (Fig. 13.8).

Metabolic Fates of Glutamic Acid

Glutamic acid is a precursor of a number of biologically active compounds (Fig. 13.28):

1. By a transamination reaction, α-amino group of glutamate becomes available for the synthesis of several **nonessential amino acids**.

2. Glutamic acid, in the presence of glutamine synthetase and ATP, reacts with ammonia and forms **glutamine** (Fig. 13.10).

3. Glutamic acid contributes in the formation of **folic acid** which is also called pteroylglutamic acid.

4. Glutamate is a component of **glutathione** (a tripeptide comprising of Gly, Cys and Glu).

5. Glutamate is an important **neurotransmitter** (Chemistry to Clinics 13.6).

6. Further, an inhibitory neurotransmitter **γ-aminobutyric acid (GABA)** is formed by decarboxylation of glutamic acid, in the brain.

7. Glutamic acid is also reversibly converted to **ornithine** as well as **proline**.

8. With acetyl CoA, glutamate forms **N-acetyl glutamate** which is required in urea synthesis.

γ-Aminobutyric Acid (GABA): It is synthesized in the brain by decarboxylation of glutamic acid by glutamic

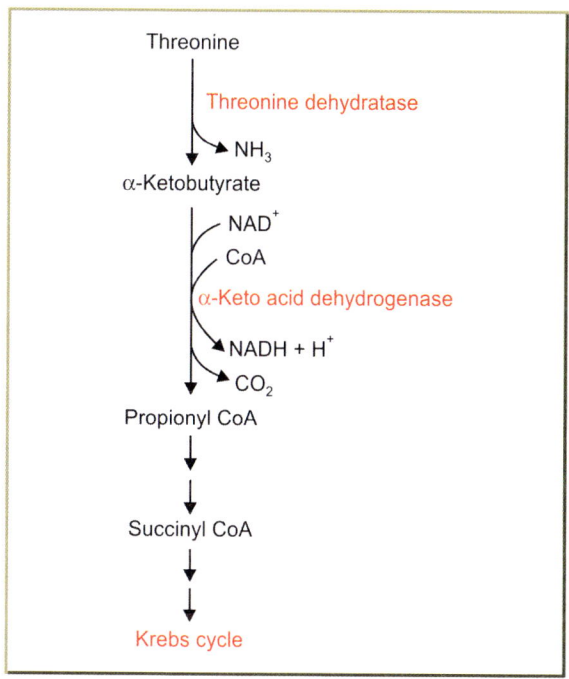

Fig. 13.27: Conversion of threonine to propionyl CoA.

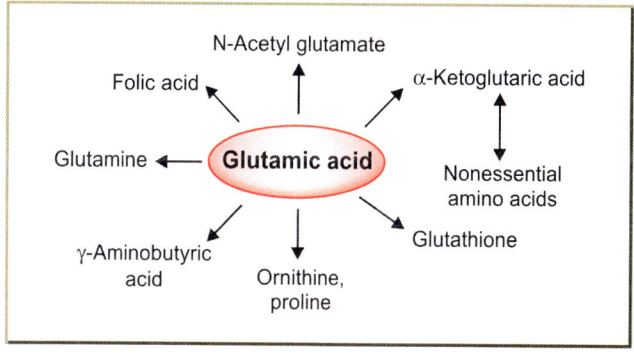

Fig. 13.28: Metabolic fates of glutamic acid.

Chemistry to Clinics 13.6: Glutamatergic Neurotransmission

N-methyl-D-aspartate (**NMDA**) receptors are ionotropic receptors associated with cationic channels in the neuronal membrane. Activation of the NMDA receptor is unique in that there is a glycine site on the NMDA receptor that must be bound along with glutamate to activate the receptor. Activation of the NMDA receptor increases Na^+ and Ca^{2+} conductance. This receptor, however, is blocked by Mg^{2+} when the membrane is in the resting state and becomes unblocked when the membrane is depolarized. Thus, the NMDA receptor is both a ligand-gated and a voltage-gated channel. Calcium gating through the NMDA receptor is crucial for the development of specific neuronal connections and for neural processing related to learning and memory. Excess entry of Ca^{2+} through NMDA receptors during **ischemic episodes** such as cerebral thrombosis and hemorrhage, is responsible for the **rapid death of neurons**.

acid decarboxylase. The reaction also requires pyridoxal phosphate as a coenzyme. Vitamin B_6 deficiency thus inhibits GABA synthesis and results in convulsions. GABA is an inhibitor of the synaptic transmission and acts as a regulator of neuronal activity. In the brain, GABA (an **inhibitory neurotransmitter**) and glutamate (an excitatory neurotransmitter) share some common routes of metabolism, in the astrocytes. After GABA is formed from glutamate, it can be transaminated with an α-keto acid and forms succinate semialdehyde. The latter is converted to succinate by succinate semialdehyde dehydrogenase and can enter the Krebs cycle (Fig. 13.29).

Glutamate and taste sensation: Four primary taste sensations have been described—sweet, sour, salty and bitter. Glutamate ions present in dietary proteins produce a 'meat-like' taste sensation by stimulating specific receptors on the tongue. This is a fifth primary taste sensation called '**umami**' or savoriness. Glutamate ions are used in the food industry as flavor enhancers in the popular food additive monosodium glutamate.

GLUTAMINE

Glutamic acid reacts with ammonia and forms its amide glutamine (Fig. 13.10). The reaction is catalyzed by the enzyme glutamine synthetase which is a mitochondrial enzyme and is found in the liver, brain, kidney and retina. This is the major pathway for the metabolic disposal of ammonia, chiefly in the brain but also in the kidney and liver.

Metabolic Fates of Glutamine

1. Glutamine is transported to the liver for the removal of its amino group as urea, and to the kidney for the excretion of its amide nitrogen as ammonia (NH_4^+), in the urine. The latter reaction is catalyzed by the enzyme glutaminase (Fig. 13.10). It thus, protects the brain by **fixing ammonia** (with glutamate), which is very toxic.
2. It is a principle source of free ammonia in the urine and thus plays an important role in the **maintenance of acid–base balance**.
3. In the central nervous system, glutamine helps in the **transport of K^+**.
4. Glutamine is important for the **synthesis of purines** in the cytoplasm and contributes to N3 and N9 of a purine ring.
5. In humans and other primates, glutamine conjugates with phenylacetate and forms **phenylacetylglutamine** (Fig. 13.30).

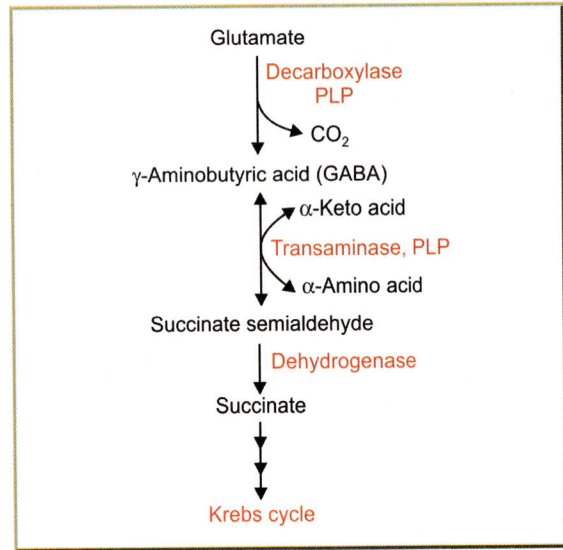

Fig. 13.29: Metabolism of GABA in astrocytes.

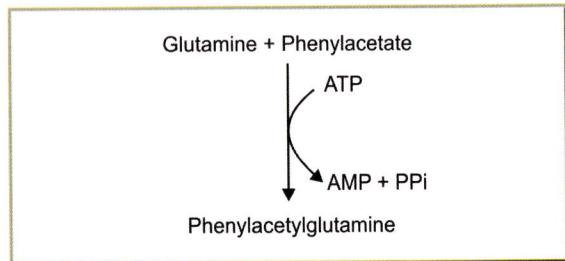

Fig. 13.30: Conjugation of glutamine.

ASPARTIC ACID

Aspartic acid is synthesized by the transamination of oxaloacetate. It is a glucogenic amino acid since its transamination yields oxaloacetate, an intermediate of Krebs cycle.

Metabolic Fates of Aspartic Acid

1. Similar to glutamic acid, aspartic acid is also important for a **transamination** reaction.
2. Aspartic acid is important for the continuation of the **urea cycle**. It combines with citrulline and forms argininosuccinic acid.
3. Biosynthesis of **carnosine** and **anserine** (Fig. 13.31).
4. Biosynthesis of **purine** (N1) and **pyrimidine ring** (C4, C5, C6 and N1) (Fig. 13.32).

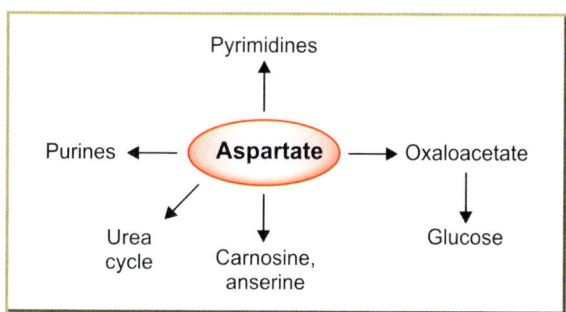

Fig. 13.31: Metabolic fates of aspartate.

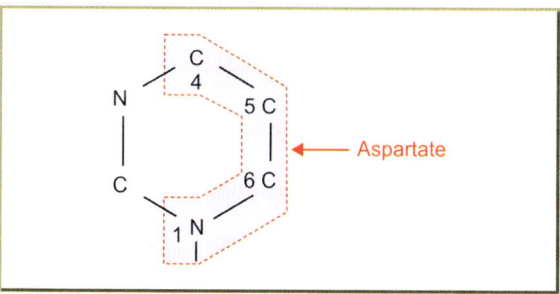

Fig. 13.32: Contribution of aspartate in a pyrimidine ring.

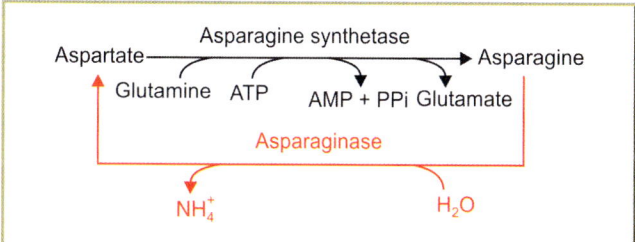

Fig. 13.33: Interconversion of aspartate and asparagine.

Chemistry to Clinics 13.7: Asparaginase and Leukemia
Asparagine is readily synthesized and degraded in most of the cells. Some leukemic cells, however, lack the ability to synthesize it. Such patients are administered with exogenous asparaginase which is useful in the treatment of leukemia.

ASPARAGINE

The amide group of asparagine comes from that of glutamine. The reaction is catalyzed by asparagine synthetase in most cells, and needs ATP (Fig. 13.33). The amide-nitrogen from asparagine is removed by the enzyme asparaginase (Chemistry to Clinics 13.7).

AROMATIC AMINO ACIDS

Phenylalanine, tyrosine and tryptophan are the amino acids with an aromatic ring, hence these three are collectively called aromatic amino acids.

PHENYLALANINE

As men and most animals cannot synthesize the aromatic ring, phenylalanine is essential in their diet. Under normal conditions, all the dietary phenylalanine that, as such, is not incorporated into the proteins, is converted to tyrosine.

Conversion of phenylalanine to tyrosine is carried out by phenylalanine hydroxylase in the presence of molecular oxygen and tetrahydrobiopterin ($B \cdot H_4$) (Fig. 13.34). In the process, $B \cdot H_4$ is converted to dihydrobiopterin ($B \cdot H_2$) and requires NADPH-dependent reductase for its regeneration.

TYROSINE

Since tyrosine can be synthesized in the body from phenylalanine, the subsequent catabolism of the two amino acids is therefore similar. Phenylalanine and tyrosine serve as precursors for a number of important biologically active compounds in different tissues (Fig. 13.35).

Metabolic Fates of Tyrosine

1. **Degradation of tyrosine in the liver**
   - Tyrosine catabolism starts with its transamination to *p*-hydroxyphenylpyruvate by tyrosine aminotransferase (tyrosine transaminase) (Fig. 13.34). It is an inducible enzyme

13

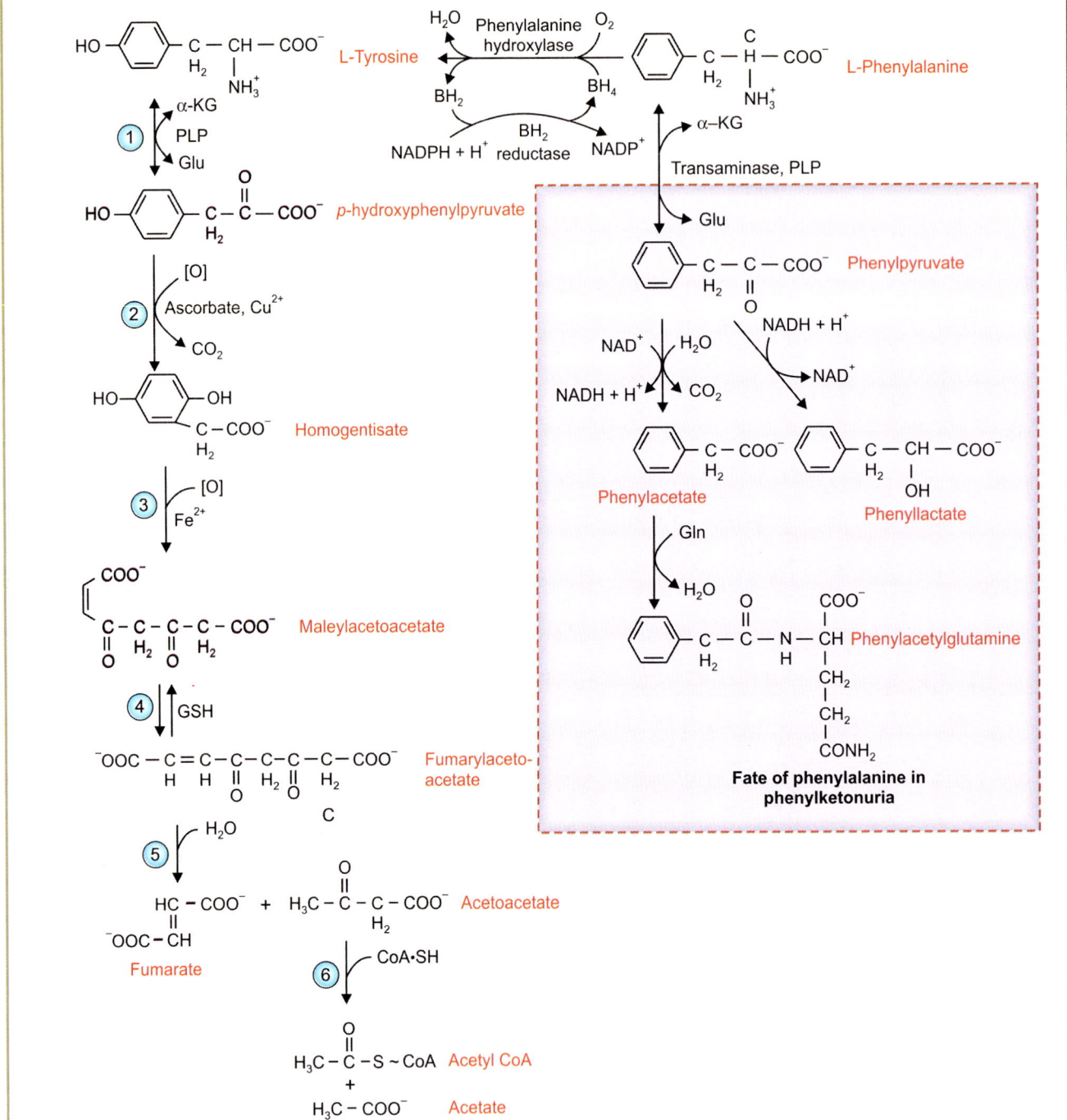

Fig. 13.34: Tyrosine catabolism. 1. Tyrosine transaminase, 2. ρ-hydroxyphenylpyruvate hydroxylase, 3. Homogentisate oxidase, 4. *Cis-, trans-*isomerase, 5. Fumaryl acetoacetate hydrolase, 6. β-ketothiolase.

whose synthesis is increased by glucocorticoids and by dietary phenylalanine/tyrosine.

- In the next step, a copper-containing enzyme complex, *p*-hydroxyphenylpyruvate oxidase converts *p*-hydroxyphenylpyruvate to homogentisic acid. The enzyme requires ascorbic acid and catalyzes decarboxylation, oxidation, migration of the carbon side chain and hydroxylation of the substrate.

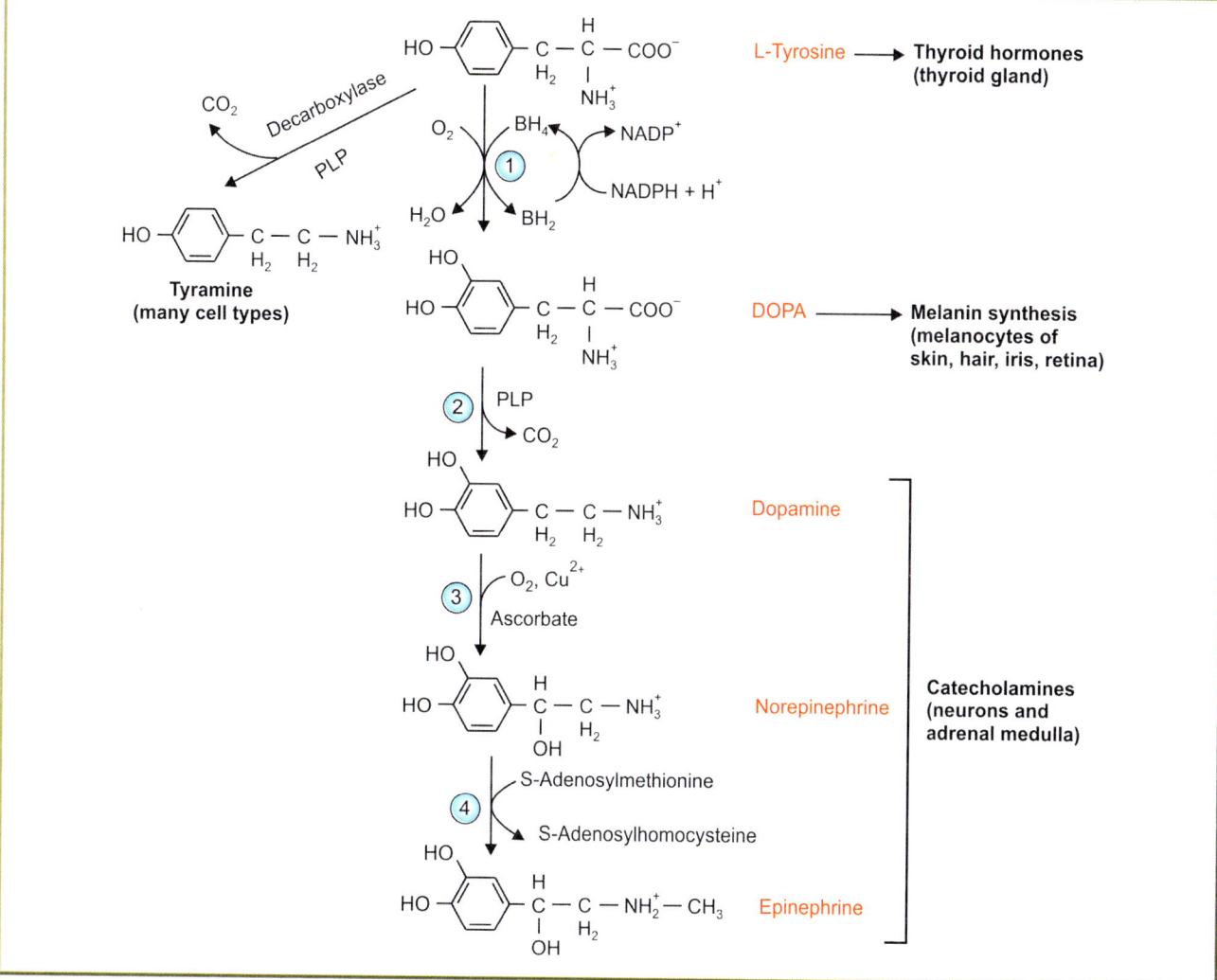

Fig. 13.35: Specialized products derived from tyrosine. 1. Tyrosine hydroxylase, 2. DOPA decarboxylase, 3. Dopamine β-oxidase, 4. Methyl transferase.

- An iron-containing enzyme homogentisic acid oxidase, oxidizes homogentisic acid.
- Subsequent reactions, catalyzed by maleyl-acetoacetate isomerase (which requires glutathione for its activity) and fumaryl-acetoacetate hydrolase, lead to the formation of the end products of tyrosine catabolism, i.e. fumarate and acetoacetate.

2. **Synthesis of catecholamines:** In the adrenal medulla, tyrosine is utilized in the synthesis of norepinephrine (noradrenaline) and epinephrine (adrenaline) (Fig. 13.35):

- Tyrosine is first converted to dihydroxy-phenylalanine (DOPA) by tyrosine hydroxylase.

- Thereafter, DOPA decarboxylase converts DOPA to dopamine which enters the storage granules as the active neurotransmitter.
- Dopamine is then converted to norepinephrine by dopamine-β-hydroxylase. Norepinephrine is a local hormone present in the sympathetic nerve endings. Its synthesis is regulated by plasma tyrosine in the CNS.
- Methylation of norepinephrine by phenyleth-anolamine-N-methyltransferase (PNMT) forms epinephrine. Active methionine (S-adenosyl methionine) is used as a methyl donor.

These aromatic amines with a **catechol ring** (3,4-dihydroxyphenyl ring), i.e. dopamine, norepine-

Chemistry to Clinics 13.8: Vanillylmandelic Acid

Catecholamines are metabolized by monoamine oxidase and catecholamine-O-methyltransferase to some excretory products, such as vanillylmandelic acid (**VMA**). Absence of this metabolite in the urine is diagnostic of a deficiency in the synthesis of catecholamines. On the other hand, catecholamine-producing tumors such as **pheochromocytoma**, result in increased urinary VMA secretion (please refer to Chapter 17 for details).

Chemistry to Clinics 13.9: Parkinson's Disease

Parkinson's disease is a degenerative condition causing '**shaking palsy**', the development of tremors that gradually interfere with motor function of the various muscle groups. It is associated with the deficiency of dopamine production in certain areas of the brain. The defect is caused by degeneration of the cells in certain small nuclei of the brain. Other symptoms include nausea, vomiting, hypotension, cardiac arrhythmias and various central nervous system symptoms. It is treated with L-DOPA which acts as a precursor of dopamine.

phrine and epinephrine are called catecholamines (Chemistry to Clinics 13.8 and 13.9).

3. **Synthesis of melanin:** In the melanocytes, tyrosine is used for the synthesis of melanin (Fig. 13.36):
   - By the enzyme tyrosinase (a copper-containing protein), tyrosine is first converted to DOPA and then to dopaquinone.
   - Subsequently, dopaquinone forms melanin, a brown-black pigment found in the skin, hair and retina. There are various types of melanins. The dark pigment, that is usually associated with melanin, is called eumelanin.

4. **Synthesis of thyroxine:** In the thyroid gland, thyroid hormones are synthesized as a result of iodination of the tyrosyl residues of the glycoprotein thyroglobulin (Fig. 13.37):
   - For iodination, iodine is first activated by peroxidase.

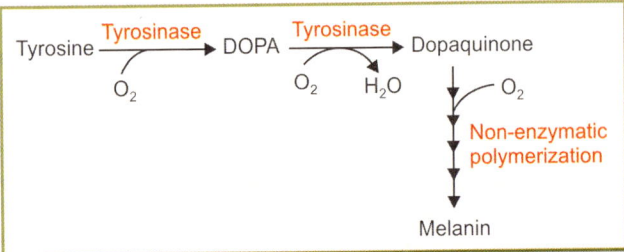

Fig. 13.36: Conversion of tyrosine to melanin.

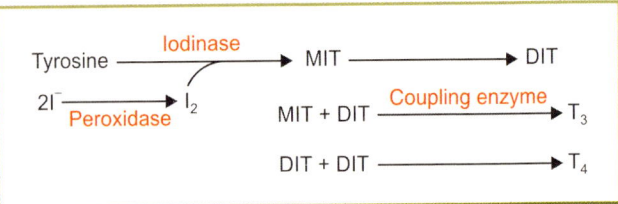

Fig. 13.37: Conversion of tyrosine to thyroid hormones.

- Subsequently, iodinase catalyzes iodination of the tyrosyl residues of thyroglobulin and converts them to monoiodotyrosine (MIT) and diiodotyrosine (DIT).
- Thereafter, coupling of either a molecule of MIT with DIT or two molecules of DIT forms triiodothyronine (T_3) or thyroxine (tetraiodothyronine or T_4), respectively. This is an intramolecular process and hormones are synthesized within the protein chain of the thyroglobulin molecule. A detailed discussion on thyroid hormone synthesis and related disorders is given in Chapter 17.

Inborn Errors of Phenylalanine/Tyrosine Metabolism

1. **Phenylketonuria**
   - Autosomal recessive deficiency of hepatic **phenylalanine hydroxylase** results in a condition called classical or type I phenylketonuria. Type II phenylketonuria is due to dihydrobiopterin reductase deficiency.
   - An excess of phenylalanine which cannot be converted to tyrosine, gets catabolized by the alternative pathway. Phenylalanine is transaminated to phenylpyruvic acid which is subsequently reduced to phenyllactic acid as well as is decarboxylated to phenylacetic acid (Fig. 13.34).
   - **Due to increased urinary excretion of phenylpyruvic acid (a phenylketone), the disease is called phenylketonuria.**
   - Increased levels of the three phenylketoacids in the blood cause **mental retardation** and **convulsions**. Besides, severe neurological symptoms and very low IQ, there is also light color of the skin and the eyes. This is due to **underpigmentation**, a result of tyrosine (and hence melanin) deficiency.

• Such infants are given **low phenylalanine diet**. Under these conditions **tyrosine becomes dietary essential**.

2. **Tyrosinemias:** A complete or partial deficiency of tyrosine aminotransferase results in tyrosinemias, a group of autosomal recessive disorders which in turn lead to the accumulation and excretion of tyrosine and its metabolites. These are of two types:

• **Type I tyrosinemia**, also called **hepatorenal tyrosinemia**, is a more serious type of the disease. It is caused by the deficiency of **fumaryl-acetoacetate hydrolase** and involves liver failure, renal tubular dysfunction, rickets and poly-neuropathy. Accumulation of fumarylace-toacetate and maleylacetoacetate, both of which are alkylating agents, can lead to DNA alkylation and carcinogenesis.

• **Type II tyrosinemia**, also called **oculocutaneous tyrosinemia**, is due to the deficiency of **tyrosine transaminase**. It results in eye and skin lesions and in mental retardation.

3. **Alkaptonuria**

• Hereditary deficiency of **homogentisic acid oxidase** causes alkaptonuria (Fig. 13.38).

• Such individuals excrete almost all of the ingested tyrosine as the colorless homogentisic acid in their urine. Homogentisic acid, in turn, gets auto-oxidized to the corresponding quinone which is subsequently polymerized to form an intensely dark colour. The **dark urine** is the only consequence of this condition in early life.

• Homogentisate is slowly oxidized to pigments that are deposited in bones, connective tissues and other organs. The condition is called **ochronosis** because of the ochre color of deposits.

4. **Albinism**

• Tyrosinase is specific for the biosynthesis of melanin in melanocytes. Lack of **tyrosinase** in melanocytes affects the synthesis of melanin and leads to the formation of white depigmented patches on the skin and iris. The condition is called albinism (Fig. 13.39).

• Lack of pigment in the skin also makes albinos more sensitive to sunlight, increases the risk of carcinoma of the skin, in addition to sunburns. Lack of pigment in the eyes may also contribute to photophobia.

Various inborn errors of phenylalanine/tyrosine metabolism are given in Table 13.5).

Table 13.5: Inborn errors of phenylalanine/tyrosine metabolism

Metabolic disorder	Deficient enzyme
Classical phenyl ketonuria Type I	Phenylalanine hydroxylase
Phenyl ketonuria Type II	Dihydrobiopterin reductase
Tyrosinemia Type I	Fumaryl acetoacetate hydrolase
Tyrosinemia Type II	Tyrosine transaminase
Alkaptonuria	Homogentisic acid oxidase
Albinism	Tyrosinase

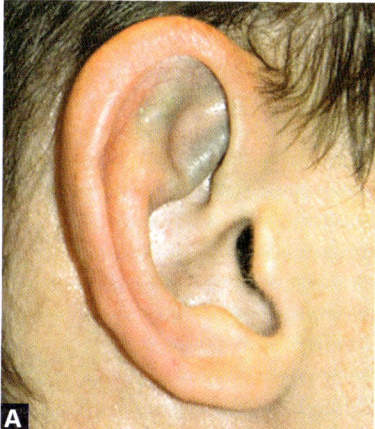 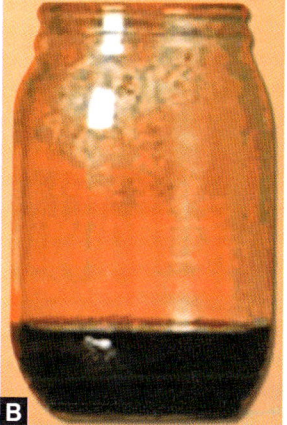 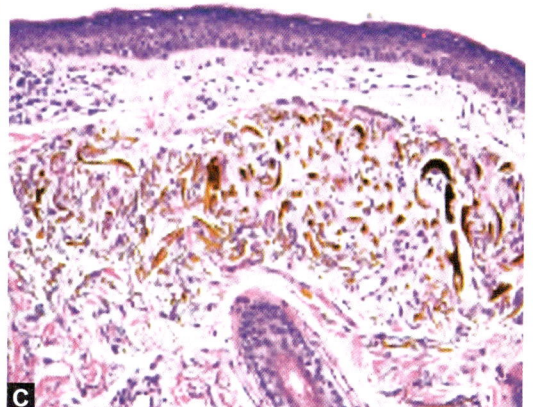

Fig. 13.38: Alkaptonuria: (A) Slate-blue **discoloration** of the **antihelix** of the ear. (B) **Darkening of the urine** on standing. (C) **Ochronosis:** Histopathology of the skin, showing sharply defined yellow-brown 'banana' shaped deposits within elastic fibers in the superficial dermis and scattered pigment-laden macrophages in the papillary dermis.

13

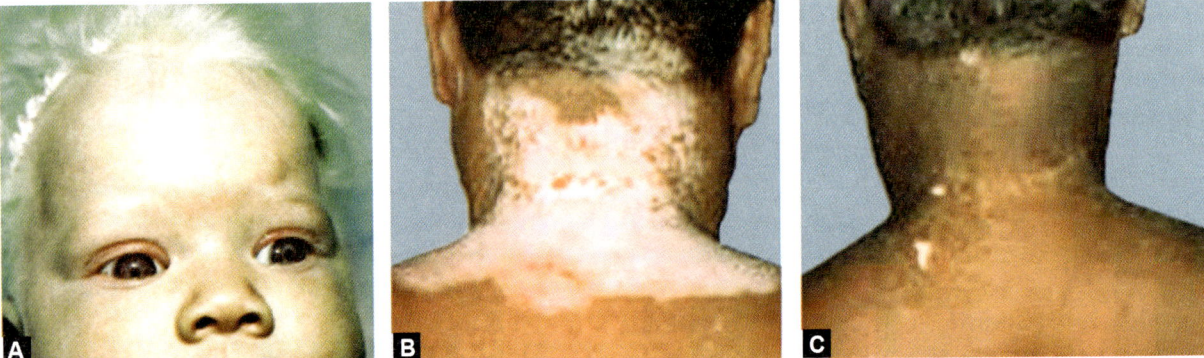

Fig. 13.39: (A) **Oculocutaneous albinism.** Hypomelanotic skin, white hair, and pink irides resulting from the **dysfunction of tyrosinase** in the melanocytes of these tissues and the subsequent lack of melanin synthesis. (B) **Vitiligo.** Hypopigmentation due to **lack of melanocytes** in the affected skin. (C) Same patient as in (B), improving **after UV-B** (the B-range of ultraviolet radiation) **phototherapy.**

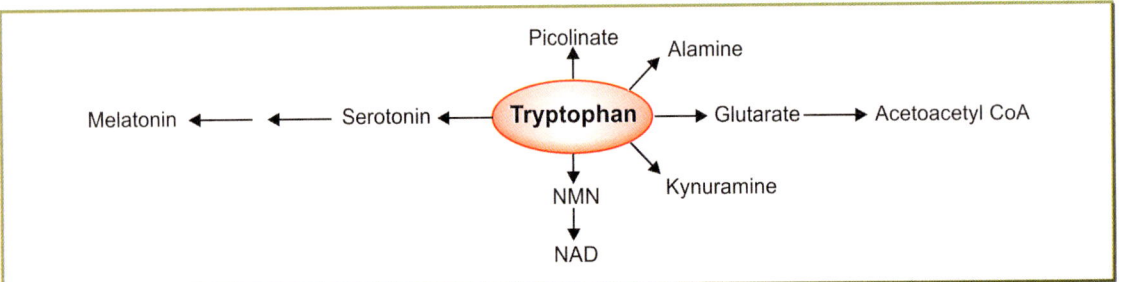

Fig. 13.40: Metabolic fates of tryptophan.

TRYPTOPHAN

Tryptophan is an essential amino acid containing indole ring.

Metabolic Fates of Tryptophan

Various metabolic fates of tryptophan are given in Fig. 13.40.

1. **Kynurenine-anthranilate pathway:** The main pathway for its degradation is called kynurenine-anthranilate pathway (Fig. 13.41). This pathway is also important for the biosynthesis of NAD:
   - In the liver, metabolism of tryptophan starts with the opening of the indole ring, leading to the formation of N-formyl kynurenine. The reaction is catalyzed by a heme-containing enzyme tryptophan dioxygenase, also called tryptophan pyrrolase. The enzyme is found in the liver and is induced by glucocorticoids as well as glucagon.
   - In the next step, formyl kynurenine is converted to kynurenine with the removal of formate by the enzyme formamidase. After this stage, the pathway has many branch points.

- In the main degradative pathway, kynurenine is hydroxylated to produce 3-hydroxykynurenine by kynurenine hydroxylase. This enzyme is inhibited by estrogen and thus women are more susceptible to pellagra (niacin deficiency disease).
- With the cleavage of alanine from the side chain by kynureninase, 3-hydroxykynurenine is converted to 3-hydroxyanthranilate. This enzyme requires pyridoxal-5-phosphate (vitamin B_6) as a coenzyme (Chemistry to Clinics 13.10).
- Subsequent oxidation of 3-hydroxyanthranilate by 3-hydroxyanthranilate oxidase forms an unstable intermediate 2-amino-3-carboxy-muconate-6-semialdehyde.

Chemistry to Clinics 13.10: Xanthurenic Aciduria

Several enzymes of the tryptophan-kynurenine pathway such as kynureninase are dependent on pyridoxal phosphate. In vitamin B_6 deficiency, kynurenine and 3-hydroxykynurenine are alternatively catabolized to kynurenic acid and xanthurenic acid, respectively. Increased excretion of xanthurenic acid imparts **greenish-yellow color to the urine** and the condition is known as xanthurenic aciduria.

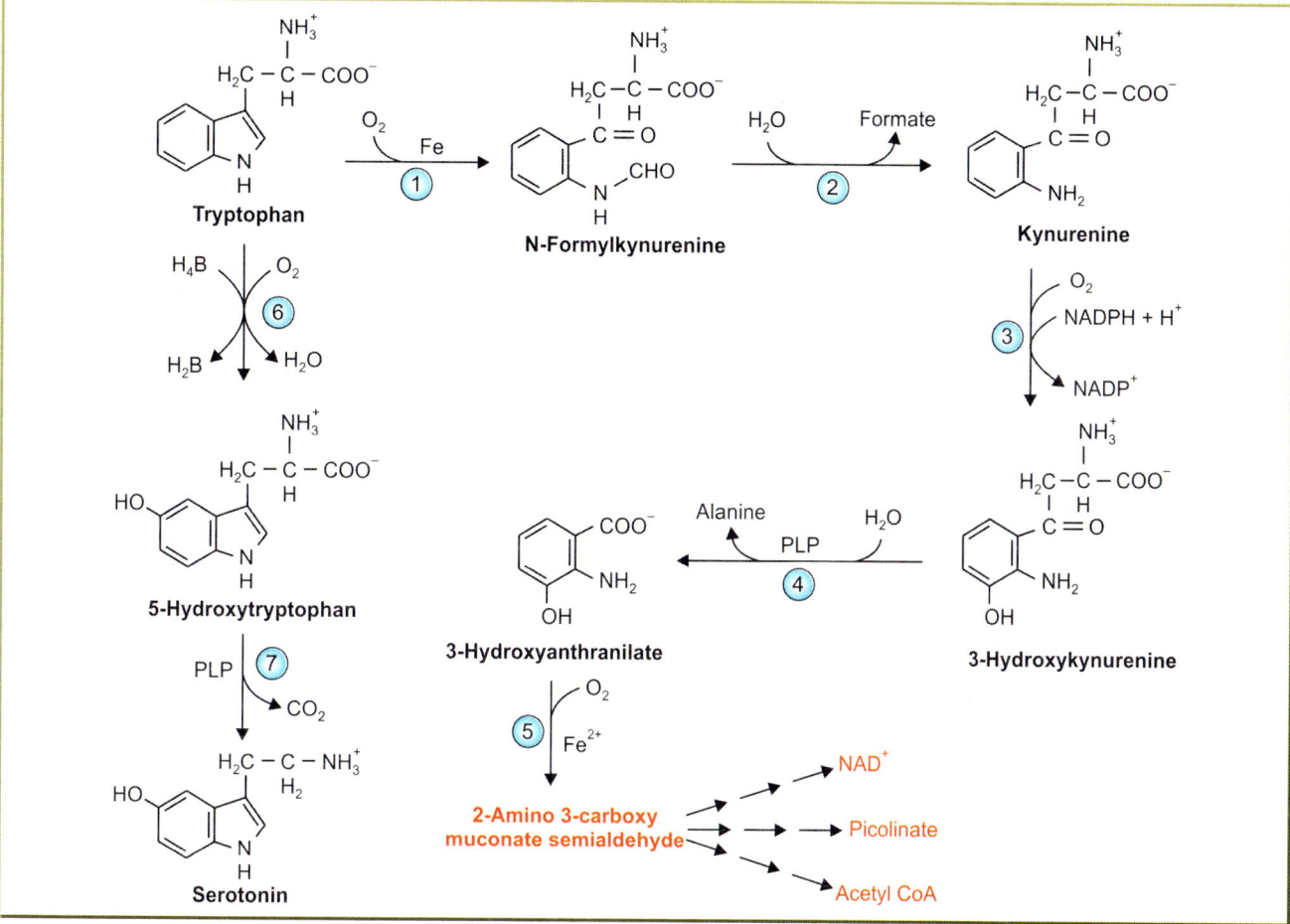

Fig. 13.41: Catabolism of tryptophan. 1. Tryptophan oxygenase, 2. Kynurenine formylase, 3. Kynurenine hydroxylase, 4. Kynureninase, 5. 3-Hydroxyanthranilate oxidase, 6. Tryptophan hydroxylase, 7. Aromatic amino acid decarboxylase.

- Through a number of steps, finally it is converted to glutarate and eventually to acetoacetyl CoA or recyclized non-enzymatically to picolinic acid which is excreted in the urine.

2. Biosynthesis of NAD:
- In the liver and some other tissues, non-enzymatic cyclization of aminocarboxymuconic semialdehyde (formed in the above pathway) converts it to quinolinic acid.
- Thereafter, quinolinate phosphoribosyl-transferase (QPRT) transfers a ribonucleotide moiety from phosphoribosylpyrophosphate (PRPP).
- Decarboxylation leads to the synthesis of nicotinate mononucleotide (a derivative of niacin) and finally to NAD. Sixty mg of tryptophan is converted to 1 mg of niacin.

In B_6 deficiency, quinolinic acid is not converted to nicotinate but to nicotinamide and its N^1-methyl derivative (N^1-methylnicotinamide). Vitamin B_6 deficiency thus results in urinary excretion of large quantities of these metabolites.

3. Synthesis of neurotransmitters: Kynurenine can also undergo transamination and condensation, and produces kynurenic acid. It is then decarboxylated to form kynuramine. Kynuramine and quinolinate have been shown to act as tryptophan-derived neurotransmitters, possibly as anti-excitotoxics and anticonvulsives.

4. Synthesis of serotonin: In platelets, brain and intestinal epithelium, tryptophan is hydroxylated by tryptophan hydroxylase to form 5-hydroxy-tryptophan that is subsequently decarboxy-lated to 5-hydroxytryptamine (serotonin) by a

Chemistry to Clinics 13.11: Malignant Carcinoid Syndrome

It results from serotonin-producing tumor cells in the intestine (Fig. 13.42). It is also called **argentaffinoma** because the tumor arises from the intestinal argentaffin cells that normally secrete serotonin. There is an increased production of serotonin that causes flushing, anxiety and gastrointestinal upset. Serotonin is normally catabolized to 5-hydroxyindoleacetic acid (**5-HIAA**). In this condition, urinary excretion of 5-HIAA is increased by more than 50 folds and establishes the diagnosis. Estimation of serum serotonin is useful to detect cases missed by urinary 5-HIAA alone.

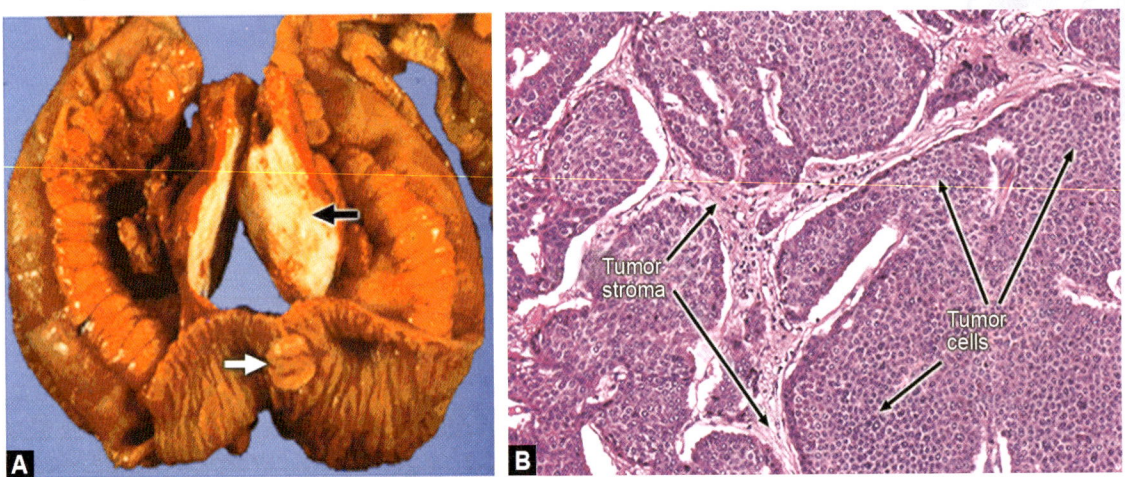

Fig. 13.42: Carcinoid tumor. (A) Small intestine has been opened disclosing a tumor (white arrow) which penetrates through the mucosa. Tumor is white, well-demarcated while the adjoining mucosa is normal with delicate transverse folds. Enlarged lymph node of mesentery has been transected (black arrow) disclosing a white metastatic tumor as opposed to the tan appearance of normal lymphoid tissue. (B) Histologically, carcinoids consist of well-defined nests of tumor cells separated by thin fibrovascular septa and populations of tumor cells with a homogeneous appearence. The tumor cells are relatively small and round with central nucleoli and abundant lightly eosinophilic and granular cytoplasm.

decarboxylase, which also needs vitamin B_6 for its activity (Fig. 13.41). Serotonin is a neurotransmitter in the brain (*see* Chapter 17 for details), a vasoconstrictor and bronchoconstrictor. Serotonin-producing tumors are known to occur (Chemistry to Clinics 13.11).

5. **Synthesis of melatonin:** The acetyltransferase present in the pineal gland and the retina catalyzes the synthesis of N-acetyl-5-methoxytryptamine, i.e. melatonin. Melatonin is a sleep-inducing substance and maintains the **circadian rhythm of sleep-wake cycle**. It also inhibits the synthesis and secretion of other neurotransmitters such as dopamine and GABA.

BRANCHED CHAIN AMINO ACIDS

Valine, leucine and isoleucine are the three essential amino acids which have aliphatic, non-polar side chains. Together, they are called branched chain amino acids (BCAA).

Degradation of Branched Chain Amino Acids

Oxidation of the BCAA is initiated in muscles since BCAA aminotransferase is present in much higher concentration in the muscles as compared to the liver. Although these three amino acids produce different products, the **first three steps in their catabolism are similar**. These include transamination, formation of CoA thioesters and their oxidation (Fig. 13.43):

1. **Transamination:** The first step in the oxidation of BCAA is the removal of α-amino group by transamination, forming the corresponding α-keto acids. The reaction is freely reversible as an α-keto acid can replace the corresponding BCAA in the diet. When BCAA are in excess than required for protein synthesis, they are transaminated to yield the corresponding α-keto acids.

Two distinct types of transaminases are known. One is valine-specific while the other acts on leucine or isoleucine (Chemistry to Clinics 13.12). Both the enzymes catalyze reversible reactions and require

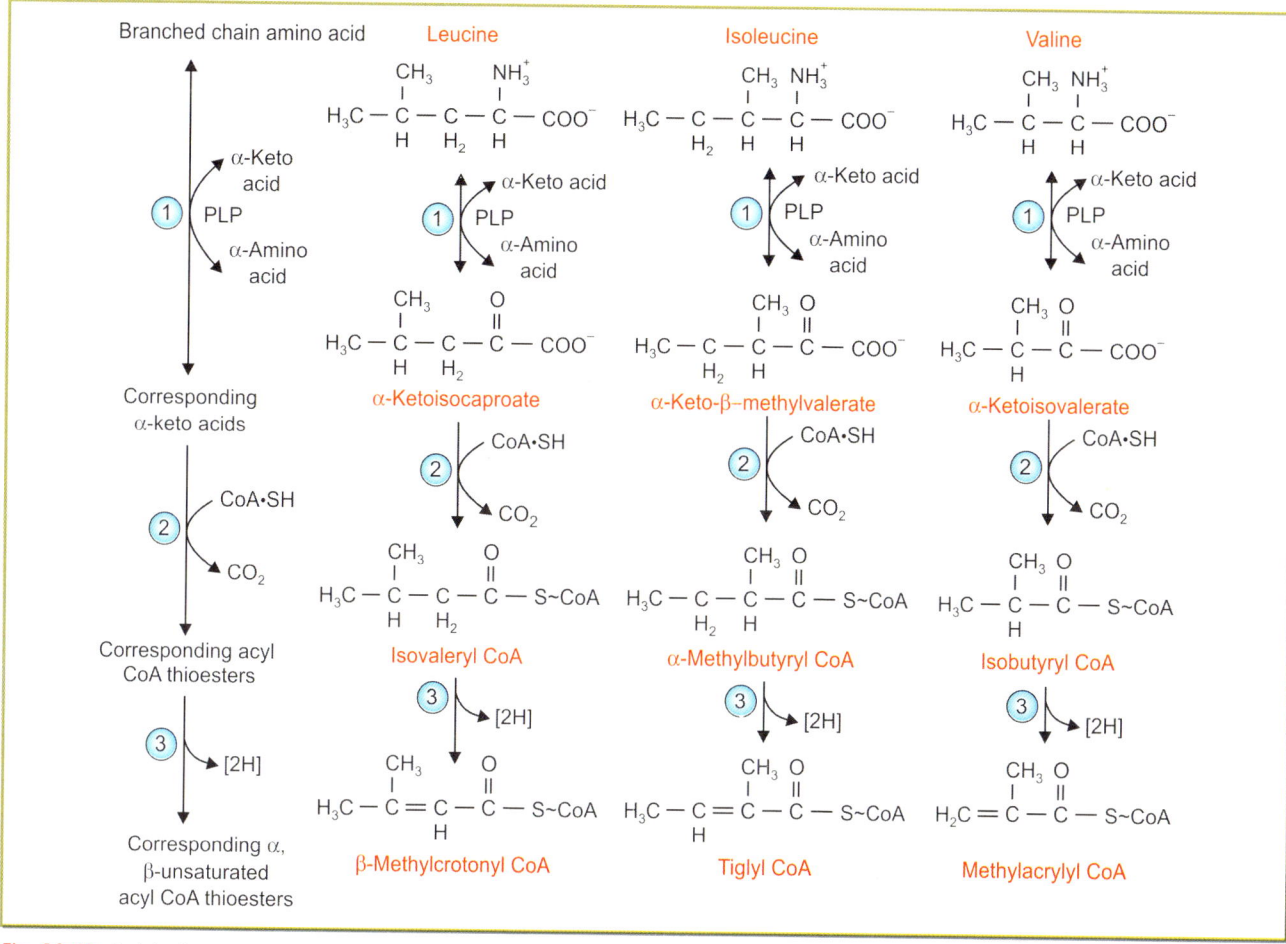

Fig. 13.43: Catabolism of branched chain amino acids: Initial three analogous reactions. 1. Transaminase, 2. Branched chain a-keto acid dehydrogenase multienzyme complex, 3. Branched acyl CoA thioester dehydrogenase.

Chemistry to Clinics 13.12: Hypervalinemia and Hyperleucine-isoleucinemia

Deficiencies of the two branched chain aminotransferases, i.e. valine aminotransferase and leucine-isoleucine aminotransferase result in hypervalinemia and hyperleucineisoleucinemia, respectively. The main clinical symptoms include vomiting, mental retardation and an abnormal electroencephalogram (EEG).

pyridoxal-5-phosphate as a coenzyme. Starvation induces muscle aminotransferases but not the liver enzymes.

2. **Oxidative decarboxylation:** Dehydrogenation of the branched chain α-keto acid is carried out by a branched chain α-keto acid dehydrogenase complex, similar to pyruvate dehydrogenase complex or α-ketoglutarate dehydrogenase complex (Chemistry to Clinics 13.13). It results in the loss of a carboxylic group, forming CoA thioester of the

Chemistry to Clinics 13.13: Maple Syrup Urine Disease

- It is an inborn error of metabolism of the 3 branched chain amino acids (valine, leucine and isoleucine).
- It is due to the deficiency of the enzyme branched chain keto acid dehydrogenase complex which is required for the oxidative decarboxylation of branched chain keto acids (Fig. 13.43).
- Branched chain keto acids derived from valine, leucine and isoleucine are excreted in the urine, giving it a typical odor of maple syrup (maple is a type of fruit) or burnt sugar, hence the disease is called maple syrup urine disease.
- The disease appears in early infancy and is characterized by ketoacidosis, severe vomiting, convulsions and early death.
- Dietary treatment (restricted intake of BCAA) to reduce the branched chain ketoacidemia is effective.

corresponding BCAA. These are called branched chain acyl CoA thioesters, and are one carbon shorter than the original BCAA.

13

The enzyme, branched chain α-keto acid dehydrogenase complex, is a high molecular weight multienzyme complex, located principally on the inner surface of the mitochondrial membrane. It has 3 subunits—α-keto acid decarboxylase, transacylase and dihydrolipoyl dehydrogenase. The complex requires several coenzymes, viz. NAD$^+$, FAD, TPP, lipoic acid and coenzyme A. The enzyme is regulated by phosphorylation-dephosphorylation. Its activity is greatly increased by dephosphorylation.

3. **Dehydrogenation:** In the next step, branched chain acyl CoA thioesters are oxidized to yield the corresponding α,β-unsaturated branched chain acyl CoA thioesters. This reaction is analogous to the dehydrogenation of straight chain acyl CoA thioesters in the catabolism of fatty acids.

Carbon skeleton of each of the branched chain amino acid now follows a unique pathway to the amphibolic end products which determine that valine is glucogenic (Fig. 13.44), leucine is ketogenic (Fig. 13.45) while isoleucine is both, i.e. ketogenic as well as glucogenic (Fig. 13.46).

SULFUR-CONTAINING AMINO ACIDS

Methionine and cysteine are sulfur-containing amino acids.

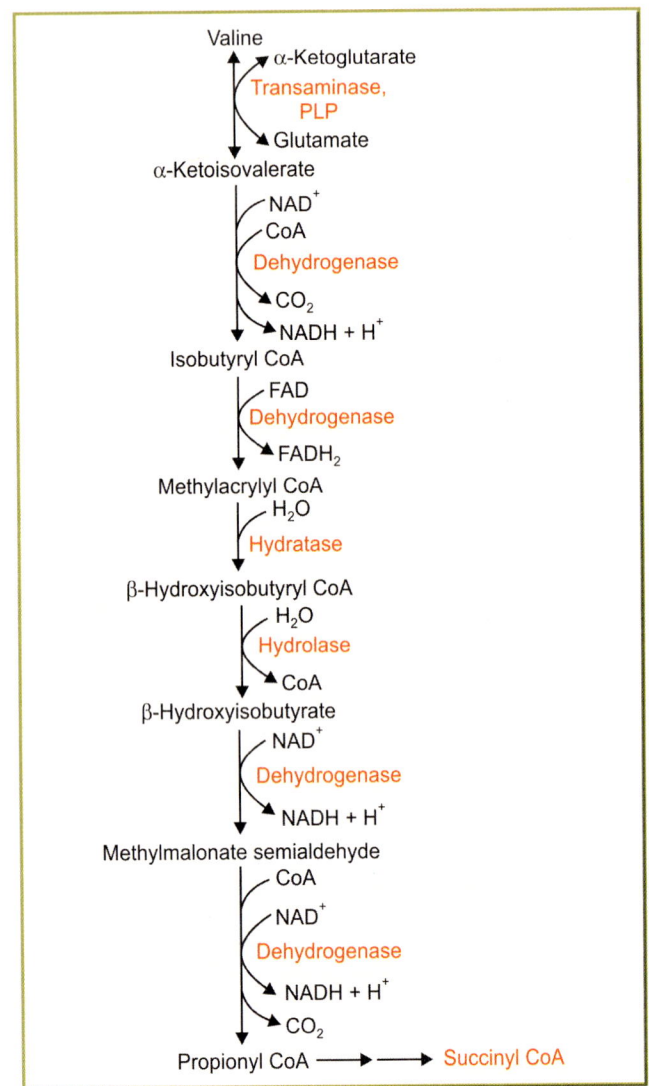

Fig. 13.44: Degradation of valine.

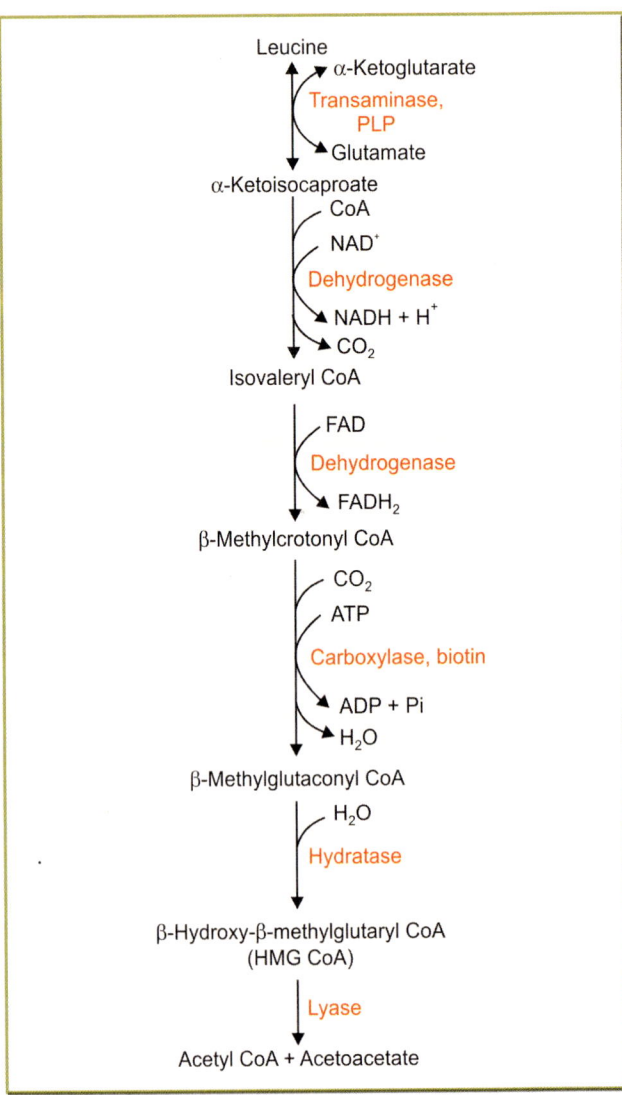

Fig. 13.45: Degradation of leucine.

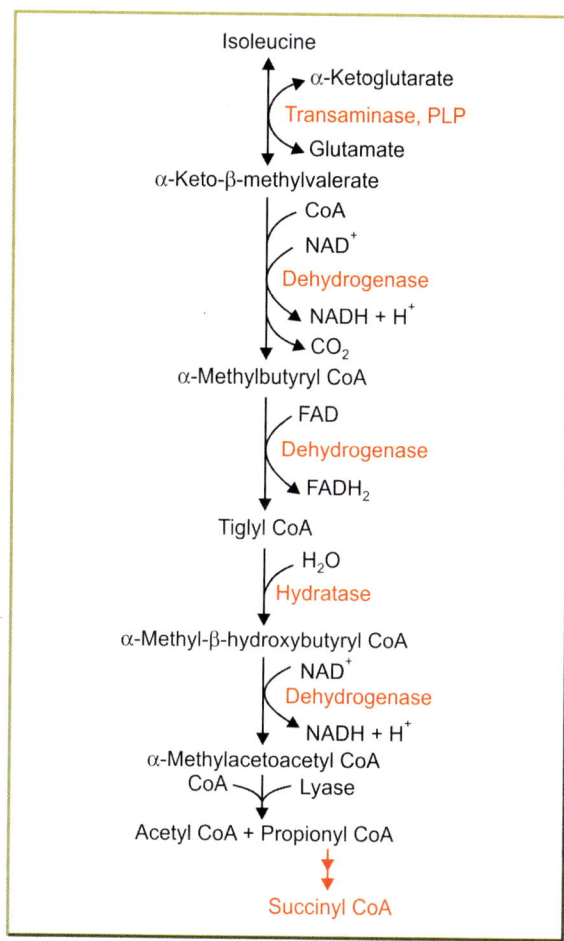

Fig. 13.46: Degradation of isoleucine.

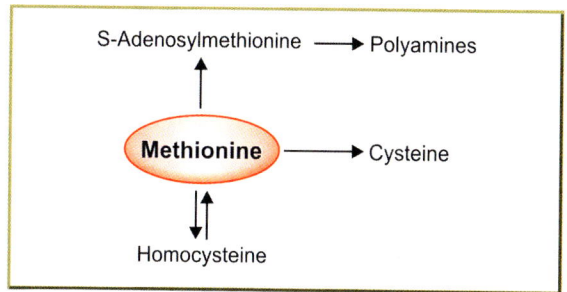

Fig. 13.47: Metabolic fates of methionine.

METHIONINE

Methionine is an essential amino acid and cannot be formed in the body. It is a glycogenic amino acid, as the end product of its catabolism is succinyl CoA. Excess of methionine thus can be used for energy. Methionine also acts as a lipotropic factor.

Metabolic Fates of Methionine

Various metabolic fates of methionine are shown in Fig. 13.47.

1. **Formation of active methionine:** The first step, in the metabolism of methionine, is catalyzed by adenosyltransferase which converts methionine to **S-adenosylmethionine (SAM) or active methionine** (Fig. 13.48), which acts as a methyl carrier and donor and helps in the synthesis of several methylated products. The methylation reactions are catalyzed by the specific methyltransferases which transfer a methyl group from SAM to an acceptor molecule. This is important in the formation of methylated products of biological significance (Table 13.6).

   S-Adenosylmethionine is also used in the biosynthesis of polyamines, i.e. spermidine and spermine.

2. **Formation of homocysteine:** After the removal of its active methyl group by a methyltransferase, SAM is converted to S-adenosylhomocysteine. Thereafter, adenosylhomocysteine hydrolase cleaves the adenosyl moiety (a molecule of adenosine) and forms homocysteine, which has one carbon more than cysteine. Homocysteine can be utilized in different ways:

Table 13.6: S-Adenosyl methionine (SAM) as a methyl group donor

Methyl group acceptor	Methylated product	Biological importance
Ethanolamine	Choline	Choline-containing phospholipids
Guanidoacetate	Creatine	Creatine phosphate, a high-energy reserve
N-acetyl serotonin	Melatonin	Neurotransmitter
Norepinephrine	Epinephrine	Catecholamine
Epinephrine	Metanephrine	Metabolite of epinephrine
Lysine residues in some proteins	Trimethyl lysine	Precursor of carnitine which shuttles activated fatty acids from cytosol to mitochondria
DNA, RNA, proteins	Methylated nucleic acids and proteins	Regulation of gene expression

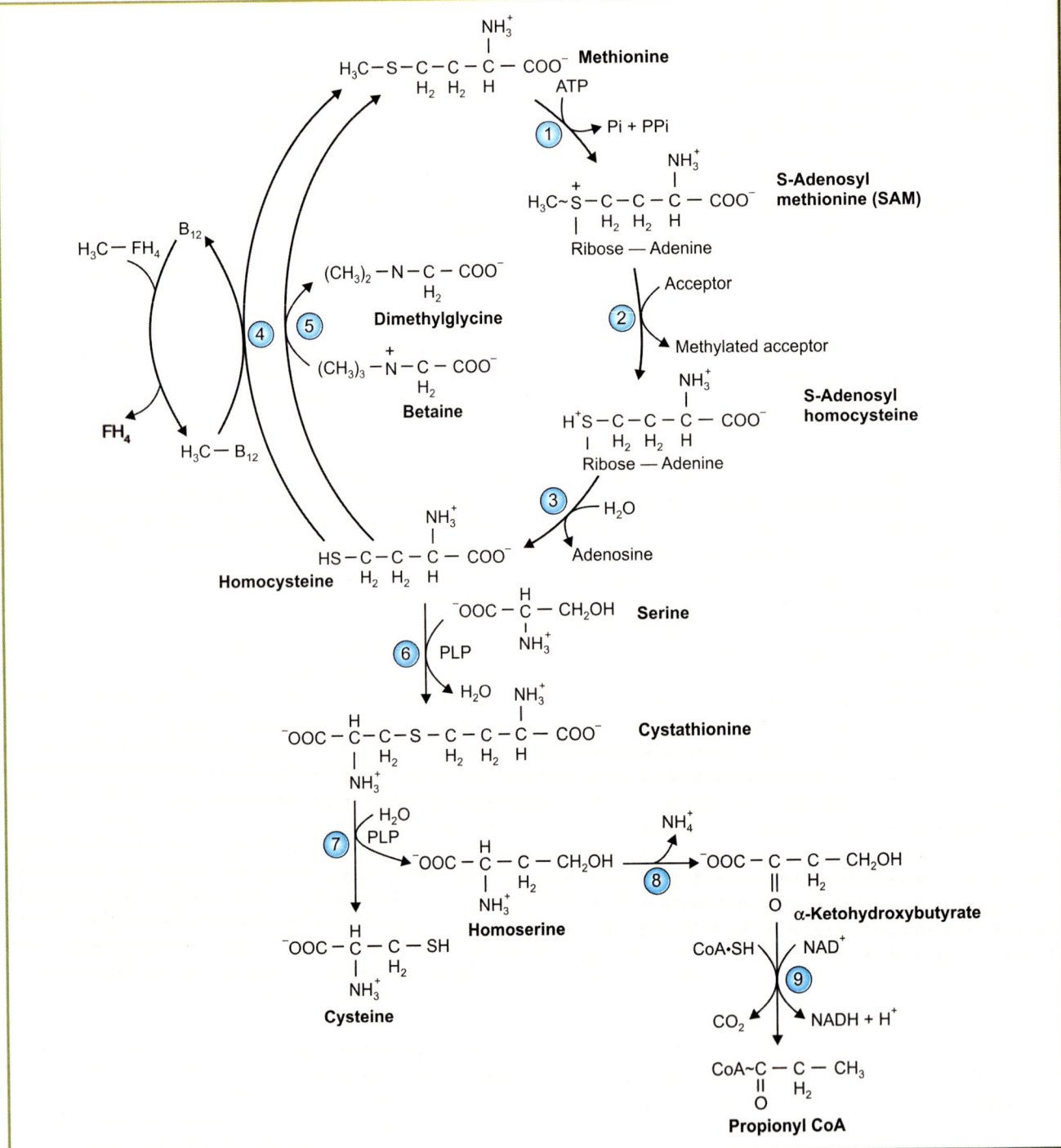

Fig. 13.48: Metabolism of S-containing amino acids. 1. Methionine adenosyl transferase, 2. Methyl transferase, 3. S-Adenosyl homocysteine hydrolase, 4. Methionine synthase, 5. Betaine hydroxymethyl transferase, 6. Cystathionine-β-synthase, 7. Cystathionase, 8. Homoserine deaminase, 9. α-Ketobutyrate dehydrogenase complex

i. **Resynthesis of methionine:** When cells need to resynthesize methionine, homocysteine methyltransferase (methionine synthase) transfers a methyl group from N^5-methyl-tetrahydrofolate (N^5-methyl·FH_4) to cobalamine, forming methyl cobalamine which

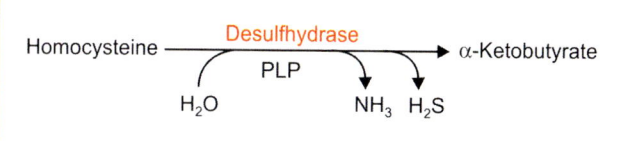

Fig. 13.49: Conversion of homocysteine to α-ketobutyrate.

can re-convert homocysteine to methionine (Fig. 13.48). Alternatively, betaine may act as a methyl donor.

ii. **Synthesis of cysteine:** Homocysteine is coupled with serine and forms cystathionine. The reaction is catalyzed by cystathionine synthase and requires pyridoxal phosphate as a coenzyme. Cystathionine is cleaved by the splitting enzyme cystathione lyase (cystathionase) and releases cysteine and α-ketobutyrate.

iii. **Amphibolic intermediates:** When there is a need for energy and not for cysteine, homocysteine can be directly degraded by homocysteine desulfhydrase to α-ketobuty-rate, NH_3 and H_2S (Fig. 13.49). α-Ketobutyrate, in turn, is oxidatively decarboxylated to form propionyl CoA which is further catabolized via methylmalonyl CoA and is finally converted to succinyl CoA.

CYSTINE

Cystine is **dicysteine**, and can be converted to two molecules of cysteine by cystine reductase which requires $NADH^+$ (Fig. 13.50). Due to the deficiency of cystine reductase, cystine may not be converted to cysteine which in turn may also impair its transport from the affected cells.

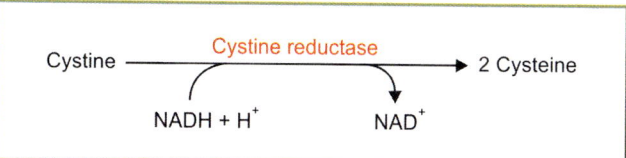

Fig. 13.50: Formation of cysteine from cystine.

CYSTEINE

Cysteine is a glucogenic amino acid. It is required for the synthesis of several proteins, particularly the scleroproteins found in the hair and keratin of nail. Cysteine also helps in maintaining the structure of

protein molecules by forming –S–S–bridges between the peptide chains such as in insulin.

Cysteine, as discussed above, can be synthesized from methionine, hence cysteine is a nonessential amino acid. Methionine thus can spare the requirement of cysteine.

Metabolic Fates of Cysteine

Cysteine may be metabolized by several routes:

1. **Formation of sulfate and active sulfate**
   - Cysteine is oxidized by the enzyme cysteine dioxygenase to form cysteine sulfinate which is decarboxylated to hypotaurine (2-aminoethane sulfate) and oxidized to form taurine.
   - Cysteine sulfinate also undergoes transamination with α-keto-glutaric acid and is converted to bisulfite and pyruvate.
   - In the presence of the hepatic enzyme sulfite oxidase, bisulfite is oxidized to sulfate which is excreted in the urine.
   - Sulfate, in the presence of ATP and the enzyme adenosine phosphosulfate pyrophosphorylase, can also be converted to 3'-phosphoadenosine-5'-phosphosulfate (**PAPS**), also called **active sulfate** (Fig. 13.51), which is used as a source of sulfate group, such as for the formation of sulfate esters of steroids, alcohols and phenols.

2. **Formation of thiocysteine:** Cysteine is also catabolised by cystathionase, which transfers the sulfur from one molecule of cysteine to the other and forms thiocysteine (Fig. 13.52).

3. **Formation of thiosulfate**
   - In the presence of an aminotransferase (cysteine α-ketoglutarate transaminase), cysteine is converted to β-mercaptopyruvate (thiolpyruvate), in the liver.
   - β-Mercaptopyruvate undergoes desulfuration, by the enzyme β-mercaptopyruvate-sulfur transferase, to form pyruvate and thiosulfate (Fig. 13.53) (Chemistry to Clinics 13.14).

4. **Formation of –SH group containing compounds:** Other sulfur containing compounds of physiological importance which can be derived from cysteine include insulin, CoA, glutathione and vasopressin.

Homocysteine versus homocystine: Total plasma homocysteine pool consists of homo-

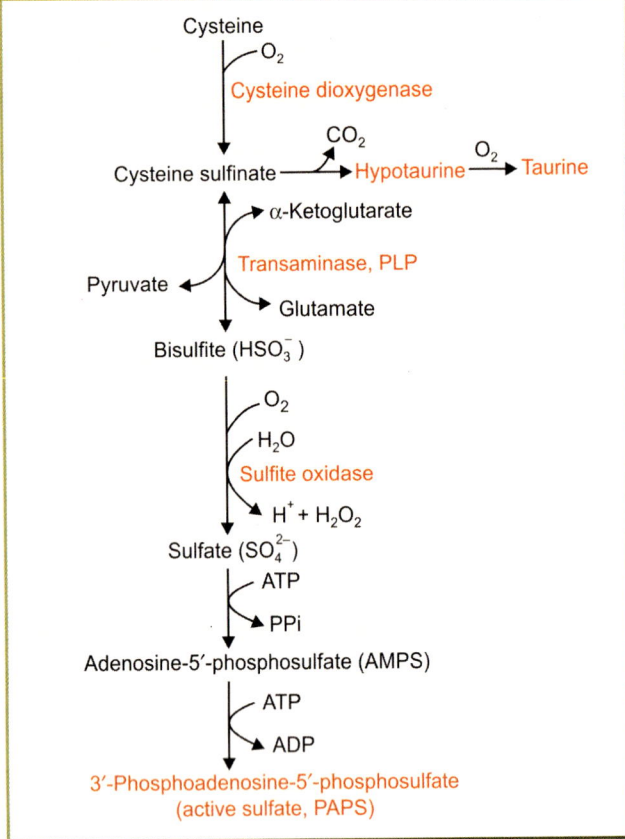

Fig. 13.51: Formation of active sulfate **(PAPS)** from cysteine.

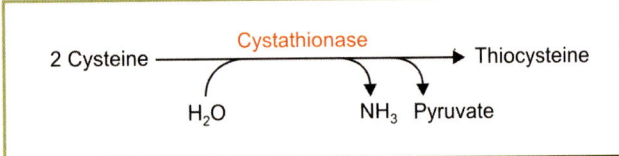

Fig. 13.52: Formation of thiocysteine.

cysteine (containing –SH group, the minor fraction), homocystine (the –S–S– form resulting from auto-oxidation of homocysteine, the major fraction) and mixed disulfides of homocysteine and cysteine.

Inborn Errors of Sulfur-Containing Amino Acids Metabolism

- **Hyperhomocysteinemia:** The disease is an autosomal recessive trait due to genetic deficiency/absence of the enzyme cystathionine-β-synthase in the liver. This, in turn, results in the accumulation of homocysteine in the blood (**hyperhomocysteinemia**) and **homocystinuria**. It is associated

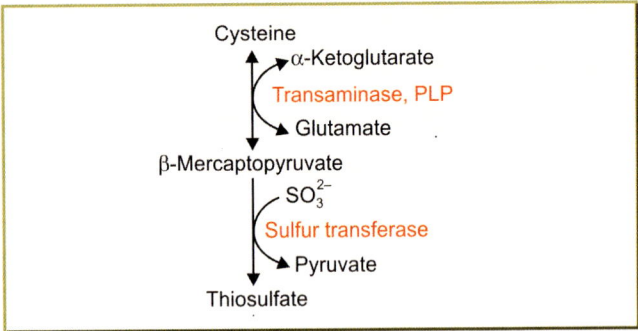

Fig. 13.53: Formation of thiosulfate.

Chemistry to Clinics 13.14: Detoxification of Cyanide

Both thiocysteine and thiosulfate can transfer sulfur to other molecules, such as cyanide ion by an enzyme called rhodanese (Fig. 13.54). This enzyme thus helps in the detoxification of cyanide to thiocyanate by using products of cysteine metabolism.

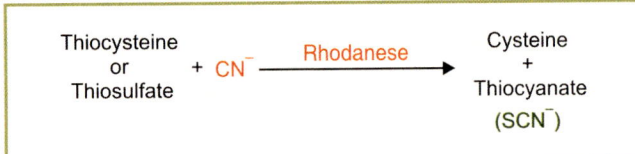

Fig. 13.54: Detoxification of cyanide.

with mental retardation, skeletal deformities involving the spine (vertebra) and thorax, seizures, and dislocation of the lens. There also occurs a defect in the synthesis of collagens since homocysteine may react with and block lysyl groups of collagens. Four different types of metabolic defects may cause homocystinuria:

- **Type I homocystinuria** is due to lack of cystathione-β-synthase and results in thrombosis, osteoporosis, dislocation of lens and mental retardation.
- **Type II homocystinuria** is due to the deficiency of N^5, N^{10}-methylenetetrahydrofolate reductase and can respond to vitamin B_6.
- **Type III homocystinuria** is due to low N^5-methyltetrahydrofolate:homocysteine transmethylase. This results in lack of methylcobalamin and does not respond to vitamin B_6.
- **Type IV homocystinuria** reflects defects in the methylation cycle due to defective intestinal absorption of cobalamin.

Hyperhomocysteinemia may also be an acquired disorder (Chemistry to Clinics 13.15).

Chemistry to Clinics 13.15: Acquired Hyperhomocysteinemia

Homocysteine lies at the junction of methionine and cysteine metabolism, linking the transmethylation and trans-sulfuration pathways (Fig. 13.48). Several B-complex vitamins such as methyl-cobalamin, tetrahydrofolate, pyridoxal phosphate, etc. are required as coenzymes in many of the reactions. Deficiency of any of these vitamins, especially in old age, may result in hyperhomo-cysteinemia. The condition is associated with increased generation of reactive oxygen species causing endothelial cell damage, often the initial event in **atherosclerosis**. It explains the occurrence of atherosclerosis and its complications in patients apparently lacking other risk factors. Further, homocysteine can form homocysteine thiolactone (a highly reactive intermediate) which thiolates free amino groups in LDL and causes their aggregation. These lipid aggregates are endocytosed by the macrophages, forming atheromas. Homocysteine is readily auto-oxidized to homocystine which aggregates due to poor solubility in plasma and causes additional endothelial damage.

- **Hypermethioninemia:** It is caused by the deficiency of methionine adenosyltransferase.
- **Cystathioninuria:** It is due to lack of β-cysta-thionase and results in mental retardation.
- **Cystinuria:** It is a defect of membrane transport of cystine and basic amino acids (lysine, arginine and ornithine). This, in turn, results in their increased renal excretion. Due to its low solubility, cystine results in the formation crystals and renal calculi (Fig. 13.55).
- **Cystinosis:** It is a hereditary disorder characterized by defective carrier-mediated transport of cystine and is thus called **cystine storage disease**. There is an excessive deposition of cystine crystals in various tissues including the kidneys, bone marrow, cornea,

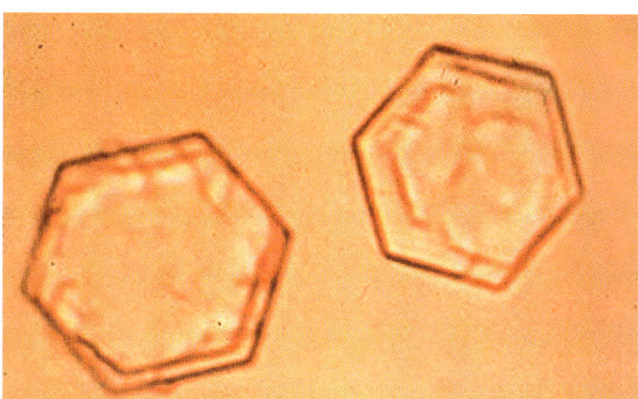

Fig. 13.55: Hexagonal cystine crystals.

conjunctiva and peripheral leukocytes. There is a generalized aminoaciduria, glycosuria and in some cases rickets or osteomalacia. The condition may appear both in children as well as in adults. Cystine crystals may result in loss of kidney function, usually causing renal failure within ten years.

LYSINE

Lysine is an entirely ketogenic amino acid since its carbons enter intermediary metabolism as acetoacetyl CoA. Lysine has two amino groups, referred to as ε- and α-amino groups.

Metabolic Fates of Lysine

1. The predominant pathway for lysine degradation in the liver proceeds via the formation of α-keto-glutarate-lysine adduct called **saccharopine**. In the initial reaction, ε-amino group of lysine conjugates with α-ketoglutarate and forms an intermediate called saccharopine which is then cleaved to glutamate and amino adipic semialdehyde. The reaction is catalyzed by a bifunctional enzyme α-amino adipic semialdehyde synthase, having lysine-α-ketoglutarate reductase activity and saccharopine dehydrogenase activity. The semi-aldehyde is then oxidized to a dicarboxylic amino acid, i.e. α-amino adipate, which through a series of reactions leads to the formation of acetoacetyl CoA (Fig. 13.56).

2. Lysyl residues in certain proteins can also be converted to **carnitine**. In the first step, there occurs trimethylation of ε-amino group of lysine side chain of the protein with S-adenosyl-methionine. The protein is then hydrolyzed to release free trimethyl-lysine which is further metabolized to carnitine.

3. Lysine residues in pro-collagens are modified post-translationally by lysyl oxidase to form **hydroxy-lysine**. The reaction requires vitamin C. The enzyme is inhibited in the disease lathyrism (Chemistry to Clinics 13.16).

Inborn Errors of Lysine Metabolism

- **Hyperlysinuria:** It is a condition where α-amino adipic semialdehyde synthase is deficient. These patients excrete lysine and saccharopine in the urine.

13

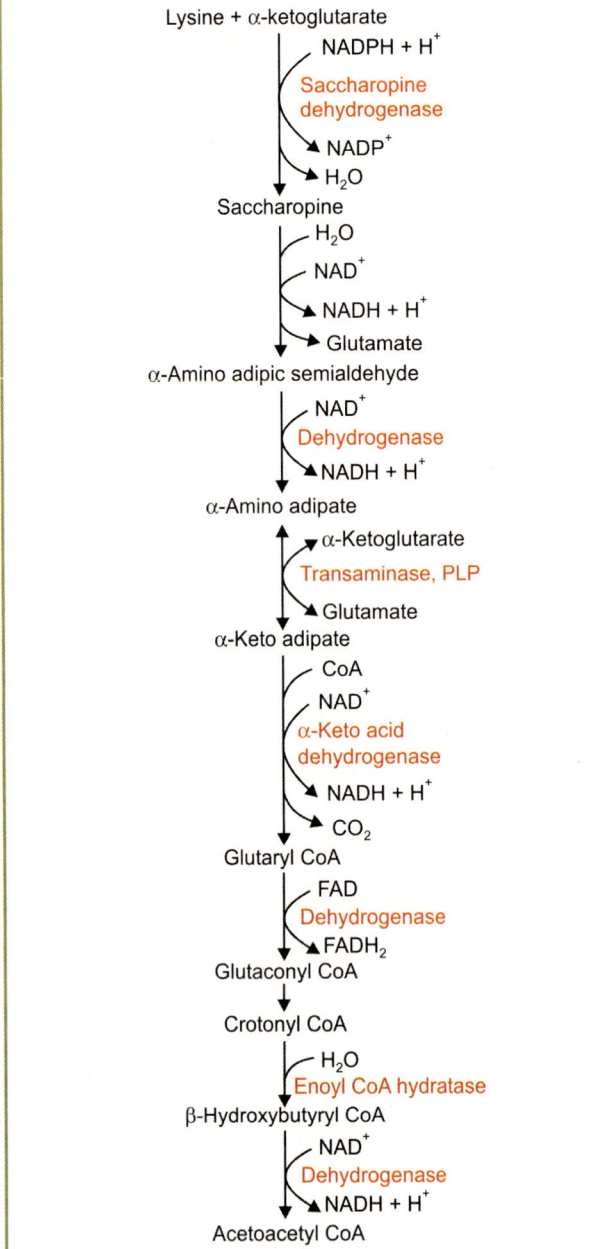

Fig. 13.56: Degradation of lysine.

• **Familial lysinuric protein intolerance:** This is due to failure to transport dibasic amino acids across intestinal mucosa and renal tubular epithelium. Plasma lysine, arginine and ornithine concentrations are reduced. There is marked hyperammonemia after a protein meal. Other features include thin hair, muscle wasting and osteoporosis.

Chemistry to Clinics 13.16: Lathyrism

It is commonly seen in people whose staple diet is the pulse *Lathyrus sativus* (popularly called 'khesari dal'). The pulse, though rich in proteins, contains a toxin called β-oxalyl amino alanine (BOAA) which inactivates lysyl oxidase thereby interfering with the proper maturation of collagens. BOAA also exerts other toxic effects. Patient presents with progressive paralysis of the lower limbs (Fig. 13.57). In the initial stages, besides elimination of the pulse from the diet, the disease is partly reversible with vitamin C supplementation in megadoses of 500–1000 mg daily.

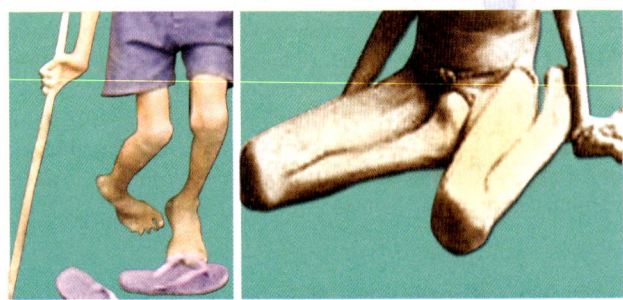

Fig. 13.57: A child crippled by **lathyrism** is forced to use a stick. Later, he may not be able to stand-up even with the help of the stick—the 'crawler' stage.

ARGININE

Arginine is a semiessential amino acid. It becomes essential in the diet when the body cannot meet the requirement, such as during growth, pregnancy and protein catabolic states. On the other hand, it is not essential for a normal adult man. Arginine is a glucogenic amino acid, as end product of arginine degradation is α-ketoglutarate. Production of arginine for protein synthesis occurs from citrulline. In the intestinal mucosa, citrulline is formed from glutamate. Citrulline, in turn, is transported to the kidney to produce arginine.

Metabolic Fates of Arginine

Metabolic fates of arginine are shown in Fig. 13.58.

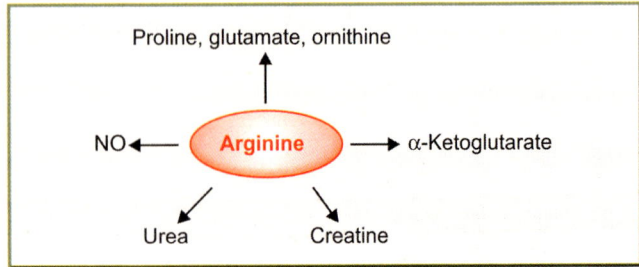

Fig. 13.58: Metabolic fates of arginine.

1. Arginine is formed in the liver via the **urea cycle**. It is catabolized, in the same cycle, by the enzyme arginase which hydrolyzes arginine to urea and ornithine. Genetic deficiency of the enzyme arginase may result in argininemia where plasma arginine level is increased and results in mental retardation.
2. Some of the arginine may also be converted to **proline** as well as to **glutamic acid** by way of ornithine (Fig. 13.59).
3. Arginine is also a source of **nitric oxide (NO)** (Fig. 13.60).
4. Arginine along with glycine and methionine contributes in the synthesis of **creatine**.
5. In the brain, arginine acts as a precursor of **agmatine**, a compound with antihypertensive properties.

Nitric Oxide

The normal vascular tone is maintained by a complex interplay between various vasoconstrictors (such as thromboxanes, angiotensin II and endothelin (Chemistry to Clinics 13.17) and vasodilators (such as prostacyclins, histamine and nitric oxide).

Nitric oxide (NO) was previously called **endo-thelium derived relaxing factor (EDRF)**.

Synthesis: It is a radical synthesized by the five-electron oxidation of amide-nitrogen of arginine, catalyzed by a family of hemoproteins called **nitric oxide synthases** (NOS, Table 13.7). Citrulline is the other reaction product (Fig. 13.60). The reaction requires five cofactors—NADPH, FAD, FMN, heme and tetrahydrobiopterin. Calmodulin, a Ca^{2+}-binding protein, is involved in the control of electron flow. The NOS was the first mammalian protein shown to contain three prosthetic groups (FAD, FMN and heme) in a single polypeptide chain.

Table 13.7: Types of nitric oxide synthases (NOS)

Type	Representation	Predominant location	Ca²⁺-dependent
1	nNOS (neuronal)	Neurons	Yes
2	iNOS (inducible)	Macrophages	No
3	eNOS (endothelial)	Endothelial cells	Yes

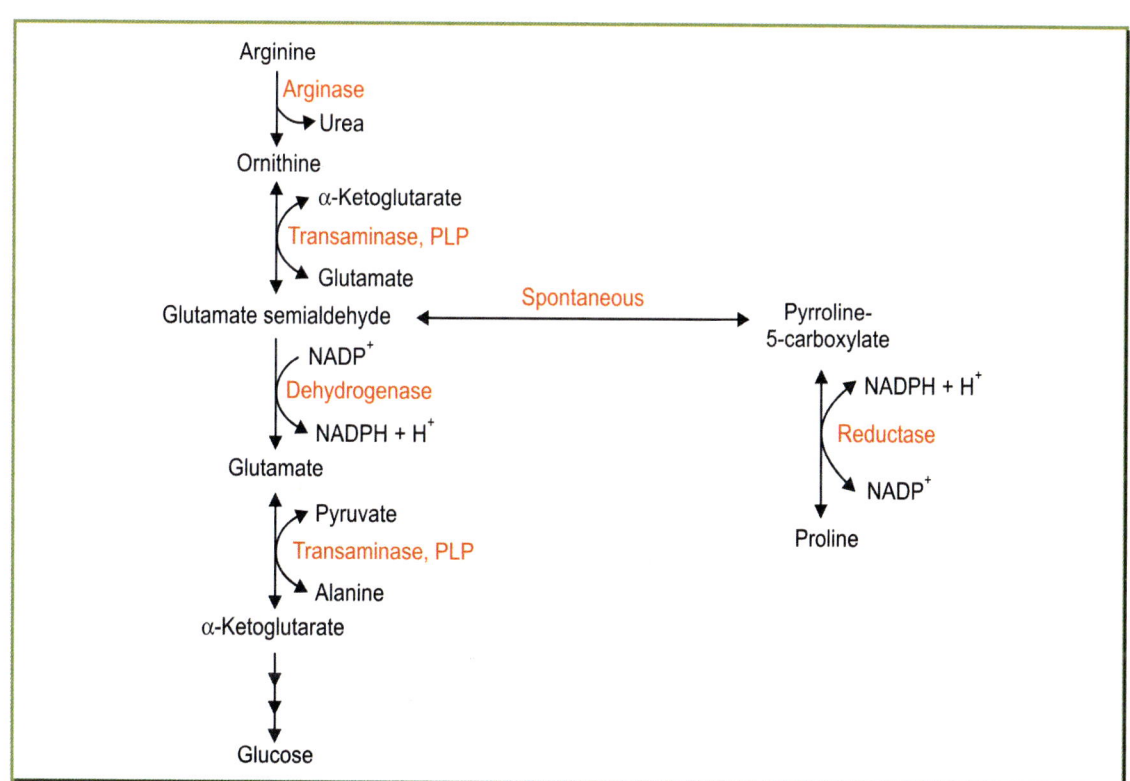

Fig. 13.59: Metabolism of arginine.

Chemistry to Clinics 13.17: Endothelin

Endothelial cells release a 21-amino acid peptide called endothelin, which is the **most potent vasoconstrictor** in the body. The vasoconstriction occurs because of a cascade of events beginning with phospholipase C activation and leading to activation of protein kinase C. Two major types of endothelin receptors have been identified and others may exist. Type A endothelin receptors cause hyperplasia and hypertrophy of vascular muscle cells and the release of NO from endothelial cells. The constrictor function of endothelin is mediated by type B endothelin receptors.

When cardiac tissue is damaged as in myocardial infarction, cardiac endothelial cells increase endothelin production which stimulates both vascular smooth muscle and cardiac muscle to contract more vigorously and induces the growth of surviving cardiac cells. However, excessive stimulation and hypertrophy of cells appear to contribute to heart failure. Further, increased formation of angiotensin II and norepinephrine during chronic heart disease stimulate endothelin production, by enhancing its gene expression. Endothelin also plays a role in renovascular hypertension, atherosclerosis, hypertension associated with insulin resistance as well as the spasmodic contraction of cerebral blood vessels after brain injury or stroke.

Mechanism of action: It is a **gaseous hormone that employs cGMP as its second messenger**.

It acts like a local paracrine hormone. It is synthesized in the vascular endothelial cells and diffuses into the inner layer, i.e. smooth muscle cells. Here it stimulates guanylate cyclase and helps to generate cGMP that in turn stimulates cGMP dependent protein kinases. This ultimately leads to muscle relaxation, i.e. **vasodilatation** (Fig. 13.60).

Biological functions

1. Vasodilatation (Chemistry to Clinics 13.18)
2. Inhibition of platelet aggregation
3. Modulation of neurotransmission
4. Insulin release
5. Immunoenhancer (Chemistry to Clinics 13.19).

However, being a radical, it is a 'double-edged sword'. It combines with superoxide anion free radical to form peroxynitrite, a source of hydroxyl free radicals.

Chemistry to Clinics 13.18: NO Donors

Treatment of angina pectoris (chest pain resulting from spasm of coronary vasculature) is largely based on the use of **'nitrate'** group of drugs (e.g. sorbitrate, monotrate, etc.) which serve as NO donors inside the body and cause vasodilatation (Fig. 13.60).

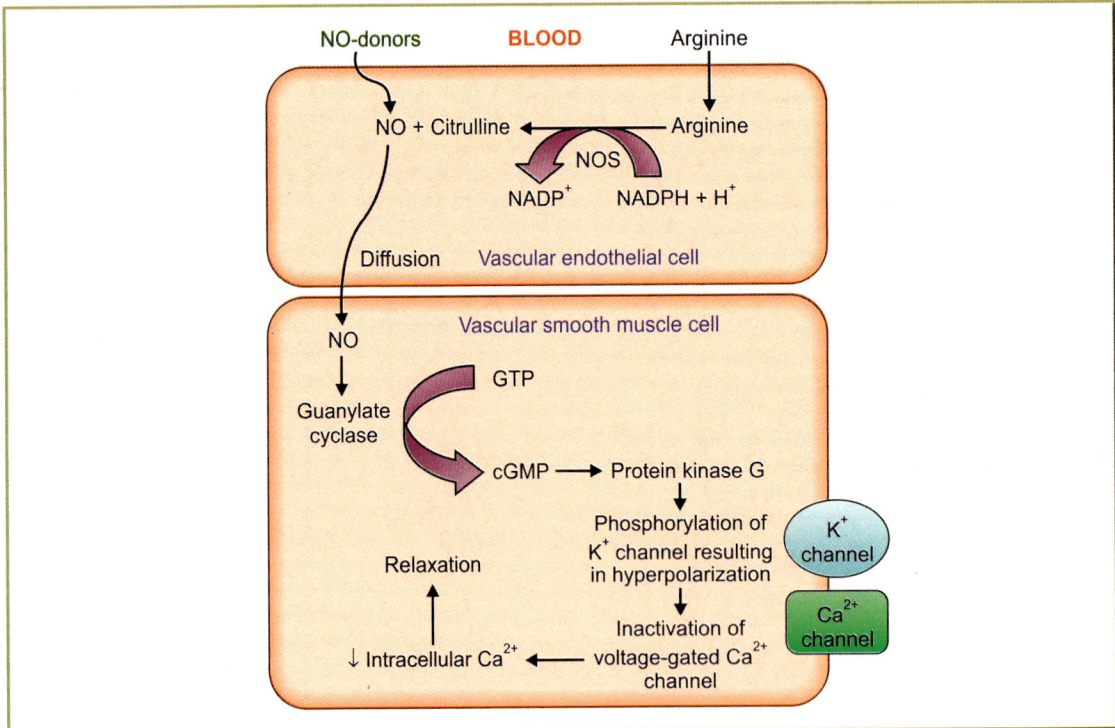

Fig. 13.60: Synthesis and mechanism of action of nitric oxide (NO). The vasomotor tone critically depends on the availability of intracellular Ca^{2+}. The NO-donors, e.g. nitrates are useful in the treatment of angina because they relax the coronary vasculature and alleviate the ischemic pain.

ORNITHINE

Ornithine is a nonessential amino acid not found in proteins.

Metabolic Fates of Ornithine

1. Ornithine by transamination is converted to glutamate-γ-semialdehyde, which is later changed to **glutamate** (Fig. 13.59).
2. Ornithine is a starting material for **urea cycle**. As described earlier, carbamoyl group from carbamoyl phosphate is transferred by the enzyme ornithine transcarbamoylase onto ornithine and forms citrulline (Fig. 13.11).
3. Ornithine is also essential for the biosynthesis of **polyamines**.

Polyamines

Examples: Putrescine, spermidine and spermine.

Synthesis: Ornithine is decarboxylated by the enzyme ornithine decarboxylase and is converted to putrescine. Subsequently, spermidine synthase transfers the propylamine group from S-adeno-

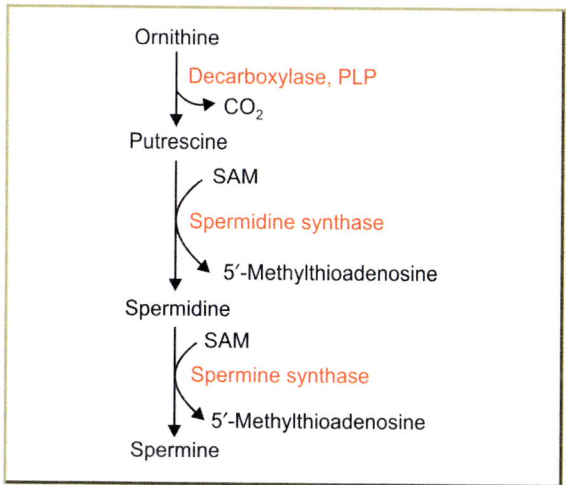

Fig. 13.61: Conversion of ornithine to polyamines.

sylmethionine onto putrescine and forms spermidine. Later, spermine synthase transfers a propylamine group form S-adenosylmethionine and forms spermine (Fig. 13.61). Most of the polyamines required by the body are synthesized by the microflora in the gastrointestinal tract or obtained from the diet, and are carried by the enterohepatic circulation.

Catabolism: These are oxidized to putrescine, and are excreted in the urine.

Properties: Highly cationic molecules that interact with DNA, and are synthesized before mitosis.

Functions
1. Essential growth factors required for regulation of gene expression, cell cycle, cell proliferation and differentiation.
2. Spermidine is also needed in protein synthesis, since butylamino group from spermidine is used for post-translational modification of one of the eukaryotic initiation factors (eIF4D).

HISTIDINE

Histidine is a semiessential amino acid like arginine as it is also essential during growth but nonessential for normal adults. Histidine is glucogenic in nature since it is converted to glutamate and finally through α-ketoglutarate can be converted to glucose. It is also important in one carbon metabolism.

Metabolic Fates of Histidine

1. Histidine **degradation** occurs mainly in the **liver**. The degradative pathway removes free ammonia, and histidine is converted to urocanic acid. The reaction is catalyzed by the enzyme histidase (histidine ammonia lyase, Chemistry to Clinics 13.20). In the next step, there is internal oxidation of the imidazole ring and reduction of the side chain with the addition of water. The reaction is catalyzed by the enzyme urocanase (urocanic acid hydratase) and requires pyridoxal-5-phosphate as a coenzyme. The imidazole ring is then hydrolytically cleaved between the nitrogen-3 and carbon-4 by the enzyme imidazolone propionase (a hydrolase), forming formiminoglutamic acid (FIGLU, Chemistry to Clinics 13.21). In the presence of tetrahydrofolic acid (FH$_4$), glutamate formiminotransferase removes the formimino group as N^5-formiminotetrahydrofolic acid, leaving L-glutamate (Fig. 13.62).

Chemistry to Clinics 13.20: Histidinemia

This hereditary disorder of histidine metabolism is due to deficiency of the enzyme histidase (histidine ammonia lyase), that converts histidine to urocanate. The enzyme is present in the skin which produces urocanate as a constituent of sweat. Due to lack of histidase, urocanate is not found in the sweat. There are elevated levels of histidine in the plasma and the urine. Some histidine may be diverted to the alternative pathway and other metabolites of histidine, i.e. imidazole pyruvate, imidazole lactate and imidazole acetate which are excreted in the urine. Besides speech defects during childhood, there is slowing of mental development. Histidine deficiency can be confirmed either by the enzyme assay in skin biopsies or by the absence of urocanate in the sweat.

Chemistry to Clinics 13.21: FIGLU Excretion Test

Formiminoglutamate (FIGLU), is an intermediate in histidine degradation (Fig. 13.62). Its formimino group is transferred to tetrahydrofolate and glutamate is produced. In patients with folate deficiency, this reaction is impaired and FIGLU is excreted in the urine. This is a diagnostic test of folate deficiency, after a test dose of histidine.

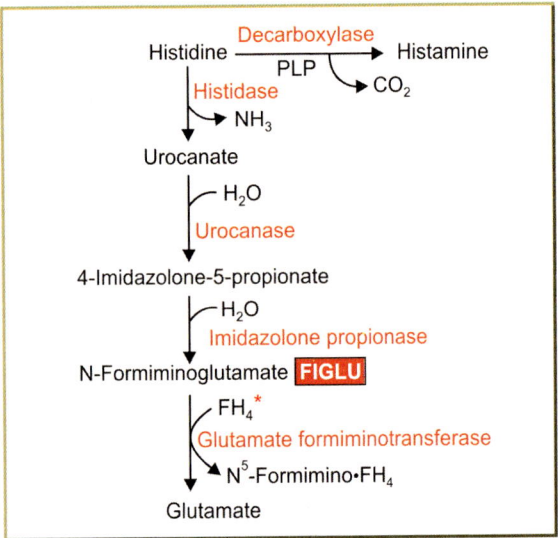

Fig. 13.62: Metabolism of histidine. *Site of block in folate deficiency.

2. Decarboxylation of histidine forms **histamine**.

   Histamine is synthesized at a significant rate in the fetal and the regenerating liver and in the healing skin wounds. Histamine is a pharmacologically active compound. It is a vasodilator, reduces blood pressure and a stimulant of gastric juice secretion. Allergic reactions increase liberation of histamine from mast cells.

   Histamine is converted to β-imidazole acetic acid by the enzyme histaminase and is excreted in the urine. Histaminase is found in most tissues but is particularly rich in lungs.

3. Histidine is a **constituent of dipeptides carnosine** (β-alanylhistidine) and **anserine** (β-alanyl-methyl-histidine) which are found in the muscle and brain. They act as intracellular antioxidants and buffers.

Pregnancy Associated Histidinuria: During pregnancy, from about fifth week until a few days post-partum, large amounts of histidine are excreted in the urine. It is probably a natural phenomenon associated with the deficiency of enzyme histidase in the liver during this period. This may be to meet the additional requirement of histidine during fetal growth. The pregnancy associated histidinuria is not observed in toxemia of pregnancy.

PROLINE

Proline is a nonessential amino acid, predominantly found in collagen. Nearly 15 to 30% of the collagen residues are proline. It can be synthesized in the body from glutamate. Conversion of glutamate to proline involves reduction of the γ-carboxylic group of glutamate to glutamate semialdehyde. This cyclizes spontaneously forming a Schiff base which is then reduced by NADPH to proline (Fig. 13.63).

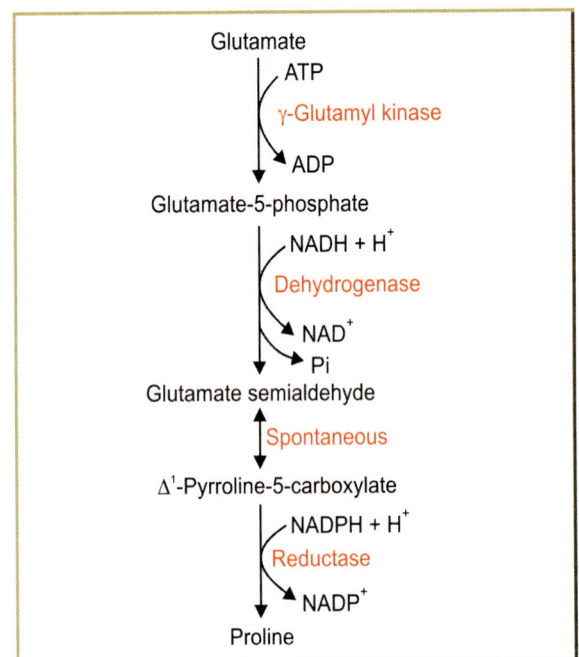

Fig. 13.63: Synthesis of proline from glutamate.

Metabolic Fates of Proline

1. Proline is converted via the Schiff base intermediate to **glutamate** (Fig. 13.64).

2. Proline via glutamate semialdehyde can also be converted to **ornithine** (Fig. 13.64).

3. By post-translational modification, proline residues, after their incorporation into a protein (e.g. collagen), are hydroxylated to **hydroxyproline**. The reaction is catalyzed by prolyl hydroxylase and requires vitamin C (Fig. 13.65).

SYNTHESIS OF SPECIALIZED PRODUCTS FROM AMINO ACIDS

CREATINE

Creatine is present in the muscle, liver, kidney and brain. It is synthesized from **glycine, arginine and methionine** (Fig. 13.66).

1. Firstly, guanidine group of arginine is transferred to glycine, to form guanidoacetic acid. The reaction is catalyzed by arginine glycine transamidinase in the **kidney**.

2. Guanidoacetate methyl transferase transfers a methyl group from S-adenosylmethionine forming creatine. This reaction occurs in the **liver**.

3. Creatine enters the blood and transported to **muscles and brain** where it is taken up by a specific transporter called 'sodium and chloride-dependent creatine transporter 1' (encoded by *SLC6A8* gene: 'Solute carrier family 6, member 8').

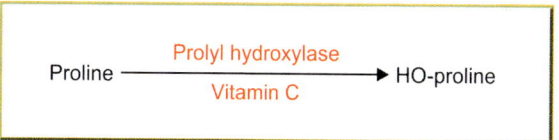

Fig. 13.65: Hydroxylation of proline.

Chemistry to Clinics 13.22: Creatine Deficiency

Recently, creatine deficiency disorders have been identified due to deficiency of arginine glycine transamidinase or guanidoacetate methyl transferase or mutated *SLC6A8*. Due to the importance of creatine phosphate in muscles and brain, the disease is characterized by muscular weakness and neurological impairment. The therapeutic benefit of creatine supplementation is being explored.

4. A high energy phosphate group is transferred from ATP and **creatine phosphate** is formed, catalyzed by creatine kinase (CK), reversibly (Chemistry to Clinics 13.22).

Importance of Creatine Phosphate

1. Creatine phosphate is the form in which high energy phosphate is stored in the muscles. It is a **phosphagen**. During exercise, ATP is used as a source of energy and is converted to ADP. During resting conditions, creatine phosphate is utilized to phosphorylate this ADP while creatine is released as creatinine. The reaction is called Lohmann reaction and is catalyzed by creatine kinase. It is a reversible reaction which can also lead to the synthesis of creatine phosphate from creatine and ATP.

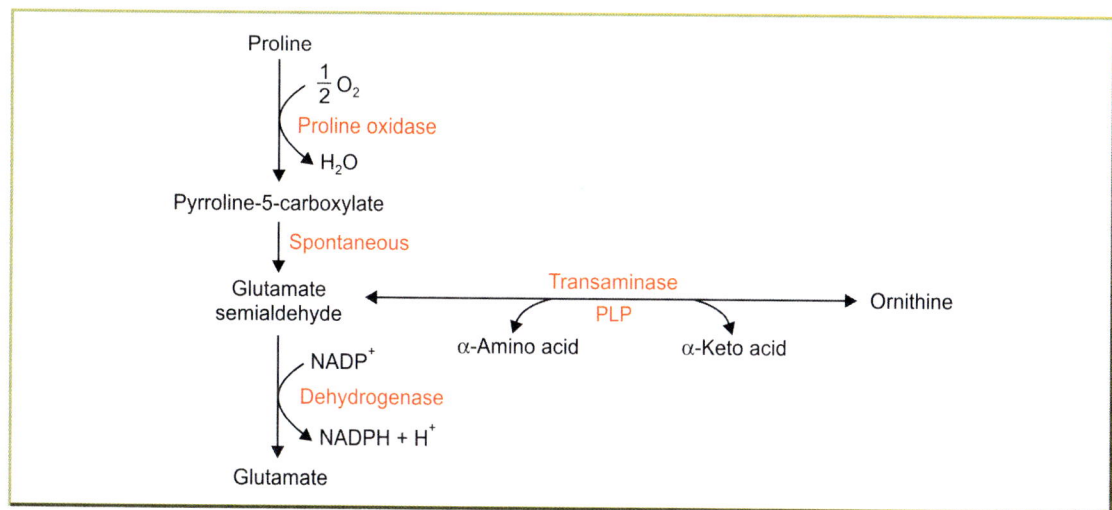

Fig. 13.64: Conversion of proline to glutamate.

13

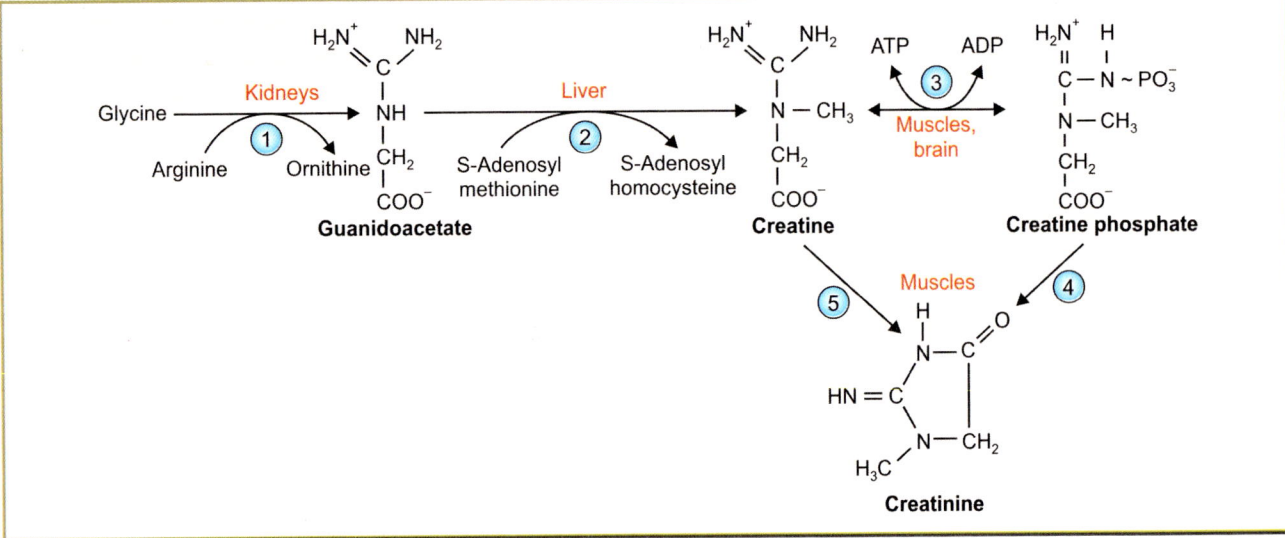

Fig. 13.66: Synthesis of creatine and creatinine. 1. Arginine glycine transamidinase **(kidneys)**, 2. Guanidoacetate methyl transferase **(liver)**, 3. Creatine kinase, CK **(muscles**, brain), 4. Non-enzymatic, spontaneous dehydration + dephosphorylation + cyclization (muscles), 5. Non-enzymatic, spontaneous dehydration + cyclization (muscles).

2. Only traces of creatine are normally present in the urine. Large quantities may be excreted in muscular dystrophies, during starvation and pregnancy.

Creatine versus creatinine: Creatinine is the **anhydride** form of creatine. It is formed in the muscle from creatine or creatine phosphate by a non-enzymatic reaction, irreversibly (Fig. 13.66).

Importance of Creatinine

1. Creatinine is one of the major **non-protein nitrogenous** excretory products after urea (others include uric acid, ammonia and traces of amino acids). Nearly 1.0–1.5 g of creatinine is excreted in the urine in 24 hours.
2. Its total excretion is independent of the amount of dietary protein but is related to **muscle mass**.
3. Serum creatinine as well as the amount of creatinine excreted by an individual remains constant from day-to-day and by calculating creatinine clearance one can **determine the renal function in terms of glomerular filtration rate**.

GLUTATHIONE

Glutathione (γ-glutamylcysteinylglycine) is a **tripeptide** synthesized by formation of the dipeptide γ-glutamylcysteine and the subsequent addition of

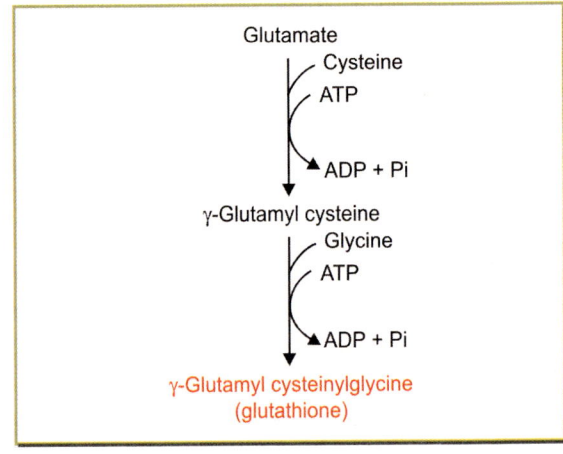

Fig. 13.67: Synthesis of glutathione.

glycine. Both the reactions require activation of carboxyl groups by ATP (Fig. 13.67). Synthesis of glutathione is largely regulated by the availability of cysteine.

Functions of Glutathione

1. Glutathione, as **antioxidant/reductant**, is important in maintaining **stability of erythrocyte membrane**.
2. **Conjugation** of various endogenous (e.g. bilirubin) and exogenous compounds (xenobiotics, e.g. drugs) by glutathione renders them more water-soluble for excretion.

3. It is involved in **group translocation of amino acids** across cell membrane through γ-glutamyl cycle.

4. It is a part of some **leukotriene** structures.

5. It is a cofactor for some **enzymatic reactions**.

6. It aids in the **rearrangement of protein disulfide bonds**.

SOME IMPORTANT QUESTIONS

1. Outline urea cycle. What is the site of urea synthesis? What is the need for urea synthesis in the body?

2. Describe various processes of the removal of ammonia from amino acids.

3. How is ammonia detoxified in our body? Outline the reactions involved in this process.

4. Explain how tyrosine is metabolized and mention the biologically important compounds formed from it.

5. What are essential amino acids? Name them. Describe various fates of phenylalanine in the body.

6. Describe digestion of proteins and absorption of amino acids.

7. Name enzymes and coenzymes of the following reactions:
   i. Synthesis of carbamoyl phosphate
   ii. Conversion of phenylalanine to tyrosine.

8. Name important biologically active compounds derived from:
   i. Glutamic acid
   ii. Tryptophan
   iii. Tyrosine
   iv. Glycine

9. Discuss briefly:
   i. Biosynthesis of creatine
   ii. Synthesis and functions of catecholamines
   iii. Transamination and its importance
   iv. Metabolic fates of carbon skeletons of amino acids
   v. Hyperhomocysteinemia
   vi. FIGLU

10. Write notes on:
   i. Alkaptonuria
   ii. Catabolism of tyrosine
   iii. Phenylketonuria
   iv. Hartnup's disease
   v. Deamination
   vi. Hyperammonemia
   vii. Glucose alanine cycle
   viii. GABA
   ix. Malignant carcinoid syndrome
   x. Maple syrup urine disease
   xi. Active methionine
   xii. Nitric oxide
   xiii. Polyamines
   xiv. Lathyrism
   xv. Primary hyperoxaluria

MULTIPLE CHOICE QUESTIONS

13

1. The following is a purely glucogenic amino acid:
   A. Isoleucine
   B. Leucine
   C. Tyrosine
   D. Methionine

2. In each urea molecule, the two nitrogen atoms are derived from:
   A. One from ammonia, one from aspartate
   B. One from ammonia, one from arginine
   C. Both from ammonia
   D. Both from glutamine

3. Deficiency of glycine cleavage complex leads to the following *except:*
   A. Hyperglycinemia
   B. Mental retardation
   C. Ketosis
   D. Death during infancy

4. Rapid neuronal death during stroke is due to increased flux of the following ions through NMDA receptors:
   A. Na^+
   B. K^+
   C. Ca^{2+}
   D. Mg^{2+}

5. Parkinson's disease is characterized by decreased neuronal synthesis of:
   A. Acetyl choline
   B. Dopamine
   C. DOPA
   D. Serotonin

6. Hepatorenal tyrosinemia is due to a deficiency of:
   A. Tyrosine aminotransferase
   B. Homogentisate oxidase
   C. Tyrosinase
   D. Fumaryl acetoacetate hydrolase

7. Increased urinary 5-hydroxy indole acetic acid (5-HIAA) occurs in tumors secreting:
   A. Melanin
   B. Serotonin
   C. Catecholamines
   D. VIP

8. In maple syrup urine disease, the typical odor of urine is due to:
   A. Branched chain amino acids
   B. Branched chain keto acids
   C. Branched chain amino acid acyl CoA
   D. Unsaturated branched chain acyl CoA

9. The second messenger for nitric oxide is:
   A. cAMP
   B. cGMP
   C. Ca^{2+}
   D. DAG

10. Daily urinary creatinine excretion is:
    A. 0.1–0.5 g
    B. 0.5–1.0 g
    C. 1.0–1.5 g
    D. 1.5–2.0 g

14

Metabolic Integration

Metabolic fuels (carbohydrates, lipids and proteins), as discussed earlier, are broken-down to as well as built up from smaller units such as glucose, fatty acids and amino acids by several metabolic pathways.

The **central theme of metabolism** is:

1. To extract energy from food.
2. Store the excess energy for future needs.
3. To maintain tissue proteins for performing various vital functions.

The body uses glucose and fatty acids as the primary fuels to obtain energy. Only under dire circumstances, amino acids are used for this purpose. Glucose can be obtained from other carbohydrates, glucogenic amino acids and the 'glycerol' portion of fat. To synthesize tissue proteins, amino acids are required. Although glucose can be channelized to make some nonessential amino acids, fat cannot serve this purpose. When energy consumed is in surplus, the body converts all the three major nutrients into stored fat.

METABOLISM OF FUEL

Carbohydrates: Glucose is stored in the body tissues, mainly in the liver and the muscle, as glycogen (glycogenesis) when blood glucose concentration is high, such as after meal. On the other hand, when blood glucose concentration is reduced, liver glycogen is degraded to release glucose (glycogenolysis). Metabolic oxidation (degradation) of glucose, called glycolysis, converts glucose to pyruvate. Besides, mammals can synthesize glucose from a variety of noncarbohydrate precursors through a series of reactions by the process of gluconeogenesis (Fig. 14.1).

Lipids: Fatty acids are released from triacylglycerols and are broken-down through β-oxidation to acetyl CoA which also serves as substrate for the synthesis of fatty acids (Fig. 14.2).

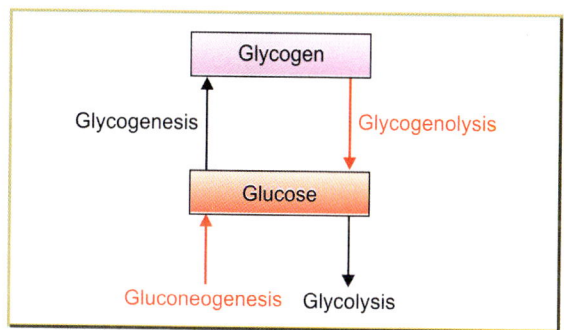

Fig. 14.1: Metabolism of carbohydrates.

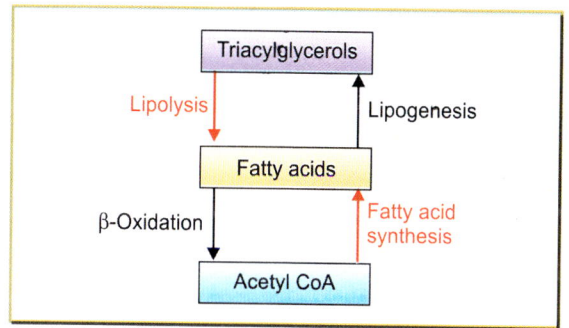

Fig. 14.2: Metabolism of triacylglycerols.

14

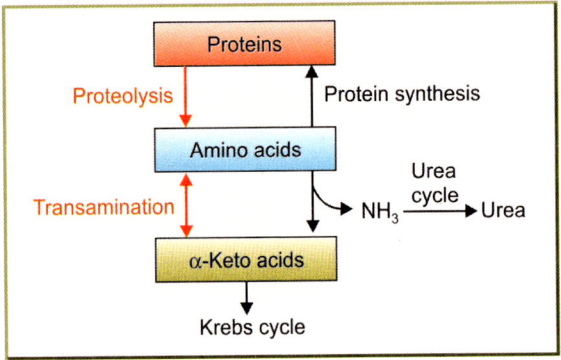

Fig. 14.3: Metabolism of proteins.

are degraded to intermediates of glycolysis and citric acid cycle while their amino group is eliminated from the body, mainly through urea cycle, as urea. On the other hand, nonessential amino acids can be formed in the body from various metabolic intermediates of the Krebs cycle (Fig. 14.3).

Key intermediates of the various catabolic processes (pyruvate and acetyl CoA) are oxidized via Krebs cycle. Coupled with the process of oxidative phosphorylation, these catabolites yield ATP.

Proteins: These are catabolized by various proteolytic enzymes to amino acids which are also used for protein synthesis by the body. Excess of amino acids

METABOLIC CHANGES IN THE ABSORPTIVE STATE

The salient features of the response of the major tissues involved in energy metabolism in the absorptive state (Fig. 14.4) include:

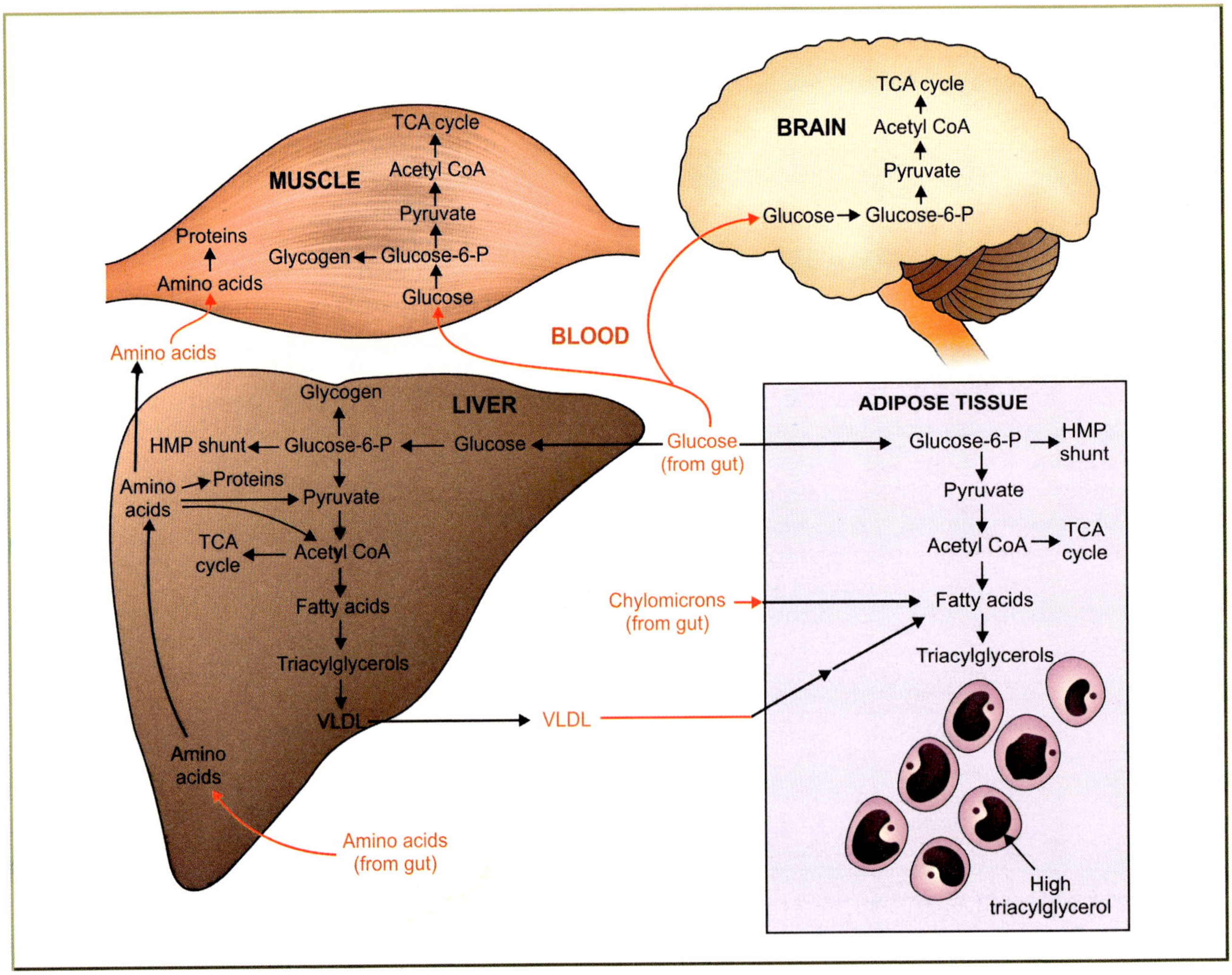

Fig. 14.4: Metabolic integration in the absorptive state.

1. The body **stores surplus energy** as:
   a. **Glycogen** in liver and muscles.
   b. **Triacylglycerol** in liver and adipose tissue.
2. **HMP shunt** is active and provides reducing power (NADPH, for reductive biosynthesis) as well as pentoses.
3. Amino acids are mainly channelized to **build tissue proteins**.
4. The **brain** utilizes **glucose** as an obligatory fuel.

METABOLIC CHANGES DURING STARVATION

Starvation may be a result of the nonavailability of food, desire to lose weight or due to certain clinical conditions, such as trauma, surgery or cancer where an individual cannot consume food (Chemistry to Clinics 14.1).

Starvation, in general, not only causes a large total weight as well as fat loss but also a substantial loss of body proteins. These changes are accompanied with the **production of ketone bodies**. Various metabolic changes, however, vary with the period of fast and can be divided into **three stages**:

Intraprandial phase: This is the early stage of starvation, the **period between meals** in a normal day. This begins 4–5 hours after a meal. After tissues take up and metabolize glucose, blood glucose concentration decreases. This, in turn:

- Stimulates the release of glucagon by the pancreas. Glucagon promotes glycogen breakdown in the liver and releases glucose. It also promotes gluconeogenesis from lactate and amino acids. The effect of glucagon thus is reverse to that of insulin.

Chemistry to Clinics 14.1: Anorexia Nervosa

Anorexia nervosa is a severe form of starvation characterized by disruption in eating behavior. This is a life-threatening psychiatric illness, found principally among adolescent girls. A person with anorexia nervosa does not eat adequate amount of food. This disease is difficult to treat successfully, particularly if diagnosis is delayed and can result in tragic death from starvation.

This mental attitude may be due to over-reaction to mild obesity, fashion cult of dieting and early menarche. Adrenal abnormality may also be a component of this condition. Nearly half of the individuals with anorexia nervosa develop **bulimia nervosa**. This is a condition, alternative to the restriction of dietary intake where some of the individuals vomit most of their food, soon after ingestion.

The reciprocal effects of the two hormones ensure that the concentration of glucose available to the extrahepatic tissues remains relatively constant.

- A fall in the circulating concentration of insulin also results in the release of free fatty acids from triacylglycerols in the adipose tissue. Peripheral muscles and adipose tissue consume progressively less glucose and switch-over to fatty acids as the main source of energy.

Postabsorptive phase: This is the second stage of starvation, i.e. the period of **overnight fast** which may vary from 12 to 24 hours. The quantity of glycogen stored in the liver, normally, cannot maintain blood glucose concentration beyond 18 hours. After liver glycogen stores begin to deplete, other metabolic changes ensure continuous supply of glucose for the brain and other tissues:

- The body begins to synthesize glucose by the process of **gluconeogenesis** from other sources, such as lactate, pyruvate, glycerol (obtained from triacylglycerols) and glucogenic amino acids.
- Amino acids for gluconeogenesis are received by the liver as a result of proteolysis of tissue proteins, mainly in the liver and muscle.
- Deamination of amino acids in the liver forms α-keto acids, such as pyruvate, oxaloacetate or some other intermediates of the citric acid cycle which are then converted to glucose by the reversal of glycolysis. Although some of the liver proteins can be used for gluconeogenesis, the main store of protein is the muscle.
- Amino acids are released, from muscle, mainly as alanine which serves as an effective substrate for hepatic gluconeogenesis. In the muscle, alanine is synthesized by transamination of pyruvate with the help of branched chain amino acids. Pyruvate is produced there either from glucose-6-phosphate via glycolysis or from the catabolism of various amino acids.

Prolonged starvation: After starvation is prolonged **beyond 48 hours**, metabolic processes are readjusted and body conserves protein. This is due to the reason that extensive depletion of body protein can severely affect several tissues. If more than one-third of the body protein is lost it may even result in death. At this stage:

14

- Glucose production is reduced to the extent that liver glucose output falls to nearly one-third.
- As the supply of glucose falls short, all tissues use fatty acids as the main source of energy. Concentration of carnitine also increases which, in turn, increases the activity of carnitine acyltransferase I and promotes β-oxidation of large quantities of fatty acids. This increases the production of acetyl CoA to the extent that it cannot be oxidized in the citric acid cycle. At the same time, on account of the conservation of glucose, synthesis of oxaloacetate from pyruvate is also greatly reduced. As a result, ketogenesis is stimulated and plasma concentration of ketone bodies is increased by more than 5 folds.

- **Ketone bodies released into the blood are used by many tissues, such as heart and skeletal muscle. Even the brain switches over to the use of ketone bodies as a source of energy**.
- Increased oxidation of ketone bodies (keto acids, i.e. acetoacetate and β-hydroxybutyrate), in turn, reduces plasma bicarbonate concentration and leads to compensated metabolic acidosis. Increased levels of keto acids also necessitates increased excretion of H^+, hence NH_4^+ excretion is also increased.
- Reduced mobilization of muscle protein also reduces nitrogen excretion which results in decreased production and excretion of urea as well as other non-protein nitrogenous (NPN)

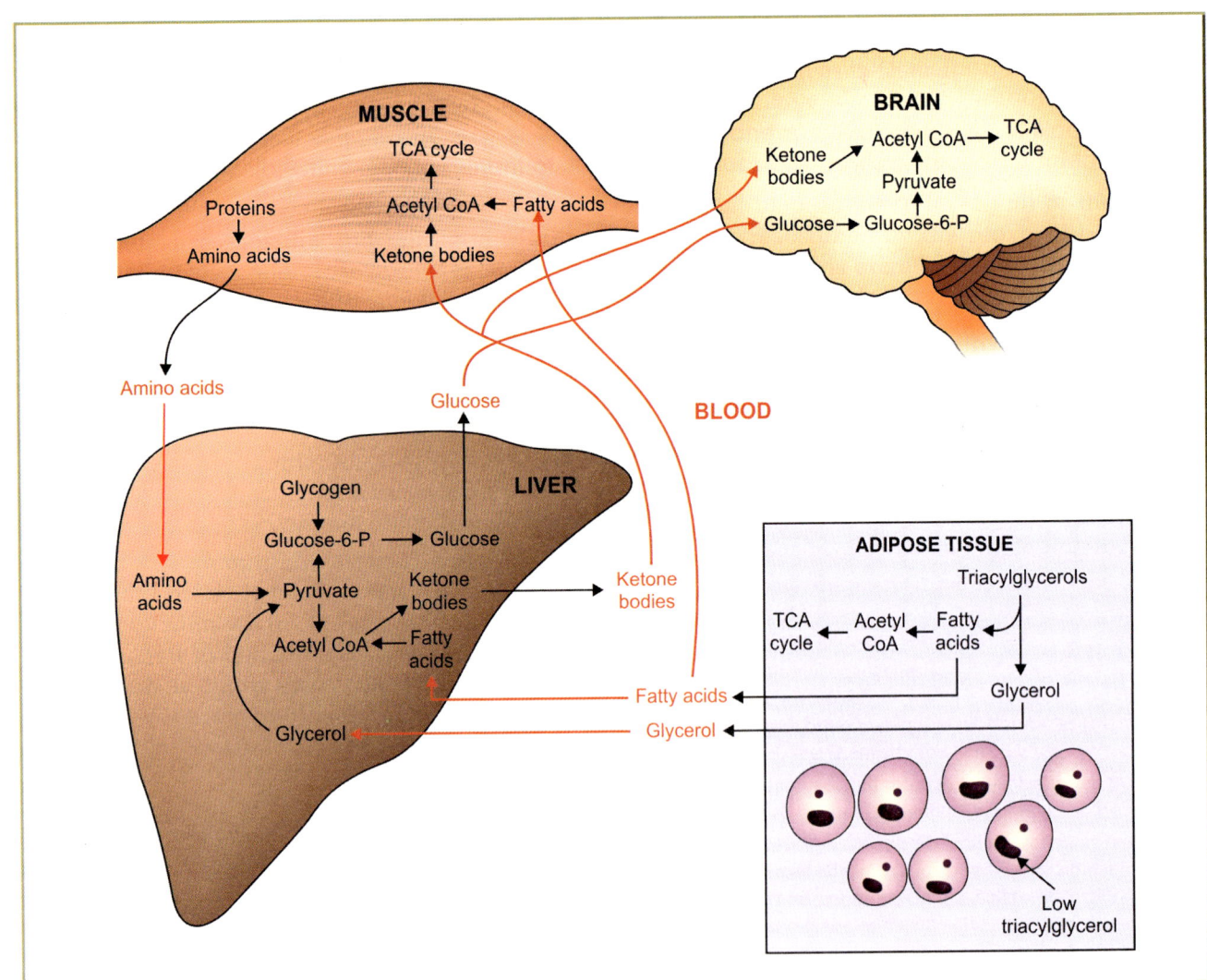

Fig. 14.5: Metabolic integration during starvation.

Table 14.1. Energy metabolism in various organs

Organ	Energy reservoir	Preferred substrate	Energy source exported
Liver	Glycogen, triacylglycerol	Amino acids, glucose, fatty acids	Fatty acids, glucose, ketone bodies
Adipose tissue	Triacylglycerol	Fatty acids	Fatty acids, glycerol
Resting skeletal muscle	Glycogen	Fatty acids	–
Exercising skeletal muscle	–	Glucose	Lactate
Heart muscle	Glycogen	Fatty acids	–
Brain	–	Glucose (ketone bodies during starvation)	–

substances from the kidney. Decreased excretion of urea also leads to reduced excretion of water and results in reduced urine volume.

- Hepatic protein synthesis is considerably reduced. Hypoalbuminemia results in water retention (edema).

Response of major tissues involved in energy metabolism during starvation is summarized in Fig. 14.5.

Energy metabolism in various organs is summarized in Table 14.1.

SOME IMPORTANT QUESTIONS

1. Discuss metabolic integration in different tissues during various stages of starvation.

2. Write notes on:
   i. Metabolic changes in the absorptive state.
   ii. Anorexia nervosa.

MULTIPLE CHOICE QUESTIONS

1. In a healthy 70 kg man, the fat content in adipose tissue is:
   A. 5 kg
   B. 15 kg
   C. 25 kg
   D. 35 kg

2. The preferred fuel substrate for adipose tissue is:
   A. Glucose
   B. Fatty acids
   C. Amino acids
   D. Ketone bodies

3. The preferred fuel substrate for exercising skeletal muscle is:
   A. Glucose
   B. Fatty acids
   C. Amino acids
   D. Ketone bodies

4. During exercise, the following is released from muscles into the circulation:
   A. Glucose
   B. Ketone bodies
   C. Lactate
   D. Glycerol

5. During starvation, the following is released from muscles into the circulation:
   A. Glucose
   B. Ketone bodies
   C. Glycerol
   D. Branched chain amino acids

Metabolism of Hemoglobin

Heme, the prosthetic group of hemoproteins, consists of one atom of ferrous ion (Fe^{2+}) and a tetrapyrrole ring called protoporphyrin IX. It though is synthesized in all mammalian tissues, its synthesis however, is most pronounced in the bone marrow and the liver because of the requirement for its incorporation into hemoglobin and cytochromes, respectively.

BIOSYNTHESIS OF HEME

In the biosynthesis of heme, **four pyrrole rings need to be formed separately** (Fig. 15.1). The organic portion of heme is derived from eight residues each of glycine and succinyl CoA. Some of the reactions occur in the mitochondria while others (the intermediate steps) take place in the cytosol (Fig. 15.2).

1. In the first step, succinyl CoA (an intermediate of the Krebs cycle) condenses with glycine and forms δ-aminolevulinic acid (ALA), in the mitochondria. The reaction is catalyzed by δ-aminolevulinic acid synthase (ALA synthase, E1) which requires pyridoxal phosphate (PLP) as a coenzyme. This is the **rate-limiting step** of heme synthesis. The enzyme is synthesized in the cytosol and is incorporated into matrix of the mitochondria.

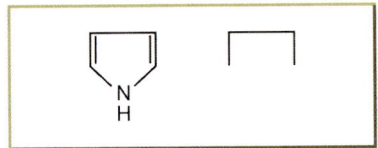

Fig. 15.1: A pyrrole ring, represented as an open rectangle for simplicity.

2. In the next step, two molecules of ALA condense asymmetrically and form porphobilinogen. This reaction is catalyzed by aminolevulinic acid dehydratase (ALA dehydratase, E2), a zinc containing enzyme present in the cytosol. It consists of eight subunits, four of which interact with the substrate. ALA dehydratase is sensitive to heavy metals, particularly **lead**. ALA levels are elevated in lead poisoning.

3. Porphobilinogen undergoes deamination by porphobilinogen deaminase (hydroxymethylbilane synthase or uroporphyrinogen I synthase, E3) and forms a linear tetrapyrrole, called hydroxymethylbilane.

4. With the ring closure catalyzed by uroporphyrinogen I co-synthase (E4), hydroxymethylbilane is converted to uroporphyrinogen I. Alternatively, uroporphyrinogen III co-synthase converts hydroxymethylbilane to uroporphyrinogen III.

   Only types I and III are found in nature. Porphyrins with **symmetric** arrangement of the substituent groups on its four rings are classified as **type I** while those with **asymmetric** substitutions are classified as **type III** porphyrins (Fig. 15.3). Under normal conditions, the uroporphyrinogen formed is almost exclusively the type III isomer. Heme is also a type III porphyrin.

5. Uroporphyrinogen I or III is converted to the respective coproporphyrinogen by uroporphyrinogen decarboxylase (E5). The enzyme is inhibited by iron salts.

6. Coproporphyrinogen III enters mitochondria and is converted to protoporphyrinogen IX. The

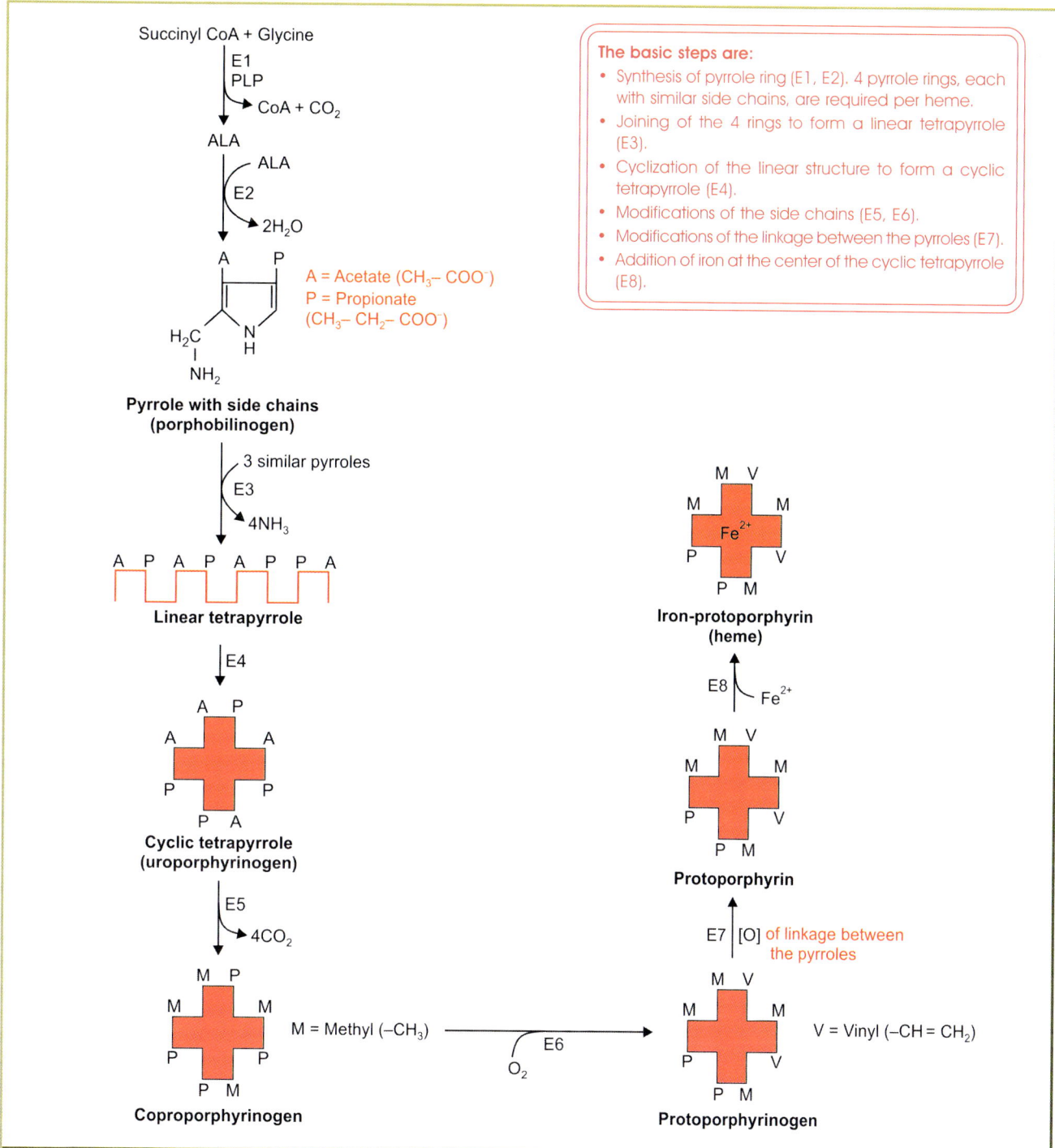

The basic steps are:
- Synthesis of pyrrole ring (E1, E2). 4 pyrrole rings, each with similar side chains, are required per heme.
- Joining of the 4 rings to form a linear tetrapyrrole (E3).
- Cyclization of the linear structure to form a cyclic tetrapyrrole (E4).
- Modifications of the side chains (E5, E6).
- Modifications of the linkage between the pyrroles (E7).
- Addition of iron at the center of the cyclic tetrapyrrole (E8).

Fig. 15.2: Heme biosynthesis.

reaction is catalyzed by coproporphyrinogen oxidase (E6) and requires molecular oxygen. The enzyme does not act on coproporphyrinogen I.

These porphyrins are identified as belonging to **series IX** since they were designated ninth in a series of the postulated isomers.

15

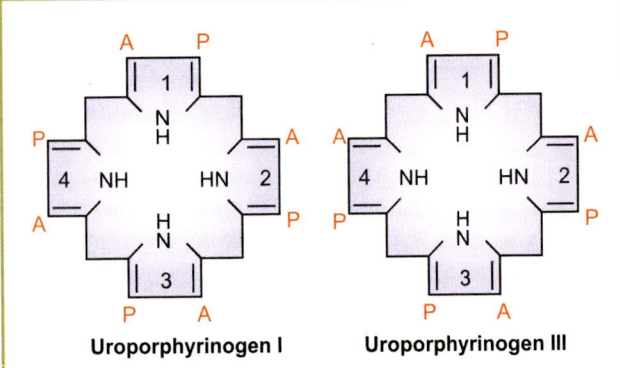

Fig. 15.3: Type I and Type III porphyrinogen.

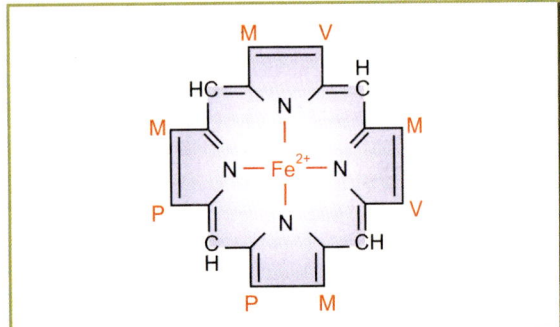

Fig. 15.4: Heme.

7. Protoporphyrinogen oxidase (E7) acts on protopor-phyrinogen IX and converts it to protoporphyrin IX, in the mitochondria. Protoporphyrin IX is water insoluble. Its excessive amounts are excreted by the biliary system into the intestinal tract.

8. In the final step of heme synthesis, ferrous iron (Fe^{2+}) is inserted into the protoporphyrin IX. The reaction is catalyzed by ferrochelatase (E8) which requires reducing substances. The enzyme is sensitive to heavy metals especially **lead**. It is also sensitive to iron deprivation.

   Thus, **heme is an 'iron-centered cyclic tetra-pyrrole'** (Fig. 15.4).

Regulation of Heme Biosynthesis

ALA synthase occurs in two forms, called the **hepatic** (ALA-S1) and the **erythrocytic** (ALA-S2) forms. ALA-S1 controls the rate limiting step of heme synthesis. Further, heme acts both as a repressor of synthesis of the enzyme as well as an inhibitor of its activity.

Salient Features of Porphyrin Biosynthesis

- **'Rule of 8':** Eight molecules each of succinyl CoA and glycine are required to synthesize one heme molecule. Eight enzymes (E1–8) participate in the process, hence eight different porphyrias can occur.
- E1,6,7,8 are mitochondrial, others are cytosolic.
- E1 catalyzes the rate-limiting step; it is repressed by heme (autoregulation) and induced by barbi-turates (sedatives), griseofulvin (antifungal) and alcohol.
- E2 and E8 are sulfhydryl enzymes that can be inhibited by inorganic lead (Chemistry to Clinics 15.1).
- Humans synthesize porphyrins with asymmetric side chains (type III).
- Porphyrin**ogens** are unstable, easily auto-oxidized in presence of light into the corresponding stable porphyr**ins**; however, E7 catalyzes the only known enzymatic conversion of a porphyrinogen to a porphyrin.
- Porphyrinogens are colorless; porphyrins are colored.
- Porphyrins exhibit characteristic absorption spectra with maximum absorbance ('Soret' band) at 400 nm.
- Porphyrins emit purple-red fluorescence upon UV exposure so that small amounts can be detected easily in biological samples.
- Synthetic porphyrins are of clinical interest (Chemistry to Clinics 15.2).

Chemistry to Clinics 15.1: Lead Poisoning

- **Inorganic lead poisoning** is an occupational hazard to workers employed in the battery and paint manufacturing industries. Further, children who are in the habit of scraping and eating wall-paints are also at risk. Inorganic lead binds to sulfhydryl proteins including ALA-dehydratase and ferrochelatase participating in heme biosynthesis, resulting in symptoms of porphyrias (an example of acquired porphyria) as well as anemia. In addition, inorganic lead displaces calcium from its various binding proteins leading to neuromuscular manifestations.
- On the other hand, **organic lead**, i.e. lead tetraethyl is added to petrol where it serves as an 'anti-knock' and protects the automobile engine. The automobile exhaust is thus rich in organic lead and is a health hazard to workers in the automobile industry. Organic lead does not result in porphyria; rather, because of its high affinity for membrane lipids it produces CNS toxicity.

Table 15.1: Types of porphyrias (Deficient enzyme is given in parantheses)

Hepatic porphyrias
- ALA dehydratase deficiency (E2)
- Acute intermittent porphyria (E3)
- Porphyria cutanea tarda (E5)
- Hereditary coproporphyria (E6)
- Variegate porphyria (E7)

Erythropoietic porphyrias
- X-linked sideroblastic anemia (E1)
- Congenital erythropoietic porphyria (E4)
- Erythropoietic protoporphyria (E8)

Chemistry to Clinics 15.2. Photodynamic Therapy

Synthetic porphyrins can be administered to cancer patients whereby they get deposited in the tumor and exert cytotoxicity upon laser exposure (cancer photodynamic therapy), e.g. porfimer used in lung cancer and esophageal cancer.

PORPHYRIAS

Porphyrias are a group of disorders due to abnormalities in the pathway of heme biosynthesis.

These can be genetic or acquired. Based on the site of overproduction, porphyrias are either **'hepatic'** or **'erythropoietic'** or sometimes **'mixed'** (Table 15.1).

Clinical Manifestations and Laboratory Diagnosis

- Deficiency of an enzyme in the heme biosynthetic pathway blocks the distal part of the pathway resulting in reduced heme synthesis. This leads to **de-repression** of ALA synthase (except when this enzyme itself is missing) and the accumulation of proximal metabolites. In fact, clinical manifestations may be triggered by intake of substances that induce ALA synthase, such as alcohol and barbiturates. In general, the clinical and laboratory features depend on whether the defect lies before the cyclization of the tetrapyrrole or after it (the cyclization is catalyzed by E4, i.e. uroporphyrinogen III co-synthase).

- In case of a **pre-cyclization defect**, there are predominantly **neurovisceral** (e.g. acute pain abdomen) and **neuropsychiatric** manifestations. It is attributed to accumulation of ALA and porphobilinogen whose increased levels are found in blood and urine.

- In case of a **post-cyclization defect**, there is enhanced synthesis of the corresponding symmetric as well as asymmetric porphyrinogens. These get converted to their respective porphyrins, which can be detected in the urine/feces. Deposition of excess porphyrins is responsible for **cutaneous** reactions (porphyrins deposited in the skin get excited on UV light exposure) and red-purple fluorescence in tissues/body fluids (Greek 'porphyria' = 'purple') (Fig. 15.5).

Management

- Avoidance of inducers of ALA synthase
- Administration of intravenous dextrose or hematin to suppress ALA synthase
- Administration of β-carotene to suppress skin reactions.

DEGRADATION OF HEME AND METABOLIC FATE OF BILIRUBIN

Degradation of heme leads to the synthesis of bilirubin whose stepwise metabolism is discussed below:

1. **Degradation of heme:** Red blood cells (RBC), as we know, have a limited lifespan of approximately 100–120 days. The senescent cells are recognized by their membrane changes, removed and engulfed by the reticuloendothelial system at the extravascular sites.

   - Degradation of the RBC occurs mainly in the **spleen, bone marrow, liver and lymph glands**. Complete degradation of heme, from hemoglobin, occurs mainly in the liver. If degradation of the RBC occurs in the tissues other than liver, hemoglobin is transported to the liver by means of the haptoglobin.

   - After an aged RBC is recognized by a macrophage, it is rapidly engulfed to form a phagosome. This, in turn, fuses with a primary lysosome and forms a secondary lysosome where cathepsins result in complete degradation of cellular proteins including globin of hemoglobin, to the constituent amino acids which are utilized for general metabolic needs.

   - Heme is released and converted to bile pigments in the endoplasmic reticulum of the cell.

2. **Synthesis of unconjugated bilirubin:** Heme is degraded in the reticuloendothelial cells to a linear tetrapyrrole, **biliverdin IXα** by a microsomal enzyme system designated as **heme oxygenase**

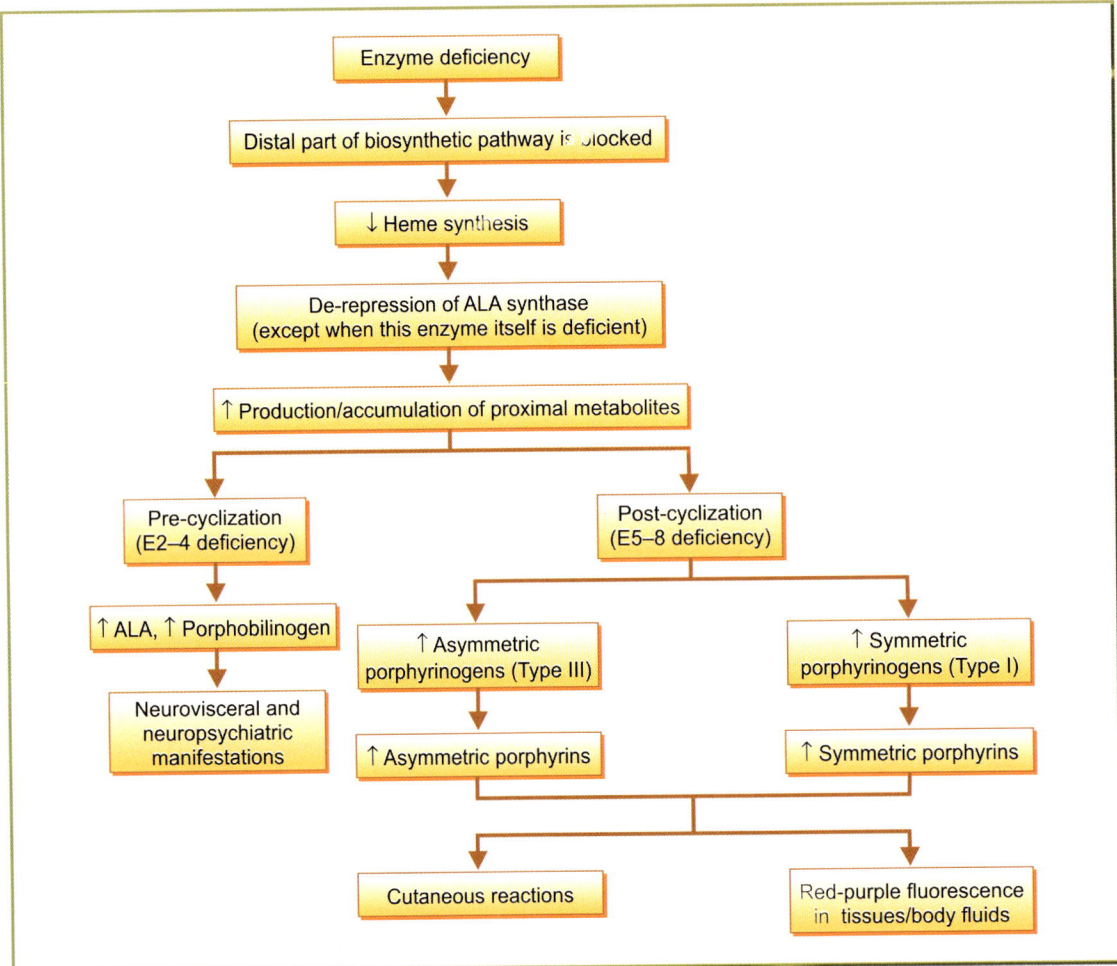

Fig. 15.5: Porphyrias: Biochemical-clinical correlations.

system. The enzyme system requires molecular oxygen and NADPH, and is induced by heme.

- The heme oxygenase system catalyzes the cleavage of the α-methenyl bridge, releasing carbon monoxide (CO) which may be trapped by hemoglobin and eventually exhaled.
- Biliverdin is reduced to **bilirubin** (also called **unconjugated bilirubin**) by biliverdin reductase (Fig. 15.6). One gram of hemoglobin yields about 35 mg of bilirubin.
- Iron released from the porphyrin ring is transferred from the cells by an iron transport protein called transferrin and is made available for the resynthesis of new hemoglobin. Besides the senescent RBC, bilirubin is also derived from the turnover of other heme containing proteins, such as cytochromes.

3. **Transport of unconjugated bilirubin in plasma:** At physiological pH, bilirubin is poorly soluble in an aqueous solution. If RBCs are degraded in the liver, further metabolism of bilirubin occurs *in situ* but bilirubin formed in other tissues is transported to the liver from where it is taken up at the sinusoidal surface of the hepatocytes by a carrier-mediated saturable system.

    Bilirubin, normally present in the blood, is bound to **albumin** and is transported to the liver. Fatty acids, thyroxine and certain drugs (such as aspirin or sulfonamide) **compete** with bilirubin for binding sites on albumin.

4. **Conjugation of bilirubin:** Hepatocytes trap bilirubin by means of a specific binding protein called **protein Y or ligandin** (a family of gluta-thione-S-transferases). Once in the hepatocytes, the

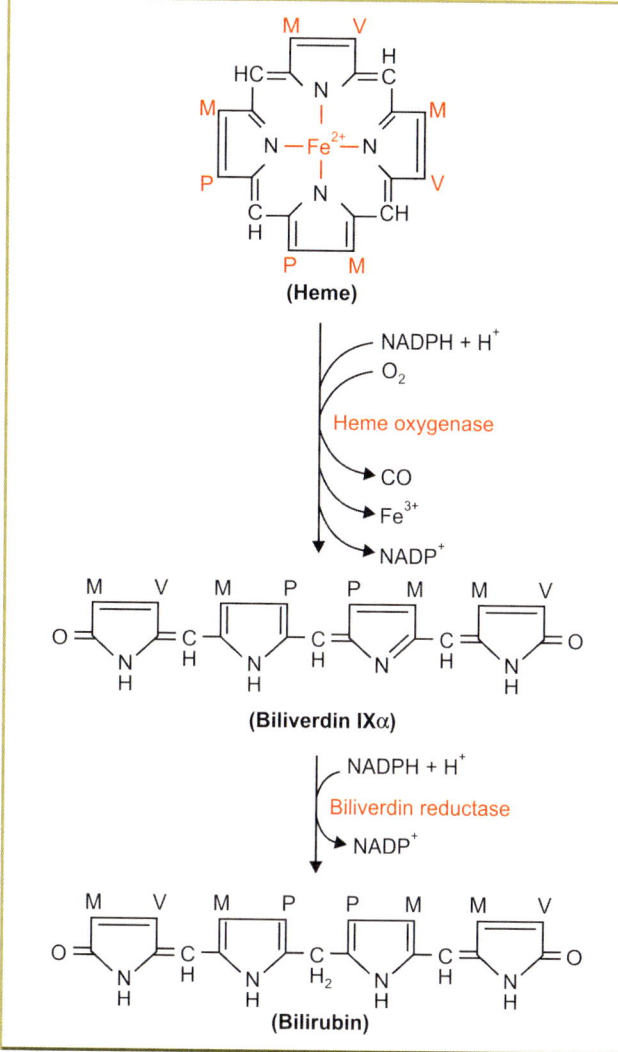

Fig. 15.6: Formation of bilirubin from heme.

propionyl side chains of bilirubin are conjugated with **UDP-glucuronate,** which is derived from the oxidation of UDP-glucose. This reaction is catalyzed by **UDP-glucuronyl transferase** and results in the formation of **conjugated bilirubin** (Fig. 15.7).

5. **Biliary secretion of conjugated bilirubin:** In the normal bile, **bilirubin diglucuronide** is the major

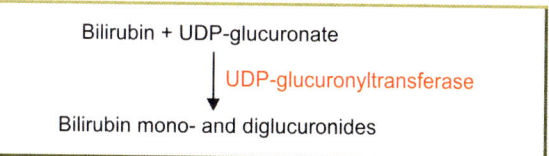

Fig. 15.7: Conjugation of bilirubin in the liver.

form of excreted bilirubin with only a small amount of the **bilirubin monoglucuronide.** As bilirubin diglucuronide is much more water soluble than free bilirubin, transferase thus facilitates excretion of bilirubin via bile duct into the intestine.

6. **Formation of urobilinogen:** As bilirubin diglucuronide is poorly absorbed by the intestinal mucosa, glucuronide residues are released in the terminal ileum and large intestine by intestinal **β-glucuronidases** and by the enzymes produced by anaerobic bacteria. The released bilirubin is reduced to colorless linear tetrapyrroles called stercobilinogen, mesobilinogen and urobilinogen. These compounds are **collectively referred to as urobilinogens.** A large portion of the urobilinogens is excreted in the feces.

7. **Enterohepatic circulation of urobilinogen:** Some of the urobilinogens (up to 2%) are also reabsorbed passively from the intestine and return to the liver via the portal venous blood. A majority of these re-circulating pigments are taken up the liver and **re-excreted** in the bile, thereby completing the enterohepatic circulation of urobilinogen (Fig. 15.8).

8. **Formation of urobilin:** Most of the reabsorbed urobilinogen is taken up by the liver and is reexcreted in the bile. A small portion of the urobilinogens (2–5%), however, escapes hepatic extraction, reaches the peripheral circulation and is excreted in the urine. The fecal and urinary urobilinogens are **auto-oxidized** to form orange-yellow colored compounds called **urobilins** or **stercobilins.**

Plasma Bilirubin and van den Bergh Reaction

In the normal state, plasma bilirubin concentration is 0.3–1.0 mg/dl. Almost all of this is **unconjugated bilirubin** bound noncovalently to albumin and does not react until it is released by the addition of an organic solvent, such as methanol. The reaction with diazonium salt yields azo dye after the addition of methanol and is called **indirect van den Bergh reaction.** Unconjugated bilirubin binds so tightly to serum albumin and lipid that it does not diffuse freely in plasma, and therefore, does not lead to an elevation of bilirubin in the urine.

In contrast, **conjugated bilirubin** is relatively water soluble and elevation of conjugated bilirubin leads to

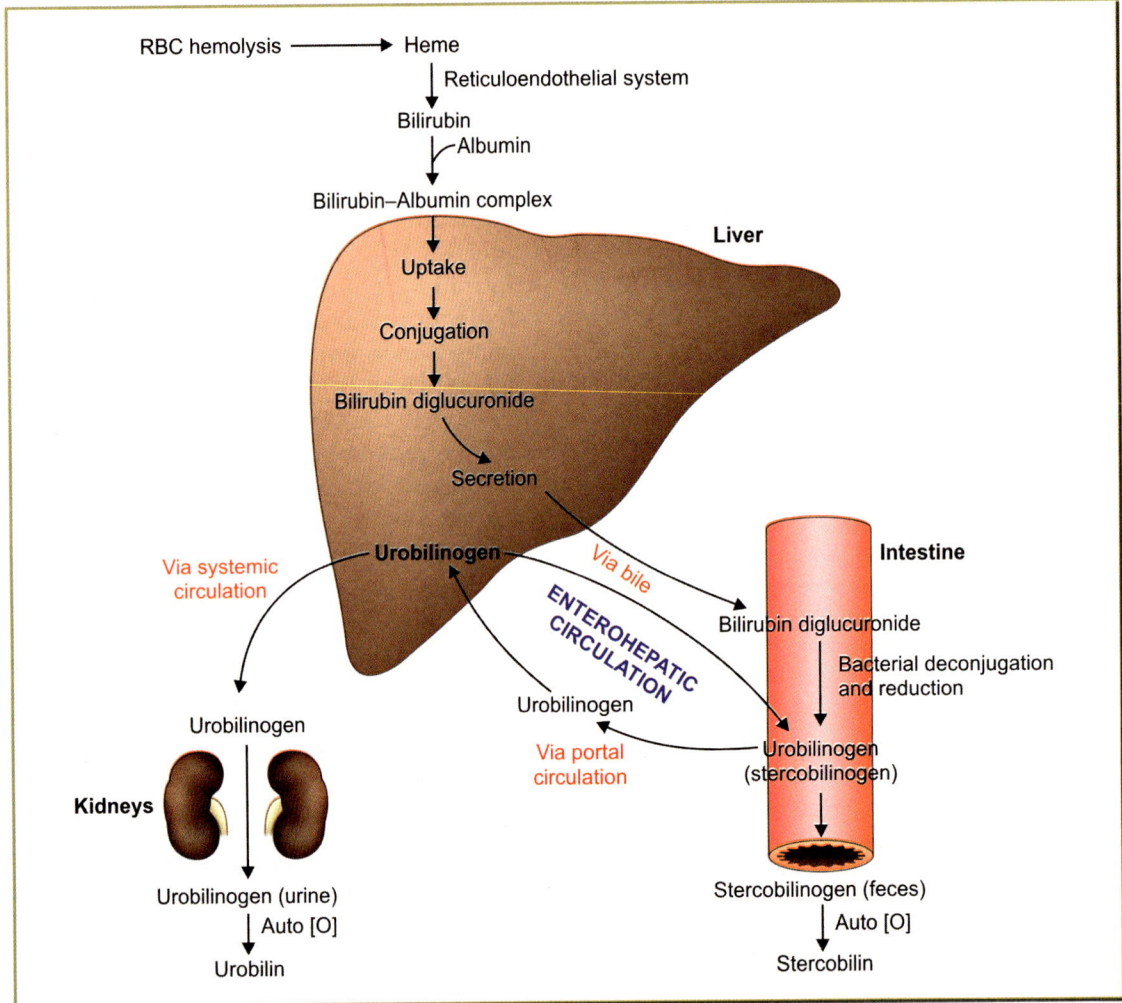

Fig. 15.8: Bilirubin metabolism.

its high urinary excretion with the characteristic deep yellow-brown color to the urine. The conjugated bilirubin is also referred to as direct bilirubin because it can be coupled readily with diazonium salt to yield azo dye. This is called the **direct van den Bergh reaction**.

Hyperbilirubinemia

A raised concentration of bilirubin in plasma is described as hyperbilirubinemia. It may be due to excessively high concentration of either free bilirubin or conjugated bilirubin. The skin, eyes and urine of the patient gradually become pigmented with a yellow to yellow-green coloration and the clinical condition is described as **jaundice** (Chapter 39).

HEME CONTAINING PROTEINS (HEMOPROTEINS)

Heme containing proteins include those proteins that contain **heme as a prosthetic group**. These include:

- Hemoglobin, transports oxygen
- Myoglobin, stores oxygen
- Cytochromes, participate in the electron transport chain
- Catalase, detoxifies hydrogen peroxide
- Peroxidases, detoxify hydrogen peroxide and organic peroxides
- Tryptophan pyrrolase, catalyzes the first step in tryptophan catabolism
- Nitric oxide synthases, catalyze the synthesis of nitric oxide

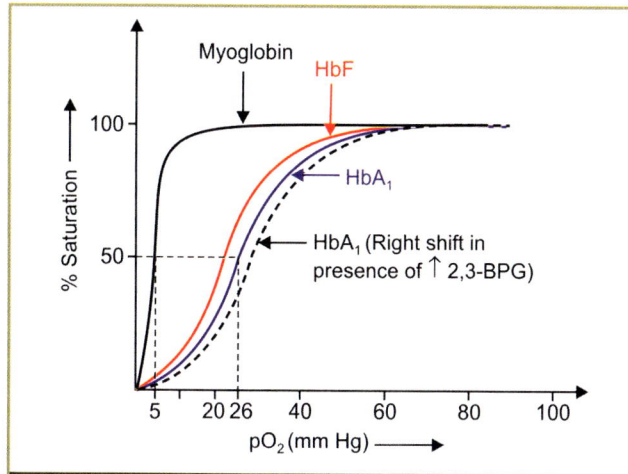

Fig. 15.9: Oxygen binding kinetics of myoglobin and hemoglobin.

- Prostaglandin synthase, catalyze the synthesis of prostaglandins.

Myoglobin

It is the hemoprotein found in **muscles**. It is made up of a **single polypeptide chain** that binds and protects the heme prosthetic group. It binds tightly to oxygen with a P50 (partial pressure of oxygen, pO_2, at which a hemoprotein is 50% saturated) of 5 mmHg (Fig. 15.9). It acts as a **reservoir of oxygen** and releases the same only when the muscle pO_2 falls to very low levels as during strenuous exercise. Its oxygen-binding kinetics is thus a rectangular hyperbola.

Hemoglobin

Hemoglobin is a globular protein present in high concentration in **RBC**. It binds oxygen in the lungs and **transports** it to the cells. It also transports CO_2 and H^+ from the tissues to the lungs. Hemoglobin also carries and releases NO in the blood vessels of the tissues. Hemoglobin molecule consists of **four polypeptide chains**, two each of different amino acid sequences.

Types of Hemoglobins

Different types of hemoglobins found at various developmental stages in normal humans are shown in Table 15.2. These include:

- **Embryonic hemoglobin:** In the first month after conception, embryonic hemoglobins appear containing two zeta chains along with either two

Table 15.2: Different types of human hemoglobins

Hemoglobin	Chain composition	Developmental stage
HbA$_1$	$\alpha_2\beta_2$	Adult
HbA$_2$	$\alpha_2\delta_2$	Adult
HbF	$\alpha_2\gamma_2$	Fetus
Hb·Gower-1	$\zeta_2\epsilon_2$	Embryo
Hb·Portland	$\zeta_2\gamma_2$	Embryo

epsilon chains ($\zeta_2\epsilon_2$) or two gamma chains ($\zeta_2\gamma_2$). These are called Hb·Gower-1 and Hb·Portland, respectively.

- **Fetal hemoglobin:** It is designated as HbF. It predominates in the blood of the human fetus. HbF contains two α chains along with two γ chains ($\alpha_2\gamma_2$). After birth, fetal hemoglobin is rapidly replaced with the adult hemoglobin whose synthesis actually starts in the late fetal life. It comprises $\approx 0.5\%$ of the total hemoglobin in adults.
- **Adult hemoglobin:** This is the major form (97%) of hemoglobin present in an adult human and consists of two α chains and two β chains ($\alpha_2\beta_2$). This is designated as HbA$_1$.
- **Minor adult hemoglobin:** Minor adult hemoglobin designated as HbA$_2$, comprises about 2.5% of the normal adult hemoglobin. It consists of two α chains and two delta chains ($\alpha_2\delta_2$).
- **Glycated hemoglobin:** It results from a covalent linkage between hemoglobin and carbohydrates (please refer to Chapter 11 for details).

Hemoglobin versus Myoglobin

Although both myoglobin and hemoglobin are oxygen-binding proteins, there are distinct structural and functional differences between the two, as highlighted in Table 15.3.

Presence of free myoglobin or hemoglobin in the urine is called myoglobinuria and hemoglobinuria respectively (Chemistry to Clinics 15.3).

Oxygenation and Deoxygenation of Hemoglobin

Role of histidine: Ferrous ion in heme can form five or six ligand bonds, depending upon whether or not O_2 is bound to the molecule. The Fe^{2+} is linked to four nitrogen atoms of the pyrrole rings of the porphyrin. It is also linked through a coordinate bond to the imidazole nitrogen of a histidine, designated as

15

Table 15.3: Comparison between myoglobin and hemoglobin

Parameters	Myoglobin	Hemoglobin (HbA$_1$)
Structural aspects		
Primary structure		
Number of amino acids	153	α-chain: 141, β-chain: 146
Molecular weight	17,000	64,500
Secondary structure		
α-helices	8 (A to H)	7 in each chain (A to G)
Proximal His F8	Present	Present
Distal His E7	Present	Present
Tertiary structure		
Shape	Globular	Globular
Size	4.5 × 3.5 × 2.5 nm	4 times larger
Surface	Polar	Polar
Interior	Nonpolar, binds heme	Non-polar, each chain binds heme
Quaternary structure	Absent (single polypeptide chain)	Present ($\alpha_2\beta_2$)
Functional aspects		
Allosteric modulation	No	Yes, mainly by 2,3-BPG
P50	5 mm Hg	26 mm Hg
Positive cooperativity	No	Yes
Kinetics	Rectangular hyperbola	Sigmoid
O$_2$-affinity	Higher	Lower
Function and location	To store oxygen and release it during exercise, hence located in myocytes	To transport oxygen from lungs to all tissues, hence located in RBC

Chemistry to Clinics 15.3: Myoglobinuria and Hemoglobinuria

Myoglobinuria refers to the presence of myoglobin in the urine; the latter turns brown ('tea colored'). Causes include extensive muscle breakdown (rhabdomyolysis), malignant hyperthermia and certain drugs such as HMG CoA reductase inhibitors (statins) and gemfibrozil used to lower serum cholesterol and triglycerides respectively. Patients who are prescribed the above drugs should be instructed to immediately report to the physician in case of unexplained shoulder pain (suggestive of rhabdomyolysis), alteration in urine color and oliguria (impending renal shut-down due to deposition of excess myoglobin in the renal tubules).

Myoglobinuria, however, cannot be differentiated from hemoglobinuria on the basis of urine color and dipstick test for blood (both give a positive test due to the presence of heme). However, serum is not discolored in case of myoglobinuria whereas it is pink-brown in case of hemoglobinuria (as compared to hemoglobin, myoglobin is cleared very rapidly from plasma). Further, serum CK-MM may be raised in case of myoglobinuria due to rhabdomyolysis.

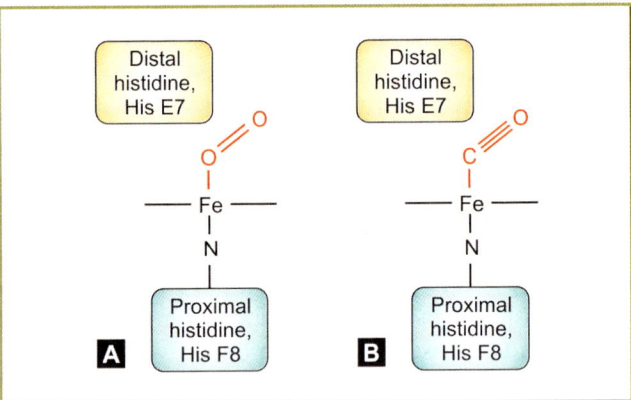

Fig. 15.10: In oxyhemoglobin (A), **oxygen** binds to the heme plane at an angle due to steric hindrance imposed by His E7. **Carbon monoxide** binds in the same stereochemical orientation (B) but with a much **higher affinity**.

the **proximal histidine or His F8** (Fig. 15.10). O$_2$, when bound to hemoglobin, forms a sixth coordinate bond with Fe^{2+}. O$_2$ gets placed between Fe^{2+} and the nitrogen of the imidazole ring of another histidine molecule, designated as the **distal histidine or His E7**. In deoxyhemoglobin, this sixth coordinated position of Fe^{2+} is unoccupied.

Heme pocket: Each polypeptide of the globin subunit contains a heme prosthetic group which is positioned within a hydrophobic pocket of the globin subunit (heme pocket). Since hemoglobin has a quaternary structure with four monomeric subunits, it has **four heme-binding sites for O_2**. Hemoglobin has a P50 of 26 mm Hg and shows sigmoidal oxygen-binding kinetics which makes it favorable for loading O_2 at a high partial pressure in the lungs, transporting it and unloading it at the low partial pressure prevailing in the metabolizing tissues (Fig. 15.9). Further, the binding of oxygen is affected by **allosteric modulators** such as 2,3-bisphosphoglycerate, H^+, CO_2, Cl^- and temperature; an increase in any of these modulators shifts the curve to the right.

T and R Conformations of Hemoglobin

Ferrous ion in deoxyhemoglobin has a slightly larger radius and gets placed in the center of porphyrin with a conformational constraint on His F8. This, in turn, results in some distortion of the porphyrin ring and the deoxy conformation of hemoglobin is thus referred to as the **tense or T conformational state**. With the binding of O_2 to the Fe^{2+}, the favorable free energy of bond formation overcomes the repulsive interaction between His F8 and porphyrin; Fe^{2+} moves into the plane of the porphyrin ring and triggers a conformational change in the hemoglobin molecule from T to the **relaxed or R conformational state** (Fig. 15.11). It is important to note that the binding of one molecule of oxygen to a polypeptide chain in hemoglobin, facilitates the sequential binding of more oxygen molecules, a phenomenon called positive cooperativity.

The T and R conformational equilibrium of hemoglobin **controls the delivery of O_2 and NO to the tissues and the transport of CO_2 away from the tissues**. Equilibrium between the T and the R state is regulated by the H^+ concentrations which are released, as T conformation is converted to the R conformation. The imidazole group of His 146 (β) is a major contributor for proton dissociation during the transition from T to R conformation.

Role of 2,3-Bisphosphoglycerate

- 2,3-Bisphosphoglycerate (2,3-BPG) is an intermediate synthesized in an **off-shoot of glycolysis**.
- It is present in small amounts in all the cells with large concentration in **RBC** (Chemistry to Clinics 15.4).

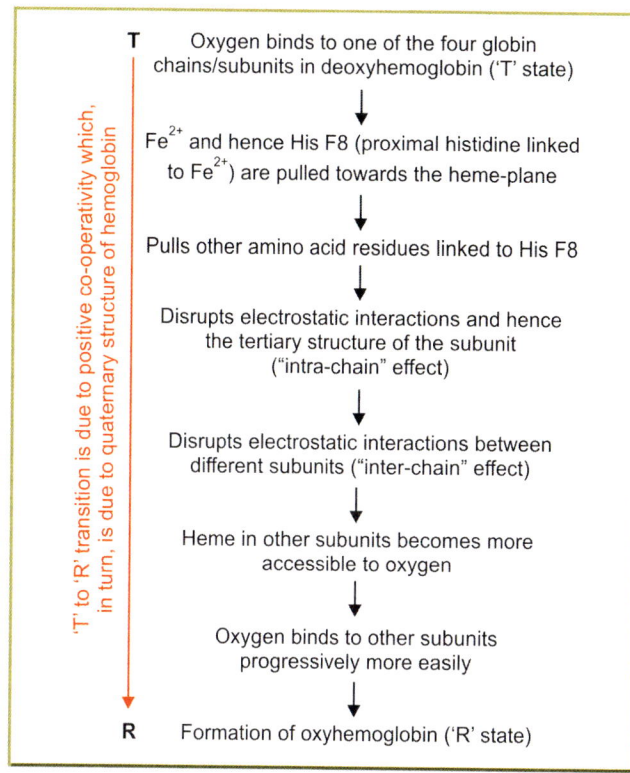

Fig. 15.11: Mechanism of oxygenation of hemoglobin in the lungs. In the peripheral tissues, the phenomenon is reversed.

Chemistry to Clinics 15.4: Importance of 2,3-BPG

- Since the binding-affinity of 2,3-BPG for heme is less in case of fetal hemoglobin (P50 = 20 mm Hg), the oxygen-dissociation curve of fetal hemoglobin is towards the left of adult hemoglobin (Fig. 15.9) which helps in the transfer of oxygen from the mother to the fetus.
- In conditions that cause hypoxia (lack of O_2, such as anemia, smoking and high altitude), the metabolism of the RBC switches over to produce more BPG.
- Prior to transfusion, blood is preserved in ACD (acid-citrate-dextrose) and with the passage of time the BPG levels fall. The blood thus fails to deliver adequate oxygen to the recipient. Hence, inosine is added to blood at the time of storage, which acts as a precursor of BPG and maintains its levels.

- It is the **most important allosteric modulator of hemoglobin**, with high affinity to the T conformation (deoxyhemoglobin) and not to the R conformation (oxyhemoglobin). It forms salt bridges through its negatively charged phosphate groups (Fig. 15.12) to the positively charged residues in the hemoglobin chains.

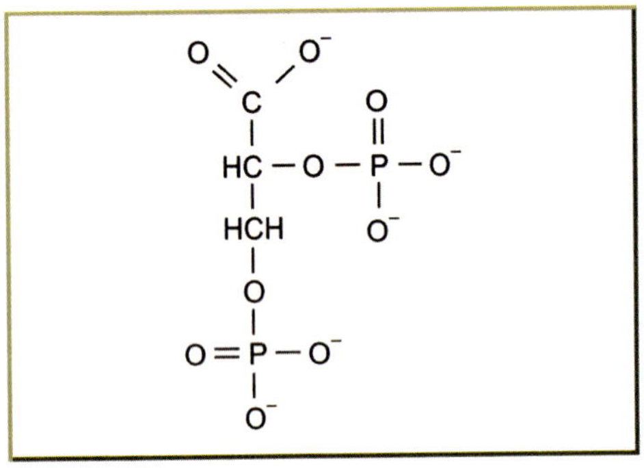

Fig. 15.12: 2,3-BPG.

- As BPG **binds tightly to T conformation**, it forces the cuarve to the right and thus the delivery of O_2 (Fig. 15.9).

Bohr Effect

The affinity of oxygen for hemoglobin is also affected by **pH**. It decreases as the pH becomes more acidic. This is known as Bohr effect. In other words, increase in acidity of hemoglobin as it binds O_2 or an increase in basicity of hemoglobin as it releases oxygen is referred to as Bohr effect. It may be expressed as shown in Fig. 15.13. It suggests that an **increase in H^+ concentration favors the release of oxygen from oxyhemoglobin**. Conversely, oxygenation of

$$HHb + O_2 \rightleftharpoons HbO_2 + H^+$$

Fig. 15.13: Bohr effect.

hemoglobin accompanies lowering of pH of the solution. Under conditions of lack of O_2, anaerobic glycolysis occurs which, in turn, produces more lactic acid and thus lowers the tissue pH. This causes more release of O_2. Thus, the combined effect of 2,3-BPG and increased acidity leads to a marked reduction in oxygen binding capacity of hemoglobin and therefore promotes oxygen release.

Transport of CO_2 from Extrapulmonary Tissues to Lungs and O_2 from Lungs to Extrapulmonary Tissues

Transport of CO_2 from tissues to the lungs, for its removal, along with the transport of O_2 from the lungs to the tissues is linked with protons generated by Bohr effect. This is achieved by two different mechanisms:

- **Isohydric transport:** The metabolizing cells utilize O_2 and produce CO_2 which diffuses from cells and enters the RBC in capillaries of tissues.

  - **Within the RBC**, CO_2 is dissolved in water and is rapidly converted to H_2CO_3, by the enzyme **carbonic anhydrase**. Spontaneously, carbonic acid is dissociated to HCO_3^- and H^+. The H^+ binds to deoxyhemoglobin, forcing the $O_2 \cdot Hb$ equilibrium from oxyhemoglobin to deoxyhemoglobin with the dissociation of O_2 which then diffuses out of the RBC to the cells of tissues. The HCO_3^- diffuses out of the RBC and is transported in plasma to the lungs (Fig. 15.14A).

  - **In the lungs**, high O_2 pressure forces the reaction in the opposite direction. It promotes the

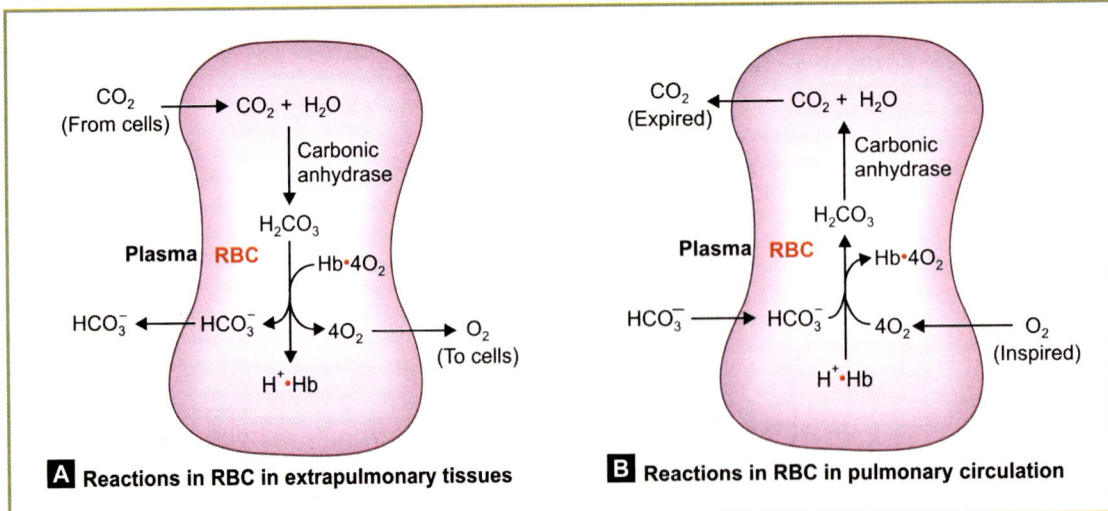

A Reactions in RBC in extrapulmonary tissues   **B** Reactions in RBC in pulmonary circulation

Fig. 15.14: Isohydric transport of CO_2 as bicarbonate.

conversion of deoxyhemoglobin to oxyhemo-globin. During this process, H^+ are dissociated, combine with HCO_3^- and reform carbonic acid. Carbonic anhydrase now catalyzes the conversion of H_2CO_3 to CO_2 and H_2O. CO_2 diffuses out of the blood into the lung alveoli and is expired into air (Fig. 15.14B).

About 80% of the cellular CO_2 is transported from tissues to the lungs by this mechanism, i.e. as HCO_3^-. This is called **isohydric transport of CO_2**.

- **Carbamino-hemoglobin:** Hemoglobin also trans-ports nearly 15–20% of the CO_2 by a second mechanism, i.e. via the formation of carbamino-hemoglobin.

  - **From cells of the tissues**, CO_2 diffuses into the RBC in capillaries and reacts with the **NH_2-terminal groups of hemoglobin poly-peptide chains** and forms carbamino-hemo-globin. This reaction also produces H^+ which promotes the dissociation of O_2 from hemo-globin. The O_2 diffuses out of the RBC to the tissues (Fig. 15.15A).

  - **In the lungs**, the high O_2 pressure forces the reactions in the opposite direction. This, in turn, leads to the expiration of CO_2 from the lungs. Free H^+ thus promotes dissociation of the carbamino group from Hb to reform CO_2 which is expired from the lungs (Fig. 15.15B).

Transport of Nitric Oxide

Nitric oxide (NO) is a potent **vasodilator**. It has a very short lifetime in the blood but is prevented from rapid destruction by hemoglobin. Hemoglobin reversibly binds NO. As hemoglobin changes from the oxy (R) conformation to the deoxy (T) conformation, it dissociates the bound NO to glutathione (GSH). NO is thus released as glutathione-nitric oxide complex (GS-NO). Glutathione not only stabilizes NO against its rapid degradation but also efficiently delivers it to the cells of the blood vessel wall and promotes relaxation of the vascular wall. This, in turn, facili-tates the transfer of gases between the blood and the cells of the tissues.

HEMOGLOBINOPATHIES

- This is a group of disorders characterized by **struc-turally and/or functionally abnormal hemoglobin** due to a **genetic** or **acquired** defect in **heme** (hemopathy) or **globin** (globinopathy) (Table 15.4).
- These hemoglobins denature easily and precipitate within the RBC, forming **Heinz bodies** (Fig. 15.16), which can damage the cell membrane.
- In some cases, the change may be clinically insignificant while in others it may cause a serious disease.
- **Anemia and reticulocytosis** are the common features. Some of the hemoglobinopathies are discussed below.

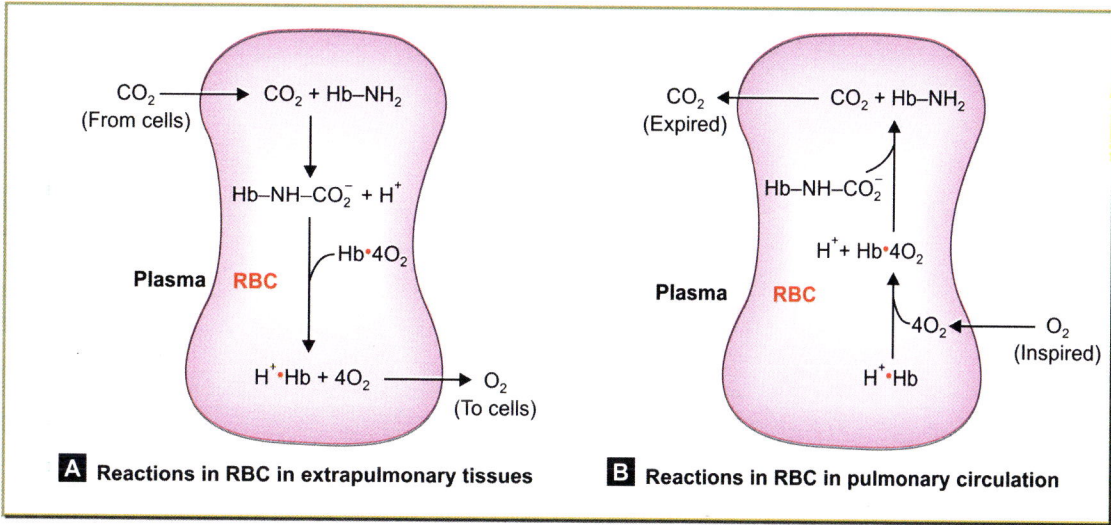

A Reactions in RBC in extrapulmonary tissues

B Reactions in RBC in pulmonary circulation

Fig. 15.15: Transport of CO_2 as carbamino-hemoglobin.

Table 15.4: Hemoglobinopathies

1. Hemopathies

  (A) Defective heme synthesis: Porphyrias, iron deficiency anemia

  (B) Defective heme function: Methemoglobinemia, CO poisoning

2. Globinopathies

  (A) Qualitative defect (globin mutated but synthesized in normal quantities): Sickle cell anemia, Hemoglobin C

  (B) Quantitative defect (globin normal but synthesized in reduuced quantities): Thalassemia, protein energy malnutrition

Methemoglobinemia

- **Methemoglobin (Met-Hb):** It is nonfunctional hemoglobin with Fe^{3+} **instead of** Fe^{2+}. Normally, Met-Hb levels are <1%. Spontaneously formed Met-Hb is reduced (regenerating normal hemoglobin) by protective enzyme systems, e.g., NADH-methemoglobin reductase (cytochrome-b5 reductase, major pathway) and NADPH-methemoglobin reductase (minor pathway) (Fig. 15.17).

- **Cause and types:** Elevated Met-Hb occurs when the mechanisms that defend against oxidative stress within the RBC are overwhelmed along with failure to reconvert Met-Hb back to oxyhemoglobin:

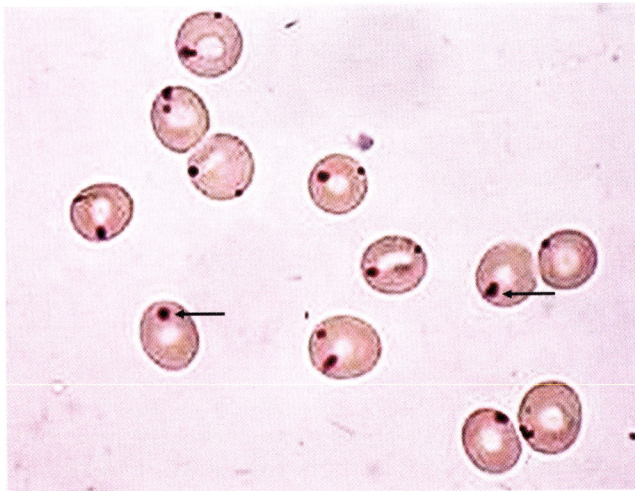

Fig. 15.16: Heinz bodies (arrows) are inclusions in the RBC composed of denatured or precipitated hemoglobin, revealed in a peripheral blood smear stained with methyl violet. They decrease cell membrane flexibility.

  – *Congenital:* Either due to deficiency of Met-Hb reductase or due to mutated hemoglobin (termed HbM) which exists in the ferric state and cannot be reduced by Met-Hb reductase.

  – *Acquired:* Exposure to certain drugs/chemicals (Table 15.5).

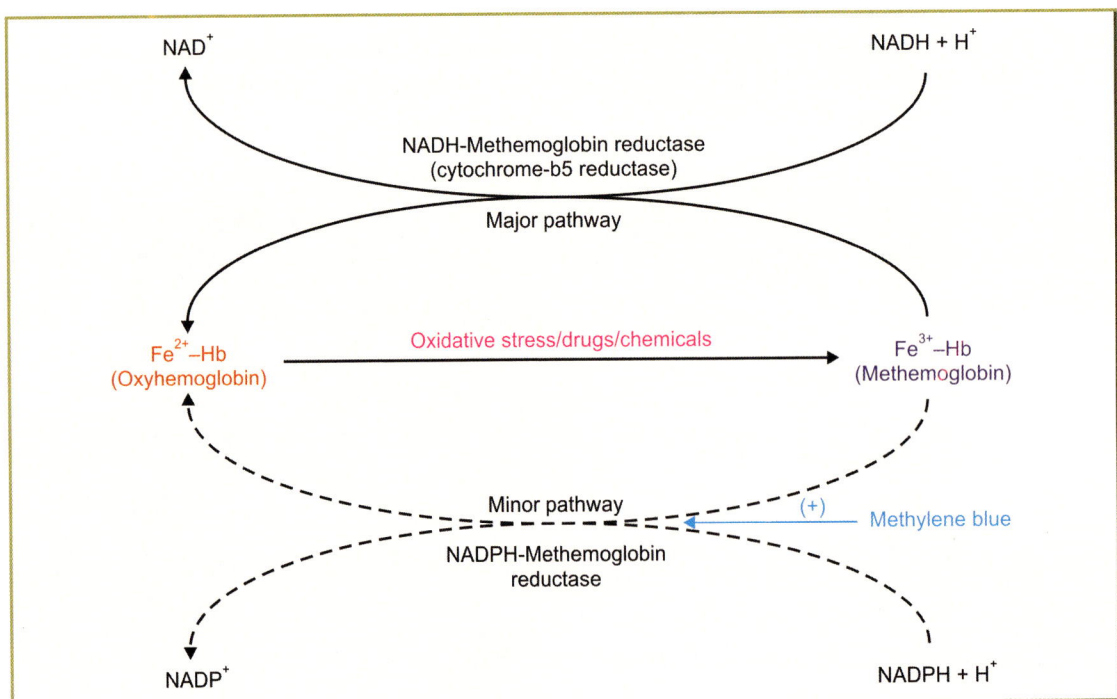

Fig. 15.17: Interconversion of oxyhemoglobin and methemoglobin.

Table 15.5: Common drugs/chemicals causing acquired methemo-globinemia

- Benzocaine: Anesthetic
- Sulfonamides: Antibiotics
- Dapsone: Treatment of leprosy
- Organic nitrates (e.g. nitroglycerin): Treatment of angina pectoris
- Inorganic nitrates: Preservatives

- **Outcome:** It reduces the ability of RBC to release oxygen to tissues, with the oxyhemoglobin dissociation **curve shifted to the left**. Hypoxia occurs due to the decreased oxygen-binding capacity of Met-Hb as well as the increased oxygen-binding affinity of other subunits in the same hemoglobin molecule which prevents them from releasing oxygen at the partial pressure of oxygen in tissues. Patients with high concentration of Met-Hb show **cyanosis** (bluish color of the skin) (Fig. 15.18A).
- **Treatment:** Intravenous **methylene blue**, which is reduced to leukomethylene blue by erythrocyte Met-Hb reductase in the presence of NADPH. Leukomethylene blue then reduces Met-Hb to oxyhemoglobin. Later, the patient may be switched over to oral methylene blue.

Carbon Monoxide Poisoning

- Carbon monoxide (CO) has 200-fold **higher affinity** for binding isolated heme (free from globin) as compared to oxygen. However, due to steric constraints imposed by His E7 (distal histidine),

this affinity is reduced substantially in the presence of globin (Fig. 15.10).
- CO-poisoning is an industrial hazard, e.g. **automobile** industry.
- It causes **cherry-red** discoloration of skin (Fig. 15.18B) and **hypoxia**.
- It can be rapidly **fatal** and requires the prompt administration of **hyperbaric oxygen**.

Sickle Cell Disease

- **Molecular defect:** The most common of all hemoglobinopathies is sickle cell disease characterized by the presence of **hemoglobin S (HbS)**. It is a variant form of the normal adult hemoglobin (HbA$_1$), in which a substitution occurs in the sixth position of the β-globin chain. Whereas in HbA$_1$, this position is occupied by a glutamic acid residue, in HbS it is substituted by valine (**β6 Glu → Val**). The molecular basis for this is a point mutation, i.e. a change in a single nucleotide within the codon from GAA or GAG which code for glutamic acid to GUA or GUG which code for valine.
- **Outcome:** Due to the presence of valine in place of glutamic acid, sickle cell hemoglobin has a lower negative charge than normal hemoglobin. As a result, HbS gets polymerized and precipitate within the RBC **particularly in the deoxygenated state**. This, in turn, makes the red blood cells assume a **sickle shape** (Fig. 15.19) instead of the normal biconcave shape. Such distorted RBC lose their deformability, resulting in higher rate of **hemolysis**

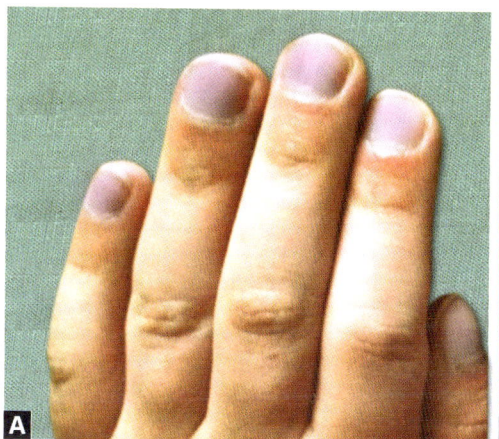
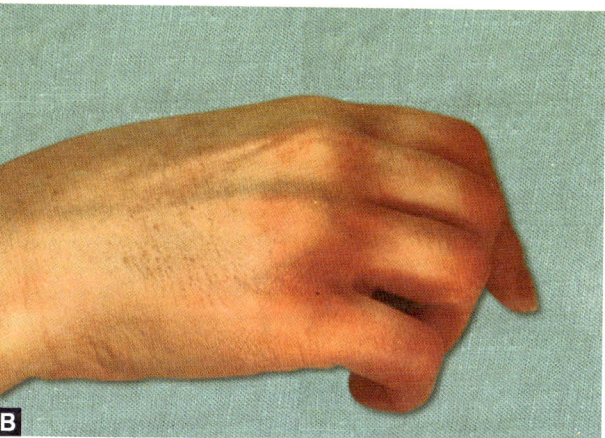

Fig. 15.18: (A) Cyanosis of nail beds in **methemoglobinemia**. (B) Cherry-red discoloration of skin in **carbon monoxide poisoning**.

15

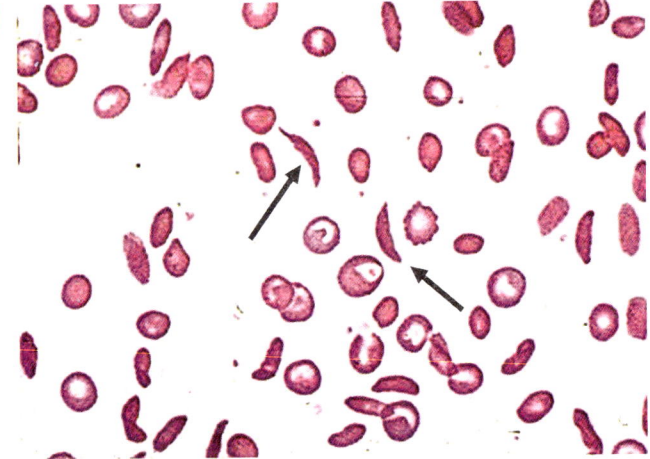

Fig. 15.19: **Sickled** red blood cells (arrows) in a peripheral blood smear.

particularly while negotiating through the microcirculation. This type of hemolytic anemia is designated as sickle cell anemia. Further, hemoglobin S though binds and releases oxygen but abnormally.

- **Sickle crisis:** During any illness such as dehydration, infection, etc. the patients are at risk of occlusion of capillaries by sickled RBC, leading to gross tissue hypoxia and damage.

- **Sickle cell trait:** Only homozygous individuals for HbS exhibit the disease. Those who are **heterozygous** for HbS do not exhibit symptoms of sickle cell anemia except under extreme conditions of hypoxia because such individuals have 50% HbA_1 and 50% HbS in their RBC. This is called sickle cell trait.

- **Diagnosis**
  1. Hemoglobin electrophoresis.
  2. Sickling test: Sickling of the RBC, on a blood film, can be induced by the addition of reducing agents such as sodium metabisulfite or sodium dithionite, and confirmed microscopically.
  3. Genetic tests (mutation analysis).

- **Treatment**
  1. Always maintain adequate hydration.
  2. Blood transfusions during acute attacks (sickle crisis).
  3. Bone marrow transplantation.

Thalassemia

- **Molecular defect:** Thalassemias are a family of related genetic disorders that arise due to the **deletion of one or more globin-like genes** in either the globin gene clusters or due to a defect in transcription and/or processing of mRNA of the globin gene (α globin gene: Chromosome 16; β globin gene: Chromosome 11).

- **Types:** If there is a reduced synthesis or total lack of synthesis of α-globin mRNA, the disease is classified **α-thalassemia**. On the other hand, if β-globin mRNA level is affected, it is called **β-thalassemia**.

- **Subtypes:** α-Thalassemia patients may be missing one to four α-globin genes. If one α-globin gene is missing, the condition is called **α-thalassemia 1 (α-thal 1)**. When two α-globin genes are missing, it is called as **α-thal 2**. Both these conditions are associated with mild to moderate anemia. If three α-globin genes are missing, it results in the formation of a tetramer of four β-globins. This condition is called **HbH disease**. When all the four α-globin genes are absent, it results in a fatal condition, called as **hydrops fetalis** (also termed Hb Barts, consisting of γ_4 chains). β-Thalassemias also exhibit different degrees of severity and can be caused by a variety of defects or deletions.

- **Thalassemia major and minor:** When the child inherits the defective gene from one parent, there are usually minor symptoms and is called **thalassemia minor** or trait (whether α or β). On the other hand, if inheritance of the defective genes is from both the parents and results in a symptomatic disease requiring treatment, it is called **thalassemia major** (α or β).

- **Diagnosis**
  1. Hemoglobin electrophoresis.
  2. Genetic tests (mutation analysis).

- **Treatment**
  1. Children require **repeated blood transfusions** for survival, which, unfortunately, results in **iron overload**, hemosiderosis and organ damage. Hence, iron chelation is required and is achieved by injections of desferoxamine or oral deferasirox.
  2. Bone marrow transplantation.

15

Hemoglobin C

Hemoglobin C is another variant of HbA_1 where $\beta6$ Glu is replaced by lysine. This, in turn, results in the formation of aggregates and reduces survival time for the red blood cells. This form of hemoglobinopathy exhibits more limited pathological effects and is commonly found among certain black African population.

SOME IMPORTANT QUESTIONS

1. Describe the biosynthesis of heme. How heme biosynthesis is regulated?

2. What is porphyria? Describe various types of porphyrias.

3. Describe how heme is degraded. Discuss the metabolic fate of bilirubin.

4. Describe:
   i. Oxygenation and deoxygenation of hemoglobin.
   ii. Isohydric transport of CO_2.

5. Compare between:
   i. Myoglobin and hemoglobin.
   ii. Myoglobinuria and hemoglobinuria.

6. Write notes on:
   i. Acute intermittent porphyria
   ii. Hyperbilirubinemia
   iii. Heme-containing proteins
   iv. Normal and abnormal hemoglobins
   v. Hemoglobinopathies
   vi. Sickle cell anemia
   vii. Thalassemia
   viii. Bohr effect
   ix. Carbaminohemoglobin
   x. Carbon monoxide poisoning
   xi. Methemoglobinemia

MULTIPLE CHOICE QUESTIONS

1. Organic lead poisoning is an occupational hazard in:
   A. Paint industry
   B. Battery industry
   C. Automobile industry
   D. All of the above

2. In the plasma, conjugated bilirubin is bound to:
   A. α_2-Globulin
   B. α_1-Globulin
   C. β-Globulin
   D. None of the above

3. In hydrops fetalis, the number of missing α-globin gene is/are:
   A. 1
   B. 2
   C. 3
   D. 4

4. The following has the highest oxygen-affinity:
   A. HbF
   B. HbA_1
   C. HbA_{1C}
   D. Myoglobin

5. Acidemia may have the following effect:
   A. Stimulate oxygen release from oxy-Hb
   B. Inhibit oxygen release from oxy-Hb
   C. No effect
   D. Inactivate oxy-Hb

Information Transfer

The human body has several means of transmitting information between cells (Fig. 16.1). These include:

1. **Short-range** or **local communication**: Direct communication between adjacent cells through gap junctions, paracrine, autocrine and juxtacrine signaling, and the release of neurotransmitters by nerve cells.

2. **Long-range** or **distant communication**: Mediated through hormones (chemical substances with regulatory functions) produced by endocrine cells.

GAP JUNCTIONS

Adjacent cells often communicate directly with each other via gap junctions, specialized protein channels in the plasma membrane of cells that are made of the protein **connexin**. Six connexin molecules assemble in the plasma membrane of one cell to form a half-channel (hemi-channel), called a **connexon**. Two connexons aligned between two neighboring cells then join end-to-end to form an intercellular channel between the plasma membranes of adjacent cells.

Functions of Gap Junctions

1. Allow the flow of **ions** (hence, electrical current) and **small molecules** between the cytosol of neighboring cells. This is critical to the function of many tissues and allows rapid transmission of electrical signals between neighboring cells in the heart, smooth muscle cells, and some nerve cells.

2. Functionally **couple** adjacent epithelial cells.

3. Control of **cell growth and differentiation** by allowing adjacent cells to share a common intracellular environment.

4. Often when a cell is injured, gap junctions **close**, isolating a damaged cell from its neighbors. This isolation process, which may result from a rise in intracellular Ca^{2+} or a fall in pH in the cytosol of the damaged cell, is followed by a controlled destruction of the cell by **apoptosis**.

PARACRINE, AUTOCRINE AND JUXTACRINE SIGNALING

Cells may signal to each other via the local release of chemical substances, called '**local hormones**'. This means of communication does not depend on a vascular system.

Paracrine Signaling

A chemical is liberated from a cell and diffuses a short distance through the extracellular fluid to act on **nearby cells**. Paracrine signaling factors affect only the immediate environment and bind with high specificity to receptors on the plasma membrane of the target cell. They are also rapidly destroyed by extracellular enzymes or bound to extracellular matrix, thus preventing their widespread diffusion. **Nitric oxide (NO)**, originally called 'endothelium-derived relaxing factor (EDRF)', is an example of a paracrine signaling molecule.

Nitric oxide: Although many cells can produce NO, it has major roles in mediating vascular smooth muscle tone, facilitating central nervous system

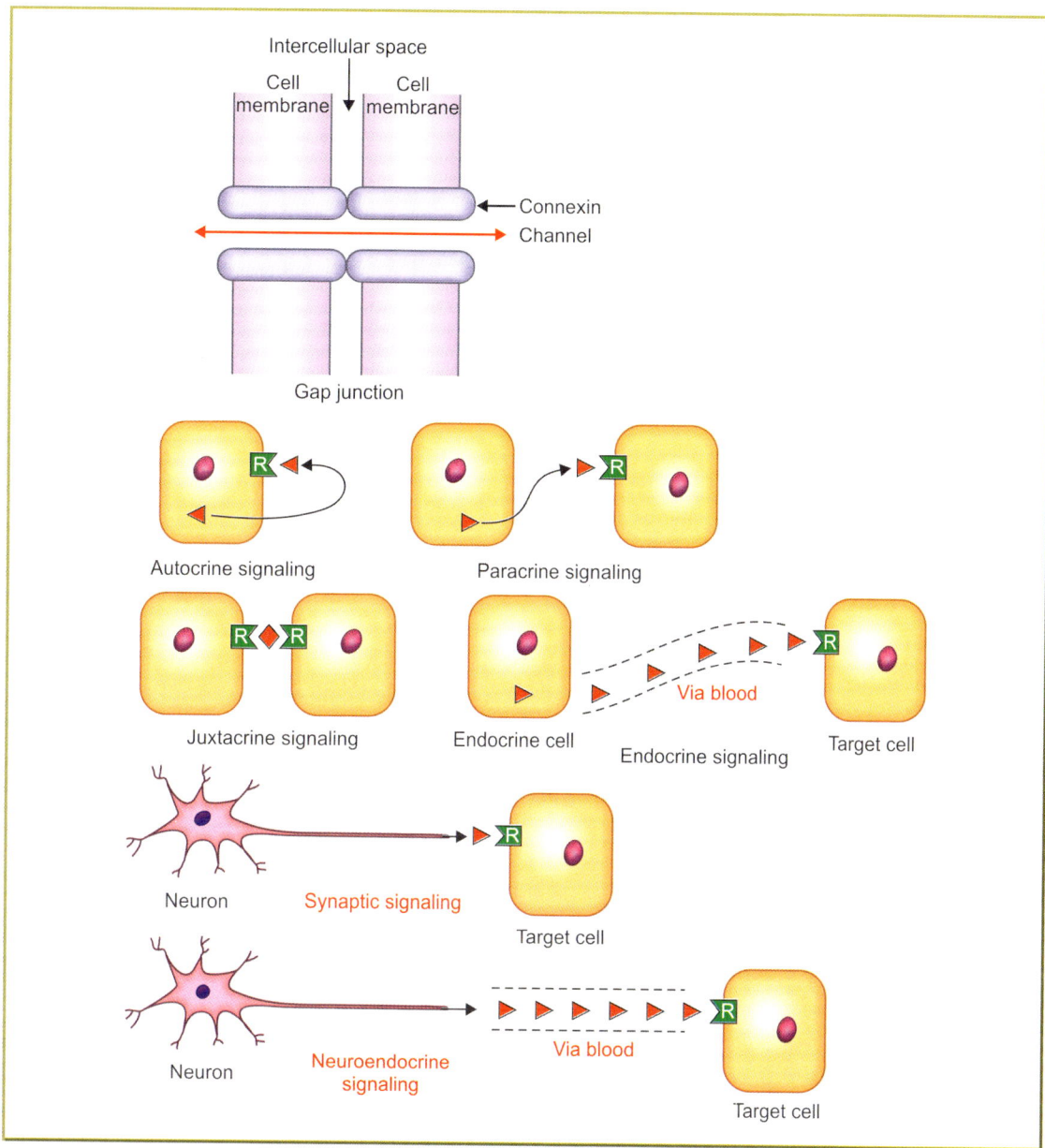

Fig. 16.1: Modes of information transfer from cell to cell.

neurotransmission activities, and modulating immune responses. The production of NO is catalyzed by nitric oxide synthase (NOS) which deaminates arginine to citrulline.

NO, produced by endothelial cells, regulates vascular tone by diffusing from the endothelial cell to the underlying vascular smooth muscle cell, where it activates its effector target, a cytoplasmic enzyme guanylyl cyclase. This is followed by an increase in intracellular cyclic guanosine monophosphate (cGMP) levels and the activation of cGMP-dependent protein kinase. This enzyme phosphorylates potential target substrates such as calcium pumps in the sarcoplasmic reticulum or sarcolemma, leading to reduced cytoplasmic levels of calcium. In turn, this deactivates the contractile machinery in the vascular smooth muscle cell and produces relaxation or a decrease of tone (*see* Fig. 13.60).

16

Autocrine Signaling

The cell releases a chemical messenger into the extracellular fluid that binds to a receptor on the surface of **the cell that secreted it**. **Eicosanoids**, e.g. prostaglandins, are examples of signaling molecules that can act in an autocrine manner. These molecules act as local hormones to influence a variety of physiological processes, such as uterine smooth muscle contraction during pregnancy.

Juxtacrine Signaling

It describes the **interaction of a membrane-bound growth factor on one cell with its membrane-bound receptor on an adjacent cell**. The ovaries provide an ideal example where all the local communication systems discussed above can be observed.

In ovarian follicles, theca and granulosa cells are exposed to different microenvironments. Vascularization is restricted to the theca layer because blood vessels do not penetrate the basement membrane. Theca cells, therefore, have better access to circulating cholesterol, which enters the cells via LDL receptors. The granulosa cells, on the other hand, primarily produce cholesterol from acetate, a less efficient process than uptake. In addition, granulosa cells are bathed in follicular fluid and exposed to autocrine, paracrine, and juxtacrine control by locally produced peptides and **growth factors**.

NEURAL COMMUNICATION

The conduction of information along nerves occurs via action potentials, and signal transmission between nerves or between nerves and effector structures takes place at a **synapse**. Therefore, nervous transmission employs a combination of 'wired' and 'wireless' communication which explains why the system is so

Table 16.1: Common examples of neurotransmitters	
Neurotransmitters	*Functions*
Acetyl choline	Control of muscle contraction
Dopamine	Control of muscle contraction
Glutamate	Sensation, learning, memory
GABA	Synaptic inhibition
Glycine	Synaptic inhibition
Norepinephrine	Response to stress
Serotonin	Regulation of sleep, temperature, sensation, memory
Melatonin	Regulation of sleep-wake cycle
Enkephalins	Inhibit pain perception
Endorphins	Inhibit pain perception
Substance P	Enhance pain perception

rapid yet highly efficient. Synaptic transmission is almost always mediated by the release of specific chemicals or neurotransmitters from the nerve terminals. Neurotransmitters are thus a special category of local hormones (Table 16.1).

Innervated cells have specialized receptors in their cell membrane that selectively bind neurotransmitters. Serious consequences occur when nervous transmission is impaired or defective (Chemistry to Clinics 16.1).

Inhibitory Neurotransmitters

Inhibitory amino acid transmitters **γ-aminobutyric acid (GABA)** and **glycine** bind to their respective receptors, causing hyperpolarization of the post-synaptic membrane. GABAergic neurons represent the major inhibitory neurons of the CNS, whereas glycinergic neurons are found in limited numbers, restricted to the spinal cord and brainstem (Chemistry to Clinics 16.2).

Chemistry to Clinics 16.1: Parkinson's Disease

Parkinson's disease (PD) is a degenerative disorder of the central nervous system that gradually worsens, affecting motor skills and speech. PD is characterized by muscle rigidity, tremors, and slowing of physical movements. These symptoms are the result of excessive muscle contraction, which is a result of insufficient dopamine, a neurotransmitter produced by the dopaminergic neurons of the brain. The symptoms of PD result from the loss of dopamine-secreting cells in a region of the brain thereby causing other neurons (secreting other neurotransmitters such as acetylcholine) to fire out of control, resulting in an inability to control or direct movements in a normal manner. Both cognitive impairment (slow reaction times) and behavioral impairment (tremors) are observed in this devastating disease.

There is no cure for PD, but several drugs have been developed to help patients manage their symptoms, although they do not halt the disease. The most commonly used drug is levodopa (L-DOPA), a synthetic precursor of dopamine. L-DOPA is taken up in the brain and changed into dopamine, allowing the patient to regain some control over his or her mobility. Current research is focusing on embryonic stem cells that are undifferentiated cells derived from embryos, and scientists may be able to encourage these cells to differentiate into neuronal cells that can replace those lost during progression of this disease.

Chemistry to Clinics 16.2: GABA Receptors

There are two types of GABA receptors: GABA$_A$ and GABA$_B$. The **GABA$_A$ receptor** is a ligand-gated Cl$^-$ channel, and its activation increases the influx of Cl$^-$ ions. The increase in Cl$^-$ conductance is facilitated by benzodiazepines such as diazepam, drugs that are widely used to treat anxiety and insomnia. Activation of the **GABA$_B$ receptor** increases K$^+$ conductance via the activation of a G protein. Drugs that inhibit GABA transmission cause seizures, indicating a major role for inhibitory mechanisms in normal brain function.

Excitatory Neurotransmitters

Excitatory amino acids, **glutamate** and **aspartate**, are the neurotransmitters for more than one-half the total neuronal population of the central nervous system. In certain pathological states, extra-neuronal concentrations of amino acids exceed the ability of the uptake mechanisms to remove them, resulting in cell death in a matter of minutes. This can be seen in severe hypoxia such as during respiratory or cardiovascular failure, and in ischemia, in which the blood supply to a region of the brain is interrupted, as in stroke. In either condition, the affected area is deprived of oxygen and glucose, which are essential for normal neuronal functions, including energy-dependent mechanisms for the removal of these amino acids from the synapse.

Excitotoxicity: The consequence of prolonged exposure of neurons to excitatory amino acids is called 'excitotoxicity'. It is largely attributed to the destructive actions of **high intracellular Ca^{2+}** brought about by stimulation of **glutamatergic receptors**. The opening of voltage-gated Ca^{2+} channels promotes the further release of glutamate leading to a vicious cycle. Cell death results from an inability of ischemic/hypoxic conditions to meet the high metabolic demands of excited neurons and the triggering of destructive changes in the cell by increased Ca^{2+} as follows:

1. Intracellular free Ca^{2+} is an activator of calcium-dependent **proteases**, which destroy microtubules and other structural proteins that maintain neuronal integrity.
2. Ca^{2+} activates **phospholipases** which break down membrane phospholipids and lead to lipid per-oxidation and the formation of oxygen-free radicals, which are toxic to cells. Another consequence of activated phospholipases is the formation of arachidonic acid and its metabolites including

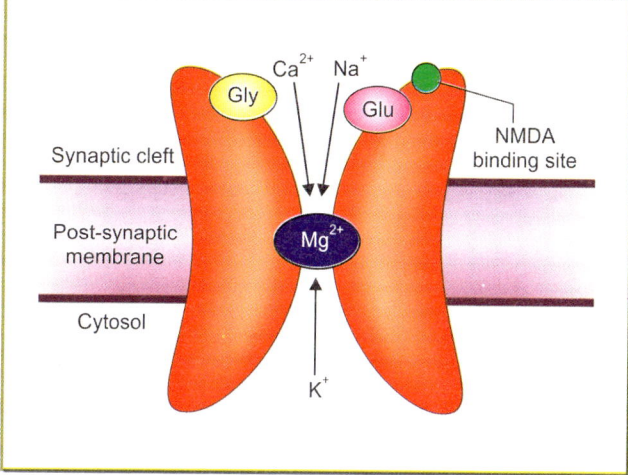

Fig. 16.2: The N-methyl-D-aspartate **(NMDA)** receptor. The binding of glutamate (Glu) and glycine (Gly) activates the receptor. It is thus a ligand-gated ion channel which permits the movement of Ca^{2+}, Na$^+$ and K$^+$ across the post-synaptic membrane. It is blocked by Mg^{2+}. The receptor is composed of multiple subunits out of which only two are shown for simplicity.

prostaglandins, some of which constrict blood vessels and further exacerbate hypoxia/ischemia.
3. Ca^{2+} activates cellular **endonucleases** leading to DNA fragmentation.
4. In the **mitochondria**, high Ca^{2+} levels induce swelling of the organelle and **impaired formation of ATP** via the Krebs cycle.

Although Ca^{2+} is the major culprit in excitatory amino acid-induced cytotoxicity, **nitric oxide (NO)** also plays an important role. Nitric oxide synthase (NOS) activity is enhanced by **N-methyl-D-aspartate (NMDA) receptor** (Fig. 16.2) activation. Neurons that exhibit NOS, and therefore, synthesize NO are protected from NO. However, NO released from NOS-expressing neurons in response to NMDA receptor activation kills adjacent neurons (Chemistry to Clinics 16.3).

Chemistry to Clinics 16.3: Drug Targets for Excitoxicity

Proposed new treatment strategies promise to enhance survival of neurons in ischemic/hypoxic disorders of the brain. These therapies include:

1. Drugs that block specific subtypes of glutamatergic receptors such as the NMDA receptor, which is mostly responsible for promoting high Ca^{2+} levels in the neurons.
2. Drugs/antioxidants that destroy oxygen-free radicals.
3. Ca^{2+} channel blocking agents.
4. NOS antagonists.

16

Opioid Neurotransmitters

Opioids are peptides that bind to opiate receptors. They are involved in the **control of pain perception** and other functions. Opioid peptides include methionine-enkephalin, leucine-enkephalin, dynorphins and β-endorphin. There are several opioid receptor subtypes: β-endorphin binds to μ receptors, enkephalins bind to μ and δ receptors while dynorphins bind to κ receptors. Many **analgesics** exploit one or more of these receptors (Chemistry to Clinics 16.4).

Chemistry to Clinics 16.4: Opioid Analgesics

Common opioid drugs include morphine, codeine, pethidine, fentanyl, pentazocine, etc. They are used to alleviate pain not responding to ordinary nonopioid analgesics, e.g. in postoperative pain, cancer pain, etc. However, they are also the common drugs of abuse.

SOME IMPORTANT QUESTIONS

1. Briefly discuss the various modes of information transfer between cells.

2. Write notes on:
    i. Autocrine signaling
    ii. Paracrine signaling
    iii. Neural communication
    iv. Nitric oxide
    v. Types of neurotransmitters
    vi. Excitotoxicity
    vii. Opioid neurotransmitters

MULTIPLE CHOICE QUESTIONS

1. **The protein connexin participates in:**
    A. Primary active transport
    B. Secondary active transport
    C. Gap junctions
    D. Synaptic transmission

2. **The following neurotransmitter enhances pain perception:**
    A. Substance P
    B. Enkephalins
    C. Endorphins
    D. Dynorphins

3. **The following is an inhibitory neurotransmitter:**
    A. Glycine
    B. GABA
    C. Both
    D. None of the above

4. **$GABA_B$ receptor is a:**
    A. Ca^{2+}-channel
    B. K^+-channel
    C. Cl^--channel
    D. Na^+-channel

5. **β-Endorphin binds to:**
    A. μ receptor
    B. δ receptor
    C. κ receptor
    D. All of the above

Endocrinology

A hormone is a **chemical messenger** that carries a signal to generate specific cellular alteration(s) by binding to its **cognate receptors**. According to the site of production and the site of action, hormones are classified into two groups:

Local Hormones

It includes the hormones that act in their immediate local environment via **paracrine/autocrine/juxtacrine signaling pathways**, and various **neurotransmitters**, as described in Chapter 16.

Endocrine (Systemic) Hormones

An endocrine or systemic hormone refers to the class of substances that arise in one tissue or gland and travel through **circulation** to reach a **target cell** which is expressing its receptors. Glands secreting these substances are called **endocrine glands**. The study of endocrine hormones, their receptors and the related disorders is referred to as **endocrinology**.

REGULATION OF HORMONE SECRETION

Most of the hormones exhibit their action through various components of the organ-system in series, referred to as the **hormone cascade system**. Hormone secretion is regulated by the hormone itself as well as by the central nervous system.

Hormonal Control

1. **Releasing hormones**: A stimulus may originate in the external environment or within the organism and may be transmitted as an electrical impulse or a chemical signal or both. In response to a signal from the central nervous system, **hypothalamus** releases specific hypothalamic releasing hormones called **liberins**. They are released in very small amounts (nanograms) and are transported down a closed **portal system** to gain access to the anterior pituitary.

2. **Tropic hormones:** In the **anterior pituitary**, the releasing hormones stimulate the secretion of specific anterior pituitary tropic hormones which are released in little higher amounts (micrograms) and circulate in the bloodstream to trigger the release of an ultimate hormone by the target gland.

3. **Ultimate hormone:** The ultimate hormone that is secreted by the **target gland** (μg to mg quantities daily), affects various target cells depending upon the number of receptors expressed by the cell.

4. **Feedback loops:** Regulation is accomplished through a series of **negative and positive feedback loops**. For example, hormones produced under the control of pituitary tropic hormones, feedback on the hypothalamic-pituitary system to regulate their own rates of secretion (Fig. 17.1). Most feedback control systems operate within minutes or hours in response to varying metabolic demands, to maintain homeostatic control within a narrow range.

Control by the Central Nervous System

Hormones secreted by the neurohypophysis and the adrenal medulla are controlled primarily by the nervous system. The hypothalamic nuclei receive

17

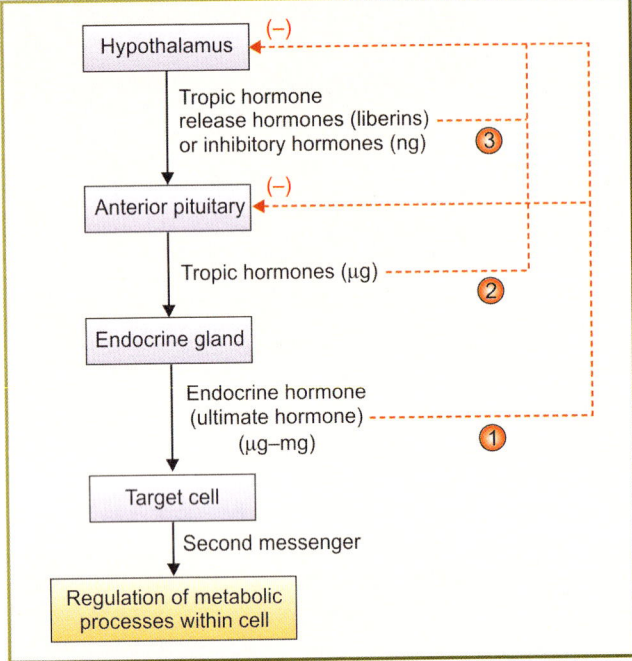

Fig. 17.1: Hormone cascade system and its regulation. 1. Long feedback loop; 2. Short feedback loop; 3. Ultra-short feedback loop.

neural signals from higher centers in the brain and fine-tune other control mechanisms.

Control by Chemical Constituents of Blood

Secretion of various hormones is also under the control of some constituents of blood, e.g. synthesis and release of insulin is regulated by the concentration of glucose present in blood. Similarly, secretion of the parathyroid hormone (PTH) is stimulated by low serum calcium levels.

Biorhythms

Certain endocrine rhythms result from cyclic activities of the **biological clock**. These include:

- **Circadian rhythm:** It occurs with a cyclic periodicity of 24 h, e.g. light-dark cycle (or sleep-wake cycle in which melatonin secreted by pineal gland plays a key role) and core body temperature (mid-afternoon peak [37.1°C] and trough/nadir [36.7°C] immediately after midnight). Many hormones follow this rhythm (Table 17.1; Chemistry to Clinics 17.1).
- **Ultradian rhythm or diurnal rhythm:** It occurs within the circadian rhythm, e.g. sleep cycles

Table 17.1: Circadian rhythm of hormones		
Hormone	*Peak*	*Trough/Nadir*
ACTH	4–8 AM	4 PM–Midnight
Cortisol	4–8 AM	4–6 PM
TSH	2–4 AM	4–8 PM
Growth hormone	Midnight	1–3 AM
PTH	2–4 PM	7–9 AM

Chemistry to Clinics 17.1: Circadian Rhythm disorders
Various disorders related to alterations in circadian rhythm include:

1. **Delayed sleep phase disorder:** Delayed sleep onset in adolescents and young adults.
2. **Advanced sleep phase disorder:** Early evening sleep onset and early morning awakening in elderly.
3. **Narcolepsy:** Excessive daytime sleepiness.
4. **Jet lag:** Due to time zone shifts.
5. **Shift work disorder:** Due to day-night work shifts.

occurring throughout night, eating and micturition (approximately every 4 h).
- **Infradian rhythm:** It occurs at longer than 24 h interval, may be weeks, e.g. menstrual cycle.

MECHANISM OF ACTION OF HORMONES

Signal Transduction

All cells have the capacity to respond to their surroundings by detecting chemical signals through receptor molecules. The sequence of steps whereby a receptor perceives the signal, a transducer relays the signal and an effector converts the signal into an intracellular response, is called **signal transduction**.

Hormones act after binding with their specific receptors which are located either intracellularly or on the cell membrane (on the extracellular aspect). **Hormone receptors** are proteins that differ by their specificity for the ligand as well as location within the cell. A hormone-receptor complex usually undergoes conformational changes due to interaction of the receptor with the hormone. There are several types of receptor systems which vary in mechanism:

1. **Intracellular receptors: Lipid-soluble hormones** such as steroids and thyroid hormones diffuse into the cell and bind to intracellular receptors which are located either in the cytosol or in the nucleus (Table 17.2). By convention, lipophilic hormones are called **class I hormones.**

Table 17.2: Hormone receptors

Type of receptor	Hormone
Intracellular Receptors	
Cytosolic	Steroids
Nuclear	Calcitriol, T_3
Cell Surface Receptors	
Linked to Tyrosine Kinase	
Intrinsic tyrosine kinase	Insulin, insulin-like growth factor-1 (IGF-1)
Recruit tyrosine kinase	Growth hormone, prolactin
G-Protein-linked Receptors	
↑Adenylate cyclase activity	ADH, epinephrine (β-adrenergic receptors), glucagon
↑Guanylate cyclase activity	ANP, nitric oxide
↑Phospholipase C activity	Oxytocin, PTH, Ca^{2+}, calcitonin, epinephrine (α_1-adrenergic receptors)

2. Membrane receptors: Water-soluble hormones such as pancreatic hormones, catecholamines, and pituitary-derived proteins/glycoproteins are hydrophilic and cannot cross the lipid barrier of the cell membrane. These hormones therefore interact with the receptors that are located on the cell surface (membrane receptors). By convention, hydrophilic hormones are called **class II hormones.**

MEMBRANE RECEPTORS

Interaction of the hormone with the cell surface receptor causes a conformational change in the receptor and other associated membrane proteins. This, in turn, activates enzymes inside the cell thereby resulting in the synthesis of a second messenger which activates the phosphorylating enzymes. There are 2 superfamilies of cell surface receptors. The first is linked to **tyrosine kinase** and the second to **G-proteins**. These receptors have 3 clearly identifiable domains:

1. **Extracellular domain (ectodomain):** It binds the hormone with high affinity.
2. **Transmembrane domain (membrane-spanning):** It is hydrophobic and varies in structure.
3. **Cytosolic domain:** It initiates the intracellular signaling cascade. This is the effector region of the receptor which may be linked with another membrane protein system, a set of enzymes that are guanosine triphosphatases (GTPases). The intracellular region may also have regulatory tyrosine or serine/threonine phosphorylation sites.

Tyrosine Kinase-linked Cell Surface Receptors

They rely upon tyrosine kinase for the initiation of downstream signals. They have a relatively simple transmembrane segment, and are of two types:

1. **Receptors with intrinsic tyrosine kinase activity:** Tyrosine kinase activity is located in the cytosolic domain. The most prominent members of this subgroup are the receptors for insulin and insulin-like growth factor-1 (IGF-1).
2. **Receptors that recruit tyrosine kinase activity:** They recruit tyrosine kinase activity after binding of the receptor with the hormone. The best known in this category are the receptors for growth hormone and prolactin.

Mechanism of Action of Insulin

Insulin receptors: Insulin receptors contain an **intrinsic (hormone-activated) tyrosine kinase activity** which serves as a direct catalyst for phosphorylation (Fig. 17.2). The receptor consists of two α- and two β-subunits. The α-subunits are on the extracellular aspect of the cell membrane and contain the insulin-binding site whereas the β-subunits possess intracellular domains containing ATP-binding sites and a catalytic kinase domain.

Signal transduction: Insulin, as we know, is secreted in response to **rising blood glucose, following a meal**. Insulin receptor binding stimulates aggregation of receptors and promotes tyrosine kinase activity in the intracellular domain of the receptors. The receptor kinase activity **autophosphorylates** its tyrosine residues, enhancing its protein tyrosine kinase activity

17

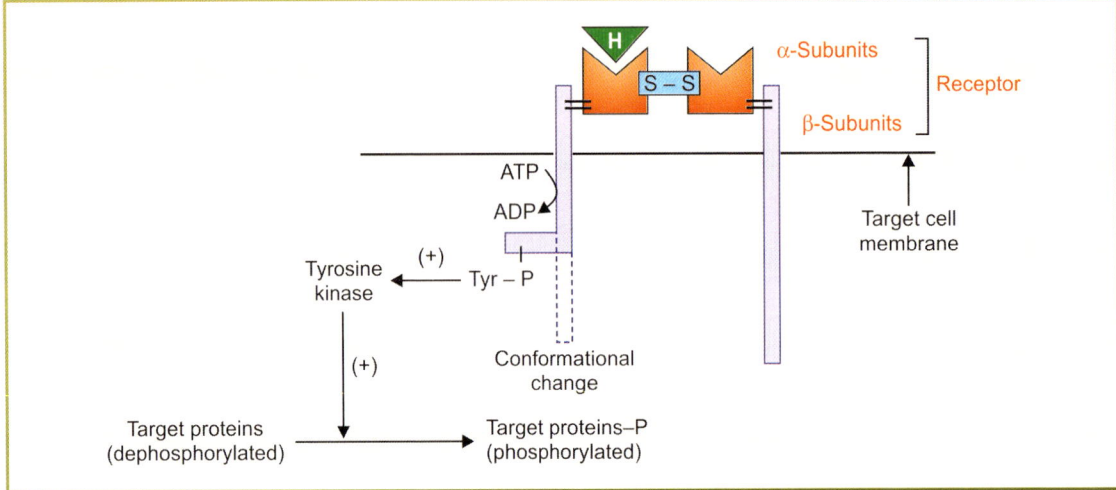

Fig. 17.2: Modulation of tyrosine kinase activity of insulin receptor. H = Hormone (insulin).

as well as phosphorylating tyrosine residues of other intracellular effector proteins called **insulin receptor substrates (IRS)**, mainly IRS-1 and IRS-2. When phosphorylated, these proteins interact with another set of proteins containing two SH2 (Src Homology 2; Src is the abbreviation for 'sarcoma' and SH2 proteins are proto-oncogenic tyrosine kinase proteins) domains, which get activated upon binding to IRS.

As a result of the binding of different signal proteins to the phosphorylated IRS, **several distinct signaling pathways become activated**. These include kinases that phosphorylate serine and threonine residues on certain proteins such as GTPase, phosphodiesterase and phosphoprotein phosphatases. Insulin dependent activation of these proteins also checks the actions of glucagon. One pathway may stimulate DNA synthesis and cell division while another may activate a transcription factor that turns-on the expression of insulin-specific genes (Fig. 17.3).

Cellular response: In muscle and adipose tissue, receptor tyrosine kinase activity induces movement of glucose transporter-4 (GLUT-4) from the intracellular vacuoles to the cell surface, thereby increasing glucose uptake. *In the muscles*, glucose is used for the synthesis of glycogen while *in the adipose tissue* glucose is used to produce glyceraldehyde-3-phosphate, which is converted to glycerol-3-phosphate for the synthesis of triacylglycerols.

The hormone-receptor complex also results in internalization and degradation of receptor molecules.

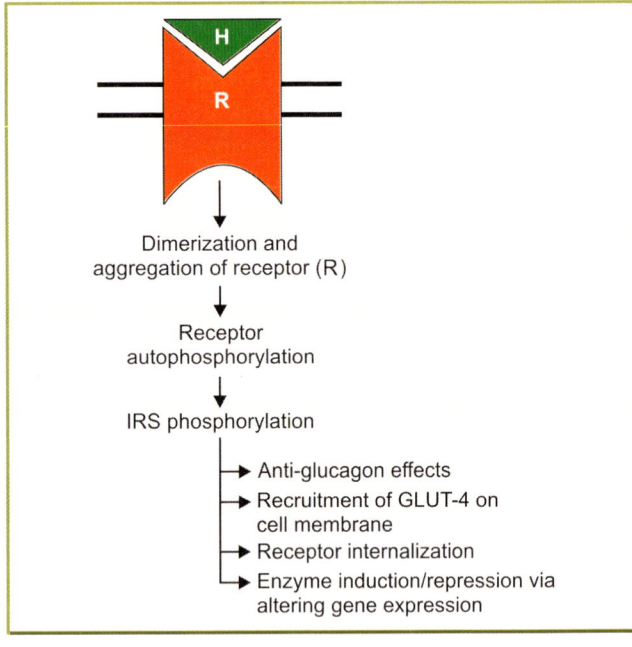

Fig. 17.3: Mechanism of action of insulin. H = Insulin hormone.

The process provides a means of regulating the effects of insulin by down-regulating its receptors.

G-Protein-linked Receptors

The second major group of cell surface receptors couples with G-proteins (**guanine-proteins**) that are associated with the inner aspect of the cell membrane. G-proteins exist as **hetero-trimeric complexes** with α, β and γ subunits in their resting state, i.e. in the absence of a hormone-occupied and activated receptor, forming a **G-protein pool** within the membrane. The β and γ subunits associate with such a high affinity that the functional units are Gα and Gβ/γ. After association of the G-protein complex with the hormone-occupied receptor, conformational changes in the α-subunit lead to increased rate of dissociation of GDP, which is replaced by GTP. This dissociates the activated G-protein from the hormone-receptor complex, releasing the α-subunit from the hetero-trimeric complex. GTP-activated α-subunit of the G-protein subsequently diffuses in the lipid bilayer and binds to the **catalytic unit** which is either adenylate cyclase or phospholipase C.

There are four major subfamilies of Gα subunit. These are $G_s\alpha$ and $G_i\alpha$ which activate or inhibit adenylate cyclase respectively; $G_q\alpha$ which activates phospholipase C; and $G_o\alpha$ which activates ion channels. Gα subunit can also function as a **GTPase** which cleaves phosphate from GTP, resulting in Gα-GDP. This switches-off the activation of the catalytic subunit and allows re-association of Gα-GDP with the Gβ/γ. This reforms a new hetero-trimer which returns to G-protein in the membrane and is **recycled** to respond to another receptor.

The most striking structural differences in G-protein-linked receptor from the tyrosine kinase-linked receptor lies in the transmembrane region which has a characteristic hepta-helical structure (i.e. it crosses the membrane bilayer seven times). Further, its cytoplasmic domain links the receptor to the signal transducing G-proteins which function as molecular switches by binding and hydrolyzing GTP to GDP. The activated protein then undergoes major structural modifications and ultimately modulates the catalytic activity of adenylate cyclase or phospholipase C. This, in turn, leads to the generation of some intracellular **second messenger** such as cAMP, IP_3, etc.

SECOND MESSENGERS

Cyclic AMP

Cyclic AMP (cAMP) is a small molecule derived from ATP by the catalytic action of the signaling enzyme adenylate cyclase (Fig. 17.4). It has a key role in the regulation of various metabolic processes.

- The **β-adrenergic** receptor is coupled to **adenylate cyclase activation** by the action of the α-subunit

of the stimulatory G-protein (G_s). $G_s\alpha$ activates membrane-bound adenylate cyclase which catalyzes the conversion of ATP to cAMP. This cyclic nucleotide acts as a potent second messenger and activates cAMP-dependent protein kinase A, which modulates multiple aspects of cell function.

- On the other hand, G-protein coupled **α-adrenergic receptors** inhibit cAMP generation via inhibitory G-protein (G_i) mediated **inhibition of adenylate cyclase**, and exhibit opposite effects.

Activation of protein kinase A by cAMP through G-protein: Inactive protein kinase A is a tetramer. It has two **regulatory subunits (R)** and two **catalytic subunits (C)**. The enzyme is activated by four molecules of cAMP which bind to the R-subunits and result in dissociation of its two C-subunits. The free C-subunit phosphorylates target proteins and produces various metabolic effects of the hormone (Fig. 17.5):

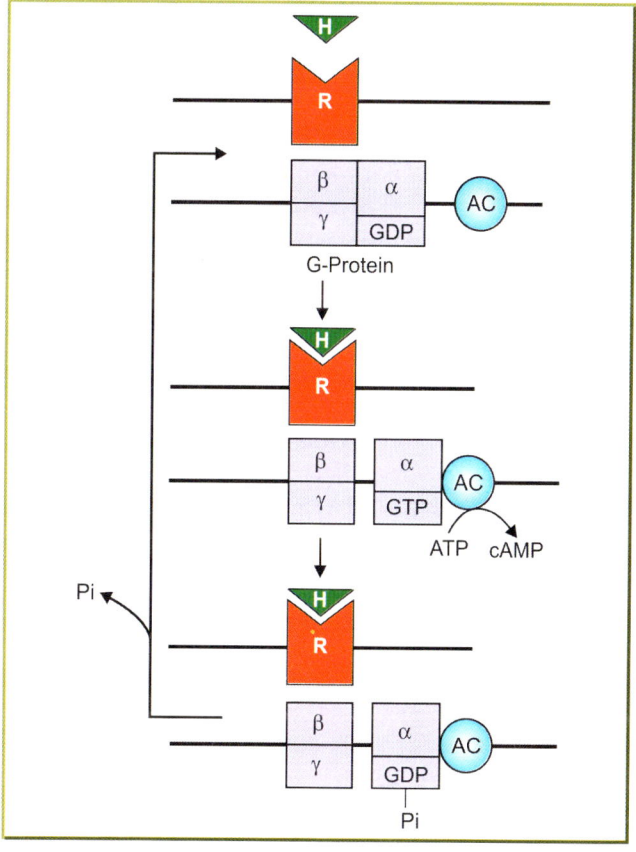

Fig. 17.4: Activation of adenylate cyclase (AC) by G-protein. H = Hormone; R = Receptor.

17

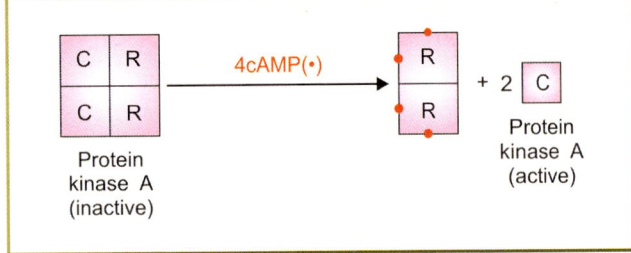

Fig. 17.5: Activation of protein kinase A by cAMP (•).

1. **Glycogen metabolism:** cAMP transduces its effects on glycogen-glucose interconversion by regulating protein kinase A, which phosphorylates target proteins on serine and threonine residues (Fig. 17.6). Two key target proteins are the enzymes phosphorylase kinase and glycogen synthase, involved in glycogenolysis and glycogenesis, respectively.

2. **Regulation of ion channels:** Protein kinase A mediated phosphorylation regulates the activity of K^+, Cl^- and Ca^{2+} channels.

3. **Cell signaling and gene regulation:** Phosphorylation regulates the activity of phosphatases that are involved in the regulation of cell signaling. In addition, translocation of protein kinase A into the nucleus allows modulation of the activity of transcription factors such as **cAMP-responsive element binding protein (CREB)**. This is then translocated into the nucleus where it binds a short palindromic sequence in the promoter region of the cAMP-regulated genes, referred to as **CRE (cAMP response element)** and thereby has a direct effect on gene transcription. Serotonin, a hormone derived from tryptophan, acts through a similar signaling pathway in the brain to regulate long-term memory (Chemistry to Clinics 17.2).

Termination of cAMP signaling: Phosphodiesterase (PDE) terminates the cAMP signal by

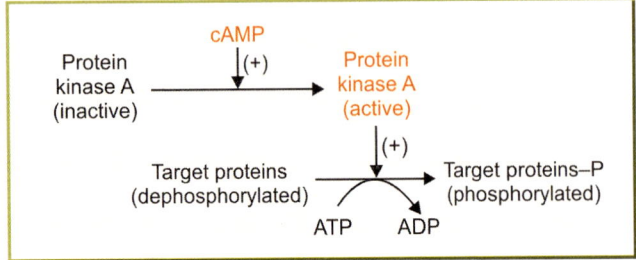

Fig. 17.6: Activation of intracellular proteins through protein kinase A.

converting cAMP to its 5′-AMP metabolite (Fig. 17.7). The PDE inhibitors are an important class of therapeutic agents (Chemistry to Clinics 17.3).

Mechanism of Action of Glucagon

Glucagon binds to its receptors on the outer surface of the target cells and stimulates breakdown of glycogen to glucose as follows:

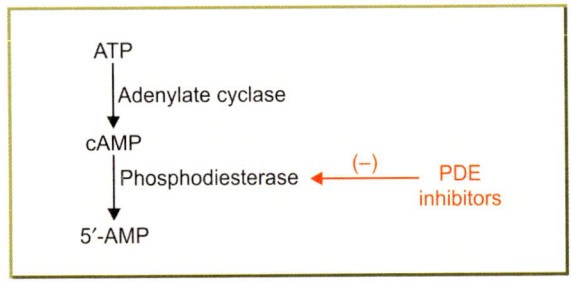

Fig. 17.7: Degradation of cAMP by phosphodiesterase (PDE), a target for PDE inhibitors.

- Binding of the hormone activates adenylate cyclase on the inner surface of the membrane, leading to the production of **cAMP**.

- This second messenger binds to the regulatory subunit of the cAMP-dependent protein kinase A, which phosphorylates phosphorylase kinase and glycogen synthase. It leads to the activation of phosphorylase kinase and inhibition of glycogen synthase.

- The activated phosphorylase kinase, in turn, **activates glycogen phosphorylase**, which initiates **glycogenolysis** leading to the production of glucose-6-phosphate that is hydrolyzed to glucose and exported to blood.

- Protein kinase A also phosphorylates inhibitor-1, a protein phosphatase inhibitor protein, which inhibits cytoplasmic phosphoprotein phosphatase.

- Other hepatic pathways including protein, cholesterol, fatty acid and triglyceride biosynthesis and glycolysis are also regulated by phosphorylation of key regulatory enzymes favoring metabolism in response to glycogen breakdown for the provision of glucose to blood, for the maintenance of vital body functions.

Guanylate cyclase receptors: Receptors for the **atrial natriuretic peptide (ANP)** and **nitric oxide (NO)** are guanylate cyclases that span the plasma membrane. Extracellular domain of the receptor binds the hormone while its intracellular domain synthesizes cGMP which serves as the second messenger for the hormone. **cGMP** mediates the action of these hormones by phosphorylating cGMP-dependent protein kinases which ultimately maintain cation channels in open conformation.

Calcium Ions as Second Messengers

Calcium ion (Ca^{2+}) is a **ubiquitous messenger** and has an important role in the transduction of signals leading to a number of cellular responses. Ligation of a wide range of hormone receptors leads to a rapid and transient increase in intracellular Ca^{2+} concentration to the micromolar range. Rapid rise and fall of Ca^{2+} is **tightly regulated** and utilizes a variety of mechanisms including cell compartmentalization. For example, intracellular Ca^{2+} can be lowered by sequestration of Ca^{2+} into the endoplasmic reticulum by Ca^{2+}-ATPase

or into the mitochondria using energy-driven electrochemical gradient. Ca^{2+} **activates several enzymes** including:

1. **Protein kinases, calmodulin-dependent kinases and some forms of protein kinase C:** Many downstream signaling events mediated by Ca^{2+} are modulated by a Ca^{2+}-sensing and binding protein, calmodulin.

2. **Phospholipase A_2:** It liberates arachidonic acid from phospholipids and thereby generates eicosanoids, precursors of important chemically related signal molecules that include thromboxanes, leukotrienes, lipoxins and prostaglandins.

3. **Cytosolic guanylate cyclase:** It catalyzes the formation of cGMP.

Inositol Triphosphate

Some hormones such as **epinephrine** and **norepinephrine** (through α-adrenergic receptors), **ADH** (via V1 receptors), **angiotensin II,** etc. bind with their receptors and result in activation of phospholipase C. This enzyme catalyzes hydrolysis of phosphatidylinositol-4,5-bisphosphate (PIP_2) to *diacylglycerol* (DAG) and *inositol-1,4,5-triphosphate* (IP_3), both of which act as second messengers (Fig. 17.8).

IP_3 diffuses into the cytosol and causes **release of intracellular Ca^{2+} from Ca^{2+}-rich organelles** such as endoplasmic reticulum (ER). Ca^{2+} interacts with calmodulin (C) and forms **Ca^{2+}-calmodulin complex** which, in turn, activates calmodulin specific kinases.

DAG activates protein kinase C that generally phosphorylates a wide range of signal transduction proteins at several residues.

Free Ca^{2+}, calmodulin specific kinases as well as protein kinase C may cause phosphorylation of the target protein(s) to exhibit physiological actions (Fig. 17.9).

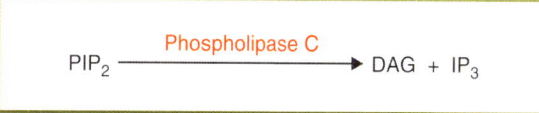

Fig. 17.8: Phospholipase C catalyzed generation of second messengers. DAG = Diacyl glycerol; IP_3 = Inositol-1,4,5-triphosphate; PIP_2 = Phosphatidyl inositol-4,5-bisphosphate.

17

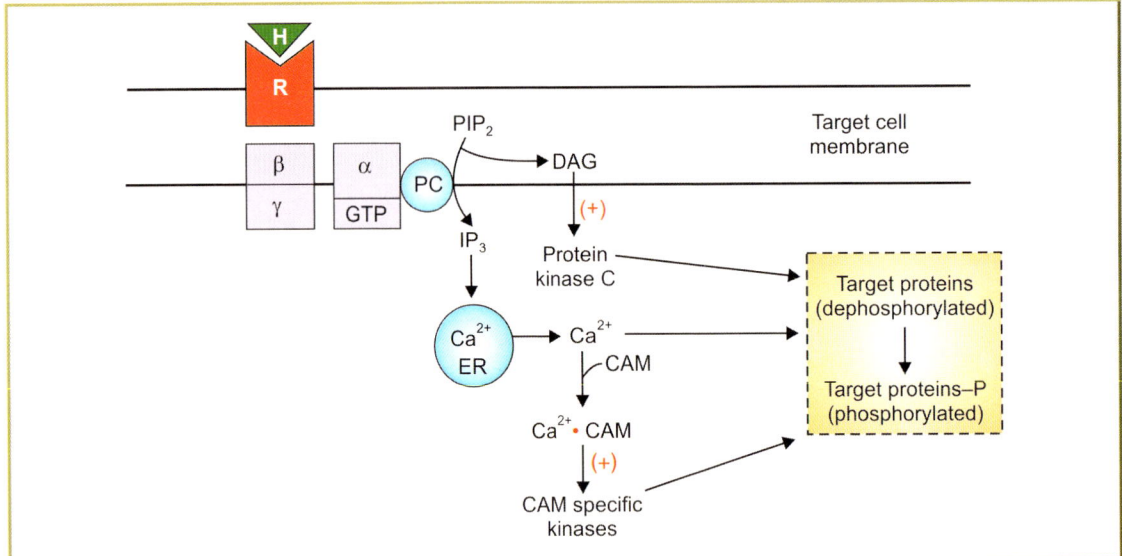

Fig. 17.9: Activation of phospholipase C (PC) by G-protein. CAM = Calmodulin; ER = endoplasmic reticulum; H = Hormone.

Mechanism of Action of Epinephrine

Epinephrine works through several distinct receptors on different cells. The best studied of these receptors are **α and β adrenergic receptors**. They bind epinephrine with different affinities and work by different mechanisms.

Action on hepatic glycogen

- Epinephrine action on hepatic **glycogenolysis via β-adrenergic receptor is similar to that for glucagon**, involving a plasma membrane epinephrine specific receptor, G-protein and cAMP. The epinephrine response augments the effects of glucagon during severe hypoglycemia.
- Epinephrine also works simultaneously through **α-receptors by a different mechanism**. Binding to α-receptors also involves G-proteins but in this case the G-protein is specific for activation of an **isoenzyme of phospholipase C**, which cleaves PIP_2 to DAG and IP_3. Both the hydrolyzed products act as second messengers.
- DAG activates protein kinase C, which, like protein kinase A, initiates a series of protein phosphorylation reactions.
- IP_3 promotes transport of Ca^{2+} into the cytosol.
- Ca^{2+} then binds to the cytoplasmic protein calmodulin, which binds to and activates phosphorylase kinase, leading to phosphorylation and activation of phosphorylase, providing glucose for blood.

- Ca^{2+}-calmodulin dependent protein kinase and other enzymes are also activated either by phosphorylation or by association with the Ca^{2+}-calmodulin complex.

Thus, a range of metabolic pathways are activated in response to stress, causing an increase in blood glucose to support a '**fight or flight**' response (discussed later).

Action on muscle glycogen: Muscles, as we know, **lack glucose-6-phosphatase** activity. Hence, muscle glycogen cannot be mobilized to replenish blood glucose. Muscle glycogenolysis is activated in response to epinephrine through β-adrenergic receptor, mediated through cAMP, providing carbohydrate for the **energy** for muscle during **prolonged exercise** (Fig. 17.10).

INTRACELLULAR RECEPTORS

Some hormones such as steroid and thyroid hormones, being **hydrophobic**, can diffuse across the plasma membrane of their target cells. The hormone diffuses into the cytosol or the nucleus where it binds either to the **cytoplasmic receptors**, e.g. glucocorticoid/mineralocorticoid receptors, or the **nuclear receptors** such as progesterone, estradiol, vitamin D_3 or androgen receptors. These receptors have two regions, i.e. a hydrophobic hormone binding region and a DNA binding region which consists of two zinc fingers, rich in cysteine and basic amino acids.

17

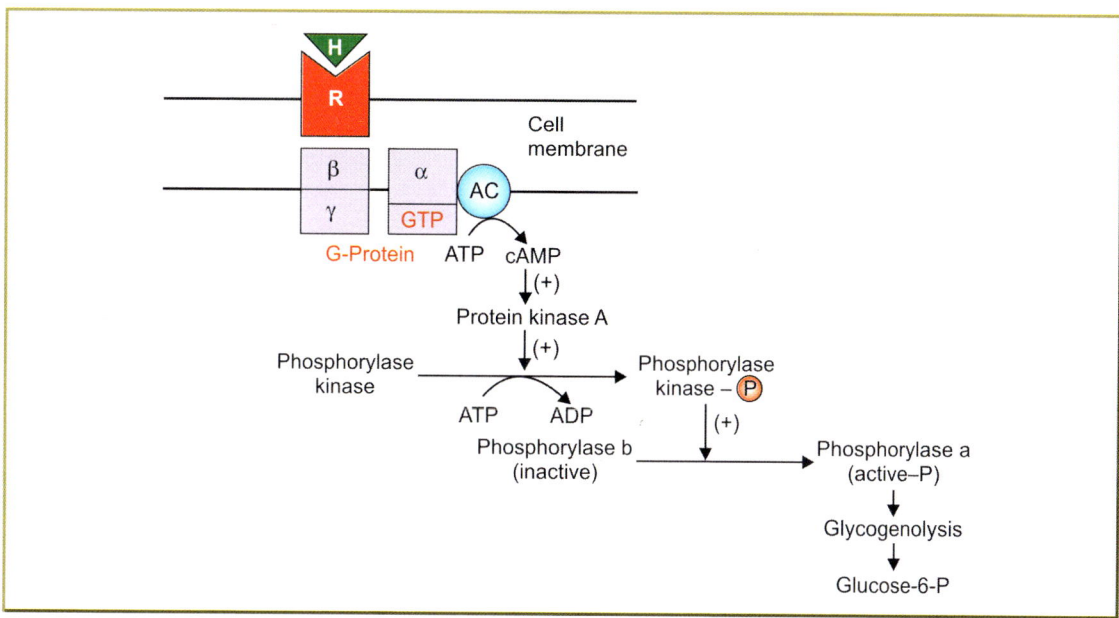

Fig. 17.10: Mechanism of action of epinephrine (H, Hormone) via β-adrenergic receptors (R) in muscle, AC=Adenylate cyclase.

Mechanism of Action of Steroid Hormones, Thyroid Hormones and Vitamin D

Binding of the hormone with the receptor causes a conformational change in the receptor and activates it. The activated receptor is thereafter translocated into the nucleus where it binds to DNA, upstream of the specific 'hormone response elements'. This, in turn, leads to the activation/repression of the transcription of the **hormone responsive genes**. The non-activated receptor cannot bind to DNA because heteromeric heat shock proteins (Hsp) block its DNA binding site (Fig. 17.11).

Regulation of Hormone Receptors

Receptor proteins are not static components of the cell. Their quantity (number/concentration of receptors) and/or quality (affinity for the hormone) may increase or decrease in response to various stimuli including the corresponding hormone itself. Hormone receptor levels undergo autoregulation. These may be downregulated or upregulated. **Downregulation** means reduction in the concentration and/or affinity of the receptor molecules while **upregulation** means increase in the concentration and/or affinity of the receptor molecules.

Many intracellular receptors are downregulated when a cell is exposed to certain amount of the hormone. The receptor gene may have a specific responsive element on its promoter whose action results in inhibition of transcription of the receptor mRNA. Downregulation of receptor by its ligand thus prevents overstimulation of the target cell when circulating hormone levels are elevated.

CLASSIFICATION OF HORMONES ACCORDING TO CHEMICAL STRUCTURE

According to the chemical structure, hormones may be divided into three groups:

1. Those containing peptide bonds, i.e. **peptide/protein hormones**.
2. Those derived from cholesterol, i.e. **steroid hormones**.
3. Those arising from the amino acid tyrosine, i.e. **catecholamines** and **thyroid hormones**.

Table 17.3 lists some of the hormones with their chemical nature, site and principal actions.

PEPTIDE HORMONES

Hormones of the hypothalamus and the pituitary are protein in nature. For their synthesis, genes encode mRNAs which are translated into protein precursors which undergo post-translational cleavage and/or processing to form the active hormone which is recognized by receptors on the target tissue.

17

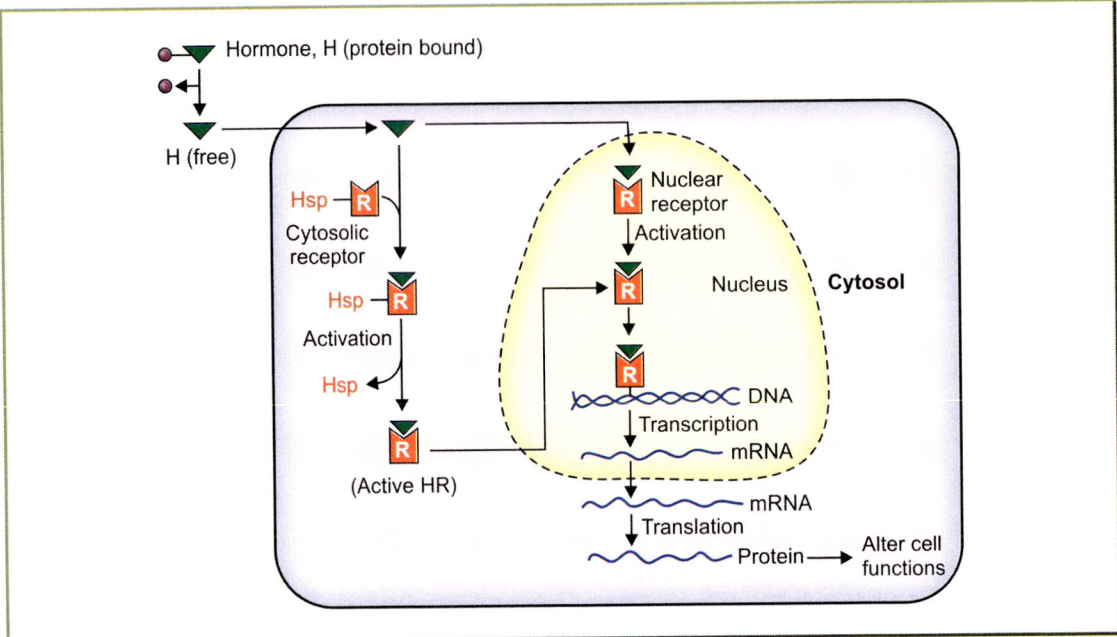

Fig. 17.11: Mode of action of hormone through intracellular receptors.

Hormones of the Hypothalamus

Hypothalamus produces a number of hormones which control secretion of the pituitary hormones (Table 17.3). These include:

- **Growth hormone releasing hormone (GHRH):** It has dominant influence on growth hormone (GH) release while somatostatin acts as **growth hormone inhibitory hormone (GHIH)**.
- **Luteinizing hormone-releasing hormone (LHRH;** also called gonadotropin-releasing hormone, **GnRH):** It plays a major role in controlling the release of luteinizing hormone (LH) and follicle stimulating hormone (FSH).
- **Thyrotropin releasing hormone (TRH):** It controls the release of thyroid stimulating hormone (TSH). It also influences the release of prolactin (PRL).
- **Corticotropin-releasing hormone (CRH):** It controls the release of adrenocorticotropin, also called adrenocorticotropic hormone (ACTH).
- **Dopamine:** It acts as prolactin inhibitory factor (**PIF**).

Various **releasing hormones (factors)** or **liberins** are synthesized in the neurons situated along the margin of the third ventricle as well as by those that are projected to other parts of the brain. Releasing factors produced by the hypothalamic neurons reach the anterior pituitary via **portal system**, to stimulate or inhibit the production of the hormone.

Hormones of the Pituitary

The pituitary gland, also designated as **hypophysis**, produces six hormones and stores additional two hormones. It is called the '**master gland**' of endocrine orchestra. It is composed of principally the anterior lobe (**adenohypophysis**) and the posterior lobe (**neurohypophysis**).

Hormones of the Anterior Pituitary

Major hormones of the anterior pituitary include GH, TSH or thyrotropin, ACTH, β-MSH, corticotropin-like intermediary peptide (CLIP), PRL, FSH and LH. Of these, all are single polypeptides except TSH, FSH and LH which are dimers and share an identical subunit. Genes for the polypeptide hormones contain coding sequence for the hormone as well as the control elements upstream of the structural gene. In some cases more than one hormone is also encoded by a gene. Some hormones of the anterior pituitary are synthesized from a large precursor referred to as pro-opiomelanocortin (POMC).

Table 17.3: Salient features of major hormones

Hormone	Chemical nature	Target (site of action)	Key functions
HYPOTHALAMUS			
Growth hormone releasing hormone (GHRH)	P	Anterior pituitary	Release of GH
Growth hormone inhibitory hormone (GHIH)	P		Suppression of GH and TSH
Luteinizing hormone releasing hormone (LHRH)	P		Release of FSH and LH
Thyrotropin releasing hormone (TRH)	P		Release of TSH and PRL
Corticotropin releasing hormone (CRH)	P		Release of ACTH and β-lipotropin
Prolactin releasing factor (PRF)	P		Release of PRL
Prolactin inhibitory factor (PIF, dopamine)	A		Suppression of PRL
ANTERIOR PITUITARY			
Growth hormone (GH)	P	Several tissues	Overall growth
Follicle stimulating hormone (FSH)	P	Ovaries	Follicular growth
Luteinizing hormone (LH)	P	Ovaries	Ovulation; secretion of progesterone
Thyroid stimulating hormone (TSH)	P	Thyroid gland	↑synthesis of T_4 and T_3
Adrenocorticotropic hormone (ACTH)	P	Adrenal cortex	↑synthesis of adrenocortical hormones
Prolactin (PRL)	P	Mammary gland, brain	Milk secretion; regulate mood and sexual behavior
β-Lipotropin	P	Adipose tissue, skin, brain	Precursor of β-MSH and endorphins; lipolysis
α-Melanocyte stimulating hormone (α-MSH)	P	Skin	Pigmentation
POSTERIOR PITUITARY			
Antidiuretic hormone (ADH, vasopressin)	P	Arterioles, distal/collecting tubules	↑Blood pressure; ↑water reabsorption
Oxytocin	P	Myometrium, mammary gland	Parturition; milk ejection
ADRENAL CORTEX			
Cortisol	S	Several tissues	Metabolism; immune regulation
Aldosterone	S	Distal tubules	Water/electrolyte balance
Dehydroepiandrosterone (DHEA)	S	Gonads	Weak androgen; estradiol precursor
ADRENAL MEDULLA			
Norepinephrine, epinephrine	A	Several tissues	↑Sympathetic activity; glycogenolysis; lipolysis
THYROID GLAND			
Thyroxine (T_4) and triiodothyronine (T_3)	A	Several tissues	Regulate metabolic rate
Calcitonin	P	Bones, kidneys	↓Plasma calcium
PARATHYROID GLAND			
Parathyroid hormone (PTH)	P	Bones, kidneys	Ca/P homeostasis

Contd...

17

17

Contd...

Hormone	Chemical nature	Target (site of action)	Key functions
PANCREAS			
Insulin	P	Several tissues	Blood glucose regulation; lipogenesis; ↑protein synthesis
Glucagon	P	Liver	Glycogenolysis
Somatostatin	P	Pancreas	↓Insulin release
GIT			
Gastrin	P	Stomach	↑HCl secretion
Secretin	P	Pancreas	↑Pancreatic HCO_3^- secretion
Cholecystokinin	P	Gallbladder	Contraction of gallbladder
Motilin (housekeeper of the gut)	P	GIT	↑GIT motility (gastric emptying and peristalsis)
Vasoactive intestinal peptide (VIP)	P	GIT	Smooth muscle relaxation (stomach, gallbladder, vascular)
Gastric inhibitory polypeptide (GIP)	P	GIT	Incretin (↑insulin secretion)
Bombesin	P	GIT	↑Gastrin release
Neurotensin	P	GIT, hypothalamus	Small intestinal contraction and secretion
Substance P	P	GIT, brain	Analgesic
KIDNEYS			
1,25(OH)$_2$D$_3$ (Calcitriol)	S	Bones, kidneys, small intestine	Ca/P homeostasis, various non-skeletal effects
Renin	P	Plasma angiotensinogen	Regulation of blood pressure; water/electrolyte balance
Erythropoietin	P	Bone marrow	↑Erythropoiesis
GONADS			
Testosterone (testes)	S	Testes	Spermatogenesis; secondary sexual characteristics
Estradiol (ovaries)	S	Endometrium, anterior pituitary	Maintain endometrium (follicular phase); ↓FSH release
Progesterone (ovaries)	S	Endometrium, anterior pituitary	Maintain endometrium (luteal phase for implantation); ↓LH release
Inhibin (ovaries)	P	Anterior pituitary	↓FSH release
ADIPOSE TISSUE			
Leptin	P	Brain	Regulation of feeding behavior
HEART			
Atrial natriuretic peptide (ANP)	P	Kidneys, adrenal cortex	Natriuresis; ↓aldosterone secretion
BLOOD VESSEL (ENDOTHELIUM)			
Nitric oxide	Gas	Vascular smooth muscle	Vasodilatation
PLACENTA			
Human chorionic gonadotropin (HCG)	P	Ovaries, uterus	Maintains corpus luteum in early pregnancy, uterine angiogenesis

P = Peptide/Protein; **S** = Steroid; **A** = Amino acid derivative

- **Pro-opiomelanocortin (POMC):** It is a polypeptide (M$_r$ 31 kD) which is encoded by a single gene (a protein hormone precursor for several hormones). *In the corticotrophs* of the anterior pituitary, it is cleaved to release **ACTH** and **β-lipotropin** as the major products into the circulation. *In the pars intermedia*, these products are further cleaved to release **α-MSH, CLIP, γ-lipotropin** and **β-endorphin**, into the circulation (Fig. 17.12).
- **Growth Hormone (GH, somatotropin):** It is secreted by somatotrophs which make up about 50% of the anterior pituitary cells. It consists of a single polypeptide chain of 191 amino acids (M$_r$ 22 kD) with two intra-chain disulfide bonds. It is cleaved from a larger precursor molecule (M$_r$ 28 kD).

Forms of GH: Multiple forms of GH exist in the circulation:

- Monomeric GH (M$_r$ 22 kD) which is the predominant form of GH.
- Large oligomeric form, the big GH (M$_r$ 44 kD).
- Smaller GH (M$_r$ 20 kD).

Somatomedins: GH is a stimulator of growth and acts indirectly by stimulating the formation of other hormones. These factors are known as somatomedins (somatotropin-mediating hormones) or insulin-like growth factors (IGFs) which are GH-dependent and are responsible for growth stimulation. **IGF-I** is the most important somatomedin for postnatal growth, produced predominantly in the liver. It is a basic protein that circulates bound to six distinct IGF binding proteins (IGF-BPs). IGF-1 is structurally similar to proinsulin and exerts insulin-like actions.

Regulators of GH: Some amino acids such as arginine are potent stimuli for GH release. Hypoglycemia is also a stimulus for GH release while an acute rise in blood sugar inhibits GH release. It may act as an insulin antagonist, to inhibit glucose uptake by the tissues. However, it complements the anabolic action of insulin on amino acid uptake. GH also increases the release of free fatty acids from the adipocytes. Increased serum free fatty acids concentration blunts GH release.

Effects of GH: GH is necessary for normal linear growth. Its secretion is low in infancy, increases during early childhood and reaches to a maximum level during puberty. GH secretion is lower in adulthood than during puberty. After the third decade, a

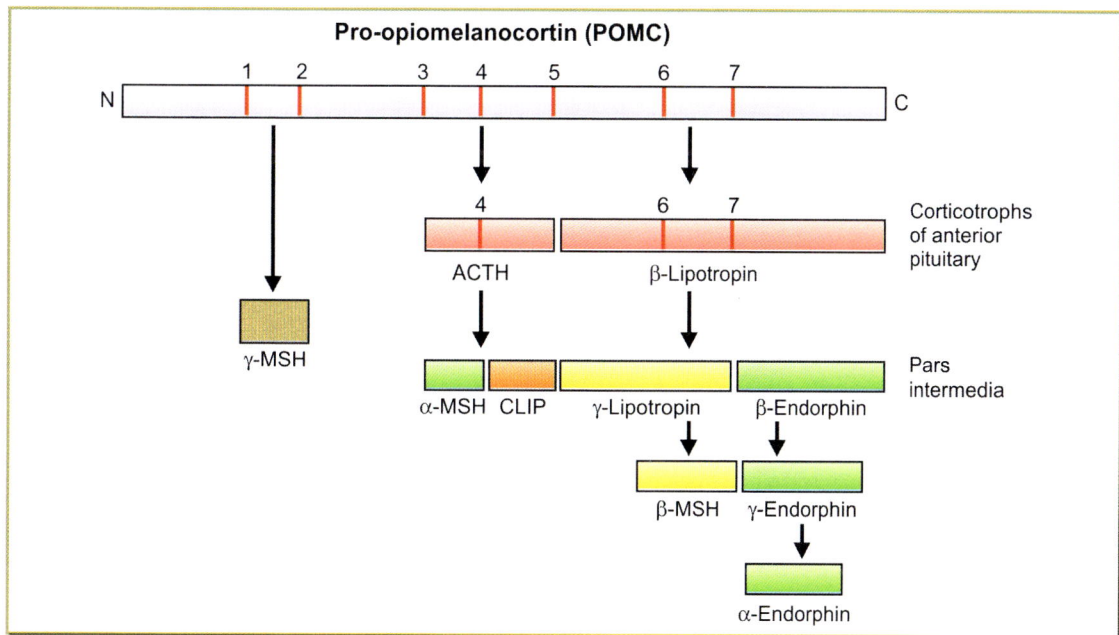

Fig. 17.12: Pro-opiomelanocortin **(POMC)** and its processing. Cleavage sites are numbered 1–7. **ACTH** regulates adrenal steroidogenesis. **CLIP** is involved in regulation of pain perception, autonomic system, biorhythms and behavior. **Lipotropins** regulate lipolysis and along with α- and β-MSH regulate skin pigmentation. γ-MSH regulates sodium balance and blood pressure. **Endorphins** modulate pain perception.

17

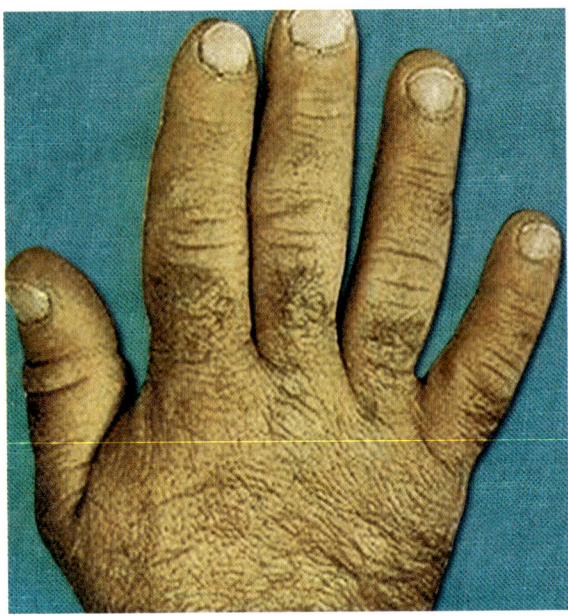

Fig. 17.13: Acromegaly. Coarse features, bony and soft tissue overgrowth. A **'moist, doughy handshake'** is characteristic.

progressive decline in secretion of GH occurs. GH also exerts various metabolic effects. It stimulates the incorporation of amino acids into proteins.

Interestingly, GH is less important in regulating fetal growth (Chemistry to Clinics 17.4). Excess of GH leads to acromegaly and gigantism while its deficiency causes short stature (dwarfism) (Chemistry to Clinics 17.5).

- **Gonadotropins:** Gonadotrophs make up about 10% of the anterior pituitary and secrete two hormones collectively referred to as gonadotropins. They are called **FSH** and **LH**. Both of these are glycoproteins

of nearly same mass (M_r 30 kD). Each of these two hormones have two chains called α- and β-chains. They have 89 amino acids in α-subunit and 115 amino acids in β-subunit. The α- and β-chains are encoded by separate genes. Both share a common α-subunit but have unique β-subunits.

FSH stimulates the growth of granulosa cells of the ovarian follicle and controls aromatase activity which is responsible for the formation of estradiol in these cells.

LH stimulates ovarian theca cells to produce androgens which diffuse to the granulosa cells where they are converted to estrogens. LH also controls testosterone production in the testis.

- **Thyroid stimulating hormone (TSH, thyrotropin):** It is produced by the thyrotrophs which constitute about 5% of the cells of the anterior pituitary. It is a glycoprotein (M_r 28 kD) composed of two dissimilar peptides, i.e. an α-subunit (89 amino acids) which it shares with LH, FSH and human chorionic gonadotropin (hCG), and a specific β-subunit (112 amino acids).

  TSH regulates biosynthesis, storage and release of thyroid hormones, and determines size of the thyroid gland. Thyroid hormones (T_4 and T_3) inhibit TSH production directly at the pituitary level.

- **Adrenocorticotropin (ACTH):** It is a polypeptide containing 39 amino acids. ACTH and a number of other peptides (lipotropins, endorphins and MSH) are processed from a large precursor, referred to as POMC. It is synthesized in the brain, anterior and posterior pituitary, and lymphocytes. It stimulates steroidogenesis via activation of the membrane-bound adenylate cyclase. First 13 amino acids of ACTH contain α-MSH sequence. Due to this reason, MSH receptors recognize and are activated by ACTH. Therefore, ACTH is an important contributing factor to skin pigmentation.

- **Prolactin (PRL):** It is secreted by the lactotrophs which constitute 15–20% of the normal pituitary and increase to 70% during pregnancy. The prolactin gene on chromosome 6 codes for a precursor molecule which is larger than the circulating hormone. PRL (M_r 23 kD) contains 198 amino acids which are arranged in a single polypeptide with three intra-chain disulfide bonds. It is essential for lactation. It also regulates mood and sexual behavior.

Hormone of the Posterior Pituitary

Oxytocin and vasopressin (antidiuretic hormone or ADH) are the hormones of the posterior pituitary. These hormones are stored in the posterior pituitary but are synthesized in separate cell-bodies of the hypothalamic neurons. Cell-bodies for the synthesis of ADH are located in the supra-optic nucleus while those for the synthesis of oxytocin are present in the

Chemistry to Clinics 17.6: Therapeutic Vasopressin

In advanced hepatic cirrhosis, the veins at the lower end of esophagus become dilated, elongated and tortuous (esophageal varices) due to portal hypertension. These varices are prone to rupture resulting in blood vomiting (hematemesis). Administration of vasopressin is beneficial in this condition as it constricts the blood vessels and minimizes blood loss.

paraventricular nucleus. Their release from the posterior pituitary occurs separately via specific stimuli acting on each of these types of the neuronal cells.

Vasopressin/ADH: It is synthesized as a pre-prohormone. It is altered in the Golgi apparatus to form a prohormone which is cleaved into vasopressin (an active hormone). Vasopressin is so called, because it is a physiological vasoconstrictor acting through V1 receptors (Chemistry to Clinics 17.6). Further, acting through V2 receptors, ADH recruits aquaporin type 2 (AQP2) channels in the apical membrane of renal distal and collecting tubules. Thus, it controls water conservation by promoting water reabsorption through AQP2. Its release is coordinated with the activity of the thirst center that regulates fluid intake. The hormone also binds to V3 receptors in the anterior pituitary as well as other parts of the brain to regulate ACTH release and other functions such as memory and body temperature. Deficiency of ADH results in diabetes insipidus (Chemistry to Clinics 17.7). Alcohol

Chemistry to Clinics 17.7: Diabetes Insipidus

It refers to the passage of large volume of dilute urine. Polyuria may be either due to the failure of ADH release in response to normal physiological stimuli (**central or neurogenic diabetes insipidus**) or failure of the kidney to respond to ADH (**nephrogenic diabetes insipidus** where the defect lies in V2 receptors or AQP2 channels of the distal and collecting tubules). Polyuria of diabetes insipidus can be distinguished from that of diabetes mellitus (Table 17.4).

Table 17.4: Biochemical distinction between diabetes insipidus and diabetes mellitus

Parameter	Diabetes insipidus	Diabetes mellitus
Urine specific gravity	Decreased (dilute urine)	Increased (presence of glucose)
Urine Benedict's test for reducing sugar	Negative	May be positive
Urine Rothera's test for ketone bodies	Negative	May be positive
Blood glucose	Normal	Increased

17

transiently suppresses ADH secretion (Chemistry to Clinics 17.8).

Oxytocin: It stimulates uterine contraction and milk ejection.

Steroid Hormones

Steroid hormones are derived from its parental precursor, i.e. **cholesterol**. They have a ring structure related to cyclopentanoperhydrophenanthrene nucleus which comprises of three 6-carbon hexane rings and a single 5-carbon pentane ring. Its carbon atoms are numbered in a sequence beginning with ring A (Fig. 17.14).

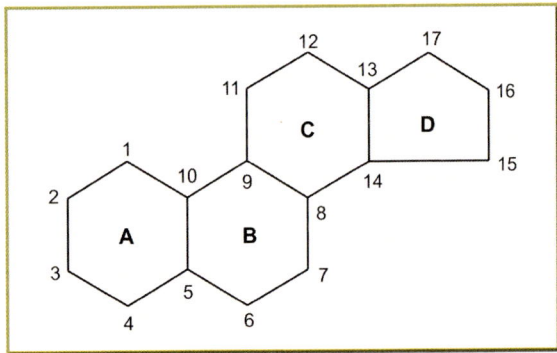

Fig. 17.14: Cyclopentanoperhydrophenanthrene (CPP) nucleus.

Biosynthesis of steroid hormones: Steroid hormones are synthesized in specific tissues in the body and are divided into two classes, i.e. the **sex and pro-gestational hormones**, and the **adrenal cortex hormones** (Table 17.5). Cholesterol (27C) derived from the diet and/or from its endogenous synthesis, is a precursor of steroid hormones. It is converted to Δ^5-pregnenolone, a common intermediate for the synthesis of various steroid hormones.

Synthesis of pregnenolone: Firstly, cholesterol undergoes side chain cleavage of a 6C aldehyde (isocaproic aldehyde), to form a common intermediate Δ^5-pregnenolone (21C) for the synthesis of various steroid hormones.

Biosynthesis of Hormones of the Adrenal Cortex

Adrenal steroids contain either 19 carbons (19C) or 21 carbons (21C):

Nineteen carbon steroids have two methyl groups at C18 and C19. These steroids also have a ketone group at C17 and are thus termed as **17-ketosteroids**. They have predominant androgenic activity.

On the other hand, the *21C steroids* have a 2-carbon side chain attached at C17 (as C20 and C21) and two methyl groups at C18 and C19. These steroids also have a hydroxyl group at C17 and are thus termed as **17-hydroxycorticosteroids** (Fig. 17.15).

Three major adrenal biosynthetic pathways lead to the production of **glucocorticoids** (e.g. cortisol), **mineralocorticoids** (e.g. aldosterone) and adrenal **androgens** (e.g. dehydroepiandrosterone). Separate zones of the adrenal cortex synthesize specific hormones. The outer zone (**zona glomerulosa**) contains enzymes for the biosynthesis of aldosterone (mineralocorticoids) while the mid-zone (**zona**

Table 17.5: Synthesis and release of steroid hormones

Steroid hormone	Second messenger	Signal	Signal system	Steroid producing cell/tissue
Aldosterone	PI, Ca^{2+}	Angiotensin II	RAAS	Zona glomerulosa
Cortisol	cAMP, PI, Ca^{2+}	ACTH	HPA cascade	Zona fasciculata
Testosterone	cAMP	LH	HPA cascade	Leydig cells
17β-Estradiol	cAMP	FSH	Ovarian cycle	Ovarian follicle
Progesterone	cAMP	LH	Ovarian cycle	Corpus luteum
Calcitriol	cAMP	PTH	Sunlight, plasma Ca^{2+}, PTH	Kidneys

PI = Phosphatidylinositol system; HPA = Hypothalamo-Pituitary-Adrenal.

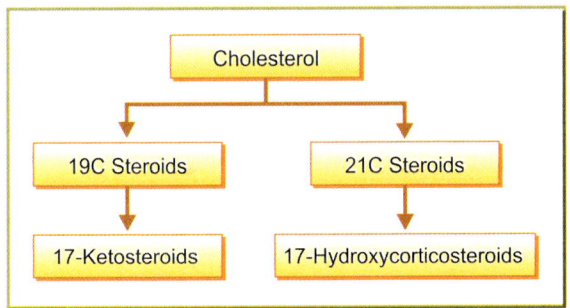

fasciculata) and the inner zone (**zona reticularis**) are the sites of biosynthesis of cortisol (glucocorticoids) and androgens respectively.

Synthesis of progesterone: Pregnenolone is converted to progesterone with the help of two cytoplasmic enzymes, i.e. 3β-ol dehydrogenase and Δ^{4,5}-isomerase. This is the end product of steroid biosynthesis in the *corpus luteum* (Fig. 17.16).

Synthesis of aldosterone: In cells of the *zona glomerulosa*, progesterone is converted to aldosterone.

This conversion requires 21-hydroxylase present in the endoplasmic reticulum and mitochondrial 11β-hydroxylase and 18-hydroxylase.

Synthesis of cortisol: In cells of the *zona fasciculata*, progesterone is converted to cortisol. This conversion requires 17α-hydroxylase present in the endoplasmic reticulum along with the mitochondrial 11β-hydroxylase and 21-hydroxylase.

Biosynthesis of Sex Hormones

Synthesis of dehydroepiandrosterone: In cells of the *zona reticularis*, Δ^5-pregnenolone is converted to dehydroepiandrosterone (DHEA). This conversion requires 17α-hydroxylase present in the endoplasmic reticulum and cytoplasmic 2C side chain cleavage enzyme (C17–20 lyase).

Synthesis of 17β-estradiol: DHEA is converted to 17β-estradiol by the action of aromatase enzyme system and 17-reductase, in the testicular Leydig cells.

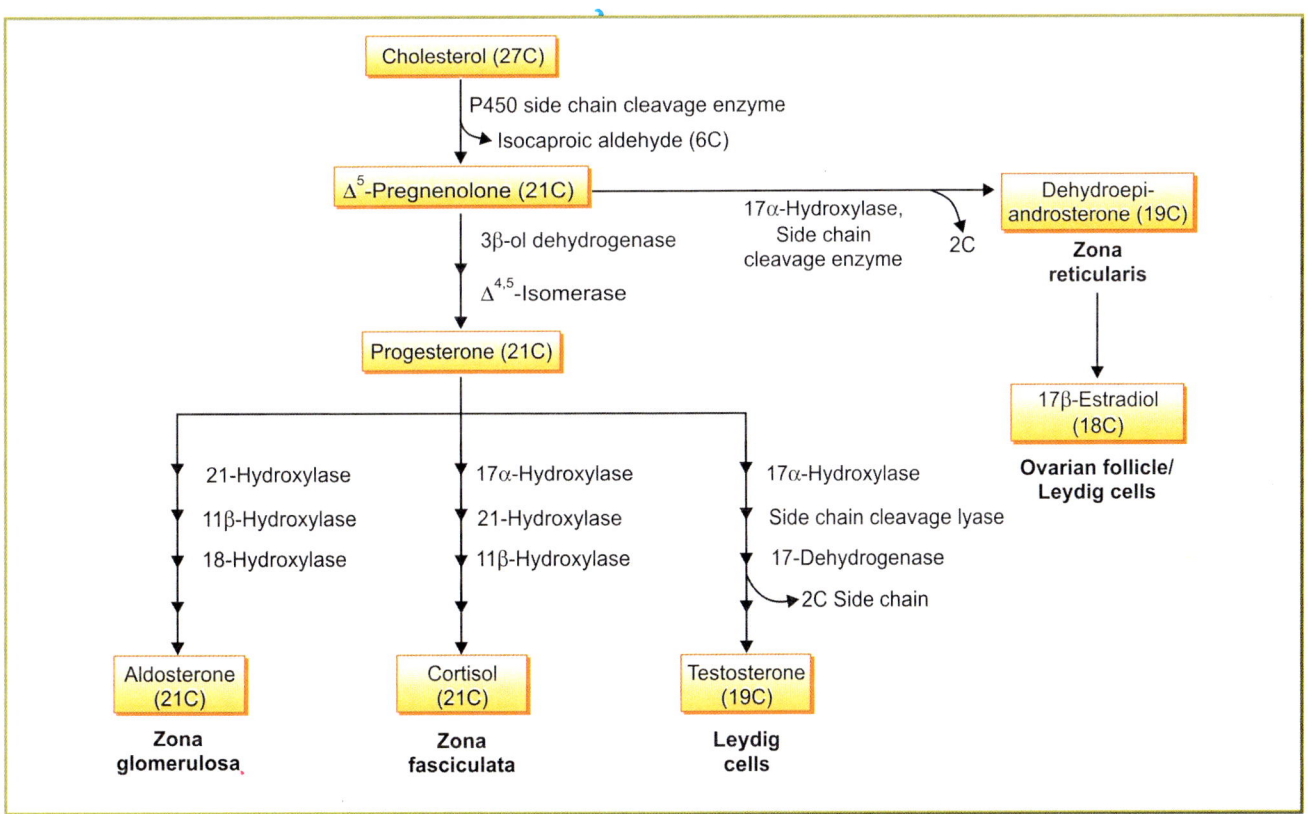

Fig. 17.16: Biosynthesis of hormones of the adrenal cortex and sex hormones. Progesterone is the end product in corpus luteum.

17

Synthesis of testosterone: In Leydig cells, progesterone is converted to testosterone, a major secretory product. This reaction is catalyzed by 17-dehydrogenase, 17α-hydroxylase and 2C side chain cleavage lyase (Fig. 17.16). Testosterone is reduced by 5α-reductase to dihydrotestosterone, the preferred ligand for the androgen receptor.

Disturbances in circulating testosterone levels are implicated in benign prostatic hyperplasia and prostate cancer (Chemistry to Clinics 17.9). Testosterone and its analogs, called anabolic steroids, are drugs of abuse particularly among body-builders and athletes (Chemistry to Clinics 17.10). Incidentally, erythropoietin (commercially available as recombinant human erythropoietin) is also abused by athletes (Chemistry to Clinics 17.11).

Chemistry to Clinics 17.10: Androgen Abuse

High blood levels of androgens have an anabolic effect on muscle tissue leading to increased muscle mass, strength and performance, a desired result for body builders and athletes. However, androgen abuse is associated with abnormally aggressive behavior and the potential for increased incidence of liver and brain tumors. Further, exogenous testosterone given to men inhibits endogenous luteinizing hormone (LH) release through a negative-feedback effect on the hypothalamic-pituitary axis. This leads to a suppression of testosterone production by the Leydig cells and a further decrease in testicular testosterone concentrations. Ultimately, testicular size decreases and infertility may occur.

Chemistry to Clinics 17.9: Prostate Cancer

An androgen is a hormone that stimulates the growth of the male reproductive tract and the development of secondary sex characteristics. Some prostate cancers (Fig. 17.17) highly depend on androgens for cellular proliferation; therefore, physicians attempt to totally ablate the secretion of androgens by the testes. Generally, two options for those patients are surgical castration and chemical castration. Surgical castration is irreversible and requires the removal of the testes whereas chemical castration is reversible. Chemical treatment is based on the use of analogs of gonadotropin-releasing hormone (GnRH), the hormone that regulates the secretion of luteinizing hormone (LH) and follicle stimulating hormone (FSH).

Long-acting GnRH agonists or antagonists reduce LH and FSH secretion by different mechanisms. The GnRH agonists reduce gonadotropin secretion by desensitization of the pituitary gonadotrophs to GnRH, leading to a reduction of LH and FSH secretion. The GnRH antagonists bind to GnRH receptors on the pituitary cells, prevent endogenous GnRH from binding to those receptors and subsequently reduce LH and FSH secretion. Shortly after treatment, testicular concentrations of androgens decline because of the low levels of circulating LH and FSH. Thus, the androgen dependent cancer cells cease to proliferate and ultimately die. Another class of the androgen-blocking drugs includes 5α-reductase inhibitors that prevent the conversion of testosterone to the highly active androgen dihydrotestosterone (these drugs are also useful in the treatment of benign hypertrophy of prostate (Fig. 17.17B) that is very common in elderly males). In addition, antiandrogens such as flutamide bind to the androgen receptor and prevent binding of endogenous androgen. Some prostate cancers are androgen-independent, and the treatment requires non-hormonal therapies including chemotherapy and radiation.

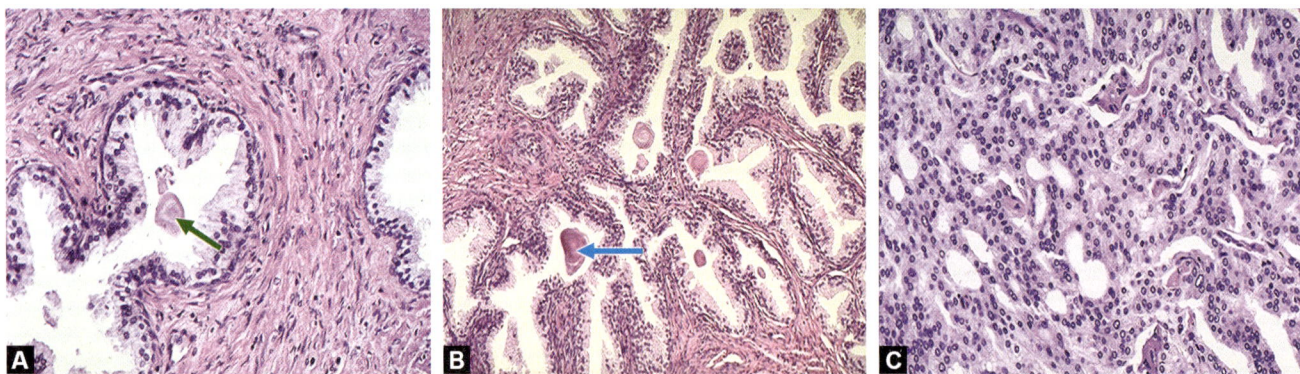

Fig. 17.17: (A) **Normal prostate.** Irregularly branching glands are lined by two cell layers: An outer low cuboidal layer and an inner layer of tall columnar mucin-secreting epithelium. These cells project inward as papillary projections. The fibromuscular stroma between the glands accounts for about half of the volume of the prostate. With aging, there may be small concretions within the glandular lumina, called corpora amylacea (arrow), representing laminated concretions) of prostatic secretions. (B) **Benign prostatic hyperplasia.** Most of the hyperplasia is contributed by glandular proliferation, but the stroma is also increased. The glands are variably sized with larger glands having prominent papillary infoldings. The columnar arrangement of cells near the gland lumina is preserved. Corpora amylacea is present. (C) **Prostatic adenocarcinoma.** Numerous infiltrating cancer cells and small back-to-back glands with no corpora amylacea and little or no intervening stroma.

Erythropoietin is a hormone of abuse in athletes particularly the cyclists. In healthy adults, RBC constitute 40–50% of the blood volume that can increase up to 60% with an injection of erythropoietin. Increase in RBC number in a fixed volume of blood increases the blood viscosity so that it imposes strain on the heart to pump harder. In a cyclist, when the heart is already pumping at its maximum, this can precipitate a heart attack.

Glucocorticoids

A glucocorticoid is a 21C steroid that acts predominantly on intermediary metabolism. The principal glucocorticoid is **cortisol** (hydrocortisone). Its effects are mediated by type II glucocorticoid receptors. The **major metabolic effects** include:

1. Increase in blood glucose level by acting as insulin antagonist since cortisol suppresses secretion of insulin, inhibits peripheral glucose uptake and promotes hepatic glucose synthesis (**gluconeogenesis**).

2. Increase in protein breakdown and **nitrogen excretion**. This is due to mobilization of glycogenic amino acid precursors from peripheral supporting structures such as bone, skin, muscle, etc. Glucocorticoids act directly on the liver and stimulate synthesis of certain enzymes, such as tyrosine aminotransferase and tryptophan pyrrolase. Increased levels of circulating amino acids, in turn, also facilitate gluconeogenesis by stimulating glucagon secretion.

3. Increased activation of cellular lipase by lipid mobilizing hormones, e.g. catecholamines and pituitary peptides. The **action of cortisol on adipose tissue differs in different parts of the body**.

4. Inhibit the synthesis of nucleic acids in most of the body tissues but RNA synthesis is stimulated in the liver.

5. **Anti-inflammatory** properties.
6. Modulate the immune response with a tendency to cause **immunosuppression**.
7. Regulate extracellular fluid volume by retarding the migration of water into cells and by promoting renal water excretion, partly by suppression of the secretion of vasopressin.
8. Enhance vascular sensitivity to catecholamines.
9. Weak mineralocorticoid-like properties.
10. Suppress the secretion of pituitary POMC and its derivative peptides, i.e. ACTH, β-endorphin and β-lipotropin as well as the secretion of hypothalamic CRH and vasopressin.
11. **Combat stress**.

Some of these properties of glucocorticoids are exploited clinically (Table 17.6).

Mineralocorticoids

A mineralocorticoid is a 21C steroid that predominantly regulates the metabolism of sodium and potassium. The principal mineralocorticoid is **aldosterone**. It has two important actions. It is a main regulator of **extracellular fluid volume** as well as **potassium homeostasis**. These effects are mediated by the binding of aldosterone to type I glucocorticoid (mineralocorticoid) receptors in target tissues.

Fluid volume is regulated through a direct effect on the collecting ducts where aldosterone causes a decrease in sodium excretion. Reabsorption of sodium causes a fall in transmembrane potential and enhances the flow of other cations such as potassium, out of the cell into the lumen. Reabsorbed sodium ions are transported out of the tubular epithelium into the renal interstitial fluid and from there into the renal capillary circulation. Water passively follows the transported sodium. Since the concentration of H^+ is greater in the lumen than in the cell, H^+ is also actively secreted.

Table 17.6: Glucocorticoids: Biochemical-clinical correlations

Normal biochemical function	Clinical application
Anti-inflammatory	Osteoarthritis (intra-articular injections)
	Bronchial asthma (inhalation/injection/oral)
Immunosuppression	Autoimmune diseases (rheumatoid arthritis, systemic lupus erythematosus) and severe allergic reactions (urticaria)
Enhance vasomotor tone and increase vascular sensitivity to catecholamines	Hypovolemic shock

17

Three major mechanisms control the release of aldosterone: Renin-angiotensin system, potassium and ACTH.

Regulation of Biosynthesis of Steroid Hormones

1. Biosynthesis of steroid hormones is under the influence of other hormones whose nature depends upon cell type and its receptor (Table 17.5). The hormone binds to cell membrane receptor and activates adenylate cyclase, mediated by a stimulatory G-protein. Activated hormone-receptor complex may directly stimulate a calcium channel or indirectly stimulate it by activating phosphatidylinositol cycle. The stimulatory response of cAMP is mediated via acute (occurring within seconds to minutes) as well as chronic effects (occurring within hours), on steroid synthesis.

   - Its acute effect is to mobilize and deliver cholesterol to the mitochondrial inner membrane. An increase in cAMP activates protein kinase A whose phosphorylation causes increased hydrolysis of cholesterol esters to free cholesterol and increases cholesterol transport into the mitochondria where cholesterol is converted to pregnenolone by the cytochrome P450 side chain cleavage enzyme.

   - The chronic effects of cAMP are mediated via increased transcription of genes. This, in turn, results in induction of a regulatory protein, designated as steroidogenic acute regulatory protein (**StAR protein**) that mediates the regulation of biosynthesis of steroid hormones (Fig. 17.18). The combination of elevated Ca^{2+} levels and protein phosphorylation as well as induction of the StAR protein, results in increased side chain cleavage and steroid biosynthesis.

2. Cortisol biosynthesis is also under the control of **ACTH** which binds to G-protein-coupled receptor. This activates adenylate cyclase and generates cAMP, leading to the activation of protein kinase A which stimulates hydrolysis of cholesterol esters by esterase. The cholesterol so formed is transported into the mitochondria by StAR and is converted to cortisol.

3. Aldosterone is a **stress hormone** and its concentration is increased in the blood during stressful situations.

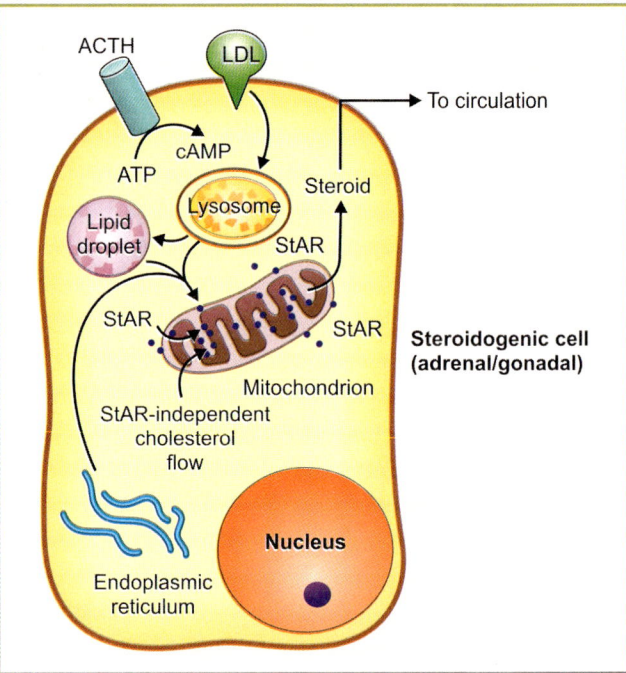

Fig. 17.18: Function of **StAR** (steroidogenic acute regulatory protein). Cholesterol from low-density lipoprotein (LDL), from cholesterol esters stored in lipid droplets, and from endogenous synthesis in the endoplasmic reticulum is transported from the outer mitochondrial membrane to the inner membrane. This transport is facilitated by StAR as well as by StAR-independent mechanisms. In the mitochondria, steroidogenesis occurs as a result of the conversion of cholesterol to pregnenolone by cytochrome P450 side chain cleavage enzyme.

4. Signals opposite to those that activate the formation of angiotensin, generate **atrial natriuretic peptide (ANP)** from the heart atria. ANP, in turn, binds to specific zona glomerulosa cell membrane receptors and activates guanylyl cyclase. Increased cGMP concentration antagonizes the synthesis and secretion of aldosterone as well as formation of cAMP by adenylate cyclase.

Renin-Angiotensin-Aldosterone System (RAAS)

This is an important system that participates in various homeostatic mechanisms such as **water balance**, **electrolyte balance** and **maintenance of blood pressure**. The main driving force for the secretion of aldosterone in adrenal zona glomerulosa cells is angiotensin II. This, is turn, is generated via RAAS under the influence of low plasma Na^+ or low blood volume or low blood pressure.

- **Renin** is a proteolytic enzyme that is produced and stored in granules of the juxtaglomerular cells of the afferent arterioles in the kidneys. It acts on its substrate **angiotensinogen** (a circulating α_2-globulin) and cleaves it to form a decapeptide **angiotensin I** which, in turn, is converted to an octapeptide **angiotensin II** by the action of angiotensin converting enzyme (**ACE**).

- Angiotensin II counteracts a decrease in mean arterial pressure by several mechanisms (Table 17.7).
- By the action of an aminopeptidase, angiotensin II is further degraded to a heptapeptide, **angiotensin III** (Fig. 17.19).
- Both angiotensin II and angiotensin III bind to angiotensin receptor and activate phosphatidyl-inositol system to generate IP_3 and DAG.
- IP_3 stimulates release of Ca^{2+} from the intracellular calcium storage vesicles. Increased cytosolic Ca^{2+} along with DAG stimulates protein kinase C. This, in turn, leads to phosphorylation of proteins that stimulate the rate-limiting steps of aldosterone biosynthesis.
- Elevated levels of the hormone are secreted into the blood, from where it enters distal kidney cells and binds to its receptor. This stimulates expression of proteins that increase transport of Na^+ from glomerular filtrate to the blood.

Control of release of renin

- *The juxtaglomerular cells*: They act as miniature pressure transducers.

Table 17.7: Mechanism of increasing blood pressure by angiotensin II

1. Powerful arteriolar vasoconstriction.
2. $\uparrow Na^+$ reabsorption by proximal tubules.
3. Release of aldosterone which promotes Na^+ reabsorption in the distal tubules.
4. Release of vasopressin (a vasoconstrictor).

- *Macula densa cells*: They function as chemo-receptors and monitor sodium and chloride load which is presented to the distal tubule.
- *Sympathetic nervous system*: It has a direct effect on the juxtaglomerular cells to increase adenylate cyclase activity.
- *Potassium*: Decreased potassium intake increases release of renin.
- *Angiotensin II*: It exerts negative feedback control on the release of renin.
- *Atrial natriuretic peptide*: It also inhibits renin release.

RAAS and hypertension: The ACE-inhibitors as well as angiotensin II receptor antagonists are important antihypertensive drugs (Chemistry to Clinics 17.12).

Disorders of Adrenal Cortex

Hyper-functioning of the adrenal cortex can result in Cushing's syndrome (Chemistry to Clinics 17.13) or hyperaldosteronism (Chemistry to Clinics 17.14).

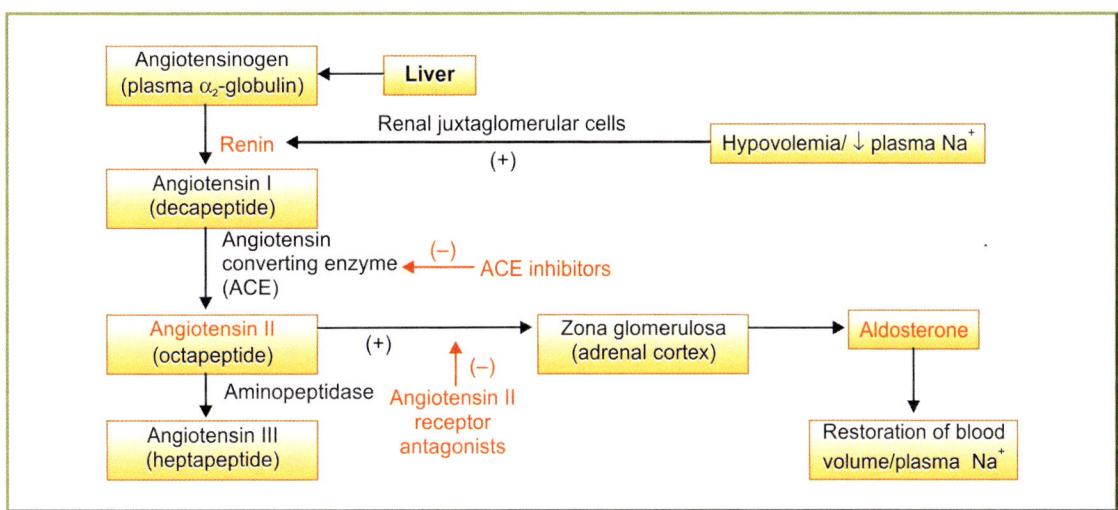

Fig. 17.19: Renin-angiotensin-aldosterone system (RAAS).

17

Many cases of hypertension are associated with an increased activity of the RAAS. This is known as renin-dependent hypertension. Drugs that break the sequence of events involved in RAAS activation are useful in treating such cases. These include ACE-inhibitors such as enalapril and angiotensin II receptor antagonists such as losartan.

On the other hand, hypo-functioning of the adrenal cortex may cause Addison's disease (Chemistry to Clinics 17.15).

Amino Acid Derived Hormones

Hormones of the **adrenal medulla** (**norepinephrine** and **epinephrine**) and **thyroid hormones** (T_3 and T_4) are derivatives of the amino acid **tyrosine**.

Norepinephrine/Epinephrine

Epinephrine and norepinephrine are synthesized from phenylalanine/tyrosine by the **chromaffin cells** of the adrenal medulla (Fig. 17.21).

Secretion of epinephrine is signaled by the neural response to stress, which is transmitted to the adrenal medulla by way of pre-ganglionic acetylcholinergic neurons. Release of acetylcholine increases the

It is a syndrome associated with hypersecretion of aldosterone (mineralocorticoids). In **primary hyperaldosteronism**, cause for excessive aldosterone production is an adenoma within the adrenal gland **(Conn's syndrome)**. The disease is characterized by hypokalemia, diastolic hypertension and muscle weakness. **Secondary hyperaldosteronism** refers to increased production of aldosterone in response to activation of the renin-angiotensin-aldosterone system. Secondary hyperaldosteronism in patients with accelerated hypertension is due to elevated plasma renin levels. In contrast, patients with primary hyperaldosteronism have suppressed plasma renin levels.

It results from progressive destruction of adrenal glands. Half of the patients have circulating adrenal antibodies. Adrenal tuberculosis is a common cause in India. The disease is characterized by weakness, anorexia, nausea and vomiting, weight loss, cutaneous and mucosal pigmentation, hypotension and hypoglycemia. Serum sodium, chloride and bicarbonate levels are reduced while serum potassium is elevated. There may also be mild to moderate hypercalcemia.

Cause: It is due to increased production of cortisol by the adrenal cortex. However, prolonged use of corticosteroids for the treatment of some diseases also result in Cushing's-like features (iatrogenic Cushing's syndrome).

Presentation: Most of the features can be explained from the known biochemical functions of cortisol (Table 17.8).

- Hypercortisolism promotes deposition of adipose tissue in characteristic sites, notably the upper face (producing typical moon-like face), the inter-scapular area (producing buffalo-hump, Fig. 17.20A) and the mesenteric bed (producing truncal obesity). The skin is thinned and weakened so that weight gain results in stretching and sometimes hemorrhages, giving the appearance of stretch marks or striae (Fig. 17.20B).
- It is also accompanied by increased hepatic gluconeogenesis and insulin resistance which, in turn, can cause impaired glucose tolerance or secondary diabetes mellitus.
- Other features include osteoporosis, diastolic hypertension, central adiposity, hirsutism and amenorrhea. Plasma and urine cortisol levels are variably elevated.
- Occasionally, hypokalemia, hypochloremia and metabolic alkalosis are present, particularly with ectopic production of ACTH.

Diagnosis: Plasma cortisol at 8 AM is >140 nmol/L (>5 µg/dl) after 1 mg dexamethasone challenge at midnight.

Table 17.8: Salient features of Cushing's syndrome

Normal biochemical function of glucocorticoids	Result of excess secretion of glucocorticoids (Cushing's syndrome) or prolonged use as a drug (iatrogenic Cushing's syndrome)
Anti-insulin action	Impaired glucose tolerance, diabetes mellitus
Protein catabolism	Muscle weakness
Lipogenesis in adipose tissue of selected body parts	Moon-like face, buffalo hump, truncal obesity
Immunosuppression	Susceptibility to infections
Weak mineralocorticoid-like activity	Water retention, edema, diastolic hypertension

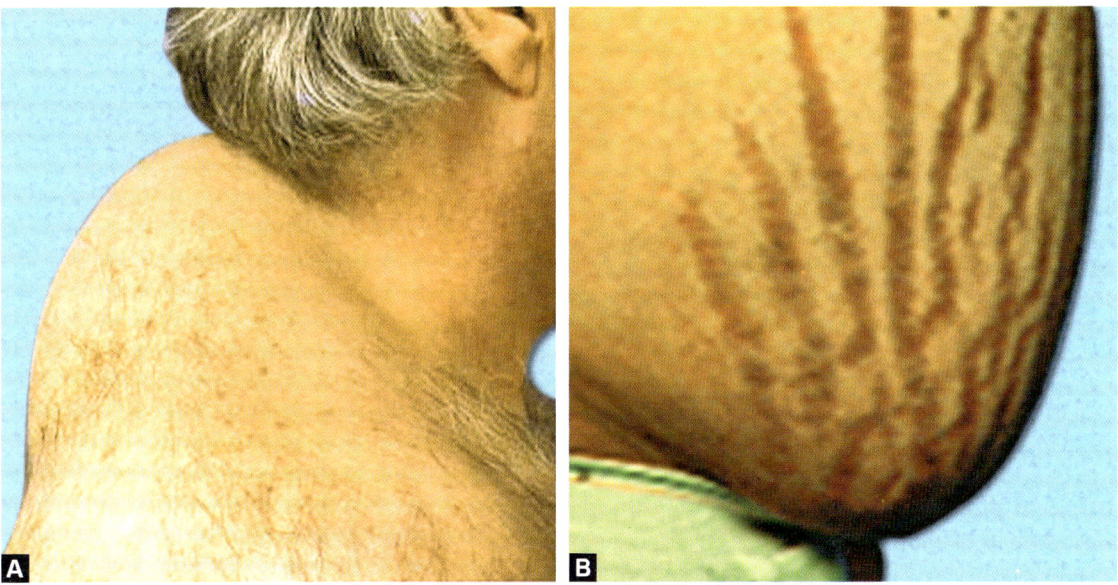

Fig. 17.20: Cushing's syndrome. (A) Buffalo hump, (B) Striae.

availability of intracellular Ca^{2+} which stimulates exocytosis and the release of hormones stored in the chromaffin granules. **Overall system of epinephrine synthesis, storage and release from the adrenal medulla is regulated by neuronal control as well as by glucocorticoid hormones (synthesized in and secreted from the adrenal cortex in response to stress).** Since cortisol is transported to general circulation through adrenal medulla, its concentration is elevated in the medulla. This, in turn, induces the enzyme phenylethanolamine-N-methyltransferase which converts norepinephrine to epinephrine. Stress, thus ensures the production of epinephrine, a critical determinant of the '**fight or flight**' response discussed below.

Once secreted into the bloodstream, epinephrine affects α receptors of hepatocytes to increase blood glucose level. It also interacts with α receptors on vascular smooth muscle cells to cause contraction and increases blood pressure.

Catecholamines: Dopamine, norepinephrine and epinephrine are collectively referred to as catecholamines. Increased production of catecholamines may result in a condition designated as pheochromocytoma (Chemistry to Clinics 17.16).

The 'fight or flight' response: This response is the classic example of the ability of the **sympathetic nervous system** to produce widespread activation of

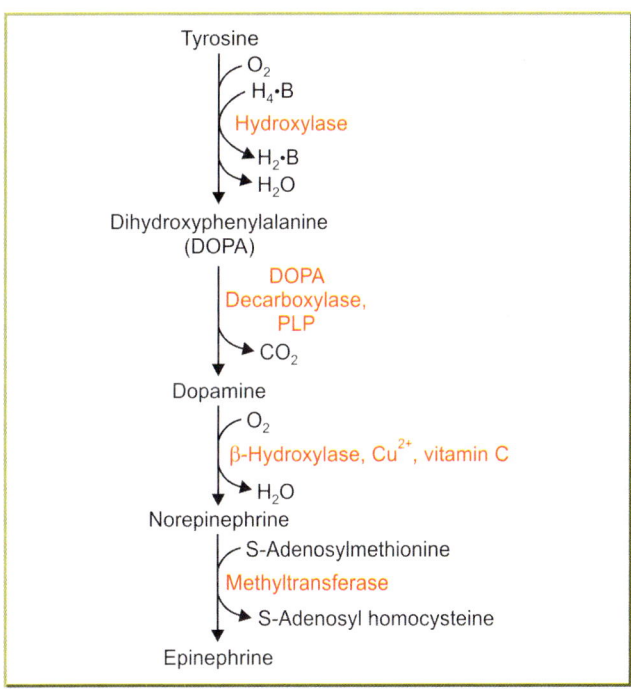

Fig. 17.21: Biosynthesis of catecholamines (dopamine, norepinephrine and epinephrine). B = Biopterin.

its effectors. The response is initiated when an organism's survival is in jeopardy and the organism may have to fight or flee. Some components of the response result from the direct effects of sympathetic activation, however, the action of **epinephrine**

Chemistry to Clinics 17.16: Pheochromocytoma

It is a tumor of the adrenal medulla. It is called the **'10% tumor'** because nearly 10% are bilateral, 10% are multiple, 10% are extra-adrenal, 10% are malignant, 10% are familial and 10% occur in children. Patients with pheochromocytoma produce, store and secrete increased amounts of catecholamines. Hypertension is the most common sign. Most of the patients secrete greater amount of norepinephrine. There is impaired glucose tolerance, elevated hematocrit and hypercalcemia in majority of the patients. Diagnosis is established by the increased urinary excretion of catecholamines or catecholamine metabolites, particularly **vanillylmandelic acid (VMA)**.

secreted by the adrenal medulla also contributes. For example:

- Sympathetic stimulation of the heart and blood vessels results in a **rise in blood pressure** because of increased cardiac output and increased total peripheral resistance.
- There is also a **redistribution of blood flow** so that the muscles and heart receive more blood, whereas the splanchnic territory and the skin receive less.
- The need for an increased exchange of blood gases is met by **acceleration of the respiratory rate** and dilation of the bronchiolar tree. The **volume of salivary secretion is reduced but the relative proportion of mucus increases**, permitting lubrication of the mouth despite increased ventilation.
- Potential demand for an enhanced supply of metabolic substrates such as glucose and fatty acids, is met by the actions of the sympathetic nerves and circulating epinephrine on hepatocytes and adipocytes. **Glycogenolysis** mobilizes stored liver glycogen, increasing plasma levels of glucose. **Lipolysis** in adipocytes converts stored trigly-cerides to free fatty acids that enter the bloodstream.
- Skin plays an important role in maintaining body temperature in the face of increased heat production from contracting muscles. The sympathetic innervation of the skin vasculature can adjust blood flow and heat exchange by vasodilation to dissipate heat or by vasoconstriction to protect blood volume. The eccrine sweat glands are important structures that also can be activated to enhance heat loss. Sympathetic nerve stimulation of the sweat glands results in the secretion of a watery fluid, and evaporation then dissipates body heat. Constriction of the skin vasculature,

concurrent with sweat gland activation, produces the **cold, clammy skin** typical of a frightened person. Sensation of **hair standing-on-end** result from activation of the piloerector muscles associated with hair follicles.

Hormones of the Thyroid Gland

The thyroid gland is composed of two lobes connected by a thin band of tissue called isthmus. Secretory units of the thyroid gland are **follicles** that consist of an outer layer of epithelial cells. These cells rest on a basement membrane and enclose an amorphous material called **colloid**, mainly composed of **thyroglobulin** which is an iodinated glycoprotein and serves as a precursor of thyroid hormones. Increased activity of the gland is characterized by a decrease in the quantity of colloid with subsequent reduction of follicular volume. During decreased glandular activity, the follicles enlarge because of the accumulation of colloid and the flattening of the follicular cells.

The thyroid gland secretes two hormones, i.e. **thyroxine** (3, 5, 3', 5'-tetraiodothyronine or T_4) and **triiodothyronine** (3, 5, 3'-triiodothyronine or T_3). Hormone synthesis in the thyroid is controlled predominantly by thyroid stimulating hormone (TSH). TSH output, in turn, is regulated by negative feedback effect of free T_3 and T_4 acting on both the hypothalamus and the pituitary. The output of TSH from the anterior pituitary is controlled by thyrotropin releasing hormone (TRH) secreted by the hypothalamus.

The thyroid gland also contains **parafollicular cells or C cells** which produce a polypeptide hormone called **calcitonin**.

Synthesis of thyroid hormones: It involves the following steps:

1. Synthesis of thyroglobulin precursor
2. Iodide uptake
3. Iodination of tyrosine residues
4. Coupling
5. Hydrolysis of thyroglobulin
6. Secretion and transport of T_4 and T_3
7. Peripheral conversion of T_4 to T_3

1. **Synthesis of thyroglobulin precursor:** The synthesis of the **protein precursor** for thyroglobulin (Tg) in the thyrofollicular cells is the first step in the formation of T_4 and T_3. The Tg is a 660 kDa

glycoprotein composed of two similar 330 kDa subunits held together by disulfide bridges. Ribosomes synthesize the subunits on the rough endoplasmic reticulum and then the subunits undergo dimerization and glycosylation in the smooth endoplasmic reticulum. The Golgi appa- ratus packages the completed glycoprotein into vesicles which **migrate** to the apical membrane of the follicular cell and fuse with it. The Tg precursor protein is **extruded** onto the apical surface of the cell where the subsequent iodination takes place (Fig. 17.22).

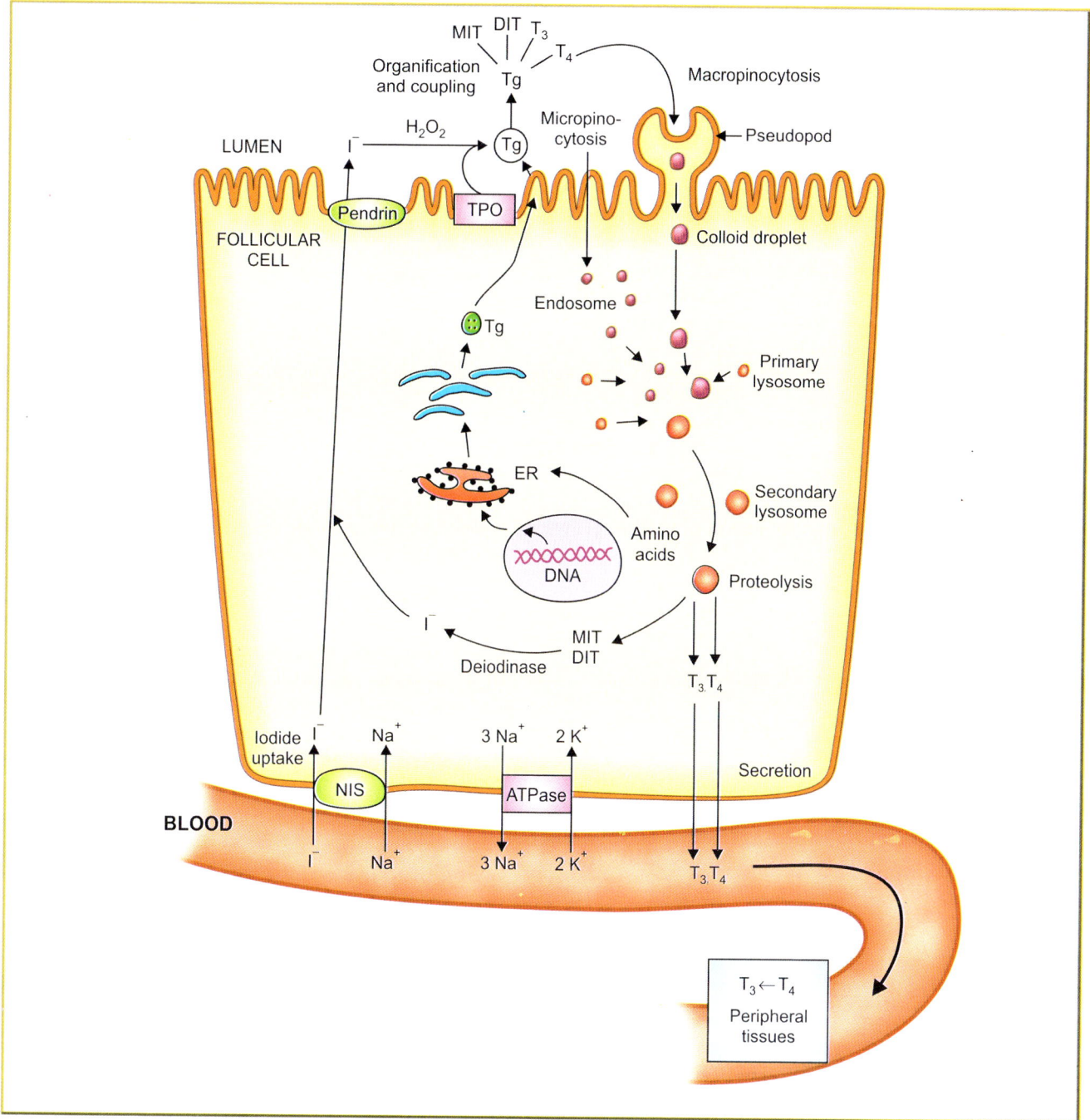

Fig. 17.22: Biosynthesis of thyroid hormones. TPO, thyroid peroxidase.

17

2. **Iodide uptake:** The iodide (I^-) required for the iodination of the Tg precursor protein comes from the blood perfusing the thyroid gland. The sodium-iodide symporter (**NIS**) located on the basal plasma membrane of the follicular cell near the capillaries that supply the follicle, uses the Na^+ gradient across the basal membrane to transport one I^- along with two Na^+ into the cytosol. Although NIS itself does not require ATP to transport I^-, the **Na^+/K^+-ATPase** is required to pump Na^+ back out of the cell and maintain the Na^+ gradient. Thus, the NIS operates on the principle of **secondary active transport**. The NIS also transports other anions such as bromide, thiocyanate and perchlorate and these can be used to reduce iodide uptake by the gland. **The follicular cell concentrates I^- many times over the concentration of I^- present in the blood.** Once inside the follicular cells, the I^- diffuse rapidly to the apical membrane where a protein called **pendrin** transports it into the follicle to be used for iodination of the Tg precursor.

3. **Iodination of tyrosine residues:** The next step in the formation of mature Tg is the addition of I^- to certain tyrosine residues in the Tg precursor protein, a process termed *'organification of iodide'*. The precursor protein contains 134 **tyrosine** residues but only a small fraction of these become iodinated so that a mature Tg molecule contains only 20–30 atoms of iodine. The enzyme **thyroid peroxidase** which is bound to the apical membrane of the follicular cells, catalyzes the iodination of Tg. The enzyme oxidizes I^- and tyrosine residue to short-lived free radicals using hydrogen peroxide that has been generated within the mitochondria of follicular cells. The free radicals then undergo addition. The product formed is monoiodotyrosine (**MIT**) which remains in peptide linkage in the Tg structure. The same enzymatic process adds the second iodide to a MIT residue forming diiodotyrosine (**DIT**).

4. **Coupling:** Iodinated tyrosine residues that are close together in the Tg precursor molecule undergo a coupling reaction which forms the iodothyronine structure. **Thyroid peroxidase**, the same enzyme that initially oxidizes iodide, catalyzes the coupling reaction through the oxidation of neighboring iodinated tyrosine residues to short-lived free radicals. These free radicals undergo addition to produce an iodothyronine residue and a dehydroalanine residue, both of which remain in peptide linkage in the Tg structure. For example, when one MIT and one DIT couple by this mechanism, **triiodothyronine (T_3)** is formed; when two DIT residues couple, **tetraiodothyronine (T_4)** is formed. However, T_3 is formed in only about one of five Tg molecules. As a result, the thyroid gland secretes substantially **more T_4 than T_3**. After being iodinated, the mature Tg molecules are **stored as part of the colloid** in the lumen of the follicle.

5. **Hydrolysis of thyroglobulin:** When the thyroid gland is stimulated to secrete thyroid hormones, vigorous **pinocytosis** occurs at the apical membranes of follicular cells. Pseudopods from the apical membrane reach into the lumen of the follicle, engulfing bits of the colloid. Endocytotic vesicles formed by this activity migrate toward the basal region of the follicular cell. The **lysosomes** fuse with the Tg-containing droplets and hydrolyze the Tg to its constituent amino acids. As a result, MIT, DIT, T_4, T_3 and amino acids are released into the cytosol. The MIT and DIT generated by the hydrolysis of Tg are rapidly **deiodinated** in the follicular cell. The follicular cell recycles the released I^- for the continued iodination of Tg. The released amino acids become part of the amino acid pool.

6. **Secretion and transport of T_4 and T_3:** The T_4 and T_3 are released from the follicular cell and enter the nearby capillary circulation. Nearly **99%** of the thyroid hormones in the circulation are bound to the plasma proteins **thyroxine-binding globulin, transthyretin and albumin**. Thus, only **1%** of the T_4/T_3 is in the **free form** and it is in **equilibrium** with the large protein-bound fraction. It is, this small amount of free thyroid hormones that interact with **target cells**.

The **protein-bound form of thyroid hormones represents a large reservoir of preformed hormone** that can replenish the small amount of circulating free hormone as it is cleared from the blood. This reservoir provides the body with a buffer against drastic changes in circulating thyroid hormone levels as a result of sudden changes in the rate of T_4 and T_3 secretion. The protein-bound hormones are also protected from metabolic inactivation and excretion in the urine. As a result, the thyroid hormones have long half-lives in the bloodstream.

Table 17.9: Comparison between T_4 and T_3

	T_4	T_3
Chemical structure	Tetraiodothyronine	Triiodothyronine
Predominant form in blood	Yes	No
Half-life in blood	7 days	1 day
Potency	Converted to T_3	Biologically active form, binds to nuclear receptors

The half-life of T_4 is about 7 days; that of T_3 is about 1 day (Table 17.9).

7. **Peripheral activation/inactivation of T_4 and T_3:** **Deiodination** reactions in the peripheral tissues both activate and inactivate thyroid hormones. The enzymes that catalyze the various deiodination reactions are regulated, resulting in different thyroid hormone concentrations in various tissues under different physiological and disease conditions (Chemistry to Clinics 17.17 and 17.18).

Although T_4 is the major secretory product of the thyroid gland, and is the predominant thyroid hormone in the blood, about 40% of the T_4 is converted to T_3 by enzymatic removal of the iodide at position 5' of the thyronine ring structure in a reaction termed outer ring deiodination (Fig. 17.23). *Type 1 deiodinase (D1)* located in the liver, kidneys and thyroid gland itself, catalyzes this reaction. The T_3 formed by this deiodination and that secreted by the thyroid gland, react with thyroid hormone receptors in target cells; therefore, T_3 **is the physiologically active form** of the

Chemistry to Clinics 17.17: 5'-Deiodination in Health and Disease

5'-Deiodination is a regulated process. Certain physiological and pathological factors influence the 5'-deiodination reaction. The result is a change in the relative amounts of T_3 and rT_3 produced from T_4. For example, the human fetus produces less T_3 from T_4 than a child or adult because the 5'-deiodination reaction is less active in the fetus. Further, 5'-deiodination is inhibited during fasting, particularly in response to carbohydrate restriction, but is restored to normal when the person is fed again. Trauma, as well as most acute and chronic illnesses, also suppresses the 5'-deiodination reaction. Under all of these circumstances, the amount of T_3 produced from T_4 is reduced and its blood concentration falls whereas that of rT_3 rises. It should also be noted that during fasting or in the disease states mentioned above, the secretion of T_4 is not increased despite the decrease of serum T_3. This is due to the fact that D2 in the CNS and pituitary is not affected under these conditions and continues to produce T_3 in quantities sufficient to maintain relatively normal hypothalamic-pituitary-thyroid axis function. It is essential to remember these facts while evaluating the serum thyroid profile of an individual.

Chemistry to Clinics 17.18: Euthyroid Sick Syndrome

Severe caloric restriction and starvation result in reduced serum T_3 levels with normal/slightly reduced T_4 and normal TSH levels. This is a result of decreased release of thyroid hormones, and reduced D1 and D2 deiodinase activity in peripheral tissues. Reductions in T_3 result in lower basal oxygen consumption, slower heart rate and attenuation of nitrogen loss—changes considered beneficial in adapting to the reduced caloric intake. In a patient who is severely ill, T_3 levels can be reduced up to 90% (i.e. almost undetectable) and rT_3 increased several-fold, with only slight reductions in T_4. In the most severe cases, release of TSH and other anterior pituitary hormones is reduced because of loss of hypothalamic input resulting from endogenous causes and, in some instances, exacerbated by therapy such as glucocorticoids that is given to ill patients. This condition is called euthyroid sick syndrome or low T_3 syndrome. Treatment of these patients with thyroid hormone supplements is controversial.

thyroid hormones. *Type 2 deiodinase (D2)* plays a similar role in other tissues such as the skeletal muscles, central nervous system, pituitary gland, and placenta. *A third deiodinase (type 3 or D3)* in the liver and kidneys catalyzes inner ring deiodination reactions during degradation of thyroid hormones. The T_4 is deiodinated at the 5' position on the inner thyronine ring to produce **reverse T_3 (rT_3)**. Because rT_3 has little or no thyroid hormone activity, this deiodination reaction is a major pathway for the metabolic inactivation or disposal of T_4. All of the deiodinases contain **selenocysteine** in the active center.

Regulation of Secretion of Thyroid Hormones

Thyroid hormones regulate their own secretion (autoregulation).

Thyroid Hormone Receptors

Target cells take up free T_4 and T_3 from the blood by carrier-mediated primary active transport. Once inside the cell, T_4 is deiodinated to T_3 that acts through its specific receptors and regulates **gene expression**. Thyroid hormone receptors are located in the **nuclei**

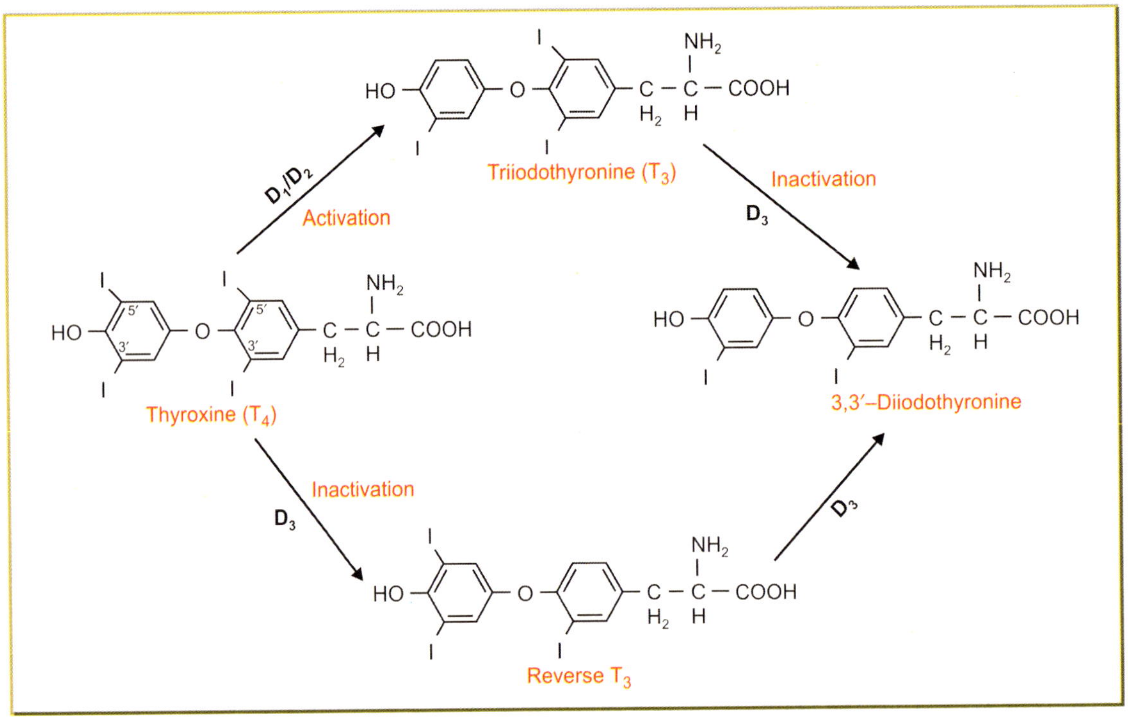

17

Fig. 17.23: Metabolism of thyroxine.

of target cells bound to thyroid hormone response elements in the DNA. The receptors are protein molecules that are structurally similar to the nuclear receptors for steroid hormones and vitamin D. Two thyroid receptor genes, **a and b**, are found on two separate chromosomes and encode several different receptor proteins (TRal, TRbl, TRb2 and TRb3). These receptors are expressed in a tissue-specific manner to impart different effects of thyroid hormones on various tissues (Chemistry to Clinics 17.19).

Functions of Thyroid Hormones

1. **Development of the central nervous system:** As we know, the human brain undergoes its most active phase of growth during the last six months of fetal life and the first six months of postnatal life. During the second trimester of pregnancy, the multiplication of fetal neuroblasts reaches a peak and then declines. Subsequently, neuroblasts differentiate into neurons and begin synapse formation that extends into postnatal life. **Thyroid hormones** first appear in the **fetal blood** during the **second trimester** of pregnancy and continue to rise

Chemistry to Clinics 17.19: Resistance to Thyroid Hormones

It results from mutations in one allele of the thyroid receptor (TRb) gene. The mutant TRb does not bind T_3 with high affinity. Patients may have features of hypothyroidism if the resistance is severe and affects all tissues. Such people are referred to as having *'generalized resistance to thyroid hormones'*.

Alternatively, patients may present with **hyperthyroidism** if the pituitary axis is more severely affected, a condition termed *'pituitary resistance to thyroid hormone'*. The hypothalamic-pituitary axis is primarily regulated by TRb and thus is more sensitive to mutations in the receptor than tissues such as the heart, in which TRa is the dominant thyroid hormone receptor. Although patients may present with symptoms of hyperthyroidism, serum TSH is normal or only slightly elevated, a finding important in differentiating between a diagnosis of thyroid hormone resistance and TSH-secreting pituitary tumor, which results in high TSH levels.

On the other hand, many patients may present with a **mixture of hypothyroid and hyperthyroid features**. Treatment is difficult because thyroid hormone supplements suppress the hypothalamic-pituitary axis and reduce the release of T_4 that can worsen the effects on the heart, which has functional TRa receptors. Development of thyroid hormone analogs that preferentially bind TRb or TRa may prove useful.

in the remaining months of fetal life. Thus, thyroid hormones are **critical** in timing the inhibition of nerve cell replication in the fetal brain, stimulate the growth of nerve cell bodies, the branching of dendrites and the rate of myelination of axons (Chemistry to Clinics 17.20).

2. **Regulation of normal body growth:** Thyroid hormones are important in regulating the growth of the entire body. Thyroid hormones **promote the general growth**, and **calcification** of the bones. Deficiency of thyroid hormones early in life leads to delayed, abnormal development of bone and can lead to dwarfism. A major way by which thyroid hormones promote normal body growth is by stimulating the expression of the gene for growth hormone (**GH**) in the somatotrophs of the anterior pituitary gland. In tissues such as the skeletal muscle, heart and liver, thyroid hormones have direct stimulatory effects on the synthesis of many structural and enzymatic proteins.

3. **Regulation of basal energy economy:** When the body is at rest, about half of the ATP produced by its cells is used to drive energy-requiring membrane transport processes. The remainder is used in involuntary muscular activity such as respiratory movements, peristalsis, contraction of the heart and in many metabolic reactions requiring ATP such as protein synthesis. The energy required to do this work is eventually released as body heat. The major site of ATP production is the mitochondria where the oxidative phosphorylation takes place. Thyroid hormones regulate the basal rate at which oxidative phosphorylation takes place in cells. As a result, they set the basal rates of body heat production and of oxygen consumed by the body, otherwise termed as the **basal metabolic rate (BMR)**. This is also called the **thermogenic action** of thyroid hormones.

Its biochemical basis is that T_3 stimulates the synthesis of cytochromes, cytochrome oxidase, Na^+/K^+-ATPase, uncoupling protein-1 (UCP-1 in brown adipose tissue) and other uncoupling proteins (UCP-2 and UCP-3) in many tissues. The effects are particularly pronounced in skeletal muscle, heart, liver and kidneys, where thyroid hormone receptors are abundant. In hyperthyroidism, oxidative phosphorylation is accelerated and body heat production and oxygen consumption are abnormally high. This can be assessed clinically by an increase in the BMR. The converse occurs in hypothyroidism.

4. **Regulation of fuel metabolism:** In addition to their ability to regulate the rate of basal energy metabolism, thyroid hormones can be viewed as **amplifiers** of cellular metabolic activity. This is mediated through the activation of genes encoding enzymes involved in metabolic pathways. They promote a **positive nitrogen balance** and synthesis of structural proteins. The effects on **carbohydrate** metabolism are **opposite to that of insulin**, hence they tend to increase blood glucose levels. They upregulate **hepatic** LDL receptors thereby favoring the **uptake of LDL-cholesterol**.

Chemistry to Clinics 17.20: Cretinism

Deficiency of thyroid hormones in the perinatal period during which the differentiation of neurons, development of neuronal circuits and myelination occurs, leads to mental retardation. Thyroid hormone replacement must be made in the first few months of postnatal life to prevent permanent mental retardation. If treatment is initiated after behavioral deficits have occurred, the retardation cannot be reversed. In addition, the physical growth of the child is also impaired. The features are collectively known as cretinism (Fig. 17.24).

On the other hand, thyroid hormone deficiency later in life also influences the functions of the nervous system. Cognitive functions including speech and memory are impaired and body movements are slow and clumsy. These changes, however, can be reversed with thyroid hormone therapy.

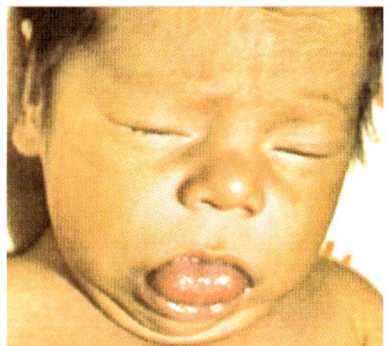

Fig. 17.24: Cretinism. Dull, puffy face and macroglossia (large, thick, protruding tongue).

Disorders of the Thyroid Gland

Autoimmune Thyroid Diseases

1. **Hashimoto's disease:** The thyroid gland is infiltrated by lymphocytes and elevated levels of antibodies against several components of thyroid tissue (e.g. antithyroid peroxidase [anti-TPO] and antithyroglobulin antibodies) are found in the serum. The thyroid gland is partly or completely destroyed, resulting in hypothyroidism.

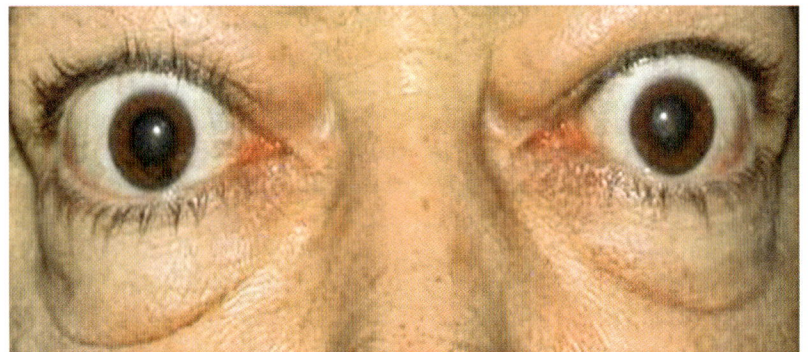
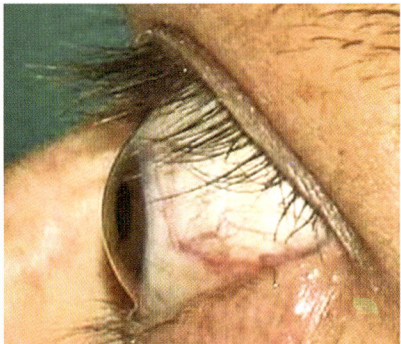

17.25: Exophthalmos in Graves' disease.

2. **Graves' disease:** Stimulatory antibodies to the thyroid-stimulating hormone (TSH) receptor activate thyroid hormone synthesis, resulting in hyperthyroidism. Bulging of eyes (exophthalmos, Fig. 17.25) is a characteristic feature due to increase in retro-ocular fibro-adipose tissue and inflammatory edema of extraocular muscles.

3. **Postpartum thyroiditis:** It usually occurs within 3 to 12 months after delivery. The disease is characterized by a transient destruction-induced thyrotoxicosis (hyperthyroidism), often followed by a period of hypothyroidism lasting several months. Many patients eventually return to the euthyroid state. The postpartum occurrence of the disorder is likely a result of increased immune system function following the suppression of its activity during pregnancy. Since 5–10% of women develop postpartum thyroiditis, it is recommended that thyroid function (serum T_4, T_3 and TSH levels) be monitored postpartum at 2, 4, 6 and 12 months in all women with thyroid peroxidase antibodies or symptoms suggestive of thyroid dysfunction.

Myxedema

In severe hypothyroidism, a slimy, myxomatous substance consisting of hyaluronic acid and chondroitin sulfate complexed with protein is deposited in the extracellular matrix of the skin, causing water to accumulate osmotically. This produces a puffy appearance of the face, hands, legs and feet, called myxedema (Fig. 17.26).

Calcitonin

Calcitonin is a polypeptide containing 32 amino acids secreted from the parafollicular **C-cells** of the thyroid

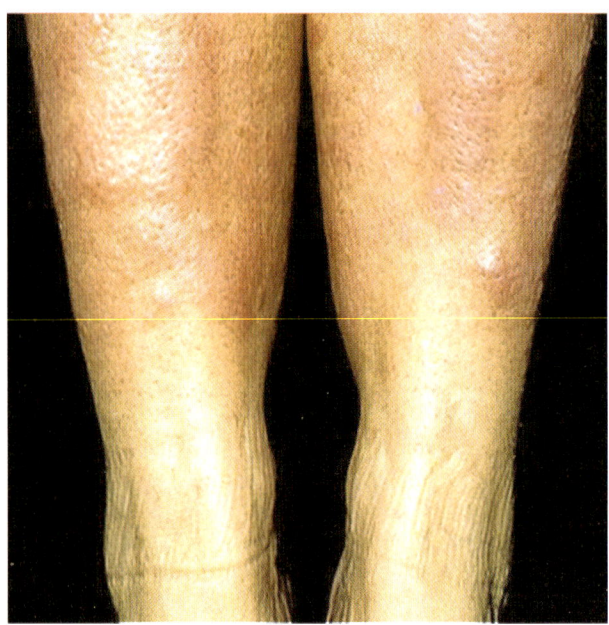

Fig. 17.26: Myxedema.

gland. It **reduces serum Ca^{2+}** by effects **opposite** to that of **parathyroid hormone** (PTH). Its secretion is under direct control of plasma Ca^{2+}. Hypercalcemia stimulates the release of calcitonin. It is a useful pharmacologic agent (Chemistry to Clinics 17.21).

Thyroid function tests are discussed in Chapter 39.

Chemistry to Clinics 17.21: Clinical Significance of Calcitonin

Diagnostic: Serum calcitonin is a tumor marker since increased levels are observed in medullary thyroid carcinoma.

Therapeutic: (i) Calcitonin inhibits osteoclastic activity, hence it is used in the treatment of osteoporosis, bone metastasis and Paget's disease. It is available in the form a nasal spray; (ii) It lowers serum calcium, hence it is used in the treatment of hypercalcemia.

PARATHYROID HORMONE

Parathyroid hormone or parathormone (**PTH**) is a polypeptide containing 84 amino acids. PTH is synthesized as **pre-proparathyroid** hormone consisting of 115 amino acids which is converted to **proparathyroid** hormone containing 90 amino acids and finally processed to PTH.

Functions of PTH: The function of PTH is to maintain the ECF calcium concentration. The hormone **acts directly on bone and kidney, and indirectly on the intestine** through its effects on the synthesis of $1, 25(OH)_2 \cdot D_3$, to increase serum calcium concentration. In turn, PTH secretion is closely regulated by the concentration of serum ionized calcium (Ca^{2+}). Any deficiency towards hypocalcemia, as might be induced by calcium deficient diet, is counteracted by an increased secretion of PTH. Hormone secretion increases steeply to a maximum value of five times the basal rate of secretion as calcium concentration falls from normal to the range of 7.5–8.0 mg/dl. This results in:

1. Increased dissolution of bone mineral thereby increasing the flux of calcium into blood.
2. Reduced renal clearance of calcium, returning more of the filtered calcium into ECF.
3. Increased efficiency of calcium absorption in the intestine.

The homeostatic role of the hormone thus serves to preserve calcium concentration in blood acutely, at the cost of bone destruction. The chronic effects of PTH cause an increase in the number of bone cells, especially osteoclasts and remodeling of the bone.

Control of PTH secretion

- **ECF calcium** level controls PTH secretion by interaction with a **calcium sensor**, G-protein-linked receptor for which Ca^{2+} act as the ligand. Stimulation of the receptor by high Ca^{2+} leads to a suppression of the rate of PTH secretion via intracellular signals generated by the active receptor. The intracellular signals may be IP_3 and DAG which are formed by the activation of phospholipase C, by the calcium sensor. The receptor is present in parathyroid glands, the calcitonin-secreting cells (C cells) of the thyroid, brain and kidney. The biological role of the receptor in tissues other than the parathyroid gland is not known.
- Besides calcium, severe **intracellular magnesium deficiency** also impairs PTH secretion.

Disorders of Parathyroid Gland

In **hyperparathyroidism**, PTH is overproduced by tumors of the parathyroid or in hyperplasia involving all parathyroid glands (generally 4 in number). Excess hormone results in hypercalcemia secondary to increased intestinal calcium absorption, reduced renal calcium clearance and increased bone calcium release. Hypophosphatemia results from the action of excessive PTH on renal tubular phosphate reabsorption.

Hypoparathyroidism causes hypocalcemia and hyperphosphatemia.

Major causes of hyperparathyroidism and hypoparathyroidism are outlined Fig. 17.27.

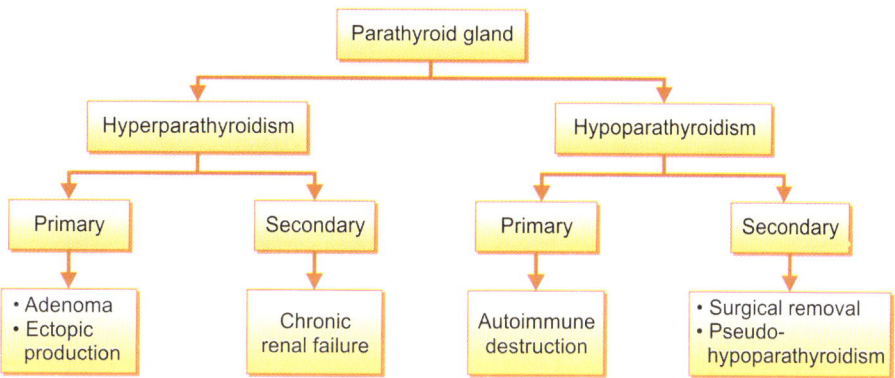

Fig. 17.27: Disorders involving the parathyroid glands. Pseudohypoparathyroidism refers to target organ resistance to PTH.

17

SOME IMPORTANT QUESTIONS

1. **What are hormone receptors? Classify them with examples.**

2. **Discuss mechanisms of hormone action.**

3. **What are hormones? Classify hormones with examples.**

4. **Describe hormones of the anterior pituitary.**

5. **Discuss:**
   i. Regulation of hormone secretion
   ii. Activation of phospholipase C
   iii. Activation of adenylate cyclase
   iv. Renin-angiotensin-aldosterone system
   v. Fight or flight response

6. **Write notes on:**
   i. Endocrine hormones
   ii. Hormone receptors
   iii. Membrane-bound receptors
   iv. Intracellular receptors
   v. G-protein
   vi. POMC
   vii. Acromegaly
   viii. Diabetes insipidus
   ix. Glucocorticoids
   x. Mineralocorticoids
   xi. Cushing's syndrome
   xii. Addison's disease
   xiii. Amino acid derived hormones
   xiv. Pheochromocytoma
   xv. Calcitonin
   xvi. Parathyroid hormone
   xvii. Hyper- and hypoparathyroidism
   xviii. Autoimmune thyroid disease
   xix. Hyper- and hypothyroidism
   xx. Catecholamines

MULTIPLE CHOICE QUESTIONS

1. **Receptors for T_3 are located in:**
   A. Cell membrane
   B. Cytosol
   C. Nucleus
   D. Mitochondria

2. **The DNA-binding region of intracellular hormone receptors is normally blocked by:**
   A. Heat shock proteins
   B. Calmodulin
   D. IP_3
   D. DAG

3. **IGF-1 is structurally similar to:**
   A. Insulin
   B. Proinsulin
   C. C-peptide
   D. Somatostatin

4. **In the corpus luteum, the end product of steroidogenesis is:**
   A. Estradiol
   B. DHEA
   C. Progesterone
   D. Aldosterone

5. **The following is abused in some sports activities:**
   A. Erythropoietin
   B. Androgens
   C. Both
   D. None of the above

6. **The following is not observed in Addison's disease:**
   A. Hypokalemia
   B. Hyponatremia
   C. Hypochloremia
   D. Hypoglycemia

7. **In the plasma, thyroid hormones are bound to:**
   A. Thyroxine-binding globulin
   B. Transthyretin
   C. Albumin
   D. All of the above

8. **In myxedema of severe hypothyroidism, the myxomatous material is composed of:**
   A. Hyaluronic acid
   B. Chondroitin sulphate
   C. Protein and water
   D. All of the above

9. **The sera of patients with Graves' disease contain:**
   A. Anti-TPO antibodies
   B. Anti-thyroglobulin antibodies
   C. Anti-TSH receptor antibodies
   D. Any of the above

10. **The kidneys synthesize the following *except*:**
    A. Angiotensin II
    B. Renin
    C. Erythropoietin
    D. Calcitriol

17

3

Molecular Biology

Metabolism of Nucleotides

Nucleotides, as discussed earlier (Chapter 7) are monomeric units of nucleic acids. These are phosphate esters of a pentose sugar (ribose or deoxyribose) which is linked through C1′ to a nitrogenous base (purine or pyrimidine base). All cells can synthesize nucleotides, either by the biosynthetic process called as *de novo* synthesis or from the degradation products of nucleic acids, i.e. free bases and nucleosides, by the **salvage pathway**.

METABOLISM OF PURINE NUCLEOTIDES

De Novo Synthesis of Purine Nucleotides

The process of synthesis of complex end product(s) in a metabolic pathway from simple precursor molecules is called as *de novo* synthesis (*de novo* = 'anew', i.e. starting 'from scratch'). A purine ring is synthesized by utilizing three amino acids (aspartate, glutamine and glycine) as carbon and nitrogen donors, besides respiratory CO_2 (HCO_3^-) and two 1C moieties (transferred via tetrahydrofolate, FH_4) as the carbon sources.

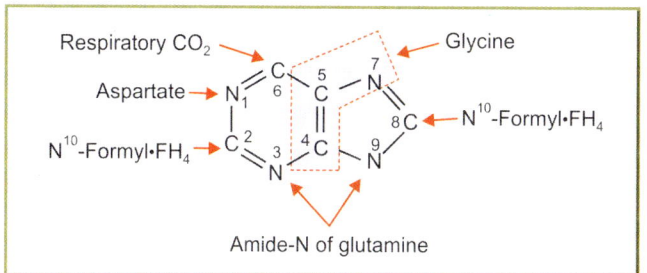

Fig. 18.1: Sources of carbon and nitrogen atoms in a purine ring.

The N1 of a purine ring is derived from the amino group ($-NH_2$) of aspartate, C2 and C8 from N^{10}-formyltetrahydrofolate (N^{10}-formyl·FH_4), N3 and N9 from amide nitrogen ($-CONH_2$) of glutamine, C6 from CO_2 (HCO_3^-), and C4, C5 and N7 from glycine (Fig. 18.1).

The purine ring is synthesized **not as a free base but as a part of the nucleotide** by a series of reactions by adding various carbon and nitrogen atoms onto ribose-5-phosphate.

Synthesis of IMP

De novo pathway for the synthesis of purine nucleotides leads to the synthesis of a nucleotide of hypoxanthine, i.e. inosine-5′-monophosphate (IMP) which in turn serves as a **precursor for AMP and GMP**:

1. The starting material for the synthesis of a purine ring is phosphoribosyl pyrophosphate (PRPP). It is synthesized by the addition of pyrophosphate from ATP, onto ribose-5-phosphate (produced in the HMP shunt). This reaction is catalyzed by phosphoribosyl pyrophosphate synthetase (PRPP synthetase), also called ribose phosphate pyrophosphokinase (Fig. 18.2). The enzyme is inhibited by both ADP and GDP.

   PRPP is used as a starting material, not only for the synthesis of purines but also for pyrimidines. PRPP is also used in the utilization of purine and pyrimidine bases by the salvage pathway.

2. The next step is the formation of 5′-phosphoribosylamine. The reaction is catalyzed by an

18

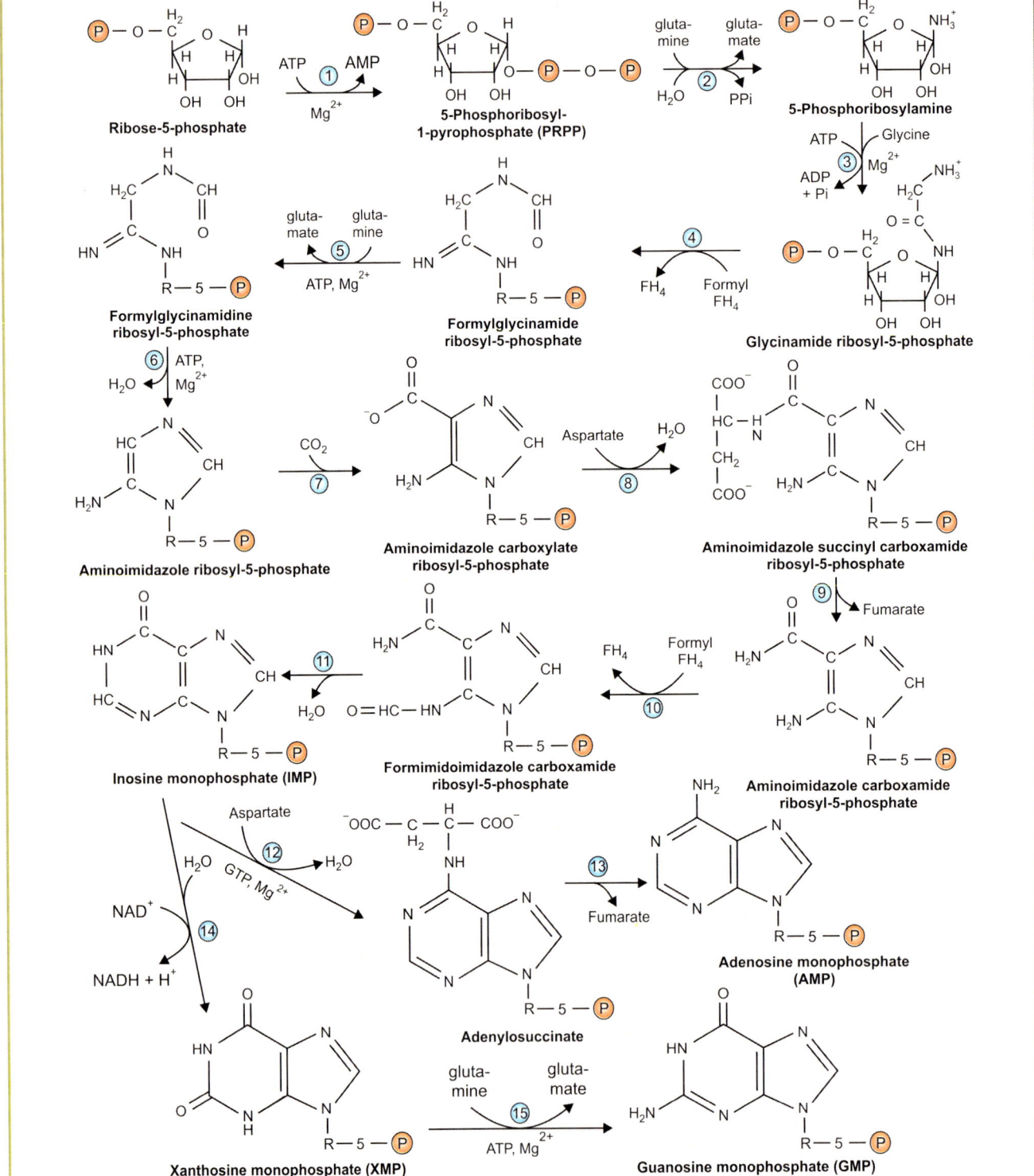

Fig. 18.2: *De novo* purine biosynthesis. 1. PRPP synthetase, 2. Phosphoribosylamine synthetase, 3. Phosphoribosyl glycinamide synthetase, 4. Formyl transferase, 5. Formylglycinamidine ribosyl-5-phosphate synthetase, 6. Amino imidazole ribosyl-5-phosphate synthetase, 7. Aminoimidazole ribosyl-5-phosphate carboxylase, 8. Succinyl carboxamide ribosyl-5-phosphate synthetase, 9. Lyase, 10. Formyl transferase, 11. IMP cyclohydrolase, 12. Adenylosuccinate synthetase, 13. Adenylosuccinase, 14. IMP dehydrogenase, 15. XMP transamidase.

amidotransferase (glutamine PRPP amidotrans-ferase), also called phosphoribosylamine synthe-tase. Pyrophosphate group is replaced by the amide nitrogen of glutamine. This, in turn, results in the acquisition of N9 of the purine ring and is a committed step. The rate of the reaction is controlled by intracellular concentrations of both the substrates, i.e. glutamine as well as PRPP.

3. In the next step, glycine gets conjugated with the amino group of phosphoribosylamine and forms 5-phosphoribosylglycinamide. The reaction is cata-lyzed by phosphoribosylglycinamide synthetase.

4. In the next reaction, N^{10}-formyl·FH_4 donates a formyl group and results in the formation of 5-phosphoribosylformylglycinamide. The reaction is catalyzed by formyl transferase or transformylase (phosphoribosylglycinamide transformylase).

5. Thereafter, through a series of reactions, **IMP** is synthesized as the **first purine nucleotide** (Fig. 18.2).

Various enzymes involved in the synthesis of a purine nucleotide are found in the **cytosol** of a cell whereas energy, to drive some of these reactions, is obtained from the hydrolysis of ATP. During this process 6 moles of ATP are utilized per mole of IMP synthesized. This implies that the *de novo* synthesis of purines is **costly** in terms of the energy investment. Hence, a purine 'salvage' pathway also exists as discussed later in this chapter.

Synthesis of AMP and GMP

The first ribonucleotide formed in the *de novo* path-way, i.e. IMP serves as a common precursor for the synthesis of AMP as well as GMP (Fig. 18.2).

• **Synthesis of AMP:** IMP reacts with aspartate and is changed to adenylosuccinate (AMPS). The reaction is catalyzed by adenylosuccinate synthe-tase. Thereafter, adenylosuccinase (adenylosucci-nate lyase) removes fumarate and forms AMP. Adenylosuccinate synthetase is a rate-limiting enzyme with AMP acting as a competitive inhibitor. GTP is used as a source of energy.

• **Synthesis of GMP:** IMP is converted to xanthosine monophosphate (XMP) by IMP dehydrogenase. Thereafter, GMP synthetase converts XMP to GMP. IMP dehydrogenase is a rate-limiting enzyme. It is regulated by GMP which acts as a competitive inhibitor for the enzyme.

Formation of GMP from IMP requires ATP as a source of energy.

Regulation of Biosynthesis of Purine Nucleotides

• Biosynthesis of IMP is regulated at the first step of the pathway by the availability of ribose-5-phosphate and hence PRPP.

• The reaction catalyzed by **amidotransferase is a committed step**, i.e. the site of metabolic regu-lation. The enzyme glutamine: PRPP amidotrans-ferase is regulated, allosterically, by the end prod-ucts of the pathway, i.e. by IMP, GMP and AMP which serve as negative effectors. On the other hand, PRPP is a positive effector for the enzyme.

• Biosynthesis of AMP and GMP from IMP is also regulated. Both, AMP and GMP each are compe-titive inhibitors of IMP in their own synthesis. From IMP to GMP, **IMP dehydrogenase is the rate limiting enzyme**. It is regulated by GMP which acts as a competitive inhibitor. Adenylosuccinate synthetase is a rate limiting enzyme in the conver-sion of IMP to AMP where AMP acts as a competitive inhibitor.

• The rate of GMP synthesis increases with the concentration of ATP while that of the AMP increases with the concentration of GTP (Fig. 18.3).

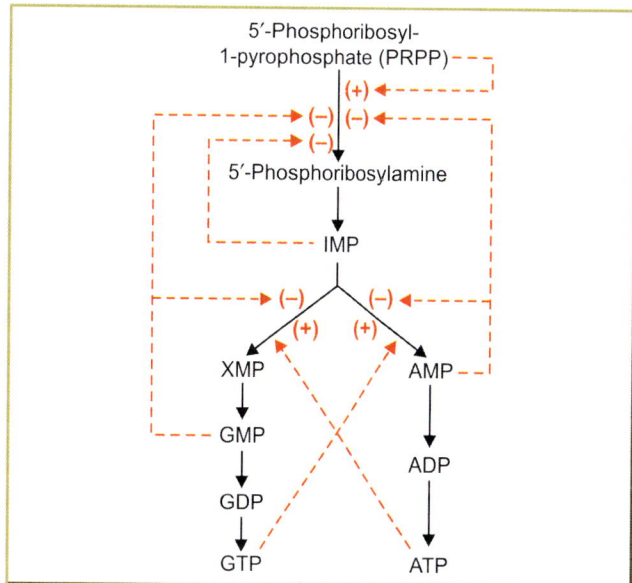

Fig. 18.3: Regulation of purine nucleotide biosynthesis. (+) = stimulation; (–) = inhibition.

18

SALVAGE PATHWAY FOR PURINES

In mammals, **free purine bases**, i.e. hypoxanthine, guanine and adenine as well as their nucleosides can also be converted to the corresponding nucleotides in the salvage pathway (Fig. 18.4). The conversion of free base to the respective nucleotide requires phosphoribosyl transferase and PRPP as a source of ribose-5-phosphate. For the salvage, adenine mainly arises from the synthesis of polyamines, i.e. from 5'-methylthioadenosine (Chapter 13). On the other hand, hypoxanthine and guanine arise from the degradation of purine nucleotides.

• **Adenine** is converted to AMP by adenine phosphoribosyltransferase (APRTase), whereas both **hypoxanthine** and **guanine** are converted to IMP and GMP respectively, by the same enzyme, i.e. hypoxanthine–guanine phosphoribosyltransferase (HGPRTase). Lack of HGPRTase activity results in a condition designated as **Lesch-Nyhan syndrome** (Chemistry to Clinics 18.1).

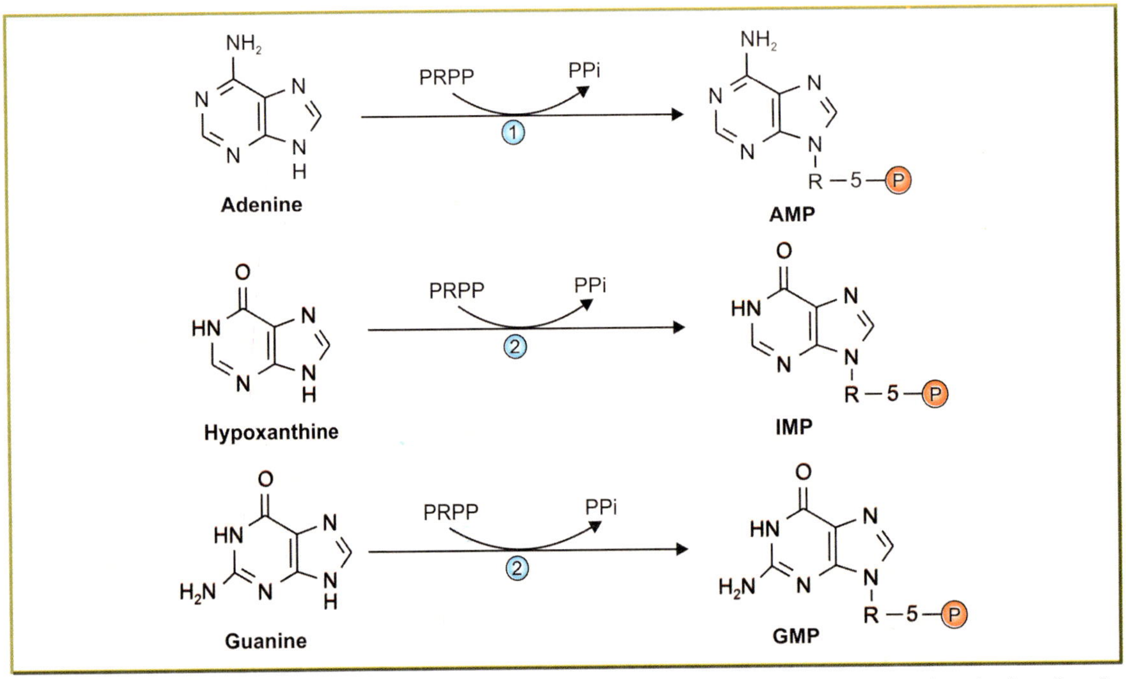

Fig. 18.4: Purine salvage pathway. 1. Adenine phosphoribosyl transferase, 2. Hypoxanthine–guanine phosphoribosyltransferase.

Chemistry to Clinics 18.1: Lesch-Nyhan Syndrome

Inability of the body to salvage hypoxanthine and guanine (Fig. 18.4) due to the complete deficiency of HGPRTase, leads to a condition called Lesch-Nyhan syndrome (partial deficiency causes Kelley-Seegmiller syndrome). Since the gene for HGPRTase is located on the X chromosome, this disease is limited to males only.

Features

1. In this condition, hypoxanthine and guanine are not salvaged. This, in turn, results in increased intracellular pool of PRPP and decreases IMP and GMP concentrations, thereby promoting *de novo* synthesis of purine nucleotides. This leads to excessive production of uric acid, hyperuricemia and gout.
2. Guanosine is an important modulator of glutamatergic neurotransmission, promoting glial reuptake of L-glutamate. A deficiency of guanosine could lead to dysregulated glutamatergic neurotransmission, including possible excitotoxic damage. This partly explains the mental retardation and some other neurological features.
3. Decreased GTP synthesis through salvage pathway reduces its availability for the enzyme GTP cyclohydrolase, an enzyme which initiates the synthesis of biopterins. The latter are essential for the synthesis of many neurotransmitters, e.g dopamine in the striatal dopaminergic pathways. This is thought to result in self-mutilation.

Diagnosis

i. Increase urinary urate/creatinine ratio.
ii. Absent/reduced enzyme activity in lymphocytes or fibroblasts.
iii. Mutation analysis of *HGPRTase* gene.

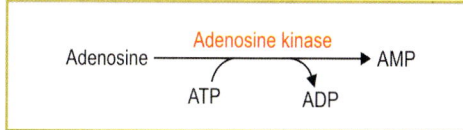

Fig. 18.5: A nucleoside kinase reaction.

- Both the phosphoribosyltransferase reactions are regulated by their end products. Whereas AMP is a competitive inhibitor of APRTase, IMP and GMP competitively inhibit HGPRTase activity.
- **Nucleosides** can be salvaged by the respective nucleoside kinases. For example, adenosine is salvaged by adenosine kinase, a 5′-phosphotransferase that utilizes ATP as the phosphate donor (Fig. 18.5).

Importance of Purine Salvage Pathway

1. The *de novo* purine synthesis is energetically expensive. Salvage reactions **conserve energy**.
2. Salvage reactions are important in cells like **erythrocytes** which lack amidotransferase and cannot synthesize 5-phosphoribosylamine.

INTERCONVERSION OF PURINE NUCLEOTIDES

To meet their need, cells can interconvert adenine and guanine nucleotides and thus maintain a balance between the two purine nucleotides. For their interconversion, GMP or AMP is first degraded to IMP which then, depending upon the need of the cell, can resynthesize any of the two nucleotides:

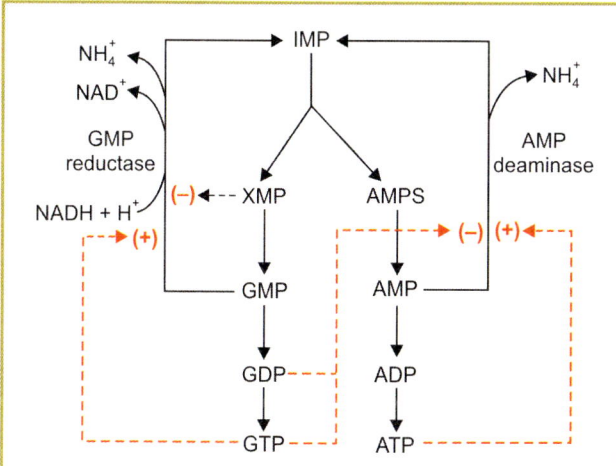

Fig. 18.6: Interconversion of purine nucleotides. (+) = Stimulation; (−) = Inhibition.

- By reductive deamination, GMP is converted to IMP. The reaction is catalyzed by GMP reductase. GTP activates this step whereas XMP competitively inhibits the reaction.
- Conversion of AMP to IMP is catalyzed by AMP deaminase (5′-AMP aminohydrolase). This reaction is activated by K^+ and ATP but inhibited by Pi, GDP and GTP (Fig. 18.6).

DEGRADATION OF PURINE NUCLEOTIDES

Degradation of purine nucleotides, i.e. AMP and GMP, leads to the formation of **uric acid**, in humans (Fig. 18.7).

Degradation of AMP

1. AMP is converted to adenosine, by 5′-AMP-nucleotidase which has high specificity for its substrate. Thereafter, adenosine deaminase (ADA) converts adenosine as well as deoxyadenosine to inosine. Alternatively, AMP deaminase, which is specific for AMP, removes ammonia and converts AMP to IMP. Subsequently, nucleotidase removes phosphoric acid and converts IMP to inosine.

   Activities of the above three enzymes, i.e. AMP-nucleotidase, ADA and AMP deaminase are several fold higher in muscle than in other tissues.
2. Purine nucleoside phosphorylase (PNP) then removes the ribose moiety from inosine and converts it to hypoxanthine.

Degradation of GMP

1. In the first step, phosphoric acid is removed by 5′-nucleotidase and GMP is converted to guanosine.
2. With the removal of the ribose moiety by PNP, guanosine is converted to guanine.
3. Guanase (an aminohydrolase), removes amino group from guanine and converts it to xanthine.

   Two distinct immunodeficiency diseases, i.e. ADA deficiency and PNP deficiency are associated with defects in the degradation of purine nucleosides (adenosine and guanosine) (Chemistry to Clinics 18.2).

Formation of Uric Acid

In human beings and other primates, the end product of purine degradation is uric acid which is excreted in the urine. Hypoxanthine and xanthine, produced

18

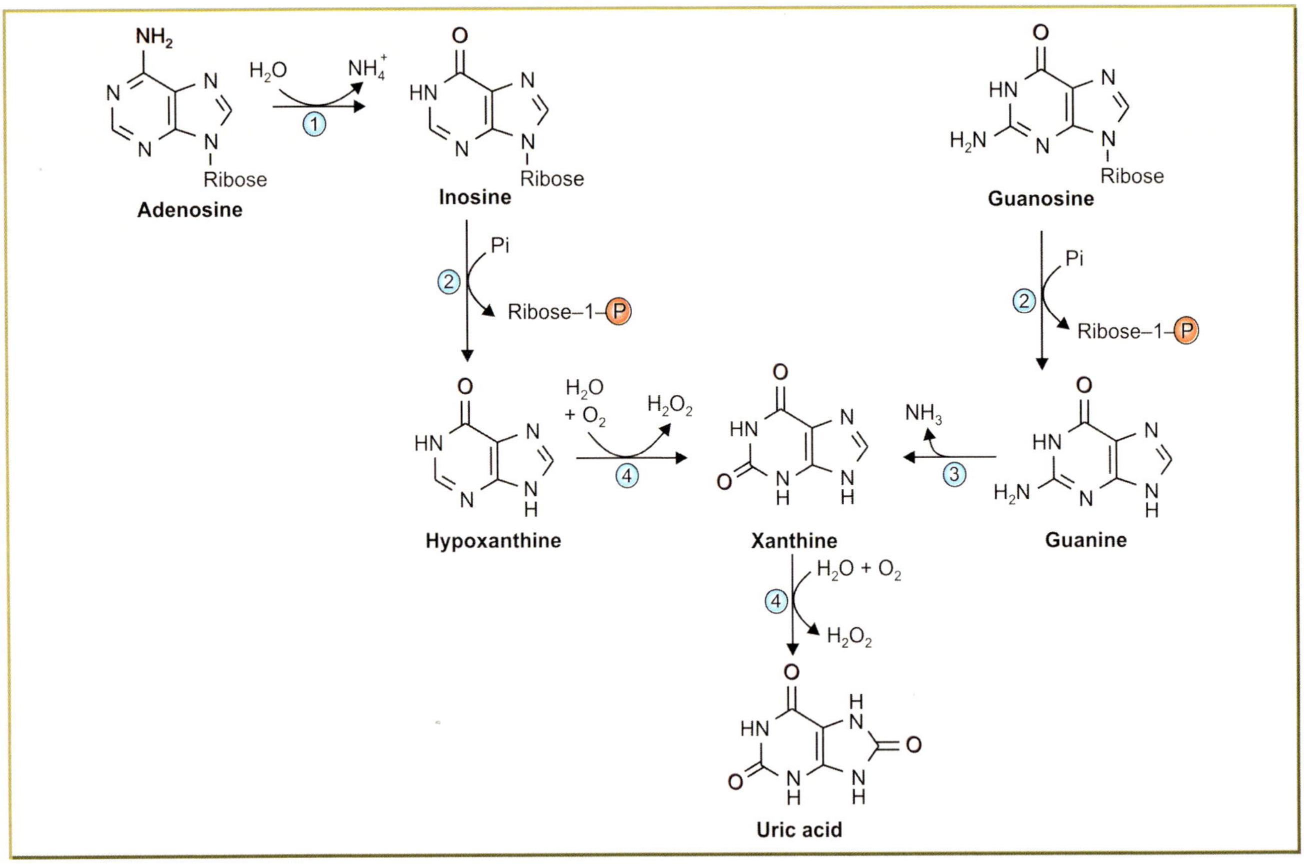

Fig. 18.7: Catabolism of purines to uric acid. 1. Adenosine deaminase, 2. Purine nucleoside phosphorylase, 3. Guanase, 4. Xanthine oxidase.

Chemistry to Clinics 18.2: Immunodeficiency Diseases Associated with Degradation of Purine Nucleosides

- **Severe Combined Immunodeficiency:** A deficiency in ADA is associated with severe combined immunodeficiency (SCID) involving both T-cell and B-cell functions. In ADA deficient patients, intracellular concentration of 2'-deoxyadenosine is increased leading to accumulation of dAMP and dATP. This not only decreases ATP synthesis but also blocks DNA replication by reducing the synthesis of other dNTPs. Thus, proliferation and differentiation of immune cells is compromised. Treatment of such children includes blood transfusion, bone marrow transplantation, enzyme replacement therapy with ADA-polyethylene glycol (the first successful application of enzyme replacement therapy for an inherited disease) and gene therapy. Recently, ADA gene has been successfully transfected into stem cells of ADA-deficient children.

- **Purine Nucleoside Phosphorylase Deficiency:** It is associated with immunodeficiency involving T-cell functions, i.e. a defective T-cell immunity but with normal B-cell functions.

In both the conditions, i.e. SCID and PNP deficiency, there is a decrease in uric acid formation which is accompanied with increased levels of purine nucleosides and nucleotides. Overwhelming infection in such children results in death within 2 years of age.

as above, are catabolized by the enzyme **xanthine oxidase** and are converted to uric acid (Fig. 18.7). This enzyme occurs in the liver and small intestinal mucosa. It is a dimeric protein which contains FAD, a Mo complex and two different FeS clusters. It also requires molecular oxygen as a substrate.

Uric acid is **sparingly soluble in an aqueous medium**. Normal serum uric acid is maintained between **3 and 7 mg/dl**. **Males** have physiologically **higher values** because of higher rate of tubular urate reabsorption, and the uricosuric effect of estrogen in females.

Hyperuricemia

Elevated level of uric acid in the serum (>7 mg/dl, called hyperuricemia) is often asymptomatic. However, it may result in its deposition as sodium urate crystals primarily in the joints, in a clinical condition, called gout (Chemistry to Clinics 18.3).

METABOLISM OF PYRIMIDINE NUCLEOTIDES

De Novo Synthesis of Pyrimidine Nucleotides

A pyrimidine ring is synthesized by utilizing two amino acids, i.e. aspartate and glutamine as carbon and nitrogen donors, and respiratory CO_2 (HCO_3^-) as

---

Chemistry to Clinics 18.3: Gout

It is a disease characterized by elevated levels of uric acid in the blood (**hyperuricemia**) and its increased excretion in the urine (**uric aciduria**) due to a variety of metabolic abnormalities. Most of the clinical conditions with hyperuricemia arise due to the poor aqueous solubility of uric acid. As a result, sodium urate crystals are deposited in joints of the extremities (**gouty arthritis**) and/or in the renal interstitial tissue (**gouty nephropathy**). The crystals activate the complement pathway resulting in the recruitment of neutrophils, macrophages, release of inflammatory mediators and free radicals. In the affected joint, hyaluronic acid is reduced both due to decreased production and increased degradation. Hyperuricemia is thus associated with recurrent attacks of painful arthritic joints and inflammation, most often of big toe (Fig. 18.8), caused by the deposition of insoluble sodium urate crystals, called **tophi**.

Primary Hyperuricemia: This is due to some metabolic defect that results in increased synthesis of purine nucleotides via *de novo* pathway, such as:

1. **Increased PRPP synthetase activity:** This results in increased intracellular concentration of PRPP which acts as a positive effector of the enzyme amidotransferase. This, in turn, increases *de novo* synthesis of purine nucleotides as well as their subsequent degradation to uric acid.

2. **HGPRTase deficiency:** Deficiency of HGPRTase, as in Lesch-Nyhan syndrome, causes a decrease in the salvage pathway of hypoxanthine and guanine to reform nucleotides. This, in turn, spares PRPP and results in overproduction of purine nucleotides and their degradation to uric acid.

3. **Glucose-6-phosphatase deficiency (glycogen storage disease I or von Gierke's disease):** It results in increased levels of glucose-6-phosphate which is diverted to HMP shunt. This, in turn, increases availability of ribose-5-phosphate and enhances the generation of PRPP. Raised levels of PRPP increase *de novo* synthesis of purine nucleotides and the overproduction of uric acid. In addition, associated lactic acidosis elevates renal threshold for urate which further leads to hyperuricemia.

Secondary hyperuricemia: It is secondary to some disease other than a metabolic disorder, such as a kidney disease or a disease associated with excessive cell turnover and increased breakdown of nucleic acids, e.g. radiation therapy/cancer chemotherapy, or psoriasis.

A better way of classifying hyperuricemia is based on its pathophysiology: Overproduction (e.g. rapidly multiplying tumors, cancer chemotherapy), underexcretion (e.g. lactic acidosis, diabetic ketoacidosis) and both (e.g. alcoholism, von Gierke's disease).

Treatment: Most effective treatment of gout includes the use of inhibitor of xanthine oxidase, such as allopurinol or its metabolite alloxanthine. Allopurinol decreases both uric acid formation as well as *de novo* synthesis of purine nucleotides.

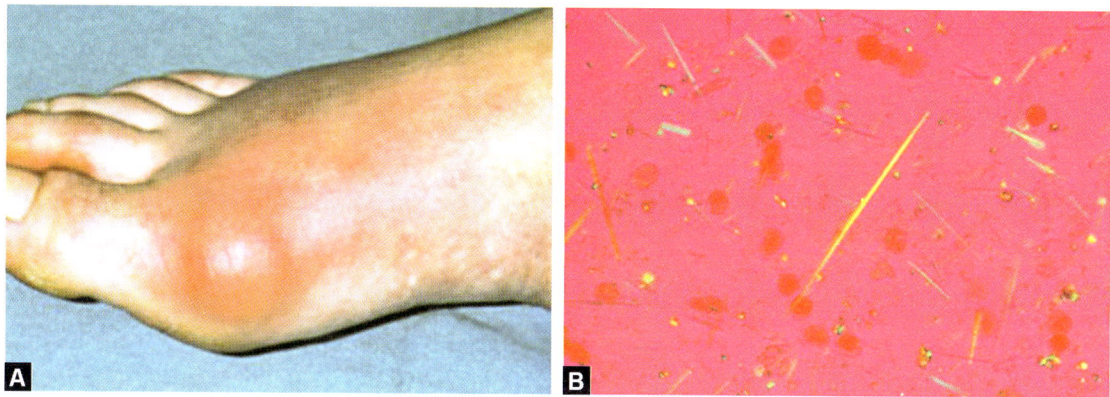

Fig. 18.8: Gout. (A) The condition most commonly affects the great toe (**first metatarsophalangeal joint**) when it is also called podagra, (B) Under polarized microscope, negatively birefringent needle-shaped monosodium urate crystals of various sizes and colors are seen in the joint aspirate.

18

a carbon donor. As shown in Fig. 18.9, N1, C4, C5 and C6 of the pyrimidine ring are derived from aspartate, C2 from HCO_3^- and N3 from glutamine.

In the *de novo* synthesis of pyrimidine nucleotides, a **pyrimidine ring is formed first**. Thereafter, ribose-5-phosphate is added via PRPP. This leads to the synthesis of UMP which serves as a precursor for other pyrimidine nucleotides (Fig. 18.10).

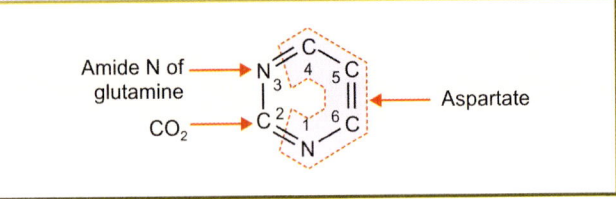

Fig. 18.9: Sources of carbon and nitrogen atoms in a pyrimidine ring.

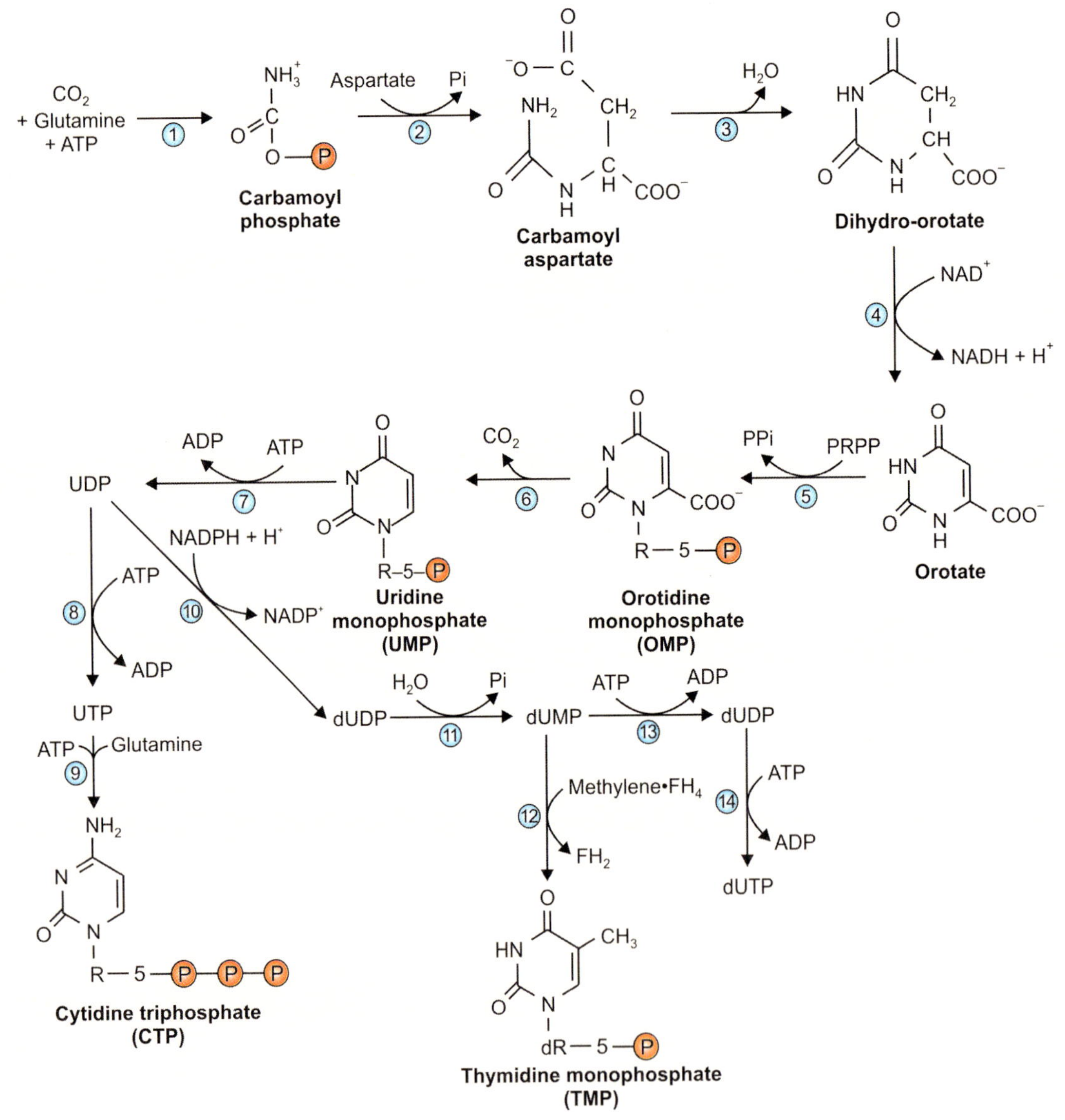

Fig. 18.10: Pyrimidine nucleotide biosynthesis. 1. Carbamoyl phosphate synthetase II (CPS II), 2. Aspartate transcarbamoylase, 3. Dihydro-orotase, 4. Dihydro-orotate dehydrogenase, 5. Orotate phosphoribosyl transferase, 6. Orotidylate decarboxylase, 7. UMP kinase, 8. UDP kinase, 9. CTP synthetase, 10. Ribonucleotide reductase, 11. dUMP synthase, 12. Thymidylate synthase, 13. dUMP kinase, 14. dUDP kinase.

Synthesis of UMP

1. The first step in the synthesis of a pyrimidine ring is the synthesis of carbamoyl phosphate from glutamine and HCO_3^-. This reaction consumes two molecules of ATP.

   This is a regulated step in the pathway and is catalyzed by carbamoyl phosphate synthetase II (**CPS II**), in the cytosol (Fig. 18.10). Remember that a similar enzyme, carbamoyl phosphate synthetase I (CPS I) uses ammonia as a source of nitrogen and synthesizes carbamoyl phosphate in the mitochondria, for the urea cycle (Chapter 13).

2. In the next step, carbamoyl phosphate condenses with aspartate and forms carbamoyl aspartate. The reaction is catalyzed by aspartate transcarbamoylase (aspartate carbamoyltransferase). This is the **committed step** in the synthesis of pyrimidine nucleotides.

3. Dihydro-orotase results in ring closure and forms dihydro-orotate. In animals, activities of the 3 enzymes, i.e. CPS II, aspartate transcarbamoylase and dihydro-orotase are present on a single trifunctional protein, termed as **CAD**.

4. Dihydro-orotate dehydrogenase, a mitochondrial enzyme, oxidizes dihydro-orotate to orotate.

5. Orotate phosphoribosyltransferase transfers ribose-5-phosphate from PRPP and converts the pyrimidine base orotate to its nucleotide, orotidine monophosphate (OMP).

6. OMP is converted to UMP by OMP decarboxylase (orotidylate decarboxylase). Orotate phosporibosyltransferase and OMP decarboxylase activities are present on a single **bifunctional protein**, termed as UMP synthase (Chemistry to Clinics 18.4).

Conversion of Nucleoside Monophosphates to Di- and Triphosphates

Various nucleoside monophosphates, i.e. AMP, GMP, CMP, UMP as well as dAMP, dGMP, dCMP and dTMP are sequentially converted to their nucleoside triphosphates.

- Firstly, a nucleoside monophosphate (NMP) is converted to the corresponding nucleoside diphosphate (NDP). The reaction is catalyzed by the base specific nucleoside monophosphate kinase.
- Thereafter, nucleoside diphosphate kinase converts a nucleoside diphosphate to the corresponding nucleoside triphosphate (Fig. 18.11).

Conversion of UTP to CTP

CTP synthetase catalyzes the formation of CTP from UTP by using glutamine as a donor of the amino group. ATP is used as a source of energy. CTP is a negative effector of the reaction (Figs 18.10 and 18.12).

Chemistry to Clinics 18.4: Orotic Aciduria

There are several types of the disease:

Type 1: It is due to a defect in *de novo* synthesis of pyrimidine nucleotides. There is a genetic deficiency of both the activities of the bifunctional protein UMP synthase, comprising of orotate phosphoribosyltransferase and OMP decarboxylase. High levels of orotic acid excretion in the urine and deficiency of enzymes in erythrocytes confirm the diagnosis.

Type 2: Reduced activity of OMP decarboxylase only.

Others

i. Ornithine transcarbamoylase (an enzyme of urea cycle) deficiency results in accumulation of carbamoyl phosphate which is channelized towards pyrimidine biosynthesis. Blood ammonia is increased whereas urea is decreased, the two features not observed in type 1 and 2 orotic aciduria.

ii. Reye's syndrome.

iii. During allopurinol therapy.

Features

Megaloblastic anemia: Deficiency of UMP (precursor of UTP, CTP and TMP) leads to decreased nucleic acid synthesis in erythroid precursors in bone marrow, and megaloblastic anemia. It does not respond to vitamin B_{12} and/or folic acid.

Physical and mental retardation: This could be due to reduced supply of pyrimidine nucleosides in the neonatal period.

Treatment: It includes feeding uridine-rich diet which reduces formation of orotate and improves anemia. Uridine is taken up by the cells, salvaged to UMP and finally to UTP which inhibits CPS II, the regulatory step in pyrimidine biosynthesis. As a result, orotic acid synthesis is decreased. Exogenous uridine thus bypasses the defective step in pyrimidine biosynthesis and by its salvage utilization, uridine supplies UTP and CTP required by the cell.

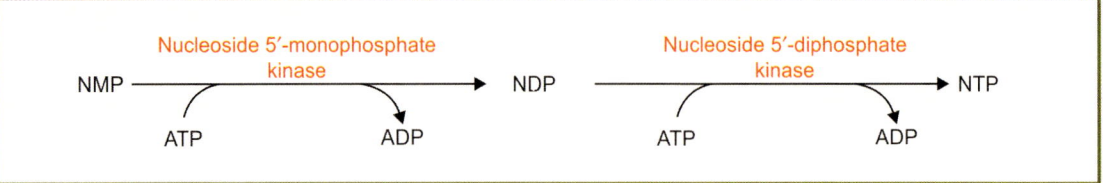

Fig. 18.11: Conversion of a nucleoside monophosphate to di- and triphosphate.

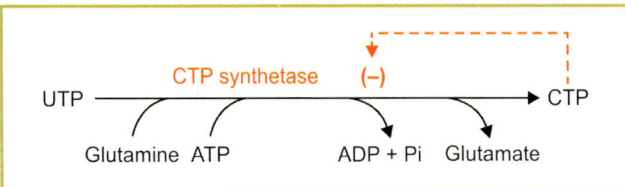

Fig. 18.12: Synthesis of CTP from UTP.

Synthesis of TMP

Both UTP and CTP can serve as precursors of TMP. The two nucleoside triphosphates are first hydrolyzed to the corresponding nucleoside diphosphates, i.e. CDP and UDP which, in turn, act as precursors of dUMP.

Thereafter, thymidylate (deoxythymidylate, dTMP or TMP) is synthesized by methylation of the deoxyuridine monophosphate (dUMP). The reaction is catalyzed by thymidylate synthase. In this reaction, N^5,N^{10}-methylenetetrahydrofolate (N^5,N^{10}-methylene·FH$_4$) is used as a source of the methyl group (one carbon moiety) and also as a reducing agent. N^5, N^{10}-methylene·FH$_4$, in turn, is converted to FH$_2$ (Figs 18.10 and 18.13). Dihydrofolate reductase

(DHFR), in the presence of NADPH + H$^+$, converts FH$_2$ back to FH$_4$.

Importance of DHFR and Thymidylate Synthase

dTMP synthesis is essentially required for rapidly proliferating cells, such as cancer cells, for DNA synthesis. Inhibition of thymidylate synthase or of DHFR blocks the synthesis of dTMP and thus kills cancer cells. Various inhibitors of these enzymes are known and are used as effective anticancer/antibacterial agents (Chemistry to Clinics 18.5 and 18.6).

Regulation of Biosynthesis of Pyrimidine Nucleotides

- Pyrimidine synthesis is regulated by CPS II. The enzyme is inhibited by CTP and is activated by ATP and PRPP (Fig. 18.14).
- OMP decarboxylase is competitively inhibited by UMP.

Chemistry to Clinics 18.5: Suicide Inhibitors

Analogs of dUMP, such as 5-fluorodeoxyuridylate (FdUMP) are irreversible inhibitors of thymidylate synthase. FdUMP binds to the enzyme thymidylate synthase like dUMP and forms an enzyme·FdUMP·FH$_4$ ternary covalent complex. This, in turn, inactivates the enzyme after undergoing some of the normal catalytic reactions. Such enzyme inhibitors are called mechanism-based inhibitors or suicide inhibitors or suicide substrates, as they force the enzyme to commit suicide.

Chemistry to Clinics 18.6: Antifolates

Antimetabolites, such as methotrexate (amethopterin), amino-pterin and trimethoprim are analogs of FH$_2$ and are called as antifolates. These drugs inhibit dihydrofolate reductase and block the regeneration of FH$_4$. This, in turn, affects dTMP biosynthesis. These drugs are used as effective anticancer agents, particularly against childhood leukemias.

Trimethoprim binds more tightly to bacterial enzymes than to mammalian cells. It is, therefore, used as an important antibacterial agent. It is an active ingredient of the popular antibiotic 'Septran'.

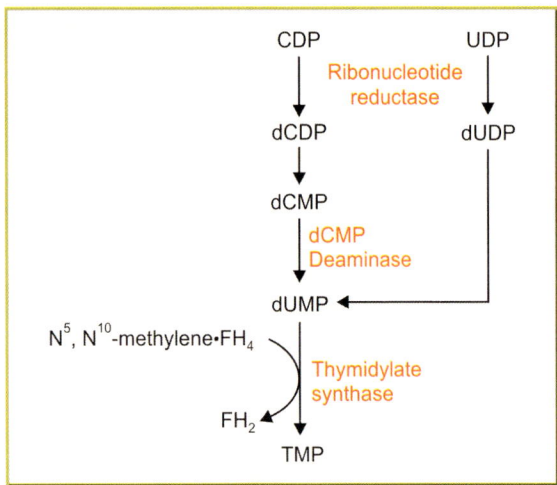

Fig. 18.13: Synthesis of TMP.

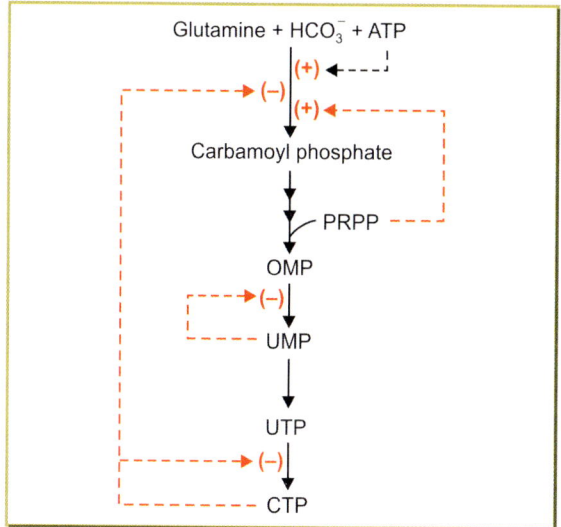

Fig. 18.14: Regulation of pyrimidine nucleotide biosynthesis. (+) = Stimulation; (–) = Inhibition.

- CTP synthetase is inhibited by CTP. This is an example of feedback inhibition. This, in turn, regulates the conversion of UTP to CTP. Cells thus maintain a balance between uridine and cytidine nucleotides.

SALVAGE PATHWAY FOR PYRIMIDINES

Pyrimidine bases orotate, uracil and thymine, but not cytosine, can be salvaged and converted to the corresponding nucleotides by pyrimidine phosphoribosyltransferase. The enzyme utilizes PRPP as a source of ribose-5-phosphate (Fig. 18.15).

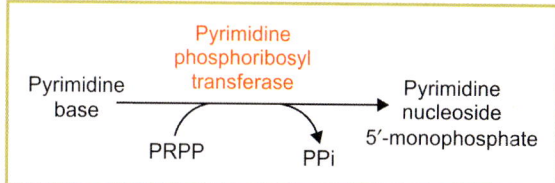

Fig. 18.15: Salvage pathway for pyrimidines.

DEGRADATION OF PYRIMIDINE NUCLEOTIDES

Pyrimidine nucleotides are first converted to free bases which are then degraded to form the end products.

Degradation of Pyrimidine Nucleotides to the Free Bases

- Pyrimidine nucleotides (CMP, UMP, dCMP and dTMP), released as a result of the turnover of nucleic acids, are converted to the corresponding nucleosides by the nonspecific phosphatases.
- Cytidine and deoxycytidine are thereafter deaminated by pyrimidine nucleoside deaminase to uridine and deoxyuridine, respectively.
- Uridine, deoxyuridine and deoxythymidine are degraded by uridine phosphorylase and result in the formation of uracil (from uridine and deoxyuridine) and thymine (from deoxythymidine) (Fig. 18.16).

Degradation of Pyrimidine Bases

Uracil and thymine produced as above are further degraded to β-alanine and β-aminoisobutyric acid (Chemistry to Clinics 18.7), respectively (Fig. 18.17).

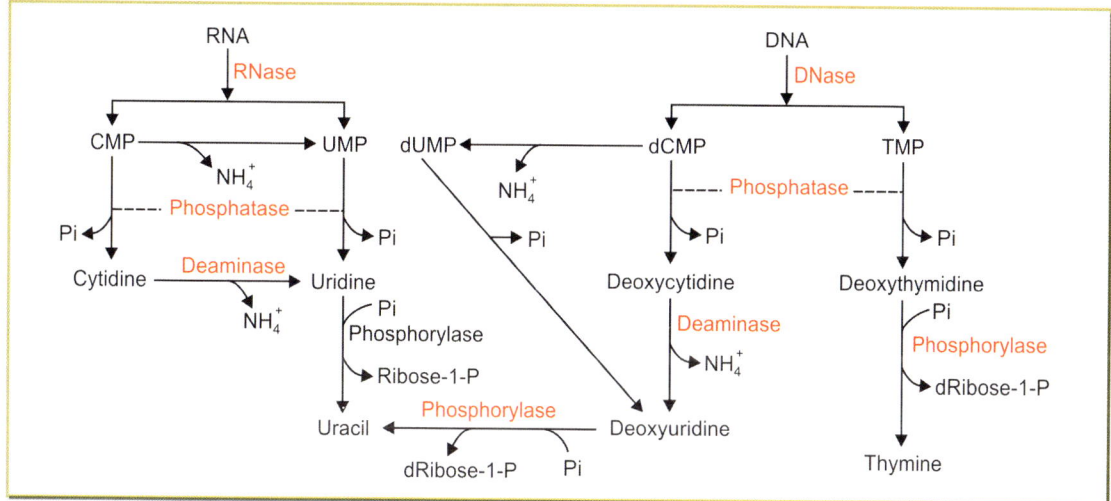

Fig. 18.16: Degradation of pyrimidine nucleotides to free bases.

Chemistry to Clinics 18.7: β-Aminoisobutyric Acid

β-Aminoisobutyric acid is excreted in the urine and is a measure of turnover of DNA or thymine nucleotides. Its urinary excretion is increased in cancer patients undergoing chemotherapy or radiation therapy, due to the increased degradation of DNA.

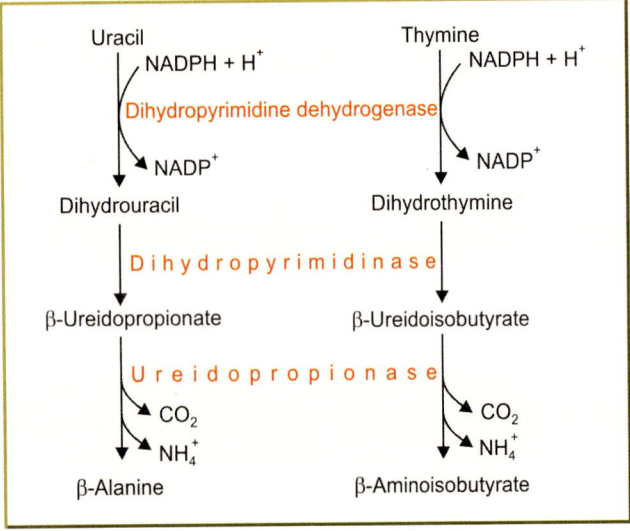

Fig. 18.17: Degradation of pyrimidine bases.

SYNTHESIS OF DEOXYRIBONUCLEOTIDES

Purine and pyrimidine ribonucleotides formed by the respective *de novo* pathways, are converted to their deoxyribonucleotides during **DNA replication**.

- Ribonucleoside diphosphates (NDPs), i.e. ADP, GDP, CDP and UDP are reduced at C2′ position to their deoxy forms, i.e. dADP, dGDP, dCDP and dUDP by ribonucleotide reductase (ribonucleoside diphosphate reductase). **Thioredoxin** (a peptide containing two cysteine residues) is used as a source of reducing equivalents. Reduced form of the coenzyme (reduced thioredoxin) gets oxidized and forms a disulfide bond.

Mammalian ribonucleotide reductase is a heterodimer. The enzyme is under allosteric regulation where the products serve as potent negative effectors of the enzyme. dATP is a potent inhibitor of the reduction of all the four nucleoside diphosphates (CDP, UDP, GDP and ADP). dGTP inhibits the reduction of CDP, UDP and GDP while dTTP inhibits the reduction of CDP, UDP and ADP.

- The oxidized thioredoxin is then reduced by thioredoxin reductase which is a flavoprotein and contains FAD as a prosthetic group. NADPH + H$^+$ serves as the terminal reducing agent (Fig. 18.18). In place of thioredoxin, **glutaredoxin** can also be used which requires glutathione and glutathione reductase.

- Phosphorylation of dNDP produces dNTP which, in turn, is used in the biosynthesis of DNA. The reaction is catalyzed by nucleoside diphosphate kinase. Any of the NTP or dNTP, such as ATP, can function as the phosphoryl donor for this reaction (Fig. 18.19).

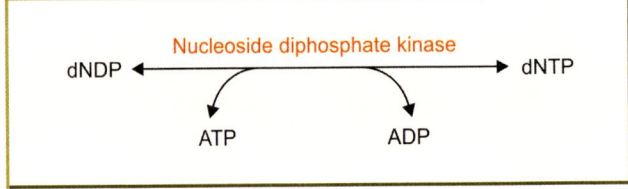

Fig. 18.19: Interconversion of dNDP and dNTP.

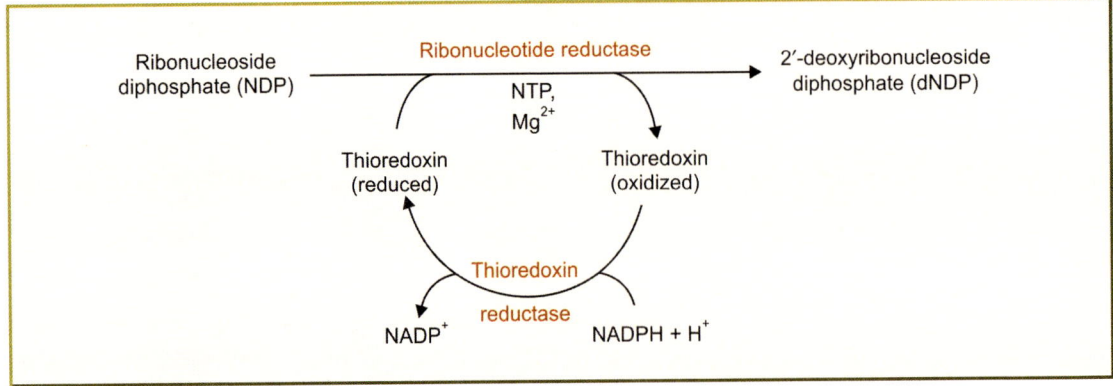

Fig. 18.18: Conversion of a ribonucleotide to deoxyribonucleotide.

SOME IMPORTANT QUESTIONS

1. What are nucleotides? Explain the process of *de novo* synthesis of purine nucleotides.

2. Describe the process of the degradation of purine nucleotides.

3. Describe the process of *de novo* synthesis of pyrimidine nucleotides.

4. Describe briefly:
   - i. Synthesis of IMP
   - ii. Regulation of purines biosynthesis
   - iii. Interconversion of purine nucleotides
   - iv. Immunodeficiency diseases related to purines degradation
   - v. Formation of uric acid
   - vi. Primary hyperuricemia
   - vii. Secondary hyperuricemia

5. Write notes on:
   - i. Salvage pathway for purines
   - ii. Lesch-Nyhan syndrome
   - iii. Severe combined immunodeficiency
   - iv. Gout
   - v. Hereditary orotic aciduria
   - vi. Suicide inhibitors
   - vii. Antifolates
   - viii. Carbamoylphosphate synthetase
   - ix. CAD
   - x. UMP synthase

MULTIPLE CHOICE QUESTIONS

1. **The first purine nucleotide synthesized *de novo* is:**
   - A. AMP
   - B. GMP
   - C. IMP
   - D. None of the above

2. **The following may be seen in Lesch-Nyhan syndrome:**
   - A. Hyperuricemia
   - B. Mental retardation
   - C. Self mutilation
   - D. All of the above

3. **Adenosine deaminase (ADA) activity is highest in:**
   - A. Muscles
   - B. Liver
   - C. Kidneys
   - D. Brain

4. **SCID is characterized by:**
   - A. Decreased T-cell function, normal B-cell function
   - B. Decreased T- and B-cell function
   - C. Normal T-cell function, decreased B-cell function
   - D. Normal T- and B-cell function

5. **Increased uric acid synthesis occurs in the following *except*:**
   - A. ADA deficiency
   - B. HGPRTase deficiency
   - C. Increased activity of PRPP synthetase
   - D. Glucose-6-phosphatase deficiency

6. **The following enzyme catalyzes the committed step in pyrimidine nucleotide biosynthesis:**
   - A. PRPP synthetase
   - B. CPS II
   - C. Aspartate transcarbamoylase
   - D. CPS I

7. **The methyl group donor in thymidylate synthesis is:**
   A. S-Adenosyl methionine
   B. Betaine
   C. N^5,N^{10}-Methylenetetrahydrofolate
   D. N^5-Methyltetrahydrofolate

8. **The following is a suicide substrate:**
   A. FdUMP
   B. Allopurinol
   C. Both
   D. None of the above

9. **The following is measured in urine to assess DNA turnover:**
   A. β-Alanine
   B. Putrescine
   C. β-Amino isobutyric acid
   D. Adenosine deaminase

10. **The following is true for sodium urate:**
   A. Poor aqueous solubility
   B. Precipitates in acidic pH
   C. Dehydration promotes precipitation
   D. All of the above

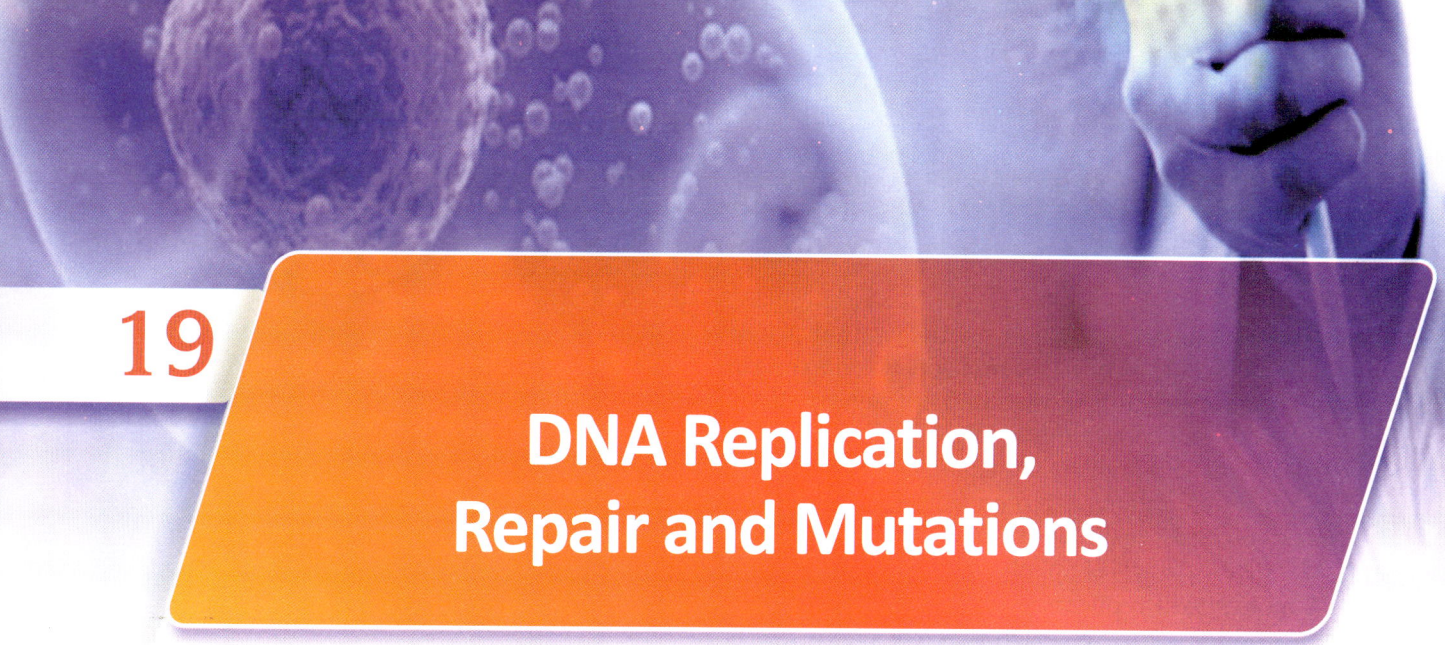

19

DNA Replication, Repair and Mutations

The process of **DNA synthesis** is called **replication**. DNA replication is carried out by enzymes known as DNA dependent DNA polymerases (DNA directed DNA polymerases) or simply referred to as **DNA polymerases**.

A SEMICONSERVATIVE PROCESS

During replication, each strand of the double-stranded DNA serves as a **template** for the synthesis of a new strand, in a very accurate manner. Since both the strands of the parental DNA double helix can serve as template and produce two daughter DNA molecules, therefore after a round of replication, each of the two newly formed double-stranded DNA molecules contain one strand from the parental double-stranded DNA while the other one is a newly synthesized complementary strand.

This process of DNA replication where after each round of replication, one strand in a double-helix is maintained intact (parental strand) and combines with the other one which is a newly synthesized daughter strand, is called as 'semi-conservative' replication (Fig. 19.1) observed in mammalian cells.

In 'conservative' replication, the two original strands remain together after serving as templates and so are the two newly synthesized strands. As a result, one of the daughter duplexes contains only parental DNA while the other daughter duplex contains only newly synthesized DNA.

In 'dispersive' replication, the parental strands are broken into fragments and the new strands are synthesized in short segments. Subsequently, the old and new segments are joined together to form a complete strand. As a result, the daughter duplexes contain strands that are composites of old and new DNA.

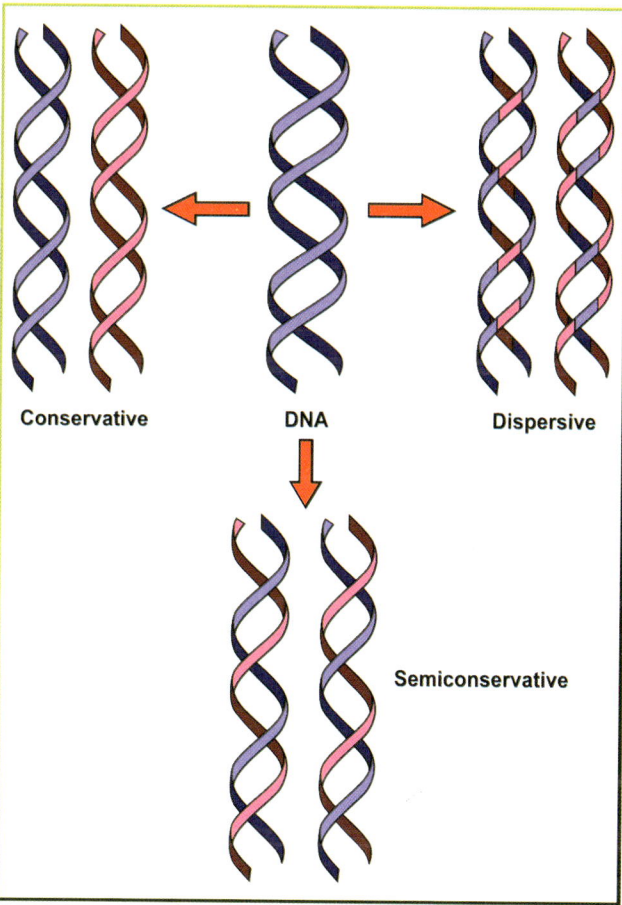

Fig. 19.1: Semiconservative replication is the biologically relevant mechanism of DNA replication.

19

THE REPLICON

The unit of DNA in which an individual act of replication occurs is called the replicon. It has an **origin** at which replication is initiated. A genome in a prokaryotic cell constitutes a single replicon, largest is that of the bacterial chromosome. Each eukaryotic chromosome contains a large number of replicons. Each replicon fires only once in each cell cycle and possesses the control elements needed for replication.

A molecule of replicating DNA, when viewed by electron microscopy, has two types of regions. It is seen as the replicated region which appears as an eye (**replication eye**) flanked by nonreplicated DNA (parental duplex). The point at which replication is occurring is called the **replication fork**, also known as the **growing point** (Fig. 19.2).

A replication fork moves sequentially along the DNA, from its starting point at the origin.

Replication may be unidirectional or bidirectional, depending on whether one or two replication forks are formed at the origin. In unidirectional replication, one replication fork leaves the origin and proceeds

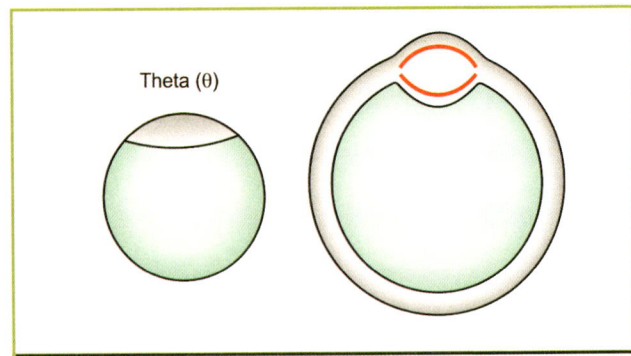

Fig. 19.4: Replication eye in prokaryotes.

along the DNA. In bidirectional replication, two replication forks are formed which proceed away from the origin in opposite directions (Fig. 19.3).

Prokaryotic replicons are usually circular where the DNA forms a closed circle with no free ends. A replication eye forms a theta (θ) structure in circular DNA (Fig. 19.4).

Origin of Replication

The site where DNA replication begins is called origin of replication. A general feature is that the overall sequence composition is **A·T-rich**. The **bacterial chromosome** is replicated bidirectionally as a single unit from **ori C**. Two replication forks initiate at ori C and move around the genome nearly at the same speed, to a meeting point.

In **eukaryotic cells**, the replication of DNA is confined to a part of the cell cycle (S phase). Replication is accomplished by dividing the chromosome into many individual replicons (Fig. 19.5).

In **yeast chromosome**, initiation of replication occurs at the locations of **autonomously replicating sequence** (ARS) elements. An ARS element also

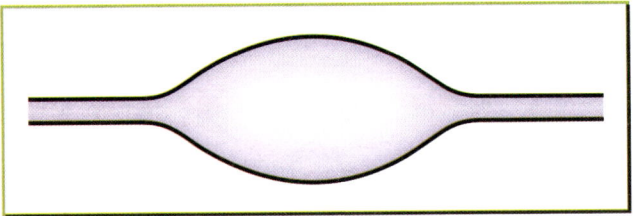

Fig. 19.2: Replication eye.

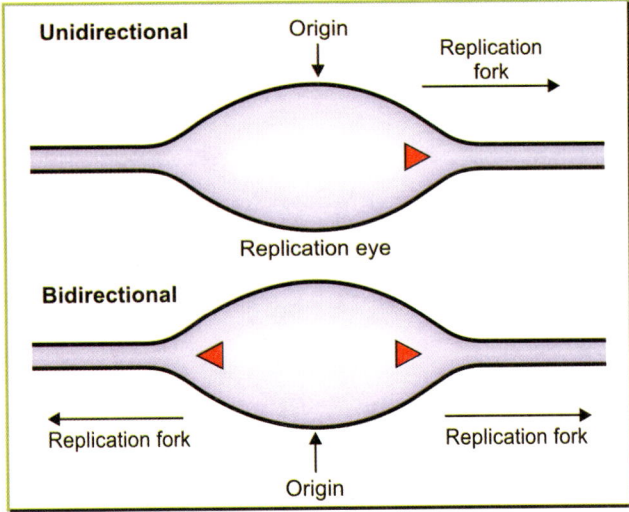

Fig. 19.3: Directions of replication.

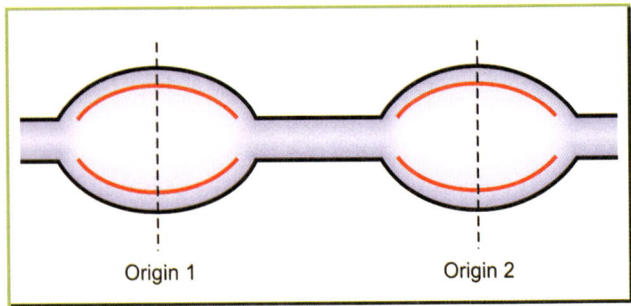

Fig. 19.5: Replication of mammalian DNA.

consists of an A·T-rich region. These ARS elements get associated with a complex of six proteins, called **origin recognition complex** (ORC).

Separation of the Two Strands

For the start of DNA replication, separation of the two strands of the parental DNA is essential so that the bases of each **template become accessible** to their complementary deoxyribonucleotides which are to be used in the construction of the new strand.

Requirement for Unwinding of the Two Strands

For the initiation of unwinding of the double helix as well as for the continuation of the separation of the two strands, various proteins and enzymes are required. These include DnaA protein, single-strand binding protein, helicase, etc.

DnaA Protein: It binds to the origin of replication and is also called **origin-binding protein**. Nearly, 20–50 monomers of DnaA bind to a specific nucleotide consensus sequence at the origin of replication (AT rich region). This requires ATP and results in separation (melting) of two strands of DNA (Fig. 19.6).

Single-strand Binding (SSB) Protein: It binds to single-strands of the DNA, preventing them from rejoining to the duplex state. SSB binds as a monomer but typically in a co-operative manner, in which the binding of additional monomers to the existing complex is enhanced. Binding of the SSB protein to the two strands neither consumes ATP nor exhibits any enzymatic activity. SSB protein also protects cleavage of the single-stranded DNA from the action of nucleases. The two strands are stripped-off the SSB protein before their replication.

In eukaryotes, the two strands (after their separation) are covered with the protein, called replication protein A (replication factor A) which is functionally equivalent to SSB protein in prokaryotes.

Helicases: It is an enzyme that separates the strands of DNA, usually using the hydrolysis of ATP. A helicase is generally a hexamer and translocates along DNA to provide multiple DNA-binding sites. It has one conformation that binds to duplex DNA and another that binds to single-strand of the DNA. Translocation between them drives the motor that melts the duplex, and requires ATP hydrolysis. A helicase initiates unwinding at a single-stranded region, adjacent to a duplex and functions with a particular polarity.

In eukaryotes, helicase activity is associated with DNA polymerase δ.

Supercoiling or Superhelicity

Chromosomes of many bacteria and viruses, as we know, exist as **coils**, i.e. they are the circular molecules of double helix DNA. When examined under an electron microscope, these circular DNA molecules (coils) have a peculiar twisted appearance and form **supercoils** (positive supercoils) during replication (Fig. 19.7).

For example, consider a two-stranded helical rope whose both ends are free. If you hold the two strands

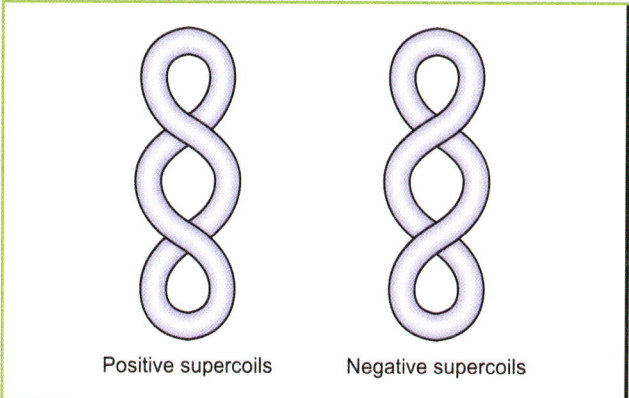

Fig. 19.7: The coiling of duplex DNA around its own axis is called supercoiling. Positive supercoils twist the DNA in the same direction as the turns of the right-handed double helix. Positively supercoiled DNA is overwound (wound more tightly). Negative supercoils twist the DNA about its axis in the opposite direction from the clockwise turns of the right-handed double helix. Negatively supercoiled DNA is underwound (and thus favors unwinding of duplex).

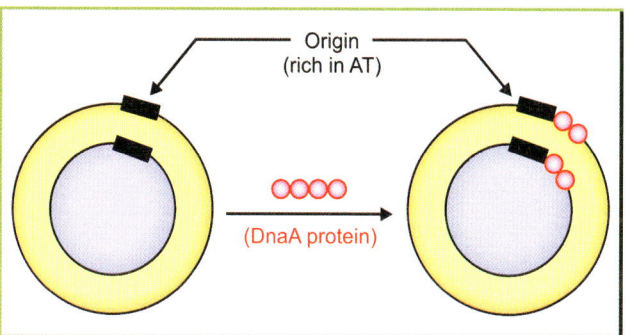

Fig. 19.6: Binding of DnaA at origin of replication.

19

at one end and begin to pull them apart, the entire fiber would rotate to resist the development of tension. If, however, the other end of the rope is fixed, the separation of the two strands at the free end would generate increasing **torsional stress** in the rope and cause the unseparated portion to become more tightly wound (Fig. 19.8). This is analogous to separation of two strands of a circular DNA (in prokaryotes) or a linear duplex DNA (in eukaryotes). However, unlike a rope which can become tightly overwound, an **overwound DNA molecule becomes positively supercoiled**.

Unwinding of a lengthy DNA at a very high speed results in **supercoiling (superhelicity)** of the helix to the extent that, if not corrected, it may stop unwinding of the parental DNA and hence DNA replication. Cells overcome these topological problems by **nicking** (cutting at a particular site, enzymatically) one or both the strands, near the replicating fork, remove the supercoils and reseal the ends with the help of a group of enzymes called **topoisomerases**. These enzymes **remove positive supercoils**.

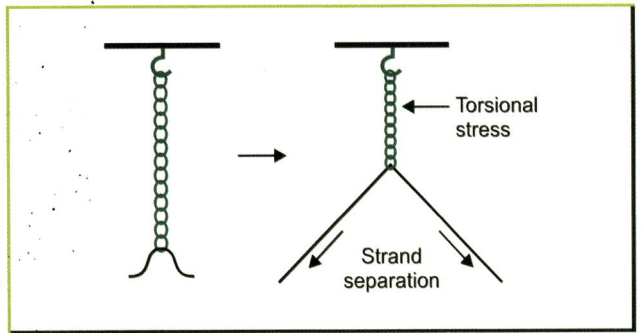

Fig. 19.8: Increasing torsional stress due to strand separation.

During this process, **negative supercoils** however, may be formed when DNA duplex is twisted in the opposite direction, i.e. in the direction opposite from the clockwise turn of the right-handed helix.

Topoisomerases: Topoisomerases are a group of **endonucleases** which alter the **topological state** of the circular DNA. The topological state of a DNA molecule is represented by **its linking number**, i.e. the number of times a DNA strand winds around the other. Topoisomerases introduce nicks in one or both the strands, remove the supercoils and reseal the ends. There are several types of topoisomerases (Table 19.1). Topoisomerase II inhibitors are in common clinical use (Chemistry to Clinics 19.1).

Polymerization of Deoxyribonucleotides

Polymerization of deoxyribonucleotides, i.e. synthesis of the new DNA strand (in the process of DNA replication and repair) is catalyzed by a family of enzymes, referred to as **DNA polymerases**. They use

Chemistry to Clinics 19.1: Topoisomerase II Inhibitors

Antimicrobials of the quinolone category such as norfloxacin, ciprofloxacin, ofloxacin, etc. and some anticancer agents such as doxorubicin and etoposide, block topoisomerase II activity. These compounds thus arrest DNA replication as well as RNA transcription, which explains the high clinical potency of these drugs. On the other hand, drugs like camptothecin, anthracycline, etc., interfere only with the enzyme catalyzed resealing of the DNA strands. They do not affect the overall activity of the enzyme but convert these topoisomerases into the DNA-breaking agents. Since DNA degradation leads to cell death, these drugs are used in the treatment of certain hematological neoplasms, e.g. leukemias and lymphomas.

Table 19.1: Topoisomerases: Salient features

Type	Target DNA	Activity		ATP required	Effects	
		Endonuclease	Ligase		Prokaryotes	Eukaryotes
I	One strand	Yes	Yes	No	Relax negative supercoils	Relax both negative and positive supercoils
II	Both strands	Yes	Yes	Yes	Relax both negative and positive supercoils. Introduce negative supercoils into relaxed DNA (gyrases)	–
III	One strand	Yes	Yes	No	Remove circular DNA products called catenates which are generated just prior to the completion of DNA replication	–
Reverse gyrase	Both strands	Yes	Yes	Yes	Found in archaebacteria: Introduce positive supercoils into DNA and prevent denaturation from high temperature and acidity	–

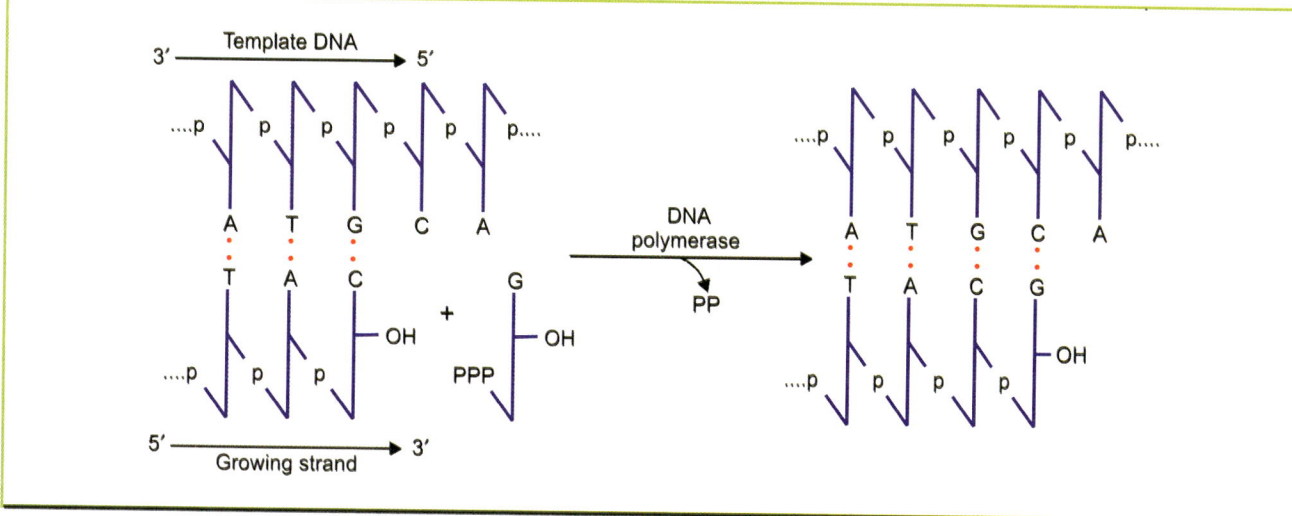

Fig. 19.9: Action of DNA polymerase.

single-stranded DNA as a template and catalyze the synthesis of the complementary strand, by using appropriate deoxyribonucleoside triphosphates. DNA polymerases add a nucleotide to the free 3'-OH group of a base-paired polynucleotide, so that the DNA chain is extended in the **5'→3' direction** (Fig. 19.9).

DNA Polymerases Versus DNA Replicases: DNA polymerases (DNA dependent DNA polymerases) are the enzymes that catalyze the synthesis of a complementary strand on a single-stranded DNA template. Some of these enzymes actually undertake replication. These are called DNA replicases. On the other hand, others are involved in subsidiary roles in replication and/or participate in repair, i.e. in the synthesis of only a segment of the DNA, to replace damaged sequences. These enzymes are referred to as DNA polymerases.

DNA Polymerases in Prokaryotes

Three distinct forms of the enzyme are found in prokaryotes. These are designated as DNA polymerases I, II and III (Table 19.2).

- **DNA polymerase I (Pol I):** It is a **processive** enzyme since it catalyzes a series of successive nucleotides polymerization steps, without releasing the single-stranded template. The enzyme has an important role in DNA replication as well as its repair in *E. coli.* The enzyme has three distinct activities, i.e. 5'→3' polymerase (synthetic) activity, and 3'→5' as well as 5'→3' exonuclease (hydrolytic) activities. Structurally, Pol I is a single polypeptide. Proteolytic cleavage of the enzyme results in the formation of two fragments, a large fragment and a small fragment. The large fragment is designated as **Klenow fragment**. It has both the 5'→3' polymerase and 3'→5' exonuclease activities. The small fragment contains 5'→3' exonuclease activity only.

  Due to its 3'→5' exonuclease activity, the enzyme edits mistakes. This proof-reading action of the enzyme ensures high fidelity in DNA replication.

  Pol I is also important in the repair of the damaged DNA.
- **DNA polymerase II (Pol II):** It has 5'→3' polymerase as well as 3'→5' exonuclease activities but

Table 19.2: Prokaryotic DNA polymerases: Salient features

Type	Activity			Effects	
	5'→3' polymerase (synthetic)	3'→5' exonuclease	5'→3' exonuclease	DNA replication	DNA repair
I	Yes	Yes	Yes	Yes	Yes
II	Yes	Yes	No	No	Yes
III	Yes	Yes	No	Yes	Yes

19

lacks 5'→3' exonuclease activity. The enzyme mainly participates in DNA repair.

- **DNA polymerase III (Pol III):** It is the **replicase** responsible for the *de novo* synthesis of new strands of DNA. It is a more complex enzyme and consists of at least ten different subunits. The catalytic core of the enzyme consists of three different subunits. These are designated as α (which contains DNA polymerase activity), ε (with 3'→5' exonuclease activity) and a θ-subunit. Besides, there are seven other subunits, five of which form a complex with the catalytic core while the other two form a clamp around the template. These are designated as β and γ-subunits. The β-subunit acts as a clamp and promotes processivity while the γ subunit helps the β-subunit to rapidly unclamp and reclamp. Hence, the **γ-subunit is also called the clamp holder**. All the ten subunits together form a labile multisubunit enzyme, known as Pol III holoenzyme.

   Pol III can polymerize a DNA strand as well as edit its mistakes but lacks nick-translation.

DNA Polymerases in Eukaryotes

Five different types of DNA polymerases have been isolated from the mammalian cells. These are designated as DNA polymerases α, β, γ, δ and ε. Each has 5'→3' synthetic activity. With the exception of polymerase γ which occurs in mitochondria, all are involved in chromosomal DNA synthesis as well as repair.

- **DNA polymerase α (Pol α):** It has 5'→3' polymerase activity but **lacks the proof-reading, exonuclease activity.** Thus, it can replicate DNA but cannot correct its mistakes. Pol α has a tightly associated **primase** activity and thus is concerned with priming (initiating) replication and is also called the **lagging strand replicase**.

   The enzyme requires frequent priming. It exhibits only a moderate processivity, i.e. Pol α synthesizes DNA at a slower speed than the prokaryotic DNA Pol III (nearly 50 nucleotides per second, compared to about 1000 nucleotides per second by Pol III).

- **DNA polymerase δ (Pol δ):** It has both 5'→3' polymerase as well as 3'→5' exonuclease (proofreading) activities. It is the nuclear replicase. Pol δ has very high processivity only when associated with a protein called **proliferating cell nuclear antigen** (PCNA, Chemistry to Clinics 19.2). Pol

Chemistry to Clinics 19.2: Proliferating Cell Nuclear Antigen (PCNA)

It is a protein (**cyclin**) which forms a trimer ring around a DNA double helix. It binds to a variety of other nuclear proteins and organizes biochemical processes at the DNA replication fork. It functions in DNA synthesis, repair, chromatin remodeling, regulation of cell cycle and apoptosis. It is a cell proliferation marker, hence a tumor with higher number of PCNA-positive cells is likely to be more aggressive and better respond to anticancer drugs. Anti-PCNA antibodies occur in many cancers as well as autoimmune diseases, e.g. systemic lupus erythematosus.

δ-PCNA complex is also designated as **leading strand replicase**.

- **DNA polymerase ε (Pol ε):** It resembles Pol δ but Pol ε is highly processive even in the absence of PCNA. It also has 3'→5' exonuclease activity that degrades single-stranded DNA to oligonucleotides instead of mononucleotides. Though Pol ε may be necessary for DNA replication *in vivo* and for filling gaps between the Okazaki fragments on the lagging strand, it is essentially involved in repairing damaged nuclear DNA.

- **DNA polymerase β (Pol β):** It is a small polypeptide. It participates in repairing damaged nuclear DNA.

- **DNA polymerase γ (Pol γ):** It occurs exclusively in the mitochondria and is involved in **mitochondrial DNA replication**.

Reverse Transcriptase

An RNA dependent DNA polymerase, designated as reverse transcriptase, is also a member of the polymerase family of enzymes. Reverse transcriptase is an essential enzyme of **retroviruses**, i.e. the RNA containing eukaryotic viruses, such as human immunodeficiency virus (**HIV**), a causative agent of acquired immunodeficiency syndrome (AIDS, Chapter 30). Reverse transcriptase **catalyzes synthesis of double-stranded DNA from single-stranded RNA template**.

   After a retrovirus infects a cell, the enzyme utilizes viral RNA as a template for the synthesis of a complementary DNA strand and results in the production of an RNA-DNA hybrid. Viral RNA strand is degraded by RNaseH and the DNA strand in turn acts as a template for the synthesis of its complementary strand. It yields a double-stranded DNA which is later integrated into the chromosome of the host cell.

Termination Sequences

Sequences that cause termination of DNA synthesis are called as termination sequences (**'ter' sites**). The ter site contains a short (nearly 23 bp) sequence which is **rich in G·T** and functions in only one orientation. The ter site is directly **opposite to the origin**.

In E. *coli,* there are two ter sites (ter E, D, A and ter G, F, B, C). Each contains multiple terminators. Each terminus is specific for one direction of fork movement.

Two replication forks that initiate bidirectional DNA replication at the origin, meet between the oppositely facing ter sites, i.e. a replication fork traveling counter-clockwise passes through ter G, F, B, C but halts at ter A, D, E. On the other hand, the replication fork which travels clockwise passes through ter E, D, A but stops at ter C, B, F, G (Fig. 19.10).

Replication of DNA in Prokaryotes

Replication of duplex DNA is a complex process which as mentioned above, requires several enzymes and other proteins. It occurs in three steps, i.e. initiation, elongation and termination.

Initiation

The major events in the initiation of DNA replication are:
- Formation of the replication fork
- Assembly of primosome and synthesis of RNA primer

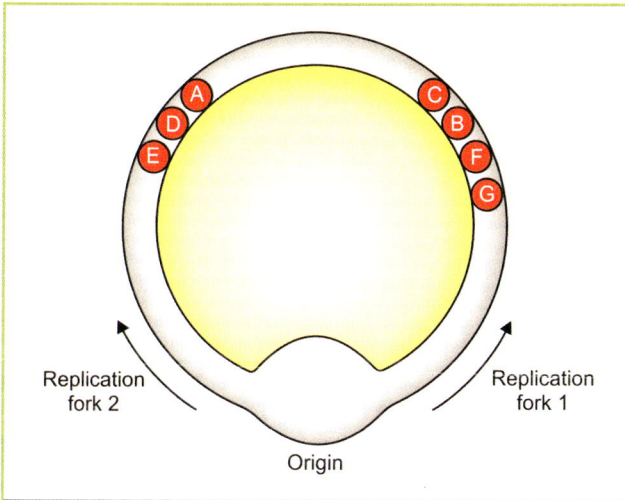

Fig. 19.10: Termination sequences.

Formation of the Replication Fork

- Replication starts at the origin which, as mentioned earlier, is referred as **ori C**, in E. *coli*. It is a sequence of nearly 250 bp that contains four sites, each with nine identical nucleotides, at which DnaA (a tetramer with 4 identical subunits) initiates stepwise assembly of the various proteins and enzymes which are required for DNA replication. Origin also contains 11 **methylation sites** recognized by Dam methylase and three **A·T-rich** direct tandem repeats, consisting of 13 bp each.

- DNA-bound DnaA protein binds additional DnaA molecules and forms DNA-protein complex. An additional factor, called HU protein (DnaC) also participates.

- DnaA and HU proteins interact with ori C and promote unwinding of DNA in the A·T-rich regions.

- **Unwinding** of the two strands is also accompanied by the displacement of DnaA protein.

- Unwinding also produces **supercoils** which are offset by the action of **DNA gyrase** (type II topoisomerase). Availability of the DnaA-binding sites at ori C or the concentration of DnaA regulates initiation.

- DnaA, with the help of DnaC also adds another protein with helicase activity, called DnaB to the above complex. The helicase activity of DnaB further unwinds DNA and creates an initiation bubble or **replication bubble or replication eye**, consisting of a few hundred nucleotide bp. Energy required for this process is provided by **ATP**. A branch point in a replication bubble at which DNA synthesis occurs is called a **replication fork**.

    A replication bubble may contain one replication fork (**undirectional replication**) or two replication forks (**bidirectional replication**).

    Formation of a replication fork initiates stepwise assembly of all the proteins and enzymes which are necessary to carry out the process of DNA replication (Fig. 19.11).

- As the helicases move in advance of each fork, two single-stranded regions are generated which are immediately covered by the **SSB-protein** which helps in keeping the two strands apart from each other.

- The two antiparallel strands of the DNA double helix are **simultaneously replicated at two**

19

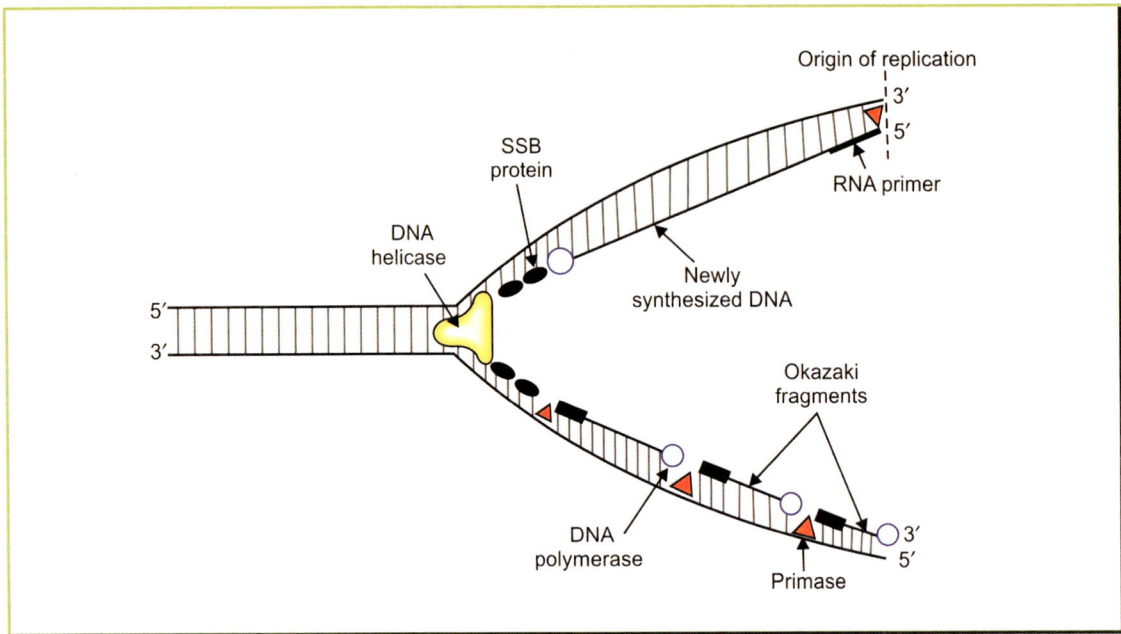

Fig. 19.11: A replication fork.

different advancing replication forks, in their 5′→3′ directions, but in different ways.

– One of the strands is **continuously** synthesized in the direction of the movement of the replication fork. It is called the **leading strand**.

– The other strand though is also synthesized in its 5′→3′ direction but **discontinuously**, in small fragments only. This strand is called the **lagging strand** and these fragments are called nascent DNA segments or precursor fragments. They are also known as **Okazaki fragments** (Fig. 19.11), based on the name of its discoverer. They vary in size from about 100–200 deoxyribonucleotides in eukaryotes, to nearly 1000–2000 deoxyribonucleotides in prokaryotes.

Primosome Assembly and Synthesis of the RNA Primer

• The assembly of DnaB-DnaC along with four other polypeptides, i.e. n, n′, n″ and i, forms a **pre-priming complex**.

• A **primase** is required to catalyze the actual priming reaction. The enzyme is a single polypeptide of 60 kD. It is an RNA polymerase that is the product of the DnaG gene. The primase is required for the synthesis of short stretches of RNA that are used as primers for DNA synthesis. DnaG primase associates transiently with the replication complex and typically synthesizes an 11–12 base primer. Whereas only one priming complex is required to initiate the synthesis of the leading strand, multiple copies of the complex are required for the synthesis of the lagging strand.

• This whole complex of primase with the pre-priming assembly is called **primosome**.

The 'n proteins' in the primosome are its specific components that are responsible for placing the primosome at the appropriate sequences. A primosome searches DNA for these specific sequences, at the expense of ATP.

• The movement of the primosome **displaces SSB proteins** and allows the primase to synthesize an RNA primer in the 5′→3′ direction.

• After promoting primer initiation at one point, the pre-priming proteins move along the template strand in order to synthesize the adjacent primer.

Characteristics of the RNA primer: As DNA polymerase cannot initiate the replication process since it is unable to assemble the first few deoxyribonucleotides, it requires an RNA primer (Table 19.3). Once a primer has been synthesized (Fig. 19.12), DNA polymerase takes over the process of DNA synthesis, may be with the involvement of a specialized

Table 19.3: Characteristics of RNA primer

- An oligonucleotide consisting of several ribonucleotides (10–60 in *E. coli*)
- Complementary and antiparallel to the DNA template.
- Starts with the sequence pppAG, opposite the sequence 3'-TC-5' in the template
- Provides a 3'-OH group to initiate the synthesis of DNA, by DNA polymerase III
- Mature DNA does not contain RNA primer

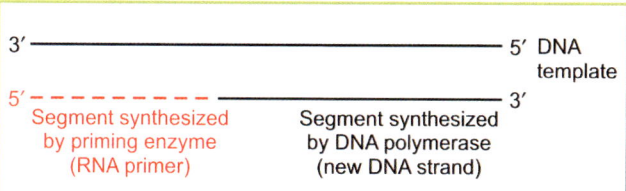

Fig. 19.12: An RNA primer.

ribonuclease called **RNase H**. The primers are eventually removed and the ribonucleotides are replaced with the deoxyribonucleotides.

Elongation

The entire assembly which carries out the process of elongation is called **replisome** (replicase system). Various components of a replisome are given in Table 19.4. A replisome exists only as a protein complex associated with the particular structure that DNA takes at the replication fork. A replisome which contains two polymerase III holoenzymes, synthesizes **both the leading strand and the lagging strand**.

Table 19.4: Components of the replisome

Protein/enzyme	Functions
DnaA	Unwinding of the two DNA strands at the origin of replication
DnaB	Helicase activity unwinds DNA to create the initiation bubble
Topoisomerase II	Removal of supercoils
SSB	Bind to single DNA strand to keep the two strands apart
DnaC	Bind to SSB protein at the origin of replication
Primase	Synthesis of RNA primer
n, n', n'' and i	Primosome assembly
DNA polymerase III	Chain elongation on the 3'-OH group of the primer
DNA polymerase I	Primer excision and gap-filling
DNA ligase	Ligation of the polynucleotide fragments

- It moves as a single unit in the 5'→3' direction along the leading strand whereas the lagging strand template loops around to permit the holoenzyme to extend the primed lagging strand.
- After completing the synthesis of an Okazaki fragment, the holoenzyme on the lagging strand is **relocated to a new primer near the replication fork** and extends the RNA primer to form a new Okazaki fragment. At each of these locations, primers are used for DNA synthesis by the DNA polymerase.
- After the polymerase reaches the end of the single-stranded template, it takes over the next primer which is annealed to the template as a **DNA-RNA hybrid** segment. Since DNA polymerase has very high processivity, it overcomes the hurdle, slides over the intervening DNA-RNA hybrid and resumes DNA replication at the 3' end of the new primer (in eukaryotes, primers may be formed at several locations determined by the nucleosome spacing).
- This results in continuous synthesis of a leading strand and several RNA primed Okazaki fragments, which are separated from each other by single-stranded nicks on the lagging strand. **Synthesis of the leading strand is always ahead of the synthesis of the lagging strand.**
- By the DNA polymerase I catalyzed nick translation, ribonucleotides (from RNA primers) are replaced with the deoxyribonucleotides and finally the nicks present in the lagging strand are sealed by DNA ligase. The enzyme requires energy which is obtained by the hydrolysis of ATP.

Termination

A protein, designated as **Tus** protein (terminator utilization substance), arrests movement of the replication fork and stops DNA synthesis.

- Tus protein acts as a **contra-helicase** and binds to a region called **ter** site. It has **G·T-rich** termination sequences.
- This, in turn, prevents advancement of the replication fork, by arresting the action of the DnaB.
- Finally, unlinking of the parent strands from the daughter strands is catalyzed by topoisomerases.

Fidelity of DNA replication: Balanced levels of dNTPs, proof-reading by polymerase I and polymerase III and the use of RNA primer, eliminate the

19

sources of error and permits accurate base-pairing and results in perfect fidelity of DNA replication.

REPLICATION OF DNA IN EUKARYOTES

DNA synthesis in eukaryotes is fundamentally similar to that in prokaryotes. All steps, such as formation of the replication fork, synthesis and removal of the primer, synthesis of Okazaki fragments, and gap-filling are similar to the corresponding steps in prokaryotes. The overall process, however, is more complex in eukaryotes.

Differences in DNA Replication between Prokaryotes and Eukaryotes

As shown in Table 19.5, DNA replication in eukaryotes differs from prokaryotes in several ways:

1. The **amount of DNA** present in a eukaryotic cell is much more than in a prokaryotic cell.

2. A eukaryotic cell contains **large number of DNA polymerase** molecules (often >20,000) as compared to small number (a few dozen) present in a prokaryotic cell. Moreover, DNA polymerase α synthesizes DNA at a slower speed than the prokaryotic DNA polymerase III. To overcome this problem, eukaryotic chromosomes contain **multiple replicating units** which are located anywhere between 5 to 300 kilo-base-pairs (Kbp).

3. Origin of replication in eukaryotes is termed as autonomous replicating sequence (**ARS**). Each sequence is nearly 100–200 bp and is characterized by A·T-rich central region. It is an 11 bp element and is designated as the ARS consensus sequence.

4. Initiation of DNA replication occurs at **several origins of replication**, simultaneously. DNA segments between two origins of replication are termed as **replicons**. An average human chromosome may contain about 100 replicons, hence replication may proceed simultaneously at nearly 200 forks.

5. Eukaryotic DNA synthesis requires replication protein A (**replication factor A**) which is the functional equivalent of prokaryotic SSB-protein.

6. In eukaryotes, helicase activity is associated with DNA **polymerase δ**.

7. As eukaryotic DNA is packed along with **histones** (as chromatin) in the nucleosomes, it is separated from histones prior to its replication, just ahead of the replication fork. After the replication, histones again get associated with the upcoming daughter duplexes and form nucleosomes.

8. Initiation of eukaryotic DNA synthesis is stringently regulated by **cyclins and cyclin dependent kinases**. The synthesis is confined to the synthetic (S phase) of the cell cycle only. This is followed by a gap period (G_1). Thereafter, cell division occurs during mitosis (M phase) which again follows a gap period (G_2). On the other hand, DNA is replicated through most of the cell cycle in prokaryotes, and cell division occurs immediately after DNA synthesis has ceased.

9. In eukaryotes, synthesis of the leading strand and the lagging strand is carried out by **different enzymes**. In prokaryotes, DNA synthesis is catalyzed by two similar but distinct subunits of the DNA polymerase III.

Table 19.5: Differences in DNA replication in prokaryotes and eukaryotes

Parameter	Prokaryotes	Eukaryotes
Start of replication	At a single site	Simultaneously at multiple sites
Strand separation	By SSB-protein	By replication protein A
Relaxation of supercoils	Only negative supercoils	Both positive and negative supercoils
Types of DNA polymerases	Three: I, II and III	Five: α, β, γ, δ and ε
Helicase activity	Specific enzyme	Associated with DNA polymerase δ
Primase activity	Specific RNA polymerase	Associated with DNA polymerase α
Synthesis of daughter strands	Both strands by DNA polymerase III	Leading strand by DNA polymerase δ, lagging strand by DNA polymerase α
Okazaki fragments	Very long	Small
Overall process	Simple, rapid, error-prone	Complex, slow, accurate

10. The ends of eukaryotic chromosomes have unusual structures called **telomeres** which are also replicated.

Telomeres

- Telomeres are 1000 or more nucleotides long **tandem-repeats** (copies of short **G and T rich** oligonucleotide sequences) present at the **3'-end** of the strand (at the end of each chromosome).
- A telomere also has a 12–16 nucleotides long single strand **overhang** (Fig. 19.13), which serves as a template for the primer that initiates the synthesis of the final Okazaki fragment on the lagging strand.
- In drosophila, the lengthening of these chromosomal ends is carried out by the transposition of DNA segments known as transposons.
- In most of the eukaryotes, telomere replication is carried out by a specialized reverse transcriptase, designated as **telomerase**.

Telomerases: These are ribonucleoproteins whose **RNA** components have enzyme activity. Such a component contains a segment that is complementary to the repeating telomeric sequence and acts as an internal template. Its function, therefore, is similar to that of reverse transcriptase.

Absence of the telomerase shortens the chromosome with each round of replication and contributes to **normal senescence** of the cell. Maintenance of the chromosomal length thus depends on the action of telomerase.

Importance of Telomeres

- Required for the **complete replication** of the chromosomes.
- To form **caps that protects** the chromosomes from nucleases and other destabilizing forces.
- **Prevent the ends** of chromosomes from **fusing** with one another.

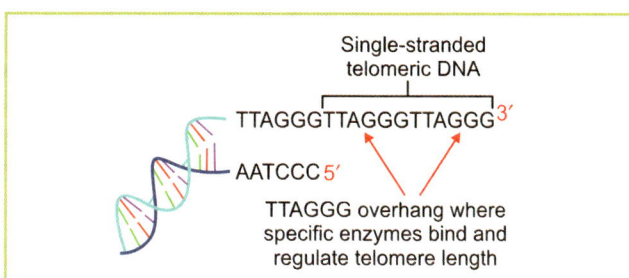

Single-stranded
telomeric DNA

TTAGGGTTAGGGTTAGGG 3'

AATCCC 5'

TTAGGG overhang where specific enzymes bind and regulate telomere length

Fig. 19.13: Telomere.

- Unlike somatic cells, **germ cells of the gonads retain telomerase activity** and telomeres of the chromosomes do not shrink after cell division. Consequently, each offspring begins life as a zygote that contains telomeres of maximum length.
- Telomere repeats gradually decrease with aging and serve as a **mitotic clock.**
- Telomere shortening plays a key role in **protecting from cancer**. Unlike normal somatic cells that lack detectable telomerase activity, majority of cancer cells contain active telomerase activity and are 'immortalized'.

Transposons

Transposons are discrete sequences in the genome that are **mobile**. These are the transposable elements, i.e. they are able to transport themselves to other locations within the genome. Transposons are found in **both prokaryotes as well as eukaryotes**. Each bacterial transposon carries gene(s) that code for the enzyme activities required for its own transposition.

Comparable systems exist in eukaryotes. The enzyme activity, **transposase**, catalyzes the excision of a transposon from a donor DNA site and its insertion at a target DNA site ('cut and paste' mechanism). **Retrotransposons**, in contrast, operate by means of a 'copy and paste' mechanism involving an RNA intermediate.

Importance of Transposons

- Generation of **moderately repeated DNA** sequences.
- **Evolution** of proteins composed of domains derived from **different ancestral genes**.
- Formation of entirely **new genes**, e.g. genes coding for telomerase, and enzymes involved in the rearrangement of antibody genes.
- Mode of **infection by retroviruses**.
- Spread of **antibiotic resistance** genes amongst pathogenic bacteria.

REPLICATION OF DNA IN MITOCHONDRIA

Mitochondrial chromosome of the mammals is a 15 Kb segment. It is **circular** and contains a 500–600 nucleotide long **D-loop** that undergoes frequent cycles of degradation and resynthesis.

- During replication of the mitochondrial DNA (mtDNA), the D-loop is extended.

19

- Replication of the mtDNA is carried out by the process in which synthesis of the leading strand precedes the synthesis of the lagging strand.
- The leading strand, in turn, displaces the lagging strand template to form a displacement loop (D-loop).
- When the D-loop has reached more than half the way around the chromosome, the lagging strand origin is exposed and its synthesis proceeds in the opposite direction around the chromosome. The synthesis of the lagging strand is thus only less than half complete by the time the synthesis of the leading strand is terminated (Fig. 19.14).

NUCLEOSOMES

Nucleosomes are the **lowest level of chromosome organization**.

- Eukaryotic DNA being large is **packed** in chromatin in association with the basic proteins called

histones, which are rich in lysine and arginine. These are positively charged molecules and form ionic bonds with the DNA which is negatively charged.

- There are five classes of histones, designated as **H1, H2A, H2B, H3 and H4**.
- Two molecules each of H2A, H2B, H3 and H4 form an **octamer-structured core** of the individual nucleosome around which a segment of the DNA double-helix is wound twice, forming a negatively super-twisted helix. These DNA segments are small (approximately 50 nucleotides), and are called **linker DNA** (Fig. 19.15).
- Histones-octamer joined by the linker DNA, forms a nucleosome (nucleofilament).
- Thereafter, H1 binds to the DNA chain, between the nucleosome beads, and helps in packaging of the nucleosome into a more compact structure. Strictly speaking, a **nucleosome** consists of **1¾ turns of DNA (≈146 bp)** around the histone-octamer, whereas when the DNA makes **two full turns (≈166 bp)**, the resulting structure is called a **chromatosome**.
- Under the electron microscope, the nucleosome core particles along with linker DNA give a '**beads on a string**' appearance (Fig. 19.16).
- Synthesis of the new histones occurs mainly during the **S phase**, simultaneously with the replication of DNA.
- Newly synthesized DNA inherits some parental histones which combine with an equal amount of the new histones, to complete the structure of the nascent nucleosomes that are formed behind the moving replication fork.

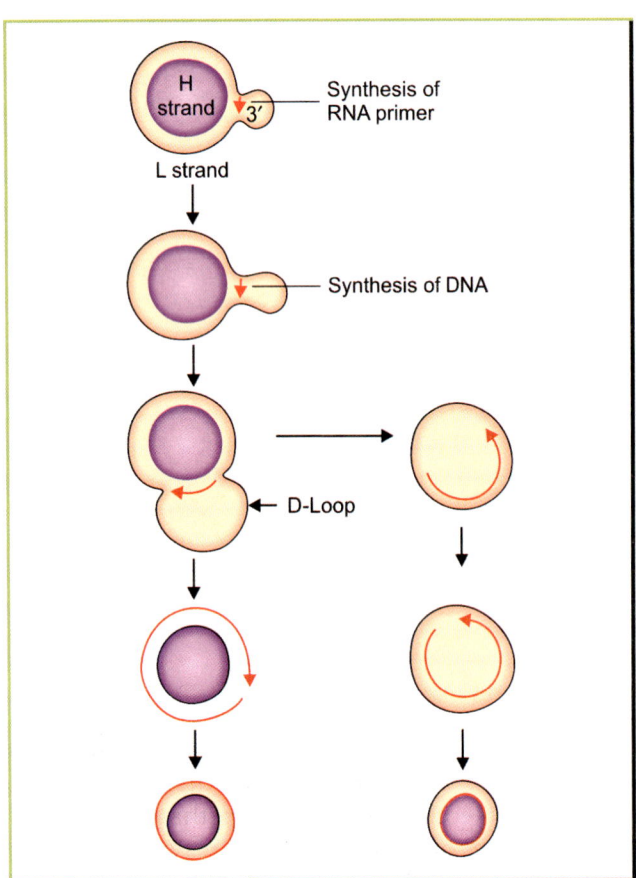

Fig. 19.14: DNA replication in mitochondria.

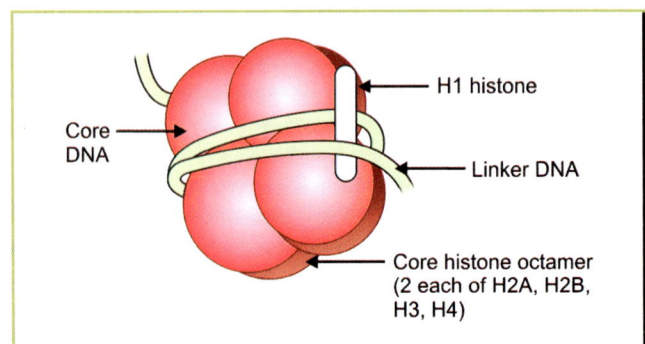

Fig. 19.15: Nucleosome/chromatosome.

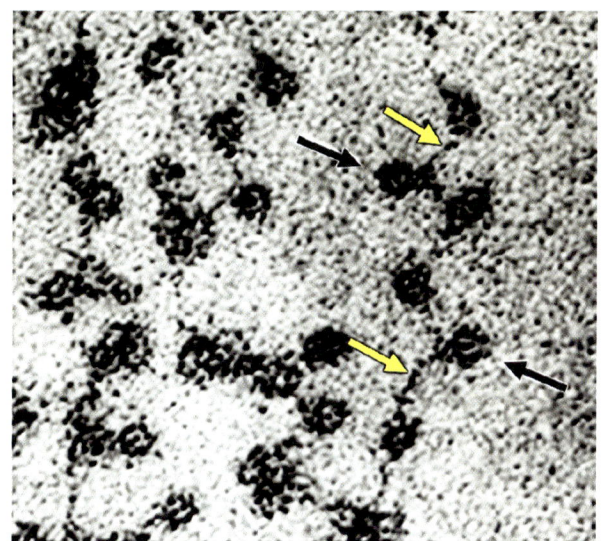

Fig. 19.16: Electron micrograph showing nucleosomes (black arrows) with linker DNA (yellow arrows): **'Beads on a string'** appearance.

DNA REPAIR

DNA is the **only macromolecule** that is repaired rather than degraded. DNA repair is a high-priority process for the maintenance of **integrity of the genetic information** and other cellular functions. It is a **very efficient** process with less than 1 out of 1000 accidental changes which may result in a **mutation**. There are several processes for DNA repair, each one of which can repair a certain type of the damage.

Replacement of Damaged Segment: Excision Repair

A segment of the damaged DNA is repaired by the process called **excision repair**. The process is catalyzed by different enzymatic systems, each one of which is specific for the repair of a specific type of damage. These repair systems are capable of recognizing and excising damaged DNA, replacing the same with newly synthesized, properly base-paired segment. The process includes incision at the site of damage, excision of the damaged segment, resynthesis of the new strand at the site of damage and ligation of the two ends. Such systems exist both in eukaryotes and prokaryotes.

Excision Repair in Prokaryotes

Excision repair is carried out by the replacement of the damaged DNA, depending upon the extent of the damage in the two strands. It includes base excision repair and nucleotide excision repair.

Base Excision Repair

It eliminates modified bases like those that have been deaminated, methylated or modified chemically.

- The modified bases are hydrolytically removed by the enzymes termed **DNA glycosylases**, e.g. deaminated cytosine (uracil) is removed by uracil DNA glycosylase. DNA glycosylases remove the damaged base by hydrolyzing the glycosidic bond.
- This, in turn, produces a deoxyribosephosphate residue, i.e. having only the sugar moiety which is linked with a phosphate but is without a base. Such a site is designated as an **apurinic-apyrimidinic site (AP site)**. Such a site may also be generated by spontaneous hydrolysis of a purine or pyrimidine. It may be called **depurination** or **depyrimidination**.
- After an AP site has been created, AP endonuclease nicks phosphodiester backbone at the AP site and excises the sugar-phosphate residue, creating a gap of one nucleotide.
- This gap is filled by the action of DNA polymerase I.
- Finally DNA ligase seals the ends (Fig. 19.17).

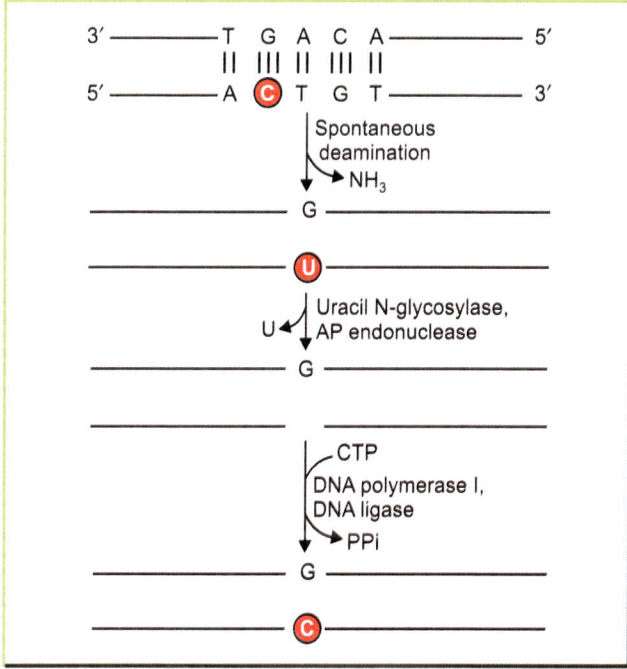

Fig. 19.17: Base excision repair in prokaryotes.

19

Nucleotide Excision Repair

It is activated when a **bulky lesion** has been produced, such as due to the interaction of DNA with a polycyclic aromatic hydrocarbon, like benzo[a]pyrene (generated by tobacco smoke). Chemotherapeutic drugs like **cisplatin** may also result in the formation of thymine-cisplatin adducts. The dimerization of the adjacent pyrimidines, induced by **UV light**, may also result in generation of a bulky lesion.

In *E. coli*, such a repair is initiated by recognition of the distortion of DNA by an endonuclease system which is a product of three genes, i.e. UvrA, UvrB and UvrC. This endonuclease system is designated as excision nuclease or **excinuclease**. In this process:

- A tetramer, consisting of two UvrA and two Uvr B proteins, is formed. This, in turn, causes local melting of DNA (at the expense of ATP) and locates the bulky lesion.
- UvrB makes 3′ incision, followed by a 5′ incision by UvrC.
- It leads to the release of an oligonucleotide including the bulky lesion, e.g. the pyrimidine dimer.
- Thereafter, UvrD (a helicase) unwinds DNA and releases the above excised oligonucleotide.
- DNA polymerase then displaces UvrB and fills the gap.
- The repair is completed by DNA ligase (Fig. 19.18).

Excision Repair in Eukaryotes

In eukaryotes, the process is similar to that in prokaryotes except that the endonuclease activity of human cells consists of 16–17 different polypeptides compared to only four proteins of *E. coli*.

- Nucleotide excision repair of human DNA begins with the binding of a protein designated as xeroderma pigmentosum A (**XP A**) to a dimer which consists of two other proteins, i.e. XP F and ERCC-1 (excision repair component). XP A binds to the dimer between XP F and ERCC-1 and forms a complex, XP F-XP A-ERCC-1. Its XPA component recognizes the damaged site and binds to it.
- Thereafter, a replication protein (HSSB) also binds to XP A and gets associated to the damaged site.
- There is also involvement of an additional enzyme complex known as general transcription factor **TFIIH**, essential for transcription initiation as well as for nucleotide excision repair. Two of its

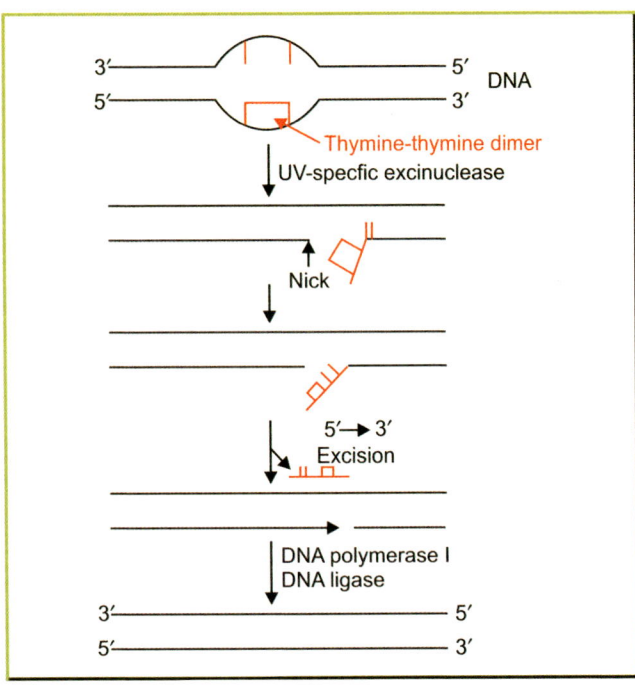

Fig. 19.18: Nucleotide excision repair in prokaryotes.

subunits, i.e. XP B and XP D are helicases and are involved in kinking and unwinding of DNA at the damaged site. The TFIIH interacts with XP C and the whole complex gets associated to the damaged site through XP A.

- Subsequently, XP G also gets associated with this complex to complete the excinuclease system.
- The 3′ nick is introduced by XP G while XP F in association with ERCC-1 makes the 5′ nick.
- This, in turn, results in excision of an oligonucleotide.
- The gap is filled by polymerases γ and ε.
- Finally, DNA ligase seals the nick.

Defects in nucleotide excision repair have been shown to result in various hereditary disorders, such as xeroderma pigmentosum, Cockayne's syndrome and trichothiodystrophy (Chemistry to Clinics 19.3).

Reversal of Damage

Some of the damages, such as formation of a dimer by the action of light, can be directly reversed by deoxyribopyrimidine photolyase, in bacteria. This enzyme disrupts the covalent bonds which hold these pyrimidine molecules together. Such an enzyme is not present in human beings.

Chemistry to Clinics 19.3: Disorders of Nucleotide Excision Repair

Xeroderma pigmentosum: This is a condition characterized by varying levels of UV sensitivity and corresponding deficiencies in DNA repair system, such as a mutation in XPV gene. These patients exhibit sunlight-induced **photodermatosis** (Fig. 19.19) characterized by severe skin reactions that range from skin ulceration to the development of skin cancer. Some forms are also accompanied by neurological abnormalities due to abnormal gene expression and DNA deterioration caused by the accumulation of the damaged DNA.

Cockayne's syndrome: This condition is associated with mutations in XP D and XP B genes. It is characterized by growth and mental retardation, neurological deficiencies and photosensitivity but not increased rate of cancer or skeletal abnormalities.

Trichothiodystrophy: This is caused by mutations in XP B, XP G and TFIIH associated excision repair subunits. These patients have scaly skin, brittle hair, short stature and neuroskeletal abnormalities.

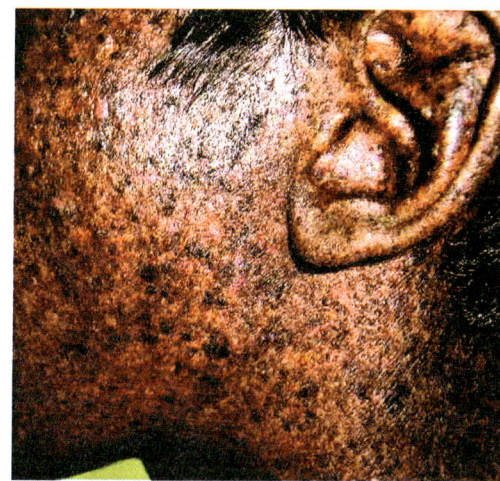

Fig. 19.19: Xeroderma pigmentosum: An inherited disease characterized by photosensitivity, epithelial atrophy and hyperpigmentation.

Mismatch Repair

If DNA polymerase makes an error, resulting in a mismatched base-pair or a small insertion or deletion, during DNA synthesis, the cell repairs the DNA by a pathway called mismatche repair. However, the cell must be able to differentiate between the template strand and the newly synthesized strand. In bacteria, DNA strands are methylated by **Dam methylase**, (Deoxyadenosine methylase), which introduces a methyl group at the N6 position of adenine in palindromic 5'-GATC sequence on the parental strand. On the other hand, immediately after replication, the DNA is hemimethylated (unmethylated). This, in turn, serves to distinguish these strands from the newly synthesized DNA strands that are methylated at a later stage.

Methylation thus, directs the repair system, for the repair of the mispaired bases.

Proteins that catalyze **mismatch repair in prokaryotes**, e.g. in *E. coli*, are designated as MutS, MutH and MutL.

- The process is initiated with the binding of MutS to the mismatch site which is followed by the addition of MutL.
- Formation of the MutS-MutL complex activates MutH which has GATC endonuclease activity and cleaves the unmethylated strand, on the 5' site of G.
- After the mismatch has been located, the unmethylated strand is unwound, degraded and replaced by the new strand. It is synthesized in the 3'→5' direction until the mismatch is reached and excised.
- The gap is filled and sealed by polymerase III and DNA ligase, respectively.

A similar mechanism exists **in eukaryotes.** Eukaryotic system, however, lacks MutH and only MutL degrades the nicked-strand.

Loss of mismatch repair activity may result in the development of tumor, such as hereditary non-polyposis colorectal cancer (**HNPCC**). Such cancers are initiated only when cells accumulate a certain mutation load.

SOS Repair

SOS repair system comprises many enzymes and proteins which are inducible and are regulated by **LexA** and **RecA** proteins. Under normal conditions, SOS repair proteins are not expressed because the repressor protein LexA binds to the promoter region and inhibits the transcription of many genes which are required for DNA repair and recombination. LexA also inhibits its own expression as well as the expression of RecA which has multiple enzymatic activities. SOS repair system is activated as a result of **severe DNA damage**.

- The binding of RecA to the exposed single-stranded DNA or damaged double-stranded DNA activates it.
- Active RecA has a proteolytic action and causes proteolysis of LexA.

- The fragmented LexA gets dissociated from DNA and allows the expression of SOS response genes.
- The products of the SOS genes assemble at the lesion and form a specialized replication system which is dependent on DNA Pol II for replicating DNA lesions. This type of replication is designated as '**lesion replication**'.
- After repair of the damaged DNA, LexA again begins to accumulate and represses the expression of SOS genes.

Post-replication Repair

Most of the DNA lesions though are repaired prior to replication, in some of the instances damage can be repaired after replication. In this process, lesions which cannot be excised are repaired by the process of recombination by using a complementary strand from another DNA (as a template).

MUTATIONS

Mutations are **inheritable, irreparable** and **permanent alterations in DNA sequence** which may be phenotypically **silent (hidden)** or **expressed (visible)**. They can be detected only by gene sequence determination.

Causes

Mutations may arise by a number of means, such as due to an error in replication during proof-reading, by UV or ionizing radiation (X-rays and γ-rays) or by a chemical mutagen (an alkylating agent). Besides, DNA may also undergo certain spontaneous changes, such as deamination of cytosine (to form uracil), depurination, etc.

Classification

Mutations are classified into two categories, i.e.:
- Point mutation, and
- Frame-shift mutation.

Point Mutation

A point mutation involves a change in a **single base-pair** in the DNA, resulting in a single base change in the corresponding mRNA. This type of mutation may also be referred to as **base substitution mutation**. This may result in *transition* or *transversion* types of mutation (Fig. 19.20).

Transition: The substitution where a **purine-pyrimidine pair is replaced by another such pair** is called transition. It may occur spontaneously, induced chemically by a base analog (e.g. 5-bromouracil) or by a mutagen (such as nitrous acid). For example, if 5-bromouracil gets incorporated into DNA (in place of a thymine), it may induce AT→GC transition. On the other hand, treatment of DNA with nitrous acid may result in both, AT→GC as well as GC→AT transitions.

Transversion: The substitution where a **purine-pyrimidine pair is replaced by a pyrimidine-purine pair** is called transversion. This may occur spontaneously and is common in human beings.

Frame-shift Mutation

Frame shift mutations are the result of **insertion or deletion** of a base-pair.

Deletion: Deletion of a base-pair from the DNA base sequence of the gene may **change its reading frame** and result in a nonfunctional gene product. For example, a frame-shift mutation as a result of base

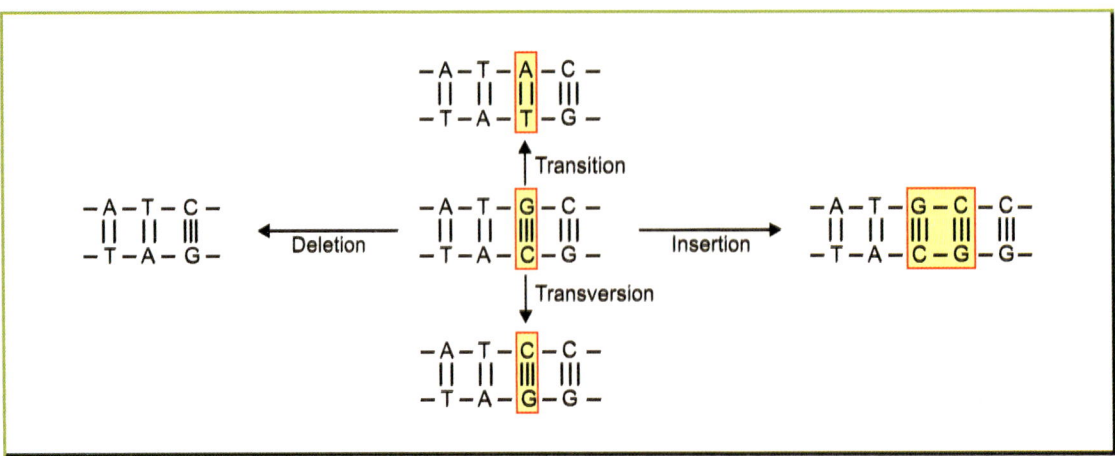

Fig. 19.20: Mutations.

deletion results in the production of abnormal hemo-globin such as **hemoglobin Wayne**. Deletion may be caused by deaminating agents.

Insertion: Insertion of a base-pair into the gene sequence can lead to the synthesis of abnormal chain length of a protein. Some insertions can be caused by mutagens, such as acridines, ethidium bromide, etc.

Effects of Mutation

Mutations may be expressed phenotypically (visible) or remain silent.

Visible Mutation

A visible or expressed mutation may be a missense mutation or a nonsense mutation.

- **Missense mutation:** It is the result of a base change that causes the incorporation of a **different amino acid** in the encoded protein. An example of missense mutation is a change in second base of the codon GAA (or GAG) which code for glutamate in the sixth position of the β-chain of hemoglobin. The change from A to U results in GUA (or GUG) which code for valine. This, in turn, results in **sickle cell anemia**, one of the most common forms of hemoglobinopathies.

- **Nonsense mutation:** It may be a result of a change in the base of the codon which may **destroy a termination codon** or result in the formation of a **new termination codon**.

  – The *formation of a new termination codon* may result in premature termination and thus reduce chain length of the protein. For example, the codon UAU or UAC normally encodes for tyrosine, as the 145th amino acid in the β-chain of hemoglobin. A single base mutation from UAU to UAA or UAC to UAG results in a termination codon, which in turn, reduces the chain length from 146 to 144 amino acids. This results in the synthesis of **hemoglobin McKees Rocks** which has a higher oxygen affinity and decreases oxygen delivery to the tissues.

  – On the other hand, *mutation of a base in the termination codon* to a codon which encodes an amino acid results in a protein that has larger chain length than the normal. For example, a normal α globin chain has 141 amino acid residues. When the stop codon UAA mutates, it results in the incorporation of an amino acid at

Chemistry to Clinics 19.4: Two-Hit Hypothesis

Polycystic kidney disease (PKD) is a disorder in which numerous cysts (fluid-filled epithelial sacs) develop in both kidneys (Fig. 19.21). The most common (85% of patients) and most severe form is autosomal dominant PKD1 (ADPKD1) and is a result of a defective gene on chromosome 16. The PKD1 gene encodes a large transmembrane protein called polycystin-1. The mutation in PKD2 gene, which accounts for about 15% of patients, encodes a transmembrane protein called polycystin-2. Normally, polycystin-1 and polycystin-2 interact with each other and are associated with the primary cilium that is present in renal tubule cells. This structure is a nonmotile sensory process located at the apical side of the cell and functions to sense changes in tubule fluid flow. In ADPKD, the primary cilium is poorly developed, suggesting a link between abnormalities in this structure and the cystic phenotype.

The phenotypic expression of ADPKD is variable. Some people show symptoms in childhood, whereas others may lead a long and healthy life with cystic kidneys detected only on autopsy. The usual pattern is for patients to develop symptoms (such as hypertension or pain in the back

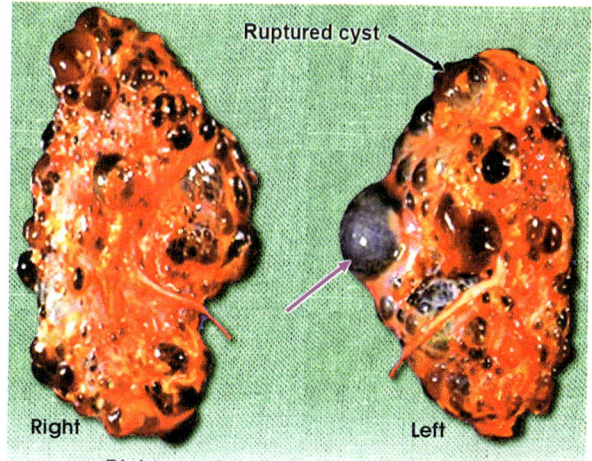

Fig. 19.21: Bilateral polycystic kidneys. Purple arrow indicates the largest cyst.

and sides) in their 30's and 40's. Extrarenal manifestations such as hepatic cysts are common. End-stage renal failure (requiring dialysis or a kidney transplantation) occurs in about 50% of patients by the age of 60. The specific gene affected, the nature of the mutation in a particular gene, the genetic background of a person and environmental factors all play a role in determining the development of the disease.

Only 1% of nephrons produce cysts in ADPKD even though every renal cell has a mutant copy of a dominant gene. The 'two-hit hypothesis' explains why the disease is so variable and why only relatively a few nephrons produce cysts. According to this hypothesis, the production of a cyst requires a second (somatic) mutation, so that the gene (allele) accompanying the inherited defective gene is also abnormal. Only when this happens does a cyst develop. Researchers have demonstrated that in many cysts in ADPKD, two abnormal genes are indeed present.

19

142nd position and increases the chain length to nearly 172 amino acids, i.e. until another stop codon is reached. Abnormally long α-globin chain has been shown to result in many instances of α-thalassemias.

Silent Mutation

This is a result of a base change that occurs in the **third position of a codon**, e.g. UUA to UUG. Since both the codons code for leucine and there is **no change in the specified amino acid**, such mutations are called silent mutations.

It is interesting to note that certain mutations which may be otherwise silent, require the presence of another mutation in a neighboring gene to become clinically manifested, as observed in polycystic kidney disease. This is called the 'two-hit hypothesis' (Chemistry to Clinics 19.4).

SOME IMPORTANT QUESTIONS

1. What is replication? Describe the process of DNA replication in prokaryotes. How does it differ in eukaryotes?

2. What are mutations? Describe different types of mutations.

3. Discuss the differences between DNA polymerases in prokaryotes and eukaryotes.

4. Describe briefly:
   i.   Origin of replication
   ii. Semiconservative replication of DNA
   iii. Topoisomerase inhibitors
   iv. Role of RNA primer in replication
   v.   Ter regions
   vi. Replication of mitochondrial DNA
   vii. Formation of nucleosomes

5. Write notes on:
   i.   DnaA protein
   ii.   Topoisomerases
   iii. DNA polymerases
   iv.   Reverse transcriptase
   v.   Replication fork
   vi.   Okazaki fragments
   vii. Primosome
   viii. Telomeres
   ix.   Histones
   x.   DNA repair
   xi.   Xeroderma pigmentosum
   xii. Single-stranded DNA-binding proteins
   xiii. DNA helicases
   xiv. Telomerases
   xv.   Point mutation
   xvi. Frame-shift mutation
   xvii. Nonsense mutation
   xviii. Silent mutation
   xix. Two-hit hypothesis

MULTIPLE CHOICE QUESTIONS

1. DNA directed DNA polymerase catalyzes the following:
   A. DNA → DNA
   B. DNA → RNA
   C. RNA → cDNA
   D. RNA → Protein

2. The site of origin of DNA replication is rich in:
   A. AT
   B. GC
   C. Any of the above
   D. None of the above

3. The following is not involved in eukaryotic nuclear DNA synthesis:
   A. DNA polymerase α
   B. DNA polymerase β
   C. DNA polymerase γ
   D. DNA polymerase ε

4. DNA glycosylases participate in:
   A. Base excision repair
   B. Nucleotide excision repair
   C. Mismatch repair
   D. SOS repair

5. An AT → GC mutation is an example of:
   A. Point mutation, transition
   B. Point mutation, transversion
   C. Frame-shift mutation, insertion
   D. Frame-shift mutation, deletion

19

20 Transcription and Post-transcriptional Modifications

Transcription is the **synthesis of an RNA molecule** using the DNA sequence of a gene as a template. In prokaryotic cells, it takes place in the ill-defined nuclear zone called the nucleoid whereas in eukaryotic cells it takes place in the well defined nucleus (transcription of nuclear DNA) or mitochondria (transcription of mitochondrial DNA).

Replication *versus* Transcription

The process of transcription is somewhat similar to DNA replication in that one strand of DNA is used as a template from which a new strand is formed. However, transcription differs from DNA replication in three important ways:

1. A **different enzyme** guides the process; whereas the enzyme used in DNA replication is DNA polymerase, the key enzyme in transcription is RNA polymerase.
2. The entire DNA molecule is duplicated in DNA replication whereas in transcription only the **small portion of DNA** molecule that includes a particular gene is transcribed.
3. DNA replication produces a double-stranded DNA molecule whereas transcription produces a **single-stranded RNA** molecule.

Sense and Anti-sense Strands

The RNAs are polymers of ribonucleoside monophosphates (**ribonucleotides**). Transcription is a strand selective process since during the process of RNA synthesis one of the strands of DNA, called the template strand, gets transcribed into RNA. The sequence of ribonucleotides in the newly synthesized

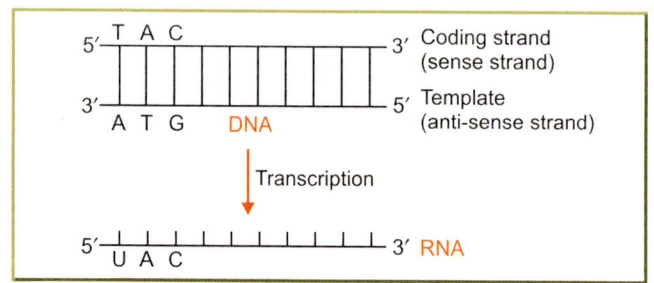

Fig. 20.1: Sense and anti-sense strands.

RNA molecule, called the **primary RNA transcript**, is **complementary** to the sequence of deoxyribonucleotides in the **template strand or the 'anti-sense' strand,** and by convention, is represented as the bottom strand of a double-stranded DNA (Fig. 20.1). Naturally, the top strand of DNA is the **'sense strand' or the coding strand** because it exactly corresponds to the sequence of a primary RNA transcript, with the only exception of 'T' for 'U'.

Modified Central Dogma of Molecular Biology

Following DNA replication, genetic information flows from **DNA to RNA to protein** in two steps, transcription and translation. This unidirectional flow is called the **central dogma of molecular biology** and is currently accepted in a **modified form** (Fig. 20.2) after the discovery of a peculiar phenomenon observed in certain RNA viruses called retroviruses. The genetic information in these viruses is present in the form of RNA which is reverse transcribed into DNA, a process called **reverse transcription** catalyzed by the enzyme reverse transcriptase.

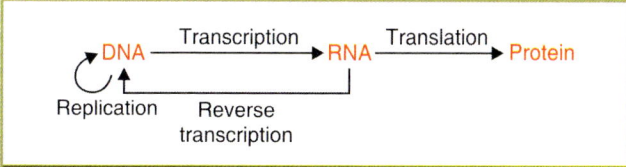

Fig. 20.2: Central dogma of molecular biology.

Types of RNAs

There are two major categories of RNA:

1. **RNA participating in transfer of genetic information:** According to their role played in the process of information transfer, many different RNA types are known:
   - *Messenger RNA* (**mRNA**) is a direct copy ('message') of the DNA sequence of a gene that is eventually provided to the ribosomes in the cytosol. Ribosomes are the subcellular entities where protein synthesis takes place.
   - A ribosome itself is made up of ribosomal proteins and RNA called *ribosomal RNA* (**rRNA**).
   - *Transfer RNA* (**tRNA**) is responsible for transferring specific amino acids in a proper sequence from the cytosolic amino acid pool to the ribosomes.
   - *Small nuclear RNAs* (**snRNA**) are 100–200 nucleotides long and form complexes with proteins called small nuclear ribonucleoprotein particles (snRNPs, pronounced '**snurps**') to participate in the processing of eukaryotic gene transcripts.
2. **Small RNAs or non-coding RNAs (ncRNA):** They are 21–28 nucleotides long and bind to DNA or other RNA molecules through complementary base pairing. They are of several types:
   - *Micro-RNAs* (**miRNA**) or small temporal RNAs (stRNA) base-pair with certain mRNA and prevent translation without degrading the mRNA itself.
   - *Small interfering RNAs* (**siRNA**) are employed in 'RNA interference' as discussed later.
   - *Small nucleolar RNAs* (**snoRNA**) act as catalysts that accomplish some chemical modifications in DNA, tRNA and rRNA.

REQUIREMENTS FOR RNA SYNTHESIS

The process of RNA synthesis requires an appropriate sequence of DNA as template, RNA polymerases and ribonucleoside triphosphates.

DNA Template

Each cycle of transcription begins as well as ends with the recognition of the specific sites in the DNA template. The sites where RNA polymerase binds are called **promoters**. Certain conserved sequences have been shown to occur in the promoter regions. These include:

Upstream/Downstream Sequences

The first nucleotide at the transcription start site is written as +1. A nucleotide in the promoter region is assigned a negative number if towards the 5′-side, i.e. prior to the **transcription start site**. It is also referred to as **upstream** to the start site. A nucleotide is assigned a positive number if present towards the 3′-side, i.e. after the transcription start site. It is called **downstream** to the start site (Fig. 20.3).

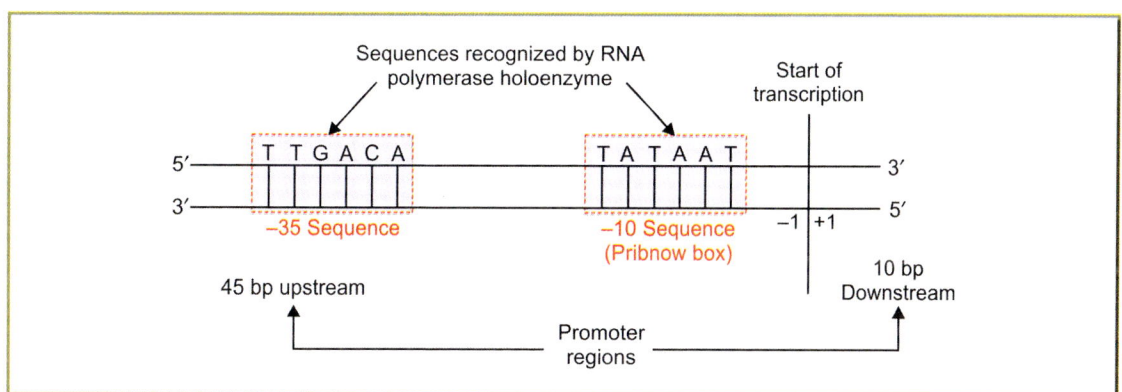

Fig. 20.3: Promoter regions in prokaryotes.

20

Promoter Regions

In prokaryotes: Prokaryotic transcription begins with the binding of RNA polymerase to a promoter on the gene. RNA polymerase holoenzyme binds to one face of the DNA extending nearly 45 base-pairs (bp) upstream and 10 bp downstream from the transcription start site. In this region there are two short oligonucleotide sequences called Pribnow box and –35 sequences. These sequences are highly conserved.

One of the sequences is located about 10 bp upstream from the transcription start site. This sequence of 6 nucleotides, i.e. TATAAT is rich in AT nucleotides and is called the **Pribnow box** or –10 box or –10 sequence (Fig. 20.3).

A second consensus sequence is located upstream from the Pribnow box. This is also an AT rich sequence containing 6 nucleotides, i.e. TTGACA. This is called **–35 sequence** since this is situated about 35 bp upstream from the transcription start site. The spacing between –35 and –10 sequences is crucial with 17 bp being highly conserved.

In eukaryotes: The promoter regions in eukaryotes are referred to as **TATA box, GC box and CAAT box**. Most mammalian genes have an AT rich consensus sequence, i.e. TATAAA, which is usually located about 25 bp before the RNA start site (25 bp upstream) and is called TATA box.

TATA box binds TATA-binding protein (TBP) which in turn, binds several other proteins called TBP-associated factors (TAF). This complex of TBP and TAF is termed as **transcription factor**, e.g. TFIID which facilitates the binding of RNA polymerase.

Two other sequences may also be found somewhere between –110 bp and –40 bp upstream, called the GC box and the CAAT box. These are the binding sites for the other transcription factors that affect polymerase function and determine the frequency of transcription (Fig. 20.4).

Enhancers

In addition to the promoter regions, transcription in eukaryotes is also affected by certain other promoter elements (sequences), called enhancers. These are gene specific sequences that stimulate the expression of a gene by nearly 100 folds. An enhancer sequence though present on the **same DNA strand** as the transcribed gene but can function in **either orientation**, i.e. either in the 5′ or the 3′ direction and may be up to 1000 bp **away from the relevant promoter**. These DNA sequences are the **binding sites for transcription factors** which modulate the binding of RNA polymerase to the promoter region.

Action of DNase

The process of transcription in eukaryotic cells is more complex since the chromatin is organized into nucleosomes and RNA polymerase cannot bind to the promoter regions as such. Hence, the **chromatin** containing the promoter sequences is made **accessible** by the action of DNase. This, in turn, ensures that transcription factors bind to the appropriate regulatory sequences.

Termination Sequences

There are also certain sites within a transcript, which may allow premature termination of transcription. Similar to the conserved sequences found in the promoter region of the DNA template, different conserved sequences are also found at the termination sites.

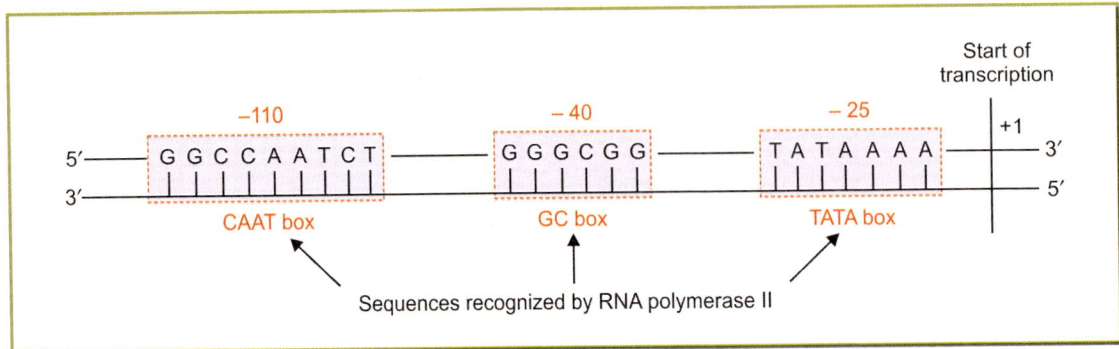

Fig. 20.4: Promoter regions in eukaryotes.

RNA Polymerases

RNA polymerases synthesize RNA in the **5'→3' direction**, using a DNA template. These enzymes initiate polymerization at the consensus sequence on a promoter site and **do not need a primer**.

In prokaryotes: In bacteria, a **single RNA polymerase** synthesizes all types of RNAs. It is a multienzyme complex. The core enzyme consists of four peptides, i.e. two α, one β and one β' subunits (Chemistry to Clinics 20.1). It cannot recognize the promoter region on the DNA template without the addition of a fifth protein, designated as the **σ subunit or sigma factor**. The binding of the σ factor to the core enzyme results in the formation of a holoenzyme which is capable of synthesizing an RNA sequence. Specific σ factors can recognize different classes of genes.

In eukaryotes: Eukaryotic RNA polymerases are inhibited by a lethal toxin, designated as α-amanitin which is synthesized by a poisonous mushroom *Amanita phalloides*. Based on the inhibition by this toxin, three types of RNA polymerases have been identified: RNA polymerase I, RNA polymerase II and RNA polymerase III. Each is capable of transcribing only a single class of RNA.

- **RNA polymerase I:** It transcribes ribosomal RNA (**rRNA**) genes which are located in the nucleolus.
- **RNA polymerase II:** It transcribes **mRNA** genes and is responsible for the synthesis of precursors of mRNAs and small nuclear RNAs (**snRNAs**). This enzyme requires specific consensus sequences, designated as the TATA box and the CAAT box. One or both of these sequences may serve as the recognition sites in the eukaryotic promoters. The rate of initiation of transcription by RNA polymerase II is also increased by the presence of enhancers which may be located upstream or downstream of the transcription start site and can be close to or thousands base-pairs away from the promoter. Very low concentration of α-amanitin inhibits the synthesis of mRNA.

Chemistry to Clinics 20.1: Rifampicin

The prokaryotic RNA polymerase is inhibited by rifampicin (also called rifampin), a front-line antibiotic used in the treatment of tuberculosis and leprosy. Rifampicin binds to the β-subunit of RNA polymerase and inhibits its activity in *Mycobacterium tuberculosis* and *Mycobacterium leprae*, the causative agents of tuberculosis and leprosy, respectively.

- **RNA polymerase III:** It produces small RNAs including various **tRNAs, 5S rRNA and other snRNAs**. The enzyme is inhibited by the higher concentration of α-amanitin.
- **Mitochondrial RNA polymerase:** In addition, there is also a mitochondrial RNA polymerase (mtRNA polymerase) which is responsible for the synthesis of mRNA, tRNA and rRNA **within the mitochondria**. This enzyme, like bacterial RNA polymerase, is inhibited by rifampicin.

THE PROCESS OF TRANSCRIPTION

The process of RNA transcription is divided into 3 steps, i.e. initiation, elongation and termination.

In Prokaryotes

Initiation of RNA Synthesis

Before the chain initiation, the **promoter region is recognized by the holoenzyme** (RNA polymerase with the sigma factor), the enzyme binds to the promoter DNA and forms a **complex**. This, in turn, results in local **opening** of about 10 nucleotide pairs of the DNA double helix, and the holoenzyme binds more tightly. The unwound DNA then binds to the initiating ribonucleotide triphosphate and the holoenzyme forms the first phosphodiester bond. A purine ribonucleotide (GTP or ATP) is usually the first to be polymerized into the RNA molecule.

Elongation of the RNA Chain

The RNA polymerase translocates to the **next position** and continues RNA synthesis. After the holoenzyme begins to synthesize a transcript, the **σ subunit is released** (Fig. 20.5). The core enzyme even without the σ factor, continues the process of RNA synthesis down the double helix and **separates** the two strands of the template. The template strand (sense strand) of the DNA, in turn, **base-pairs** with the growing RNA chain.

Topoisomerases, the components of the transcription complex, help the process of unwinding and restoring the DNA double helix.

Termination of RNA Synthesis

The RNA polymerase complex also recognizes the ends of the genes. Transcription termination can occur in either of the two modes, i.e. either the enzyme RNA

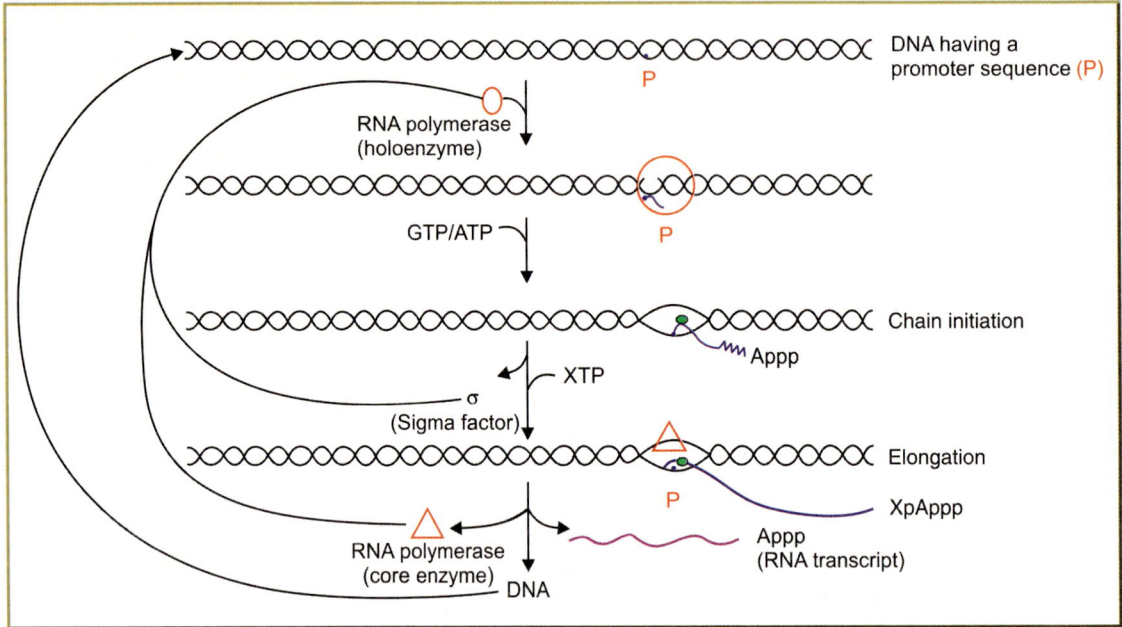

Fig. 20.5: The process of RNA transcription.

polymerase itself recognizes the termination region on the DNA template which is referred to as the rho (ρ)-independent termination, or the termination may require an additional protein designated as the ρ factor, for the release of the RNA product, termed as ρ-dependent termination.

- **Rho-independent termination:** Like the consensus sequence at the promoter region, transcription termination signals also have a distinct consensus sequence, about 40 bp in length and contains **GC rich hyphenated-inverted repeats**. This is followed by a series of AT base-pairs. The GC rich palindrome (inverted repeat) precedes a sequence of 6–7 U residues in the RNA chain. As transcription proceeds through the hyphenated-inverted repeat, the general transcript forms an intra-molecular hairpin structure which is crucial for the termination of the process. This, in turn, facilitates separation of the newly synthesized RNA from its DNA template (Fig. 20.6).
- **Rho-dependent termination:** It requires participation of an additional protein designated as the **rho (ρ) factor** which is a hexameric protein possessing an **RNA dependent ATPase activity**. The ρ-dependent termination region lacks the sequence of repeated adenylates in the template but has a short sequence that is transcribed to form a hairpin. The nascent RNA wraps around the

ρ-factor and ATP hydrolysis, in turn, dissociates the RNA transcript from the DNA template.

In Eukaryotes

Transcription in eukaryotes is more complex than the process in prokaryotes. Whereas transcription in prokaryotes requires only an appropriate sequence of DNA as template, RNA polymerase holoenzyme and ribonucleoside triphosphates as the substrate, transcription initiation in eukaryotes requires several **additional molecular events**:

1. **Chromatin** though is organized in nucleosomes, some of its part containing promoter sequences is not well-organized and is not accessible to the transcription machinery. It requires **DNase** activity for the **proper access** to the transcription machinery.
2. Certain gene specific sequences referred to as **enhancers** are needed. These sequences stimulate transcription as well as binding of the various transcription factors.
3. As discussed earlier, besides RNA polymerase, certain other proteins called **transcription factors** are also required. They bind to certain sequences in the promoter region for the initiation of the transcription process. These transcription factors, in turn, also facilitate the binding of RNA polymerase.

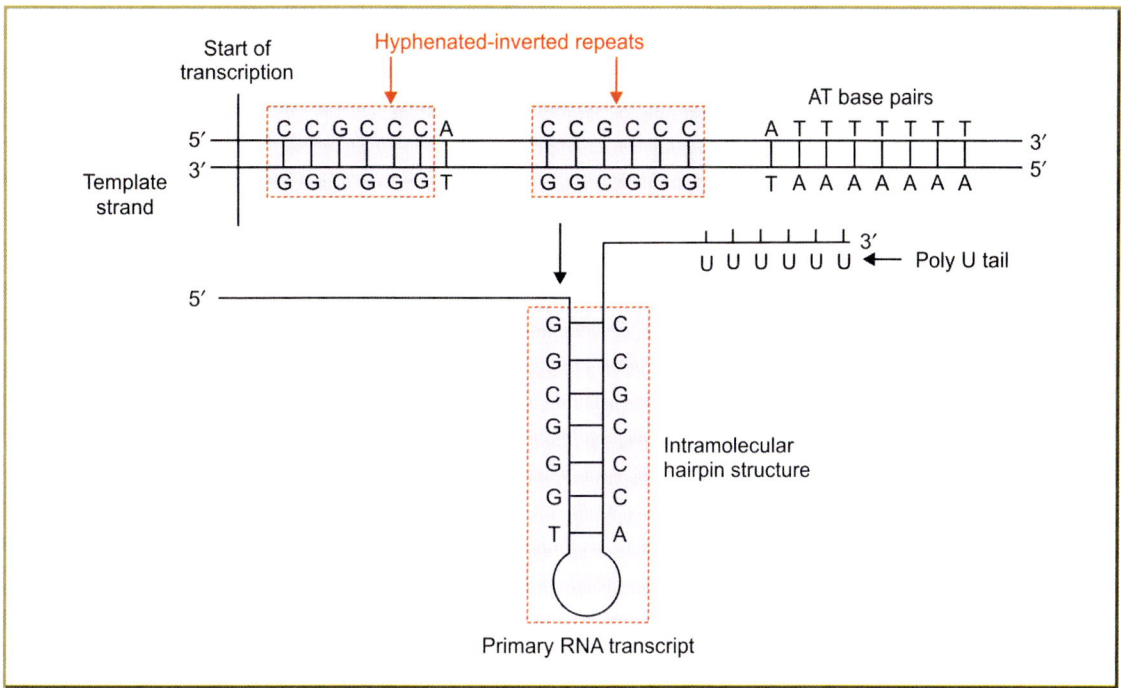

Fig. 20.6: Rho-independent termination of transcription.

4. Eukaryotes have **three distinct RNA polymerases**, each one of which is specific for transcribing a particular class of RNA only.

Transcription of mRNA

The genes for mRNA are located within the nucleus and are transcribed by **RNA polymerase II**.

- The enzyme initiates transcription by recognizing several consensus sequences upstream from the initiation site, e.g. the TATA box and the CAAT box. As mentioned above, these consensus sequences require the binding of specific transcription factors which recognize the nucleotide sequence of the appropriate controlling sequence element. The transcription factors bind with each other and with the RNA polymerase II to activate transcription. DNA binding and activation activities of the factors are located in separate domains of the protein. Mutations in the genes of several transcription factors occur in cancer (Chemistry to Clinics 20.2).

- During transcription by RNA polymerase II, there also occurs the **addition of 7-methylguanosine cap**. As the transcription complex moves along the DNA, the capping enzyme-complex modifies the 5′ end of the nascent mRNA. The addition of GTP

Chemistry to Clinics 20.2: Transcription Factors and Cancer

Several transcription factors have been shown to be mutated in various cancers:

1. NF-κB (nuclear factor kappa-light-chain-enhancer of activated B-cells): Hepatocellular cancer in patients with chronic hepatitis B.
2. GATA1 (binds to DNA GATA-containing sequences): Megakaryoblastic leukemias in patients with Down syndrome.
3. CTCF (DNA **CCCTC**-binding **f**actor): Prostate cancer.

is catalyzed by a guanylyl transferase while its methylation is carried out by guanine-7-methyltransferase. This **5′-capping facilitates the initiation of translation and helps in stabilizing the mRNA** (Fig. 20.7).

- After initiation and cap synthesis, RNA polymerase continues transcription of the gene until a **polyadenylation signal sequence**, i.e. AAUAAA is reached. This consensus sequence is present in the mature mRNA and signals **cleavage of the nascent mRNA precursor**, about 20 nucleotides downstream.

Transcription of tRNA

Transcription of tRNA is carried out by **RNA polymerase III**. Transcription factors bind to DNA

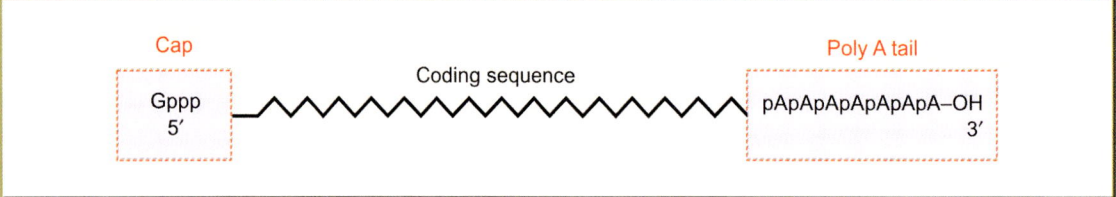

Fig. 20.7: Eukaryotic mRNA with 5'-cap and 3'-poly A tail.

and direct the action of RNA polymerase III. It does not require a specific sequence other than the factor binding sequence which is located at the 5' region of the gene, i.e. preceding the transcribed sequences within the DNA sequence, encoding the RNA.

Transcription of rRNA

The genes for rRNA are located in the nucleolus and are transcribed by **RNA polymerase I**.

- In a eukaryotic cell, **several hundred copies of each rRNA gene are tandemly repeated** in the DNA, within a specific region of a chromosome. Each repeat unit transcribes a primary transcript which contains a copy of each of the rRNA sequence, i.e. 28S, 5.8S and 18S RNAs. This, in turn, ensures the synthesis of **equimolar amounts of the three rRNAs**. The repeat units are separated from each other by the nontranscribed spacer region where the promoter and the enhancer sequences are located. The size of the nontranscribed spacer and the position of the enhancer element, however, vary from one organism to another.

- The promoter sequences are located between –40 to +10 bp and –150 to –110 bp positions. A transcription factor binds to the promoter and directs RNA polymerase I for recognition of the promoter sequence. In human ribosomal DNA, the enhancer element is located about 250 bp upstream from the promoter.

- Termination of transcription also occurs within the nontranscribed spacer region, before RNA polymerase I reaches the promoter of the next repeat unit.

Differences in transcription between prokaryotes and eukaryotes are given in Table 20.1.

POST-TRANSCRIPTIONAL MODIFICATIONS

Prokaryotic mRNA is generally identical to its primary transcript. In eukaryotes, mRNA genes are transcribed as pre-mRNA primary transcripts which are extensively modified post-transcriptionally. The primary transcripts of tRNAs and rRNAs are processed post-transcriptionally, both in prokaryotes and eukaryotes.

hnRNA and mRNA

The primary transcripts of RNA molecules synthesized by RNA polymerase II are called as **pre-mRNA**. These molecules are very large and their nucleotide sequences are very heterogeneous because they represent the transcripts of many different genes. Therefore, they are called **heterogeneous nuclear RNA (hnRNA)**. They are processed post-transcriptionally and modified to the functional mRNAs as follows (Figs 20.7 and 20.8):

1. Shortly after transcription is initiated, the 5'-end of the growing transcript is capped by addition

Table 20.1: Differences in transcription between prokaryotes and eukaryotes

Parameter	Prokaryotes	Eukaryotes
Nucleosomal organization	Not required; chromatin easily accessible to the transcription machinery	Required; DNase ensures proper access to the transcription machinery
Promoter region	Single, binds RNA polymerase	Complex, binds RNA polymerase and other transcription factors
RNA polymerase type(s)	One only	Three, one for each class of RNA
Introns in the primary transcript	Rare	Common
Post-transcriptional modifications	Restricted to tRNA and rRNA	Occur in all the three classes of RNA

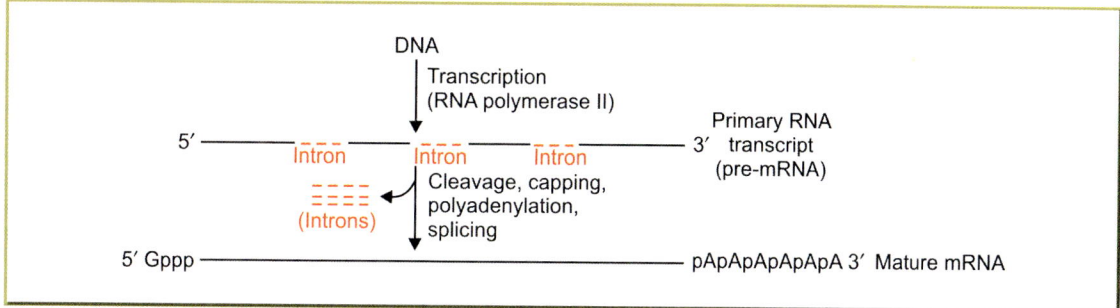

Fig. 20.8: Post-transcriptional processing of mRNA.

of guanylyl residue. This is called **5'-capping**. Subsequently, the cap is **methylated**.

2. The poly A tail of 40 to 200 adenine nucleotides is added to the free 3'-end by a soluble polymerase. **Polyadenylation** does not require a template. The poly A tail helps in stabilizing the mRNA and facilitates its exit from the nucleus.

3. Several non-coding sequences are present within the pre-mRNA but not in the mature mRNAs and are called intervening sequences or **introns**. The expressed or retained sequences are called **exons**. As pre-mRNA is extruded from the RNA polymerase complex, it is rapidly bound by small nuclear ribonucleoproteins (**snRNPs** or snurps), e.g. U1 RNA, U2 RNA, etc. Different snurps bind to the RNA precursor and form a large complex termed **spliceosome**. This, in turn, carries out the dual step of **RNA splicing**, i.e. breakage of the intron at the 5' site and joining of the upstream and downstream exon sequences together.

After the removal of all introns, fully functional mature mRNA which is ready to direct protein synthesis leaves the nucleus and passes into the cytosol (Chemistry to Clinics 20.3). **Mutations in the β-globin gene interfere with intron removal and lead to β-thalassemia**.

rRNA

Ribosomal RNAs are synthesized from long precursor molecules called **pre-rRNAs** or **45S RNAs**

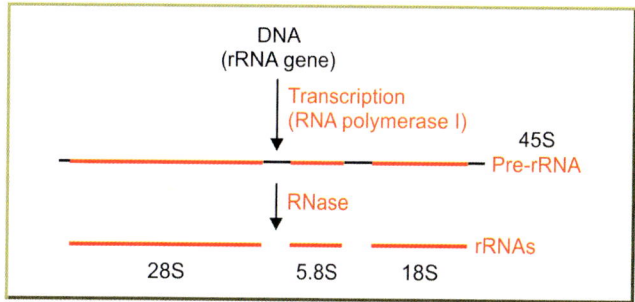

Fig. 20.9: Post-transcriptional processing of eukaryotic rRNA.

which contain sequences for 28S, 5.8S and 18S rRNAs. Each pre-rRNA molecule is **cleaved** to yield the required rRNA species (Fig. 20.9). Some of the proteins destined to become components of the ribosomes, also get associated with the pre-rRNAs prior to and during post-transcriptional modification in the nucleolus.

tRNA

The tRNA molecules undergo following changes:

1. The primary transcript of a tRNA gene has a large number of **extra-nucleotide sequences** on both 5' as well as 3' ends, and is trimmed nonspecifically. The **5' extension** is cleaved by the **endonucleolytic cleavage** by ribonuclease P (a ribozyme) while the **3' extension** is cleaved by the **exonucleolytic cleavage**.

2. Sometimes, the primary transcript may also contain **introns which are removed** by a two component enzyme system where one of the enzymes removes introns while the other rejoins the remaining exon chains.

3. Each functional tRNA, both in the cytoplasm as well as in the mitochondria, has a sequence of three nucleotides, i.e. **CCA at the 3' terminus**. These three

20

nucleotides are added sequentially by tRNA nucleotidyltransferase.

4. Each tRNA molecule also has several **modified nucleotides**. Modifications may be found in the nitrogenous bases as well as in the ribose moiety. These modifications are completed before the tRNA precursors are cleaved to mature tRNAs by various enzymes which are either site specific or nucleotide sequence specific.

RNA INTERFERENCE

Specific cellular mRNAs can be degraded by introducing mammalian cells to a double-stranded RNA (**dsRNA**, derived from a virus or a transposon or artificially prepared in the laboratory) in which one of the strands is complementary to the mRNA being targeted. Inside the cell, the dsRNA forms a 'small interfering RNA' (**siRNA**) and the phenomenon is called RNA interference (**RNAi**) (Chemistry to Clinics 20.4).

It is employed in '**post-transcriptional gene silencing**' or '**gene knock-down**' (different from 'gene knock-out', i.e. disruption or removal of a gene itself) as follows (Fig. 20.10):

- A dsRNA is introduced into a target cell. One strand of the dsRNA is designed to be an antisense RNA because its sequence is complementary to the RNA transcript of the gene selected for silencing.
- Inside the cell, an ATP-dependent RNase III called '**dicer**', catalyzes the cleavage of both strands to produce a double-stranded small interfering RNA (**ds-siRNA**), 21–23 nucleotides long and having 2-nucleotides long 3'-overhangs on each strand.

Chemistry to Clinics 20.4: RNA Interference

The siRNAs can be used as therapeutic agents. Several potential clinical applications of RNAi are currently being evaluated, e.g. treatment of cancer, AIDS and other infections. Further, RNAi is currently the method of choice for eukaryotic gene inactivation. The consequences of loss of gene function reveal the role played by the gene product (RNA or protein) in the cell.

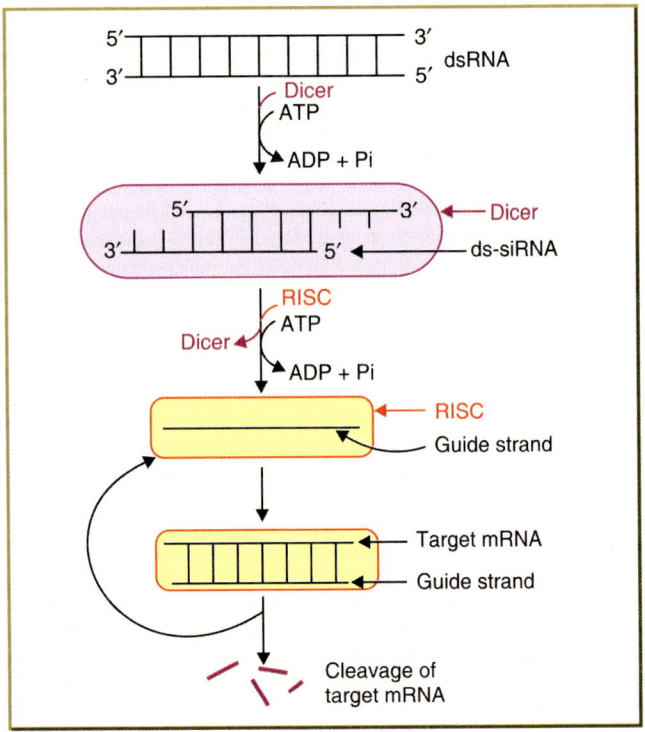

Fig. 20.10: RNA interference.

- The ds-siRNA is passed onto another protein complex called RNA-induced silencing complex (**RISC**).
- In an ATP-dependent manner, RISC unwinds the ds-siRNA and selects the antisense strand, now called the '**guide strand**'. The other strand called the '**passenger strand**' is discarded.
- RISC pairs the single guide strand with a complementary region on the target gene transcript (mRNA).
- The RNase H activity of RISC performs its '**slicer**' function by cleaving the RNA transcript so that it can no longer be translated by ribosomes.
- The guide strand remains associated with RISC, hence it can be used for **multiple cycles** of mRNA cleavage, i.e. post-transcriptional gene silencing.

SOME IMPORTANT QUESTIONS

1. Differentiate structural and functional features of three types of RNA.

2. Describe the process of transcription in prokaryotes. How does it differ from eukaryotes?

3. Differentiate between RNA polymerases found in prokaryotes from those of eukaryotes.

4. Differentiate between the promoter regions in prokaryotes and eukaryotes.

5. Write notes on:

i. Promoter regions

ii. RNA polymerases

iii. Post-transcriptional modifications

iv. DNA template

v. Upstream nucleotide sequence

vi. Pribnow box

vii. TATA box

viii. Enhancers

ix. Rho-dependent termination of transcription

x. Rho-independent termination of transcription

xi. RNA interference

MULTIPLE CHOICE QUESTIONS

1. Rifampicin binds to the following subunit of prokaryotic RNA polymerase:

A. α

B. β

C. β'

D. σ

2. In eukaryotes, the following enzyme is inhibited by high concentration of α-amanitin:

A. RNA polymerase I

B. RNA polymerase II

C. RNA polymerase III

D. mtRNA polymerase

3. The following enzyme participates in processing eukaryotic hnRNA:

A. Guanylyl transferase

B. Guanine-7-methyl transferase

C. Adenylate polymerase

D. All of the above

4. Human mitochondrial RNase P is a:

A. Ribozyme

B. Ribonucleoprotein

C. Protein

D. RNA-DNA hybrid

5. RNA interference is not equivalent to:

A. Post-transcriptional gene silencing

B. Gene knock-down

C. Gene knock-out

D. Aptamer-based gene silencing

Translation and Post-translational Modifications

Genetic information, as discussed earlier, is stored in cells in the form of linear sequences of nucleotides in DNA which uses simple four letter alphabets, A, C, G and T. This information of DNA is encoded (transcribed) in four letter alphabets, A, C, G and U in mRNA from where it is expressed (translated) in twenty letter language of amino acids in proteins. The mRNA is translated from **5'-end to 3'-end**, producing a protein which is synthesized from the **amino terminal end to the carboxyl terminal end**. **Protein biosynthesis** is thus the biochemical translation of the genetic information, from the **four-letter language of nucleic acids** into the **twenty-letter language of proteins**. The process of protein biosynthesis, therefore, is also called as **translation**.

THE GENETIC CODE

The genetic code is a dictionary that gives the correspondence between a sequence of four nucleotide bases found in mRNA to the sequence of twenty amino acids known to occur in polypeptides. Each individual word in the code is composed of **three nucleotide bases**. This is due to the reason that if one nucleotide encodes for an amino acid, four nucleotides will code for $(4)^1$, i.e. four amino acids only. If there are two nucleotides in a code it will translate into $(4)^2$, i.e. 16 amino acids only. Hence, a 3:1 correspondence of nucleotides to amino acids with $(4)^3$, i.e. 64 different combinations is essential to encode all the 20 amino acids. These three-base genetic words are called **codons**, present in the mRNA language as nucleotides (U, C, A and G) and are written in a sequence from 5'-end to the 3'-end. Codons are thus the **permutations of four bases taken in sets of threes**. The 64 different combinations of three-base words (codons) comprise the **genetic code** (Table 21.1).

Salient Features of the Genetic Code

- **Punctuation:** Out of 64 codons, **61 code for different amino acids** and are designated as amino acid codons whereas the other three which do not code for any amino acid are called as nonsense codons. These **three nonsense codons**, i.e. UAG, UAA and UGA are the *stop signals*. These are also known as termination codons. On the other hand, AUG is the start signal and specifies methionine. The four codons, i.e. the start signal (AUG) which codes for methionine and the three stop signals (UAG, UAA and UGA) thus function as punctuation, signaling the start and the stop of protein biosynthesis.
- **Degeneracy:** Only two amino acids are designated by the single codons, i.e. methionine as AUG and tryptophan as UGG. Other amino acids are designated by two, three, four or six codons. **Multiple codons thus encode for a single amino acid**. This is called degeneracy in the code.
- **Universality:** The genetic code is nearly universal, i.e. **same codes are used** in all living organisms with the **exception in the mitochondria**. Non-universal codon usages have been found in the mammalian mitochondria, e.g. UGA which usually is a termination code, codes for tryptophan in mitochondria. Similarly, AGA and AGG which usually code for arginine, are the termination codons in mitochondria.

21

Table 21.1: Genetic code

5'-Base	Middle-base							3'-Base
	U		C		A		G	
U	UUU		UCU		UAU		UGU		U
	UUC	Phe	UCC		UAC	Tyr	UGC	Cys	
	UUA		UCA		UAA		UGA	Stop	
	UUG		UCG	Ser	UAG	Stop	UGG	Trp	
C	CUU		CCU		CAU		CGU		C
	CUC		CCC		CAC	His	CGC		
	CUA		CCA		CAA		CGA		
	CUG	Leu	CCG	Pro	CAG	Gln	CGG	Arg	
A	AUU		ACU		AAU		AGU		A
	AUC		ACC		AAC	Asn	AGC	Ser	
	AUA	Ile	ACA		AAA		AGA		
	AUG	Met/Start	ACG	Thr	AAG	Lys	AGG	Arg	
G	GUU		GCU		GAU		GGU		G
	GUC		GCC		GAC	Asp	GGC		
	GUA		GCA		GAA		GGA		
	GUG	Val	GCG	Ala	GAG	Glu	GGG	Gly	

Salient features of the genetic code are given in Table 21.2.

REQUIREMENTS FOR PROTEIN BIOSYNTHESIS

Protein biosynthesis requires mRNA, ribosomes, tRNAs, several protein factors and ATP as a source of energy.

Table 21.2: Salient features of the genetic code

Degeneracy	Multiple codons code for same amino acid
Unambiguous	A specific codon codes for only a single amino acid
Non-overlapping	Reading of the genetic code occurs without overlapping
Punctuation	Message is read continuously without any break between the sequence of codons until a non-sense codon is reached
Universality	The same codon is used in all the living organisms, with only few exceptions in the mitochondria

Messenger RNA

- Messenger RNA (mRNA) is the **carrier of information present in DNA**.
- In eukaryotes, mRNAs are usually synthesized as large precursor molecules (heterogeneous nuclear RNA, **hnRNA**) which are **processed** prior to their export from the nucleus.
- The 5'-end of the mRNA is **capped** with 7-methyl-guanosine triphosphate (Fig. 21.1). There is also a 5'-nontranslated region which separates the cap from the translation initiation signal (an AUG codon for methionine).
- An uninterrupted 5'→3' nucleotide sequence specifies a polypeptide which is followed by a specific translation termination signal. This stop codon is followed by a 3'-untranslated sequence of about 200 nucleotides and a long **polyadenylate tail**.
- Eukaryotic mRNA is **monocistronic**, i.e. it encodes a single polypeptide. In prokaryotes, most mRNAs

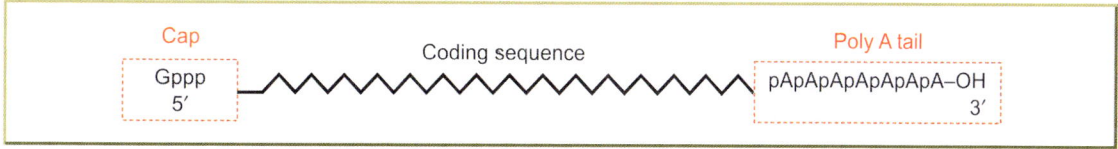

Fig. 21.1: Eukaryotic mRNA with 5'-cap and 3'-poly A tail.

21

are polycistronic (encoding several polypeptides) and there is no polyadenylate tail.

Ribosomes

- Ribosomes are work-benches for **protein biosynthesis**.
- They are large complexes with two dissimilar subunits, i.e. a **large subunit** and a **small subunit**. There relative sizes are given in terms of the sedimentation coefficient (S or Svedberg values).
- Some ribosomes occur **free in the cytosol** but many are **bound to the membrane of the rough endoplasmic reticulum**. Free ribosomes synthesize proteins that remain within the cytosol or become targeted to the nucleus, mitochondria or some other organelle. Membrane-bound ribosomes synthesize proteins that are to be secreted from the cell and function in other cellular membranes or vesicles.
- A **eukaryotic** ribosome particle is **80S** molecule with two subunits of **60S** and **40S**. The large subunit

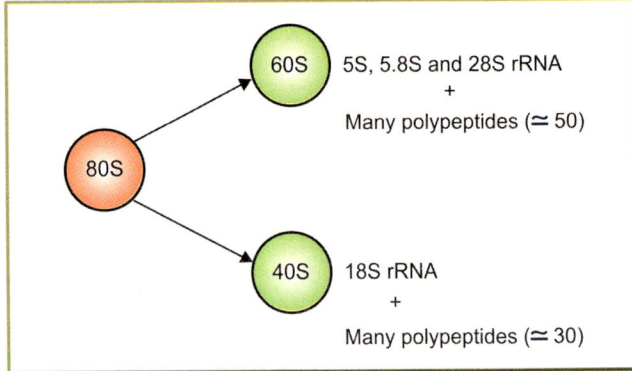

Fig. 21.2: Mammalian ribosomes.

contains 3 molecules of rRNA (5S, 5.8S and 28S rRNA) and nearly 50 protein molecules. The small subunit has 18S rRNA and about 30 polypeptides (Fig. 21.2). A **prokaryotic** ribosome is **70S** molecule with two subunits of **50S** and **30S**. The 50S subunit contains 5S and 23S rRNAs, and 32 polypeptides whereas the 30S subunit has 16S rRNA and 21 protein molecules.

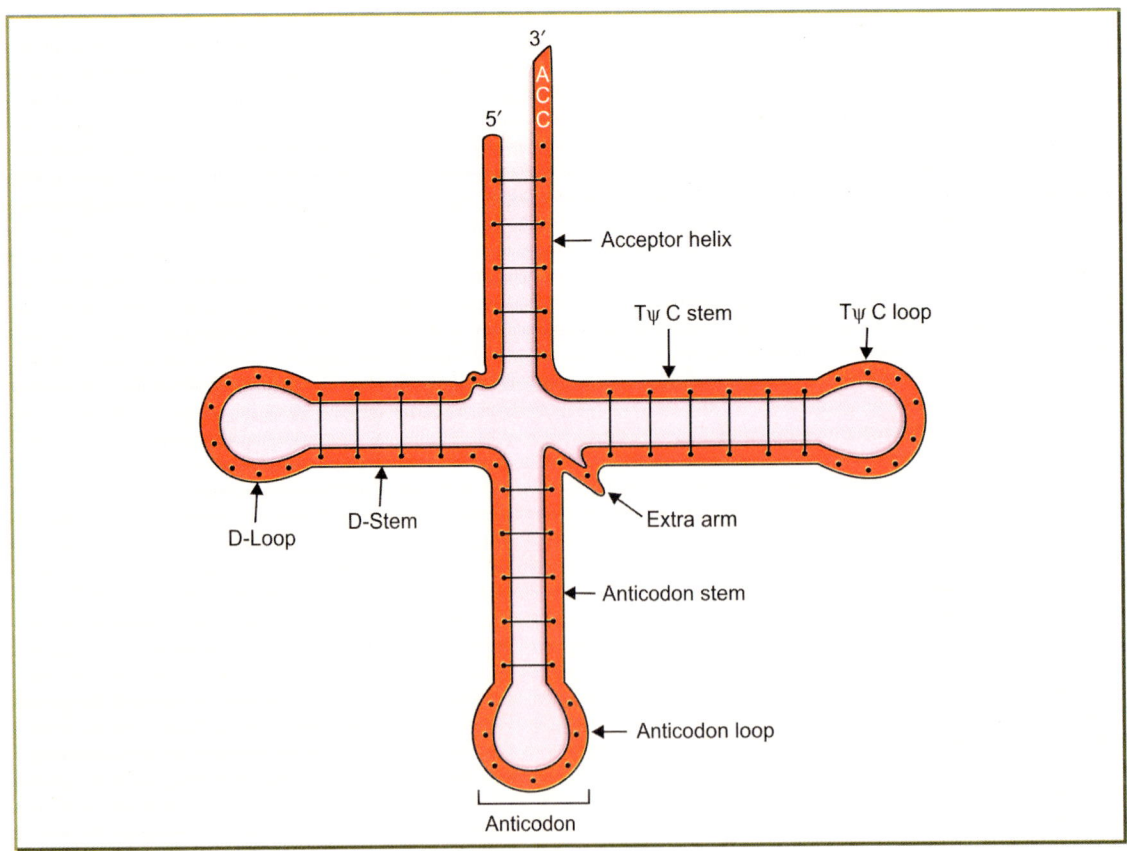

Fig. 21.3: Clover-leaf model of tRNA.

21

- A ribosome has two binding sites for tRNA. These sites are called as the **A site** and the **P site**. During translation, an incoming aminoacyl-tRNA, as directed by the codon, binds at A site. This codon specifies the next amino acid to be added to the growing peptide chain. The P site is occupied by the peptidyl-tRNA which carries an upcoming polypeptide chain.

Transfer RNAs: Codon-Anticodon Interaction

- Transfer RNAs (tRNAs) act as the **bilingual translators**.
- Most of the cells have ≈**50 different types** of tRNAs.
- All tRNA molecules have several common structural characteristics, i.e. each has a **3'-terminal CCA** sequence to which an amino acid binds and a **clover-leaf like secondary structure** (Fig. 21.3).
- Each tRNA molecule also has a three-base nucleotide sequence called **anticodon**. The anticodon specifies the insertion of an amino acid, carried by that tRNA onto the growing polypeptide chain. Hence, tRNAs are also called **adaptor molecules** because of their ability to carry a specific amino acid

for its incorporation into the growing polypeptide chain (Fig. 21.4).

- Translation of the codons of mRNA involves their direct interaction with the complementary anticodon sequences in tRNA. Binding of the tRNA anticodon to the codon on the mRNA follows the *rule of complementarity* and *antiparallel binding*, i.e. the mRNA codon is read in the 5'→3' direction by an anticodon, pairing in the 3'→5' orientation.

THE PROCESS OF PROTEIN BIOSYNTHESIS

Besides the activation of amino acids, protein biosynthesis involves initiation, elongation and termination along with the release of a polypeptide. **Formation of each peptide bond consumes 4 molecules of ATP.**

Activation of Amino Acids

For the incorporation of amino acids into a polypeptide chain, amino acids are first activated and get linked to their appropriate tRNA carriers. This linkage of an amino acid to the tRNA **requires energy** and is catalyzed by **aminoacyl-tRNA synthetase**.

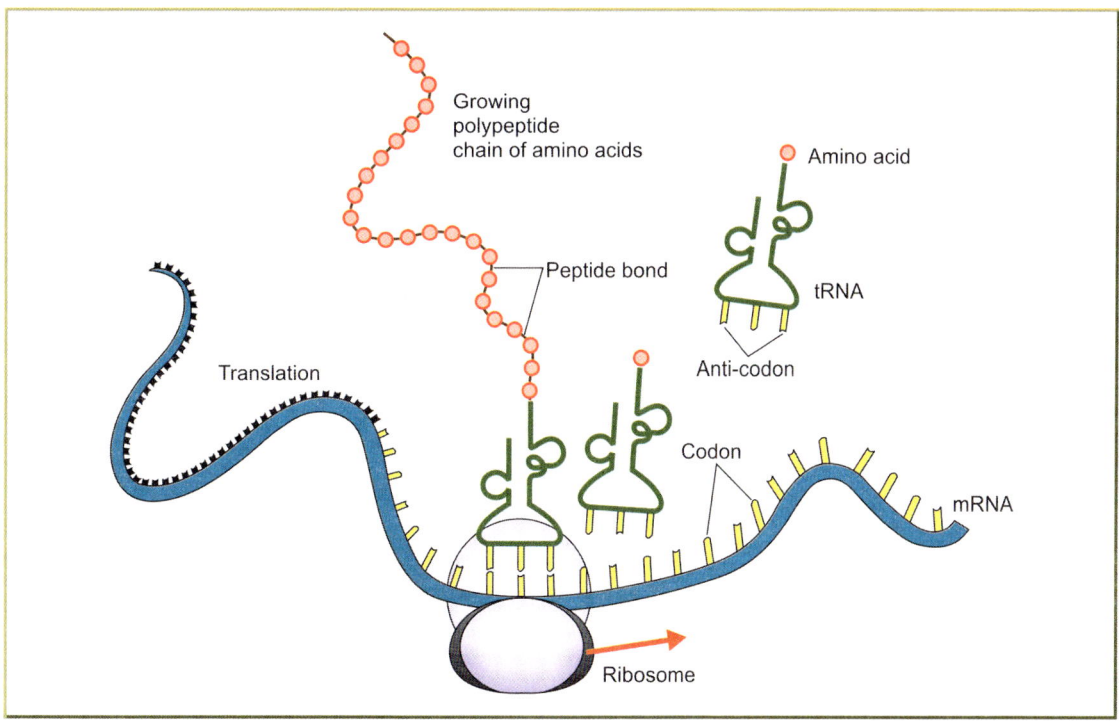

Fig. 21.4: Codon-anticodon interaction: The **'adapter'** role of tRNA.

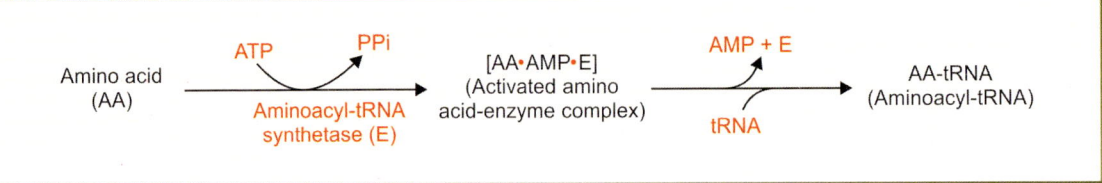

Fig. 21.5: Formation of amino acyl-tRNA.

Aminoacyl tRNA synthetases are a group of enzymes, each one of which is **specific for a single amino acid and its appropriate tRNA species**.

During the process, a high energy complex, i.e. **amino acid-AMP-enzyme complex** is formed as an intermediate. Each synthetase then recognizes a tRNA and transfers amino acid from the amino acid-AMP-enzyme complex onto the corresponding tRNA (Fig. 21.5). Aminoacyl tRNA synthetases not only carry the correct amino acid but also **edit protein synthesis**. A misacylated tRNA is recognized and removed (deacylated).

During translation, mRNA sequences are written as well as read in the **5′→3′ direction** whereas due to the codon-anticodon interaction, amino acid sequences are written as well as synthesized from the **amino-terminal to the carboxy-terminal end**.

Wobble hypothesis: As mentioned above, each tRNA species carries a unique amino acid and has a specific three-bases anticodon sequence. At the same time, we know that there are 61 codons which designate an amino acid while most cells have nearly 50 tRNA species. This, in turn, suggests that certain variations from the standard base-pairing, in codon-anticodon interactions, do occur and that all the codons may not be used equally. Some codons may be read more efficiently by one anticodon than the other while some may be used very rarely suggesting that many amino acids can be carried by more than one tRNA species as well as degenerate codons can be read by more than one tRNA (but always one carrying the correct amino acid).

The possibility by which **one anticodon recognizes more than one codon for a specific amino acid** is described by a hypothesis given by Crick and is referred to as Wobble hypothesis. This explains that the **base at the 5′-end of the anticodon (the first base of the anticodon or the third base of the codon) is not as well-defined** with respect to its spatial configuration as the other two bases, i.e. the first two positions of a codon predominate in tRNA selection and the **degenerate (third) position is less important**.

Initiation of Protein Biosynthesis

Requirements: Initiation of protein synthesis involves the assembly of various components of the translation system, i.e. two ribosomal subunits, the mRNA to be translated, the aminoacyl-tRNA specified by the first codon in the message, GTP and several initiation factors that facilitate assembly of the initiation complex.

In **eukaryotes**, several initiation factors (**eIF**) participate in initiation. The **initiation codon AUG is** first recognized by a special initiation tRNA that carries **methionine**. This recognition is facilitated by eIF-2 in humans.

Ternary complex

- As a first step, eukaryotic initiation factor 2a (eIF-2a) binds to GTP and methionyl-tRNA (Met-tRNA$_i^{Met}$), and forms a ternary complex (Fig. 21.6).
- The second step requires 40S ribosomal subunit associated with eIF-3. Mammalian eIF-3 is a complex protein and has 8 different polypeptides. eIF-3 is also called as anti-association factor since it blocks the association of 40S with the 60S subunit.

Pre-initiation complex

- A complex, comprising of eIF-2a·Met-tRNA$_i^{Met}$·GTP, eIF-3·40S, eIF-4c and some other protein factors, is formed.
- This complex, in turn, binds to mRNA and forms a pre-initiation complex.
- In addition, eIF-4a and eIF-4b are required to unwind the secondary structure in mRNA.
- It also requires eIF-4f (also called cap-binding protein) which helps to place the message on the 40S subunit. During this process, a molecule of ATP is hydrolyzed and helps to locate and place the initiation AUG sequence in the mRNA.

The final pre-initiation complex thus includes 40S ribosomal subunit, eIF-2a·Met-tRNA$_i^{Met}$·GTP ternary complex, correctly oriented mRNA, and several protein factors.

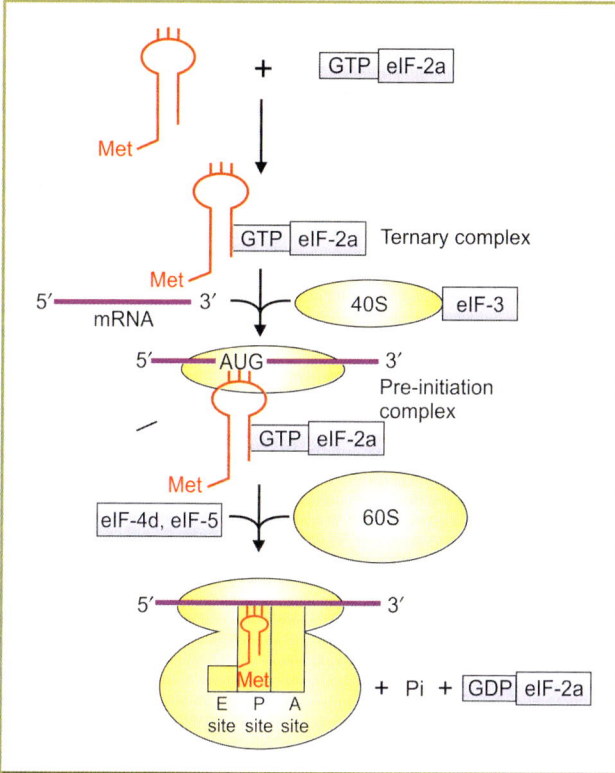

Fig. 21.6: Initiation of protein synthesis.

Initiation complex

- The eIF-5 interacts with the pre-initiation complex, GTP is hydrolyzed and eIF-2·GDP, eIF-3 and other factors are released.
- The 40S·Met-tRNA$_i$^{Met}·mRNA complex interacts with the 60S subunit and initiation factor eIF-4d, to generate an 80S ribosome with the mRNA initiator tRNA correctly positioned on the ribosome.
- The eIF-2·GDP so released interacts with the guanine nucleotide exchange factor eIF-2b and GTP to regenerate eIF-2a·GTP for another round (Fig. 21.6).

In prokaryotes: Three initiation factors (IF) are known, called IF-1, IF-2 and IF-3.

Prokaryotes utilize a specific initiation tRNA whose **methionine is modified by formylation of its amino group**. This fMet-tRNA$_i$^{Met} is rcognized by IF-2. The IF-3 forms a complex with the 30S subunit and binds to mRNA.

Shine-Dalgarno sequence: Shine-Dalgarno discovered that in *E. coli*, a purine-rich sequence of about 10 nucleotides is located upstream of the initiation

AUG codon in the mRNA. The sequence, designated as Shine-Dalgarno sequence, forms complementary base pairs to the pyrimidine-rich sequence of 8 nucleotides on 3'-end of the 16S rRNA and facilitates binding and positioning of mRNA on the 30S ribosomal subunit, in prokaryotes.

Chain Elongation

Requirements: Stepwise elongation of the peptide chain results in the formation of a polypeptide. At each step, ribosomal **peptidyl transferase** transfers the growing polypeptide from its carrier tRNA to the α-amino group of the amino acid residue of the aminoacyl-tRNA specified by the next codon. The process requires certain nonribosomal proteins called **elongation factors**, which utilize the energy liberated by GTP hydrolysis. This, in turn, **ensures the selection of proper aminoacyl-tRNA** and the movement of the mRNA and associated tRNAs through the decoding region of the ribosome.

Specific sites span ribosomal subunits: During translation, up to three tRNA molecules may be bound at the specific sites that span the two ribosomal subunits. The initiating methionyl-tRNA is placed in such a position that it occupies the donor site, also called the peptidyl site or **P site** of the ribosome, in the way that its methionyl residue may be donated (transferred) to the free α-amino group of the incoming aminoacyl-tRNA (Fig. 21.7). The aminoacyl-tRNA, specified by the next codon of the mRNA, is bound at the acceptor site, also called the aminoacyl site or **A site** of the ribosome. The initiating methionyl-tRNA and the incoming aminoacyl-tRNA are now appropriately positioned in the manner that their anticodons are paired with the successive codons of the mRNA in the P and A sites of the 40S subunit while their amino acids are besides one another at the peptidyl transferase site of the 60S subunit. After the transfer of the methionine to the amino group of the aminoacyl-tRNA, the anticodon of the deacylated tRNA remains in the small subunit P site while its acceptor end is located in the large subunit exit site, referred to as **E site**.

Ternary complex

- The EF-lα component of EF-1 first forms a ternary complex with aminoacyl-tRNA and GTP.
- This EF-lα·aminoacyl-tRNA·GTP complex binds to the ribosome and **if codon-anticodon interactions**

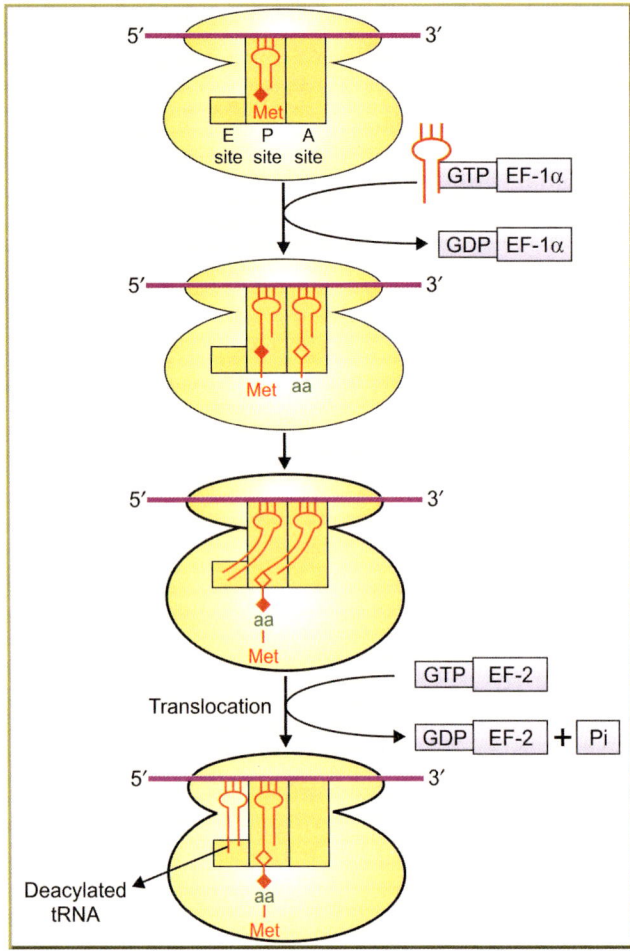

Fig. 21.7: Elongation of peptide chain.

are correct, the aminoacyl-tRNA is placed at the A site.
- GTP is hydrolyzed and EF-lα·GDP complex is dissociated.
- The initiating methionyl-tRNA and the incoming aminoacyl-tRNA are now properly positioned on the ribosome. Their anticodons are paired with the successive codons on the mRNA, in the decoding region of the small subunit and their amino acids are besides one another, at the peptidyl transferase site of the large subunit.

Formation of a peptide bond: Peptidyl transferase catalyzes attack of the α-amino group of the amino-acyl-tRNA onto the carboxyl carbon of the methionyl-tRNA. This results in the transfer of methionine to the amino group of the aminoacyl-tRNA which then occupies a hybrid position on the ribosome, i.e. the anti-codon remains in the 40S on the A site while the

acceptor-end along with the attached peptide are in the 60S on the P site.

Chemical nature of peptidyl transferase: It was initially thought that peptidyl transferase was one of the proteins of the ribosome. It has, however, now been conclusively proved that this enzyme activity resides in the rRNA of the large ribosomal subunit. Therefore, peptidyl transferase is a good example of a **ribozyme**.

Translocation

- The anticodon of the deacylated tRNA remains in the 40S on the P site while its acceptor is located in the 60S towards the upper end, called the exit site (**E site**).
- The mRNA and the dipeptidyl-tRNA at the 40S A site are now repositioned by elongation factor 2 (EF-2), also called **translocase**, for another elongation cycle to begin.
- The EF-2 moves mRNA and the dipeptidyl-tRNA, in codon-anticodon register, from the A site to the P site. During this process, GTP is hydrolyzed and the A site is fully vacated.
- As the dipeptidyl-tRNA is moved to the P site, the deacylated donor (methionine) tRNA is also moved to the E site which only exists in the 60S subunit. The ribosome can now enter a **new cycle** (Fig. 21.7).

In prokaryotes: Elongation factors are different from those in eukaryotes, designated as EF-Tu, EF-Ts and EF-G (GTP-dependent translocase).

Termination

Requirements: Termination of the process of protein biosynthesis requires a stop codon. A chain-termi-nating codon (UAG, UAA or UGA) in the A site does not promote binding of any tRNA species.

Hydrolysis and polypeptide release
- A non-ribosomal protein called releasing factor (**eRF**), binds the ribosome as an eRF·GTP complex (Fig. 21.8).
- The peptide-tRNA ester linkage is cleaved through the action of peptidyl transferase (a hydrolase) and the polypeptide is released from its carrier tRNA.
- Dissociation of eRF from the ribosome requires hydrolysis of GTP and releases the ribosome to dissociate into its two subunits which can the re-enter the cycle, at the initiation stage.

In prokaryotes: Instead of eRF, three release factors, i.e. RF-1, RF-2 and RF-3 are required. RF-1 acts in

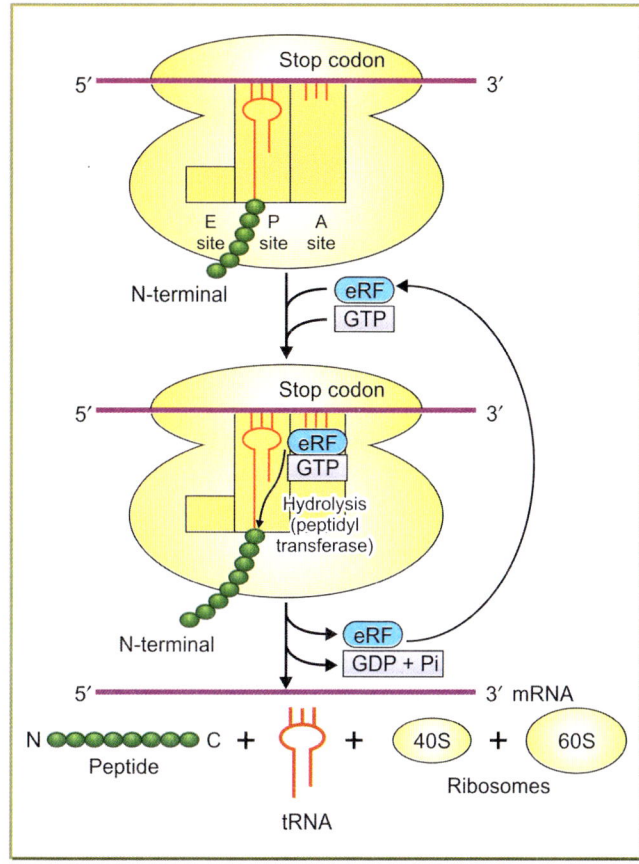

Fig. 21.8: Termination of protein synthesis.

response to UAG or UAA whereas RF-2 is required in response to UGA or UAA. The RF-3 has a GTPase activity and activates RF-1 and RF-2.

Differences in protein biosynthesis between prokaryotes and eukaryotes are given in Table 21.3.

PROTEIN BIOSYNTHESIS IN MITOCHONDRIA

Mitochondria have an independent apparatus for protein synthesis which includes RNA polymerase, aminoacyl-tRNA synthetases, tRNAs and ribosomes. Its salient features include:

1. The number of tRNA species in mitochondria is small and the genetic code, as mentioned earlier, is slightly different.
2. Mitochondrial ribosomes are smaller and rRNAs are shorter.
3. An initiator Met-tRNA$_i^{Met}$ is modified by a trans-formylase that uses N^{10}-formyltetrahydrofolate to produce fMet-tRNA$_i^{Met}$.

INHIBITORS OF PROTEIN BIOSYNTHESIS

Many antibiotics and toxins inhibit protein biosynthesis most of which are useful in clinical practice (Table 21.4).

Antimicrobials which Interfere with Initiation

- **Streptomycin:** It binds to the small subunit of prokaryotic ribosomes, interferes with the initiation of protein biosynthesis and causes misreading of mRNA.
- **Neomycin and gentamicin:** They interact with the small ribosomal subunit and cause mistranslation.
- **Tetracycline:** It binds directly to the ribosomes and interferes in aminoacyl-tRNA binding.

Antimicrobials which Interfere with Elongation

- **Puromycin:** It structurally resembles an aminoacyl-tRNA. It thus binds at the ribosomal A site and acts as an acceptor in the peptidyltransferase reaction. Hence, puromycin prematurely terminates translation leading to the release of peptidyl-puromycin complex.
- **Chloramphenicol:** It directly inhibits peptidyl transferase (Chemistry to Clinics 21.1).
- **Clindamycin:** It binds to 50S subunit, overlaps A and P sites, blocks peptidyl transferase activity.

Table 21.3: Differences in protein synthesis between prokaryotes and eukaryotes

Parameter	Prokaryotes	Eukaryotes
mRNA	Polycistronic	Monocistronic, contains poly(A) tail
Ribosomes	Free, 70S in size comprising of 30S and 50S subunits	Free as well as bound to endoplasmic reticulum, 80S in size comprising of 40S and 60S subunits
Initiation factors	Three	At least nine
Initiation tRNA	Formylated (N-formylmethionyl-tRNA)	Non-formylated (Met-tRNA)
Elongation factors	EF-Tu, EF-Ts, EF-G	EF-1, EF-2
Releasing factors	RF-1, RF-2, RF-3	eRF

21

Antibiotic/Inhibitor	Inhibitory effect in		Inhibits the process of
	Prokaryotes	Eukaryotes	
Streptomycin	30S subunit	—	Initiation, and misreading of the mRNA
Tetracyclin	30S subunit	40S subunit	Binding of aminoacyl-tRNA
Puromycin/Chloramphenicol	70S ribosome	80S ribosome	Peptide transfer
Erythromycin	50S subunit	—	Translocation
Fusidic acid	EF-G	—	Translocation
Cycloheximide	—	80S ribosome	Elongation
Diphtheria toxin	—	60S subunit	Translocation
Ricin	—	60S subunit	Multiple processes in protein synthesis
α-Sarcin	—	60S subunit	Multiple processes in protein synthesis
Colicin E3	30S subunit	—	Initiation

Table 21.4: Inhibitors of protein biosynthesis

Chemistry to Clinics 21.1: Chloramphenicol

Once it was the drug of choice in enteric fever (e.g. typhoid fever caused by *Salmonella typhi*). Its popularity decreased because in rare patients it caused aplastic anemia. Later, better drugs such as the quinolones (e.g. ciprofloxacin, ofloxacin) became available. At present, chloramphenicol is mostly employed in topical ophthalmic preparations.

Chemistry to Clinics 21.2: Diphtheria Toxin

The bacterium *Corynebacterium diphtheriae* harbors the bacteriophage *corynephage β*. Diphtheria toxin is a phage-encoded enzyme secreted by the bacterium. It is an NAD-dependent ADP-ribosylase. It ribosylates and thus inactivates eukaryotic translocation factor, eEF-2. This factor contains a modified histidine residue called diphthamide which gets ribosylated.

- **Erythromycin:** It blocks 50S subunit causing premature peptidyl-tRNA dissociation in prokaryotes.
- **Fusidic acid:** It interferes in the translocation by inhibiting the EF-3 (GTP-dependent translocase), in prokaryotes.
- **Cycloheximide:** It inhibits translocation of peptidyl-tRNA in eukaryotes.
- **Diphtheria toxin:** It is a protein produced by *Corynebacterium diphtheriae* and inhibits eukaryotic translocation (Chemistry to Clinics 21.2).

Toxins that attack RNAs

- **Ricin:** It is obtained from castor bean and cleaves the adenine from an rRNA in the large subunit, and thus inactivates the ribosome.
- **α-Sarcin:** It is a fungal toxin which cleaves an rRNA at a single site within the large subunit of the ribosome and inactivates the ribosome.
- **Colicin E3:** It is obtained from *E. coli*. It has ribonuclease activity. It cleaves 16S rRNA of the 30S ribosomal subunit near the mRNA-binding sequence and the decoding region. It thus

inactivates the small subunit of the ribosome and stops protein synthesis.

POST-TRANSLATIONAL MODIFICATIONS

Several proteins undergo a variety of modifications, after the synthesis of a polypeptide chain. Since these modifications occur **after translation**, such changes are referred to as post-translational modifications. These include selective partial proteolysis of the translated sequence or covalent addition of one or more chemical groups on the amino acids, in a protein chain.

Selective Partial Proteolysis

Some proteins, destined for secretion from the cell, are initially synthesized as large precursor molecules that are not functionally active. A portion of such a protein is removed by specialized endoproteases. This, in turn, results in the release of a biologically active protein molecule. Some of these precursor proteins are cleaved in the endoplasmic reticulum or the Golgi apparatus while others in the developing secretory vesicles or after secretion. For example:

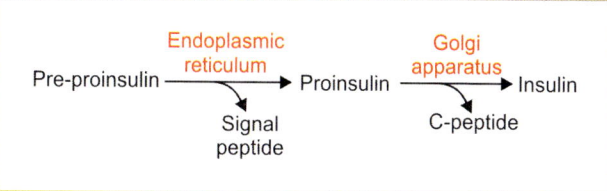

Fig. 21.9: Conversion of pre-proinsulin to insulin.

1. **Conversion of pre-proinsulin to insulin:** Insulin is synthesized as pre-proinsulin which enters the endoplasmic reticulum lumen. Signal peptidase cleaves the signal peptide from it and generates pro-insulin which is transported to the Golgi apparatus where it is packed into the secretory granules. The C peptide (an internal connecting peptide) is removed by proteolysis and the mature insulin is secreted (Fig. 21.9).

2. **Activation of a zymogen:** Proteolysis also leads to zymogen activation, such as digestive proteases. Inactive zymogen precursors are packed in storage granules and are activated by proteolysis upon secretion, e.g. trypsinogen is cleaved to give trypsin or chymotrypsinogen is converted to chymotrypsin.

Covalent Modifications

1. **Phosphorylation:** It may occur on the hydroxyl group of a serine or a threonine residue in a protein, e.g. glycogen phosphorylase and glycogen synthase.

2. **Glycosylation:** Proteins of the plasma membrane or those which are to be secreted from the cell, have carbohydrate chains attached to the hydroxyl group of the serine or threonine by the O-linkage, or to the NH_2 group of asparagine by the N-linkage. Stepwise addition of these sugar molecules (glucose, galactose, mannose, fucose, etc.) occur in the endoplasmic reticulum and the Golgi apparatus. Glycosylation of proteins thus forms a glycoprotein.

3. **Methylation:** Methylation of the ε-amino group of lysine occurs in histones. This, in turn, modulates their interaction with the DNA.

4. **Hydroxylation:** Proline and lysine residues of collagen, the most abundant protein present in the human body, are extensively hydroxylated in the endoplasmic reticulum. **Collagens are an ideal example** of proteins that undergo **extensive post-translational modifications** as discussed in Chapter 37.

Table 21.5 lists some important conditions related to abnormal post-translational modifications of proteins.

Table 21.5: Conditions related to abnormal post-translational modifications

- Familial hyper-proinsulinemia: An autosomal dominant condition; abnormally processed insulin (pro-insulin) enters the circulation.
- Acute pancreatitis: Premature activation of pancreatic zymogens.
- Cancer: Abnormal histone methylation alters their DNA binding and hence gene regulation.
- Scurvy: Vitamin C deficiency leading to abnormal processing of collagens.

SOME IMPORTANT QUESTIONS

1. Give a brief account of protein biosynthesis.

2. Explain the significance of post-translational modifications with examples.

3. Write notes on:
   i. Genetic code
   ii. Wobble hypothesis
   iii. Shine-Dalgarno sequence
   iv. Peptidyl transferase
   v. Inhibitors of protein biosynthesis
   vi. Diphtheria toxin

MULTIPLE CHOICE QUESTIONS

21

1. **The number of amino acid codons in the genetic code is:**
   A. 64
   B. 63
   C. 62
   D. 61

2. **The function of amino acyl-tRNA synthetase is:**
   A. Activate a specific amino acid
   B. Transfer amino acid to the corresponding tRNA
   C. Deacylation of misacylated tRNA
   D. All of the above

3. **The peptidyl transferase activity resides in:**
   A. tRNA
   B. mRNA
   C. rRNA of large ribosomal subunit
   D. rRNA of small ribosomal subunit

4. **Chloramphenicol inhibits:**
   A. Amino acyl-tRNA synthetase
   B. Peptidyl transferase
   C. Elongation factor 1
   D. Elongation factor 2

5. **The target for diphtheria toxin is:**
   A. Amino acyl-tRNA synthetase
   B. Peptidyl transferase
   C. Elongation factor 1
   D. Elongation factor 2

Regulation of Gene Expression

A gene is a sequence of DNA that codes for a product which may be a protein as in the case of the majority of genes or RNA as in the case of genes that code for tRNA and rRNA. The crucial feature, however, is that the product diffuses away from its site of synthesis to act elsewhere. The process by which a gene gives rise to a product is called **gene expression**.

Gene expression is **controlled by several factors** that interact specifically as well as nonspecifically with DNA, such as various environmental factors. For example, supply of nutrients can affect the rate of synthesis of some of the proteins in bacteria. Similarly, cells of the multicellular organism change substantially in shape, growth rate and other characteristics in response to several hormones and growth factors.

ORGANIZATION OF GENOME

Genome is a **complete set** of genetic instructions, i.e. the number, organization and functions of various genes in an organism. The apparent number of genes, like the overall quantity of DNA, roughly parallels complexity of the organism, e.g. *E. coli* has nearly 4300 genes whereas the total number of genes is nearly 40,000 in humans. A large part of the genome consists of the potential **protein-coding sequences** with open-reading frames that are not interrupted by the stop codons. On the other hand, many of the genes have no known function. Such genes are referred to as **orphan genes**.

Gene Cluster

Genes are randomly distributed in a genome, i.e. no discrete proportion of the genome contains relatively more genes or genes related to a particular function than any other portion of the genome. However, genes with related functions are found close together, i.e. in **clusters**. A set of genes descended by duplication and variation, from some ancestral gene, is called a **gene family**. Its members may be clustered together or dispersed on different chromosomes. Some gene families consist of identical members.

Clustering is a prerequisite for maintaining identity between genes, although clustered genes are not necessarily identical. Gene clusters range from extremes where **duplication** has generated an adjacent related gene, to the cases where hundreds of identical genes lie in a **tandem array**. Extensive tandem repetition of a gene may occur when the product is needed in unusually large amounts, e.g. the genes for rRNA and histone proteins. rRNA gene clusters code only for a single rRNA precursor.

Non-transcribable DNA

DNA, in a gene, contains two types of sequences called the control sites and the coding regions.

The part of the DNA that is expressed via the production of mRNA, to synthesize a protein, is called the **coding region**. The **non-coding region** of the DNA contains several sequences that are called **non-transcribable sequences**. These sequences include the **regulatory sequences** which separate individual genes and the sites that govern origin

22

and termination of replication. The proportion of non-transcribed sequences varies greatly. For example, it may be about 10–20% in *E. coli* to as much as **98% in humans**. Much of the non-transcribed DNA in eukaryotes consists of **repetitive sequences**.

Repetitive Sequences

Sequences that are present in **>1 copy in each genome** are called repetitive sequences. Repetitive DNA components consist of families of sequences that are not exactly the same but are related. DNA of most of the higher organisms contains several repetitive sequences. Repetitive DNA sequences may be of two types:

- **Highly repetitive sequences:** These are simple sequences that occur in tandem, ranging from 5 to 300 base-pairs (bp). They are repeated several times and occupy more than 50% of the total DNA. They are sometimes called **satellite DNA**. High concentration of repetitive DNA is located at the **centromeres** (the regions of the eukaryotic chromosomes that are attached to microtubular spindle during mitosis) and **telomeres** (ends of chromosomes). Highly repetitive DNA often forms discrete clusters.

- **Moderately repetitive sequences:** They are longer sequences and range from one-hundred to several-thousand bp in length and are quite variable. Some are clustered in one region of the genome while others are scattered throughout the DNA. Sometimes, a sequence is highly conserved from one repeat to another while on the other hand, different repeat units of the same sequence may have considerable divergence. Moderately repetitive component includes a total length of 6×10^5 bp of DNA, repeated nearly 350 × per genome. Since they have no known function, these sequences form a part of the **selfish or junk DNA**.

  Neither of these classes represents a protein. These unexpressed sequences accumulate mutations at a greater rate than the expressed sequences.

The Operon

An operon is a **coordinated unit of gene expression**, i.e. a set of clustered genes, **in bacteria**. An operon includes:

- The adjacent **structural genes** that code for the related enzymes or associated proteins.

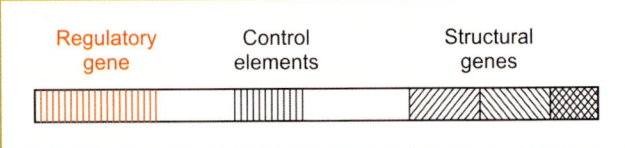

Fig. 22.1: General structure of an operon.

- A **regulatory gene** that encodes a repressor protein which binds to the operator site. The binding of the repressor to the operator prevents transcription of the structural genes.
- **Control elements** that are the sites on the DNA near the structural genes, at which regulatory proteins act (Fig. 22.1).

TYPES OF REGULATION OF GENE EXPRESSION

There are two types of regulation:

Induction: It is the process of increase in expression of genes in response to the presence of a specific substrate called an **inducer**.

Repression: It is the process of turning-off transcription of a gene in response to the presence of a specific substrate called a **repressor**.

REGULATION OF GENE EXPRESSION IN PROKARYOTES

Several systems of gene expression are known to exist in prokaryotes.

1. LAC OPERON

- The lac operon (lactose operon) contains three adjacent structural genes, designated as **lac Z**, **lac Y** and **lac A** (Fig. 22.2). Lac Z codes for β-galactosidase, lac Y for permease and lac A for transacetylase. All the three genes are transcribed to give a single mRNA molecule that encodes three proteins.
- Lac operon also contains a regulatory gene, referred to as **lac I**, that encodes a protein called **repressor**. Lac I is located just in front of the controlling elements for the structural genes, i.e. the ZYA gene-cluster.
- Lac operon also has an operator site (**lac O**) and a promoter site (**lac P**). These are the two control elements, located in front of the three structural

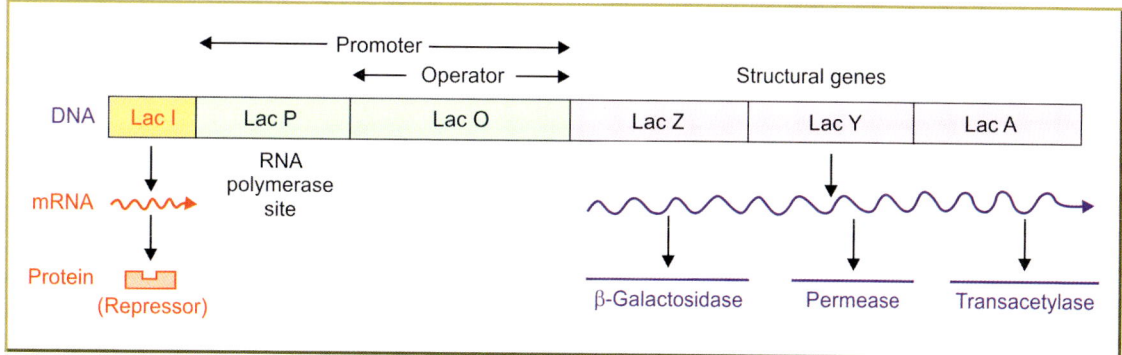

Fig. 22.2: Lac operon.

genes of the operon. Operator sequence is continuous with the promoter as well as structural genes while the promoter is located immediately in front of the operator sequence. The promoter contains a recognition site for RNA polymerase, and in turn, directs the enzyme to occupy the correct transcription initiation site.

Bacteria such as *E. coli,* usually depend upon glucose as the source of carbon and energy. However, when glucose is lacking, *E.coli* can use lactose as the source of carbon. An essential enzyme in the metabolism of lactose is β-galactosidase that converts lactose into its monosaccharides (glucose and galactose). When *E. coli* is grown in a medium in the absence of lactose, it does not require β-galactosidase. On the other hand, when lactose is the sole source of carbon, several-fold increase in β-galactosidase occurs in the cell. Bacteria thus respond to the need, to metabolize lactose, by increasing the synthesis of β-galactosidase. Also, if lactose is removed from the medium, synthesis of the enzyme stops.

Besides β-galactosidase, two other proteins namely, galactoside permease and thiogalactoside trans-acetylase are also synthesized. Permease is required for the transport of lactose across the bacterial cell membrane. On the other hand, though transacetylase is not essential for lactose metabolism, it plays an important role in acetylation and detoxification of the metabolite.

This ability of bacteria to produce a series of proteins, only when needed for the utilization of a substrate, allows the bacteria to **adapt to the environment** without any need to continuously synthesize large quantities of the enzymes when these are not required.

Lac Repressor

The lac operon, as discussed above, contains a regulatory gene lac I. The product of expression of this gene is a protein called repressor which inhibits the synthesis of the three enzymes. Repressor forms a tetramer, an active form of the protein.

In the absence of lactose, repressor recognizes the operator and binds to it. Binding of repressor to operator, prevents binding of RNA polymerase and thus blocks transcription of structural genes. As a result, only a small quantity of the enzymes is produced (Fig. 22.3). Addition of lactose to the medium leads to the formation of 1,6-allolactose, an analog of lactose (where galactose and glucose are linked by α-1,6 linkage instead of β-1,4 linkage). It is a side product of the β-galactosidase reaction and acts as an **inducer**. Inducer binds to repressor and forms an **inducer-repressor complex** which cannot bind to the operator. The operator remains unoccupied and allows the transcription and subsequent translation of the enzymes (Fig. 22.4).

Lactose or its metabolite since acts as an **inducer**, it enhances the synthesis of the three enzymes.

All the three structural genes are coordinately expressed, i.e. either all the three are equally transcribed or none of these is transcribed. The repressor thus inhibits (represses) the transcription, until the presence of lactose.

Catabolite Repression

Besides a binding site for RNA polymerase, promoter also contains a recognition site for another protein called **catabolite activator protein** (CAP). It is a DNA-

22

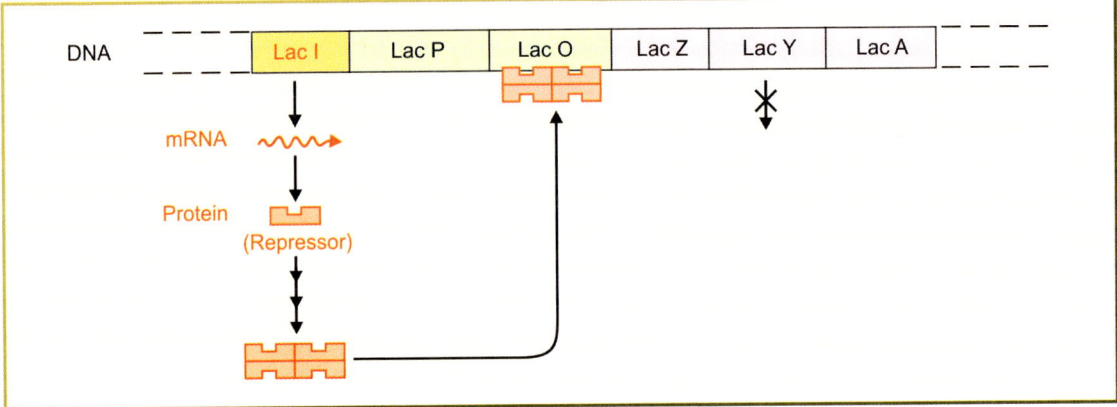

Fig. 22.3: Expression of lac operon in the absence of inducer.

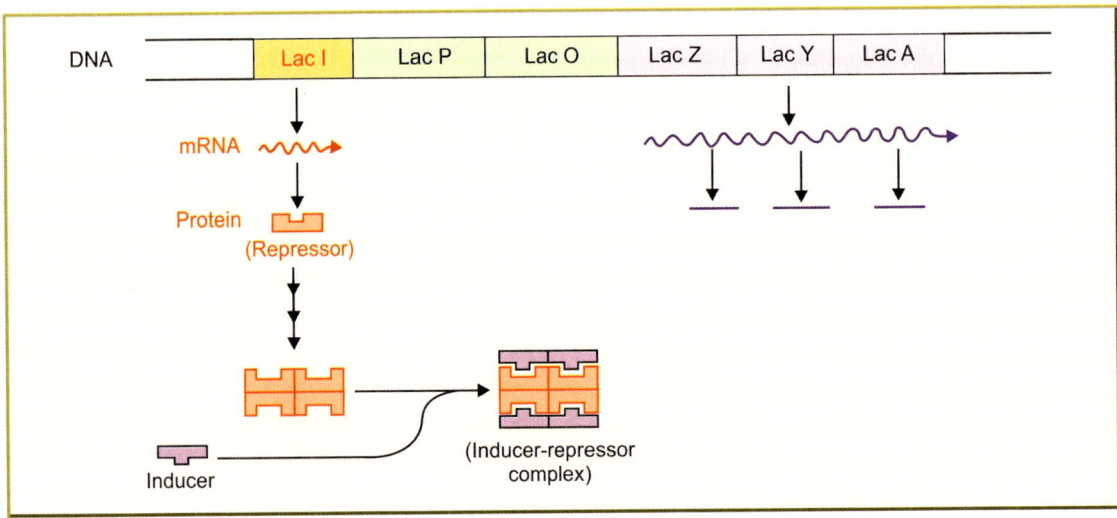

Fig. 22.4: Expression of lac operon in the presence of inducer.

binding protein, also called **cAMP-response protein** (CRP), since CAP can bind to cAMP and form a complex with it. It is the CAP-cAMP complex that binds to the promoter and not the CAP alone.

As mentioned earlier, *E. coli* prefers glucose as a metabolic fuel instead of other sugars. For example, if both glucose and lactose are present in the medium in equal concentrations, bacteria will preferentially metabolize glucose. Only after all the glucose has been utilized, it will start utilizing lactose. This is because **glucose lowers the intracellular concentration of cAMP**.

When glucose is absent from the medium, cAMP level increases. The CAP undergoes conformational changes and forms **CAP-cAMP complex** that binds

to the promoter and exerts a positive control on transcription. The binding also facilitates the binding of RNA polymerase to the promoter and thereby results in transcription (Fig. 22.5). On the other hand, when glucose is present, it inhibits the synthesis of cAMP whose level is reduced (Fig. 22.6). The CAP-cAMP complex cannot be formed and a positive effect on RNA polymerase does not occur.

It is, therefore, clear that glucose, a catabolite of lactose, interferes with the induction of lac operon and this effect is called **catabolite repression**. The **CAP is a positive regulator** since it turns the transcription 'on', in contrast to the **lac repressor which is a negative regulator** and turns the transcription 'off'.

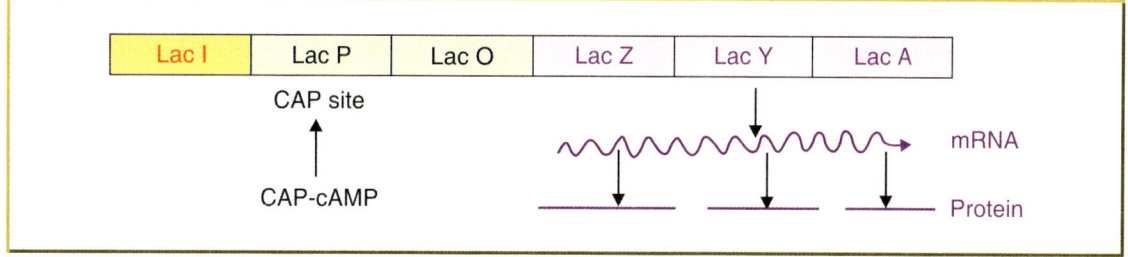

Fig. 22.5: Catabolite repression.

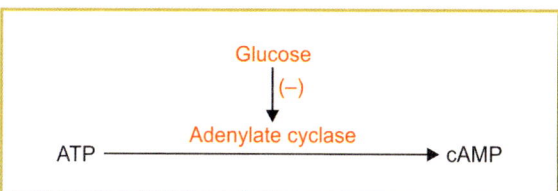

Fig. 22.6: Inhibition of cAMP synthesis by glucose.

2. TRYPTOPHAN OPERON

In *E. coli*, tryptophan is synthesized from chorismic acid in five steps which are catalyzed by three different enzymes (two of these enzymes, i.e. anthranilate synthetase and tryptophan synthetase, each have two different subunits).

- For the synthesis of these five proteins, tryptophan operon (**trp operon**) contains a cluster of five structural genes, designated as **trp A, trp B, trp C, trp D and trp E.**

- Upstream from this cluster of genes, is a promoter (**trp P**) where transcription begins and an operator (**trp O**) to which a repressor protein binds (Fig. 22.7).

  Repressor is a product of the R gene which is unlinked to tryptophan operon. It is a tetramer of four identical subunits and forms a complex with the co-repressor which is a small molecule, such as L-tryptophan. **Repressor-co-repressor complex,** in turn, binds to the operator and physically blocks the binding of RNA polymerase to the promoter. This, in turn, results in decreased rate of transcription. Besides, repressor is also known to regulate the transcription of its own gene, i.e. the R gene. Thus, when trp operon is actively transcribed, it is said to be derepressed, as the repressor alone cannot prevent the binding of RNA polymerase with the promoter. On the other hand, when repressor complexes with the co-repressor, trp operon gets repressed. Repression causes nearly 70-fold reduction in the rate of trp operon transcription.

- Trp operon also contains additional regulatory elements that impose further control on transcription. One of these additional control sites is a secondary promoter which is located within the coding sequence of the trp D gene and is designated as trp P_2. This secondary promoter is not regulated by the repressor but transcribes an mRNA that

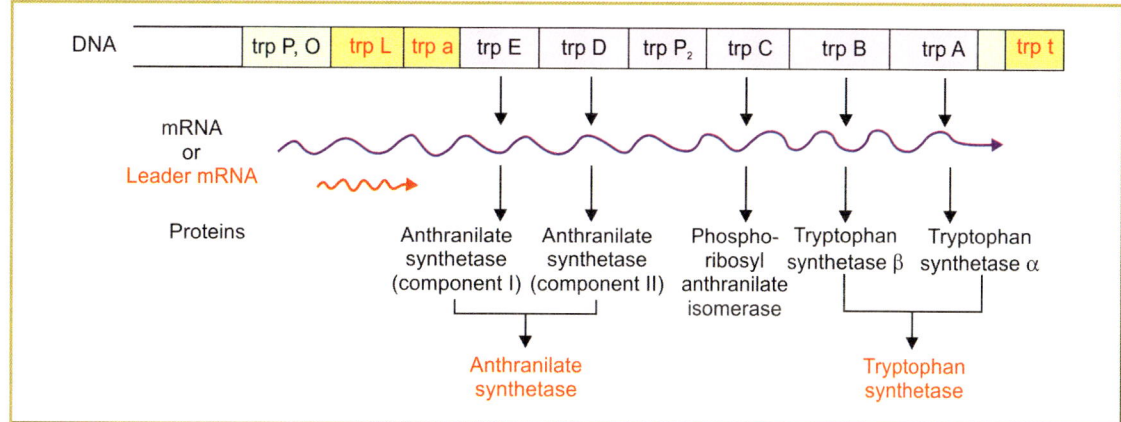

Fig. 22.7: Tryptophan operon of *E. coli.*

22

contains coding sequence for the last three genes of the operon (trp CBA).

- Besides, there also exists an additional transcriptional control element, located upstream of the trp E gene, in the leader sequence (**trp L**). This control element is termed as **attenuator**.

Regulatory elements of the tryptophan operon thus are: The primary promoter (trp P), operator (trp O), attenuator (trp a), secondary internal promoter (trp P_2) and terminator (trp t).

Attenuation

Attenuation is a prokaryotic mechanism for regulating transcription through modulation of the nascent RNA secondary structure. The **attenuator** is a short openreading frame encoding a 14-amino acid **leader peptide** which contains two adjacent tryptophan residues in positions 10 and 11. RNA sequence of the attenuator region contains four complementary segments, referred to as segments 1, 2, 3 and 4, respectively. These can adopt several possible secondary structures. Segments 3 and 4 together with the succeeding residues constitute a **transcription terminator** (a GC rich hairpin, followed by several U residues). Transcription rarely proceeds beyond this site (termination site) unless tryptophan is in short supply.

During tryptophan deficiency, the entire polycistronic mRNA, inclusive of the trp L sequence, is synthesized. After tryptophan synthesis starts, rate of transcription decreases since tryptophan binds to trp repressor. Tryptophan, in turn, results in premature termination of transcription. As a result of it, mRNA transcribes only the trp L segment.

Attenuation thus regulates trp operon transcription according to the supply of tryptophan.

3. BACTERIOPHAGE λ

One of the regulatory systems that controls the lifecycle of *E. coli* is bacteriophage λ. Soon after entering the host, the linear phage DNA with its complementary single-stranded ends called the cohesive ends (**cos sites**), circularizes and starts directing the replication process. At this stage, the virus has a choice of two alternative pathways, i.e. the **lytic mode** or the **lysogenic mode**. This, in turn, depends upon a complex system that regulates the transcription of phage genes (Fig. 22.8).

Lytic Pathway

In the lytic mode, phage DNA directs its own replication and the synthesis of the viral proteins, resulting in the lysis of the host cell and release of about 100 progeny phage particles. In the lytic mode of replication of the phage, proper timing is essential.

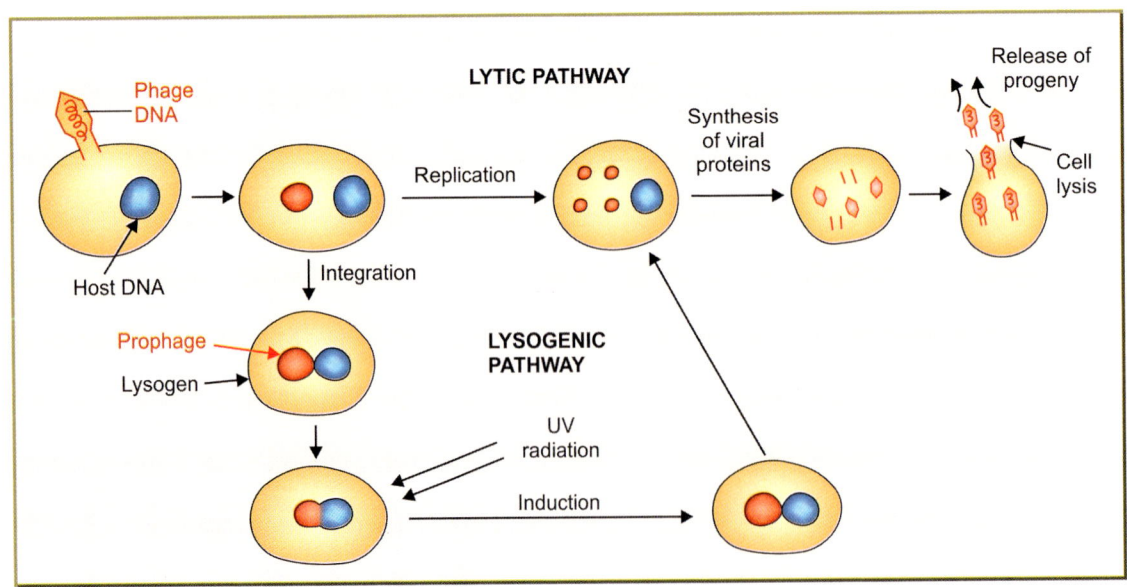

Fig. 22.8: Lytic/lysogenic cycle of bacteriophage λ.

Lysogenic Pathway

In the lysogenic pathway, phage DNA is integrated at a specific site in the host chromosome in such a way that the phage DNA passively replicates with the host cell. The phage is then designated as a **prophage** and the host is called **lysogen**. DNA damage, e.g. by UV radiation can induce excision of the prophage from the lysogenic bacterial chromosome and cause the phage to take up the lytic cycle. Phage DNA can be excised from the host DNA even after many bacterial generations to initiate a lytic cycle. However, when the host DNA is damaged, the phage enters the lytic mode and escapes the host.

Phage integrity is mediated by integrase, the product of int gene which acts as a type I topoisomerase. It nicks and reseals one strand of the double-helical DNA. Integrase functions with excisionase in removing prophage from the host DNA, in the lytic pathway.

REGULATION OF GENE EXPRESSION IN EUKARYOTES

Gene regulation in eukaryotes is more complex than in prokaryotes due to the reason that most of the DNA is packed in inaccessible structures called chromatin. Moreover, a vast majority of DNA in multicellular organisms is not transcribed. In eukaryotes, gene expression is regulated at three distinct levels:

1. Transcriptional level
2. Processing level
3. Translational level.

These aspects are briefly discussed below.

Regulation at Transcriptional Level

Transcriptional control mechanisms determine whether or not a gene is transcribed and if so, how often. It is important to realize that **all the differentiated eukaryotic cells retain all of the genetic information; however, different genes are expressed at different stages of development by cells in different tissues, and by cells exposed to different stimuli.**

Transcription of a particular gene is **controlled by transcription factors (TF)** which are proteins that bind to specific sequences located beyond the gene's coding region. The closest upstream regulatory sequence is the TATA box which is also the site of assembly of the pre-initiation complex. The activity of proteins at the TATA box depends on interactions with other proteins

bound to other sites (e.g. various 'response elements' or 'enhancers'). Proteins bound to enhancers or promoters are brought into contact by loops in the DNA. Further, TF contain at least **two domains**, one whose function is to recognize and bind to a specific DNA sequence, and another whose function is to regulate transcription (stimulate or inhibit) by interacting with other proteins. The TF bind to DNA as homo- or heterodimers with the help of unique structural DNA-binding motifs/domains.

DNA-binding Domains

Transcription factors contain many common types of motifs that are responsible for their binding to DNA. These DNA-binding domains are usually quite short and comprise only a small part of the protein structure. Several types of DNA-binding motifs exist:

Zinc finger motif: It is a small group of conserved amino acids with a characteristic pattern of cysteine and histidine residues that constitute the zinc binding site (Fig. 22.9). Zinc finger motifs are found in two

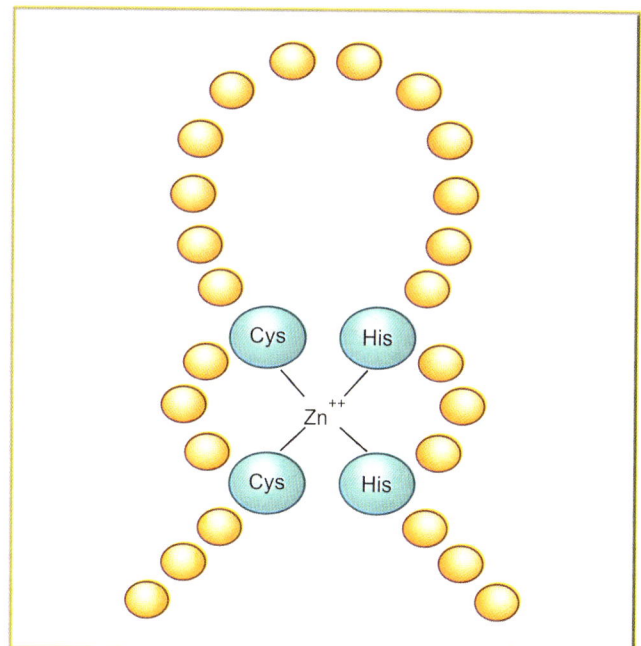

Fig. 22.9: A zinc finger. The motif takes its name from the loop of 12 amino acids (yellow) that protrudes from the zinc-binding site. Either 2 cysteine and 2 histidine residues (a cysteine-histidine zinc finger) or 4 cysteine residues (a cysteine-cysteine zinc finger) coordinate a zinc ion. The loop intercalates directly into the DNA helix. It was originally found in the factor TFIIIA, required for RNA Pol III to transcribe 5S rRNA genes.

22

types of DNA-binding proteins, such as the zinc finger proteins (e.g. TFIIIA) and some of the steroid receptors (e.g. estrogen receptors).

Steroids such as estrogen, due to their hydrophobic nature, diffuse across the cell membrane. Within the cell, estrogen binds to the highly specific soluble receptor proteins (eukaryotic transcription factors), called as nuclear hormone receptors. They have two highly conserved domains, i.e. a DNA-binding domain and a ligand-binding domain. DNA-binding domain lies towards the center of the molecule and provides these receptors with sequence-specific DNA binding sites. **Zinc ions stabilize the structure of these domains**, hence such domains are often referred to as zinc finger domains. Estrogen receptors bind to specific DNA sites referred to as estrogen response elements (EREs) that contain a consensus sequence. The second highly conserved region of the nuclear receptor proteins is referred to as the ligand-binding site. On binding of the ligand (signal molecule), ligand-receptor complex modifies the expression of the specific genes, by binding to control elements in the DNA.

Steroid receptors: Most of the steroid receptors such as the glucocorticoid receptors have several independent domains. These are the members of a superfamily of transcription factors, each one of which is activated by binding to a particular receptor molecule. Each of these small molecules binds to its specific receptor that activates gene expression.

Homeodomains: These domains bind related targets in DNA. The C-terminal region of the homeodomain, present in proteins of many eukaryotes, is homologous with the helix-turn-helix motif of prokaryotic repressors. Homeodomain proteins contain a sequence of 60 amino acids which can be either transcriptional activators or repressors. The homeodomain particularly identifies genes concerned with the developmental regulation.

Helix-loop-helix motif: The amphipathic helix-loop-helix motif is found in some developmental regulators and in genes coding for the eukaryotic DNA-binding proteins. Each amphipathic helix presents a face of hydrophobic residues on one side and charged residues on the other side. The length of the connecting loop varies from 12 to 28 amino acids. The motif enables proteins to dimerize and a basic region near

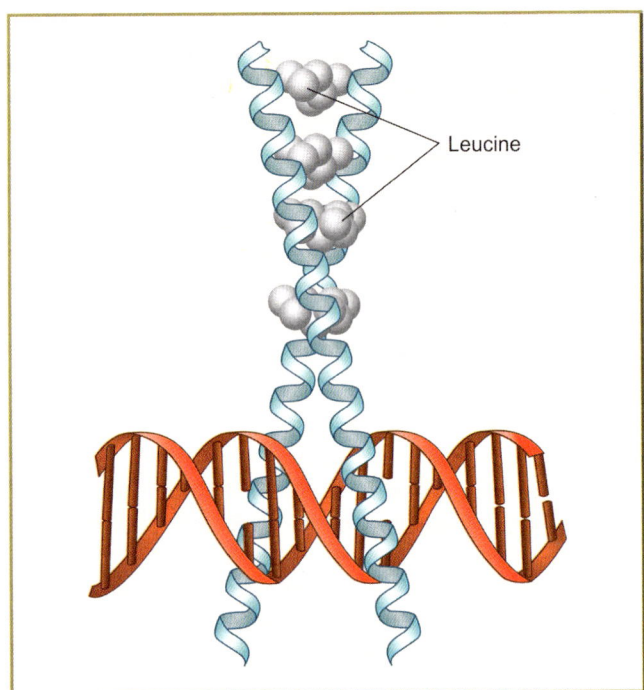

Leucine

Fig. 22.10: The leucine zipper is a stretch of amino acids rich in leucine residues (grey) providing a dimerization motif. The zipper forms an amphipathic helix in which the leucines of the zipper on one protein (blue) protrude from the α-helix and interdigitate with the leucines of the zipper of another protein in parallel to form a coiled coil domain. The region adjacent to the leucine repeats is highly basic in each of the zipper proteins, comprising a DNA-binding site. The 2 leucine zippers form a Y-shaped structure, in which the zippers comprise the stem, and the 2 basic regions bifurcate symmetrically to form the arms that bind to DNA (red).

this motif contacts DNA. These protein motifs thus interact by combinatorial association.

Leucine zippers: Leucine zippers consist of a stretch of amino acids with a leucine residue in every seventh position (Fig. 22.10). A leucine zipper in one polypeptide interacts with a zipper in another polypeptide to form a dimer. Adjacent to each zipper is a stretch of positively charged residues that is involved in its binding to DNA. Leucine zippers are found in the factors jun and fos, the products of the gene c-jun and c-fos respectively.

Co-activators and Co-repressors

Activation/repression of transcription is mediated by a number of large complexes that function as co-activators/co-repressors. They serve as bridges between TF bound at upstream regulatory sites and the basal transcription machinery bound at the core

Chemistry to Clinics 22.1: HATs as Drug Targets

A potential role of HATs in the pathology of cancer, asthma, chronic obstructive pulmonary disease (COPD) and viral infection has been described. Thus, specific HAT inhibitors may find therapeutic applications.

Chemistry to Clinics 22.3: DNA Methyltransferase Inhibitor

Decitabine is a new anticancer drug which acts as false substrate to inhibit DNA methyltransferase. Reduced DNA methylation results in enhanced expression of anti-oncogenes thereby suppressing tumor growth.

promoter. Other specialized co-activators include histone acetyl transferases (**HATs**) responsible for acetylation of core histones resulting in transcriptional activation, and chromatin remodeling complexes causing nucleosomes to slide along DNA.

Histone acetyl transferases (HATs): As nucleosomes bind DNA tightly, it is not possible for RNA polymerase and its associated transcription factors to get access to promoter of the gene, to initiate transcription. In order to alter the structure of chromatin and make it accessible for the transcription machinery, histones are acetylated in a controlled fashion. The ε-amino groups of Lys residues near the N-termini of histones H3 and H4 are acetylated by cytoplasmic HATs. There are two groups of HATs: **Group A** describes those enzymes that are involved with transcription while **group B** describes the enzymes which are involved with nucleosome assembly. Acetylation of histones thus occurs at both replication and transcription (Chemistry to Clinics 22.1).

Histone acetylation decreases the affinity of histones for DNA, making additional genes accessible for transcription. On the other hand, a family of **histone deacetylases** removes the acetyl groups which were activated by histone acetylation. This silencing of genes facilitates the recruitment of RNA polymerase to other genes, so as to limit the amount of chromatin for scanning by the transcription factors. Deacetylation, in turn, contributes to transcriptional repression and conversely, repressors may be associated with deacetylases.

Methylation/Demethylation of DNA

In mammals, **transcriptionally silent DNA is highly methylated** than the DNA that is transcribed

(Chemistry to Clinics 22.2). About 70% of the 5'-CpG-3' sequences in mammalian genomes are methylated at the C5 position of cytosine. However, the distribution of these methylated cytosines varies depending upon the cell type. Methylation is catalyzed by **DNA methyltransferases** (Chemistry to Clinics 22.3).

The methyl group of 5-methylcytosine is projected into the major groove where it interferes with the binding of proteins that stimulate transcription. Relative absence of the 5-methylcytosine, near the start site, is referred to as **hypomethylation/under-methylation**. Only few sites are methylated in tissues in which the gene is expressed suggesting that an active gene may be undermethylated. The region of undermethylation coincides with the region of maximum sensitivity to DNase1. Demethylation at the promoter may be necessary to make it available for the initiation of transcription and is carried out by demethylases. The nucleosomes at the CpG-rich unmethylated islands in the 5' regions also have a reduced content of histone H1.

Another phenomenon associated with DNA methylation is '**genomic imprinting**'. Certain genes are active or inactive during early developmental stage depending solely on whether they were brought into the zygote by the sperm or the egg/ovum, i.e. the genes are 'imprinted' according to their parental origin. Genomic imprinting is an '**epigenetic**' phenomenon because the difference between alleles is based on parental inheritance and not on DNA sequence. It is the result of selective DNA methylation of one of

Chemistry to Clinics 22.2: DNA Methylation in Health and Disease

DNA methylation is an epigenetic modification of the genome that is involved in embryonic development, transcription, X chromosome inactivation, genomic imprinting, maintaining chromatin structure and chromosome stability. Altered DNA methylation is common in many conditions including cancer.

Chemistry to Clinics 22.4: Syndromes Related to Genomic Imprinting

In Prader-Willi syndrome, several genes on chromosome 15 of paternal origin are non-expressed or deleted. The maternal copy of the genes is imprinted and silenced. Children present with disturbances in physical and sexual development besides eating disorders. The converse, i.e. non-expressed genes on chromosome 15 of maternal origin and imprinted/silenced paternal copy of genes results in Angelman syndrome characterized by developmental delay, speech impairment and an apparently happy expression.

22

the two alleles. Examples of imprinted genes include- gene encoding a fetal growth factor called insulin-like growth factor 2 (**IGF 2**) is active only on the chromosome transmitted from the father whereas gene encoding a specific K-channel (**KVLQT1**) is only active on the chromosome transmitted from the mother. Disturbances in imprinting patterns are associated with specific diseases (Chemistry to Clinics 22.4).

Riboswitches

It refers to conserved sequences of some mRNAs in the 5′ or 3′ untranslated region. These regions bind specific metabolites and regulate gene expression in response to changing concentrations of those metabolites.

Regulation at Processing Level

Gene expression is regulated at the processing level by alternative splicing or RNA editing.

Alternative splicing: It is a process whereby a single gene can encode two or more related proteins. Many primary transcripts can be processed by more than one pathway, producing **mRNAs containing different combinations of exons**. An example of alternative splicing occurs during the synthesis of a protein **fibronectin** found in blood as well as the extracellular matrix (ECM). Fibronectin produced by fibroblasts and retained in the ECM contains two extra peptides compared to the one produced by hepatocytes and secreted into the blood. The extra peptides are encoded by portions of the pre-mRNA that are retained during processing in the fibroblast but are removed during processing in the hepatocyte.

RNA editing: It involves changes in an RNA transcript by **deaminating a base**. For example, an 'A'→'I' change (adenine to inosine; deamination at 6-position in a purine ring) can be catalyzed by adenosine deaminase. This changes the coding possibilities since 'I' pairs with 'G' (instead of 'A' pairing with 'U', if editing had not occurred). Editing of RNA transcripts of **cerebral glutamate receptors** by this mechanism dramatically alters their ion-conductance properties. Another example is a 'C'→'U' change (cytosine to uracil; deamination at 4-position in a pyrimidine ring) catalyzed by cytosine deaminase. This again changes the coding possibilities since 'U' pairs with 'A' (instead

of 'C' pairing with 'G', if editing had not occurred). Editing of apo B-100 transcripts by this mechanism changes codon 2153 from CAA (encoding glutamine) to UAA (a stop codon), resulting in a shorter protein product apo B-48. This is the reason why **apo B-100** is formed in the **liver** and secreted in **VLDL** whereas **apo B 48** (consisting of only the N-terminal 48% of apo B 100) is formed in the **small intestine** and secreted in **chylomicrons**.

Regulation at Translational Level

Gene expression is regulated at the translational level by various processes including **mRNA localization, control of translation of existing mRNAs, and mRNA longevity**. For example, in eukaryotes, genes encoding proteins that transport and store **iron** are regulated at the translational level. Iron response elements (IRE) present in certain mRNAs are bound by an IRE-binding protein when this protein is not bound with iron. Location of the IRE regulates expression of the gene, in response to changes in iron status of the cell.

Expression levels of ferritin (an iron storage protein found primarily in the liver and the kidney) and transferrin (a transport protein that carries iron in the serum) receptors, are reciprocally related in their responses to changes in iron level. When iron is deficient, the amount of transferrin receptors increases and little or no new ferritin is synthesized. An increase in the cellular iron level leads to the destruction of transferrin-receptor mRNA and hence, a reduction in the production of transferrin receptor protein. The extent of mRNA synthesis for these proteins, however, does not change correspondingly. Instead, regulation takes place at the level of translation.

The **major regulatory points** of eukaryotic gene expression are highlighted in Fig. 22.11.

GENE EXPRESSION IN PROKARYOTES VERSUS EUKARYOTES

The overall control of gene expression is much more complex in eukaryotes and the major differences are presented in Table 22.1.

1. The genome being regulated is significantly **larger** in eukaryotes, e.g. the E. coli genome consists of a single circular chromosome containing 4.6×10^6 bases, compared to approximately 40,000 genes containing 3000×10^6 bases in human DNA.

22

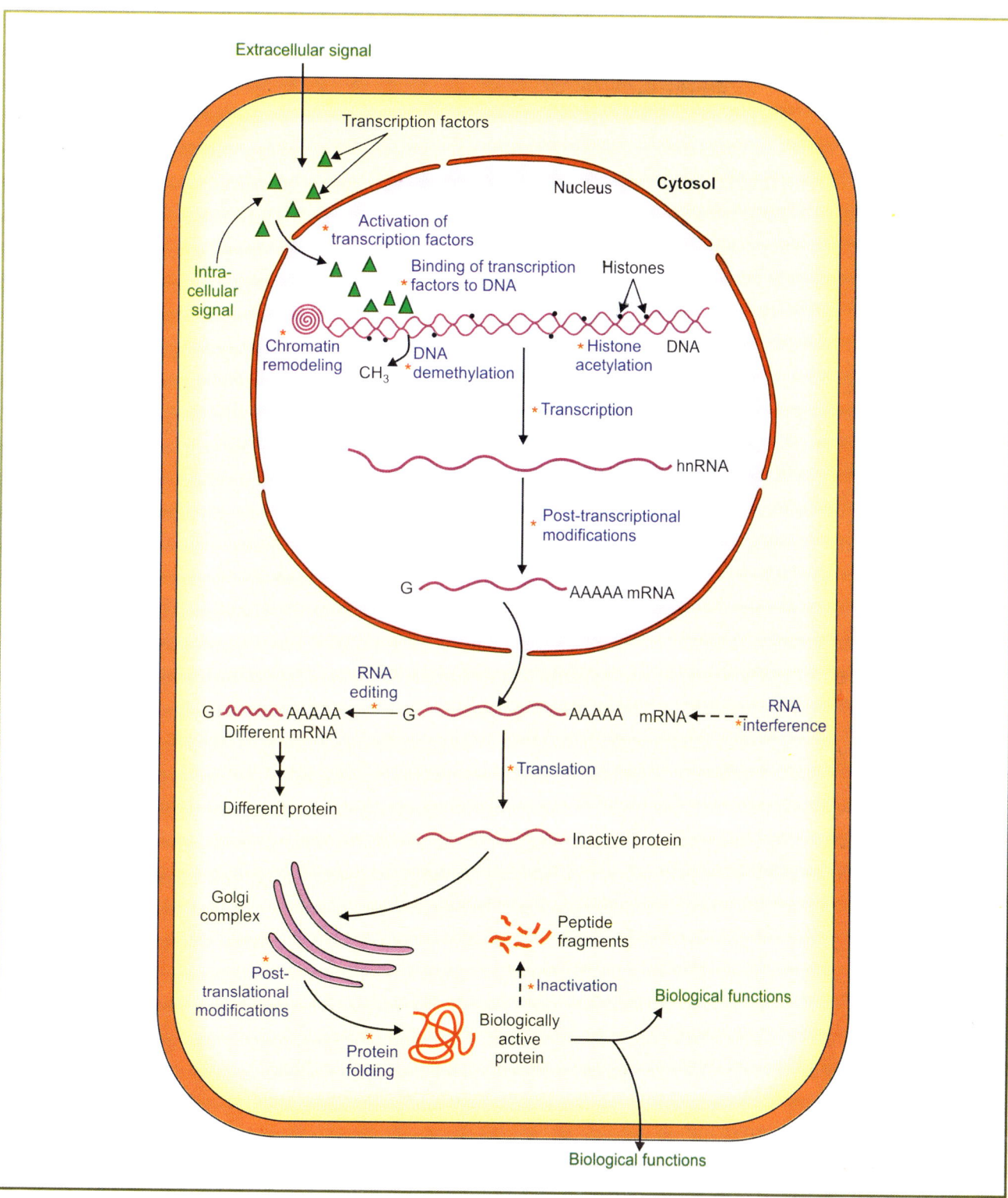

Fig. 22.11: Various steps (*) of regulation of eukaryotic gene expression: Chromatin remodeling, histone acetylation, DNA demethylation, activation of transcription factors, binding of transcription factors to DNA, transcription, post-transcriptional modifications, RNA editing, RNA interference, translation, post-translational modifications, protein folding and degradation.

22

Table 22.1: Differences in regulation of gene expression in prokaryotes and eukaryotes

Parameter	Prokaryotes	Eukaryotes
Genome size	Smaller; 4.6×10^6 bases in *E. coli*	Larger; 3000×10^6 bases in humans
Cell types	Usually a single type	Different cell types (e.g. liver cells, pancreatic cells); each contains the same set of genes but in different cells they are differentially expressed
Operons	Present	Absent
Transcription and translation	Coupled	Uncoupled
Untranscribed DNA	Very small amount	Large amount
Overall control of gene expression	Simple	Complex

2. Many eukaryotes have **different cell types**, e.g. the liver cells and the pancreatic cells, etc. These cells differ from others as their genes are differentially expressed.
3. Eukaryotic genes are **not organized into operons** but are spread widely across the genome.
4. In prokaryotes, transcription and translation are tightly coupled, i.e. protein synthesis starts on mRNA templates well before the mRNA has been completely synthesized. In eukaryotes, transcription and translation are distinct processes occurring in the nucleus and cytoplasm respectively. Thus, **transcription and translation are uncoupled** in eukaryotes.
5. A large amount of **non-transcribable DNA** is present in eukaryotes.

SOME IMPORTANT QUESTIONS

1. Describe regulation of gene expression in prokaryotes. How it differs from eukaryotes?

2. Discuss:
    i. Types of regulation of gene expression
    ii. Lac operon
    iii. Catabolite repression
    iv. Attenuation
    v. Chromatin remodeling

3. Write notes on:
    i. Gene cluster
    ii. Non-transcribable DNA
    iii. The operon
    iv. Lac repressor
    v. Tryptophan operon
    vi. Replication of bacteriophage λ
    vii. DNA-binding domains
    viii. Genomic imprinting

MULTIPLE CHOICE QUESTIONS

1. **The non-transcribable DNA constitutes:**
   A. Regulatory sequences
   B. Origin and termination of replication
   C. Centromeres and telomeres
   D. All of the above

2. **The following is not a product of structural genes in lac operon:**
   A. β-Galactosidase
   B. Permease
   C. Lac repressor
   D. Transacetylase

3. **Following histone acetylation, the affinity of histones for DNA:**
   A. Remains unchanged
   B. Decreases

   C. Increases
   D. Any of the above

4. **The commonest methylated base in transcriptionally silent mammalian DNA is:**
   A. Adenine
   B. Thymine
   C. Guanine
   D. Cytosine

5. **The difference between apo B-48 and apo B-100 is due to:**
   A. Genomic imprinting
   B. Alternative splicing
   C. Frame shift mutation
   D. RNA editing

22

Genetic Engineering

23

Recombinant DNA is a DNA molecule having different fragments from different sources. The science of various techniques used in the dissection of complex genomes into defined fragments, with complete analysis of the nucleotide sequences and functions is called **recombinant DNA technology** or **molecular cloning** or **genetic engineering**. The technology makes it possible to isolate, amplify and modify specific DNA sequences. This, in turn, allows the removal of a piece of DNA out of a larger molecule such as the genome of a virus or a human being and its amplification.

Palindrome

In a palindromic DNA segment, the sequence of nucleotides is the same in each strand when the two strands of the palindrome are read in opposite directions, i.e. it has **two-fold symmetry**. These sequences are four to six nucleotides long and are the sites which are recognized and cleaved by restriction endonucleases. The recognized sequences are **completely symmetrical inverted repeats**, known as palindromes (Fig. 23.1). They also serve as recognition sites for methylases that modify the host DNA by introducing methyl groups into two bases of a palindrome. Once these bases are methylated, the palindrome cannot be recognized by the corres-

ponding restriction endonuclease and thus the DNA gets protected from cleavage.

Restriction Endonucleases

Restriction endonucleases (**restriction enzymes**) are the enzymes that recognize and cleave specific DNA sequences which are symmetrical inverted repeats, known as palindromes. Their salient characteristics include (Table 23.1):

- Highly **specific** enzymes which make **two cuts**, one in each strand of the double-stranded DNA and generate a 3'-OH terminus and a 5'-p terminus. They are named according to the bacterial source from which they are isolated: The first letter of the genus and first two letters of the species of the bacterium that produces it, followed by its serotype or strain, if any. There may also be a Roman numeral if the bacterium contains more than one type of the restriction enzyme.
- Classified into **three categories**, i.e. as types I, II and III. Types I and III make cuts in the vicinity of the recognition sites in an unpredictable manner. Type II specifically cuts DNA within the recognition sequences. Type II enzymes are very useful in the

Table 23.1: Salient features of restriction endonucleases

- Isolated from bacteria
- Recognize and cleave specific DNA sequences (palindromes)
- Generate sticky ends or blunt ends
- Some are isoschizomers
- Used to prepare restriction digest
- Used to prepare restriction map

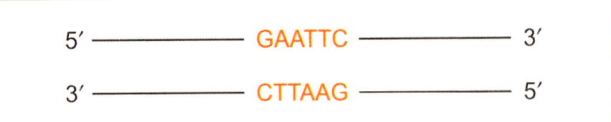

Fig. 23.1: A palindrome.

laboratory for the reconstruction of a genetic map. A large number of restriction enzymes with various recognition sequences have been characterized, such as EcoRI, the enzyme isolated from *E. coli* RY13.

- Most of the restriction endonucleases cleave two strands of a DNA in a staggered manner and produce fragments with single-stranded regions at their 5' and 3' ends, called as the **sticky-ends or cohesive ends**. DNA fragments generated from different molecules with the same restriction endonuclease have complementary single-stranded ends which can be annealed and covalently linked together with a DNA ligase, producing a recombinant DNA molecule.

    Some of the restriction endonucleases cut both the strands symmetrically and produce restriction fragments with base-paired ends, called as the **flush-ends or blunt-ends**. Enzymatically, a poly (dA) tail is added to one of the species of the blunt-ended DNA while a poly (dT) tail is added to the blunt-ended DNA of the other species. These two DNA fragments with complementary tails can then be annealed and ligated (Fig. 23.2).

- Confer **protection** to the host bacteria against invading bacteriophages (viruses that are specific for bacteria). Bacterial DNA sequences normally recognized by a restriction endonuclease may be protected from cleavage by methylation of certain nucleotide specific sequences of its own DNA (enzyme recognized palindromes) by methylases. On the other hand, viral DNA that has not been methylated on at least one of its two strands is recognized as foreign and is hydrolyzed by the restriction endonuclease.

- Sometimes, different restriction enzymes recognize and cleave within identical target sequences. They are referred to as **isoschizomers**, meaning that they cut at the same site. For example, EcoRII and AtuI are isoschizomers cutting at ↓CCAGG.

- Treatment of the DNA molecule with a restriction endonuclease results in the production of a series of precisely **defined fragments** that can be separated according to their size by gel electrophoresis and visualized by an appropriate technique, such as staining, fluorescence or radioactive labelling. A particular enzyme thus generates a unique family of fragments for any given DNA molecule. The product of fragmentation is called 'restriction digest'.

- Restriction endonucleases are used to construct a new type of genetic map, referred to as a **restriction map**.

RESTRICTION MAP

Restriction map is a **diagrammatic representation** of a DNA molecule, showing the sites recognized by restriction endonuclease. It is constructed by the analysis of the fragments which are generated by the digestion of the DNA with a restriction endonuclease. In a restriction map, sites of the enzymatic cleavage within the DNA are also defined (Fig. 23.3).

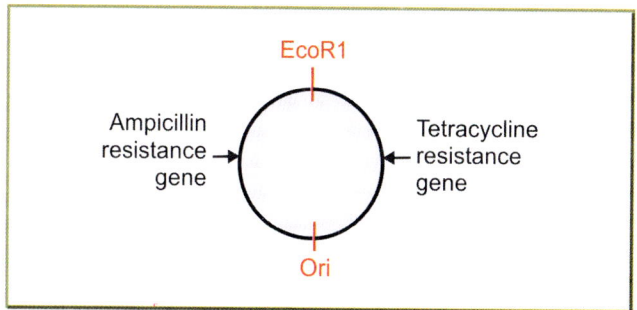

Fig. 23.3: A restriction map.

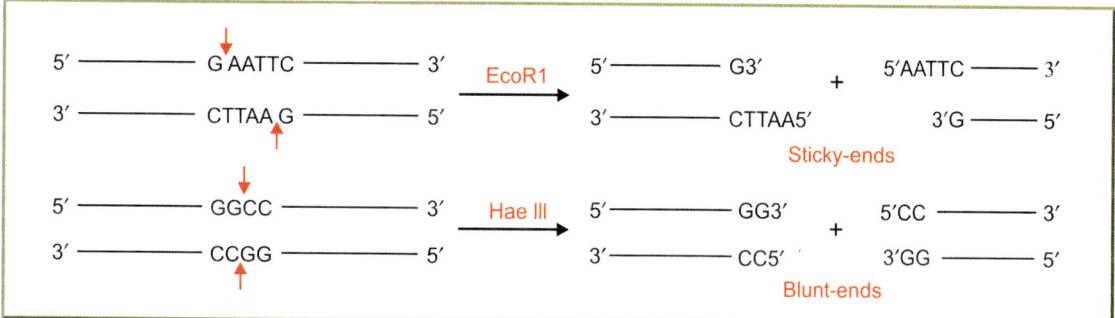

Fig. 23.2: Action of type II restriction endonucleases.

23

Technique: For the restriction endonuclease mapping of DNA, the purified DNA is subjected to a restriction endonuclease digestion for varying times which generates partially-to-fully cleaved DNA fragments. These fragments are separated by agarose gel electrophoresis and stained with ethidium bromide. Sizes of the DNA fragments are determined by their relative migration through the gel. DNA bands are visualized with a UV light source and photographed. The relative size of each fragment within the DNA molecule is deduced from the size of the incompletely hydrolyzed fragments.

Uses of restriction maps: Restriction maps are the convenient frameworks locating particular base sequences on a chromosome, and for comparing different chromosomes. Restriction maps can be used to:

- Demonstrate **sequence diversity** of the organelles DNA, such as mitochondrial DNA within the species.
- Detect **deletion mutations**.
- For **cloning and sequencing** of the genes and their flanking DNA regions.

CLONING

A clone is the collection of identical cells arising from a common ancestor. Cloning is a technique for the production of **multiple identical copies** of a DNA segment or a cell of an organism that contains the desired DNA. Various small autonomously replicating DNA molecules are used as cloning vectors.

Vector

A vector (a cloning vector) is a molecule of **carrier DNA** to which the fragment of foreign DNA, to be cloned, can be attached. A vector must:

- Be capable of autonomous replication.
- Contain at least one specific nucleotide sequence recognizable by a restriction endonuclease.
- Carry at least one gene that confers its ability as a vector.

Commonly used vectors include a plasmid, a bacteriophage, a cosmid, or yeast artificial chromosome.

Plasmid: Plasmids are small circular DNA molecules of only a few thousand base-pairs, found in **prokaryotes**. Plasmids replicate independently of replication of the main bacterial chromosome. They replicate easily, carry genes that confer resistance to one or more antibiotics and have several restriction sites where foreign DNA can be easily inserted. Bacterial plasmids are most suited as recombinant DNA vectors. These are, however, useful to clone DNA segments of up to 10 Kb-pairs only.

Bacteriophage λ: Bacteriophage λ (phage λ) is a type of **virus** (phage particle) that infects and replicates in bacteria. It is a cloning vector that can accommodate DNA inserts of up to 16 Kb-pairs. The λ phage selectively infects bacteria and can replicate by either a lytic or a lysogenic (nonlytic) pathway. It contains a self complementary 12 bases long single-stranded tail, called the cohesive termini (cos sites) at both the ends of its double-stranded DNA molecule.

During infection by the phage, DNA contained in the head of the phage particle enters the bacteria where it is replicated nearly hundred-times and packaged to form progeny phage particles. The part of the phage particle which is not required for infection can be replaced by foreign DNA. Such a recombinant DNA, also called chimeric DNA, is packaged into phage particles and can be introduced into the host cell.

Cosmid: Cosmid vectors are a **cross between plasmid and bacteriophage**. Cosmids contain an antibiotic resistance gene for the selection of a recombinant DNA molecule, an origin of replication for propagation in bacteria and a cos site for packaging of the recombinant molecules in the bacteriophages. A cosmid vector can accommodate foreign DNA insert of up to nearly 45 Kb-pairs.

Yeast artificial chromosomes: Yeast artificial chromosomes are linear DNA molecules that contain all the chromosomal structures required for normal replication and segregation, during **yeast cell division**. Much large DNA segments (up to several hundred Kb-pairs) can be cloned in these vectors.

GENOMIC LIBRARY

Genomic library is a **set of cloned DNA fragments representing the entire genome of the organism**. When a complex mixture of thousands of genes, arranged on different chromosomes (such as in the human genome), is subjected to hydrolysis with a single restriction endonuclease, it results in the generation of a large number of DNA fragments. These DNA fragments are annealed with a vector which has also been cleaved with the same restriction enzyme. Usually, only one of the DNA fragment out of the large number, is inserted into each vector. Bacteria are transformed with the recombinant molecules in such a way that only one plasmid is taken up by a single bacterium. Each recombinant molecule gets replicated within the bacterium. Since each bacterium progeny carries multiple copies of the recombinant DNA, the total population of bacteria now contains fragments of DNA that may represent the entire human genome.

Complementary DNA and cDNA Library

Transcription of a functional eukaryotic mRNA with the use of RNA dependent DNA polymerase (**reverse transcriptase**) in the presence of the four dNTPs, results in the formation of a complementary strand of DNA, called complementary DNA (cDNA). The collection of cloned cDNAs synthesized from the total mRNA, in a given tissue or cell type is called a cDNA library, such as liver cDNA library, reticulocyte cDNA library, etc. A cDNA library thus **represents the population of mRNAs** in a tissue.

cDNA libraries are prepared by first isolating all the mRNAs in a tissue and then copying these molecules into double-stranded DNA using the enzymes reverse transcriptase and DNA polymerase. For the construction of a recombinant DNA, the cloning vector and the foreign DNA are cut by the same restriction endonuclease. The complementary ends of the two DNAs, i.e. the vector and the foreign DNA fragments, form base-pairs (anneal) and are covalently joined (ligated) by the action of DNA ligase. This, in turn, results in the formation of a chimeric DNA containing a portion of the foreign DNA inserted into the vector (Fig. 23.4).

Directional Cloning versus Shotgun Cloning

DNA molecules whose ends have different overhangs can be used to form chimeric constructs in which the foreign DNA can enter the plasmid in only one orientation, not randomly. For this, the **foreign DNA** is digested with **two different restriction enzymes**. The **same two enzymes** are used to digest the **plasmid** followed by ligation. This is **directional cloning**.

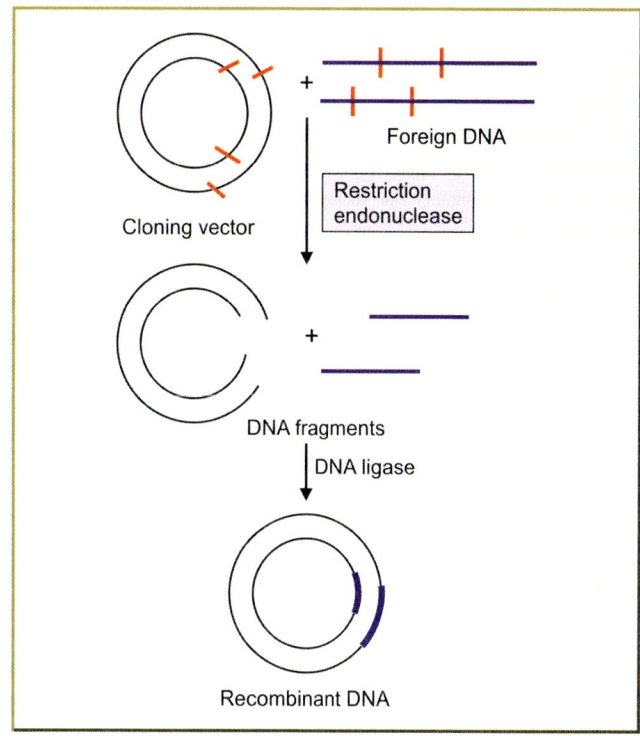

Fig. 23.4: Construction of a recombinant (chimeric) DNA.

A particular gene constitutes a very small part of the genome so that it is cumbersome to attempt to recover such sequences from the isolated DNA. Instead, a genomic library is prepared by isolating total DNA, digesting it into fragments of suitable sizes and cloning them into an appropriate vector. This approach is called **shotgun cloning,** because it does not target a particular gene but instead **clones all the genes at one time**. The idea is that at least one clone will contain at least some part of the gene of interest. For this, the DNA is only partly digested so that not every restriction site is cleaved in every DNA molecule. Therefore, even if the gene of interest contains a susceptible restriction site, some intact genes are still present in the digest.

Functional Cloning versus Positional Cloning

In a disease, if an **abnormal protein is already identified**, functionally characterized and sequenced, it is possible to develop probes which can identify and locate the corresponding gene on the chromosome. This is **functional cloning** through which the **gene for hemophilia A** was identified.

On the other hand, the **abnormal protein may be unknown** but genetic mapping in affected families

23

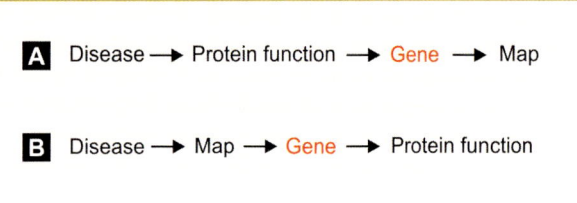

A Disease ⟶ Protein function ⟶ Gene ⟶ Map

B Disease ⟶ Map ⟶ Gene ⟶ Protein function

Fig. 23.5: Functional cloning (A) and positional cloning (B).

identifies the chromosomal position of the gene and ultimately the gene itself. Thus, the amino acid sequence may be deduced followed by its functional characterization and link with the disease. This is **positional cloning** through which the gene and **mutated protein for cystic fibrosis** was identified (Fig. 23.5).

STEPS IN RECOMBINANT DNA TECHNOLOGY

Recombinant DNA technology involves several steps:
1. A fragment of DNA of the appropriate size is generated by using restriction endonuclease.
2. The fragment is isolated and incorporated into another DNA molecule known as a vector which contains sequences necessary to direct DNA replication.
3. The vector, with the DNA of interest, is introduced into the cells where it is replicated.
4. Finally, cells containing the desired DNA are identified.

RESTRICTION FRAGMENT LENGTH POLYMORPHISM (RFLP)

The human genome is extremely heterogeneous. A variation which affects **<1%** of a population is called a 'genetic variant' whereas that affecting **≥1%** of the population is termed as **'genetic polymorphism'**. A high degree of genetic polymorphism describes individuality in human and other species. There are inherited differences in DNA sequences among the members of the same species. These differences, in turn, lead to variations in the sites of cleavage of DNA by particular restriction endonucleases producing DNA fragments of different lengths.

The length of the restriction fragment is altered if the genetic variant alters the DNA so as to create or abolish a site of restriction endonuclease cleavage. RFLPs can be used to detect human genetic defects, e.g. in prospective parents or in fetal tissue. As homologous human chromosomes differ in sequences, these genetic differences result in different restriction sites. For example, whole human genomic DNA isolated from two individuals and digested with a restriction endonuclease when transferred (blotted) to a nitrocellulose filter and hybridized with a probe showed different pattern of bands. Individual A presented a normal pattern while individual B had a high molecular weight band (Fig. 23.6). The action of a restriction enzyme on two homologous chromosomes (DNA) thus results in the formation of

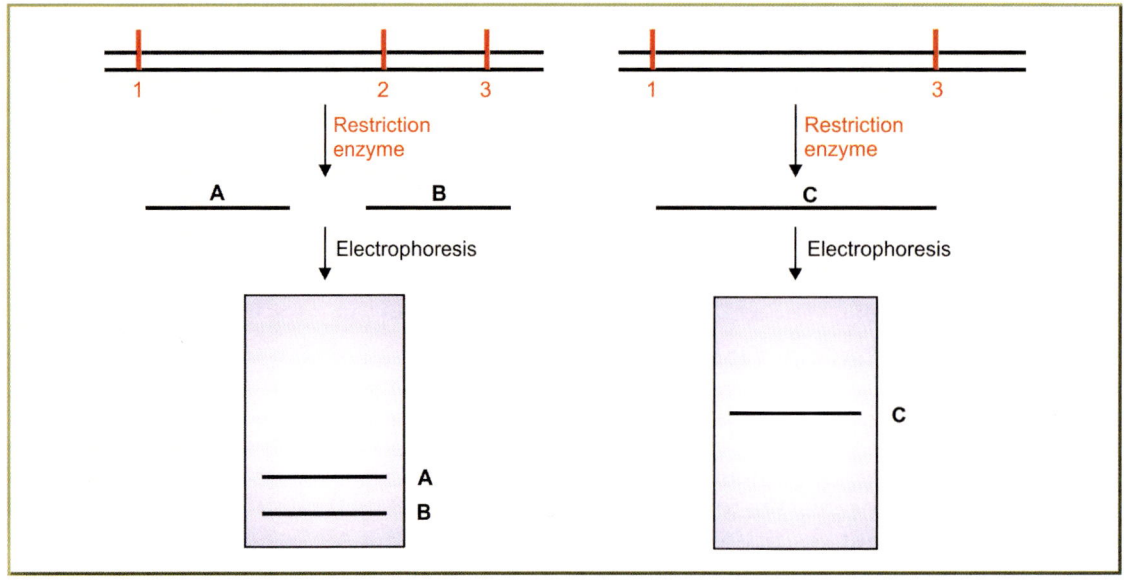

Fig. 23.6: RFLP analysis of two homologous chromosomes.

Chemistry to Clinics 23.1: Restriction Fragment Length Poly-morphism (RFLP)

RFLP is useful in the diagnosis of those inherited disorders for which a molecular defect is not known, such as to define the clonal origin of tumors. If a particular RFLP is closely linked to a defective gene, the detection of such an RFLP in an individual indicates high probability of inheritance of such a defective gene.

fragments with different lengths due to the altered DNA, i.e. the two DNA molecules show restriction fragment length polymorphism (RFLP) (Chemistry to Clinics 23.1).

CHROMOSOME WALKING

The technique is used either to analyze long stretches of DNA or when the sequence is known but the **location of a particular gene is unknown**. It involves the following steps (Fig. 23.7):

- A clone is selected from a genomic library and a small fragment from one end is subcloned.
- The subclone is hybridized with other clones and a second clone is identified that hybridizes with the previous subclone.
- The end of the second clone is then subcloned and used similarly for hybridization.
- The process is repeated and restriction map of each selected clone is constructed at each step and

compared to know the region of overlap, equivalent to **'walking along the chromosome'**. The **cystic fibrosis gene** was identified by this technique.

DNA SEQUENCING

The process of determining the **sequence of nucleotides** in DNA is designated as DNA sequencing. The sequence, in turn, also highlights the sequences of their encoded proteins. DNA sequencing also reveals information about the regulation of genes. Once known, a nucleic acid sequence can be duplicated, modified and expressed. This facilitates the study of proteins that could not otherwise by obtained in large quantities.

For determining the sequence of a small polynucleotide, it is partially digested with snake venom phosphodiesterase which breaks phosphodiester bonds between the nucleotide residues starting at the 3′ end of the nucleotide. This, in turn, results in a mixture of fragments of all lengths which can be separated. By comparing the base composition of a pair of fragments that differ in length by one nucleotide, the identity of the 3′-terminal nucleotide in the larger fragment can be established. Analysis of each pair of fragments thus reveals the sequence of the original polynucleotide (Fig. 23.8).

POLYMERASE CHAIN REACTION

Polymerase chain reaction (**PCR**) is a procedure for **amplifying a segment of DNA by repeated rounds of replication** centered between primers that hybridize with the two ends of DNA segment of interest.

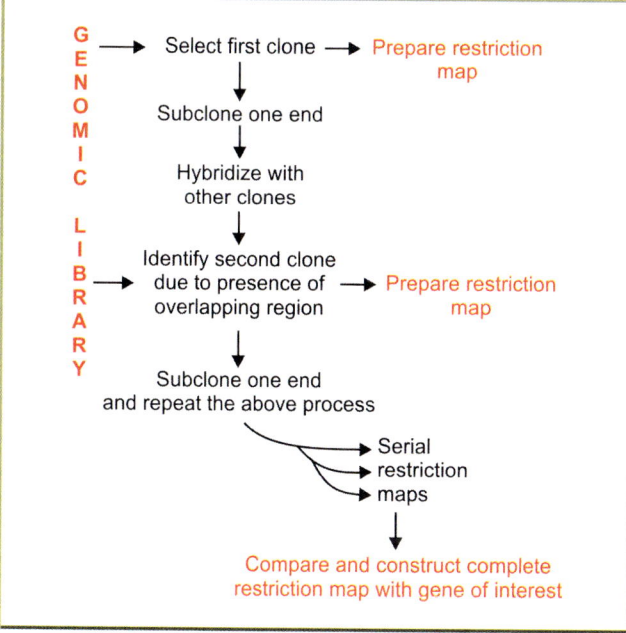

Fig. 23.7: Chromosome walking.

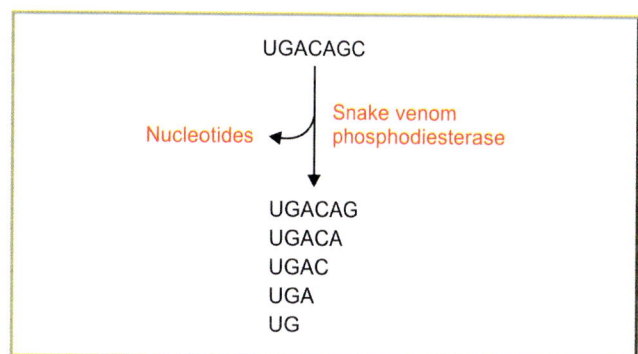

Fig. 23.8: DNA sequencing.

23

The process of PCR

The PCR requires two nucleotide oligomers that can hybridize to the complementary DNA sequences in a region of interest. These oligomers serve as primers for DNA polymerase, the enzyme that extends each strand:

- In order to initiate the process, DNA sample is heated to 90°C to dissociate the two strands of DNA and cooled in the presence of excess amounts of two different complementary oligomers that hybridize to the known vector DNA, flanking the foreign DNA insert.
- A new cycle of DNA replication is initiated in the presence of DNA polymerase and all the four dNTPs.
- In the presence of sufficient quantities of dNTPs, DNA polymerase directs the synthesis of the complementary strands. DNA polymerase used for DNA amplification by PCR is a heat-stable DNA

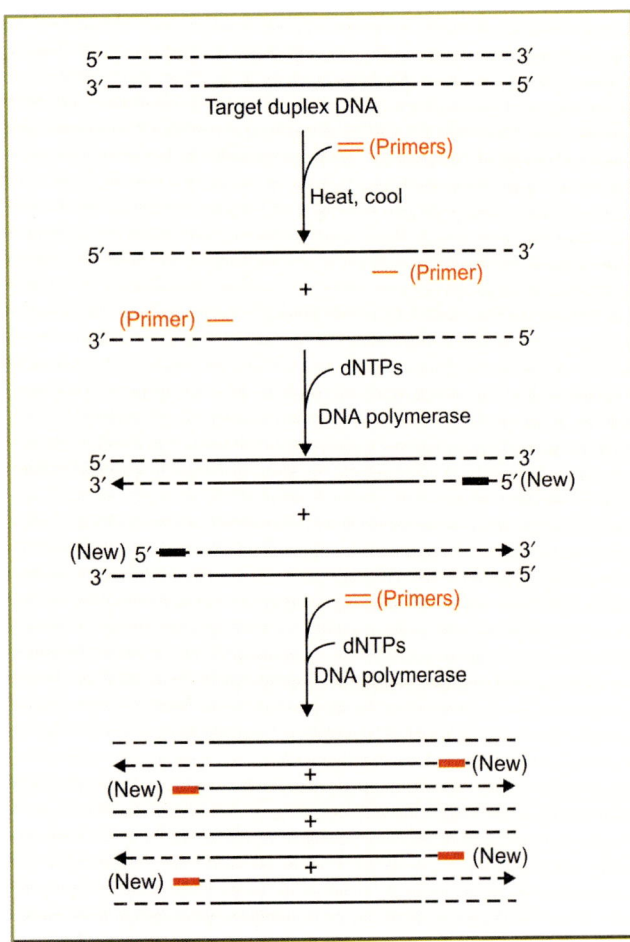

Fig. 23.9: Polymerase chain reaction (PCR).

Chemistry to Clinics 23.2: Applications of Polymerase Chain Reaction (PCR)

1. PCR amplification of potential DNA sequences from various infectious pathogens, such as *Mycobacterium tuberculosis*, human immunodeficiency virus, Hepatitis B virus, etc. helps in identification of the infectious agent.
2. To detect rare pathological changes, such as mutations leading to cancer.
3. In forensic investigations where only a very small quantity of the DNA is available, such as a drop of dried blood, semen or a single hair. The DNA from such a material is amplified by PCR and its RFLPs can be used to identify the source/donor with the preserved biological material.

polymerase such as Taq DNA polymerase which is isolated from *Thermus aquatics*. Being heat stable, this enzyme eliminates the need for fresh enzyme after each cycle.

- The product of PCR is a double-stranded DNA molecule and the reaction is completed in each cycle when all of the template molecules have been copied (Fig. 23.9).
- Multiple cycles of this process, each doubling the amount of the target DNA, geometrically amplify DNA to the extent that twenty cycles of PCR increase the amount of the target sequence by nearly one million-fold.

Advantages of PCR

1. PCR amplification has become an indispensible tool in biotechnology with several applications (Chemistry to Clinics 23.2).
2. PCR amplification of a specific DNA sequence can be accomplished with a purified DNA sample or a small region within a complex mixture of DNA.
3. The major advantages of PCR over cloning, as a mechanism of amplifying a specific DNA sequence, are its sensitivity and speed.

Reverse Transcriptase Polymerase Chain Reaction (RT-PCR) and Real Time PCR (qRT-PCR or Q-PCR)

Reverse transcriptase polymerase chain reaction (**RT-PCR**) is a variation of the basic PCR method and is useful when the nucleic acid to be amplified is **RNA instead of DNA**. The enzyme **reverse transcriptase** is employed to synthesize a cDNA strand complementary to the RNA and this cDNA serves as the template for further cycles of conventional PCR. However, it has several **drawbacks** as:

- It is time consuming

Table 23.2: Advantages of real time PCR (Q-PCR)

- Completely automated process and minimizes user intervention
- Time-saving
- Sensitive
- In-built controls avoid false-positive diagnosis
- Provides a quantitative estimate of amplification in every cycle
- Applicable to detect and quantify DNA as well as RNA (qRT-PCR)

- It has low sensitivity
- It is semiquantitative

These drawbacks are circumvented by employing another version of the technique called real-time RT-PCR (**qRT-PCR or Q-PCR** which should not be confused with RT-PCR). The Q-PCR enables detection with simultaneous quantification besides numerous other **advantages** (Table 23.2).

PROBE

The probe is a **labeled single-stranded DNA or RNA** segment whose sequence is **complementary** to a portion of the DNA of interest (**target DNA**). A probe is used to pick up a specific gene/DNA sequence of interest, out of the large number of DNA fragments which are obtained after cleavage of the large DNA molecule by restriction endonucleases. A probe may be a synthetic oligonucleotide of 20 to 30 nucleotides, usually labeled with a radioisotope, an antibody or a nonradioactive biotin-coupled oligonucleotide.

The probe, in turn, hybridizes with the target DNA or RNA of interest in a screening procedure. After washing away the unbound probe, presence of the probe on the nitrocellulose is detected by a technique such as autoradiography. Only those colonies or plaques containing the desired gene bind the probe and are detected. Using this technique, a human genomic library of nearly one million clones can be readily screened for the presence of one particular DNA segment.

Probes are used in laboratory diagnosis of many genetic diseases such as sickle cell anemia phenylketonuria, or certain types of cancers.

DNA CHIP TECHNOLOGY (DNA MICROARRAY TECHNOLOGY)

It is a small device in which thousands of nucleotide sequences are attached to a chip in a **grid pattern**. The chip has a solid surface of glass or silicon (gene chip) and contains a chemical matrix of polyacrylamide or lysine to which the sequences are covalently linked by a technique called **surface engineering**. These sequences act as probes to detect whether a test sample contains a particular DNA or RNA sequence. For example:

- mRNAs are isolated from normal and suspected cancerous tissue and processed as shown in Fig. 23.10.
- By reverse transcription, cDNAs are prepared and labeled with separate colored fluorescent labels. The labeled cDNAs are mixed and added to the chip containing an array of 60,000 or more different DNA sequences, each single-stranded and nearly 20 nucleotides long. Thus, each strand represents a tiny but unique region of a gene in the genome.
- The cDNAs that are complementary to the probes on the chip hybridize and adhere to that location. Unbound cDNAs are washed away.
- A scanner detects the **patterns of hybridization** by sensing the **color signals which differ** depending on the presence or absence of specific cDNAs (Fig. 23.10) (Chemistry to Clinics 23.3).

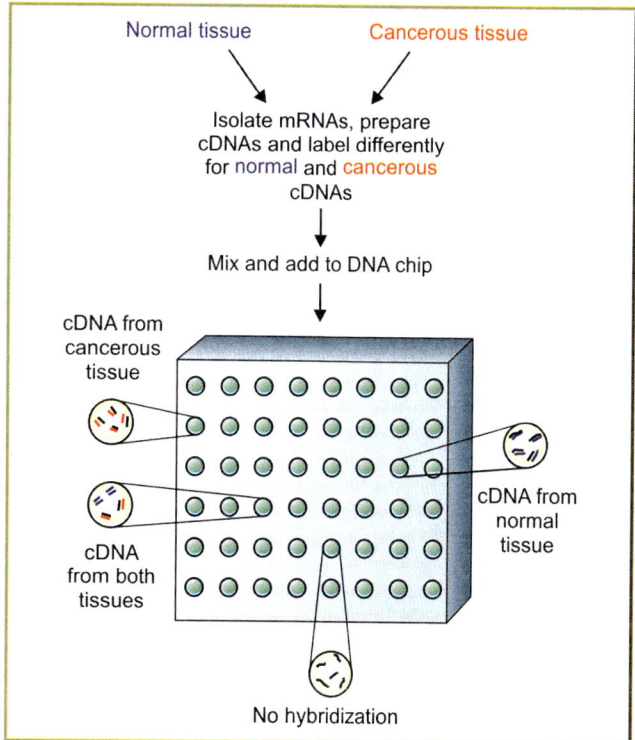

Fig. 23.10: DNA chip technology.

Chemistry to Clinics 23.3: Applications of DNA Microarray

- Each area of the chip represents a known DNA sequence corresponding to a known gene, hence the identities of the hybridizing cDNAs reveal which genes are expressed in cancerous versus normal tissue.
- Based on the genes expressed, specific treatment strategies can be planned.
- Many genetic tests can be performed rapidly and in parallel.

PEPTIDE NUCLEIC ACIDS (PNA)

These are **analogs of DNA or RNA** where the sugar-phosphate backbone is replaced artificially by a **peptide backbone** made up of repeating units of N-(2-aminoethyl)-glycine residues linked by peptide bonds. The PNA are resistant to nucleases as well as proteases and are therefore **highly stable**. They are used as **probes** that bind to specific DNA/RNA sequences. They are also used for **'antisense' drug therapy**.

SOUTHERN BLOTTING

Southern blotting is a procedure for **identifying a DNA sequence** after electrophoresis, through its ability to **hybridize** with a complementary single-stranded segment of the labeled DNA or RNA. This technique is used to detect mutations in DNA and involves the use of restriction enzyme in combination with the DNA probes. The technique is named after its inventor Edward Southern.

- DNA is extracted from the cells, e.g. a patient's leucocytes, and is cleaved into several fragments by using a restriction endonuclease.
- These fragments are separated on the basis of their size, by **electrophoresis** as the large fragments move slower than the smaller fragments.
- The fragments of interest are identified by a probe.
- The DNA is denatured and transferred onto the nitrocellulose membrane. Radioactive probe hybridizes with the restriction fragments and produces dark bands on the exposed X-ray film (Fig. 23.11).
- The patterns observed on Southern blot analysis depend upon the specific restriction endonuclease as well as the probe used to visualize the restriction fragments. The presence of a mutation affecting a restriction site causes the pattern of bands to differ from those seen with a normal gene.

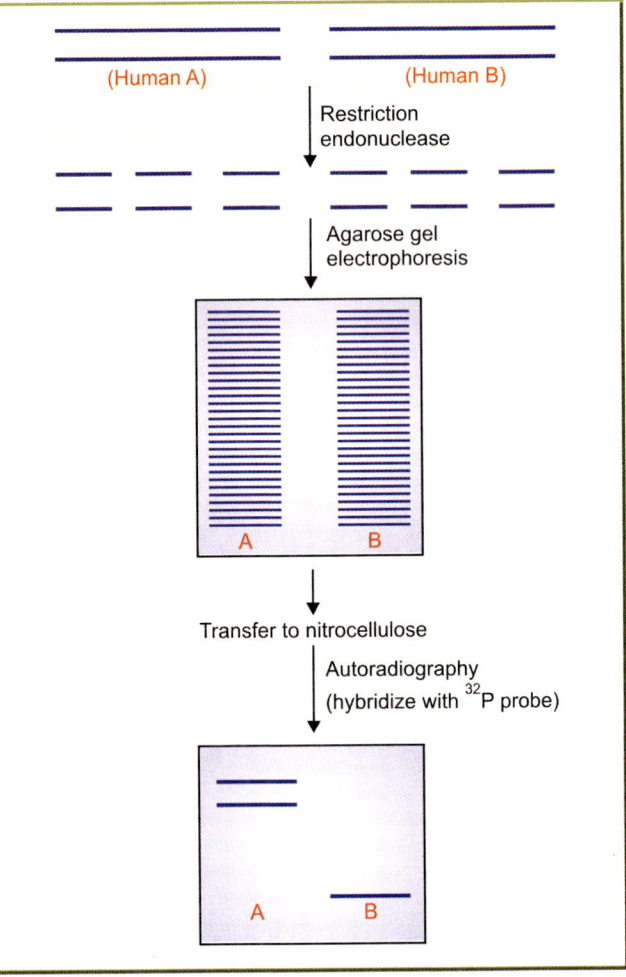

Fig. 23.11: Southern blotting.

NORTHERN BLOTTING

Specific **RNA sequences** are detected through a variation of the Southern blot, by the technique referred to as Northern blotting. It is a procedure for identifying RNA containing a particular base sequence through its ability to hybridize with a complementary single-stranded segment of the DNA or the RNA.

WESTERN BLOTTING

A specific **protein** is analogously detected by the technique called Western blotting. Immunoblotting is a technique in which a molecule immobilized on a membrane filter can be detected through its ability to bind to an antibody directed against it. A Western blot is an **immunoblot** to detect an immobilized protein after electrophoresis.

23

Northern blot or Western blot, however, do not relate to the name of an individual like the Southern blot but are referred only traditionally.

TRANSGENIC ANIMALS

Animals that develop from a fertilized egg when foreign genes are inserted into the genome of a fertilized egg, carry that gene in every cell. Such multicellular organisms expressing a foreign gene (gene from another organism) are said to be transgenic and the foreign gene which is transplanted is called **transgene**. For the change to be permanent, a **transgene gets integrated into the germ cell** of the organism. Transgenic mice and other animals as well as transgenic plants have been developed successfully. Transgenic animals are useful for:

- Analysis of tissue-specific gene expression.
- Studying results of gene overexpression/silencing.
- Discovering genes involved in development.
- Correction of genetic deficiencies.

DNA FINGERPRINTING

The use of **DNA restriction analysis to identify individuals** is called DNA fingerprinting. It is a variation of RFLP analysis in which the probe hybridizes to sequences between restriction enzyme sites that are highly polymorphic. These highly polymorphic sites are called **hypervariable regions** and are made up of tandem repeats of short sequences of 10–60 bp. The number of repeats may vary considerably between individuals and often are called **variable number of tandem repeats** (**VNTRs**). The sequence of each repeat may be unique and detected by a single locus probe or have core regions common to many other hypervariable regions that may be detected by a multilocus probe.

The hybridization pattern detected by a **Southern blot** analysis (Fig. 23.11) with different probes is generally specific to an individual, just like a fingerprint. The hypervariable regions show a high degree of variability between individuals. This, in turn, can serve as a **DNA fingerprint** that is **unique to the individual**.

DNA fingerprinting can be used for forensic identification, identifying parentage or for the evaluation of the success of bone marrow transplants.

DNA FOOTPRINTING

It is a technique to **identify the nucleotide sequence in DNA where a specific protein binds**, e.g. the promoter sequence bound by RNA polymerase holoenzyme. The DNA is suitably labeled at one end and the labeled-DNA-protein complex is incubated with DNase1. Subsequently, the DNA is denatured and the sets of labeled fragments are subjected to **gel electrophoresis**. Labeled naked DNA (without bound protein) is treated similarly for comparison. The protein binding site is revealed by the **absence of some fragments on the gel** (Fig. 23.12). Functional aspects of promoters can be studied by using reporter genes.

REPORTER GENE

Regulatory sequences such as promoters can be investigated by placing them into plasmids upstream of a gene, called a reporter gene, whose expression is easy to measure. Such chimeric plasmids are introduced into cells of choice to assess the function of the promoter sequence because the expression of the reporter gene serves as a 'report' on the effectiveness of the promoter.

Applications of Recombinant DNA Technology

Recombinant DNA methodologies are useful for numerous biological disciplines, such as in the study of evolution, forensic biology, clinical medicine and agriculture. Some of its major applications are discussed below:

1. **Understanding gene structure and function:** Treatment of a particular DNA segment with a specific restriction endonuclease produces a set of fragments. Analysis of fragments produced by different enzymes gives a 'restriction map' of the gene. In this way, the structure of the globin gene was determined (Fig. 23.13).

2. **Molecular analysis including pedigree analysis:** It has become possible to determine the cause of many diseases at the 'grass-root' level, i.e. the fundamental molecular defects leading to disease processes and often being inheritable (Fig. 23.14).

3. **Restriction fragment length polymorphism (RFLP), DNA fingerprinting and chromosome walking:** The techniques are used to:
   - Establish the **perfect genetic identity** of an individual in medicolegal cases to identify criminals and settle issues of disputed paternity.

23

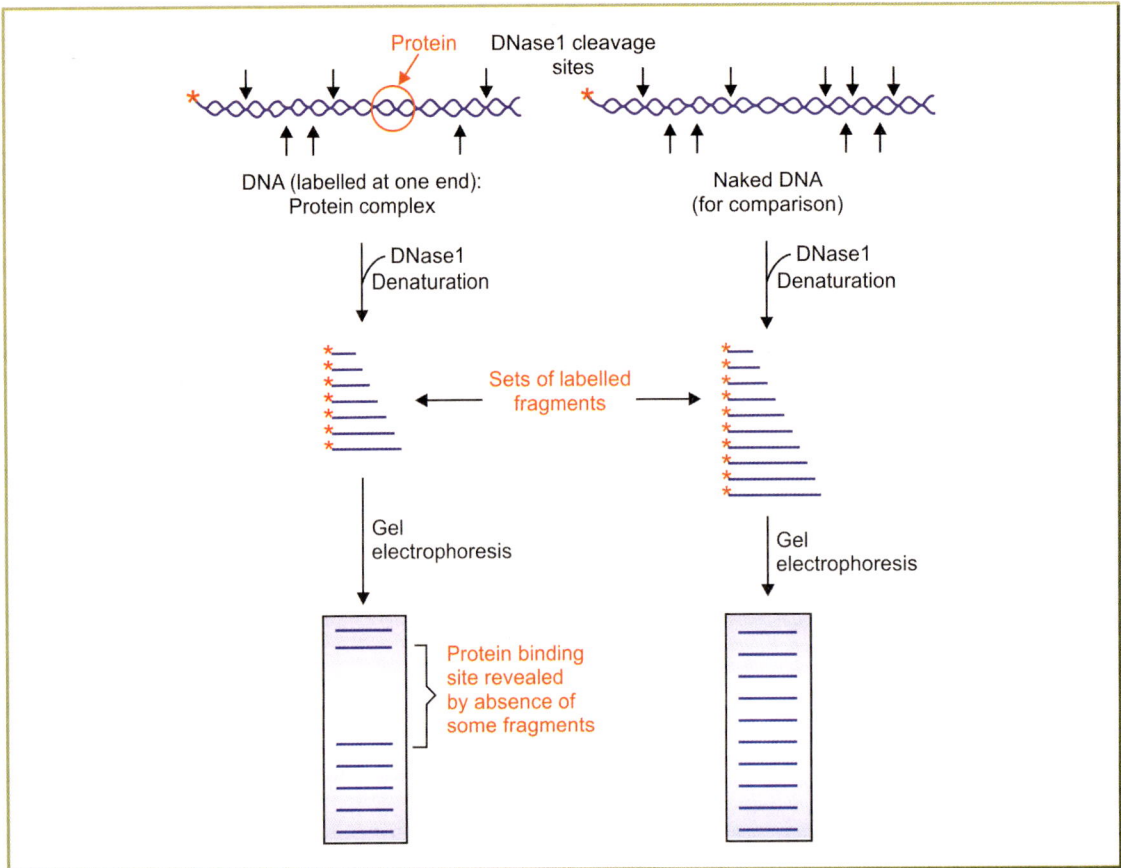

Fig. 23.12: DNA footprinting.

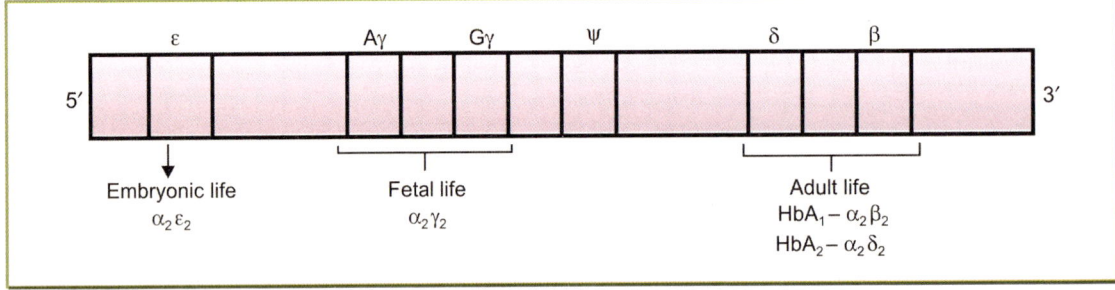

Fig. 23.13: Structure of globin gene.

- Study various races and ethnic populations, i.e. **population genetics**.
- Perform **linkage studies** in cases where the exact genetic defect in a disease is unknown. For example, linkage analysis in patients from many families affected with cystic fibrosis revealed two RFLPs flanking a particular gene comprising 1.5 million base pairs on chromosome 7. By chromosome walking, the exact mutation site was identified, i.e. ΔF508 leading to a malfunctioning cystic fibrosis transmembrane receptor (CFTR) protein. A similar approach proved that Duchenne muscular dystrophy was due to a mutation in dystrophin gene on the X-chromosome. Other examples include α-thalassemia (chromosome 16), β-thalassemia

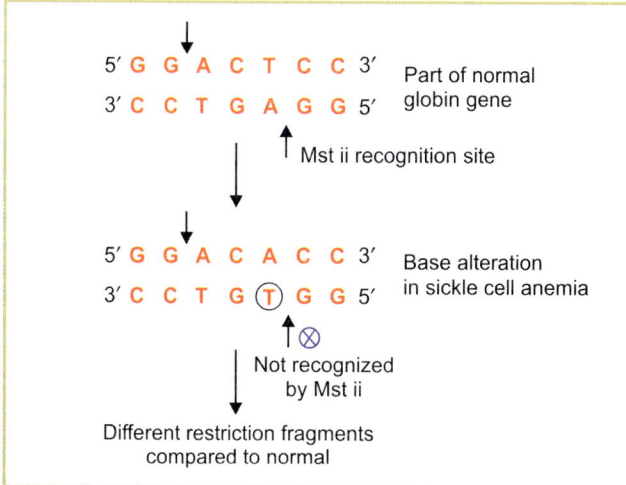

5′ G G A C T C C 3′   Part of normal
3′ C C T G A G G 5′   globin gene

Mst ii recognition site

5′ G G A C A C C 3′   Base alteration
3′ C C T G (T) G G 5′   in sickle cell anemia

Not recognized
by Mst ii

Different restriction fragments
compared to normal

Fig. 23.14: Molecular diagnosis of sickle cell anemia.

(chromosome 11), adenosine deaminase deficiency (chromosome 20) and phenylketonuria (chromosome 12).

4. **Disease prevention:** This has been achieved through:

- **Preclinical diagnosis** and carrier detection in case of hepatitis B, AIDS and tuberculosis.
- **Prenatal diagnosis** where the disease is detected in the unborn (fetus), providing an option to the parents to terminate the pregnancy if deemed necessary. Genetic markers are available for several diseases (Table 23.3).

5. **Recombinant DNA products:** A cloned gene is inserted into an expression vector (plasmid) that contains properly positioned transcriptional and translational control sequences. A genetically engineered organism thus can produce large quantities of the desired protein. Such organisms are called as **over-producers**. A wide range of proteins are commercially being produced to ease the life of patients suffering from many diseases (Table 23.4).

Table 23.3: Diseases where prenatal diagnosis is possible

Autosomal dominant	Autosomal recessive	X-linked
Myotonic dystrophy	Cystic fibrosis	Hemophilia
Huntington's chorea	Phenyl ketonuria	Duchenne muscular dystrophy
		Becker's dystrophy
		Fragile X mental retardation syndrome

Table 23.4: Diseases being treated by recombinant DNA protein products

Recombinant protein	Target disease
Human insulin	Diabetes mellitus
Human growth hormone	Dwarfism
Somatostatin	Acromegaly
Tissue plasminogen activator	Myocardial infarction
Coagulation factors VIII and IX	Hemophilia A and B
Erythropoietin	Anemia of chronic renal failure
Colony stimulating factor	Severe immunodeficiency
Growth factors	Extensive non-healing wounds
Interferons, interleukins	Cancer, advanced viral infections
Monoclonal antibodies	Cancer
Superoxide dismutase	Reperfusion injury in cardiac surgery
Vaccines	Hepatitis B

6. **Gene therapy:** It is the transfer of genetic material to the cells of an individual in order to produce a therapeutic effect. Gene therapy retains considerable promise for treating >4000 known genetic diseases, particularly those with no alternative treatment.

Guidelines for gene therapy

- Only somatic cells should be employed to avoid alterations in germ cell lines.
- Lethal genetic diseases should be selected.
- The normal gene must be identified and cloned.
- Single-gene disorders should be chosen.
- Feasibility and benefits should be documented in properly conducted animal experiments prior to undertaking human trials.

Types of gene therapy

i. **Gene replacement:** To replace the defective gene with the normal gene.

ii. **Gene augmentation:** It is the most popular technique involving the introduction of a foreign gene into the cell to mask the results of the defective gene. Methods of augmentation therapy include:

- Calcium-DNA precipitates
- Electroporation
- Microinjection
- Retroviral vectors
- Adenoviral vectors
- Plasmid-DNA complexes

23

- Naked DNA (DNA vaccines)
- Site-directed recombination

iii. **Genome editing:** It refers to correction of mutation by selectively removing and replacing defective lengths of DNA. Zinc finger nucleases (artificial restriction enzymes prepared by fusing a zinc finger DNA-binding domain to a DNA-cleavage domain) are employed to target the desired DNA sequence. By taking advantage of the usual DNA repair mechanisms, the sequence is successfully altered. Compared with simple gene replacement therapy, genome editing carries lower risk of random insertion into the genome.

Disease candidates for gene therapy

- **Globin chain disorders:** Hemoglobinopathies.
- **Immunodeficiency disorders:** AIDS, adenosine deaminase (ADA) deficiency, nucleoside phosphorylase deficiency, leucocyte adhesion deficiency. Gene for ADA has been successfully introduced into children with ADA deficiency.
- **Metabolic disorders:** Urea cycle enzyme deficiency, Lesch-Nyhan syndrome, phenylketonuria, lysosomal storage diseases, familial hypercholesterolemia, atherosclerosis.
- **Organ-system disorders:** Duchenne muscular dystrophy, cystic fibrosis, α_1-antitrypsin deficiency, Huntington's disease, cancers.
- **Coagulation disorders:** Hemophilia A and B.

7. Miscellaneous uses:

- Introduction of recombinant DNA products into plants provide more nutritious and higher yielding crops that are more resistant to environmental stresses, and reduce the need to add agricultural chemicals. Genetic engineering also provides plant products suited for specific purposes (Chemistry to Clinics 23.4).
- Enzymes produced by this technology are used to prepare detergents, sugars, cheese, etc.
- Engineered proteins are used as food additives.
- Engineered microbes are used to extract oil and minerals from ground deposits, to digest oil spillage as well as to detoxify hazardous waste dumps and sewage.

Chemistry to Clinics 23.4: Genetically Engineered Coffee
Caffeine synthase, the enzyme that catalyzes the final two steps in the caffeine biosynthetic pathway in the coffee plant, can be inactivated by genetic engineering techniques. Thus, 100% caffeine-free coffee can be produced that still retains the flavor and aroma since caffeine itself is tasteless and odorless. Although this coffee lacks the caffeine-dependent CNS stimulatory effects, it is preferred by coffee lovers who are prone to caffeine-dependent side effects such as increase in blood pressure, insomnia, anxiety, tremors, palpitations and gastrointestinal upset. The unique advantage of genetic engineering over the traditional decaffeination process is that the latter neither results in 100% decaffeination nor it preserves the flavor and aroma.

SOME IMPORTANT QUESTIONS

1. What is recombinant DNA technology? Discuss its applications.

2. Describe briefly:
   i. Restriction endonucleases
   ii. Cloning
   iii. Complementary DNA and cDNA library
   iv. RFLPs
   v. DNA sequencing
   vi. Polymerase chain reaction

3. Write notes on:
   i. Palindrome
   ii. Restriction map
   iii. Vector
   iv. Plasmid
   v. Cosmid
   vi. Genomic library
   vii. Southern blotting
   viii. Probe
   ix. Northern blotting
   x. Western blotting
   xi. Immunoblot
   xii. Transgenic animals
   xiii. Gene therapy
   xiv. DNA fingerprinting
   xv. DNA footprinting

MULTIPLE CHOICE QUESTIONS

1. The small size of cloned DNA fragments is a major limitation with:
   A. Yeast artificial chromosomes
   B. Bacteriophages
   C. Plasmids
   D. Cosmids

2. When the DNA sequence is known but the location of the gene is unknown, the following is the most suitable approach to find the same:
   A. Shotgun cloning
   B. RFLP analysis
   C. SNP analysis
   D. Chromosome walking

3. An RNA sequence may be determined by:
   A. Southern blot
   B. Northern blot
   C. Western blot
   D. Any of the above

4. Prenatal diagnosis is possible for:
   A. Myotonic dystrophy
   B. Huntington's chorea
   C. Cystic fibrosis
   D. All of the above

5. The principles of gene therapy include the following *except:*
   A. Normal gene must be identified and cloned
   B. Lethal genetic disease should be selected
   C. Germline cells must be employed
   D. Single gene disorders should be chosen

24

Human Genome Project

BASIC OBJECTIVES AND IMPACT

The human genome contains DNA with 3×10^9 **base-pairs located on 23 pairs of chromosomes** that determine the genetic characteristics of every cell in the human individual. Efforts to determine the nucleotide sequence of the entire human genome were officially declared in the **'Human Genome Project'** (Fig. 24.1). The project was approved by the US Congress in 1991 and has extensive international collaboration.

In February 2001, the first draft of the human genome sequence was published. It was the crowning achievement of 20th century biology in the start of the new millennium. Knowing the entire sequence of the human genome amounts to knowing the **blueprint that dictates every biochemical process in our body**. All of us have genomes that are **99.9% identical and 0.1% different**. Collectively, these are responsible for not just how our body performs in the present but also in the future and even our overall lifespan.

GENETICS VERSUS GENOMICS

- Genetics is the study of individual genes and how they are expressed and transmitted in cells and organisms. Genomics is built on that platform of genetics, seeking to understand the structure and

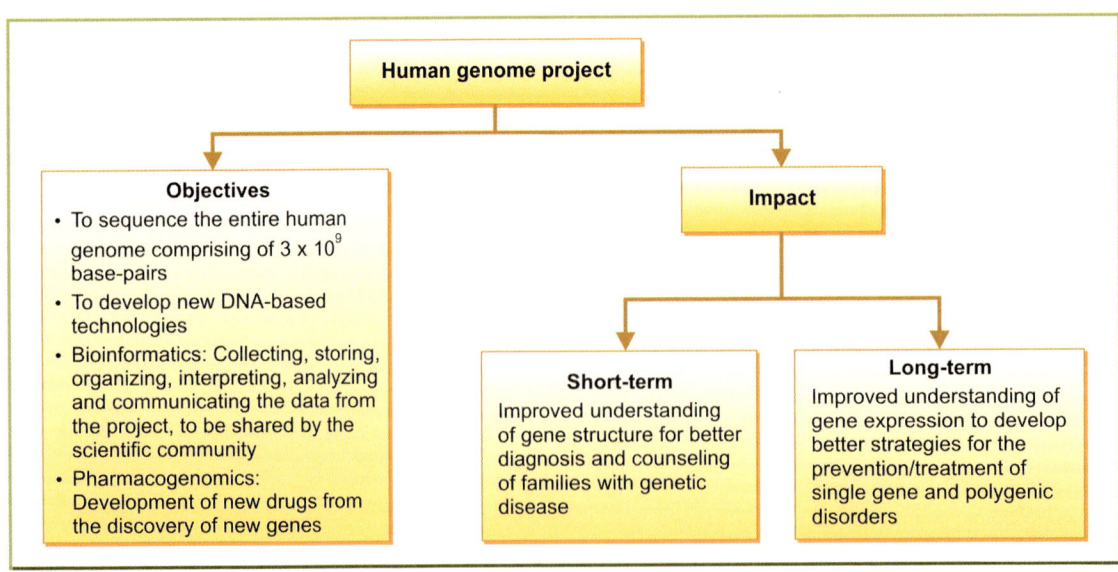

Fig. 24.1: Objectives and impact of human genome project.

Table 24.1: Chronological sequencing of various genomes

Organism	Genome size (millions of base-pairs)	Predicted number of genes
Bacterium *Haemophilus influenzae*, 1995	1.8	1740
Budding yeast *Saccharomyces cerevisiae*, 1996	12	6000
Bacterium *Escherichia coli*, 1997	4.6	3240
Nematode worm *Caenorhabditis elegans*, 1998	97	19100
Flowering plant *Arabidopis thaliana*, 2000	125	25500
Fruit fly *Drosophila melanogaster*, 2000	180	13600
Human *Homo sapiens*, 2001	3200	30000–40000

expression of entire genomes and how they change during evolution. The successful sequencing of the human genome depended on several earlier efforts to sequence the genomes of other organisms (Table 24.1).

- Genetics focuses on individual genes and how they function, either alone or together with a limited set of other genes, to control a phenotype. Genomics take a far more comprehensive approach, monitoring the coordinated activities of all the genes in the genome.

- Simple experiments such as cross-breeding and others developed by Mendel are important tools to uncover the role played by specific genes in inheritance as well as to produce a particular trait or phenotype. The study of genomics requires more sophisticated and complex experimental designs to analyze the expression of genes in the whole genome.

Some of the critical discoveries and events that finally led to the sequencing of the human genome are outlined below:

- **4th century BC:** Hippocrates, the father of medicine, noted that **signs of disease could appear throughout a family**, even over successive generations. Aristotle declared that **parents pass biological information to their offspring**.

- **1677:** Antonie van Leeuwenhoek **invented the microscope** and revealed the **existence of sperm**. He speculated that offspring arose from interacting cells contributed by both parents.

- **1865:** Gregor Mendel studied inheritance in garden pea and defined the basic laws of heredity: **Equal segregation and independent assortment**.

- **1909:** Thomas Morgan established that **genes are arranged on chromosomes** in linkage groups.

- **1928:** Frederick Griffith demonstrated that a **'transforming factor'** of unknown identity can convert harmless bacteria into lethal ones.

- **1944:** Avery, Macleod and McCarty identified the **'transforming factor' as DNA**, the possible biochemical basis of heredity.

- **1952:** Hershey and Chase proved that **DNA is the hereditary material**, by using viruses to infect bacteria.

- **1952–1953:** Rosalind Franklin performed **X-ray crystallographic studies** that proved critical in understanding DNA structure.

- **1953:** James Watson and Francis Crick discovered the **double helical structure of DNA**.

- **1960–1970:** Establishing the **genetic code** and the **central dogma of molecular biology**: flow of genetic information from DNA to RNA to protein.

- **1972:** Paul Berg created the **first recombinant DNA molecule** by linking the sequences from two different viruses.

- **1977:** Sanger, Maxam and Gilbert developed **DNA sequencing** techniques.

- **1987:** Applied Biosystems Inc. launched the **first machine for automated DNA sequencing**.

- **1990:** National Institutes for Health (USA) and Department of Energy (USA) **established the** publicly funded **Human Genome Project**, with James Watson as the Director. An international consortium of sequencing centers was scheduled to completely sequence the human genome by 2005. Later, Watson resigned due to disagreements

24

on the patenting of genes and Francis Collins became the new Director.

- **1995:** Craig Venter reported the **first complete genome sequence** of a free-living organism, the bacterium *Haemophilus influenzae*. A controversial method called 'whole-genome shotgun sequencing' was used.

- **1996:** The Human Genome Project reported the **complete genome sequence** of the budding yeast *Saccharomyces cerevisiae*. The conventional method of 'map-based sequencing' was used.

- **1998:** Craig Venter established an independent private company called Celera Genomics, **targeting the sequencing of the entire human genome** by 2001.

- **2001:** The Human Genome Project and Celera Genomics independently **published the complete human genome sequence** in the journal '*Nature*' and '*Science*' respectively. However, this does not mean that the genome was 100% sequenced. Like other eukaryotic genomes, the human genome contains stretches of repetitive DNA that are difficult to sequence. These regions, however, contain very few genes or regulatory sequences that continue to be sequenced.

GENOMICS AND PROTEOMICS

- **Structural genomics:** Advances in protein crystallization, X-ray diffraction and nuclear magnetic resonance spectroscopy along with genome sequencing has made it possible to undertake large-scale **analysis of protein structure** (and hence function). This has boosted the development of new drug targets.

- **Functional genomics:** It refers to the **study of all the genes that are expressed during major metabolic shifts**. For example, the set of genes expressed during aerobic conditions are quite different from those expressed during anaerobic conditions. The same holds true for genes expressed during embryogenesis as compared to postnatal life.

- **Proteomics:** It refers to the **study of all the proteins (protein profiling) synthesized by a particular cell under specified conditions**. It provides an indirect assessment of gene expression under those conditions.

ANALYSIS AND INTERPRETATION OF THE SEQUENCED HUMAN GENOME

The **major facts** emerging from the sequenced human genome are briefly discussed below:

1. **True genes:** Previously, it was held that approximately 100,000 different genes are required to encode the entire phenotype of a human individual. Now, it has been realized that the number is between 30,000 and 40,000. It is clear that genes occupy **only 2–3% of the human genome**.

2. **Organism complexity:** The above mentioned information suggests that, surprisingly, humans require only ten times the number of genes needed by the bacterium *E. coli*. In other words, are humans only a little more complex than bacteria? To answer this question, the various factors determining the complexity of the two organisms should be compared:

   - Firstly, assuming that a given gene can adopt one of two opposite states, i.e. 'on' or 'off', the number of possible RNA products in humans with 40,000 genes is $2^{40,000}$ compared with 2^{3240} for *E. coli* having 3240 genes.

   - Secondly, the variable removal of introns from human RNA means that a single gene can produce many different RNA transcripts. In case of *E. coli*, each gene produces only one RNA product due to lack of introns.

   - Thirdly, different mechanisms of regulating gene expression make humans far more complex than simple bacteria like *E. coli*.

3. **Evolutionary insights:** Comparison of human genome sequence and their protein products with that from other organisms provides evolutionary insights. For example, nearly 60% of human proteins are similar to proteins found in fruit flies and worms. These are the proteins participating in the core processes required for life, such as DNA synthesis enzymes, transcription factors, metabolic enzymes, receptors, etc. Therefore, such proteins were established early in the process of evolution.

4. **Biological clock:** The knowledge about the evolutionary conservation of genes and their corresponding proteins as discussed above provides another advantage. Understanding how these genes function in other organisms sheds light on the functions of their human counterparts. For example, when we fly on an airplane across several

time zones, our sleep pattern gets disturbed. The phenomenon, called 'jet lag', is due to a disruption of our 'biological clock'. Various clock genes regulate the daily cycling of many physiological events including sleep. Earlier studies in the fruit fly *Drosophila* had already provided clue to the existence of such clock genes.

5. **Genetic screening:** The link between mutation(s) in a given gene and the likelihood of developing a disease forms the basis for genetic screening. Today, people have the option of testing themselves or even their unborn for several such diseases. However, knowledge of the human genome sequence and the availability of new genomic techniques have gone one step further in detecting diseases involving multiple genes and their interactions, e.g. breast cancer.

6. **Single nucleotide polymorphisms (SNPs):** Single base-pair differences, known as 'single nucleotide polymorphisms' (SNPs), are one important source of genomic variation. If one could associate the presence of one or more SNPs with susceptibility to a particular disease, individuals possessing the specific 'SNP profile' could be forewarned of the oncoming disease allowing timely treatment/prevention (Chemistry to Clinics 24.1).

7. **Personalized medicine:** The SNP profiles provide insights into how an individual will respond to

Chemistry to Clinics 24.1: SNP Profile

A particular SNP in the apolipoprotein E (*apoE*) gene is associated with an enhanced risk of developing Alzheimer's disease whereas another *apoE* SNP reduces the risk. Thus, by determining the SNP profile for the *apoE* gene, a person can predict whether or not there is a risk for Alzheimer's disease later in life.

Chemistry to Clinics 24.2: Personalized Medicine

Interferon therapy is frequently employed in patients suffering from hepatitis C, a form of viral hepatitis notorious for complications like hepatic cirrhosis and even cancer. Paradoxically, even at equivalent doses, there is a wide and unpredictable variation in terms of the efficacy of the drug and its side effects. DNA analysis has now revealed that patients harboring a single base change, i.e. C (cytosine) instead of T (thymine) in a tiny DNA segment near the interleukin-28 gene (IL28B), are more likely to respond to treatment with fewer adverse effects. The ability to predict who will respond and who might be resistant thus requires knowledge of single nucleotide polymorphism (SNP) in an individual, and is a part of 'personalized medicine'.

drug therapy and the development of 'personalized medicine' (Chemistry to Clinics 24.2). For example, certain plasma membrane proteins pump anti-cancer drugs out of the cells resulting in the need for higher drug doses. Knowing the SNP profile of genes encoding such proteins would identify persons requiring higher or lower drug doses.

8. **Potential misuse:** Since the SNPs can help to create highly personalized genetic profiles, there is potential for their misuse and genome-based discrimination between individuals. For example, health insurance companies will be tempted to raise the premiums for persons who are at higher risk for a disease in future. In fact, the risk for a serious disease might lead to a denial for insurance. Susceptibility to alcoholism, schizophrenia, etc. might prevent individuals from getting certain types of jobs. Thus, to prevent the misuse of SNP profiles, new guidelines for personal privacy must be established to secure the ethical, legal and social issues surrounding the genetic information.

SOME IMPORTANT QUESTIONS

1. What is Human Genome Project?

2. Explain the terms genetics, genomics and proteomics.

3. Write notes on:
   i. SNP
   ii. Personalized medicine

24

MULTIPLE CHOICE QUESTIONS

1. **The number of base-pairs in the human genome are:**
   A. 3×10^3
   B. 3×10^5
   C. 3×10^7
   D. 3×10^9

2. **The 1st genome to be completely sequenced was:**
   A. *Homo sapiens*
   B. *Haemophilus influenzae*
   C. *Escherichia coli*
   D. *Saccharomyces cerevisiae*

3. **In the human genome, true genes constitute:**
   A. 2–3%
   B. 12–13%
   C. 20–30%
   D. 95–98%

4. **Single nucleotide polymorphism in a tiny DNA segment near IL28B gene results in a differential response to pegylated interferon therapy in:**
   A. Hepatitis C
   B. Parkinson's disease
   C. Alzheimer's disease
   D. Multiple sclerosis

5. **Functional genomics refers to the study of:**
   A. All the proteins that are synthesized by a particular cell under specified conditions
   B. All the genes that are expressed during major metabolic shifts
   C. Large scale analysis of protein structure
   D. Individual genes and how they are expressed and transmitted in cells.

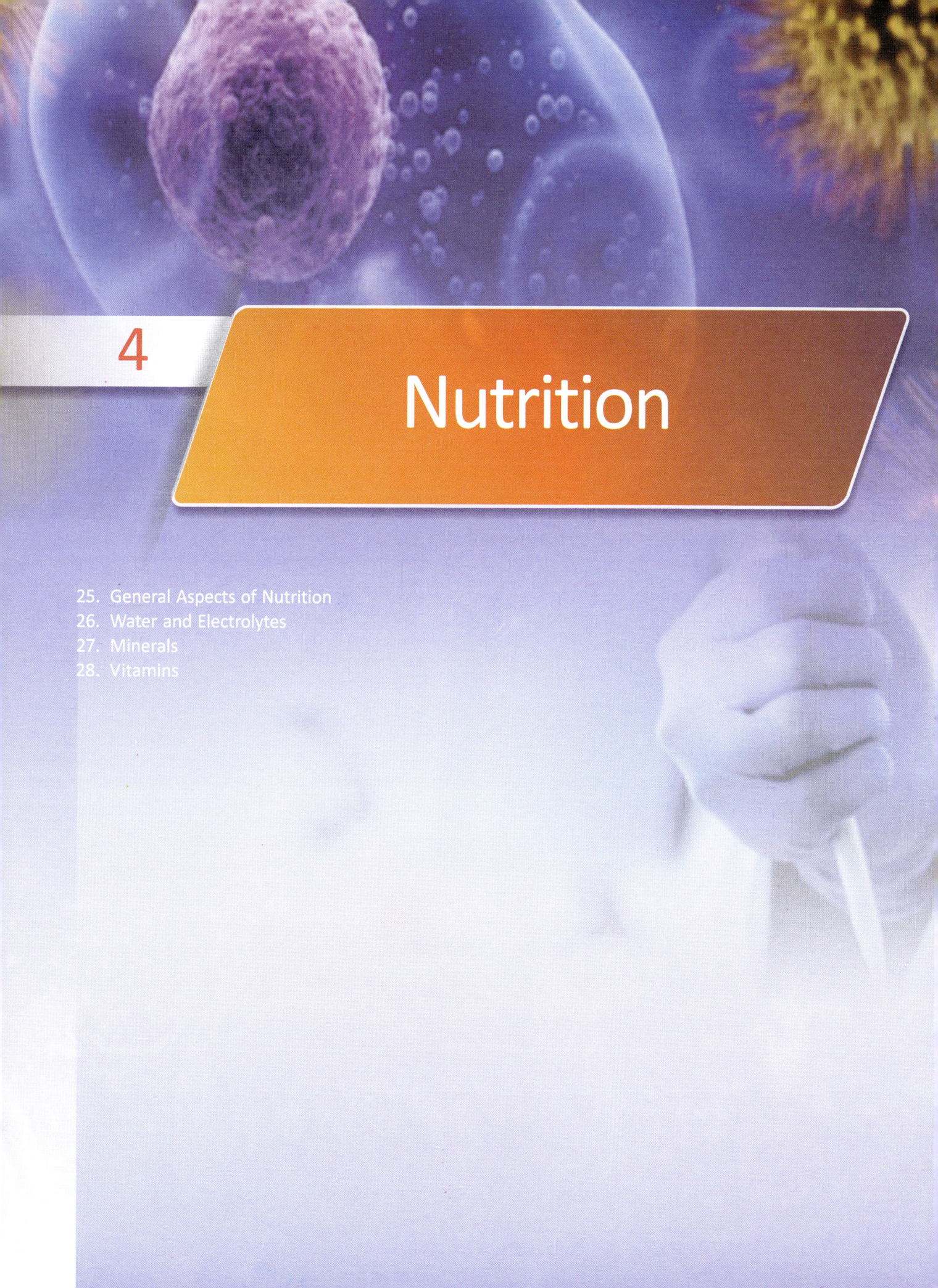

4

Nutrition

General Aspects of Nutrition

The study of the **qualitative** as well as **quantitative** requirements of the various **proximate principles** of food, to maintain good health is known as nutrition.

PROXIMATE PRINCIPLES OF FOOD

Proximate principles of food include:

1. **Carbohydrates, lipids and proteins:** These are the sources of **energy** in the diet, hence also called caloric principles. The chemical energy stored in these macromolecules is harvested in the form of high energy phosphate bond (~P) such as present in ATP, creatine phosphate, etc. Proteins, in addition to energy, also supply specific amino acids and nitrogen for growth and maintenance of the tissues.

2. **Vitamins and minerals:** These nutrients although do not yield energy but form an essential part of chemical mechanisms for the **utilization of energy** and are essentially required for the **synthesis of various metabolites**. Further, some of the minerals are also incorporated into the structure of various tissues or play an important role in acid–base balance.

3. **Water:** Essential for providing an aqueous medium.

ENERGY

Energy stored in various foodstuffs since is ultimately converted to heat, energy output can therefore be measured as the heat output from the body. The energy content of the food is therefore represented in terms of calories, the unit of heat.

A **calorie** is defined as the amount of heat required to raise the temperature of 1 g of water by 1°C, i.e.

from 14.5° to 15.5°C. The international unit of energy is joule; 1 calorie = 4.18 joule. A joule (J) is defined as the amount of heat required to move a mass of 1 kg, by 1 meter distance, by a force of 1 newton.

The amount of heat released by combustion of food is actually expressed in terms of kilocalories (**kcal or C**) since the unit of calorie is very small; 1 kcal (C) = 1000 calories = 4.18 kJ.

CALORIMETRY

As daily heat output from the body has to be replaced by supplying equivalent amount of calories in the food, calories requirement can thus be estimated by measuring calories output. The technique of the measurement of energy expenditure is known as calorimetry which is of two types:

Direct calorimetry: It is the **most accurate** method, though easy in theory, but **difficult and costly** in practice. A subject is placed in an insulated chamber, around which a weighed quantity of water is circulated at a known rate and temperature. All the heat produced is measured directly by recording the total amount of heat which is transferred to the circulating water.

Indirect calorimetry: Here, the quantity of heat produced by the body as a result of combustion of food is calculated from the **quantity of oxygen consumed**. Technically, it is a **simpler** procedure than the direct measurement of heat output. Under normal conditions, one liter of O_2 consumed accounts for approximately 4.82 kcal of energy spent by the body.

25

In addition to O_2 utilized and CO_2 produced, the amount of nitrogen excreted during a given period of time can also be measured. Since each g of urinary nitrogen represents 6.25 g of protein, the approximate amount of the protein metabolized can also be calculated.

Respiratory Quotient

Combustion of all organic substances consumes O_2 and results in the liberation of CO_2. The **ratio of the volume of CO_2 expired to the volume of O_2 utilized** is known as respiratory quotient (RQ) (Fig. 25.1).

$$RQ = \frac{\text{Volume of } CO_2 \text{ expired}}{\text{Volume of } O_2 \text{ utilized}}$$

$$RQ \text{ (Glucose)} = \frac{6CO_2}{6O_2} = 1.0$$

$$RQ \text{ (tristearin)}_2 = \frac{114CO_2}{163O_2} = 0.7$$

Fig. 25.1: Calculation of respiratory quotient (RQ).

RQ for the oxidation of **carbohydrates** is 1.0, since on its complete oxidation the volume of CO_2 eliminated is equal to the volume of O_2 consumed. For example, for the oxidation of a molecule of glucose, six volumes of CO_2 are expired at the expense of six volumes of O_2:

$$C_6H_{12}O_6 + 6O_2 \longrightarrow 6CO_2 + 6H_2O$$

Its RQ, is therefore, equivalent to 1 (Fig. 25.1).

Oxygen content of **lipids** is lower than its carbon content; lipids therefore require more O_2 for their oxidation. For example, for the oxidation of two molecules of tristearin, 114 volumes of CO_2, are liberated while 163 volumes of O_2 are required:

$$2C_{57}H_{110}O_6 + 163O_2 \longrightarrow 114CO_2 + 110H_2O$$

Therefore, its RQ is equivalent to 0.7 (Fig. 25.1)

Hence, the RQ for lipids is 0.7.

Oxidation of **proteins** though cannot be so readily expressed due to their variable chemical structures, the RQ value of proteins has been reported to be 0.8.

As varying proportions of carbohydrates, lipids and proteins are consumed in the diet, each having its own RQ, the RQ for a mixed food is taken as 0.82.

At this value, every liter of O_2 consumed represents an energy expenditure of 4.82 kcal.

Table 25.1: Caloric value of major foodstuffs

Foodstuff	Caloric value (kcal/g)	
	In a bomb calorimeter	*In the body*
Carbohydrates	4.1	4.0
Lipids	9.4	9.0
Proteins	5.4	4.0

ENERGY CONTENT OF FOOD

Energy content of the food, as mentioned earlier, is generally described in terms of kcal (Calories).

Different foodstuffs release different amounts of heat. This is expressed in terms of the **caloric value of food** which is defined as the amount of heat (energy) produced on complete combustion of 1 g of the foodstuff in the presence of O_2. From the metabolic oxidation of carbohydrates and lipids, the heat of combustion in a bomb calorimeter as well as the amount of energy available in the human body are nearly the same (Table 25.1). This is because their oxidation is complete, both outside as well as within the body. Since actual caloric values for carbohydrates and lipids **are not much different under the two conditions, for simplicity these values are taken as 4 kcal/g for carbohydrates and 9 kcal/g for lipids**.

For **proteins**, the actual heat output as obtained in a calorimeter is 5.4 kcal/g whereas the value obtained in the body is only **4.0 kcal/g**. The caloric value of a protein in a person is therefore less than that observed in a bomb calorimeter. This is due to the reason that proteins are not completely oxidized in the body and that the nitrogenous end products of protein catabolism (urea, ammonia, etc.), still have some energy though it is not available for the body.

The quantity of heat produced by the body as a result of combustion of different foodstuffs can thus be calculated if the quantity of each foodstuff present in the diet is known.

The caloric value of alcohol is 7 kcal/g while that of wheat is 3.5 kcal/g.

Basal Energy Requirement

An individual even at complete physical and mental rest requires some energy for the following basal metabolic processes:

1. Energy-dependent membrane transport. In fact, the activity of Na^+/K^+-ATPase accounts for nearly 50% of basal energy requirements.

2. Thermoregulation.
3. Involuntary muscle contractions of heart, respiratory muscles and intestine (peristalsis).
4. Gastrointestinal and other body secretions.
5. Renal tubular reabsorption.
6. Conduction of nerve impulses.

The energy required for these processes is known as the basal requirement. Average basal requirement per 24 hours is taken as 1500 kcal for an adult male and 1300 kcal for a female. The basal requirement is determined as the rate of metabolic activities of the body in resting conditions, better known as the **basal metabolic rate**.

BASAL METABOLIC RATE (BMR)

It is defined as the rate of energy utilization in the resting state. It is determined experimentally when the subject is lying down at **complete physical and mental rest** (with closed eyes but awaken), wearing light cloths, at a room temperature of around 20–25°C, and at least 12 hours after the last meal, i.e. in the post-absorptive state. BMR is proportional to lean body weight and thus to surface area. It is expressed as $kcal/m^2/hr$ and is determined with the help of **indirect calorimetry**.

Oxygen consumption is measured at complete resting state for 6 min. The value is then multiplied by ten and thus the O_2 consumption per hour is calculated. By multiplying this value with 4.82 (the amount of heat produced per litre of O_2 consumed), the amount of heat produced per hour (kcal/hr) is calculated. This is then divided with the surface area to obtain the value of BMR.

Average value for a normal adult male is 40 kcal/m^2/hr and for a female is 36 kcal/m^2/hr.

BMR of an individual can also be expressed as a percentage of the normal value. Values between –15% and +20% of the normal value are considered to be within the normal limits.

Factors Affecting BMR

1. **Age:** Age reflects growth as well as lean muscle mass. Infants and children require more energy for growth. This, in turn, is reflected in terms of a higher BMR. Thus, BMR is high in actively growing children upto 5 years of age. BMR again increases thereafter at puberty. Since muscle tissue is gradually replaced with fat and water during the aging process, adults have reduced BMR. There is nearly 2% decrease in BMR per decade in adults.

2. **Sex:** Since women have a smaller percentage of lean muscle mass than men and due to the effect of female hormones on metabolism, women have lower BMR.

3. **Surface area:** The effect of surface area is simply related to the rate of heat loss by the body, e.g. greater the surface area, the greater is the rate of heat loss. A lean individual actually has a greater surface area and thus a greater BMR than an obese individual of the same weight.

4. **Climate:** BMR is lower in the temperate (warm) climate than the cold climate.

5. **Physiological state:** BMR is increased in severe stress and after trauma. BMR remains unaltered during early pregnancy but after first half of pregnancy, an increase in BMR is observed. This is due to the additional BMR of the fetus.

6. **Diet:** Vegetarians have a lower BMR. BMR is lowered in undernutrition and during starvation, where BMR can decrease up to 50%. Caffeine, nicotine and alcohol increase BMR.

7. **Hormones:** Thyroxine, sex hormones, growth hormone, epinephrine and corticosteroids increase BMR. Thyroxine is the most important hormone in this regard. In fact, the measurement of BMR is used in the assessment of thyroid function. BMR is increased up to 75% in hyperthyroidism and reduced up to 50% in hypothyroidism. BMR is also increased in hyperactivity of the adrenals. In adrenal tumors and Cushing's syndrome BMR is increased. It is decreased in Addison's disease. BMR is also increased in hyperfunctioning of the anterior pituitary.

8. **Clinical disorders:** BMR is increased during fever as well as in certain infectious and hypercatabolic states. During fever, increase in BMR is usually proportional to rise of body temperature. For every 1°C rise in body temperature, there is nearly 12% increase in BMR. Due to increased metabolic activity of the cell, BMR is increased in leukemia, polycythemia, anemia, cardiac failure and hypertension.

SPECIFIC DYNAMIC ACTION OF FOOD

- **Specific dynamic action (SDA):** It is defined as the **extra heat production, over and above the actual** caloric value of the food when it is metabolized by the body. This stimulant action of food is also known as the **thermogenic effect** or the **calorigenic action** of food. These terms describe the effect of food in raising metabolic rate above the value found during fasting.

- **SDA depends on the type of food:** Protein food increases various metabolic processes by as much as 30%, whereas lipids by about 12% only. Carbohydrate meal also increases metabolic activities but to the least of all the foodstuffs, i.e. by about 5% only. For a mixed food, the SDA value is taken as 10% of the basal requirement.

  When we consume 25 g of protein, though theoretically we should get 100 kcal as per calorific value of 4 kcal/g, but ingestion of protein raises the metabolism by 30%, thus 25 g of protein actually releases 130 kcal of heat in the body. This extra 30 kcal generated from 25 g of proteins is actually the amount of heat body has spent for the catabolism of 25 g of protein and is regained back, as the product of SDA.

- **Significance of SDA**
  1. The cause of the calorigenic action though remains uncertain, however, it can partly account for the various activities being performed by the body such as for secretion of gastric juice, etc. The high value of SDA on feeding a diet rich in proteins and amino acids is actually due to the **requirement of energy for various metabolic activities** such as deamination of amino acids and synthesis of urea, etc. This energy is derived by the oxidation of other metabolites present within the tissues.

  2. High SDA of protein is also an important factor in the **regulation of body temperature**, as one feels satisfied after food, particularly after a protein rich meal in winter.
  3. The allowance for SDA should be added during **diet planning**.

ENERGY REQUIREMENT FOR PHYSICAL ACTIVITY

Energy requirement is also determined in a large part, by the extent and type of the physical activity which an individual performs over a period of time (Table 25.2). According to the physical activity, the whole population can be divided into three types of workers:
1. Those individuals who perform light type of physical activity are called **sedentary** workers, e.g. a shopkeeper, a carpenter, a painter, etc.
2. **Moderate** category of workers include those individuals who are performing both physical as well as mental activities, like a student, a farmer doing mechanized farming or a soldier, etc.
3. Jobs, such as the work of a plumber, the work in coal-mining, stone-crushing, rickshaw-pulling, etc. are included in the **heavy** category of physical activity.

On an average, a moderate male worker, e.g. a student requires nearly 2800 kcal per day while a female performing the same type of work needs only about 2200 kcal/day.

Average daily calorie requirement for different category of workers is given in Table 25.3.

BALANCED DIET

A balanced diet is defined as a diet which provides, quantitatively as well as qualitatively, adequate

Table 25.2: Calorie requirements for some of the physical activities

Physical activity	Average calorie requirement (kcal/hr)
Reading/sitting/standing	35
Tailoring/typing/writing	70
Household work	105
Carpentary/painting	140
Slow walk	200
Moderate walk	250
Walking downstairs	350
Walking fast/running/swimming	450
Walking upstairs	1000

Table 25.3: Average calorie requirement for different categories of workers

Category	Requirement (kcal/day)			
	Basal	SDA	For activity	Total (approximate)
Male				
Sedentary	1500	150	800	2400
Moderate	1500	150	1200	2800
Heavy	1500	150	2400	4000
Female				
Sedentary	1300	130	500	1900
Moderate	1300	130	800	2200
Heavy	1300	130	1600	3000

amounts of all the proximate principles of food for maintaining an optimum health. As a general rule, the following criteria should be met in a balanced diet:

1. **Calorie distribution:** Nearly 65–75% of the calories should be derived from carbohydrates, 15–20% from lipids and 10–15% from proteins.
2. **Carbohydrates:** It should include both digestible as well as indigestible (fibers) carbohydrates.
3. **Lipids:** It should mainly be from the vegetable sources. It should be rich in polyunsaturated fatty acids (PUFAs) but low in cholesterol.
4. **Proteins:** It should be of high biological value and easily digestible.
5. **Vitamins and minerals:** Green-leafy vegetables, fruits and milk should be included to provide the required amounts of vitamins and minerals.
6. **Water:** Adequate water intake is a must for all the aspects of metabolism besides elimination of toxic wastes.
7. **Economy:** The diet should have a variety of items from different sources, best possible within one's own budget.

Average dietary requirement for various nutrients is given in Table 25.4.

Role of Carbohydrates in Balanced Diet

Dietary carbohydrates are classified into:

1. **'Available' or 'digestible' carbohydrate:** It is digestible by enzymes in the GIT and thus serves as source of energy. Carbohydrates are at the forefront and most efficient sources of energy. From 65 to 75% of the energy should be derived from this source. Any carbohydrate in excess of that needed for energy is converted to glycogen and triacylglycerols for storage in the body. Carbohydrate containing foods, such as cereals and pulses, are the cheapest sources of energy and hence should form a greater part of the required calories in a diet. Principal sources of carbohydrates in the diet include starch (cereals, pulses and potatoes), lactose (milk), and sucrose (table sugar). Glucose though is specifically required by many tissues but may not form an essential part of the diet since starch and other dietary carbohydrates are readily converted to glucose in the body. A significant source of starch is potato. Compared to potato, the

starch content of wheat is about 70% while that of pulses is 60%.

2. **Dietary fibers:** 'Unavailable' or 'indigestible' carbohydrate that is **not digestible** by enzymes in the GIT and thus does not serve as source of energy is called 'dietary fibre' or 'non-starch poly-saccharides', which is again of two types:

   i. **Crude/insoluble fibre or 'roughage'**, e.g. cellu-lose and hemicellulose. Their functions include:
      - Retention of water during intestinal transit thereby preventing constipation.
      - Binding various dietary toxins thereby reducing the incidence of colon cancer.
      - Imparting a sense of early satiety (fullness of stomach) thereby helping to reduce calorie intake and thus to control obesity and diabetes mellitus.

      Insoluble fibers are abundant in vegetable grains. It is worth mentioning that insoluble fibres also include some non-polysaccharides, e.g. lignins (carrots, strawberry seeds), cutins and tannins.

   ii. **Soluble fiber**, e.g. gums and pectins found in legumes, fruits and oats. Their functions include:
      - Binding cholesterol and bile salts thereby reducing their enterohepatic circulation and enhancing the conversion of cholesterol into bile salts, lowering plasma cholesterol levels.
      - Reducing gastric emptying thereby delaying the postprandial rise in blood glucose of diabetic patients.

3. **Resistant starch:** Small fractions of starch that escape digestion and absorption are called 'resistant starch', found in whole legumes, raw potatoes and unripe bananas. Like fibers, they promote bowel movement in the colon but unlike fibers, they do not reduce blood cholesterol since they cannot bind to bile salts.

Role of Lipids in Balanced Diet

Dietary lipids include triglycerides, cholesterol, phospholipids and other complex lipids. As lipids are the **concentrated source of energy** and provide more than twice the energy supplied by carbohydrates or proteins per unit weight (9 kcal/g from lipids compared to 4 kcal/g from carbohydrates or proteins), lipids thus reduce bulk of the food. Dietary lipids are also important for their palatability, ability to impart

25

Table 25.4: Recommended daily allowance (RDA) of different nutrients

	Calories (kcal)	Protein (g)	Ca (mg)	Iron (mg)	Vitamins								
					A* (mg)	D (IU)	B_1 (mg)	B_2 (mg)	NE** (mg)	B_6 (mg)	Folic acid (µg)	B_{12} (µg)	C (mg)
Infants (<1 year)	100–200/ kg	1.7–2.3/ kg	500–600	1.0/kg	300–400	–	50–60/ kg	60–70/ kg	0.7–0.8/ kg	0.2–0.4	25–30	0.2	20–30
Children	1200–1400	20–25	400–500	20–25	250–300	200	0.6–0.7	0.7–0.8	8–9	0.6–0.7	50–100	0.2	30–50
Moderate workers													
Adult male	2500–3000	55–60	500–700	20–25	600–700	200	1.2–1.5	1.4–2.0	17–20	1.4–2.0	50–100	0.5–1.0	30–50
Adult female	2000–2200	45–50	500–700	30–35	600–700	200	1.0–1.1	1.0–1.2	12–14	1.0–1.1	50–100	0.5–1.0	30–50
Additional requirement													
During pregnancy	300	20	400	10	–	–	0.2	0.2	2	0.5	200	0.5	10
During lactation	500	25	400	–	400	–	0.4	0.4	5	0.5	50	0.5	40

* Retinol equivalents
**Niacin equivalents

a sense of satiety, forming membrane structures, absorption of lipid soluble vitamins, etc.

As lipids from vegetable sources are rich in poly-unsaturated fatty acids, it serves as a source of **essential fatty acids** for the body. **Phospholipids** and other complex lipids are also essential for the functioning of the nervous tissue. **Cholesterol** is present in the food of animal origin only and is an important precursor of vitamin D, steroid hormones and bile acids.

It is recommended that lipids should provide about 20% of the daily energy requirement. Out of this, about 10% of the calorie intake should be from invisible fat, such as from milk, cereals, pulses and legumes (pulses and legumes can provide nearly 5% fat). The remaining 10% of the calories may be added in the form of visible fat, such as from ghee, butter or oil, etc. provided no contraindications exist. *Trans* **fat should be avoided**.

Plant Fat versus Animal Fat: Fats included in the diet should preferably be derived from vegetable sources. This is not only lower in cost but also superior in quality as compared to the animal fat because **vegetable fat contains more of the PUFAs**. Sun-flower oil, cottonseed oil, wheat-germ oil, soya bean oil and corn oil are some of the vegetable oils in common use. These oils have more than 50% of the fat as PUFAs. Hydrogenation of the vegetable oil reduces the quantity of PUFAs, originally present in the oil.

Predominant fatty acids in animal fat, such as in meat, are saturated. **Excess consumption of saturated fat**, such as from animal sources and of cholesterol, such as from eggs is associated with **hyperchole-sterolemia** and **atherosclerosis**. Eggs have highest concentration of cholesterol. Cholesterol content of the skimmed-milk is lower than the whole milk. Pulses do not contain cholesterol. Besides atherosclerosis, excess cholesterol can also result in the formation of **biliary stones** leading to obstructive jaundice and fat indigestion. High fat intake is also associated with **cancer** of the breast and the colon.

Compared to the cost of carbohydrates which are the cheapest sources of energy, dietary fats are costlier. Thus, it is appropriately said that people who require more fat cannot afford it but those who can afford it should not consume it.

Essential Fatty Acids: Three polyunsaturated fatty acids have been recognized as essential in the diet of most animals. These are **linoleic acid, linolenic acid and arachidonic acid**, and are called as essential fatty acids.

These fatty acids are needed for lowering serum cholesterol, for maintaining the function and integrity of membrane structure, and for the synthesis of eicosanoids. The most common symptom of essential fatty acids deficiency is a scaly dermatitis.

Role of Proteins in Balanced Diet

Proteins serve many roles:

1. They are essential **structural components** of the cell.
2. Proteins are important for maintaining output of essential secretions, such as digestive **enzymes** and peptide or **protein hormones**.
3. Amino acids, the hydrolyzed product of protein, are required for the synthesis of **plasma proteins** which are essential for the maintenance of osmotic balance, transport of substances through blood and for maintaining immunity.
4. Excess of the protein may be used as a source of **energy**. Normally, the contribution of protein to energy value in a balanced diet should be 10 to 15% of the total calorie intake.
5. Protein is a source of both **essential as well as nonessential amino acids**.

Daily protein requirement for an adult man is nearly 0.8–1.0 g/kg body weight. During pregnancy and lactation, protein requirement is increased by about 10–25 g/day. Protein requirement also increases during growth or recovery from prolonged illness. Children may require 2.0–2.5 g of protein/kg of body weight.

Among the various dietary sources, meat, eggs, soya bean and milk are good choices.

'Protein Sparing' Effect of Carbohydrates and Lipids in Balanced Diet: Dietary intake of carbohydrates and lipids are also important in determining daily protein requirement. As energy content of the diet from carbohydrates and lipid increases, the need for protein decreases. This is referred to as protein sparing. **Carbohydrate is more efficient in protein sparing than lipid** since carbohydrate can be used as an energy source by all cells whereas lipid cannot be used by some of the cells, such as RBC. Excess protein is used as a source of energy, with the glucogenic amino acids being converted to glucose while the

25

ketogenic amino acids being converted to fatty acids and ketone bodies.

Assessment of Dietary Protein Quality: A good quality protein should not only be rich in **all the essential amino acids** but should also be **easily digestible**. Quality of the dietary protein can be assessed by several criteria such as biological value, digestibility, net protein utilization, amino acid score or chemical score. Biological value, digestibility or net protein utilization can be assessed by knowing the amount of protein-nitrogen that is ingested, absorbed and retained by the body. For example, if a person ingest 'I' g of protein-nitrogen out of which 'A' g is absorbed and 'R' g is retained by the body. Accordingly:

- **Biological value (BV) of the protein** refers to the proportion of the absorbed protein nitrogen retained by the body, i.e. BV - R/A. It is usually expressed as a percentage.
- **Digestibility (D)** refers to the proportion of the ingested protein nitrogen absorbed by the body, i.e. D = A/I.
- **Net protein utilization (NPU)** refers to the proportion of the ingested protein nitrogen retained by the body, i.e. NPU - R/I, or NPU = BV × D.
- **Amino acid score:** It refers to the total amino acid content in the protein relative to that present in the same quantity of a reference protein, expressed as percentage.
- **Chemical score:** It refers to the content of each essential amino acid in the protein relative to that present in the same quantity of a reference protein, expressed as percentage.

Nitrogen Balance: Protein status of the body can be assessed by calculating the nitrogen balance of an individual. Nitrogen balance is a comparison between intake of nitrogen as protein and its excretion through various routes, chiefly as undigested protein in feces, and urea and ammonia in urine (Fig. 25.2). A subject is said to be in nitrogen equilibrium, i.e. **zero nitrogen balance** when daily nitrogen intake equals excretion, i.e. the output through the urine, feces and skin.

A growing child should be in a **positive nitrogen balance**. Other conditions like pregnancy, lactation and convalescence (recovery from metabolic stress or acute illness) should also be associated with positive nitrogen balance. On the other hand, injury, chronic diseases (such as tuberculosis, rheumatoid arthritis, cancer), increased muscular activity, inadequate protein intake, lack of essential amino acids and increased metabolic stress lead to a **negative nitrogen balance** (Table 25.5).

Essential Amino Acids, Complete and Incomplete Proteins: Dietary protein is also an important source of amino acids required for the growth in children and

Table 25.5: Nitrogen balance and its alterations

N-balance	Protein intake (I)/ output (O)	Condition
Equilibrium	I = 0	Normal/healthy
Positive	I > 0	Growth, pregnancy, convalescence
Negative	I < 0	↓ Protein intake, trauma, chronic illness (e.g. tuberculosis)

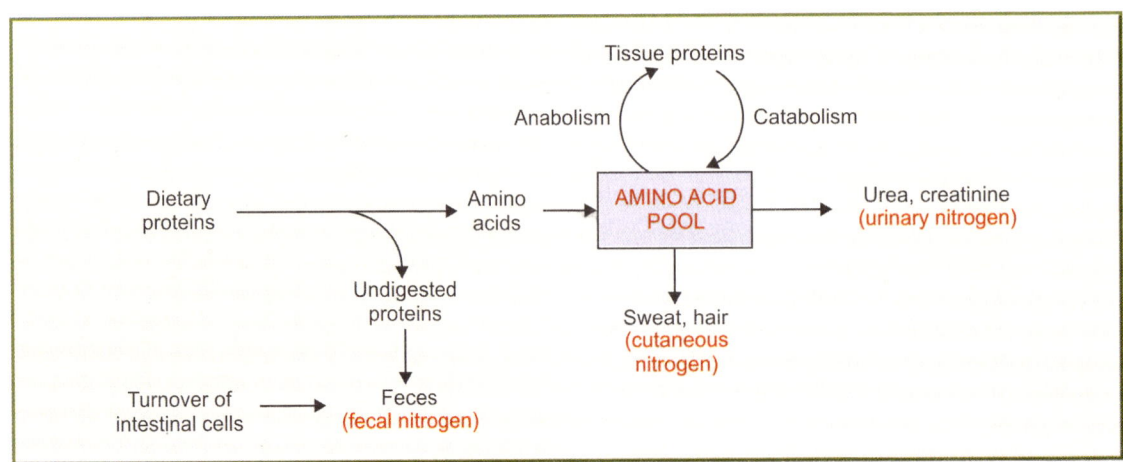

Fig. 25.2: Nitrogen balance.

for the maintenance of nitrogen balance in adults. As growth slows down, the need for protein declines. The requirement of protein is not only with respect to the quantity of protein in the diet but also the quality. An adult human body can maintain its nitrogen equilibrium on a mixture of 8 amino acids as the sole source of nitrogen. These are called **essential amino acids** and include isoleucine, leucine, lysine, methionine, phenylalanine, threonine, tryptophan and valine. In addition, histidine and arginine are also needed in extra amounts by infants during growth, and by females during pregnancy and lactation. These two amino acids are called **semiessential amino acids**.

Generally, most animal proteins such as **egg albumin, milk casein**, etc. contain **all the essential amino acids** and are called **complete proteins**. **Vegetable proteins**, e.g. wheat often lack one or more essential amino acids, and are called **incomplete proteins**.

Supplementary Action of Proteins: For vegetarians, though pulses are an important source of protein but, as mentioned above, most of the **vegetative proteins** are of **poor biological value** because they are **limiting** in some of the essential amino acids, such as wheat is limiting in lysine, pulses in methionine while maize in lysine, methionine as well as tryptophan.

Cereals in general are deficient in lysine and threonine. Cereals however, contain sufficiently high amounts of methionine. On the other hand, legumes and pulses are good sources of lysine and threonine but are poor in methionine. Therefore, the amino acids present in excess in pulses can effectively supplement the limiting amino acids of cereals and vice versa. This is known as **supplementary action of proteins**. It also provides a strong biochemical basis for the **traditional Indian dietary habit** of taking rice or wheat-bread with pulses.

PROTEIN ENERGY MALNUTRITION (PEM) OR PROTEIN CALORIE MALNUTRITION (PCM)

It is a **malnutrition-spectrum** whose extreme forms are known as kwashiorkor and marasmus (Fig. 25.3). **Kwashiorkor** usually occurs in the post-weaning period when diet is **adequate in energy but severely deficient in protein**. Clinical features include muscle wasting, edema, anemia, dry and brittle hair, diarrhea, dermatitis of various forms and retarded growth. On the other hand, **marasmus** occurs due to the **deficient**

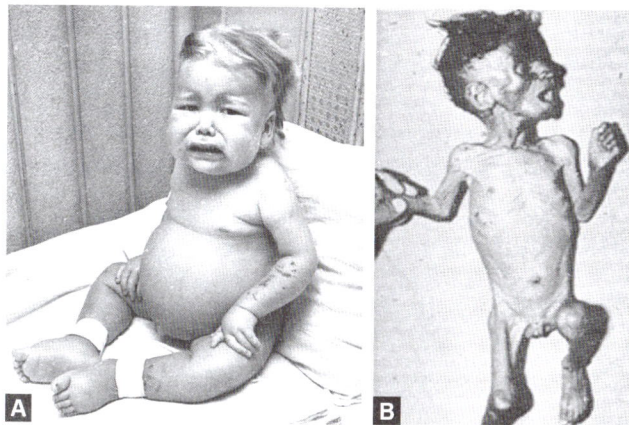

Fig. 25.3: The two extremes of the spectrum of protein-energy malnutrition. (A) Kwashiorkor, (B) Marasmus.

intake of both protein and calories, i.e. total food, generally due to early weaning. It differs from kwashiorkor with respect to the subcutaneous fat which disappears in marasmus but not in kwashiorkor. A marasmic infant thus generally has a thin, wasted appearance and is small-for-age. Some important features of kwashiorkor and marasmus are shown in Figs 25.4 and 25.5, and compared in Table 25.6.

Preservation of Vitamins

The days are gone when people used to buy food items and consume most of them on the same day. Our cooking, eating and drinking habits have changed markedly so that particular attention needs to be focused on preserving vitamins in food prior to consumption:

- Refrigerate fruits and vegetables to slow the degradation of nutrients.
- Cut fruits and vegetables should be wrapped airtight prior to refrigeration to prevent oxidation especially of vitamin C.
- Avoid prolonged exposure to UV light (sunlight and fluorescent light) that may degrade riboflavin.
- Rinse fruits and vegetables before (not after) cutting to minimize losses of water soluble vitamins.
- Avoid high temperature and long cooking time that may destroy thiamin.
- Use minimum water for cooking and then use it in other dishes.
- Avoid microwave for milk products and meat since microwave destroys vitamin B_{12}.

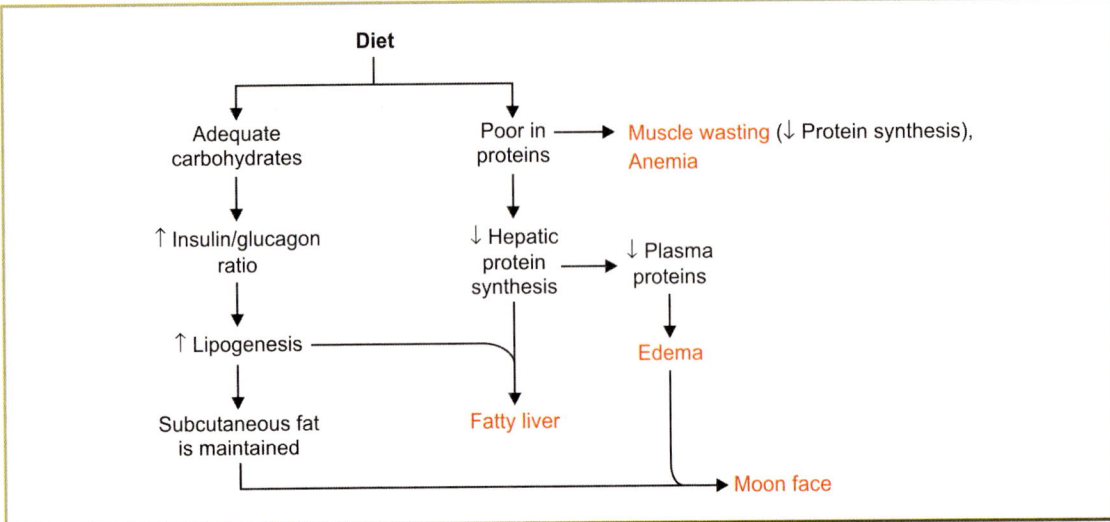

Fig. 25.4: Biochemical-clinical correlations in kwashiorkor.

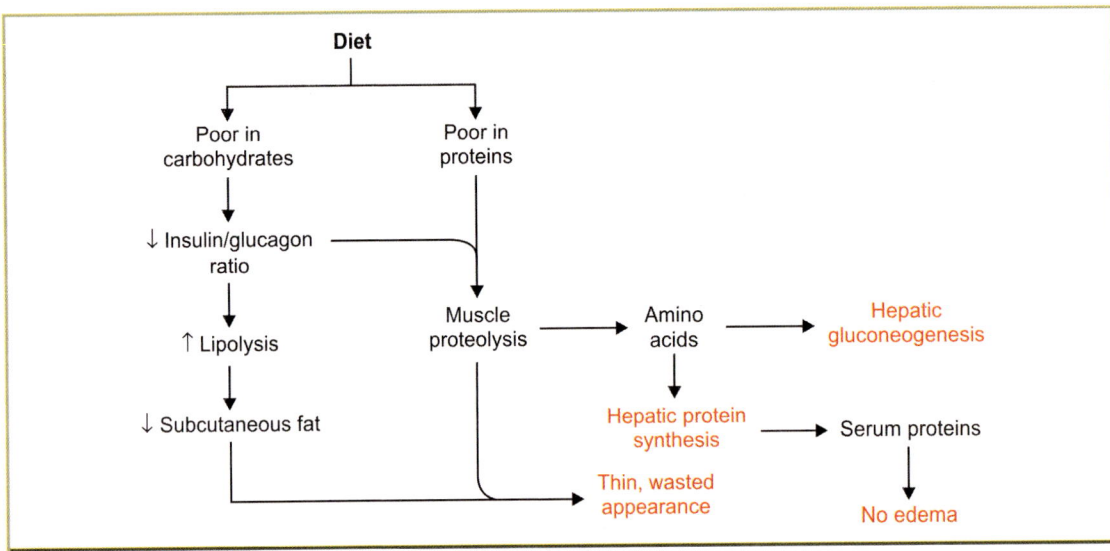

Fig. 25.5: Biochemical-clinical correlations in marasmus.

NUTRITIONAL SIGNIFICANCE OF SOME OF THE FOODSTUFFS

Milk

Milk is a good source of proteins, particularly that of all the essential amino acids, besides, lactose, vitamin A, calcium and phosphorus. Milk however, is poor in iron, vitamin C and essential fatty acids.

Egg

Egg is rich in cholesterol, saturated fatty acids and calcium but poor in vitamin C and essential fatty acids. Egg-yolk contains cholesterol.

Consumption of raw egg can result in biotin deficiency due to the presence of avidin.

Meat

Meat provides protein (rich in essential amino acids), iron, zinc, but lacks essential fatty acids.

Soya Bean

It is a good source of proteins especially for vegetarians. Further, it is rich in fibers, and is cholesterol-free.

Table 25.6: Comparison between kwashiorkor and marasmus

Kwashiorkor	*Marasmus*
Occurs in the post-weaning period (1–3 years)	Occurs due to early weaning (<1 year)
Deficiency of dietary proteins	Deficiency of dietary proteins plus energy
Rapid /acute onset	Slow/chronic development
Moderate weight loss; child is 60–80% weight-for-age	Severe weight loss; child is <60 weight-for-age
Moderate muscle wasting with retention of some body fat	Severe muscle wasting with practically no body fat
Edema is a conspicuous feature	No edema
Enlarged fatty liver	Liver is normal
Face reflects irritability and misery	Face shows apathy and anxiety
Loss of appetite	Good appetite possible
Hair shows color changes ('flag sign', Fig. 25.6) and becomes straight	Hair is sparse, thin and dry
Skin may develop lesions (flaky paint dermatitis)	Skin is dry, thin and easily wrinkles

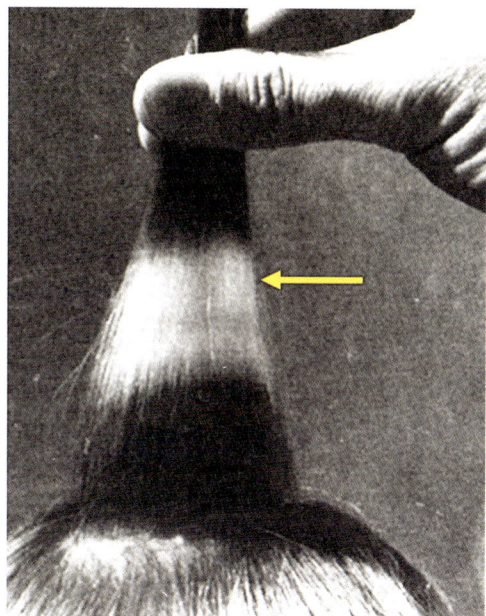

Fig. 25.6: '**Flag sign**' in kwashiorkor: Bands of depigmented (arrow) and normal hair caused by alternating periods of poor and relatively adequate protein intake.

COMMON NUTRITIONAL DISORDERS

As each nutrient is required by the body in only an appropriate amount, excessive intake or dietary deficiency of a nutrient may be harmful for the body. This, in turn, may result in a disorder. Some of the common nutritional disorders are given in Fig. 25.7. PEM was discussed above. Obesity, the commonest form of malnutrition today, is discussed in Chapter 12.

NUTRITIONAL ASPECTS OF ALCOHOLISM

Ethanol provides **empty calories** (7 kcal/g) and following prolonged consumption, its metabolism is associated with many deleterious consequences (Fig. 25.8):

- Increased formation of acetaldehyde is associated with facial flushing and headache especially in sensitive individuals, i.e. those having a higher activity of alcohol dehydrogenase. Further, acetaldehyde forms adducts with the amino groups of proteins resulting in loss of biological function of these proteins.
- Increased generation of reactive oxygen species/reactive nitrogen species result in oxidative/nitrosative stress with damage to cellular lipids, carbohydrates, proteins and DNA with carcinogenic potential.
- Increased $NADH/NAD^+$ ratio in the hepatocytes reduces fatty acid oxidation, promotes lipogenesis with accumulation of triacylglycerols, fatty liver and if untreated, cirrhosis. Further, it inhibits gluconeogenesis causing hypoglycemia especially in the undernourished, and promotes accumulation of lactate and lactacidosis.
- Deficiency of micronutrients causing neurological manifestations, anemia, etc.

DRUG-NUTRIENT INTERACTIONS

Nutritional disorders can also result from the prolonged use of certain drugs (Table 25.7) thereby demanding appropriate nutritional supplementations.

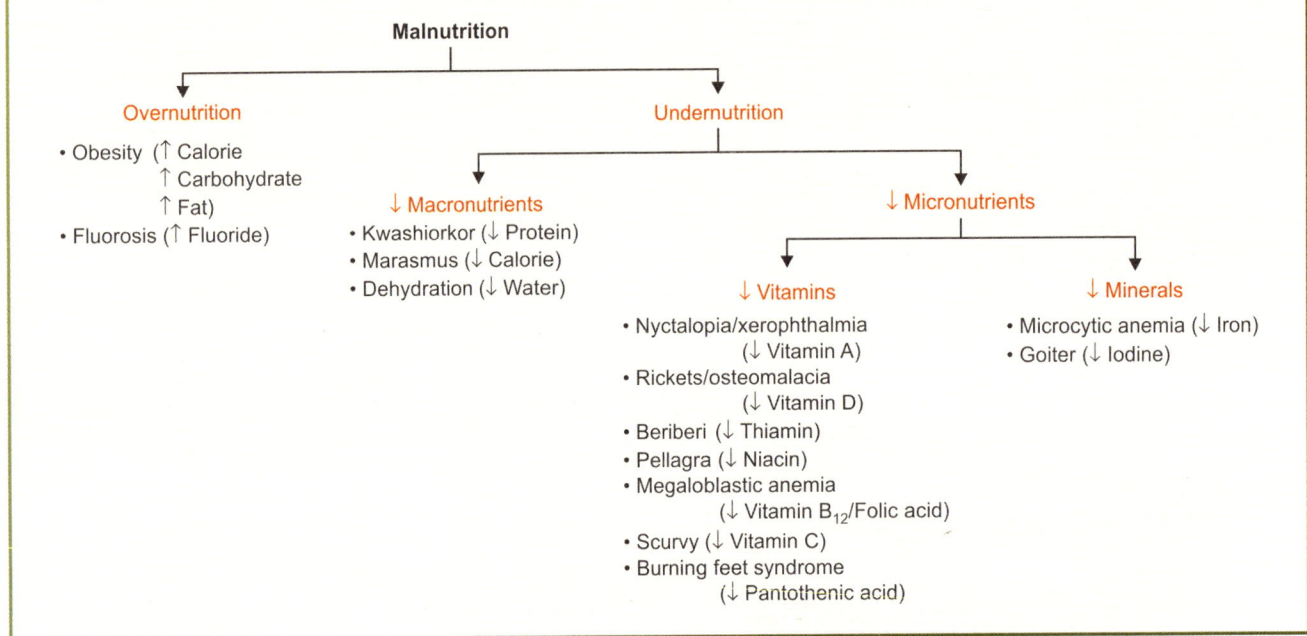

Fig. 25.7: Some common nutritional disorders.

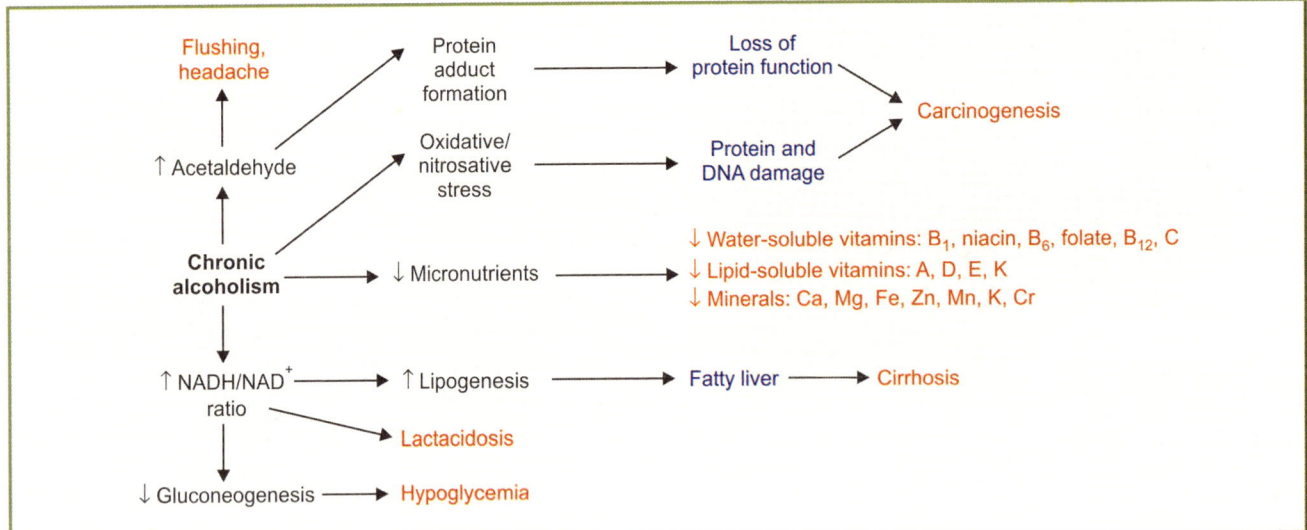

Fig. 25.8: Nutritional implications of chronic alcoholism.

Table 25.7: Drug-nutrient interactions

Drug	Indications	Nutrient deficiency
Phenytoin	Epilepsy	Vitamin D, folate, vitamin K
Cholestyramine	Hypercholesterolemia	Lipid-soluble vitamins, Iron
Corticosteroids	Autoimmune diseases, connective tissue disorders, etc.	Vitamin D, calcium, zinc, potassium
Thiazide diuretics	Hypertension with edema	Potassium, zinc
Isoniazid	Tuberculosis	Pyridoxine
Oral contraceptives	Birth control	Pyridoxine, folate, vitamin B_{12}

SOME IMPORTANT QUESTIONS

1. Define basal metabolic rate. Discuss various factors influencing BMR.

2. Describe the role of different components of a balanced diet for a male student.

3. Discuss:
   i. Role of crude-fiber in diet
   ii. Importance of carbohydrates in human nutrition
   iii. Supplementary action of proteins
   iv. Protein energy malnutrition
   v. Nutritional aspects of alcoholism

4. Write notes on:
   i. Biological value of proteins
   ii. Balanced diet
   iii. Respiratory quotient
   iv. SDA
   v. Essential fatty acids
   vi. Essential amino acids
   vii. Calorimetry
   viii. Nitrogen balance
   ix. Drug-nutrient interactions

MULTIPLE CHOICE QUESTIONS

1. The RQ is least for:
   A. Carbohydrates
   B. Lipids
   C. Proteins
   D. Mixed diet

2. The caloric value of ethanol is:
   A. 0.7 kcal/g
   B. 7.0 kcal/g
   C. 70.0 kcal/g
   D. 700.0 kcal/g

3. Most of the basal energy requirement is used for:
   A. Active membrane transport
   B. Nerve impulse transmission
   C. Involuntary muscle contraction
   D. Thermoregulation

4. The BMR is not increased in:
   A. Addison's disease
   B. Hyperthyroidism
   C. Cushing's syndrome
   D. Pheochromocytoma

5. Prolonged consumption of cholesterol-rich diet may be associated with:
   A. Cancer of breast and colon
   B. Biliary stones
   C. Atherosclerosis
   D. Any of the above

6. Juvenile-onset obesity is mainly:
   A. Hypoplastic
   B. Hyperplastic
   C. Atrophic
   D. Hypertrophic

7. Metabolic syndrome includes:
   A. Obesity and dyslipidemia
   B. Insulin resistance
   C. Hypertension
   D. All of the above

8. The following is a popular prescription for the purpose of weight reduction in obesity:
   A. Pancreatic lipase inhibitor
   B. Pancreatic amylase inhibitor
   C. Salivary amylase inhibitor
   D. All of the above

9. Edema, enlarged fatty liver and hair 'flag sign' are characteristic of:
   A. Marasmus
   B. Obesity
   C. Nephrotic syndrome
   D. Kwashiorkor

10. The following is required more during pregnancy than during lactation:
    A. Iron
    B. Calcium
    C. Vitamin D
    D. Vitamin A

26

Water and Electrolytes

Adequate hydration (water) and normal levels of electrolytes are important for proper functioning of the body.

METABOLISM OF WATER

Water is a very special kind of nutrient since

- Water is consumed at more frequent intervals and in greater amounts as compared to other nutrients.
- It is the most abundant substance present in the body.
- It is more important than food, as if one is given water but no food, the individual may survive for several weeks inspite of the loss of most of the body fat and 50% of the tissue proteins. On the other hand, a loss of about 10% of the body water may cause illness whereas a further loss of 10% of body water may even cause death.
- Increased fluid intake is very beneficial for individuals with renal calculi, urinary tract infections and chronic obstructive respiratory disease.

Human body consists of about 50–70% of its weight as water. At birth, about 75% of total body mass is water which is reduced to nearly 60% for an average adult male. The value falls to about 50% thereafter. Due to relatively high fat content, females have nearly 5% less water.

Most tissues contain more than 70% water though bone and adipose tissue contain relatively lesser amounts. This is due to the reason that the proportion of water in a tissue or in the whole body depends upon the proportion of fat in the tissue (Table 26.1).

Table 26.1: Average water content of different tissues

Tissue	Water content (% of total weight)
Whole body	60–70
Muscles	75–80
Nervous tissue	70–85
RBC	60
Bones	25
Adipose tissue	20

Physiological Functions of Water

Water is needed for various physicochemical processes in the body:

1. It is a common solvent in which most of the chemical reactions of the body occur.
2. It participates in various metabolic processes within the cell.
3. It transports vital substances via blood, lymph and other body fluids.
4. It is also essential for the elimination of waste products from the body.
5. Water intake helps to maintain water content of the feces and thus promotes regular bowel movement.
6. Increased water intake prevents urinary tract infections and kidney stones by increasing the flow of urine.
7. It helps to provide lubrication in various strategic locations of the body, e.g. synovial fluid between the joints, mucus in the respiratory passage, etc.
8. As the latent heat of evaporation of water is high, it assists in the regulation of body temperature.

Distribution of Water in Different Compartments

Total body water can be divided into two major compartments—intracellular fluid (ICF) and extracellular fluid (ECF).

- The **ICF** is composed of the fluid within the trillions of cells in our body.
- The **ECF** is composed of fluid outside the cells. In a young adult man, two-thirds of the body water is in the ICF and one-third is in the ECF (Fig. 26.1).

These two fluids differ strikingly in terms of their electrolyte composition. Their total solute concentrations (osmolalities), however, are equal because of the high water permeability of most cell membranes so that an osmotic difference between cells and ECF rapidly disappears.

The **ECF** can be further subdivided into two sub-compartments, which are separated from each other by the endothelium of blood vessels.

- The **plasma** is the ECF found within the vascular system. It is the fluid portion of the blood in which blood cells are suspended. The plasma water comprises of about 3.5 L for an average 70 kg man (Fig. 26.1).
- The **interstitial fluid and lymph** are considered together because they cannot be separated easily. Both are ultrafiltrates of plasma. The interstitial fluid directly bathes most body cells and the lymph is the fluid within lymphatic vessels. The water of the interstitial fluid and lymph comprises of 10.5 L of the ECF.

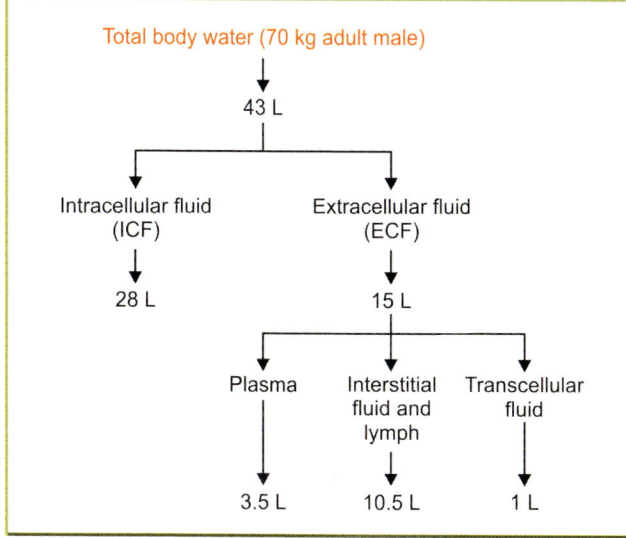

Fig. 26.1: Distribution of body water.

Chemistry to Clinics 26.1: Shock
In pathological conditions causing shock such as bacterial sepsis, extensive burns, the permeability of the vascular endothelium increases. This, in turn, results in leakage of albumin and a reduction in the effective circulating volume leading to hypotension.

The plasma, interstitial fluid and lymph are nearly identical in composition except for the higher protein concentration in the plasma. Plasma is separated from the interstitial fluid by the endothelial lining of the capillaries which acts as a semipermeable membrane and allows the passage of water and diffusible solutes but not the large molecular weight substances, such as proteins (Chemistry to Clinics 26.1).

Transcellular fluid: An additional ECF compartment, the transcellular fluid (Fig. 26.1), is small but physiologically important, amounting to 1–3% of body weight. It includes the cerebrospinal fluid, aqueous humor, secretions of the gastrointestinal tract and associated organs (saliva, gastric juice, bile, pancreatic juice, intestinal juice, etc.), renal tubular fluid and bladder urine, synovial fluid and sweat. In these cases, the fluid is separated from the plasma by an epithelial cell layer in addition to a capillary endothelium. The epithelial layer modifies the electrolyte composition of the fluid so that transcellular fluids are not plasma ultrafiltrates (as are interstitial fluid and lymph). There is a constant turnover of transcellular fluids; they are continuously formed and absorbed or removed. Impaired formation, abnormal loss from the body or blockage of fluid passage can have serious consequences.

The composition of ICF differs markedly from that of the ECF, as these compartments are separated from each other by a cell membrane. These differences in composition in the two compartments are a consequence of the Gibbs-Donnan equilibrium (Chapter 3).

Sources and Requirement

Most of the foods, beverages, and many fruits and vegetables are good sources of water. Water is also available to the body as a result of metabolic breakdown of food for energy. The amount of water produced by the oxidation of nutrients however, depends upon the type of the nutrient used in the body, e.g. 100 g of fats produce 107 ml, 100 g of carbohydrates produce 56 ml while 100 g of proteins produce 41 ml of water. On an average, the amount of endogenous water produced by an individual is nearly 300 ml per day.

Daily need for water varies widely with variations in several characteristics of the person, e.g. body surface area, amount of body fat, metabolic rate, physical activity and environmental factors, as temperature, humidity, altitude, clothing, etc. The minimum requirement for a resting healthy 70 kg adult man, at moderate environmental temperature and humidity, is about 1700–1800 ml/day. Normal activity increases this requirement by 700–800 ml/day. Thus, a total of about 2500 ml of water is required daily. This, in turn, suggests that under normal circumstances about 1 ml/kcal is a reasonable allowance for an adult. A higher requirement, $\approx$1.5 ml/kcal, is recommended for healthy infants.

Regulation of Body Water

In a normal adult, the quantity of water intake is balanced by that which is eliminated from the body everyday, thus maintaining a state of equilibrium (Fig. 26.2). Water balance is thus regulated by two mechanisms, i.e. by its intake as well as output.

Water intake: Volume of the liquid ingested is regulated by thirst which is under the control of thirst center. Minimum requirement for water, however, is highly variable and depends upon several other factors such as:

- **Obligatory losses:** There is an obligatory but variable loss of water in insensible perspiration, breath and feces. Sweating can greatly increase fluid loss and thus its demand.
- **Disease conditions:** Fluid intake is also associated with physical condition and injury, e.g. fluid loss increases due to watery diarrhea or blood loss, etc. Human body has receptors in the right atrium, called baroreceptors which are sensitive to changes in osmotic pressure and blood volume. During

certain pathological conditions, e.g. congestive heart failure, hepatic cirrhosis, nephrotic syndrome, etc. baroreceptors detect a decrease in blood volume despite an overall expansion of the ECF. This excess fluid in the ECF compartment gets collected in the tissues and cause edema.

- **Dietary factors:** Sodium tends to hold water so extra sodium (salt) intake may increase water content of the body. Carbohydrate content of the diet affects both sodium and water balance. Increased amount of carbohydrate in the diet increases water retention while a low carbohydrate intake results in a loss of body fluid. Serum proteins influence water balance by their osmotic effect since proteins draw water from the interstitial fluid into the blood. If a low protein diet is consumed for a longer duration, serum albumin levels fall to such an extent that fluid accumulates between the cells and thus total body water is increased.

Water output: Water is removed from the body in the form of urine, feces, perspiration and expiration (Fig. 26.2):

- **Urine:** It is an important medium for the elimination of water present in the body in excess of its requirement. Normally, about 1.2 to 1.5 liter of water is excreted in the form of urine, daily.
- **Feces:** Normally, about 80–150 ml of water is excreted in the feces of an adult, daily. The value may increase considerably on a high vegetable diet, particularly in the presence of diarrhea.
- **Perspiration:** The amount of water lost in the perspiration varies enormously. When the environmental temperature or humidity increases, sweat glands become active and thus in summer excessive water is lost via perspiration. Sweat removes a hypotonic solution which in addition to water also contains Na^+ and Cl^-. *Insensible perspiration* is the process whereby the body loses water continuously from the skin surface and lungs. Contrary to the *visible perspiration* which removes hypotonic solution, insensible perspiration consists solely of water. Normally, from an adult human being about 300–700 ml of water is eliminated by this route, daily.
- **Expiration:** Nearly 500 ml of water is lost daily in the exhaled air.

Failure to regulate water balance results in dehydration (Chemistry to Clinics 26.2) or edema (Chemistry to Clinics 26.3).

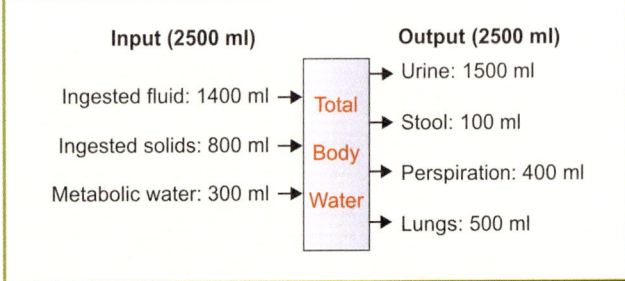

Fig. 26.2: Water homeostasis.

Chemistry to Clinics 26.2: Dehydration

Water deficit or volume depletion is referred to as dehydration. However, pure water deficit is rare and hence in clinical practice, the term 'dehydration' indicates water plus electrolyte deficit. Several conditions such as diarrhea, uncontrolled diabetes mellitus, diabetes insipidus, overdose of diuretics, heat stroke, etc. may lead to dehydration. Fluid and electrolyte status of these patients should be corrected at the earliest by employing suitable oral (oral rehydration solution) or intravenous (isotonic saline, dextrose-saline, Ringer lactate) fluids.

Chemistry to Clinics 26.3: Edema

Due to the retention of water alongwith sodium, both of these move from the blood to the interstitial fluid allowing maintenance of a relatively normal blood volume. When fluid retention is observable, the condition is called edema which takes the form of puffiness in the fingers and ankles or sometimes of the entire body (anasarca). Retention of sodium and water, as occurs in patients with congestive heart failure, increases workload on the heart and may precipitate an acute failure. A serious consequence of acute heart failure may be congestion in the lungs (pulmonary edema) and thus may lead to respiratory distress.

Diet modifications, particularly reducing sodium intake often in conjunction with diuretic therapy is helpful in the treatment of conditions associated with excessive retention of sodium and water. However, when diuretic therapy is used along with sodium restriction, special attention should also be paid towards the need of potassium and other minerals whose excretion is also affected by the diuretics. For example, the use of diuretics such as furosemide and thiazides, may cause depletion of potassium, magnesium and zinc.

Any fluid intake below 2000 ml daily is considered to be a restriction. Sodium-restricted diet though is very helpful in preventing fluid accumulation; sometimes it is necessary to restrict both water as well as Na^+ intake. The restricted intake of water and Na^+ is termed as fluid restriction. In congestive heart failure, cirrhosis of the liver with ascites or any other disease in which intravascular volume is increased, fluid restriction may be employed to promote diuresis or to prevent life-threatening hyponatremia.

METABOLISM OF ELECTROLYTES

Major electrolytes are the ionic forms of essential minerals, specifically sodium (Na^+), potassium (K^+), calcium (Ca^{2+}), magnesium (Mg^{2+}), chloride (Cl^-) and phosphates (HPO_4^{2-}). Electrolytes are distributed unevenly between ICF and ECF. Different concentrations of electrolytes in the two compartments are vital for the normal physiological processes.

Metabolism of calcium, magnesium and phosphorus is being discussed separately in the next chapter. The metabolism of Na^+, K^+ and Cl^- is being discussed here.

Table 26.2: Electrolyte distribution in various fluid compartments

Electrolyte	Concentration (mmol/L)	
	Intracellular fluid	Plasma
Total anions	**205**	**154**
Cl^-	2	103
HPO_4^{2-}	148	4
Others	55	47
Total cations	**205**	**154**
Na^+	10	142
K^+	160	4
Others	35	8

Table 26.2 gives the differences in chemical composition of the ICF and plasma. Since interstitial fluid and plasma are nearly similar in composition, they are considered together. Even though there are marked differences in the composition of ICF and ECF, their osmolarity is essentially the same.

Tonicity, Osmolarity and Osmolality

Tonicity takes into account the concentration of only impermeable solutes in a solution while osmolarity refers to the total concentration of permeable plus impermeable solutes. Osmotic concentration or **osmolarity** is the number of osmoles of solute per liter of solution, expressed as Osm/L. On the other hand, **osmolality** is the number of osmoles of solute per kg of solvent, expressed as Osm/kg.

Electrolyte Balance

Various mechanisms operate to maintain a normal electrolyte balance in body fluids (Fig. 26.3). Table 26.3 lists functions of electrolytes.

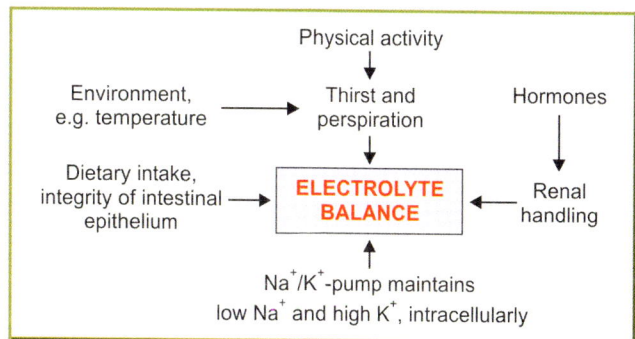

Fig. 26.3: Electrolyte balance. Aldosterone, secreted by the adrenal cortex, facilitates the retention of Na^+ and excretion of K^+ by the kidneys. Hypofunctioning of the adrenal cortex **(Addison's disease)** results in hyponatremia with hyperkalemia while hyperfunctioning of the adrenal cortex **(Cushing's syndrome)** results in hypernatremia with hypokalemia.

26

SODIUM

The adult human body contains ≈100 g of sodium, as sodium ions (Na^+). About half of this is found in the extracellular fluid while the remaining half in the cells and bone. Sodium is the **major cation in the ECF**. It exists in the body in association with several anions such as chloride, bicarbonate, phosphate, lactate and proteinate. High concentration of Na^+ along with low K^+ in the extracellular fluid is maintained by Na^+/K^+-ATPase (Na^+/K^+-pump).

Na^+/K^+-ATPase (also called Na^+/K^+-pump): It transports **Na^+ from inside to outside** of the cell, actively against an electrochemical gradient. Transport of **$3Na^+$** is coupled with the transport of **$2K^+$ in the opposite direction**. The pump is present in the cell membrane and derives its energy from ATP. The pump consists of a large transmembrane catalytic subunit which has a binding site for ATP along with a binding site for Na^+ on the internal surface and for K^+ on the external surface. This active transport of Na^+ results in maintaining high concentration of Na^+ and Cl^- extracellularly (in the ECF), and K^+ intracellularly (in the ICF).

Table 26.3: Functions of major body electrolytes

Sodium
1. Regulation of osmotic pressure of extracellular fluid
2. Regulation of acid–base balance of extracellular fluid
3. GI and renal absorption of monosaccharides and amino acids
4. Maintenance of neuromuscular irritability and excitability
5. Maintenance of blood viscosity
6. Cofactor for Na^+/K^+-ATPase

Potassium
1. Regulation of intracellular osmotic pressure
2. Regulation of intracellular acid–base balance
3. GI secretions
4. Maintenance of neuromuscular irritability and excitability
5. Storage of proteins and glycogen
6. Cofactor for enzymes, e.g. Na^+/K^+-ATPase, pyruvate kinase, etc.

Chloride
1. Regulation of osmotic pressure of extracellular fluid
2. Regulation of acid–base balance of extracellular fluid
3. Component of gastric juice (HCl)
4. Component of innate immunity (HOCl)
5. Chloride shift helps in maintaining electrical equilibrium between intracellular and extracellular fluids
6. Cofactor for enzymes, e.g. salivary amylase

Absorption and Excretion

Sodium is completely absorbed by the gastrointestinal tract. It is mainly excreted by the kidneys. Under normal physiological conditions, its daily urinary excretion is equal to its intake, since only less than 2% of the ingested sodium is eliminated in the feces. It is freely filtered by the glomerulus. About 70% of the filtered sodium is reabsorbed by the proximal tubules, 15% by the loops of Henle, 5% by the distal convoluted tubules and about 10% by the collecting ducts. Active reabsorption of Na^+ in the proximal tubule results in the passive reabsorption of Cl^- and HCO_3^- along with water. This helps to maintain electrical neutrality of the extracellular fluid while the reabsorption of water ensures normal osmotic pressure. Sodium homeostasis is influenced by several general factors (Fig. 26.3).

Natriuretic Hormones

1. **Atrial natriuretic peptide (ANP):** It is a 28-amino acid peptide synthesized and stored in myocytes of the cardiac atria. It is released on stretch of the atria, e.g. following volume expansion. This hormone has several actions that increase Na^+ excretion. ANP acts on the kidneys to increase glomerular blood flow, the filtration rate and inhibits Na^+ reabsorption by the inner medullary collecting ducts. The second messenger for ANP in the collecting duct is cGMP. ANP directly inhibits aldosterone secretion by the adrenal cortex; it also indirectly inhibits aldosterone secretion by diminishing renal renin release. ANP is a vasodilator and therefore lowers blood pressure. Some evidence suggests that ANP inhibits AVP secretion.

2. **Urodilatin (kidney natriuretic peptide, KNP):** It is a 32-amino acid peptide derived from the same prohormone as ANP. It is synthesized primarily by intercalated cells in the cortical collecting duct, is secreted into the tubule lumen and inhibits Na^+ reabsorption by inner medullary collecting ducts via cGMP.

3. **Brain natriuretic peptide (BNP):** It was first isolated from the brain but is also produced by myocytes in the cardiac ventricles. Increased plasma levels serve as a marker of cardiac injury. Recombinant BNP is used to promote renal Na^+ excretion in patients with decompensated congestive heart failure.

4. Guanylin and uroguanylin: These are peptide hormones produced by the small intestine in response to salt ingestion. They activate guanylyl cyclase and produce cGMP as a second messenger, as their names suggest, and induce a natriuresis.

5. Bradykinin: It is produced locally in the kidneys and inhibits Na^+ reabsorption.

6. Prostaglandin E_2 and I_2 (prostacyclin): These are local hormones produced in the kidneys from arachidonic acid, and increase renal Na^+ excretion.

Sources and Requirement

The most important source of sodium is the common **table salt**, i.e. sodium chloride. Meat, seafoods, milk, cheese and bread are its good sources. Plant sources are usually low in sodium. Daily intake of sodium as sodium chloride, varies from 5 to 15 g depending upon the climate.

Alterations in Sodium Homeostasis

Hyponatremia

It is defined as plasma Na^+ concentration **<135 mEq/L**. It is the most common disorder of body fluid and electrolyte balance. Most often it reflects a problem of too much water, not too little Na^+, in the plasma. Drinking large quantities of water rarely causes hyponatremia because of the large capacity of the kidneys to excrete dilute urine. If, however, plasma antidiuretic hormone (ADH) is not decreased when plasma osmolality is decreased or if the ability of the kidneys to dilute the urine is impaired, hyponatremia may develop even with a normal water intake.

Because Na^+ is the major solute in the plasma, it is not surprising that hyponatremia is usually associated with hypo-osmolality. However, hyponatremia may also occur with a normal or even elevated plasma osmolality.

- **Hyponatremia and hypo-osmolality** can occur in the presence of a decreased, normal or even increased total body Na^+ (Chemistry to Clinics 26.4).
- **Hyponatremia and increased plasma osmolality** is seen in hyperglycemic patients with uncontrolled diabetes mellitus. In this condition, the high blood glucose causes the osmotic withdrawal of water from cells and the extra water in the ECF space leads to hyponatremia. Plasma Na^+ falls by 1.6 mEq/L for each 100 mg/dl rise in blood glucose.
- **Hyponatremia and normal plasma osmolality** are seen in the so-called **pseudohyponatremia**. This occurs when plasma lipids or proteins are greatly elevated. These molecules do not significantly elevate plasma osmolality. However, they do occupy a significant volume of the plasma and because the Na^+ is dissolved only in the plasma water, the Na^+ measured in the entire plasma is low.

Hypernatremia

Hypernatremia is defined as plasma Na^+ concentration **>150 mEq/L**. It is **always hyperosmolar** and is characterized by edema, azotemia and anemia.

Chemistry to Clinics 26.4: Hyponatremia and Hypo-osmolality

- **Hyponatremia and decreased total body Na^+:** It is seen with increased Na^+ loss such as with vomiting, diarrhea and diuretic therapy. The decrease in ECF volume stimulates thirst and ADH release. More water is ingested but the kidneys form osmotically concentrated urine, resulting in plasma hypo-osmolality and hyponatremia.
- **Syndrome of inappropriate ADH secretion (SIADH):** It occurs with neurological disease, severe pain, certain drugs (such as hypoglycemic agents) and with some tumors.
- **Hyponatremia and increased total body Na^+:** It is seen in edematous states such as congestive heart failure, hepatic cirrhosis and nephrotic syndrome. The decrease in effective arterial blood volume stimulates thirst and ADH release. The excretion of dilute urine may also be impaired because of decreased delivery of fluid to diluting sites along the nephron and collecting ducts. Although both Na^+ and water are retained by the kidneys in the edematous states, relatively more water is conserved leading to a dilutional hyponatremia.
- **General symptoms:** Muscle cramps, lethargy, fatigue, disorientation, headache, anorexia, nausea, agitation, hypothermia, seizures and coma. These symptoms, mainly neurological, are a consequence of the swelling of brain cells as plasma osmolality falls. Excessive brain swelling may be fatal or may cause permanent damage.
- **Treatment:** Identify and treat the underlying cause. If Na^+ loss is responsible for the hyponatremia, isotonic or hypertonic saline or NaCl by mouth is usually given. If the blood volume is normal or the patient is edematous, water restriction is recommended. Hyponatremia should be corrected slowly and with constant monitoring because too rapid correction can be harmful, resulting in central pontine myelinolysis.

26

It is generally accepted that abnormal retention of salt (NaCl) by the kidneys is the major contributor to hypertension. Both the Na^+ and Cl^- in salt are critical; if chloride is replaced by bicarbonate or citrate ions in the diet then hypertension does not develop. Nonetheless, it is common to focus on Na^+ as the culprit because it is actively reabsorbed by the kidneys and the Cl^- usually just follows along. Salt retention leads to water retention and hence, higher volume and pressure in the vascular system. Dietary salt restriction and the use of diuretics, i.e. drugs that promote salt and water excretion, are highly effective in treating salt sensitive hypertension.

Multiple genes and environmental factors contribute to hypertension. Many of the implicated genes affect blood pressure by changing salt and water reabsorption by the kidneys. A good example is Liddle syndrome, an autosomal dominant disorder in which patients develop early and severe hypertension. In these patients, the renal epithelial Na^+ channel is constitutively activated, leading to excessive Na^+ and water reabsorption. They also develop hypokalemia caused by excessive renal loss of K^+. The hypertension can be effectively treated by a low-salt diet and the use of a diuretic drug, amiloride, which specifically blocks the overactive Na^+ channel.

Accumulation of Na^+ in the body has been shown to result in a concomitant rise in blood pressure referred to as essential hypertension (Chemistry to Clinics 26.5).

Symptoms are primarily neurological which include tremors, irritability, confusion and coma.

POTASSIUM

Potassium is the **chief cation in the ICF**. Its functions are outlined in Table 26.3. Potassium homeostasis is influenced by several general factors (Fig. 26.3).

Absorption and Excretion

Potassium is completely absorbed from the gastrointestinal tract. Less than 10% of the potassium is eliminated in feces. It is freely filtered at the glomerulus. Its active tubular reabsorption occurs throughout the nephron. Potassium is normally excreted almost entirely by the kidneys.

Sources and Requirement

Potassium is widely distributed in plants as well as animals, as the chloride, phosphate and carbonate salts of inorganic acids, organic acids and proteins. The good sources of potassium are coffee, cocoa, dried beans, wheat bran, most of the vegetables such as potato, tomato, dairy products, fish, eggs, meat and fruits like banana, peach and orange. Though the normal intake of potassium has been recommended as about 4 g daily, the daily requirement in sodium to potassium ratio of 1:1, on a molar basis, has been suggested.

Alterations in Potassium Homeostasis

Disorders of acid–base balance, water balance and administration of some drugs are often accompanied by alterations in potassium balance: Either potassium deficit (hypokalemia) or excess (hyperkalemia).

Hypokalemia

- Hypokalemia is defined as serum potassium concentration **<3.5 mEq/L**.
- It is seen in individuals taking potassium losing diuretics (carbonic anhydrase inhibitors, loop diuretics and thiazides), those with severe liver disease, gastrointestinal losses, and metabolic alkalosis. Hyperaldosteronism can cause excess excretion of potassium accompanied by increased retention of Na^+ which leads to depletion of plasma K^+. Prolonged hypokalemia, in turn, further causes damage to the kidneys.
- Both cardiac and skeletal muscles are affected by hypokalemia. Deficiency symptoms include muscular weakness, mental apathy, cardiac arrhythmias (irregular heart beat), tachycardia (heart beat more rapid than usual), hypotension, paralysis, bone fragility, etc.
- It can be corrected by oral KCl supplements and, if necessary, by suitable intravenous electrolytes.

Hyperkalemia

- Hyperkalemia is defined as serum potassium concentration **>5.5 mEq/L**.
- Hyperkalemia arises when K^+ excretion by the kidney is depressed such as in acute renal failure.
- Acidosis causes leakage of K^+ from the cell which may increase plasma K^+ while leaving the cells depleted of K^+.
- Potassium-sparing diuretics may lead to hyperkalemia.
- Early signs of cardiac damage include arrhythmia followed by a slowing of the heart rate, ventricular fibrillation and arrest in diastole.

- Hyperkalemia may lead to CNS depression, mental confusion, numbness or tingling of extremities and weakness of respiratory muscles resulting in difficulty in breathing and speech. High concentration of potassium is also toxic to the muscles and may cause paralysis.

- Under such situations, K^+ is excluded from the diet. Insulin and glucose promote the uptake of K^+ into the cells and this treatment is used for patients suffering from life-threatening hyperkalemia.

CHLORIDE

Chloride (Cl^-) is the **most abundant anion in the ECF**. Normal plasma chloride concentration varies between 95 and 107 mEq/L. The highest concentration of chloride is found in the CSF. Its functions are outlined in Table 26.3.

Alterations in plasma Cl^- concentration generally parallel with those in plasma Na^+ except in the presence of some acid–base disturbances. The determination of plasma Cl^- concentration thus is useful in the differential diagnosis of acid–base disturbances, for calculating the anion gap.

Anion Gap

In a normal individual, the sum of the concentrations of Na^+ and K^+ is greater than the sum of the concentrations of Cl^- and HCO_3^-. This difference is called the anion gap. It represents other plasma anions such as phosphates, sulfates, protein and organic acids which are not routinely measured.

Anion gap = $[Na^+ + K^+] - [Cl^- + HCO_3^-]$. Its normal value is in the range of 12–16 mEq/L.

The anion gap is most commonly used to establish a **differential diagnosis for metabolic acidosis**. In metabolic acidosis, with an increased anion gap, H^+ rises in the body with some anion other than Cl^-. Metabolic acidosis (without an increase in anion gap) is due either to accumulation of H^+ with Cl^- or to a decrease in the concentration of sodium bicarbonate.

Chloride Shift

At the normal pH (7.4) of blood, carbonic acid (a constituent of the bicarbonate buffer) dissociates into H^+ and HCO_3^- (bicarbonate ions). Some of the HCO_3^- combine with K^+ present in the red blood cells and form potassium bicarbonate while the remainder is diffused from the cell to the plasma. The electro-

neutrality of plasma, caused by the shifting of HCO_3^- from the red blood cells is balanced by the shift of Cl^- from plasma into red blood cells. This process is known as chloride shift.

Absorption and Excretion

Chloride is readily absorbed from the gastrointestinal tract. Excretion of chloride is mainly through urine and is parallel to that of Na^+. Daily excretion of Cl^- is 5–8 g.

The chloride of blood is secreted in the gastric juice in the form of HCl. On a diet low in salt, the content of chloride in the blood and urine drops down.

In patients with cystic fibrosis, Cl^- excretion is greatly increased in the sweat (Chemistry to Clinics 26.6).

Sources and Requirement

The most important source of chloride in the diet is the common **table salt** (sodium chloride). Seafoods, milk, meat and eggs are good sources. Most of the dietary chloride is taken with sodium. Daily requirement for adults is 5–15 g.

Alterations in Chloride Balance

Hypochloremia

Decrease in plasma Cl^- concentration, called hypochloremia, occurs in:

- **Persistent diarrhea and prolonged vomiting**. The chloride content of the gastric juice is normally about 150 mmol/L. Patients who lose large volumes of gastric secretion, e.g. due to pyloric stenosis, often show a marked fall in plasma Cl^-. Loss of HCl, in turn, results in compensatory increase in plasma HCO_3^-. Hence, these patients develop metabolic alkalosis, and are often dehydrated.

- **Metabolic acidosis** such as diabetic ketoacidosis and renal failure.

- In **respiratory alkalosis** due to hyperventilation which leads to elimination of CO_2 with consequent increase in blood HCO_3^- and a compensatory decrease in Cl^-.

- **Extreme sweating**.

- **Salt-losing nephritis**, e.g. chronic pyelonephritis, which is probably due to defective tubular reabsorption.

- In patients with **Addison's disease**, due to reduced renal tubular reabsorption of chloride.

26

Chemistry to Clinics 26.6: Cystic Fibrosis

Exocrine glands: These are responsible for secreting mucus, tears and digestive juices onto the body's internal surfaces (e.g., lungs and gut) and sweat on the external surface (skin). Normal mucus forms a gel-like barrier that protects the lining of cells. In the lungs, mucus also functions as a mucociliary transport system that removes dust, pollen, bacteria and other particulate matter out of the lungs to prevent infection.

Pathophysiology: Cystic fibrosis is a genetic disease involving the exocrine glands.

- Patients have excess mucus production as well as altered mucus proteins that cause the mucus to become thick and sticky, thereby obstructing airflow in the small airways. This not only makes breathing difficult but also allows bacterial infection and inflammation to occur.
- In response, neutrophils are recruited to fight infection in the lungs; as they die, they release elastase and their DNA into the mucus, which further thickens the mucus and exacerbates the situation. Thus, a vicious cycle is set up causing more airway obstruction.
- Patients with cystic fibrosis frequently cough and require daily chest and back clapping to dislodge the mucus from the plugged airways.
- Pancreatic function is lost as a result of thick secretion clogging the pancreatic ducts.
- Consequently, most patients with cystic fibrosis have an insufficient amount of digestive enzymes for normal digestion.
- Cystic fibrosis also affects the reproductive organs causing infertility.

Molecular defect: The genetic defect responsible for cystic fibrosis is the mutation in a gene called the cystic fibrosis transmembrane conductance regulator (CFTR) which results in nonfunctional CFTR proteins in the exocrine glands (Fig. 26.4). Normally, in the lungs and pancreas, the protein functions to pump Cl^- out of the cells while in cystic fibrosis Cl^- is retained within the cells. Consequently, the cells take up water from the surrounding mucus by osmosis, making it highly viscid. On the other hand, in the sweat gland ducts, the protein normally moves Cl^- into the cells. Hence, in cystic fibrosis, sweat Cl^- fails to get absorbed. Millions of people carry one copy of the defective gene responsible for the disease. Fortunately, these people are asymptomatic because they must inherit two defective genes, one from each parent, to develop the symptoms of cystic fibrosis.

Complication: *Pseudomonas* bacteria are the leading cause of lung infection and death among cystic fibrosis patients.

Diagnosis: High sweat Cl^- and DNA analysis to detect the mutation (the commonest mutation is $\Delta F508$ resulting in deletion of phenylalanine at position 508 in CFTR protein).

Treatment

- Until recently, bacterial infections of the lung were treated intravenously with antibiotics. Systemic treatment required high doses of antibiotics so that the drug reaches the lung. These high systemic doses are not only expensive but more importantly, cause irreversible damage to hearing and to kidney function.
- Recently, a nanomist device has been developed to deliver the antibiotics as an aerosol to the peripheral airways. This new procedure requires less drug dosage, reduces the cost and eliminates the systemic side effects.
- A second aerosol device being developed is a DNase atomizer. A naturally occurring enzyme called DNase can cut long DNA molecules into shorter strands. Giving DNase as an aerosol cuts the DNA strands that are released from neutrophils that die while fighting bacterial infection. The aerosolized DNase thins the mucus and makes it less sticky, thus making it easier to cough up.

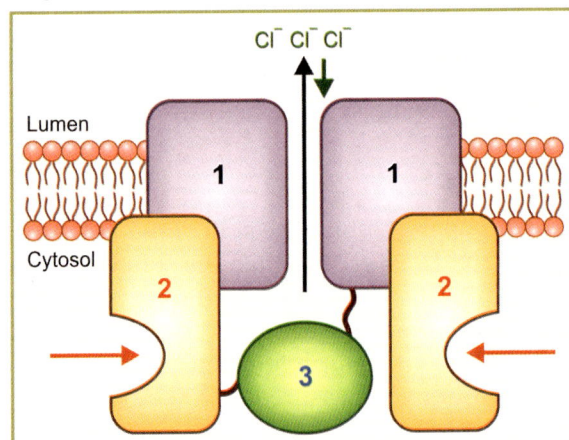

Fig. 26.4: Normal cystic fibrosis transmembrane conductance regulator **(CFTR)**. The **direction of Cl^- movement is cell-specific**, e.g. in sweat gland duct, it serves to absorb sweat Cl^- (green arrow) whereas in lungs and pancreas it serves to secrete Cl^- (black arrow). 1. Transmembrane domain, 2. Nucleotide-binding domain (red arrows indicate ATP-binding sites), 3. Regulatory domain. The chloride channel is blocked due to mutated CFTR in cystic fibrosis so that the concentration of Cl^- in the sweat increases. Conversely, lack of Cl^- secretion makes the secretions viscid in the lungs and pancreas.

Hyperchloremia

Increased plasma Cl^- concentration called hyperchloremia, occurs with dehydration, in patients with acute renal failure, renal tubular acidosis, metabolic acidosis associated with prolonged diarrhea and loss of sodium bicarbonate, diabetes insipidus, and adrenocortical hyperfunction (Cushing's syndrome).

Some increase in plasma chloride may also occur in patients who develop respiratory acidosis.

In severe diarrhea, there is a loss of HCO_3^- while in respiratory acidosis there is retention of CO_2 due to shallow breathing. Thus, reduced levels of HCO_3^- result in compensatory hyperchloremia.

SOME IMPORTANT QUESTIONS

1. What are the important physiological functions of water in the body?

2. Discuss various factors responsible for the regulation of body water.

3. Describe physiological functions of sodium and its regulation.

4. Discuss important physiological functions of potassium and its regulation.

5. Describe physiological functions of chloride and its regulation.

6. Write note: on:
    i. Intracellular fluid
   ii. Extracellular fluid
  iii. Electrolytes
   iv. Na^+/K^+-ATPase
    v. Hyponatremia
   vi. Hypernatremia
  vii. Hypokalemia
 viii. Hyperkalemia
   ix. Anion gap
    x. Chloride shift
   xi. Hypochloremia
  xii. Hyperchloremia
 xiii. Dehydration
  xiv. Edema
   xv. Cystic fibrosis
  xvi. Natriuretic hormones

MULTIPLE CHOICE QUESTIONS

1. **Water content is least in:**
   A. Adipose tissue
   B. Bones
   C. Muscles
   D. Nervous tissue

2. **Maximum water is produced by the oxidation of:**
   A. Carbohydrates
   B. Proteins
   C. Lipids
   D. Nucleic acids

3. **The major extracellular cation is:**
   A. K^+
   B. Na^+
   C. Ca^{2+}
   D. Mg^{2+}

4. **Hyponatremia along with decrease in total body sodium may occur in:**
   A. Vomiting
   B. Diarrhea
   C. Diuretic therapy
   D. All of the above

5. **Highest concentration of Cl⁻ is in:**
    A. Gastric juice
    B. CSF
    C. Pancreatic juice
    D. Saliva

6. **Normal anion gap is:**
    A. 2–6 mEq/L
    B. 12–16 mEq/L
    C. 22–26 mEq/L
    D. 0.2–0.6 mEq/L

7. **Cystic fibrosis affects the following ion channel:**
    A. Na^+
    B. K^+
    C. Cl^-
    D. HCO_3^-

8. **In Addison's disease, serum Cl^- level is generally:**
    A. Increased
    B. Normal
    C. Decreased
    D. May be increased or decreased

9. **Hyperchloremia may occur in:**
    A. Cushing's syndrome
    B. Acute renal failure
    C. Renal tubular acidosis
    D. All of the above

10. **In case of life-threatening hyperkalemia, the fastest way to lower serum K^+ is:**
    A. Intravenous dextrose-insulin
    B. Albuterol inhalation
    C. Intravenous loop diuretics
    D. Oral $NaHCO_3$

Minerals

In addition to carbohydrates, lipids, proteins, vitamins and water, body also needs small amounts of a number of inorganic substances called minerals and trace elements. These are classified into 3 categories based on their daily requirements (Fig. 27.1).

CALCIUM

Amongst various minerals, calcium (Ca) is found in **highest concentration in the body** and is needed by all the cells. Adult human body contains nearly 1.0 to 1.2 kg of calcium. About 99% of it is present in the skeletal tissue, i.e. in the bones and teeth while the remaining is found in the soft tissues, such as the muscle and the nervous tissue. Normal serum calcium level is 9–11 mg/ 100 ml. It is present in blood in three different forms:

1. About 45–50% of the total serum calcium is present in the **ionized form** as Ca^{2+} ions. It is freely exchangeable between the soft tissues, the extracellular fluid and the blood.
2. Nearly equal amount, i.e. 45–50% is **bound to proteins**.
3. The remaining 5–10% is present in the form of **salts**, with citrate, phosphate, etc.

Biological Functions

Calcium performs several functions such as:

1. Calcification of the growing bones and teeth, and maintenance of the mature bones.
2. Activator of a number of enzymes, e.g. adenylate cyclase, ATPases, protein kinases, etc. Ca^{2+} activates phosphorylase kinase through its binding to calmodulin and thus increases the rate of glycogen breakdown. It activates pyruvate dehydrogenase phosphatase which, in turn, activates pyruvate dehydrogenase complex to produce acetyl CoA.

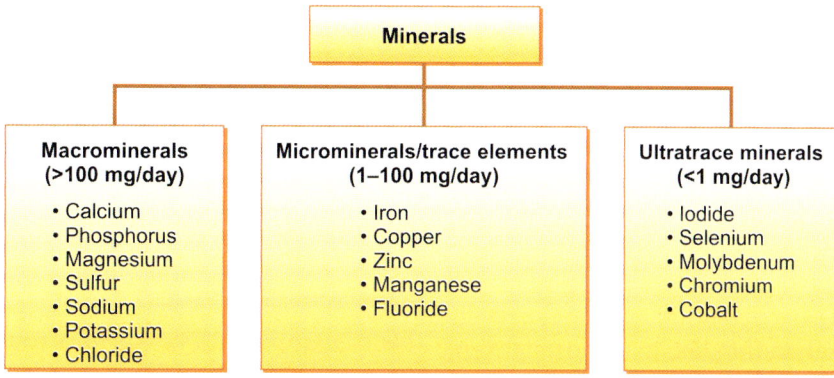

Fig. 27.1: Classification of minerals based on daily requirements. Sodium, potassium and chloride are discussed in Chapter 26.

Ca^{2+} also regulates the enzymes of citric acid cycle, at several steps. For example, Ca^{2+} also activates isocitrate dehydrogenase and α-ketoglutarate dehydrogenase. Thus, Ca^{2+} stimulates the production of ATP.

3. Clotting of blood.
4. Contraction of muscles (excitation-contraction coupling).
5. Regulates the permeability of the capillary walls and excitability of the nerve fibres.
6. Secretion of various hormones and acts as a second messenger.
7. Decreases fluidity of the membranes.

Absorption and Excretion

Only about 10–30% of the dietary calcium is normally **absorbed**. It is absorbed throughout the small intestine but mostly in the duodenum where pH is close to 7; as the pH increases towards the jejunum and ileum, absorption decreases. Both passive diffusion and calcitriol-mediated active transport are responsible for calcium uptake. Absorption depends upon several factors, such as calcium content of food, presence of interfering substances and the presence of vitamin D:

1. In vitamin D deficiency, calcium absorption is impaired.
2. Excess of phosphate lowers calcium absorption.
3. Phytic acid and related substances, present in unrefined cereals, interfere with the absorption of calcium.
4. Excessive amounts of fat, fiber and oxalate in the diet reduce calcium absorption, due to the formation of insoluble salts.
5. Higher amounts of dietary protein, lactose and acidic pH promote calcium absorption.

Calcium is **excreted** in the feces, urine and sweat:

- Dietary calcium, which is not absorbed in the intestine, is excreted in the feces. Excretion in the feces continues even when its intake is low, thereby resulting in negative calcium balance.
- Depending upon its dietary absorption, amount of calcium excreted in the urine varies from 50 to 200 mg/day. Urinary excretion is increased (hypercalciuria) by ingestion of the excessive amount of protein in the diet, in acidosis, thyrotoxicosis, hypoparathyroidism and restricted physical activity.
- In tropical climate, calcium excretion is increased in sweat.

Calcium homeostasis: Maintenance of serum calcium level within the normal limit is called calcium homeostasis. As mentioned above, nearly 45–50% of the serum calcium is present in the ionized form (Ca^{2+}). This form of calcium is freely exchangeable between the soft tissues, the extracellular fluid and the blood, and is called **diffusible calcium**. Most of the functions of calcium are performed by the ionized form (Ca^{2+}) only. Serum Ca^{2+} level is regulated in a complex manner by parathyroid hormone (PTH), vitamin D and calcitonin (Fig. 27.2).

- **Parathyroid hormone:** If serum Ca^{2+} concentration falls, secretion of PTH is increased. The hormone:
  - Acts directly on osteoclasts and increases dissolution of bone mineral. This process is called *bone resorption*.
  - Increases reabsorption of Ca^{2+} from the kidney tubules. The overall effect of the two processes is to elevate serum Ca^{2+} level.
  - Stimulates 1-α-hydroxylase activity in the kidney which, in turn, activates vitamin D and converts it to 1,25-dihydroxycholecalciferol, also called *calcitriol* or *active vitamin D*.
- **Active vitamin D:** It increases serum Ca^{2+} concentration by promoting intestinal absorption of Ca^{2+} as well as its renal tubular reabsorption.
- **Calcitonin:** It is secreted when serum Ca^{2+} level rises. Its action is to lower serum Ca^{2+} level by promoting deposition of calcium, by the osteoblasts. It also promotes renal Ca^{2+} loss.

  Thus, PTH and calcitonin act in **opposite** directions in regulating serum calcium.

Calmodulin: It is a eukaryotic **Ca^{2+}-binding protein** that participates in numerous cellular regulatory processes. Calmodulin functions as a Ca^{2+}-sensor and Ca^{2+}-buffer in the cell, responding to changes in intracellular Ca^{2+} concentration which, in turn, affects the activities of a number of enzymes and acts as a second messenger for hormonal action.

Requirement and Sources

Daily requirement of calcium varies from individual to individual, due to the existence of several factors which affect availability of calcium. The RDA is nearly

27

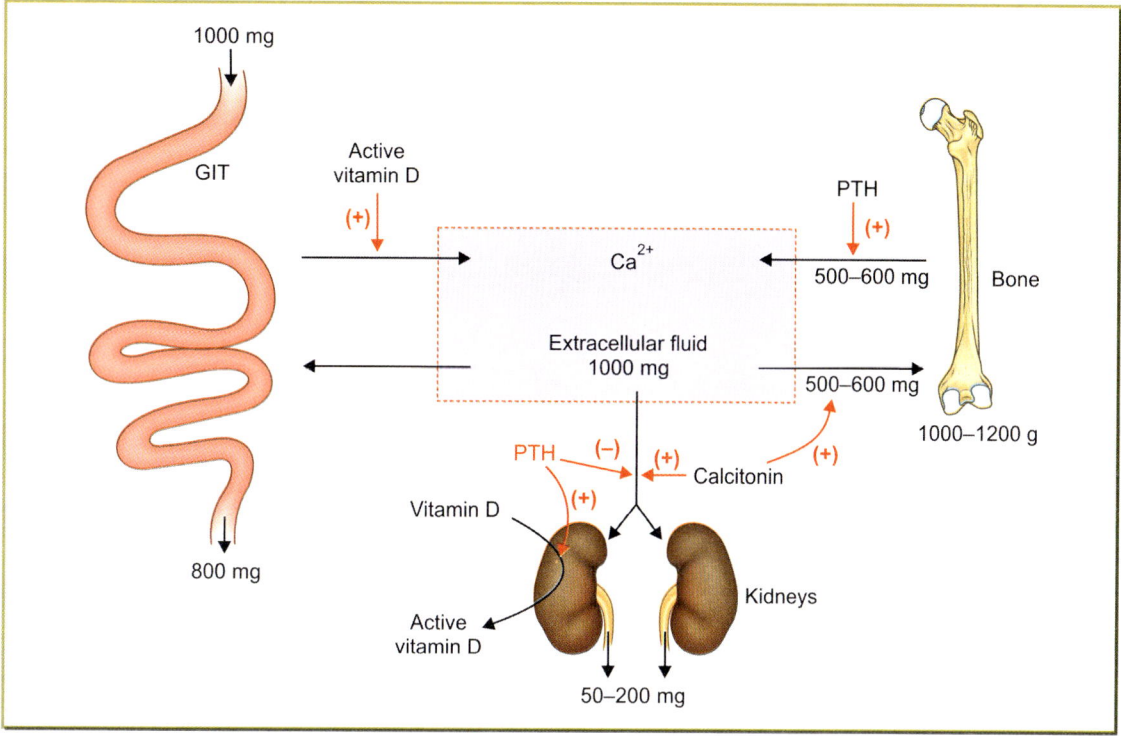

Fig. 27.2: Calcium homeostasis.

800 mg in an adult. During pregnancy and lactation, its requirement is increased to about 1.2 g/day.

Milk and milk products are rich sources of calcium. Besides milk, egg yolk, dry fruits, legumes, cabbage, cauliflower and leafy vegetables are good sources of calcium.

Deficiency Disorders

A decrease in Ca^{2+} concentration in serum results in hypocalcemia. It may be due to increased pH, decreased intake or increased excretion of calcium. Hypocalcemia may also be caused by the deficiency of vitamin D or in hypoparathyroidism. Prolonged hypocalcemia may lead to faulty calcification of bone similar to that observed in rickets in children and osteomalacia in adults. Hypocalcemia may also contribute to osteoporosis.

Hypocalcemia affects motor nerves which become oversusceptible to stimuli, resulting in neuromuscular hyperexcitability and epileptiform convulsions. This is known as tetany (Chemistry to Clinics 27.1).

Osteoporosis: Decreased calcium intake, particularly during/after menopause leads to increased fragility and fractures of bones, mainly of the extremities and pelvis. This is due to **reduced bone density** (bone mass per unit volume) called osteoporosis. It is characterized by the loss of bone matrix and progressive demineralization. Thus, in contrast to osteomalacia where mineralization fails to occur on a normal osteoid matrix, in osteoporosis, **both the matrix formation and**

Chemistry to Clinics 27.1: Tetany

Causes: It may arise from various causes such as severe hypocalcemia (total serum calcium <7 mg/dl; ionized Ca^{2+} <2.5 mg/dl), hypoparathyroidism (may occur accidentally during thyroid surgery), hypomagnesemia, hyperphosphatemia, and alkalosis (at higher pH, more calcium is bound to albumin thus decreasing ionized calcium). Under these conditions, the membrane permeability for Na^+ increases leading to rapid, successive, spontaneous depolarization.

Presentation: Neuromuscular excitability with painful muscle spasm is the chief symptom in adults and convulsive seizures in children.

Complication: Death may occur due to laryngospasm.

Emergency treatment: Intravenous calcium gluconate (preferred over calcium chloride because it causes less tissue necrosis if extravasated); correct the abnormalities in magnesium and pH simultaneously.

27

the subsequent calcification are at fault. Increased supply of calcium in the food or oral supplementation of calcium along with the estrogen therapy in postmenopausal woman retards osteoporosis.

Besides calcium, vitamin C, vitamin K, magnesium, phosphorus, copper, zinc, manganese and boron are also important in bone formation. Vitamin D is also essential for the absorption and utilization of calcium. Therefore, an adequate diet sufficient in all the nutrients along with regular exercise is important for preventing osteoporosis.

Hypercalcemia

Hypercalcemia may be due to increased intake of calcium (Chemistry to Clinics 27.2), raised levels of plasma albumin or increased renal reabsorption of Ca^{2+}. It may also by caused by hyperactivity of the parathyroid gland (hyperparathyroidism) or hyper-vitaminosis D. Hypercalcemia may lead to the formation of stones (calculi), loss of appetite, vomiting, constipation, weakness of muscles and sluggish reflexes.

PHOSPHORUS

Phosphorus (P) is widely distributed in most of the tissues. A normal adult body contains nearly 600–800 g of phosphorus. About 75% of it is present in combination with calcium in the bones, teeth and skeletal tissues. The blood, muscle and the nerve tissue also contain fairly good amounts.

Biological Functions

Phosphorus is present in two forms, i.e. as inorganic phosphorus and organic phosphorus, both of which perform different functions.

A. Inorganic phosphorus

1. It is essential with calcium, for the mineralization of bones and teeth. It is a part of the crystal, hydroxyapatite, which is laid down on collagen in the ossification process of bone formation.
2. Maintenance of acid–base balance. In the renal system, phosphate functions in the excretion of hydrogen ions. Filtered phosphate reacts with the secreted H^+ and releases Na^+ which gets reabsorbed through the renal tubules, under the influence of aldosterone.

B. Organic phosphorus

It is the phosphorus found in the form of esters of various organic compounds, such as in phospholipids, nucleic acids, coenzymes, etc.

1. In the form of *phospholipids*, phosphorus is essential for the transport and metabolism of lipids and also forms an integral part of the cell membrane.
2. In the form of *nucleic acids*, it forms an important constituent of the cell nucleus and is essential for cell multiplication and protein synthesis.
3. *Organic esters* of phosphoric acid such as ADP, glucose-6-phosphate, etc. are necessary for metabolism and in the production of energy-rich compounds (ATP, creatine phosphate).
4. As a component of several coenzymes (TPP, $NADP^+$), it also participates in various enzyme catalyzed reactions.
5. It also acts as an activator for enzymes involved in phosphorylation/dephosphorylation processes.

Absorption and Excretion

Depending upon the presence of other constituents, about 10–40% of the dietary phosphorus is **absorbed** as inorganic phosphate in the small intestine.

- Organic phosphate is hydrolyzed in the intestinal lumen and released as inorganic phosphate, through the action of pancreatic/intestinal phosphatases, e.g. alkaline phosphatase.
- Phosphorus present in animal foods, such as in milk and eggs, is absorbed to a greater extent than that is available from cereals and legumes, due to their high phytic acid (hexaphosphoinositol) content.
- Absorption of phosphorus also depends upon the dietary content of phosphorus (absorption of phosphorus is increased when its intake is low), as well as calcium and vitamin D.
- An increase in dietary magnesium also results in reduction in phosphate absorption.

Serum phosphorus: Absorbed phosphate exists in plasma in two forms, i.e. as phospholipids and in the inorganic form. The inorganic form, like calcium, can be either protein bound or free. In normal adult human beings, serum phosphorus (as inorganic phosphorus) varies from 2.5 to 4.5 mg/100 ml. Circulating phosphates are in equilibrium with the skeletal and cellular inorganic phosphates, as well as the organic phosphates. PTH and serum calcium regulate the level of phosphorus in the serum as well as its reabsorption by the renal tubules.

About two-thirds of the dietary phosphorus is **excreted** in the urine, while the remaining one-third is excreted in the feces. PTH increases excretion of phosphate by inhibiting its tubular reabsorption.

Requirement and Sources

Daily requirement of phosphorus is nearly 50% higher than calcium. It varies from 1.0 to 1.5 g/day. Phosphorus is found in food containing phosphoproteins, nucleoproteins, phospholipids and glycerophosphates as well as inorganic phosphates chiefly of Ca and Na. Calcium-rich diets, e.g. milk, cheese and beans are also rich sources of phosphorus. Besides, eggs, cereals, fish and meat are also good sources of phosphorus.

Deficiency Disorders

Deficiency of phosphorus may lead to several neuro-muscular, skeletal and renal manifestations. Low serum phosphorus concentration may be a result of vitamin C deficiency and causes defective bone calcification. Similar to hypocalcemia, hypophosphatemia may also lead to rickets in children and osteomalacia in adults; in these conditions, the product of serum calcium and inorganic phosphorus which is normally 40 (10 mg calcium × 4 mg phosphorus), may decrease to <30.

MAGNESIUM

Adult human body contains nearly 20–25 g of magnesium (Mg). Nearly 75% of it is combined with calcium and phosphorus and is present in the bones. Bone magnesium is divided between the crystal lattice and the exchangeable surface pool. The remaining is present in the soft tissues, such as the muscle and the nervous tissue and in body fluids. In blood, most of the magnesium is intracellular.

Biological Functions

1. Component of bone structure.
2. Nerve impulse transmission.
3. Magnesium ions (Mg^{2+}) act as activator for several enzymes, particularly those requiring ATP, such as glucokinase, hexokinase, acyl CoA synthetase, alkaline phosphatase, DNA polymerase, RNA polymerase, etc.
4. Formation of cAMP and thus in mediating the effects of numerous hormones.
5. Electron transfer and stabilization of the redox centres.
6. Stabilizes the complex structures assumed by many RNAs.
7. Free nucleotides, which are anionic in nature, are usually associated with Mg^{2+} in the cells, e.g. Mg^{2+} provides stability to ATP.
8. Muscle contraction.

Absorption and Excretion

Nearly 50% of the dietary magnesium is absorbed from the small intestine. High intake of fat, calcium and phosphorus reduce magnesium absorption. An alkaline food also diminishes its absorption.

Magnesium is excreted both in the feces as well as in the urine. Intake of alkaline food reduces its intestinal absorption as well as urinary excretion.

Requirement and Sources

Average daily requirement is 250–300 mg. It is widely distributed in several animal tissues and vegetables. Whole grain, cereals, potato, seafoods, coffee, tea and cocoa are good sources.

Deficiency Disorders

Magnesium deficiency (hypomagnesemia) is often observed in:

1. Alcoholics
2. Patients treated with certain types of diuretics
3. Metabolic acidosis
4. Uremia
5. Children suffering from kwashiorkor
6. Pregnancy (particularly during toxemia of pregnancy)
7. Rickets
8. Diarrhea and vomiting.

27

Deficiency symptoms include tremors, depression, hyperirritability, cardiac arrhythmias, muscular weakness and convulsions. Low levels of serum magnesium may also produce tetany (Chemistry to Clinics 27.1).

Toxicity

Toxicity may be observed due to increased use of magnesium containing laxatives and antacids (Chemistry to Clinics 27.2). Chief symptoms include drowsiness, lethargy and weakness.

IRON

The total quantity of iron (Fe) in normal adult human body is about 4 g. Most of it is present as a component of hemoglobin and myoglobin. Iron binds to different proteins either by its incorporation into a protoporphyrin ring or its interaction with other protein ligands. In the protoporphyrin ring, iron may be incorporated as Fe^{2+} or Fe^{3+} iron. The Fe^{2+}-protoporphyrin complex is called **heme** while Fe^{3}-protoporphyrin complex is designated as **hematin**.

Biological Functions

Iron forms a component of several heme and non-heme proteins:

1. Hemoproteins
- Hemoglobin is required for the transport of O_2 and CO_2.
- Myoglobin is an oxygen-storage protein in muscles.
- Cytochromes are required in the electron transport chain and oxidative phosphorylation.
- Cytochrome P450 system is responsible for many biotransformation reactions.

- Several enzymes contain heme iron, as a part of their prosthetic group, e.g. catalase, peroxidase, tryptophan pyrrolase, nitric oxide synthases, prostaglandin synthase, etc. As a component of the lysosomal enzyme myeloperoxidase, iron is required for phagocytosis and thus killing of bacteria by the neutrophils.

2. Non-heme proteins: Transferrin, ferritin and iron-sulfur proteins (ferridoxins).

Ferridoxins: These are non-heme iron proteins called *iron-sulfur centers* or iron-sulfur proteins. These consist of equal number of iron and sulfide ions and occur as prosthetic groups and are coordinated with cystine-sulfhydryl groups of proteins. Due to the presence of iron, Fe-S centers occur in the oxidized as well as the reduced state. Regardless of the number of Fe atoms present in them, the redox states of Fe-S clusters differ by one formal charge only.

Ferridoxins are involved in various enzymatic oxidation processes, such as in the mitochondrial electron transport chain. For example, complex I which passes electrons from NADH to CoQ, contains one molecule of FMN and 6 to 7 Fe-S clusters that participate in the electron transport.

Absorption of Iron

Iron metabolism is unique in the sense that it operates largely as a closed system, i.e. it is regulated mainly at the absorption level (Fig. 27.3). Whatever is absorbed is utilized by the body very efficiently and its losses are minimal. Thus, iron is called a '**one-way substance**'.

Absorption of iron mainly occurs in the stomach, duodenum and upper part of the small intestine. Normally, only about 10% of the dietary iron is

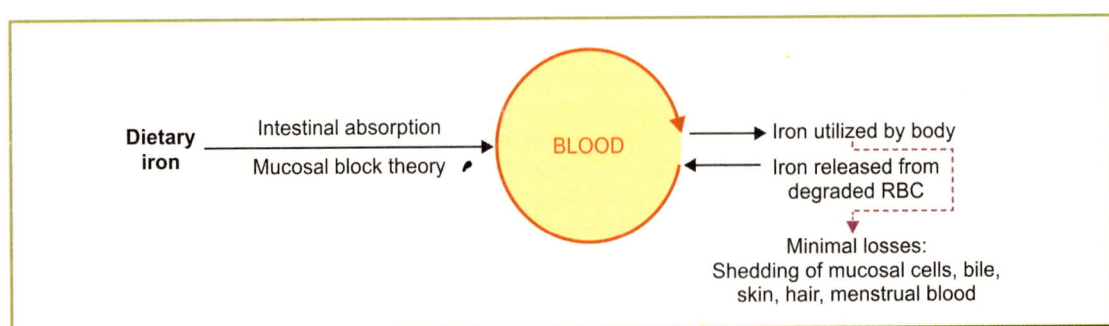

Fig. 27.3: Iron: A 'one-way substance'.

absorbed. Unabsorbed iron is excreted in the feces. Efficiency of absorption is increased up to 30% during severe iron deficiency.

Factor Affecting Iron Absorption

1. **Body iron status versus iron intake:** Absorption of dietary iron varies inversely with the iron stores of the body. Thus, iron absorption increases with its intake but up to a limit.
2. **Chemical form of dietary iron:** Heme iron is well absorbed. Iron in the ferrous form (Fe^{2+}) is more effectively absorbed than the ferric form (Fe^{3+}). The protein mucin in the duodenal lumen helps to solubilize and absorb Fe^{3+}.
3. **Reducing substances:** Amino acids, specially cysteine and the presence of various other reducing substances, such as vitamin C in the diet maintain the Fe^{2+} state of iron and thus promote its absorption.
4. **Complexing agents:** Iron from vegetables and cereals is poorly absorbed due to the presence of oxalates, phosphates, carbonates, phytates and fibre.
5. **Gastric hydrochloric acid:** It enhances iron absorption by stimulating pepsin-mediated digestion of dietary protein which, in turn, releases protein-bound iron.

Mucosal-Block Theory of Iron Absorption

Mechanism: Iron may be absorbed as intact heme, Fe^{2+} and/or Fe^{3+}.

- Brush border of enterocytes contain a multi-protein complex called **paraferritin complex** (Fig. 27.4). One of the proteins, called *divalent metal transporter-1* (DMT-1), transfers Fe^{2+} from the lumen to the cytosol.
- On the other hand, **mucin** in the duodenal lumen helps to solubilize Fe^{3+} and makes it available for binding with a transmembrane protein called *integrin*, which interacts with another protein *mobilferrin* responsible for transferring iron from the luminal to the cytoplasmic surface of the cell accompanied by its reduction to Fe^{2+} by NADPH-dependent *ferri-reductase*.
- In the mucosal cells, Fe^{2+} is again oxidized to Fe^{3+} form by a copper-containing protein called **ferroxidase I** or **ceruloplasmin**. The subsequent fate of iron depends on the total iron status of the body:

Chemistry to Clinics 27.3: Anemia of Chronic Disease
Hepcidin binds to ferroportin-1 and internalizes it within the enterocytes. This results in the retention of iron within cells, and a reduction in plasma iron levels. Hepcidin is thus the 'master regulator' of iron metabolism. It is partly responsible for the *anemia of chronic disease* (tuberculosis, rheumatoid arthritis, etc.); where hepcidin is released from the liver in response to inflammatory cytokines which results in an increased hepcidin concentration and a consequent decrease in plasma iron levels.

- **If body iron stores are optimum or in excess:** Majority of the Fe^{3+} combines with **apoferritin** and is stored as mucosal **ferritin**. With the normal cell turnover, ferritin (and hence iron) is lost in the feces.
- **When the body needs iron:** Majority of the mucosal iron is delivered across the cells to the blood (via a membrane protein called **ferroportin-1** which shuttles Fe^{2+} followed by its simultaneous oxidation to Fe^{3+} by another membrane protein called **hephaestin**) where it is trapped by **transferrin**, the iron-transport protein, to be delivered to the rest of the body. Importantly, ferroportin-1 is inhibited by a plasma protein called **hepcidin** (Chemistry to Clinics 27.3).

Ferritin: The Mucosal Iron Receptor

Ferritin is an iron containing protein involved in the **storage of iron**. The protein component is called **apoferritin** which consists of 24 subunits of the H chains and the L chains arranged spherically. All the 24 units may be composed entirely of the H forms or the L forms or a mixture of the H and the L forms. In the heart apoferritin, the H form tends to predominate whereas in the liver and spleen, apoferritins are composed mainly of the L form. The L form is also the main constituent of ferritin under conditions of iron overload. Their synthesis is regulated by the concentration of free intracellular iron. In a normal healthy adult, nearly 1500–2000 atoms of iron are bound in the whole ferritin complex. This ratio of iron to the polypeptide however, is not constant since the apoprotein has the ability to gain and release iron, according to the physiological needs of the body:

- Uptake of iron is associated with the oxidation of Fe^{2+} to Fe^{3+}.
- Intake of iron also regulates the rate of synthesis of apoferritin so that more protein is available for iron binding when the intake is high.

27

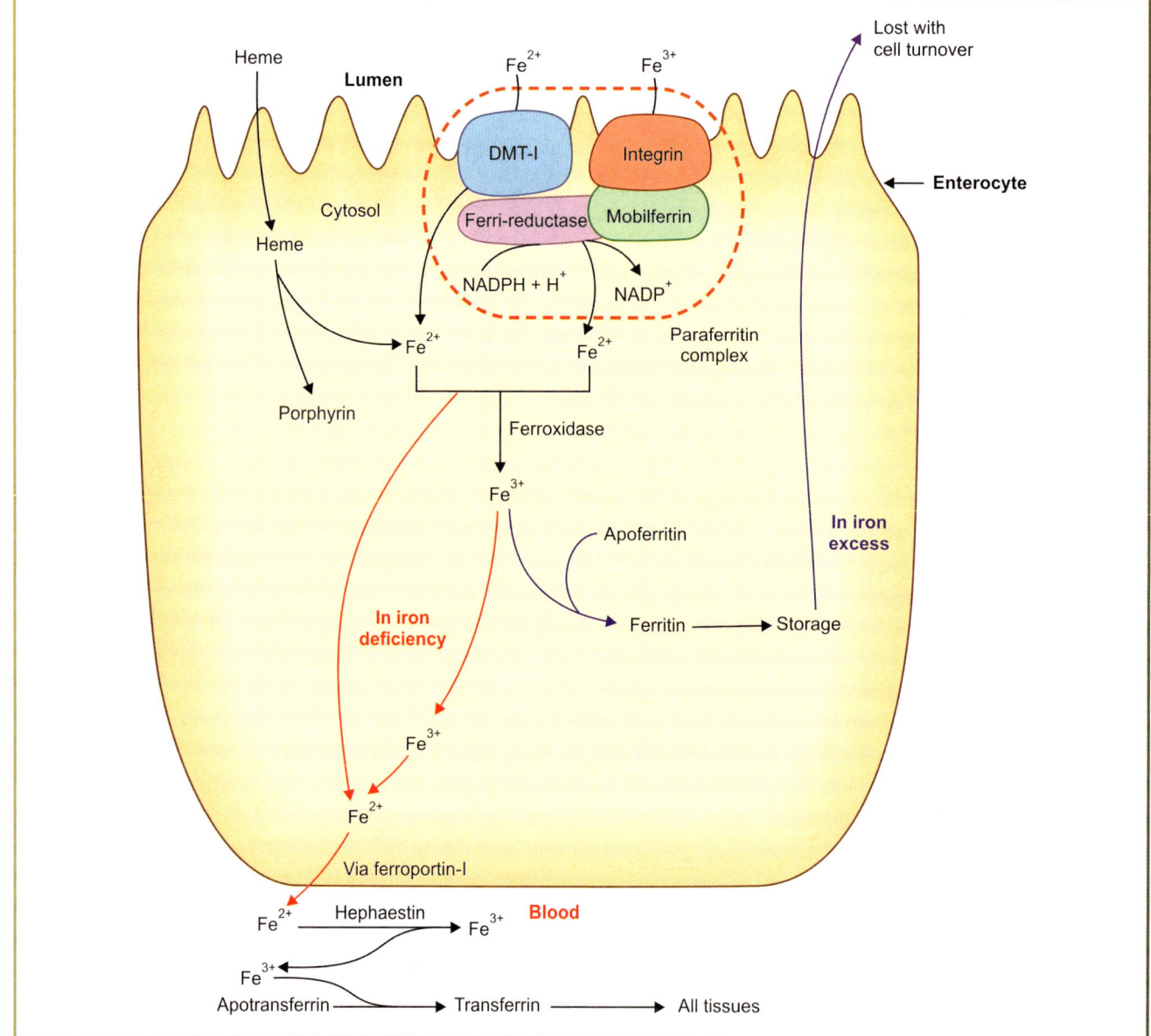

Fig. 27.4: Mechanism of iron absorption and mucosal block theory.

Therefore, ferritin acts both as a sink for iron during its excess intake as well as its source during iron deprivation. Apoferritin, also called the **'mucosal iron-receptor' protein** in the upper small intestine, thus controls the absorption of iron as it has a very rapid turnover.

Ferroxidases (Multi-copper Oxidases)

The Fe^{2+} (reduced) and Fe^{3+} (oxidized) forms of iron are physiologically important since iron in hemo-globin is present in the Fe^{2+} state while it is transported in transferrin and stored in ferritin in the Fe^{3+} state. Oxidation requires copper-containing proteins designated as multi-copper oxidases or **ferroxidases**.

Ferroxidase I is identical with plasma **cerulo-plasmin**, a copper-containing protein. Interconversion of Fe^{2+} to Fe^{3+} forms of iron is essential for its absorption and incorporation into various iron-containing proteins. The role of ferroxidases also points to the significance of copper in iron metabolism.

Table 27.1: Key proteins participating in iron homeostasis

Paraferritin complex

- **Divalent metal transporter-1** (DMT-1): Transfers Fe^{2+} from the intestinal lumen to the cytosol of enterocytes.
- **Integrin**: Receives Fe^{3+} from lumen and transfers it to mobilferrin.
- **Mobilferrin**: Cytosolic shuttle for Fe^{3+}.
- **Ferrireductase**: Reduction of absorbed Fe^{3+} to Fe^{2+} in the cytosol.

Mucin: Solubilizes Fe^{3+} in the duodenal lumen and makes it available for binding with integrin.

Multi-copper oxidases (ferroxidases, e.g. ceruloplasmin, hephaestin): Oxidation of Fe^{2+} to Fe^{3+} in the cytosol/plasma.

Apoferritin: Intracellular iron storage as ferritin; 'mucosal iron-receptor'.

Ferroportin-1: Exit of Fe^{2+} from enterocytes into blood.

Hephaestin: Oxidation of Fe^{2+} to Fe^{3+} during its exit (via ferroportin-1) from enterocytes into blood.

Hepcidin: Inhibitor of ferroportin-1; 'master regulator' of iron absorption.

Apotransferrrin: Transport of Fe^{3+} in plasma as transferrin.

Hemosiderin: Intracellular storage form of excess iron.

Table 27.1 summarizes various proteins involved in iron homeostasis.

Iron Response Elements

The synthesis of receptors of transferrin and ferritin are reciprocally related to the cellular iron content. Specific untranslated sequences in the mRNA for both the proteins are designated as 'iron response elements' (**IRE**) which interact with the iron response element-binding protein (IRE-binding protein). Thus, when plasma iron levels are high, cells synthesize more ferritin while the mRNA for the transferrin receptor is degraded. On the other hand, when iron levels are low, mRNA for the transferrin receptors synthesizes more of the transferrin receptors while mRNA for the ferritin receptors becomes inactive.

Storage and Transport

From the mucosal cells, as discussed above, Fe^{2+} passes into blood where it is oxidized to Fe^{3+} and is incorporated into **apoferritin**. Some of it is also incorporated into another serum protein called **apotransferrin** which binds two Fe^{3+} and is converted to transferrin (Fig. 27.4).

Transferrin and Total Iron-binding Capacity (TIBC)

Transferrin is a non-heme iron-containing serum glycoprotein (β_1-globulin) synthesized in the liver. It **transports iron** to the sites where it is required, such as in the bone marrow. The apoprotein part of transferrin is designated as apotransferrin. There are two iron-binding sites in an apotransferrin molecule. Though several metals can bind to apotransferrin, it has highest affinity for Fe^{3+}. **Iron is always transported in the Fe^{3+} form.** Although Fe^{2+} may be bound to apotransferrin, it rapidly gets oxidized to the Fe^{3+} form.

In a normal healthy adult, nearly one-third of the iron-binding sites are occupied. Thus, total iron-binding capacity (TIBC) of the serum is directly related to its transferrin concentration. TIBC is reduced in iron deficiency anemia but is increased in pernicious anemia and hemochromatosis. In iron overload, serum transferrin may be fully saturated. About 45% of the circulating transferrin is in the iron-free form and is called **unsaturated transferrin**.

There are specific receptors on the surface of many cells, for transferrin. **Transferrin receptor** is a transmembrane protein consisting of two subunits. Transferrin binds to its receptors and is internalized by the **receptor-mediated endocytosis**. The acid pH inside the lysosome causes iron to dissociate from the complex. After the release of iron, receptor-apotransferrin complex returns to the cell surface where apotransferrin is released for reutilization, i.e. to pick up more iron for its delivery to the site where needed. Plasma transferrin is in equilibrium with hemoglobin (the Fe^{2+}-containing hemoprotein) in the bone marrow erythroid precursors, as well as with ferritin in the liver.

- In the bone marrow, the Fe^{3+} is again reduced to Fe^{2+} and is incorporated into heme for the synthesis of hemoglobin.
- On the other hand, when there is a need for iron by the body, such as after hemorrhage, liver and spleen release their stores (ferritin). After ferritin reaches a low level, another iron storage protein, called **hemosiderin** releases iron.

Hemosiderin

Hemosiderin is an iron storage protein found as brownish granules in the cells. Excess of iron, such as during iron overload, stimulates the storage

27

capacity of the newly synthesized apoferritin which may be partially degraded by proteolytic enzymes of the lysosomes. It is followed by the release of iron oxide micelles which form insoluble aggregates and get trapped in the secondary lysosomes. These insoluble aggregates of amorphous iron are designated as hemosiderin. In a normal healthy subject, very little hemosiderin is detectable. The quantity of hemosiderin **increases during iron overload**.

Excretion

As mentioned above, only about 10% of dietary iron is absorbed but once absorbed, a very little of it is excreted (Fig. 27.3). Hence, iron is called a 'one-way substance', a unique feature that is not shown by any other micronutrient.

Nearly 1% of the red blood cells are continuously degraded in the reticuloendothelial system each day. In an adult human being, this results in the release of about 25 mg of iron, majority of which is conserved and reused.

- An adult male or a non-menstruating female loses only about 1 mg of iron everyday.
- Nearly 50–60% of this is lost from the gastrointestinal tract, either in the bile or by the shedding of the mucosal cells.
- The remaining is lost from the skin and the hair with practically no loss in the urine.
- In females, there is an additional loss of iron through menstruation, ranging from 1 to 3 mg/day.

Requirement and Sources

Assuming about 10% efficiency of absorption, the recommended dietary allowance for iron is about 10 mg for normal adult males. The RDA is nearly 20 mg/day for non-pregnant females, during the reproductive stage of their life. This is on account of the increased loss during menstruation. Due to the increasing iron-demand of the body during pregnancy and lactation, the RDA is increased to nearly 30 mg/day.

Foods cooked in iron cook-wares are the best sources of iron. Animal foods such as meat, fish and eggs are good sources of heme iron. Green-leafy vegetables, cereals and legumes (whole grains) are good sources of non-heme iron. However, due to the presence of oxalates and phytates, iron from vegetable sources is poorly absorbed. **Milk is a poor source of iron.**

Chemistry to Clinics 27.4: Iron Deficiency Anemia

Causes

- *Inadequate intake*: Malnutrition, pregnancy (increased fetal demand).
- *Poor absorption*: Prolonged gastroenteritis, complete/partial gastrectomy.
- *Increased losses*: Excessive blood loss during menstruation, gastrointestinal hemorrhage, hookworm infections.

Presentation: It is the commonest disorder of iron metabolism and the commonest form of nutritional anemia. It is a common feature in children, adolescent girls and females of the child-bearing age, particularly in the developing countries.

- Children become dull, inactive, lose appetite and have poor growth.
- Deficiency of iron in females also reduces their work capacity. On exertion, such women get breathless and remain fatigued.
- Iron deficiency is also associated with decreased immuno-competence and susceptibility to infections.

Diagnosis: Low plasma iron and ferritin, increased plasma total iron binding capacity (TIBC), low transferrin saturation (percent) and microcytic hypochromic blood picture (Fig. 27.5).

Treatment: Oral iron supplementation (parenteral iron in severe cases).

Deficiency Disorders

The commonest disorder is iron deficiency anemia (Chemistry to Clinics 27.4).

Anemia

Anemia is a condition which is characterized by a reduced number of circulating erythrocytes or reduced amount of hemoglobin in them, or both. Based on the RBC size and the hemoglobin content, anemia is of three types:

1. **Microcytic hypochromic anemia:** The erythrocytes are much smaller in size and have reduced hemoglobin content. Their number may also be reduced but to a smaller extent. It is caused by iron deficiency (Fig. 27.5).

2. **Macrocytic hyperchromic/normochromic anemia:** The size of the erythrocytes is increased while their number is reduced, presenting the characteristic blood picture of megaloblastic anemia including pernicious anemia. It is caused by the deficiency of vitamin B_{12} and/or folic acid.

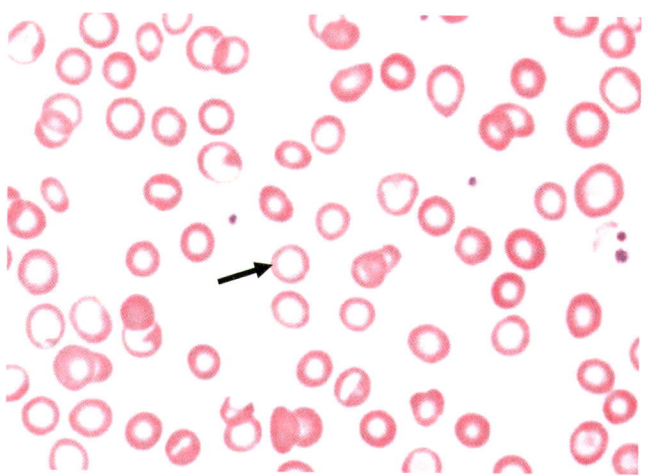

Fig. 27.5: Iron deficiency anemia morphologically characterized by variable degrees of **microcytosis** and **hypochromia** which results in widening of the central pallor accounting for >1/3rd of the total RBC diameter (arrow).

3. **Normocytic normochromic anemia:** The size as well as the hemoglobin content of the erythrocytes remains normal but number of the circulating erythrocytes is reduced. It is usually a result of internal or external hemorrhage.

Toxicity

Iron overload is toxic (Chemistry to Clinics 27.5).

COPPER

The human body contains 100–150 mg of copper (Cu), out of which nearly 50% is found in the muscles and about 25% in bones.

Chemistry to Clinics 27.5: Hemosiderosis and Hemochromatosis

Excess of iron in the body, results in its deposition as hemosiderin in various tissues such as liver, spleen, skin and cardiac muscles. It is called **hemosiderosis** (Fig. 27.6) which increases the risk of cardiovascular disease, besides hepatomegaly, pancreatitis and skin pigmentation. Repeated blood transfusions as required in thalassemia major, can lead to hemosiderosis. Other causes include alcoholic cirrhosis and chronic pancreatitis. A genetic susceptibility to iron overload is due to a failure of the regulation of iron absorption and leads to a condition called **hemochromatosis**, whose features are like hemosiderosis.

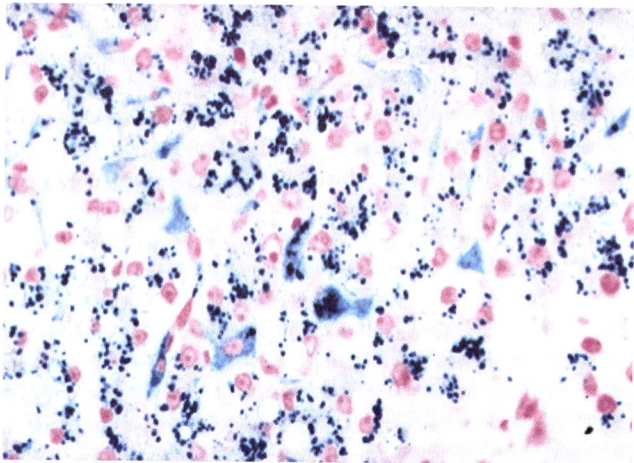

Fig. 27.6: Hemosiderosis: Prussian blue stain (for iron) of the liver to demonstrate large amounts of hemosiderin in the cytoplasm of hepatocytes and Kupffer cells.

Biological Functions

1. Copper is a component of many enzyme systems of metabolic importance (Table 27.2).

Table 27.2: Copper-containing enzymes and their metabolic importance

Enzymes	Metabolic importance
Multi-copper oxidases (ferroxidases)	Iron metabolism: Tissue-specific conversion of intracellular Fe^{2+} to Fe^{3+} to facilitate its storage or exit from cells, e.g. ferroxidase I (ceruloplasmin in enterocytes, liver, plasma), glycosylphosphatidylinositol-ceruloplasmin (brain), hephaestin (enterocytes), zyklopen (placental trophoblasts)
Cytochrome oxidase	Electron transport chain
δ-Amino levulinate synthase	Synthesis of heme
Lysyl oxidase	Synthesis and maturation of collagen and elastin
Ascorbic acid oxidase	Interconversion of L-ascorbate (active vitamin C) and dehydroascorbate
Tyrosinase	Synthesis of melanin pigments
Dopamine β-oxidase	Synthesis of catecholamines
Superoxide dismutase (SOD)	Antioxidant
ATP7A	Intestinal copper absorption
ATP7B	Secretion of copper from hepatocytes into bile

27

2. It is also an important constituent of several proteins, such as erythrocuprein, cerebrocuprein and hepatocuprein which are present in the bone marrow, brain and liver, respectively.

Absorption and Excretion

About one-third of the dietary copper is absorbed primarily from the duodenum. Phytate, zinc, ascorbic acid and certain amino acids inhibit copper absorption.

- **ATP7A** (ATPase, Cu^{2+}-transporting α-polypeptide) is required for the intestinal uptake of dietary copper.
- Inside the intestinal mucosal cells, copper binds to another low molecular weight metal-binding protein called **metallothionein**. Copper absorption thus depends upon the availability of these proteins.
- In all tissues except the liver, another isoform of ATP7A is present in the Golgi complex where it regulates the availability of copper for its incorporation into copper-containing enzymes. However, if copper levels are elevated, this protein shuttles to the cell membrane and removes excess copper from the cell.
- After absorption, copper enters the plasma where almost all of it is present in the bound form. While some of it is loosely bound to albumin (called the direct reacting copper or the transport form of copper), most of it is bound to a specific copper-binding protein called **ceruloplasmin** (Fig. 27.7).

After absorption, copper is stored in the liver and is excreted via bile. The secretion of copper from the hepatocytes into the bile requires the enzyme **ATP7B** (ATPase, Cu^{2+}-transporting β-polypeptide). Very little copper is excreted in the urine.

Ceruloplasmin: It is a **copper containing α₂-globulin present in the plasma**. It is **synthesized in the liver** in the form of an apoprotein called **apoceruloplasmin**. After 6–8 atoms of copper are incorporated per molecule of apoprotein, it is converted into ceruloplasmin (Fig. 27.7). Ceruloplasmin is also called **ferroxidase I** and is an example of multi-copper oxidase (Table 27.2). It helps in the oxidation of ferrous iron (Fe^{2+}) to the ferric iron (Fe^{3+}) for its incorporation into transferrin and ferritin. Thus, copper, through ceruloplasmin, **helps in iron metabolism**.

It should be remembered that plasma ceruloplasmin levels are raised non-specifically during any ongoing acute inflammatory process in the body. Hence, ceruloplasmin is called an **'acute phase reactant'**.

Requirement and Sources

A normal adult requires 2–3 mg of copper per day. Copper is widely distributed in various types of foods. Nuts, leafy vegetables, dried legumes, egg-yolk, fish and meat (liver) are good sources.

Milk is a poor source of copper.

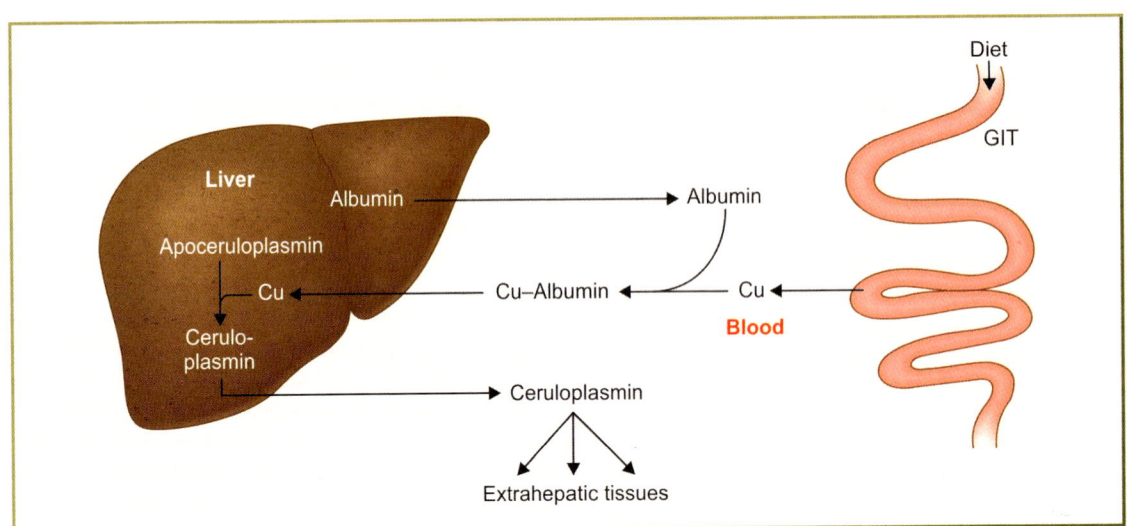

Fig. 27.7: Absorption and transport of copper.

27

Deficiency Disorders

Some of the symptoms of copper deficiency include hypercholesterolemia, demineralization of bones, leukopenia, demyelination of the neural tissue and alopecia (loss of hair). There is also microcytic normochromic anemia which cannot be cured by iron supplementation alone, since copper, as ferroxidase, is essential for the intestinal absorption of iron and in its metabolism. Copper deficiency in infants has been found to be associated with a condition described as Menkes disease (Chemistry to Clinics 27.6).

Toxicity

Copper toxicity may manifest as diarrhea, blue-green discoloration of the saliva, hemolysis, proteinuria and renal failure. Increased amount of copper is deposited in the liver and brain in Wilson's disease (Chemistry to Clinics 27.7).

IODINE

About 20–30 mg of iodine is present as iodide (I^-) in adult human body. Nearly two-thirds of it is present

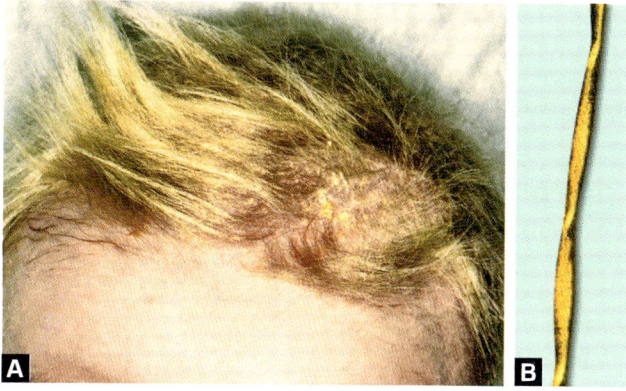

Fig. 27.8: Copper deficiency results in defective keratinization: (A) **Menkes** kinky hair which feels like steel wool (steely hair syndrome). (B) Pili torti: Twisting of the hair shaft on its own axis.

Chemistry to Clinics 27.7: Wilson's Disease (Hepatolenticular Degeneration)

Cause: It is an autosomal recessive inherited disorder in which there is a positive copper balance due to deficient synthesis of ceruloplasmin in the liver. There is a defect in the incorporation of Cu^{2+} into newly synthesized apoceruloplasmin, to form ceruloplasmin. Besides, a defect in the ATP7B protein in the hepatocytes (responsible for copper-efflux into bile) is also a culprit. The net result is free Cu^{2+} accumulation to highly toxic levels mainly in the liver and the basal nuclei of the brain which promotes the generation of free radicals leading to extensive cell damage.

Presentation: Liver failure, neurological disturbances and characteristic Kayser-Fleischer rings in the cornea (Fig. 27.9).

Diagnosis

- Decreased plasma ceruloplasmin levels.
- Increased urinary excretion of copper which, in turn, causes renal tubular damage with hemoglobinuria and generalized aminoaciduria.
- Increased hepatic copper content on liver biopsy.
- Mutation analysis of *ATP7B* gene.

Treatment: Repeated administration of copper-chelating agents such as penicillamine.

Chemistry to Clinics 27.6: Menkes Disease

It is an X-linked hereditary disease due to failure of copper absorption across the serosal membrane of intestinal mucosal cells. The molecular defect lies in the enterocyte membrane transport protein ATP7A. This, in turn, leads to low concentrations of copper in the plasma and the liver. Further, a defective ATP7A in other extrahepatic tissues results in deficiency of various copper containing oxidases (tyrosinase, lysyl oxidase, etc.) leading to various systemic manifestations such as skeletal malformation, mental retardation, defective thermoregulation and immunodeficiency. Menkes disease is also called **'kinky-hair syndrome'** due to the failure to keratinize hair which become kinky and steel-grey (Fig. 27.8).

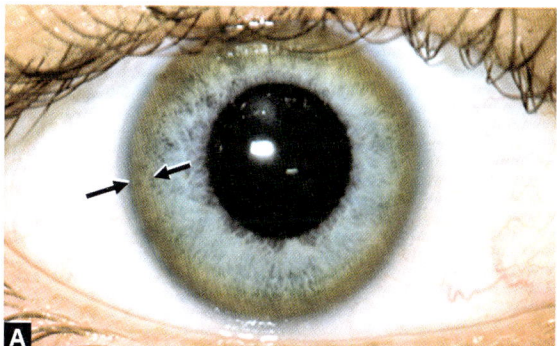

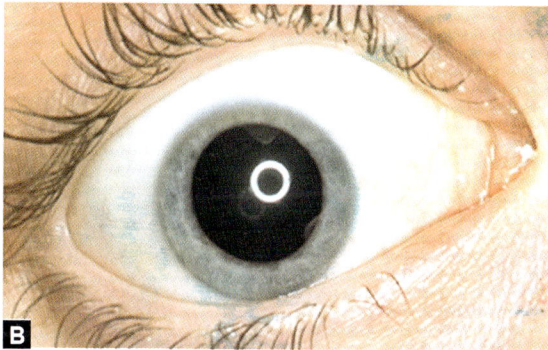

Fig. 27.9: Wilson's disease: (A) Kayser-Fleischer ring (arrows), (B) Complete resolution following **copper-chelating** (penicillamine) treatment.

27

in the thyroid gland as free I^- as well as in the form of monoiodotyrosine, diiodotyrosine, T_3 and T_4.

Biological Functions

The important function of iodine is synthesis of the iodine-containing hormones, i.e. thyroxine (T_4) and triiodothyronine (T_3), the physiologically active substances that are formed by the thyroid gland. These hormones regulate basal metabolic rate throughout life, and during growth and development in children.

Absorption and Excretion

Iodine is quickly absorbed from food and water as inorganic iodide (I^-) from the small intestine.

Depending upon the activity of the thyroid gland, a portion of the absorbed I^- is taken up by the gland (Chemistry to Clinics 27.8).

In the epithelial cells of the thyroid gland, it is oxidized and gets conjugated with the thyroglobulin bound tyrosine residues, resulting in the formation of T_3 and T_4.

Nearly 90% of the plasma I^- is in the organic form, i.e. bound to protein and is called protein-bound iodine (PBI).

About 10% of the circulating organic iodine is excreted in the feces. Inorganic iodide is mostly excreted in the urine and partly through bile and saliva.

Requirement and Sources

Daily requirement of iodine is about 50–100 μg and is mostly fulfilled from drinking water. To ensure adequate supply of dietary iodine, it is desirable to use iodized salt. Seafood, fruits, vegetables, cereals and meat are good sources. Iodine content of the food depends upon the iodine content of the soil in which these are grown.

Chemistry to Clinics 27.8: Goitrogens

Some of the ingredients present in foodstuffs may prevent utilization of iodine by the thyroid gland. Such substances are called goitrogens, e.g. thiocyanate, perchlorate, goitrin, isoflavones, etc., and are abundant in cabbage, turnip, mustard-seeds, peanuts, sweet potatoes, soya beans, etc. Goitrogens are inactivated by heating/cooking. Hence, from a practical point of view, consumption of raw goitrogenic foods in large quantities over a long duration carries a risk of producing goiter.

Deficiency Disorders

Iodine deficiency may lead to goiter. The term **'goiter'** simply refers to a diffuse enlargement of the thyroid gland due to any cause and it may be associated with overactivity or underactivity of the gland.

Endemic Goiter

Endemic goitrous belt: Iodine deficiency is common in some parts of the world. In India, certain sub-Himalayan regions contain less iodine in the soil. This part of the country is called the goitrous belt.

Mechanism of goiter: Dietary iodine deficiency causes depletion of thyroid iodine stores and therefore reduces output of the thyroid hormones. A decrease in serum T_4 stimulates release of pituitary thyroid stimulating hormone (TSH), resulting in hyperplasia of the thyroid gland. This, in turn, traps and processes the available iodine more efficiently. The gland returns to its normal size after sufficient amount of dietary iodine is available. This is called **simple goiter or colloid goiter**. Long-standing cases of simple goiter may lead to the development of nodules which are localized areas of cellular proliferation within the gland. This condition is called **nodular goiter**.

Presentation: The most characteristic feature is enlargement of the thyroid gland, to the extent that a large nodule can be visible in the neck (Fig. 27.10).

Complications: Severe deficiency of iodine in children may result in growth retardation, called cretinism, and myxedema in adults (Chemistry to Clinics 27.9).

Prevention: Intake of sufficient iodine which may be accomplished by adding inorganic iodides to the source of drinking water or by the addition of iodides to the table-salt.

Toxicity

Iodine toxicity may result in thyrotoxicosis.

FLUORIDE

Fluoride (F^-) is present in traces in human tissues, mainly in bones, teeth, thyroid gland and skin.

Biological Functions

Fluoride promotes normal bone development, increases retention of calcium and phosphorus, and

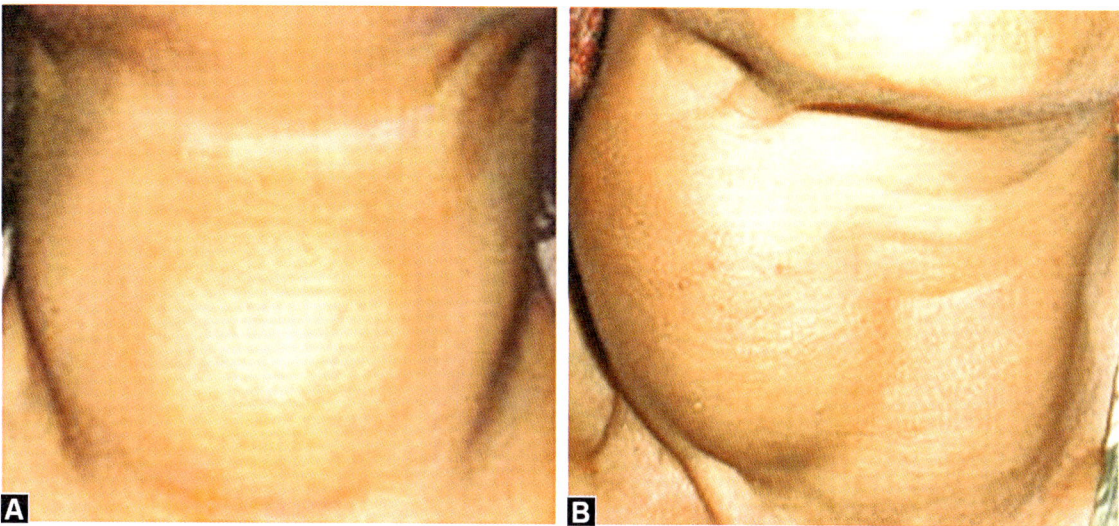

Fig. 27.10: (A) Simple colloid goiter, (B) Multinodular goiter.

Chemistry to Clinics 27.9: Cretinism and Myxedema

Cretinism: It is a condition of hypothyroidism in infants and children which, in turn, affects growth. A cretin child is a dwarf, has a thick tongue and skin, and is mentally retarded and sexually underdeveloped. The deficiency coincides with the critical perinatal period when thyroid hormones are required for neuronal development.

Myxedema: Severe hypothyroidism in adults leads to a condition called myxedema. The skin becomes thick and puffy, due to the deposition of mucous like slimy, viscous material (myxomatous material, mucopolysaccharides) in the skin of the face, hands and legs. Body weight is increased due to the retention of water and NaCl. There is mental dullness and hypersensitivity to cold. It is an emergency requiring intravenous thyroid hormone replacement and corticosteroids.

Chemistry to Clinics 27.10: Dental Caries

Dental caries is characterized by destruction of the tooth enamel as a result of the action of the microorganisms (normally present in the oral cavity) on carbohydrates, particularly during the formation of teeth (Fig. 27.11). Breakdown of the enamel, in turn, exposes the dentine and leads to the development of caries (Fig. 27.12).

prevents osteoporosis during aging. It imparts stability to bones and enamel, due to formation of the highly insoluble **fluoroapatite** from hydroxy-apatite. Hardening of dental enamel makes it resistant to acids.

Absorption and Excretion

Soluble fluorides are maximally (about 90%) absorbed through gastrointestinal tract. Absorption from drinking water is almost complete. After absorption, fluoride is distributed throughout the extracellular fluid. Only a small amount of it is deposited in dental enamel and the bones.

Fluoride is mainly excreted through urine.

Requirement and Sources

Daily requirement has been defined as 2–3 mg. Though fluoride is present in almost all foods in small quantities, drinking water is an important source of fluoride in a human diet. Fluoride content of water depends upon fluoride content of the soil. One part per million (1 PPM) of fluoride in drinking water supplies nearly 1–2 mg of fluoride/day which is sufficient to meet the requirement.

Tea is also a good source of fluoride.

Deficiency Disorders

Deficiency of fluoride promotes the development of **dental caries** in children (Chemistry to Clinics 27.10) and **osteoporosis** in adults, particularly in post-menopausal women.

Toxicity

Large intake of fluoride results in **fluorosis** (Chemistry to Clinics 27.11).

27

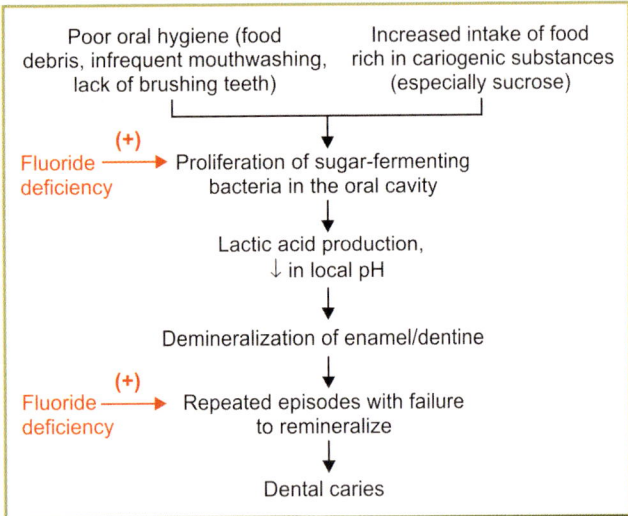

Fig. 27.11 flow chart:

Poor oral hygiene (food debris, infrequent mouthwashing, lack of brushing teeth)   Increased intake of food rich in cariogenic substances (especially sucrose)

Fluoride deficiency (+) → Proliferation of sugar-fermenting bacteria in the oral cavity

↓

Lactic acid production, ↓ in local pH

↓

Demineralization of enamel/dentine

↓

Fluoride deficiency (+) → Repeated episodes with failure to remineralize

↓

Dental caries

Fig. 27.11: Dental caries aggravated by fluoride deficiency.

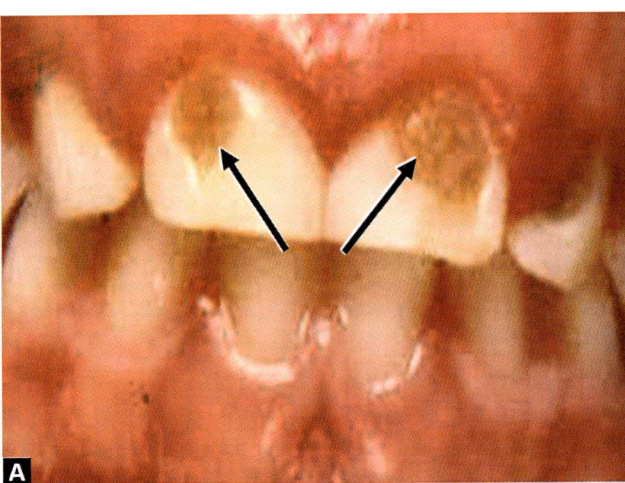

A

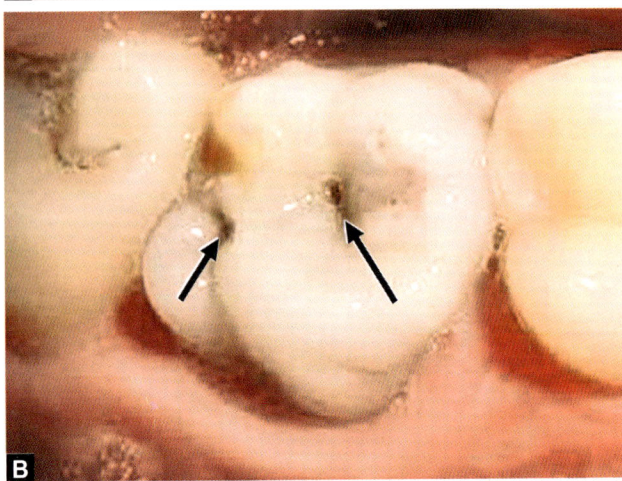

B

Fig. 27.12: Dental caries. (A) Characteristic lesions (arrows) on the enamel, (B) Cavities (arrows) in a neglected case of caries.

Chemistry to Clinics 27.11: Endemic Fluorosis

Though some amount of fluoride is necessary for normal metabolism of the bones and teeth, large doses may be toxic and may lead to fluorosis which is an important public health problem in many parts of the world. High content of fluorosis in rocks may result in increased levels of fluoride in groundwater and its entry into the body.

Presentation: Muscle wasting (inhibition of protein biosynthesis) and impairment in energy metabolism (inhibition of enolase in glycolysis). Fluoride toxicity may manifest in two major forms, i.e. as dental fluorosis and skeletal fluorosis which together constitute endemic fluorosis:

- **Dental fluorosis:** It occurs mainly in children who are exposed to high fluoride intake before completion of mineralization of the tooth enamel. The teeth exhibit mottled enamel. Mottling is confined to permanent teeth and is characterized by multiple, minute white flecks and yellow/brown spots which are scattered irregularly over the tooth surface (Fig. 27.13).
- **Skeletal fluorosis:** The clinical features include pain, inflammation and restricted movement of the joints and stiffness of the spine. Further, significantly higher intake of fluoride (more than 3 mg/L, in drinking water) results in a variant of severe form of the skeletal fluorosis called 'genu valgum' (knock-knee) (Fig. 27.14). Besides the features of dental and skeletal fluorosis, these individuals also exhibit extensive osteoporosis of the limb bones.

Prevention: Defluoridation of water and dietary interventions.

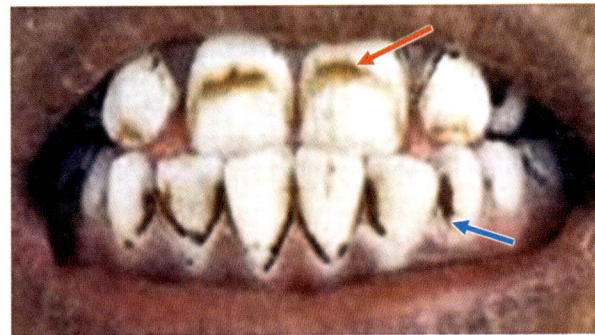

Fig. 27.13: Dental fluorosis: The teeth of the upper jaw (the two central incisors) show mottling and discoloration (red arrow) horizontally aligned on the enamel surface, away from the gums. It cannot be cleaned by a dentist. However, the teeth of the lower jaw show discoloration along the gums (blue arrow) due to dirty teeth (not fluorosis), which can be cleaned by a dentist.

MANGANESE

Total body manganese (Mn) content of an adult human is about 10–12 mg. It is mainly concentrated in the bones, liver and kidney. Most of it is present in the mitochondria and plays an important role in biological oxidation.

27

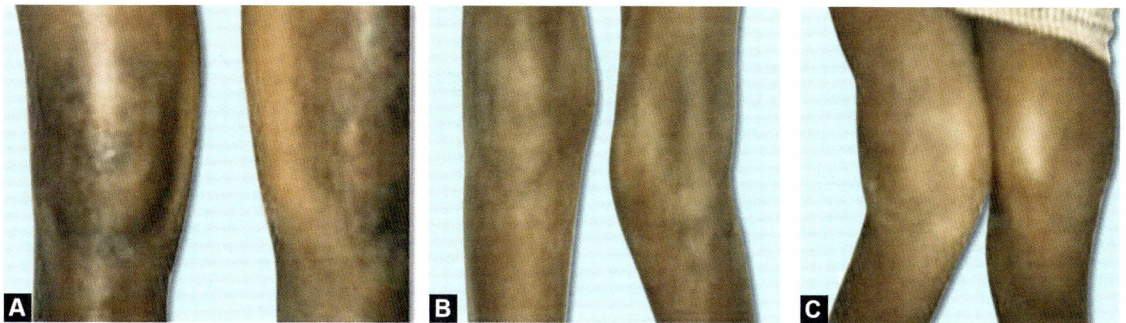

Fig. 27.14: Skeletal fluorosis. (A) **Stage I:** Swollen, painful and rigid knee joints. (B) **Stage II:** Deformed but mobile joints. (C) **Stage III:** Patient is crippled with severe restriction of movement.

Biological Functions

1. Cofactor for various enzymes such as hydrolases, decarboxylases and transferases, e.g. phosphorylases and phosphotransferases.
2. Synthesis of glycoproteins and proteoglycans, in the cartilages.
3. Stimulates biosynthesis of cholesterol and long-chain fatty acids.
4. Prevents lipid peroxidation and exhibits lipotropic effects.

Absorption and Excretion

Only about 5% of the dietary manganese is absorbed. Ethanol increases while dietary calcium, phosphorus and iron reduce its absorption.

Manganese is mainly excreted via bile, in the feces. Only a small fraction of it is excreted in the urine.

Requirement and Sources

Daily requirement is about 2–5 mg. It is widely distributed in nuts, whole grain cereals, legumes and leafy-vegetables. Tea is a rich source of manganese.

Deficiency Disorders

Manganese deficiency leads to bone deformities, poor growth and ataxia in several animal species. Its deficiency has also been shown to decrease the synthesis of oligosaccharides, glycoproteins and proteoglycans.

Toxicity

Manganese is relatively nontoxic but toxicity can occur in manganese-ore mine workers. Inhalation poisoning produces severe psychotic symptoms and parkinsonism.

CHROMIUM

Total body chromium (Cr) content of adult humans is between 5–10 mg. It is present in two forms, i.e. in the trivalent form (Cr^{3+}) and the hexavalent form (Cr^{6+}). **The trivalent form of chromium is biologically active.** An organic compound of chromium is termed as glucose tolerance factor (Chemistry to Clinics 27.12).

Biological Functions

1. Chromium, as a component of glucose tolerance factor, is important in the regulation of blood glucose.
2. Chromium is also important in the metabolism of lipoproteins and maintains normal level of cholesterol in the blood.

Absorption and Excretion

Chromium is poorly absorbed. After its absorption, it combines with plasma β-globulin.

It is excreted in traces in the urine.

Chemistry to Clinics 27.12: Glucose Tolerance Factor

- It is a naturally occurring coordination complex between chromium (Cr^{3+}), nicotinic acid and glutathione (a tripeptide of three amino acids, i.e. glycine, glutamate and cysteine).
- It helps in the storage of insulin in the granules of the pancreatic β-cells as well as its secretion. It may also potentiate the effects of insulin by facilitating its interaction with the receptors and thus it is important in the removal of ingested glucose from the circulation.
- Chromium-picolinate is available commercially and is prescribed as an auxiliary drug to patients suffering from diabetes mellitus.

27

Requirement and Sources

Daily requirement is about 50–100 µg. Brewer's yeast, mushrooms, black pepper, meat (liver), cereals (whole-grains), nuts and cheese are good sources.

Deficiency Disorder

Chromium deficiency can impair glucose tolerance.

Toxicity

Chromium toxicity may be observed on occupational exposure to chromium dust which, in turn, may induce lung cancer.

SELENIUM

Selenium (Se) though is widely distributed in all the tissues but is present in higher amounts in the renal cortex, pancreas, pituitary and liver.

Selenoproteins

Selenoproteins are selenium containing proteins which have selenocysteine (**SeC**) residues. The SeC is incorporated into the peptide chain during its synthesis by the ribosomes, as the 21st amino acid, as a result of some variation in the standard translational machinary. The SeC residues participate in redox reactions, such as those catalyzed by glutathione peroxidase which is a selenoprotein.

Biological Functions

1. An essential component of selenoproteins such as **glutathione peroxidase**, which protects the cells against the damage caused by H_2O_2. Thus, Se is an **antioxidant**. Further, it acts as a synergistic antioxidant with vitamin E and protects the cell membrane against free radicals.
2. Required in some of the immune mechanisms.
3. Biosynthesis of ubiquinone and thus essential for ATP biosynthesis in the mitochondria.

Absorption and Excretion

Selenium is absorbed mainly in the duodenum.

It is excreted mainly in the feces and the expired air.

Requirement and Sources

The RDA is 50–100 µg. Plant-foods, cereals, fish and meat are rich sources of selenium. Food content of selenium however, depends upon the selenium content of the soil.

Deficiency Disorders

Selenium deficiency may be observed when its soil content is low. Deficiency may also be observed in protein energy malnutrition. Selenium deficiency may lead to liver necrosis, muscular dystrophy, cardio-myopathy and dilatation of the heart.

Toxicity

Very high intake of selenium may result in its toxicity and the condition is called as **selenosis**. Its toxicity has been observed in workers in the paint, glass and ceramic industries. These individuals have difficulty in breathing due to inhalation of excessive selenium. High selenium intake may induce weight loss, hair loss, dermatitis, diarrhea, emotional disturbances (irritability) and garlic-like odor in breath.

Patients with primary neoplasms of the reticulo-endothelial system show high levels of selenium in their sera. Excess of selenium as SeC may replace sulfur in tissues and inhibits SH-containing enzymes.

ZINC

Total body content of zinc (Zn) in an adult is about 2.0 g. The choroid of the eye, liver, pancreas, prostate gland and prostatic fluid contain high concentrations of zinc.

Biological Functions

Zinc performs diverse biological functions (Table 27.3).

Absorption and Excretion

Only about 20% of the dietary zinc is absorbed. Absorption of zinc occurs in the duodenum and the ileum. Phytate and dietary fiber decrease its absorption. They lower the availability of dietary zinc and thus increase its excretion in the feces. Zinc absorption is directly proportional to the levels of metallothionein in the intestinal mucosal cells.

Zinc is excreted through pancreatic juice.

Enteropancreatic circulation: Many digestive enzymes secreted from the pancreas contain zinc. Therefore, the gastrointestinal tract receives zinc from two sources during meals—one from food and the

Table 27.3: Functions of zinc

1. **Component of several enzymes**
   - Carbonic anhydrase
   - Lactate dehydrogenase
   - Alcohol dehydrogenase
   - Alkaline phosphatase
   - DNA and RNA polymerases
   - Retinene-retinal reductase
   - Cytosolic superoxide dismutase
2. **Blood glucose regulation:** Zinc forms a complex with insulin, helps in its storage and release from the β-cells of the pancreas.
3. **Maintains plasma vitamin A levels**: By stimulating the release of vitamin A from the liver into the blood.
4. **Taste sensation:** Zinc is a constituent of gustin, a salivary polypeptide necessary for the normal development of taste buds.
5. **Regulation of gene expression:** Essential component of zinc-finger motifs of various regulatory DNA binding proteins.
6. **Enhances immunity**
7. **Normal growth and reproduction.**

other from the pancreatic secretions. The zinc circulates in the body from the pancreas to the small intestine and back to the pancreas via blood, thus completing the enteropancreatic circulation.

Requirement and Sources

Daily intake of about 10–15 mg is sufficient to meet its requirement. Good dietary sources are meat, seafoods, egg, legumes and milk. Colostrum is a very rich source of zinc.

Deficiency Disorders

Since body stores of zinc are small, dietary deficiency can therefore produce symptoms promptly, particularly when its soil content is low (Chemistry to Clinics 27.13).

Chemistry to Clinics 27.13: Zinc Deficiency

Severe zinc deficiency is seen in alcoholics, chronic renal disease, severe gastroenteritis and malabsorption, and protein-energy malnutrition. Clinical manifestations include:

1. Poor wound healing, loss of appetite, poor growth and alopecia (loss of hair).
2. Impairment of sexual development in children.
3. Impairment in brain functions.
4. Certain fetal abnormalities during pregnancy besides hypogonadism, dwarfism (stunted growth) and gross skin lesions with severe acrodermatitis.
5. Delayed recovery from diarrhea.
6. Zinc deficiency affects spermatogenesis, parturition and lactation in experimental animals.

Toxicity

Zinc, when consumed in excessive amounts, produces toxic effects, such as acute gastrointestinal irritation, gastric ulcers, nausea and vomiting. It also interferes with the utilization and functions of copper, and may also cause anemia. Zinc-containing multivitamin cocktails are widely available commercially and need to be used with caution.

COBALT

Adult human body contains only 2–3 mg of cobalt (Co), mainly concentrated in the liver and the kidney.

Biological Functions

1. Cobalt is an important constituent of **vitamin B$_{12}$ (cobalamin)**, about 4% by weight. Vitamin B$_{12}$ is the only compound of cobalt which is nutritionally effective in human beings and other monogastric animals.
2. Cobalt also acts as a cofactor for some enzymes, such as glycylglycine dipeptidase found in the intestinal juice.
3. Cobalt stimulates the production of erythropoietin which, in turn, promotes erythropoiesis.

Absorption and Excretion

Absorption and metabolism of cobalt is similar to that of vitamin B$_{12}$. It is stored in the liver and excreted via bile.

Requirement and Sources

The RDA is 1–2 μg. Its requirement can be met from dietary B$_{12}$. Foods from the animal origin are good sources of cobalt. Meat (liver) is a rich source.

Deficiency Disorders

Cobalt deficiency is not generally observed in human beings. Its deficiency may cause pernicious anemia, as seen due to the deficiency of vitamin B$_{12}$.

Toxicity

Higher doses of cobalt may produce several toxic effects, such as polycythemia (increased erythrocytes in the blood), hypothyroidism, cardiomyopathy and heart failure.

27

MOLYBDENUM

An adult human body contains nearly 5 mg of molybdenum (Mo). Though it is present in all the tissues, liver and kidney contain large amounts.

Biological Functions

Molybdenum is an integral part of several flavoprotein containing oxidase systems, e.g. xanthine oxidase, aldehyde oxidase and sulfite oxidase. Thus, it helps in the transport of electrons. These enzymes contain a substituted pterin ring (molybdopterin) in which molybdenum is bound to two sulfur atoms.

Absorption and Excretion

About 50% of dietary molybdenum is readily absorbed in the small intestine.

It is mainly excreted in the urine. Its excretion increases with high protein intake, particularly with a cysteine-rich diet.

Requirement and Sources

Daily requirement is about 100–200 µg. Pulses, cereals, green-leafy vegetables and meat are good sources. Dietary content of molybdenum depends upon molybdenum content of the soil.

Deficiency Disorders

Molybdenum deficiency, due to the deficiency of molybdenum containing enzymes, may lead to reduced food consumption and mental retardation. Decreased xanthine oxidase activity may increase excretion of xanthine and decreases uric acid excretion.

Toxicity

Toxicity may occur on a high molybdenum diet. Molybdenum toxicity causes **molybdenosis** which is characterized by weight loss, anorexia, anemia, severe diarrhea and skeletal deformities. Very high amount

Table 27.4: Minerals and trace elements, their important biological functions, sources, daily requirements, deficiency disorders and toxicity symptoms

Mineral/trace elements	Biological functions	Sources	Daily requirements	Deficiency disorders	Toxicity
Calcium (Ca)	Calcification of teeth and bone, blood clotting, and cofactor for enzymes, such as adenylate cyclase, glycogen synthase, etc.	Milk and milk products, legumes, and dry fruits	800–1200 mg	Tetany, osteoporosis	Renal stones
Phosphorus (P)	Calcification of teeth and bone, component of nucleic acids, regulation of blood pH, and activator for enzymes involved in phosphorylation/dephosphorylation	Milk and milk products, eggs, meat, legumes, and cereals	1.0–1.5 g	Neuromuscular, skeletal, and renal manifestations	–
Iron (Fe)	Component of heme and nonheme proteins, e.g. hemoglobin, catalase, cytochromes, etc.	Meat, green-leafy vegetables	10–20 mg	Anemia	Hemosiderosis
Copper (Cu)	Component of many enzymes, such as cytochrome oxidase, ceruloplasmin, tyrosinase, etc., also helps in iron metabolism	Meat, eggs, and legumes	2–3 mg	Menkes disease, anemia, neutropenia	Wilson's disease
Zinc (Zn)	Cofactor for various enzymes, such as carbonic anhydrase, DNA and RNA polymerases, alkaline phosphatase; also has role in insulin secretion and taste development	Meat, seafoods, and legumes	10–15 mg	Poor wound healing, growth retardation	Gastrointestinal irritation
Iodine (I$_2$)	Synthesis of thyroid hormones	Iodized salt, seafoods	50–100 µg	Endemic goiter, myxedema, cretinism	Thyrotoxicosis

(Contd.)

Mineral/trace elements	Biological functions	Sources	Daily requirements	Deficiency disorders	Toxicity
Fluoride (F⁻)	Promotes normal bone and teeth development	Drinking water and tea	2–3 mg	Dental caries	Fluorosis
Magnesium (Mg)	Component of the bone structure, in nerve impulse transmission, also acts as cofactor for various ATP-dependent enzymes	Cereals, seafoods, tea and coffee	250–300 mg	Depression, muscle weakness, and tetany	Drowsiness and lethargy
Manganese (Mn)	Cofactor for various enzymes, such as hydrolases, decarboxylases, trans-ferases, etc.	Nuts, wholegrains, and tea	2–5 mg	Bone deformities	Psychotic symptoms
Chromium (Cr)	Regulation of blood glucose	Mushrooms, nuts, and black pepper	50–100 µg	Glucose intole-rance	Lung cancer
Selenium (Se)	Component of selenoproteins, such as glutathione peroxidase	Cereals, fish, and meat	50–100 µg	Liver necrosis	Hair loss
Cobalt (Co)	Component of vitamin B_{12}	Liver	1–2 µg	Pernicious anemia	Polycythemia, hypothyroidism
Molybdenum (Mo)	Component of flavoprotein contain-ing oxidases, such as xanthine oxidase	Pulses and cereals	100–200 µg	Affects growth, causes mental retardation	Anorexia and diarrhea

of molybdenum also inhibits the absorption and utilization of copper.

As shown in Table 27.4 , each of the minerals/trace elements has specific biological functions, and its deficiency as well as excess may lead to undesirable consequences. An overview of the biochemical assessment of micronutrient status is given in Table 27.5.

Table 27.5: Biochemical assessment of micronutrient status

Lipid soluble vitamins	Vitamin A	Serum retinol, serum retinol binding protein
	Vitamin D	Serum vitamin D
	Vitamin E	Serum α-tocopherol, RBC hemolysis
	Vitamin K	Serum vitamin K, plasma prothrombin, prothrombin time
Water soluble vitamins	Vitamin B_1	RBC transketolase, RBC thiamine pyrophosphate (TPP)
	Vitamin B_2	RBC glutathione reductase
	Vitamin B_3	Urinary N-methyl nicotinamide/2-pyridine ratio
	Vitamin B_6	Plasma B_6, RBC transaminase, urinary xanthurenic acid
	Biotin	Urinary biotin, urinary 3-hydroxy isovaleric acid
	Folic acid	RBC folate
	Vitamin B_{12}	Serum vitamin B_{12}, urinary methylmalonic acid
	Vitamin C	Plasma and leukocyte vitamin C
Minerals	Sodium	Serum Na^+
	Potassium	Serum K^+
	Chloride	Serum Cl^-
	Magnesium	Serum Mg^{2+}
	Calcium	Serum Ca^{2+}
	Phosphorus	Serum PO_4^-
	Copper	Serum copper and ceruloplasmin, RBC superoxide dismutase
	Zinc	Plasma and hair zinc
	Iodine	Urinary iodine, serum thyroxin, serum TSH
	Selenium	RBC selenium, RBC glutathione peroxidase
	Iron	Hb, hematocrit, serum ferritin, serum total iron binding capacity, serum iron, serum transferring saturation, RBC protoporphyrin

27

SOME IMPORTANT QUESTIONS

1. Describe dietary sources, daily requirement and functions of calcium in the human body.

2. Describe the role of calcium and phosphorus metabolism in relation to calcitonin, parathyroid hormone and 1,25-dihydroxycholecalciferol.

3. Name iron containing proteins and explain their functions. How iron metabolism is regulated? Mention disorders related to iron metabolism.

4. Describe in brief:
   i. Absorption and transport of iron
   ii. Osteoporosis
   iii. Calcium homeostasis
   iv. Fluoride as a nutrient
   v. Role of copper in iron metabolism
   vi. Significance of zinc-containing proteins in the body

5. Write notes on:
   i. Copper toxicity
   ii. Biological functions of selenium
   iii. Wilson's disease
   iv. Fluorosis
   v. Dental caries
   vi. Biochemical role of calcium
   vii. Calmodulin
   viii. Tetany
   ix. Ferredoxins
   x. Ferritin
   xi. Ferroxidases
   xii. Transferrin
   xiii. Hemosiderin
   xiv. Anemia
   xv. Hemochromatosis
   xvi. Ceruloplasmin
   xvii. Menkes disease
   xviii. Cretinism
   xix. Myxedema
   xx. Selenoproteins
   xi. Molybdenosis

6. Discuss:
   i. Biochemical role of magnesium
   ii. Mucosal-block theory of iron absorption
   iii. Endemic goiter
   iv. Biochemical role of manganese
   v. Glucose tolerance factor
   vi. Biochemical significance of zinc
   vii. Biochemical role of cobalt
   viii. Biochemical assessment of micronutrient status.

MULTIPLE CHOICE QUESTIONS

1. **Calcium absorption is decreased by all of the following** *except:*
   A. Acidic pH
   B. Phosphates
   C. Oxalates
   D. Alkaline pH

2. **Tetany may occur in all of the following** *except:*
   A. Hypocalcemia
   B. Hypomagnesemia
   C. Acidosis
   D. Alkalosis

3. **The normal serum 'Ca × P' product (each expressed in mg/dl) is:**
   A. 10–20
   B. 20–30
   C. 30–40
   D. 40–50

4. **Magnesium toxicity may occur with:**
   A. Excessive use of Mg-containing antacids
   B. Treatment with diuretics
   C. Metabolic acidosis
   D. Uremia

5. **In iron deficiency anemia, TIBC:**
   A. Increases
   B. Decreases
   C. Remains unchanged
   D. Cannot be calculated

6. **Hemosiderosis may be observed in:**
   A. Multiple blood transfusions for thalassemia major
   B. Chronic pancreatitis
   C. Alcoholic cirrhosis
   D. All of the above

7. **'Kinky hair syndrome' is due to a genetic deficiency of:**
   A. Keratin
   B. Collagen
   C. Elastin
   D. ATP7A

8. **Goitrogens include:**
   A. Thiocyanate and perchlorate only
   B. Goitrin and isoflavones only
   C. Perchlorate and goitrin only
   D. All of the above

9. **Glucose tolerance factor consists of:**
   A. Cr^{3+}, nicotinic acid, GSH
   B. Zn^{2+}, nicotinic acid, GSH
   C. Cr^{3+}, pyridoxine, GSH
   D. Zn^{2+}, pyridoxine, GSH

10. **Insulin storage and release requires:**
    A. Zn
    B. Ca
    C. Fe
    D. Mn

Vitamins

Vitamins are organic constituents of food, called 'protective accessory food factors'. These are essential for life and well-being. Vitamins, in general, cannot be synthesized by the body and have to be supplied in the diet though in very small quantities. Thus, they are **micronutrients**. Vitamins are divided into two groups:

1. Lipid soluble vitamins, and
2. Water soluble vitamins

1. LIPID SOLUBLE VITAMINS

Lipid soluble vitamins are vitamin A, vitamin D, vitamin E and vitamin K. Their general properties include:

- Dietary lipid soluble vitamins are absorbed from the gastrointestinal lumen, in the presence of **lipids and bile salts**.
- Their precursors are called **provitamins** and are found mostly in plants.
- Due to their lipid solubility, they are **stored** in the liver, adipose tissue, etc.
- Because they can be stored, a dietary **deficiency takes time** to become manifest.
- Large doses, for a fairly long duration, may result in toxic symptoms (**hypervitaminosis**).

VITAMIN A (ANTI-NIGHTBLINDNESS FACTOR)

Vitamin A has a characteristic 6-membered ring known as β-ionine ring attached with a long hydrocarbon side chain (Fig. 28.1).

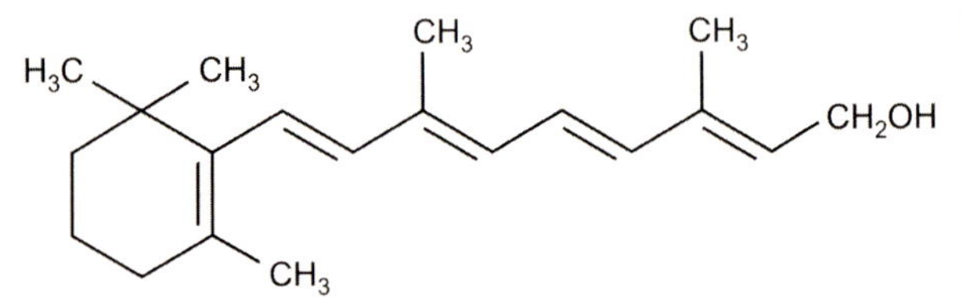

Fig. 28.1: Vitamin A alcohol (retinol).

Vitamin A is an alcohol (**retinol**) but it may be converted into an aldehyde (**retinal**, also called retinene) or an acid (**retinoic acid**). All the three forms are found in different tissues. The main, naturally occurring form of vitamin A though contains a β-ionine ring, a dehydro form, with two double bonds in the ring is also known to occur. This is called vitamin A_2. The β-ionone ring of vitamin A_2 thus contains two double bonds. The aldehyde form of vitamin A_2 is designated as 3-dehydroretinal.

Provitamin A

Carotenoids are called provitamin A. These are found in plants and depending upon the presence of additional ionine ring(s), these provitamins are designated as α, β or γ-carotenes. Rich sources of carotenes are yellow-colored fruits and vegetables such as carrots, pumpkin, papaya, mango, etc. **Polar bear is the richest animal source.**

β-Carotene has highest vitamin A activity of all the natural carotenoids. Cleavage of the carotenes give rise to vitamin A in the intestinal wall. Whereas

28

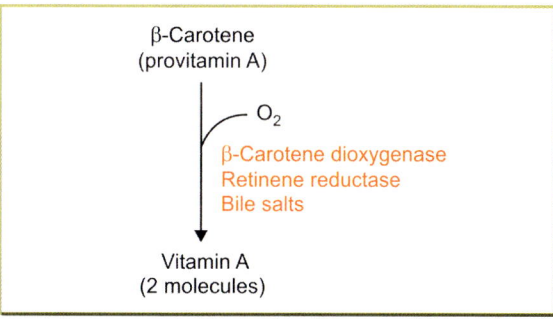

Fig. 28.2: Conversion of β-carotene to vitamin A.

β-carotene gives 2 molecules, α- and γ-carotenes each give rise to only one molecule of vitamin A (retinol). Conversion of β-carotene into retinal requires β-carotene dioxygenase, retinene reductase, molecular oxygen and bile salts (Fig. 28.2).

Conversion of carotenes into vitamin A: Provitamins (carotenoids) are, as such, absorbed in the gastrointestinal lumen and are converted into retinol in the intestinal epithelium. After its entry into the intestinal mucosa, retinol is re-esterified with long chain fatty acids and enters the lymphatics, in chylomicrons as retinyl esters. Most of the vitamin A esters are **stored in the liver**. When needed, retinol is released from the liver and is transported in the blood vessels bound to **retinol-binding protein (RBP)**. In the serum, RBP-retinol complex combines with transthyretin, another protein, which is also synthesized in the liver. Retinol-binding protein can transport retinol, retinoic acid and carotenes. Some of the retinoic acid is also transported, in circulation, by albumin.

The retinol is removed from the serum and is utilized by the target cells, such as retinol photoreactors and epithelial linings. In the retina, it is converted to retinal which is essential in visual functions whereas in the epithelial tissues, retinol is converted to retinoic acid which is required for maintaining epithelial functions, i.e. growth and differentiation.

Absorption and Metabolism

Nearly 50–90% of vitamin A is absorbed in the intestine and is released into the lacteals. The vitamin is absorbed in the esterified form (retinyl esters) in the presence of bile. Dietary absorption of vitamin A and its main metabolism is shown in Fig. 28.3.

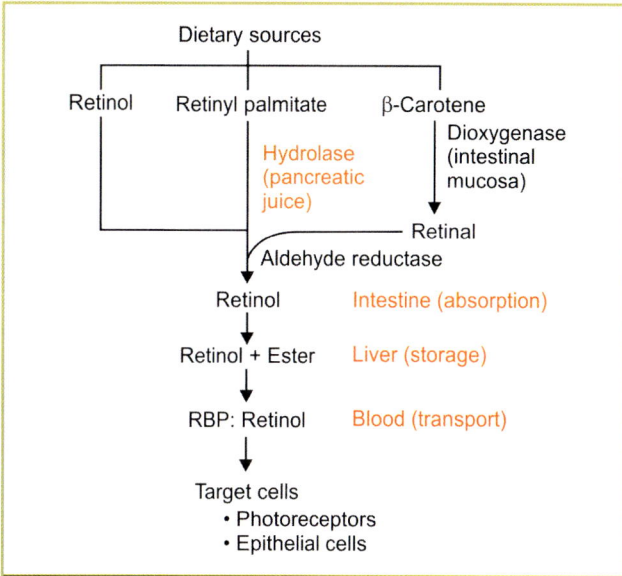

Fig. 28.3: Vitamin A metabolism.

Biological Functions

Various biological functions of vitamin A are performed by retinol, retinal and retinoic acid.

1. Vision: Vitamin A is essential for the functioning of the rods as well as the cones, in the retina.

Biochemical aspects of vision: White light represents a fusion or mixture of individual colored lights called monochromatic light. By shining a beam of white light through a glass prism, white light can be resolved into its constituents. This is the **visible spectrum** (Fig. 28.4).

On the basis of differences in the biochemical series of events, vision is of two types—scotopic and photopic.

Scotopic vision: It refers to vision in **dim light** that depends on the **rod cells** in the retina. Rods are of one type only and provide **monochromatic vision**. They contain a photopigment called **rhodopsin** made up of the glycoprotein opsin and the aldehyde derivative of vitamin A called retinal. In dim light or darkness, retinal has a bent shape and is called 11-*cis*-retinal, which fits with opsin. When it absorbs light, the molecule straightens to form all-*trans*-retinal. This *cis* to *trans* conversion (isomerization) is the first step in converting light to an electrical signal in the retina. In darkness, an enzyme reverses the process. The chain of events in the cells of the retina are known as **Wald's visual cycle** and are shown in Fig. 28.5.

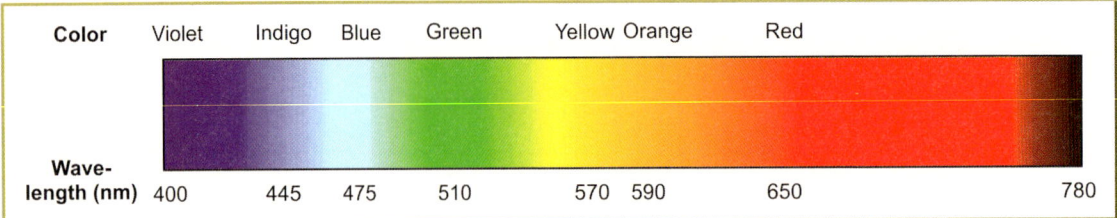

Fig. 28.4: The visible spectrum.

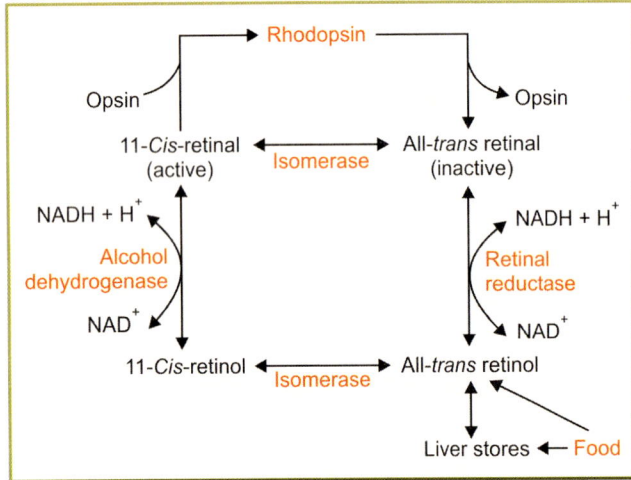

Fig. 28.5: Wald's visual cycle in rod cells.

When light falls on the retina, rhodopsin is bleached and generates all-*trans* retinal which cannot form a complex with opsin. Visual excitation further changes the structural configuration of opsin, which in turn, generates nerve impulses. All-*trans* retinal is immediately reduced to all-*trans* retinol by the enzyme, all-*trans* retinal dehydrogenase (retinal reductase). All-*trans* retinol is then transported to and stored in the liver where it is isomerized to 11-*cis* retinol by an isomerase. After its delivery to the retina, 11-*cis* retinol is again changed to 11-*cis* retinal which can conjugate with opsin to form rhodopsin, in dark.

Photopic vision: It refers to vision in **bright light** that depends on the **cone cells** in the retina. Cones are of three types and provide **trichromatic vision**. Each cone type contains a specific photopigment made up of retinal and one of three opsins which filter the light before it reaches retinal. The 'red' photopigment (**porphyropsin**) responds best to yellow-orange light (558 nm), the 'green' photopigment (**iodopsin**) responds best to green light (531 nm) and the 'blue' photopigment (**cyanopsin**) responds best to blue light

Chemistry to Clinics 28.1: Color Blindness

Color blindness is a genetic disease; however, severe vitamin A deficiency may result in acquired defects in the functioning of cones. However, it may be clinically difficult to diagnose because by this time, the corneal damage already interferes with vision. Chronic malabsorption is a frequent cause which is often overlooked, though it readily responds to vitamin A supplementation.

(420 nm). Although each cone type responds maximally to a particular wavelength, it does respond to other wavelengths as well. This means that for any given wavelength, all the three cone types get excited to different degrees. The final color sensation is determined by the pattern of the frequency of impulses generated by the three cone systems. When white light falls on the retina, they are stimulated in roughly equal proportions. As the intensity of light is reduced, the cones cease to respond and the rods take over. The various types of **color blindness** can be explained in terms of the absence or deficiency of one or more of the specific cone cell type (Chemistry to Clinics 28.1).

Light/dark adaptation: When a person passes from darkness to bright light he is dazzled, but shortly thereafter he sees well again. This adjustment or decrease in sensitivity on exposure to bright light is called light adaptation but is, strictly speaking, the disappearance of dark adaptation.

2. Cell growth and differentiation: Vitamin A, as **retinoic acid**, plays a key role in:
  i. Synthesis of membrane glycoproteins.
  ii. Synthesis of glycosaminoglycans that are important constituents of the extracellular matrix.
  iii. Formation of intercellular gap-junctions required for proper cell-to-cell communication.
  iv. Controlling the stepwise formation of particular cell types from precursor cells, i.e. differentiation.

Collectively, these actions ensure the maintenance of epithelial integrity.

3. Immunity: Since vitamin A is required to maintain the integrity of the tissues lining the eyes, the gastrointestinal tract, the genitourinary tract, the respiratory system, and skin, it ensures an optimal functioning of the immune system.

4. Antioxidant: Both vitamin A and β-carotene detoxify free radicals, and are therefore, lipid-phase antioxidants.

5. Anticancer: The ability of vitamin A to maintain epithelial integrity, to strengthen the immune response, to act as an antioxidant, and to regulate cell growth and differentiation, makes it an important anticancer vitamin.

6. Intermediary metabolism: Vitamin A favors synthesis of the steroid hormones particularly corticosterone and cortisol that, in turn, favor gluco-neogenesis. Vitamin A also plays a role in cholesterol biosynthesis, i.e. in the final stage of cyclization of squalene to cholesterol.

Deficiency Diseases

Vitamin A deficiency is primarily due to its low dietary intake. It is aggravated by infections which reduce its absorption and utilization.

1. Vitamin A deficiency though affects many tissues, it is most detrimental for the **eyes** (Chemistry to Clinics 28.2).
2. Deficiency of vitamin A results in **xerosis and keratinization of various extraocular epithelial surfaces** including the mucous membrane: Skin (becomes dry and rough), urogenital tract (chances of urolithiasis, infertility, degeneration of the testes, abortion and production of malformed off-springs), etc.
3. Increased susceptibility to infections, free radical mediated cytotoxicity and carcinogenesis.

Chemistry to Clinics 28.2: Ocular Effects of Vitamin A Deficiency

Deficiency of vitamin A results in **xerophthalmia**, i.e. drying of the conjunctiva and the cornea, followed by destruction of the cornea and blindness. The various stages are shown in Fig. 28.6. It should be remembered that the initial symptoms (night blindness) are due to retinol/retinal deficiency in the visual pigments whereas the later manifestations (Bitot's spots onwards) are due to a deficiency of retinoic acid and a consequent failure to maintain epithelial integrity.

Xerophthalmia occurs when body stores of vitamin A are exhausted and supply fails to meet requirement. The first symptom of xerophthalmia is **night blindness**, i.e. an individual cannot see to get around after dark or in a dark room. Since retinal is essential for the synthesis of rhodopsin by the rods, vitamin A deficiency interferes with the production of rhodopsin, impairs rod functions and results in night blindness. It responds rapidly to vitamin A therapy.

If untreated, **Bitot's spots** develop: Accumulation of foamy/cheesy material on the conjunctiva. Although these spots may differ in size, location and shape, they have a similar appearance. When the cornea becomes dry, the condition is called as xerosis. If the disease is not treated, it can progress within hours to an ulcer of the cornea. A **corneal ulcer** can lead to melting or wasting of the cornea, called **keratomalacia**. It indicates destruction of a part or of the complete corneal stroma, resulting in permanent structural alteration. Keratomalacia can lead to perforation of the cornea. At this stage, a **corneal scar** remains in the eye. The sooner the disease is treated, the smaller the ulcer and smaller the scar which however, remains forever.

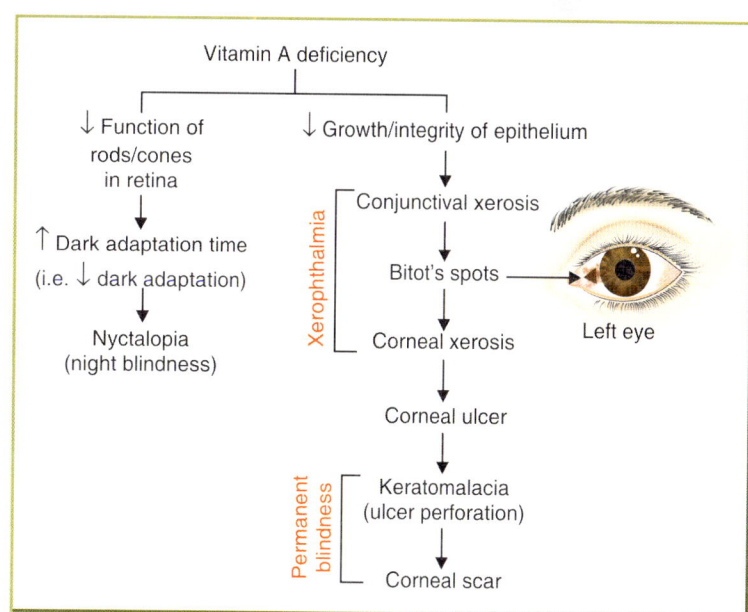

Fig. 28.6: Effect of vitamin A deficiency on the eyes.

28

4. Vitamin A deficiency also affects osteoblastic activity and results in defective resorption of the bone thereby affecting growth of children.

Sources and Requirement

Liver oil (especially fish-liver oil), eggs, milk and milk products are good sources of **vitamin A**.

Papaya, carrots, sweet potatoes and green-leafy vegetables are good sources of **carotenes**.

The recommended daily allowance (RDA) of vitamin A for an adult is 2000–2500 IU (750–1000 µg).

Daily requirement of β-carotene is 4000–6000 IU (about 2000 µg).

One IU of vitamin A is the activity present in 0.3 µg of retinol.

One retinol equivalent is the activity present in 1 µg of retinol or 6 µg of β-carotene.

Hypervitaminosis A

Since vitamin A is a lipid soluble vitamin and is stored in the liver, so if taken in large quantities for a long period, it may be toxic. **Vitamin A toxicity** (hypervitaminosis A) includes dry and rough skin, scaly dermatitis, besides headache, nausea, vomiting, loss of appetite, hepatomegaly, painful joints and bone abnormalities. In high doses, preformed vitamin A or retinol can be even teratogenic. It can cause birth defects (craniofacial abnormalities) and spontaneous abortions if taken during early stages of pregnancy. Because body converts carotenoids into vitamin A only when necessary, thus taking large quantities of carotenes do not cause vitamin A toxicity and there is no risk of its overdose.

VITAMIN D (CALCIFEROL, ANTI-RICKETS FACTOR, SUNSHINE VITAMIN)

Vitamin D is a **sterol** and a **prohormone,** present in nature in several forms. Two common forms are:

- **Vitamin D$_2$ (ergocalciferol):** It is of **plant origin,** obtained from the ergot plant. It can also be synthesized in the laboratory, by irradiating ergosterol. Note that vitamin D$_1$ is a complex of ergocalciferol and lumisterol.

- **Vitamin D$_3$ (cholecalciferol):** It is of **animal origin** (Fig. 28.7), the natural substance obtained from fish oil or derived from 7-dehydrocholesterol by ultraviolet irradiation in the skin. Interestingly,

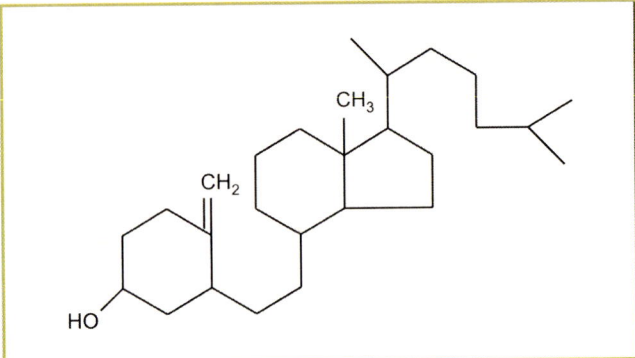

Fig. 28.7: Vitamin D$_3$ (cholecalciferol).

vitamin D$_3$ and its active metabolites have also been obtained from some plant sources, particularly from tomato leaves.

Both vitamin D$_2$ and D$_3$ are **secosteroids** (steroid with an open 'B' ring) and are metabolically activated to carry out their functions.

Provitamin D and Previtamin D

7-Dehydrocholesterol is a precursor of vitamin D$_3$ in animals and is called as **provitamin D$_3$.** It is synthesized in human beings in the intestinal mucosa. By the action of UV light in the skin, 7-dehydrocholesterol is converted into an intermediate called **previtamin D$_3$** which is spontaneously isomerized to vitamin D$_3$ (cholecalciferol) (Fig. 28.8). In this process (photobiogenesis), the UV rays of sunlight with a wave length of **290–315 nm** (the UV-B range), initiates photoconversion.

On the other hand, ergosterol is the provitamin D$_2$ in plants. In the presence of light, by the process of photolysis, ergosterol is converted to previtamin D$_2$ which is isomerized to ergocalciferol (vitamin D$_2$).

Absorption and Metabolism

In addition to its endogenous synthesis, vitamin D is also absorbed from diet. Maximum absorption of

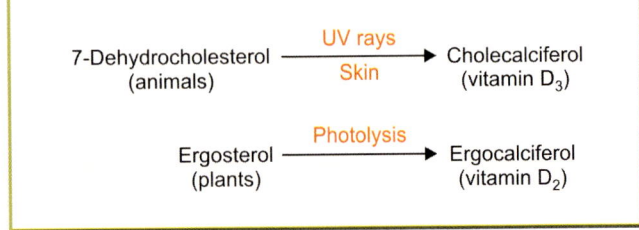

Fig. 28.8: Conversion of provitamin D to vitamin D.

vitamin D_3 occurs in the jejunum. After its absorption from the intestine or following formation in the skin, vitamin D_3 binds to a specific globulin termed as **vitamin D binding-protein (DBP, also called transcalciferrin)** in the plasma and transported to the liver.

Metabolic Activation of Vitamin D

Activation of vitamin D takes place partly in the liver and partly in the kidney.

The first metabolic step occurs in the liver where vitamin D is hydroxylated by the cytochrome P_{450}-dependent enzyme 25-hydroxylase, to 25-hydroxycholecalciferol [$25(OH)\cdot D_3$]. This is also the storage form of the vitamin in the liver. The circulating level of **$25(OH\cdot D_3)$** also reflects **vitamin D nutritional status**. It is an immediate precursor of the **active vitamin D (calcitriol)**.

From liver, 25-hydroxycholecalciferol is transported to the kidneys, where it is further hydroxylated at position 1, by the mitochondrial enzyme 1-α-hydroxylase, and is converted to 1,25-dihydroxycholecalciferol

[$1,25(OH)_2\cdot D_3$]. This is the **physiologically active form of the vitamin**. This metabolite functions as a hormone and is essential in calcium homeostasis. Further, due to the presence of 3-OH groups, active form of vitamin D, i.e. $1,25(OH)_2\cdot D_3$ is also called **calcitriol**. Alternatively, $25(OH)\cdot D_3$ may also be converted to the inactive $24,25(OH)_2\cdot D_3$ (Fig. 28.9).

Regulation of 1-α-hydroxylase: The enzyme 1-α-hydroxylase is present in renal tubules, bone and placenta. The enzyme is regulated by parathormone (parathyroid hormone or **PTH**), which is required for the conversion of 25-hydroxycholecalciferol to calcitriol. Besides PTH, 1-α-hydroxylase is also regulated by serum **phosphorus** as well as by calcitriol itself (**autoregulation**). The production of $1,25(OH)_2\cdot D_3$ is also enhanced or suppressed under the conditions of low or high serum calcium, respectively.

Biological Functions of Calcitriol

1. **Skeletal effects:** The most important biological role of calcitriol is the regulation of serum calcium and

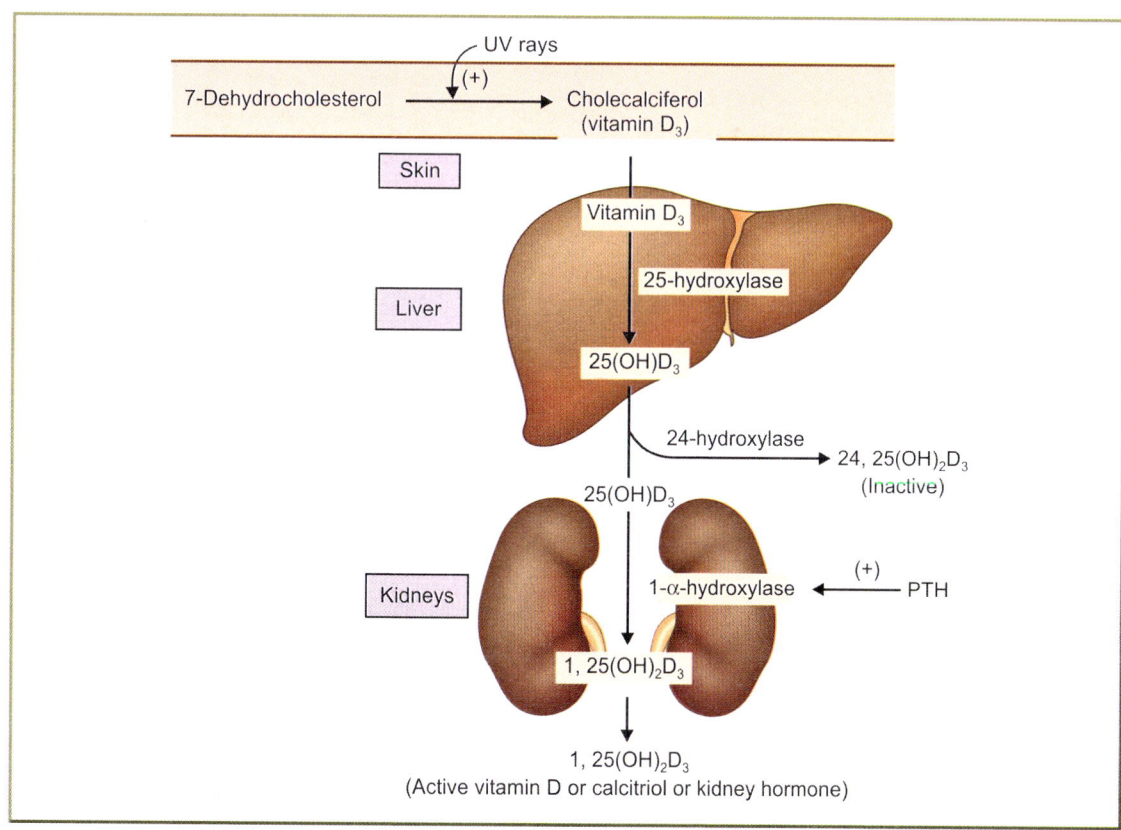

Fig. 28.9: Activation of vitamin D.

28

phosphorus levels. The net result is achieved through its action in the intestine, bone and kidneys:

- *In the intestine*: Calcium absorption from the intestine occurs in **three steps**: release of calcium from its bound forms in the food such as calcium phosphate; sequestering calcium in the cytosol by binding it to specific proteins; and energy-dependent exit of calcium from the cells into the circulation. Calcitriol induces the synthesis of alkaline phosphatase, calcium binding proteins such as calmodulin, and Ca^{2+}-dependent ATPase to increase the efficiency of absorption of calcium as well as phosphorus at each step.

- *In bones*: Bone remodeling is a **dynamic and continuous** process. Bone formation is carried out by cells called osteoblasts whereas the opposite process, bone resorption, is performed by osteoclasts. Calcitriol stimulates the synthesis of the proteins osteocalcin and osteopontin in the osteoblasts; these proteins become a part of the bone matrix (osteoid) and bind calcium. Thus, calcitriol favors mineralization when serum calcium is normal or rising (as after a meal). However, when serum calcium tends to fall, calcitriol promotes the differentiation of pre-osteoclasts to osteoclasts which in turn mobilize calcium from the bone, i.e. causes demineralization of the bone and restores normocalcemia.

- *In kidneys*: Calcitriol increases the tubular reabsorption of calcium and excretion of phosphorus.

  The overall effect of calcitriol therefore is to maintain **calcium/phosphorus homeostasis** and its actions on individual target tissues are dictated by the serum calcium/phosphorus levels. It should be remembered that calcitriol always works in **collaboration with PTH and calcitonin**.

2. **Non-skeletal effects:** Contrary to popular belief, the non-skeletal actions of vitamin D are **as important** as the skeletal ones. The major aspects regulated by vitamin D include:
   - Cell proliferation and differentiation
   - Insulin release
   - Action of growth hormone
   - Immune response
   - Fertility

Significance of 25-hydroxyvitamin D: Serum $25(OH) \cdot D_3$ is an indicator of an individual's **vitamin D**

status in the body; normal range 25–30 ng/ml although some consider that it should be >30 ng/ml.

Deficiency Diseases

Deficiency of vitamin D generally does not occur as it can be synthesized in the body. Deficiency may however, occur due to lack of sunshine.

Skeletal effects of vitamin D deficiency: A deficiency of vitamin D leads to **rickets in children** (Fig. 28.10) and to **osteomalacia in adults**. Rickets is of several types and osteomalacia is different from osteoporosis (Table 28.1 and Fig. 28.11). Please refer to Chapter 27 for details of osteoporosis.

It should be remembered that serum alkaline phosphatase is normally elevated in growing children and may also be raised in unrelated diseases in adults because of the existence of isoenzymes, hence it is useful to measure calcium × phosphate product (Chemistry to Clinics 28.3).

Non-skeletal effects of vitamin D deficiency: Vitamin D deficiency may also lead to defects in insulin secretion and impaired glucose tolerance; impaired immunity; carcinogenesis, etc.

Sources and Requirement

Vitamin D can be synthesized in the body by the action of ultraviolet light on the skin: 10–20 minutes of daily exposure to the midnoon/afternoon sunshine is adequate to meet the daily needs of vitamin D. However, some researchers recommend a much longer exposure.

Rich dietary sources are milk, butter, egg yolk, fish oil and liver oil. The RDA is 200 IU (5 mg cholecalciferol; 40 IU = 1 mg). Doses in elderly should be higher and individualized as per their vitamin D status.

Hypervitaminosis D

Extremely large doses of vitamin D (hypervitaminosis D) can cause hypercalcemia, hyperphosphatemia,

---

Chemistry to Clinics 28.3: Calcium × Phosphate Product
Product of serum calcium and inorganic phosphorus which is normally 40 (10 mg calcium × 4 mg phosphorus), may decrease to <30 in rickets and osteomalacia. Administration of vitamin D in therapeutic doses and/or exposure to sunlight corrects the deficiency.

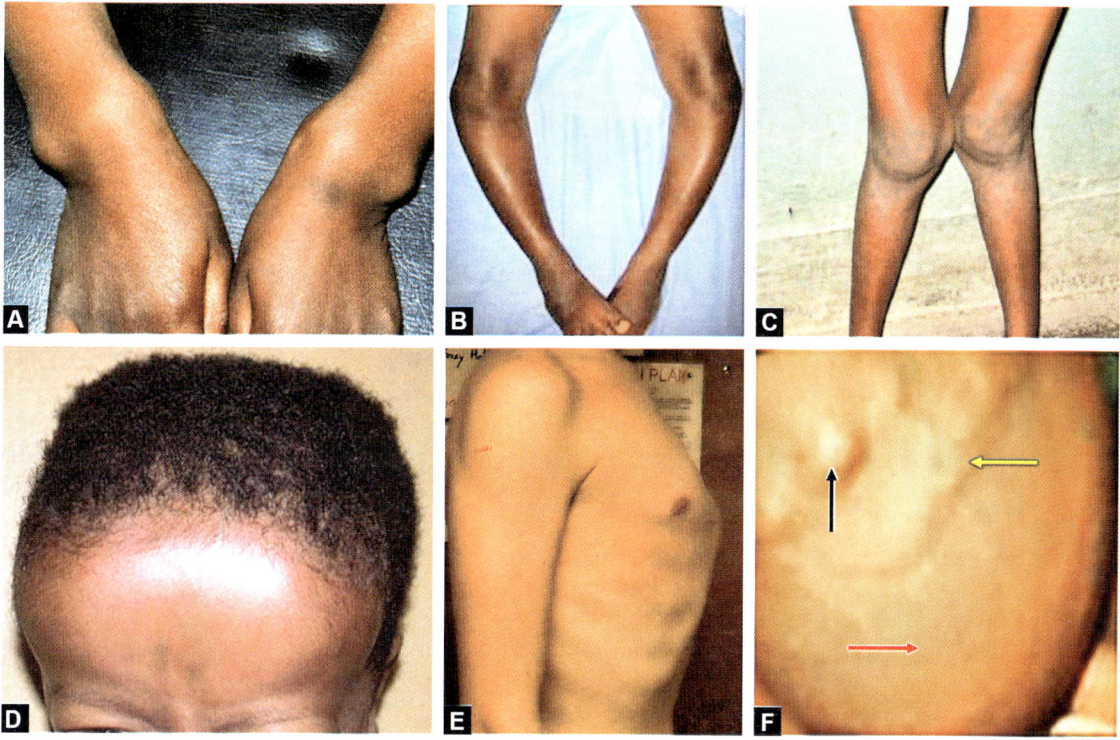

Fig. 28.10: Salient clinical features of **rickets**. (A) Enlarged wrists, (B) Bow legs (genu varum), (C) Knock-knees (genu valgum), (D) Frontal bossing, (E) Pigeon chest (pectus carinatum, protrusion of the sternum and ribs), (F) Rachitic rosary (prominence of costochondral junctions, black arrow), Harrison's sulcus (horizontal groove corresponding to the indentation of lower ribs at the diaphragmatic attachment, yellow arrow) and pot belly (red arrow).

Table 28.1: Comparison between the various types of rickets, osteomalacia and osteoporosis

Parameter	Vitamin D responsive rickets	Vitamin D-resistant rickets	Renal rickets	Osteomalacia (adult rickets)	Osteoporosis
Inherited/acquired	Acquired	Inherited	Acquired	Acquired	Acquired
Age	Infancy/childhood	Infancy/childhood	Any	Adult and elderly	Adult and elderly
Cause	↓Dietary vitamin D and/or ↓exposure to sunlight	↓Renal 1α-hydroxy-lase	↓Functional renal mass, e.g. chronic renal failure due to diabetes mellitus, hypertension, etc.	↓Dietary vitamin D and/or ↓exposure to sunlight (females during pregnancy and lactation; women who are protected from sun-light, such as those observing purdah; prolonged bed-ridden patients)	Multifactorial-↓dietary calcium, ↓estrogen, prolonged bed-ridden patients, drug induced, e.g. corticosteroids
Bone structure	Osteoid matrix of developing bone fails to get properly mineralized	As in vitamin D-responsive rickets	Bone healthy initially; demineralization of osteoid later in life, coinciding with the phase of renal disease	Bone healthy since childhood; extensive demineralization of normal osteoid later in life, coinciding with the phase of vitamin D deficiency	Bone healthy since childhood; ↓osteoid formation plus ↓mineralization leads to ↓bone density (mass per unit volume) later in life

Contd...

28

Contd...

Parameter	Vitamin D-responsive rickets	Vitamin D resistant rickets	Renal rickets	Osteomalacia (adult rickets)	Osteoporosis
Common clinical presentation	Enlarged wrists and ankles, bowed-legs, knock-knees, delayed dentition	As in vitamin D-responsive rickets	Features of the specific disease that resulted in chronic renal failure	Weakness, bone pain, delayed parturition (in females due to pelvic bone deformities)	Weakness, bone pain, fracture(s)
Biochemical findings in serum	↓Calcium, ↓vitamin D, ↓Ca × P product, ↑alkaline phosphatase, ↑PTH	As in vitamin D-responsive rickets	As in vitamin D-responsive rickets; plus features of the specific disease that resulted in chronic renal failure	As in vitamin D-responsive rickets	Normal calcium and vitamin D, normal or ↑alkaline phosphatase, normal PTH, ↓estrogen (postmenopausal)
Treatment	Vitamin D, sunlight	Calcitriol	Calcitriol	Vitamin D, sunlight	Calcium, vitamin D, estrogen replacement (postmenopausal)

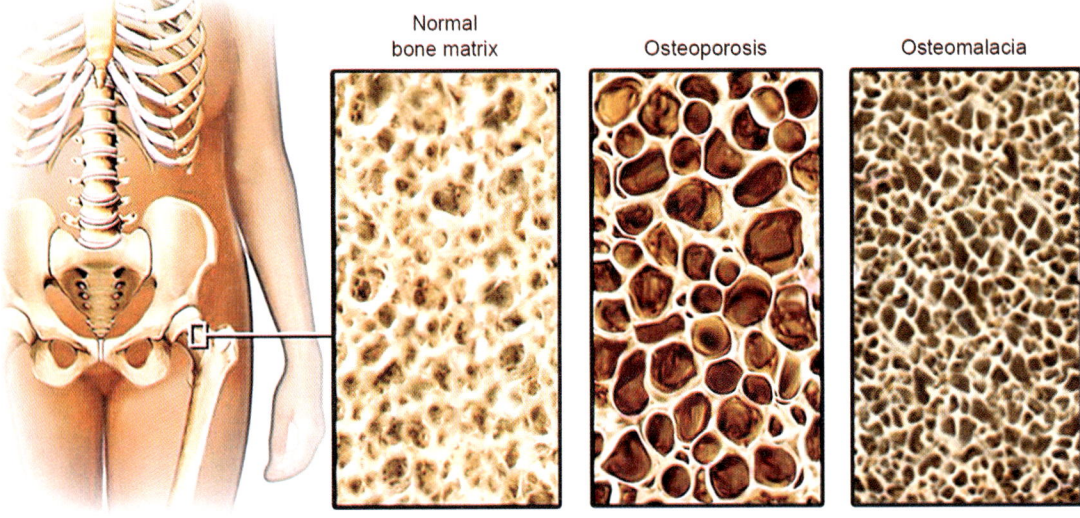

Fig. 28.11: Osteoporosis is characterized by a decrease in bone density (mass per unit volume) and occurs in a fully developed bone. It appears like 'pores' in the bone, hence the name. **Osteomalacia** is a defect in bone mineralization in a developing or developed bone. The osteoid is generally preserved. It is the adult counterpart of rickets.

anorexia, nausea, vomiting and diarrhea, besides bone pain and metastatic calcification of the soft tissues including the kidney, the myocardium, the pancreas and the uterus.

VITAMIN E

Several compounds belonging to the group of **tocopherols**, such as α, β, γ and δ tocopherols have been shown to exhibit vitamin E activity but **α-tocopherol has the highest biological activity** and widest distribution. α-Tocopherol is an alcohol

which has phytol and trimethylhydroquinone in its structure (Fig. 28.12).

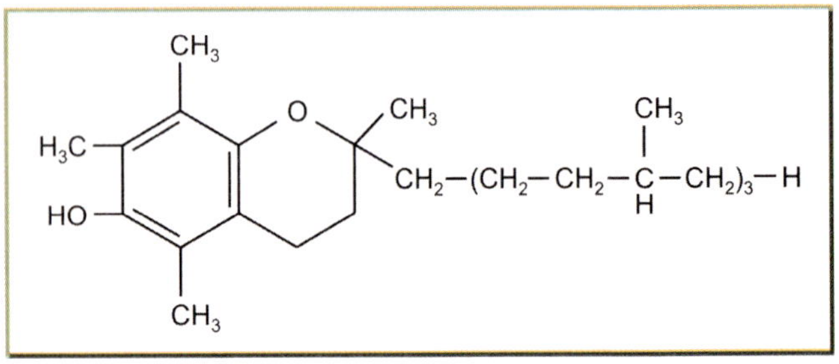

Fig. 28.12: α-Tocopherol (vitamin E).

Commercially, vitamin E is available both as a natural substance as well as a synthetic compound. Natural vitamin E is d-α-tocopherol and is a single stereoisomer. On the other hand, synthetic vitamin E is dl-α-tocopherol which is produced commercially.

Absorption and Metabolism

Vitamin E is readily absorbed from the gastrointestinal tract with the dietary lipids and is transported in lipoproteins to the liver and peripheral tissues. Compared to synthetic vitamin E, natural form is retained better by the body. It is also concentrated in phospholipids. The levels of vitamin E in plasma lipoproteins and phospholipids depend upon the dietary levels of vitamin E, various pro- and anti-oxidants, selenium and sulfur-containing amino acids. High doses of vitamin C may decrease vitamin E absorption.

Biological Functions: Chain-Breaking Antioxidant

- All **unsaturated fatty acids** especially those containing more than two double bonds, are sensitive to the attack by oxygen and form lipid peroxides. The process, designated as peroxidation, is initiated by free radicals (please refer to Chapter 34 for details). Once initiated, **lipid peroxidation process is a chain reaction** and is a potential source of damage to the cell membrane and other components. The products of lipid peroxidation, such as

malondialdehyde can cross-link several biological molecules. Vitamin E is the major lipid soluble antioxidant in cell membrane that breaks the chain of lipid peroxidation (Fig. 28.13).

- It protects readily oxidizable molecules in the cells, such as polyunsaturated fatty acyl components of phospholipids of the cell membrane, and vitamin A esters.

- Through its ability to quench free radicals generated by metabolic processes and environmental pollutants, vitamin E can help protect cells and other components of the body from several diseases, such as cancer, heart diseases and premature aging.

Deficiency Diseases

Unlike other vitamins, deficiency of vitamin E does not produce a specific disease with rapidly progressing symptoms. Instead, the results of vitamin E deficiency usually take years to develop:

1. Low blood levels of vitamin E have been reported in acne, anemia, infections, cancers, periodontal disease, neuromuscular diseases and Alzheimer's disease.

2. Vitamin E deficiency is seen in patients with abetalipoproteinemia. Such individuals are unable to form chylomicrons and VLDL, as a consequence of which vitamin E is neither absorbed nor distributed.

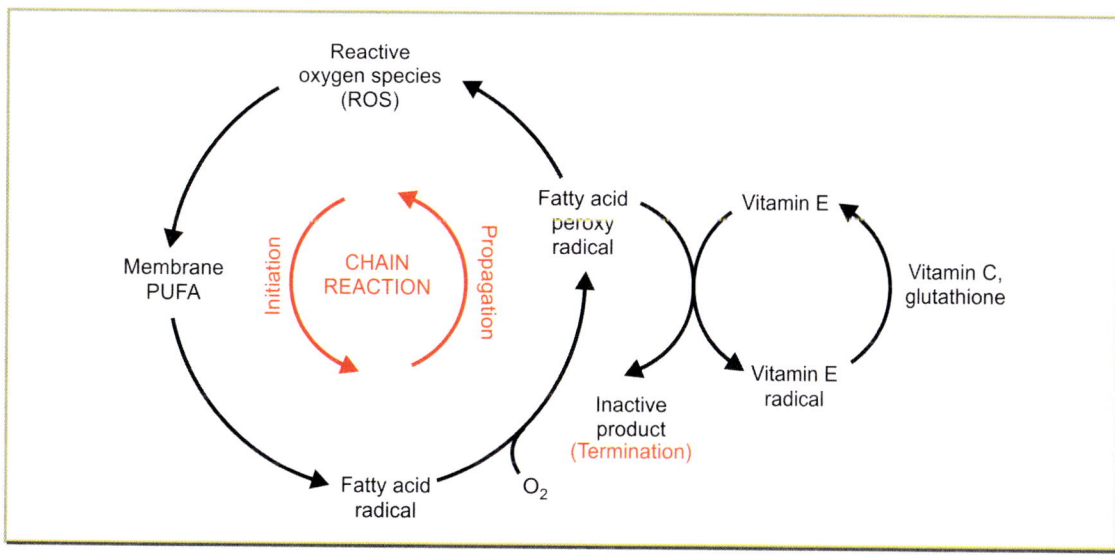

Fig. 28.13: Vitamin E: A chain-breaking antioxidant.

28

3. Deficiency of vitamin E is seen in children with fat malabsorption. In newborn infants, sprue, creatinuria, peptic ulceration, red cell hemolysis, etc, is common. Such children show signs of severe progressive neuropathy and retinopathy.

4. Other deficiency symptoms, observed in various animal species include certain reproductive defects such as sterility, degeneration of the testes, regression in the fetal resorption besides hepatic necrosis, muscular dystrophy and vascular system defects. Axonal degeneration of the large myelinated axons results in posterior column and spinocerebellar symptoms such as ataxia, decreased vibration and position sensation.

Selenium and vitamin E: Some of the symptoms of vitamin E deficiency can be cured by giving high doses of selenium. Selenium (as **selenocysteine**) forms a part of the active center of the enzyme **glutathione peroxidase**. This enzyme protects cellular components against peroxidases and utilizes glutathione, which in turn, gets oxidized.

Clinical use of vitamin E: Contrary to common practice, clinical use of vitamin E should be limited (Chemistry to Clinics 28.4).

Sources and Requirement

Oils such as corn oil, cotton seed oil and sunflower oil are the richest sources of vitamin E.

Tocopherols are present in small quantities in green-leafy vegetables (spinach and lettuce), milk, milk products and egg yolk.

Requirement of vitamin E however, varies from individual to individual, depending on the level and nature of activity, diet, exposure to psychological stress and polluted environment, and on the intake of polyunsaturated fatty acids (PUFA). Normally, 0.4 mg

Chemistry to Clinics 28.4: Prescribing Vitamin E

The common practice of prescribing vitamin E as a general health supplement should be discouraged. Since a clear-cut clinical deficiency of vitamin E is not seen, its use is limited and may show response in:

1. Fibrocystic breast disease (episodes of tightness or pain in the breasts at specific periods of the menstrual cycle).
2. Intermittent claudication (episodes of tingling, numbness and pain in the legs due to ischemia).
3. Patients at high risk of free radical-mediated injury (prescribed along with other antioxidants).

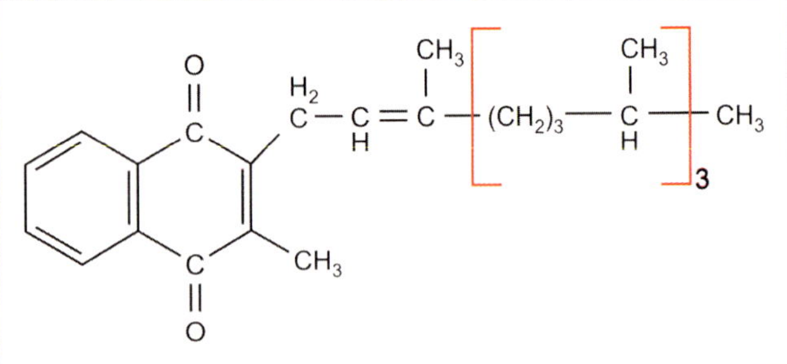

Fig. 28.14: Vitamin K_1 (phylloquinone).

of vitamin E is required per g of PUFA. The RDA of vitamin E in adults is 15 mg.

VITAMIN K

The name vitamin K (**Koagulation** factor) has been derived from the Danish word Koagulation since it has an important role in blood clotting. Various compounds related to 2-methyl-1,4-naphthoquinone have been described to have vitamin K activity.

The most important form which occurs naturally is **vitamin K_1** (phylloquinone). It is found in **plants** and has a phytyl side chain (Fig. 28.14).

Vitamin K_2 (menaquinone or farnequinone) is synthesized by the **intestinal bacteria** and has a farnesyl side chain (the chain with 7 isoprenoid units).

Vitamin K_3 (menadione) is a **synthetic** compound available commercially for therapeutic uses. It is water soluble and gets easily absorbed on parenteral administration.

Absorption

Vitamin K is absorbed with dietary lipids in the presence of bile salts and is utilized in the liver.

Biological Functions

Vitamin K is essential for the maintenance of normal levels of some of the blood clotting factors such as **factor II (prothrombin), factor VII, factor IX and factor X**. These proteins are synthesized in the liver in their **inactive forms** and are converted into their **biologically active forms** in the presence of vitamin K.

Prothrombin is rich in glutamate residues (**Glu**). During post-translational changes, several of the Glu are carboxylated into γ-carboxyglutamate (**Gla**) and

Chemistry to Clinics 28.5: Vitamin K Antagonists

Due to structural similarity to vitamin K, dicumarol and warfarin act as antagonists to vitamin K (Fig. 28.15). They act as competitive inhibitors of the enzymes concerned with the activation of prothrombin and other coagulation factors which require vitamin K as the coenzyme. Warfarin inhibits the conversion of vitamin K epoxide to vitamin K as well as the conversion of preprothrombin precursor to active prothrombin.

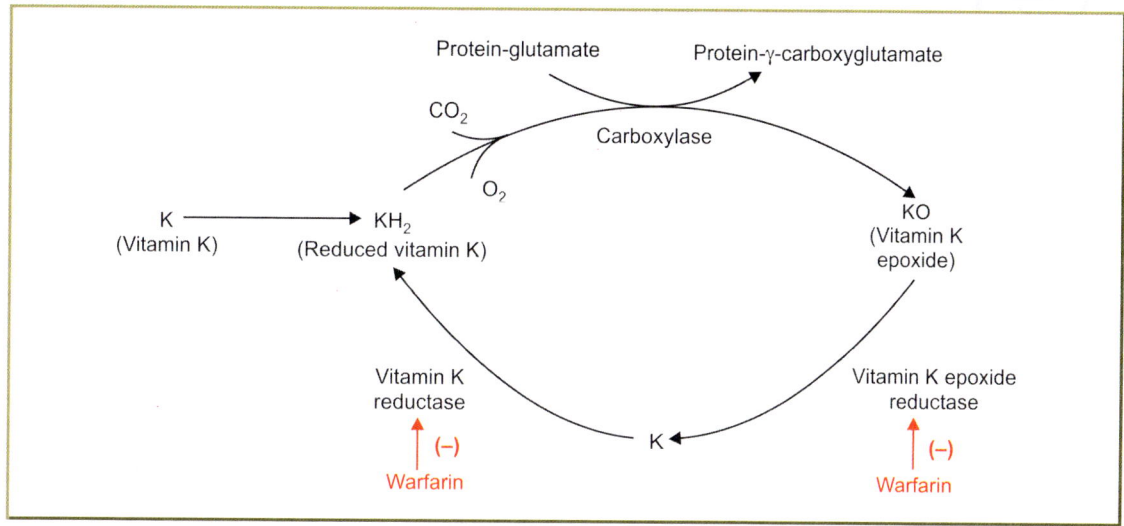

Fig. 28.15: Vitamin K cycle.

form the sites of Ca^{2+} binding on a prothrombin molecule. The reduced form of vitamin K is essential for the introduction of carboxylate groups into Glu and thus converts them into Gla. For this process, O_2 is also necessary. Vitamin K, in turn, gets oxidized to vitamin K epoxide, which is reduced back by epoxide reductase (Fig. 28.15).

Besides prothrombin, clotting factors VII, IX and X also undergo carboxylation of their Glu.

Deficiency Diseases

Deficiency of vitamin K is seen in newborns due to sterile intestine, particularly the premature infants. It is also common in patients with malabsorption (sprue), obstructive jaundice, advanced hepatic damage (liver carcinoma, cirrhosis, etc.), in subjects on prolonged antibiotics or anticoagulant therapy (Chemistry to Clinics 28.5).

Common deficiency symptoms include cutaneous and intramuscular **hemorrhages** with bluish-red coloration in different parts of the body. There is a decrease in the levels of plasma vitamin K. **Prothrombin time is increased**.

Sources and Requirement

Vitamin K is found in abundance in green-leafy vegetables such as spinach, lettuce and cabbage. Besides, fish, liver and skeletal muscle are also good sources of vitamin K.

The RDA is 20 to 100 µg. However, it is advised to administer a **single prophylactic dose of 1 mg of vitamin K_3 to the newborn on the first day of life**.

Table 28.2 lists various lipid-soluble vitamins, their functions and RDA.

2. WATER SOLUBLE VITAMINS

Water soluble vitamins include vitamin B complex and vitamin C. Their general properties include:

• Dietary water soluble vitamins are absorbed rapidly from the gastrointestinal lumen, **irrespective of the presence of lipids**.

• Most of them are converted into **coenzymes** for various metabolic reactions.

• Vitamin status of the body can be **assessed** by measuring one or more **enzyme activities** in the **isolated red blood cells**.

Table 28.2: Lipid-soluble vitamins, their biological functions and RDA

Vitamin	Provitamin	Biological functions	Deficiency disorders	Sources	RDA
A (Retinol)	Carotenoids (Carotenes)	In vision, epithelial integrity	Night blindness, disorders of epithelium and mucus membrane	Animal, fish and vegetable oils	2000–2500 IU
D (Calciferol)	7-Dehydro-cholesterol	Calcium/phosphate homoeostasis	Rickets, osteomalacia	Fish oil, UV rays	200 IU
E (Tocopherol)	–	As antioxidant	Hemolytic anemia in infants	Plant oils	15 mg
K	–	In blood coagulation	Bleeding disorder	Plant oils, intestinal bacteria	20–100 µg

- Due to their water solubility, they **cannot be stored** to any significant extent.
- Because they cannot be stored, a dietary **deficiency quickly becomes manifest**. Typical deficiency symptoms for most of the water soluble vitamins, particularly those of vitamin B complex, include dermatitis, glossitis, cheilosis and diarrhea besides some of the neurological symptoms, such as peripheral neuropathy and malaise.
- Large doses are excreted in the urine and **rarely result in toxicity**.

VITAMIN B COMPLEX

Vitamins of the B complex group include a group of compounds, most of which can also be synthesized in the gastrointestinal tract by the microbial flora. Most of the components of vitamin B complex group are **heat stable, except vitamin B_1 which is heat labile**.

THIAMIN (ANTIBERIBERI FACTOR, ANEURINE)

Thiamin is the first member of the vitamin B complex and therefore is known as **vitamin B_1**. Due to its role in the prevention of beriberi, it is also called **antiberiberi factor**. Since the vitamin has an important role in the nervous system, it is also called **aneurine**. Structurally, a thiamin molecule consists of a pyrimidine ring, which in turn, is linked to a thiazole ring (Fig. 28.16). Thiamin occurs as thiamin hydrochloride. Though thiamin is heat labile, it is quite stable in the acidic medium. Tea, coffee, raw-fish and shellfish contain **thiaminase** which can destroy the vitamin.

Coenzyme Form

Thiamin in its diphosphorylated form, i.e. as thiamin pyrophosphate (**TPP**) acts as a coenzyme. It is

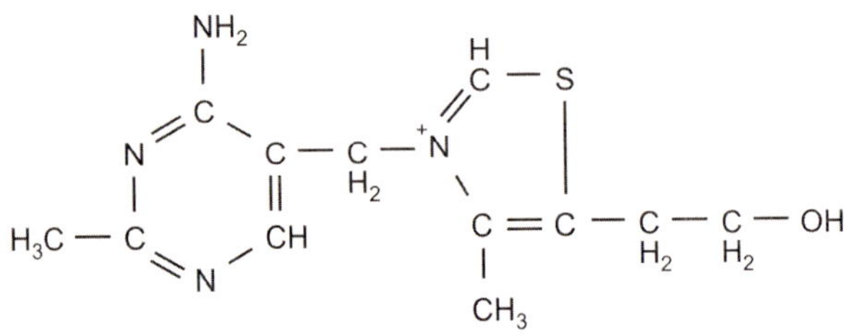

Fig. 28.16: Thiamin (vitamin B_1)

important in carbohydrate metabolism. The reactions where TPP is used as a coenzyme include:

1. **Oxidative decarboxylation** of α-ketoacids, e.g. of pyruvate to acetyl CoA by pyruvate dehydrogenase complex, and α-ketoglutarate to succinyl CoA by α-ketoglutarate dehydrogenase complex, in the citric acid cycle.
2. TPP is also a coenzyme for **transketolase** in the hexose monophosphate shunt. RBC transketolase activity is measured to assess thiamin status of the body.

Deficiency Disorder

Thiamin deficiency results in beriberi (Chemistry to Clinics 28.6).

Sources and Requirement

Thiamin though is widely distributed, its rich sources are cereal grains, yeast, liver, kidney and heart. The RDA depends upon carbohydrate intake of the individual and has been defined as 0.4–0.5 mg/1000 kcal. Its requirement is increased in fever, hyperthyroidism, alcoholics and pregnant woman.

Deficiency of thiamin commonly occurs in:

1. Areas where people consume polished-rice; it results in loss of available thiamin. The loss can be decreased by using unpolished or parboiled rice or whole wheat flour.
2. Consumption of raw fish in large quantities
3. Chronic alcoholics.

Deficiency of thiamin causes beriberi. Signs and symptoms, however, vary according to duration and severity of the disease as well as the predominant organs involved. It is classified into:

1. **Wet beriberi:** It affects the cardiovascular system, and results in edema and dilated heart.
2. **Dry beriberi:** It affects the nervous system and causes peripheral neuropathy with myelin degeneration, leading to foot-drop, wrist-drop and sensory changes.
3. **Wernicke's encephalopathy:** Alcoholic patients with chronic thiamin deficiency may also have CNS manifestations, ophthalmoplegia, cerebeller ataxia and mental impairment.

RBC transketolase activity is reduced in beriberi. Blood pyruvic acid concentration is raised.

RIBOFLAVIN (LACTOFLAVIN)

Riboflavin (**vitamin B$_2$**) is also called as lactoflavin due to its high content in milk. The vitamin is sensitive to light and ultraviolet irradiation but is stable in acidic and neutral medium. The structure contains an isoalloxazine ring with a ribitol side chain (Fig. 28.17).

Coenzyme Forms

Riboflavin with phosphoric acid forms flavin mononucleotide (FMN) which is a coenzyme form of the vitamin. The other coenzyme form of riboflavin is flavin adenine dinucleotide (FAD). It is a dinucleotide of FMN and AMP (Fig. 28.18).

Biochemical Role

The two coenzymes form an integral part of the flavoprotein containing enzymes and are important in oxidation-reduction reactions, requiring **oxido-**

reductases. The isoalloxazine ring serves as an acceptor of the two hydrogens, and in turn, gets reduced (Fig. 28.19).

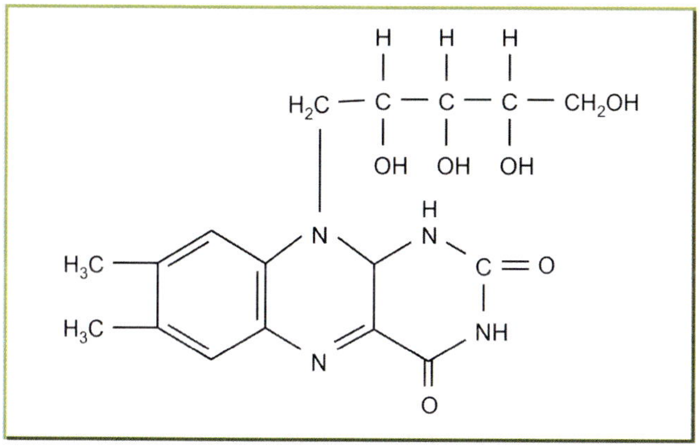

FMN is an important coenzyme of cytochrome c reductase and L-amino acid oxidases. FAD is a coenzyme of succinate dehydrogenase, glycerol-3-phosphate dehydrogenase, xanthine oxidase, glycine oxidase, sphingosine reductase and D-amino acid oxidases. It is an integral part of acyl CoA dehydro-genase. It is thus important in the metabolism of carbohydrates, lipids as well as proteins.

Deficiency Disorders

It is uncommon but may be associated with niacin or iron deficiency. Symptoms include cheilosis (lesions

Fig. 28.17: Riboflavin (vitamin B$_2$).

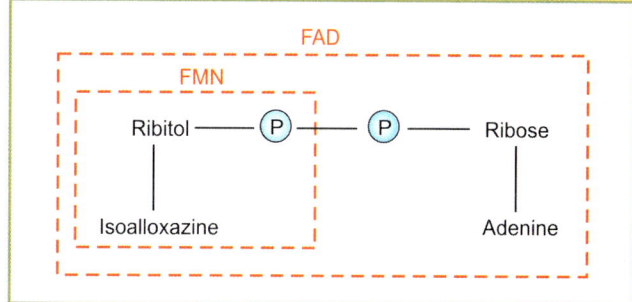

Fig. 28.18: Vitamin B$_2$ coenzymes.

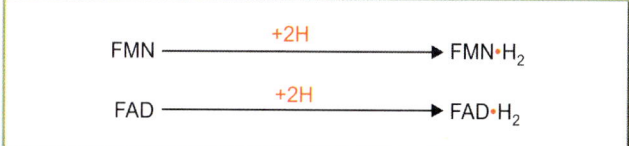

Fig. 28.19: Reduction of vitamin B$_2$ coenzymes.

28

of the angles of the mouth), glossitis, dermatitis, photophobia and lacrimation.

Sources and Requirement

It is though widely distributed in nature, milk, liver and kidneys are rich sources of riboflavin. The RDA is 0.5–0.6 mg/1000 kcal.

NIACIN (ANTI-PELLAGRA FACTOR)

Niacin (B_3) is also known as **pellagra preventive factor** or anti-pellagra factor because of its role in the prevention of pellagra. Niacin is a generic name given to two compounds having pyridine ring with a carboxyl group-**nicotinic acid** (Chemistry to Clinics 28.7) and its amide called **nicotinamide** (Fig. 28.20).

Besides its absorption by the intestine, niacin is also synthesized in the body from an essential amino acid **tryptophan**.

Coenzyme Forms

Niacin is an important constituent of two coenzymes, i.e. nicotinamide adenine dinucleotide (NAD^+) and its

phosphorylated form called nicotinamide adenine dinucleotide phosphate ($NADP^+$). Both the coenzymes contain two nucleotides (each of pyridine and adenine), which are linked together. In both the forms, i.e. NAD^+ as well as $NADP^+$, since the nitrogen atom of the pyridine ring is in the oxidized state, they have a positive charge. These coenzymes are important in **oxidation-reduction reactions** and are used with dehydrogenases where they act as electron acceptors (Fig. 28.21).

Biochemical Role

NAD^+ is used as a coenzyme with malate dehydrogenase (in the conversion of malate to oxaloacetate) and lactate dehydrogenase (LDH) which converts lactate to pyruvate. $NADP^+$ is used as a coenzyme with isocitrate dehydrogenase and glucose-6-phosphate dehydrogenase. Glutamate dehydrogenase, however, can use both, i.e. either NAD^+ or $NADP^+$ (Fig. 28.22).

Deficiency Disorder

Niacin deficiency results in pellagra (Chemistry to Clinics 28.8).

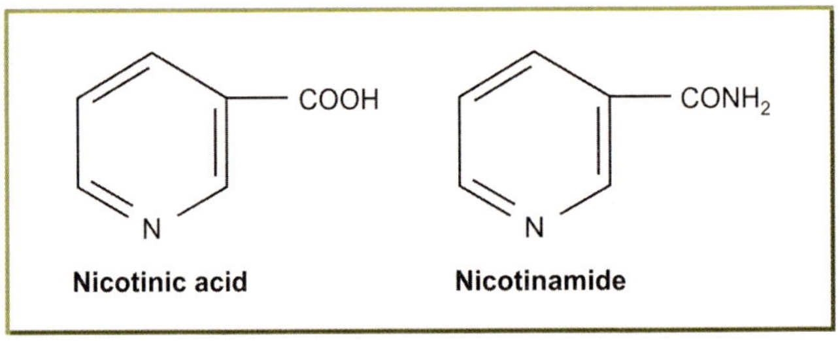

Chemistry to Clinics 28.7: Niacin Flush

Nicotinic acid, derived from the vitamin niacin, is clinically used as a hypolipidemic agent to reduce high blood cholesterol levels. Large amounts of nicotinic acid dilate the capillaries so that the patient may complain of tingling sensations that could be painful. This is known as 'niacin flush'. Interestingly, another niacin derivative called nicotinamide, neither exhibits niacin flush nor it reduces blood cholesterol.

Fig. 28.20: Niacin vitamins.

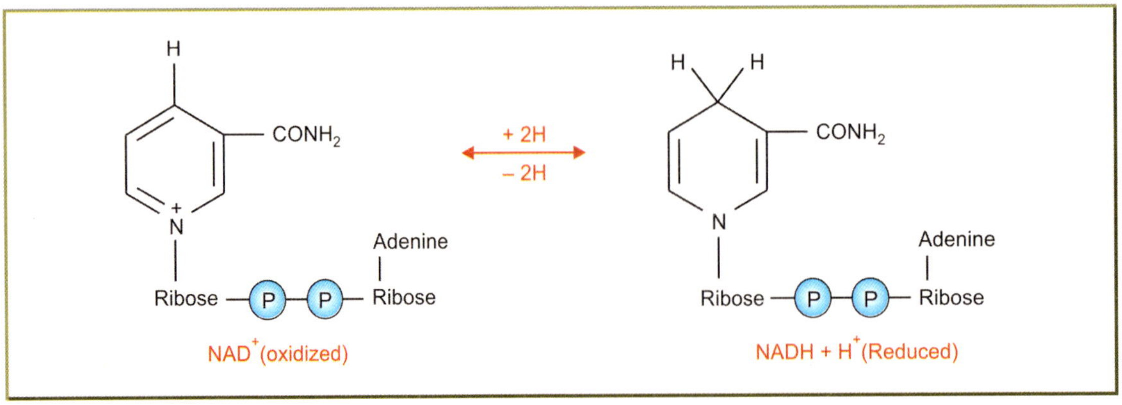

Fig. 28.21: Role of niacin in an oxidation-reduction reaction.

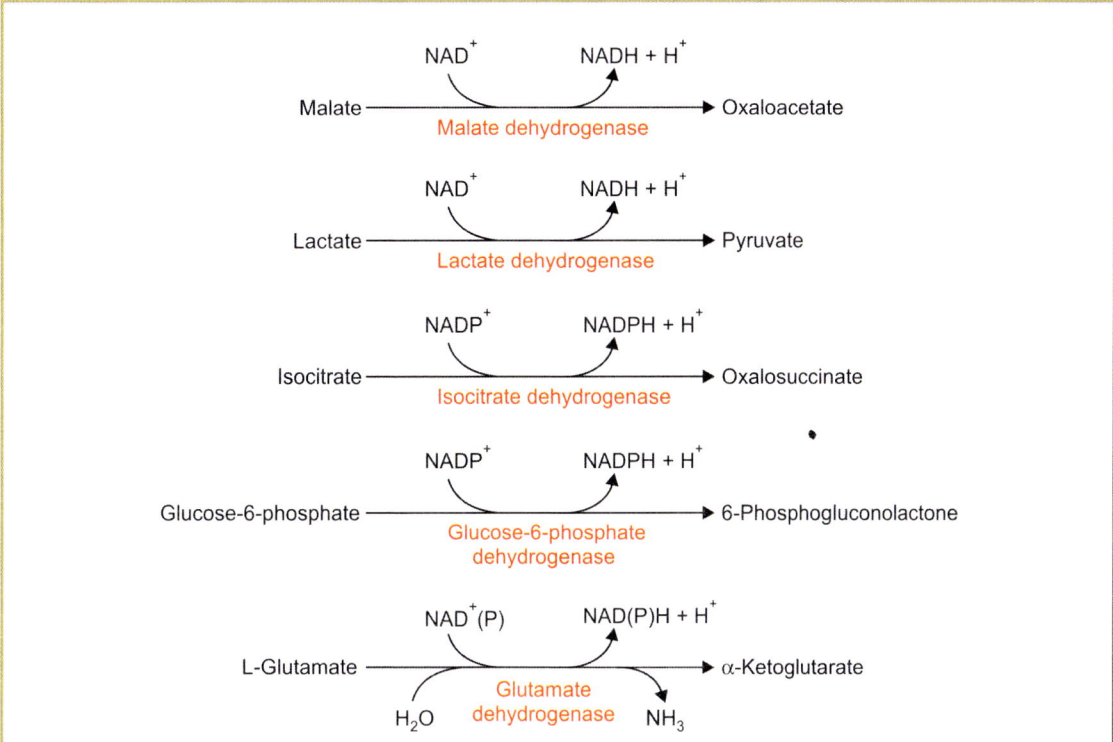

Fig. 28.22: Some examples of reactions requiring niacin coenzymes.

Chemistry to Clinics 28.8: Pellagra

Deficiency of niacin is not usually observed since it can be synthesized in the body from tryptophan (an essential amino acid). Its deficiency, however, may occur in:

1. People whose staple food is maize or sorghum (jowar). These cereals are rich in leucine but are deficient in tryptophan; the amino–acid imbalance affects tryptophan-niacin pathway, and in turn, reduces the biosynthesis of niacin (normally 60 mg tryptophan forms 1 mg niacin). Leucine itself also inhibits endogenous biosynthesis of niacin.

2. Patients taking isonicotinic acid hydrazide (INH), an antitubercular drug (along with the deficiency of vitamin B$_6$).

3. Patients with Hartnup's disease which is due to a defect in tryptophan absorption.

Deficiency of niacin leads to pellagra, a disease characterized by 3Ds, i.e. **d**ermatitis, **d**iarrhea and **d**ementia:

1. **D**ermatitis: It results in pain in those parts of the body which are exposed to sunlight, such as face, neck, hands and feet. These parts become bronze-colored resembling sunburn and later become thickened (Fig. 28.23).

2. **D**iarrhea: It is accompanied with anorexia and other abdominal discomforts.

3. **D**ementia: It is due to impaired ability of the brain to utilize carbohydrates. Symptoms like depression, confusion and psychosis are commonly observed which are due to decreased synthesis of tryptophan-derived neurotransmitters.

Prolonged deficiency of niacin may ultimately result in **d**eath, the fourth 'D' of pellagra.

Sources and Requirement

Rice polish, yeast, liver, poultry and green vegetables are good sources of niacin. Milk and milk products though are not common sources of niacin but are important pellagra preventive factors due to their high content of tryptophan. Daily requirement of niacin is related to the intake of tryptophan. The RDA is 5.5–6.5 mg/1000 kcal.

Niacin can be synthesized by human beings from tryptophan provided other B complex vitamins are adequate in the diet. Biosynthesis of niacin requires

28

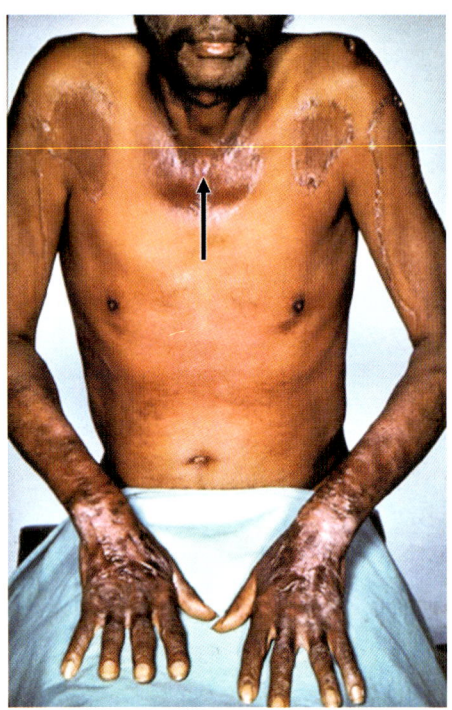

Fig. 28.23: Pellagra with characteristic dermatologic features: Desquamation, erythema, scaling and keratosis of sun-exposed parts. The skin lesion may surround the neck, the so-called Casal's necklace (arrow).

pyridoxal phosphate. **Sixty mg of tryptophan can form one mg of niacin.**

PYRIDOXINE

Pyridoxine is also called **vitamin B₆.** It is a group of 3 compounds—**pyridoxine, pyridoxal and pyridoxamine,** which contain a pyridine ring (Fig. 28.24).

Coenzyme Form

The vitamin is transported in the blood in its coenzyme form, i.e. pyridoxal-5-phosphate or **PLP** (Fig. 28.25).

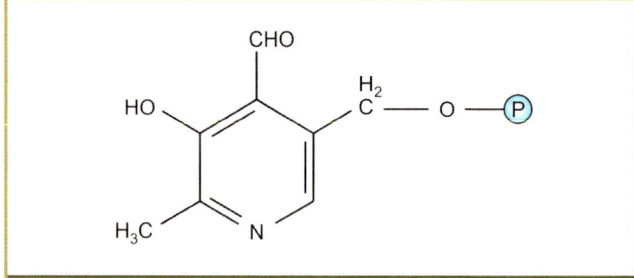

Fig. 28.25: Pyridoxal-5-phosphate (PLP).

Biochemical Role

1. **Transamination:** With transaminases, PLP acts as an acceptor of the amino group from an amino acid thereby forming the corresponding α-keto acid and pyridoxamine phosphate. Followed by reversal of the process, pyridoxamine releases amino group to the other α-keto acid, for the formation of the corresponding amino acid (Fig. 28.26).

   During this process, PLP forms a Schiff's base with α-amino acid through a bond between aldehyde group of PLP and α-amino group of the amino acid.

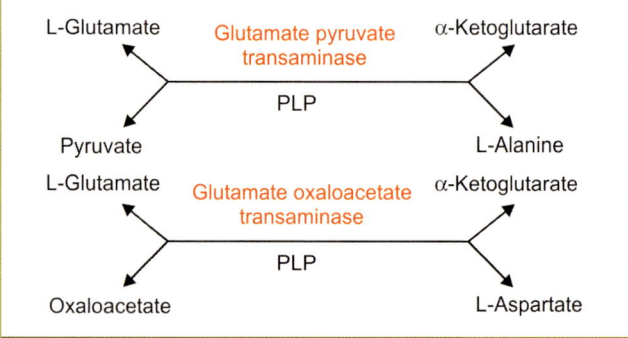

Fig. 28.26: Role of PLP in transamination reactions.

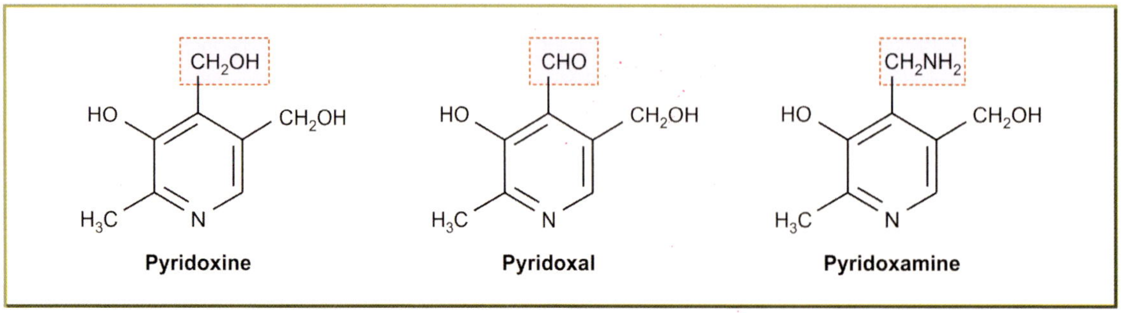

Fig. 28.24: Vitamin B₆.

Pyridoxal phosphate is used as a coenzyme for glutamate pyruvate transaminase (GPT) also called alanine aminotransferase (ALT), glutamate oxaloacetate transaminase (GOT) also called aspartate aminotransferase (AST), tyrosine transaminase, etc.

2. **Dehydratases and desulfhydrases:** These enzymes require PLP for the metabolism of hydroxyamino acids and sulfur-containing amino acids.

3. **Decarboxylation:** Pyridoxal phosphate is a coenzyme for decarboxylases. The PLP thus regulates neuronal activity since it is important in the synthesis of many biogenic amines that are neurotransmitters (Table 28.3).

4. **Niacin synthesis:** Pyridoxal phosphate, as a coenzyme is required for kynureninase in the conversion of tryptophan to niacin. In pyridoxine deficiency, instead of niacin, tryptophan is converted to xanthurenic acid which is excreted in the urine. Deficiency of pyridoxine thus can be **diagnosed by measuring urinary excretion of xanthurenic acid**, following a test dose of tryptophan.

5. **Heme synthesis:** Pyridoxal phosphate is required as a coenzyme in the synthesis of heme, i.e. for the formation of δ-aminolevulinic acid from glycine and succinyl CoA, by δ-aminolevulinic acid synthase. It is also important for the incorporation of iron into hemoglobin. Hence, PLP is an accessory hemopoietic vitamin.

6. **Glycogen metabolism:** Pyridoxal phosphate is essential in glycogen metabolism in muscle and liver since it acts as a coenzyme for phosphorylase.

7. **Fatty acid chain elongation:** Vitamin B_6 is essential in chain elongation of unsaturated fatty acids, e.g. in the conversion of linoleic acid to arachidonic acid.

8. **Amino acid absorption:** Vitamin B_6 is required for the absorption of dietary amino acids.

Deficiency Disorders

Deficiency symptoms include cheilosis, glossitis and hypochromic anemia. In infants, deficiency of B_6 affects central nervous system and results in convulsions, demyelination of the peripheral nerves and degeneration of axons. Practically, however, the important causes include:

1. **Tuberculosis:** Deficiency of vitamin B_6 may occur in patients with tuberculosis who are taking the antitubercular drug isonicotinic acid hydrazide (isoniazid or **INH**) which acts as an antagonist to vitamin B_6 (Fig. 28.27).

2. **Oral contraceptive pills (OCP):** In the past, the use of OCP with high estrogen content led to a vitamin B_6 deficiency state. This is because estrogen stimulates tryptophan catabolism, that in turn, requires vitamin B_6. Currently, OCP are formulated with low to moderate estrogen content.

Clinical uses of pyridoxine: Several clinical situations mandate the use of pyridoxine (Chemistry to Clinics 28.9).

Sources and Requirement

Rich sources are egg, fish, green-leafy vegetables and cereals. Besides, it is also produced by microflora of the intestinal tract. Since vitamin B_6 is important in the metabolism of several amino acids, its requirement

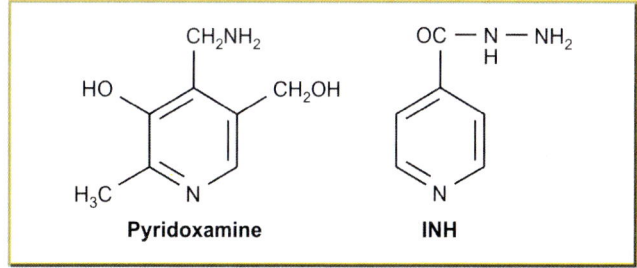

Fig. 28.27: Pyridoxamine and its antagonist INH (an antitubercular drug).

Table 28.3: Neurotransmitters (biogenic amines) synthesized by vitamin B_6-dependent decarboxylation reactions

Substrate	Enzyme	Product (neurotransmitter)
Glutamic acid	Glutamate decarboxylase	γ-Aminobutyric acid (GABA)
DOPA	DOPA decarboxylase	Dopamine
5-Hydroxytryptophan	5-Hydroxytryptophan decarboxylase	5-Hydroxytryptamine (serotonin)
Histidine	Histidine decarboxylase	Histamine
Tyrosine	Tyrosine decarboxylase	Tyramine
Kynurenic acid	Kynurenic acid decarboxylase	Kynuramine

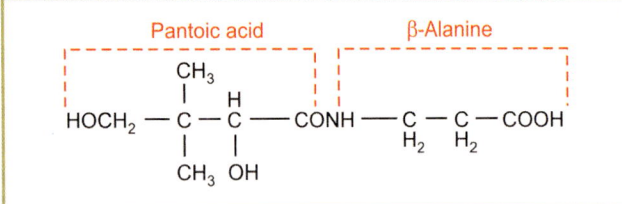

Fig. 28.28: Pantothenic acid.

depends upon dietary intake of protein. The RDA is 1–2 mg.

PANTOTHENIC ACID

Pantothenic acid contains a molecule of pantoic acid and β-alanine (Fig. 28.28). It is heat stable in acidic medium.

Coenzyme Form

Pantothenic acid is an important constituent of **coenzyme A** (Fig. 28.29). Besides pantothenic acid, coenzyme A contains a nitrogenous base adenine in the form of its nucleotide (AMP). Formation of coenzyme A therefore requires ATP. Coenzyme A also has a sulfhydryl group (–SH) which is contributed by β-mercaptoethanolamine (thioethanolamine). Due to the presence of –SH group, coenzyme A is also written as **HS-CoA** or simply as **CoA**.

Biochemical Role

1. The most important function of CoA is that it acts as a carrier for acetate by forming **acetyl CoA (active acetate)**.

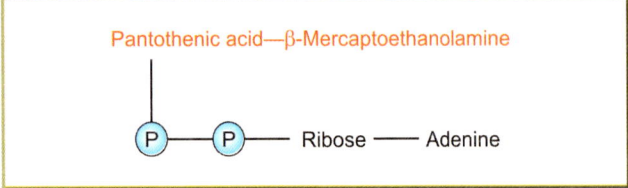

Fig. 28.29: Coenzyme A.

- Active acetate is used in the synthesis of citrate and enters Krebs cycle.
- Active acetate is also used in the synthesis of acetylcholine, a neurotransmitter.
- Acetyl CoA is also a precursor of cholesterol and steroid hormones in the adrenal cortex.

2. Pantothenic acid, as 4-phosphopantothenic acid, forms a prosthetic group of the acyl carrier protein and thus participates in fatty acid synthesis.
3. Activation of fatty acids to form fatty acyl CoA and for their subsequent oxidation to give 2-carbon fragments (acetyl CoA).
4. Oxidative decarboxylation of pyruvate which is converted to acetyl CoA and enters Krebs cycle.
5. Metabolism of branched chain amino acids (valine, leucine and isoleucine) and forms CoA derivatives of their α-keto acids.
6. Activation of succinic acid, and therefore, is also used in the biosynthesis of heme. Hence, pantothenic acid is an accessory hemopoietic vitamin.

Deficiency Disorders

Pantothenic acid deficiency in human beings affects both, the nervous system as well as the digestive system. Its deficiency has also been shown to result in adrenal insufficiency. Deficiency symptoms include headache, fatigue, impaired motor activity, muscle cramps and gastrointestinal disturbances.

It has been used with limited success in the treatment of **burning feet syndrome** and in the healing of ulcers and bed sores.

Sources and Requirement

Pantothenic acid occurs in all animals and plant tissues. Rich sources are yeast, liver, egg, potato, whole cereals and legumes. The RDA is 5–10 mg.

BIOTIN (ANTI-EGG WHITE INJURY FACTOR)

Biotin is also called anti-egg white injury factor since it protects animals against the toxicity of raw-egg white. Raw-egg white contains a protein **avidin** which acts as an antagonist to biotin and forms avidin-biotin complex. On cooking the egg white, avidin gets inactivated and cannot bind biotin.

Structurally, biotin is a cyclic derivative of urea with a thiophene ring (Fig. 28.30).

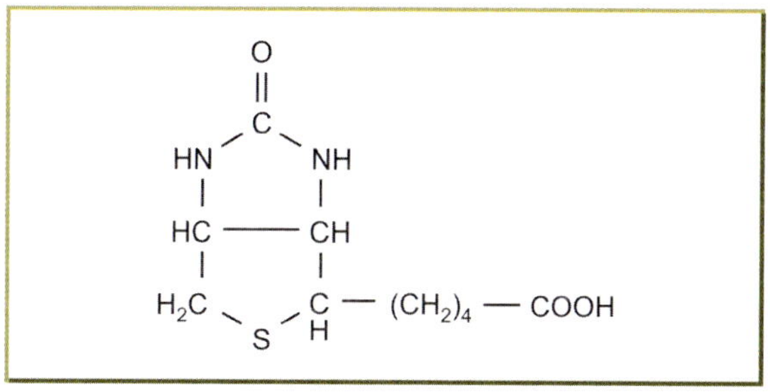

28

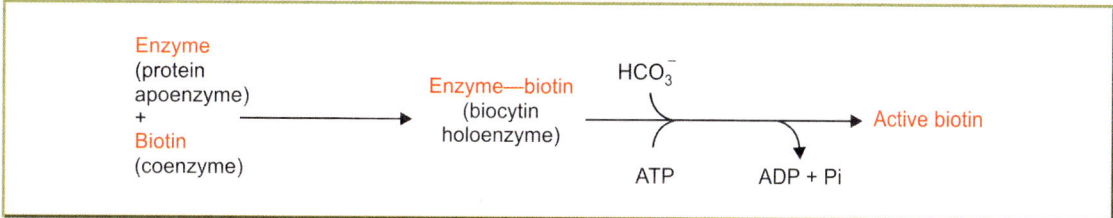

Fig. 28.30: Biotin.

Coenzyme Form

Biotin coenzyme, as a prosthetic group, binds by an amide linkage to the ε-amino group of the lysyl residue of the apoenzyme and forms biotin-enzyme complex (holoenzyme), called **biocytin**. Biocytin accepts carboxylate group from bicarbonate and forms **carboxy biocytin-enzyme complex**, called **active biotin** (Fig. 28.31).

Biochemical Role

Biotin (as active biotin) is required as a coenzyme by **carboxylases** and is important in several reactions involving CO_2 fixation, such as:
- In the carboxylation of pyruvate to form oxalo-acetate with the enzyme pyruvate carboxylase.
- For the conversion of propionic acid (propionyl CoA) to succinic acid via methylmalonyl CoA with the enzyme propionyl CoA carboxylase.
- In the conversion of acetyl CoA to malonyl CoA (required in the formation of long-chain fatty acids) with the enzyme acetyl CoA carboxylase.
- In transcarboxylation reaction, i.e. in the catabolism of branched chain amino acids.

Deficiency Disorders

Biotin deficiency is not generally seen as it can be synthesized by the intestinal flora. Consumption of raw-egg white, however, can produce neurological abnormalities by inhibiting the absorption of biotin. Deficiency may cause mild dermatitis, nausea, loss of appetite, muscular pain and anemia.

Sources and Requirement

Rice polish, whole cereals, milk, yeast and meat (liver, kidney) are good sources of biotin. The RDA is 150–300 μg.

CHOLINE

Choline is trimethylethanolamine (Fig. 28.32).

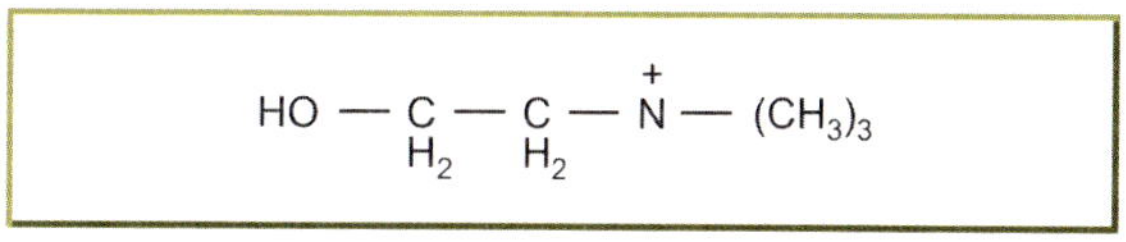

$$HO - \underset{H_2}{C} - \underset{H_2}{C} - \overset{+}{N} - (CH_3)_3$$

Fig. 28.32: Choline.

Biochemical Role

Choline has several important biochemical functions in the body:
- It is converted to betaine which is used as a methyl group donor for several transmethylation reactions.
- Choline is acetylated and is converted to acetyl-choline, a neurotransmitter.
- It has lipotropic activity and thus prevents fatty liver (accumulation of abnormal quantities of fat in the liver).

Deficiency Disorders

Choline deficiency is not generally observed since it is widely distributed in nature, as a constituent of phospholipids. Moreover, it can also be synthesized in the liver if adequate amounts of methyl donors, such as betaine and methionine are present. Deficiency may be associated with fatty liver and hemorrhagic necrosis of kidneys.

Choline as a drug: As choline salicylate, it is a part of topical preparations for the treatment of **aphthous ulcers** (small, painful mouth sores).

Enzyme (protein apoenzyme) + Biotin (coenzyme) → Enzyme—biotin (biocytin holoenzyme) → HCO_3^- ATP → ADP + Pi → Active biotin

Fig. 28.31: Activation of biotin.

28

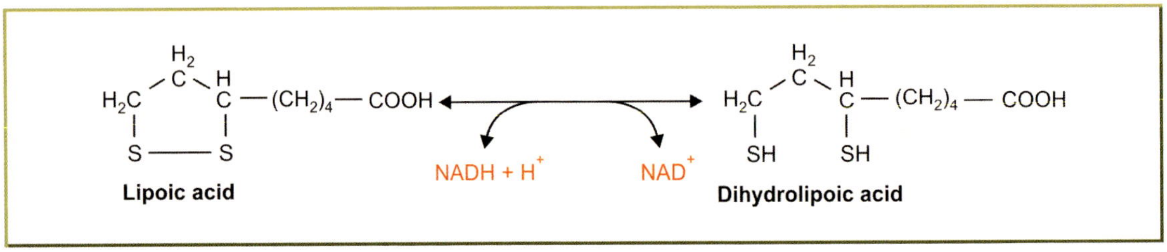

Fig. 28.33: Lipoic acid.

Sources and Requirement

Egg yolk, several animal tissues, cereals and vegetables are good sources. The RDA is 0.3–1.0 g.

LIPOIC ACID

Chemically, lipoic acid is a **sulfur**-containing fatty acid and is also called **thioctic acid** (Fig. 28.33).

Biochemical Role

Lipoic acid mediates the transfer of electrons and activated acyl group which is released after decarboxylation and oxidation of α-keto acids, within the multienzyme complex. Lipoic acid, in turn, undergoes reversible oxidation and reduction. It is reduced to **dihydrolipoic acid** which acts as an acceptor of the activated acyl group.

Lipoic acid is used as a coenzyme with several other coenzymes, such as TPP, NAD^+, FAD, and CoA, in the oxidative decarboxylation of α-keto acids, e.g. in the conversion of pyruvate to acetyl CoA by pyruvate dehydrogenase complex or in the conversion of α-ketoglutarate to succinyl CoA by α-ketoglutarate dehydrogenase complex, in the citric acid cycle.

Sources and Requirement

Since lipoic acid is widely distributed in all natural foods, deficiency symptoms as well as requirements have not been well established.

FOLIC ACID

Folic acid and related compounds with folic acid activity are given the generic name **folacin**, a word derived from 'folium' meaning leaf. Folic acid is also called **pteroylglutamic acid**. It contains a pteridine nucleus, a molecule of p-aminobenzoic acid (PABA) and 1, 3 or 7 glutamate molecules (Fig. 28.34).

Coenzyme Form

Folic acid (folate) is reduced to its coenzyme form called **tetrahydrofolic acid (FH_4)**. Firstly, folate is reduced by folate reductase to dihydrofolate (FH_2) and subsequently by dihydrofolate reductase to the active coenzyme, i.e. FH_4 (Fig. 28.35). The reactions are NADPH dependent.

Biochemical Role: One Carbon Metabolism

Tetrahydrofolate (FH_4) serves both as acceptor as well as donor of one carbon (1C) unit, in a variety of

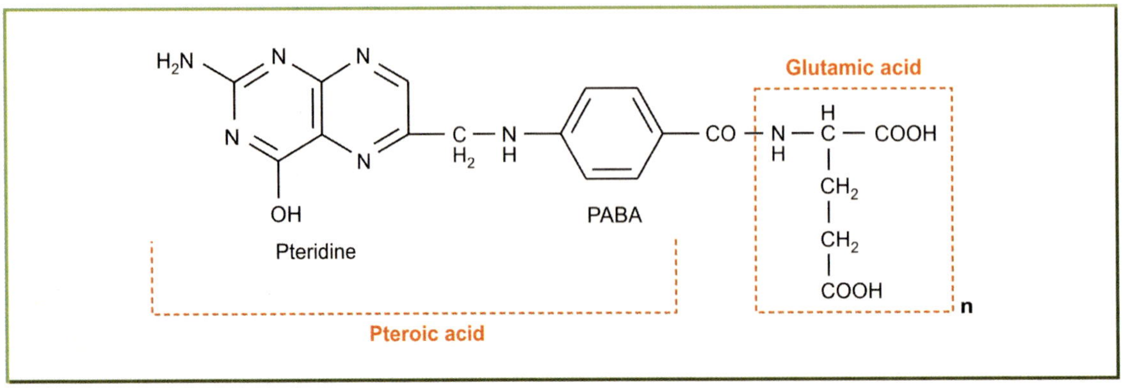

Fig. 28.34: Folic acid (pteroyl glutamic acid).

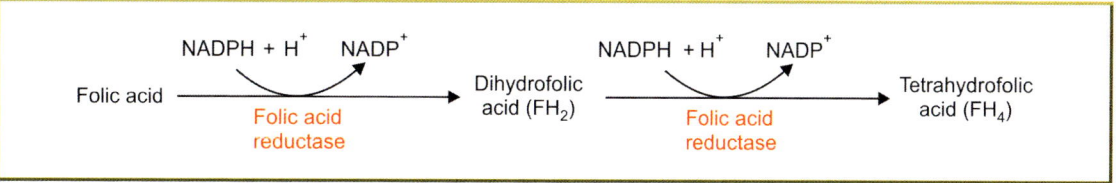

Fig. 28.35: Formation of active folate (FH$_4$).

reactions involved in amino acid and nucleotide metabolism:

1. Folic acid is converted to N^5-formyltetrahydrofolic acid (N^5-CHO·FH$_4$) or folinic acid in the liver and is thus used in the transfer of one carbon group (one carbon moiety) from a donor to the acceptor molecule (Fig. 28.36).

Besides formyl (–CHO), 1C moiety may participate in the form of formate (–HCOO$^-$), methenyl (=CH–), methylene (–CH$_2$–), methyl (–CH$_3$), hydroxymethyl (–CH$_2$OH) or formimino (–CH=NH) groups. The various forms are inter-convertible to one another by NADP$^+$ or NAD$^+$ dependent dehydrogenases.

The sources of one carbon moiety may be histidine (formimino group), β-carbon of serine (hydroxymethyl group) or choline, thymine and methionine (methyl group).

2. One carbon moiety carried by FH$_4$ may be utilized in many reactions, such as it acts as a donor of carbon atom 2 and 8 in the biosynthesis of a purine ring, in the conversion of glycine to serine, uracil

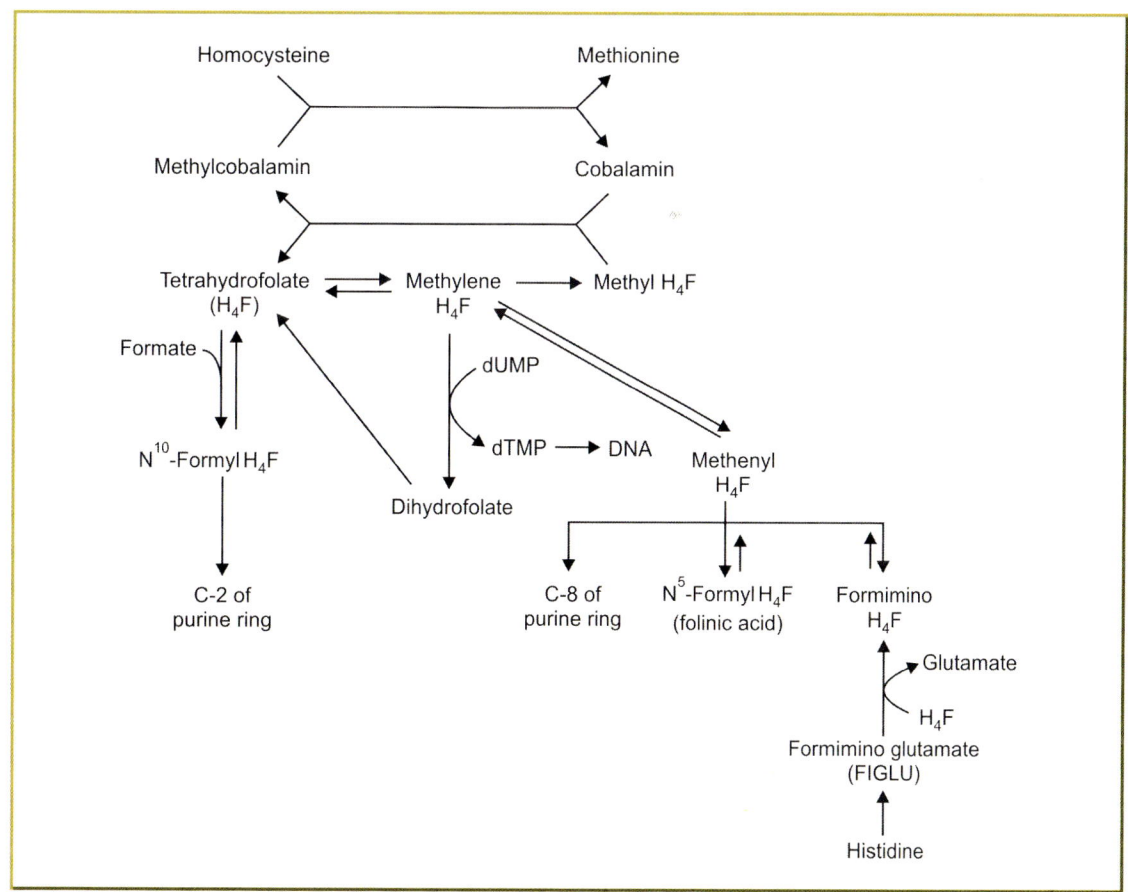

Fig. 28.36: Interrelationships between cobalamin, folate and 1 'C' metabolism.

28

to thymine, homocysteine to methionine, and in the biosynthesis of choline.

In some of these reactions, vitamin B_{12} (cobalamin) is also required.

Deficiency Disorders

Folic acid deficiency is not generally observed as it can be synthesized by the intestinal flora. Deficiency may occur in stressful conditions, during pregnancy, intestinal malabsorption (such as steatorrhea or due to antibiotic therapy) and may result in:

Macrocytic (megaloblastic) anemia: It may be accompanied by leucopenia. It is based on the 'methyl folate trap hypothesis' (discussed later under 'HEMOPOIETIC VITAMINS').

Neural tube defects: Folic acid deficiency in early pregnancy has been implicated in neural tube defects. Folate deficiency impairs nucleotide biosynthesis, hence, it reduces the efficiency of both DNA as well as RNA synthesis and thus affects growth. Folic acid supplementation is therefore routinely done in pregnant women.

Deficiency of folic acid can be **diagnosed by measuring urinary excretion of formiminoglutamic acid (FIGLU)** (Chemistry to Clinics 28.10). Interestingly, folate antagonists are useful anticancer drugs (Chemistry to Clinics 28.11).

Sources and Requirement

Folic acid is present in green-leafy vegetables such as spinach and cabbage, besides yeast, liver and kidney. The RDA is 150–300 μg.

Chemistry to Clinics 28.10: FIGLU Test

Histidine is catabolized in the liver and releases formiminoglutamic acid (FIGLU), which in the presence of FH_4, forms N_5-formimino-tetrahydrofolic acid and glutamic acid (Fig. 28.36). In folic acid deficiency, FIGLU is excreted in large quantity in the urine following a test dose of histidine.

Chemistry to Clinics 28.11: Folic Acid Antagonists

Certain compounds interfere with the metabolic functions of folic acid and are called folic acid antagonists. Most potent of these are aminopterin and amethopterin. These are the competitive inhibitors of dihydrofolate reductase and are used as anticancer agents, e.g. in childhood leukemias.
Aminopterin (4-aminofolic acid) inhibits the conversion of folic acid to folinic acid and thus blocks the biosynthesis of nucleic acids.
Amethopterin (N^{10}-methylfolic acid or methotrexate) inhibits folic acid reductase, thus affects the conversion of folic acid to FH_4.

VITAMIN B_{12} (CASTLE'S EXTRINSIC FACTOR, CYANOCOBALAMIN)

Vitamin B_{12} is also known as **cyanocobalamin** due to the presence of a cyano group and a cobalt atom. The central ring structure of vitamin B_{12} has a corrin nucleus which is similar to a porphyrin but with a central cobalt atom. Cobalt is linked to a cyano group and to a nitrogen of the imidazole ring which is esterified through aminopropanol and propionic acid to ring IV of the corrin nucleus (Fig. 28.37).

The cyano group may be replaced by nitrate ($-NO_2$) or hydroxyl group ($-OH$) to give **nitrosocobalamin** or **hydroxycobalamin**, both of which are hemo-poietically active forms of the vitamin.

Absorption, Storage and Transport

Dietary cobalamin (Cbl) initially binds to specific '**R-proteins**' in the stomach in the presence of HCl. There are two sources of R-proteins: The saliva and the gastric secretions. Another protein, **Castle's intrinsic factor** (IF), is secreted from the gastric parietal cells which replaces R-proteins and binds to Cbl (the '**extrinsic factor**') in the duodenum. The IF-Cbl complex is carried over to the ileum where it is recognized by specific receptors. Here, Cbl is absorbed leaving IF in the lumen. In pernicious anemia, autoantibodies interfere with the handling of Cbl resulting in Cbl deficiency despite adequate dietary intake of Cbl (Fig. 28.38).

Vitamin B_{12} is transported in the blood by two proteins which are designated as transcobalamin I and transcobalamin II. They deliver Cbl from the liver to various tissues as hydroxycobalamin which is either converted to methylcobalamin or to deoxyadeno-sylcobalamin. **Vitamin B_{12} activity is thus present in methylcobalamin, nitrosocobalamin as well as hydroxycobalamin.**

Vitamin B_{12} is excreted in the urine as well as in the feces.

Coenzyme Forms

Both **methylcobalamin** as well as **deoxyadenosyl-cobalamin** act as B_{12} coenzymes and are called **cobamides**.

Biochemical Role

1. **Collaborative action with folic acid (as methyl-cobalamin):** Required for the formation of

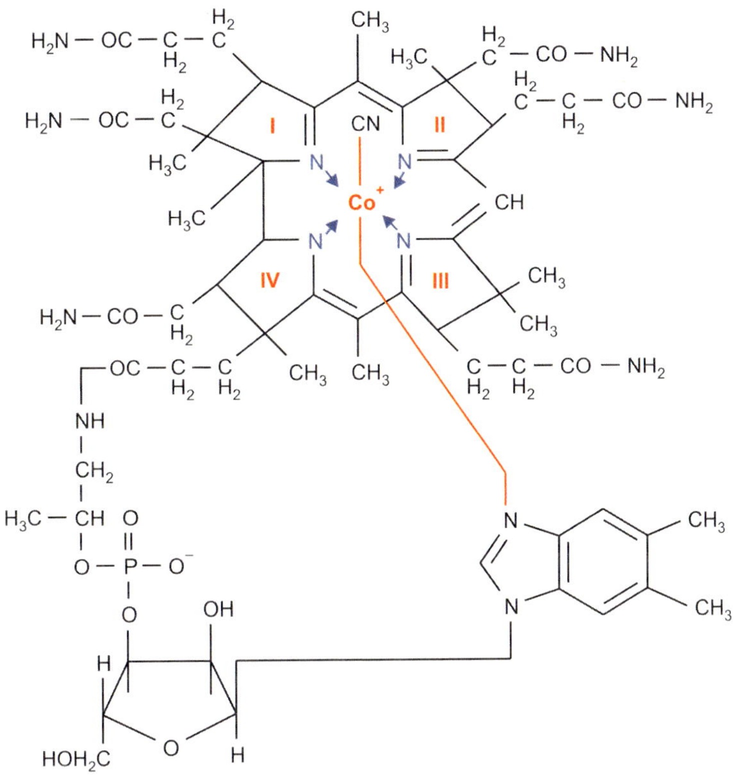

Fig. 28.37: Vitamin B_{12} (cyanocobalamin).

methionine from homocysteine (Fig. 28.36). The vitamin thus maintains methionine stores in the body and spares FH_4 for the biosynthesis of purine and pyrimidine bases for nucleic acids.

2. **Metabolism of branched chain amino acids (as deoxyadenosylcobalamin).**
3. **Metabolism of fatty acids containing odd number of carbon atoms (as deoxyadenosylcobalamin):** Required for the conversion of methylmalonyl CoA to succinyl CoA catalyzed by methylmalonyl CoA isomerase.

Deficiency Disorders

Vitamin B_{12} deficiency is not generally observed, due to its widespread distribution in animal tissues and synthesis by the microbial flora, except in geriatric cases or in strict vegetarians because plants do not synthesize vitamin B_{12}.

- Deficiency can occur because of prolonged reduced intake, intestinal malabsorption, atrophy of the gastric mucosa or deficiency of the intrinsic factor (e.g. in **pernicious anemia**). In pernicious anemia,

any of three different types of antibodies may be found in the serum (Fig. 28.38).

- The clinical outcomes are **megaloblastic anemia** and **subacute combined degeneration of the spinal cord** (discussed later under 'Hemopoietic vitamins').
- Vitamin B_{12} deficiency also results in **methyl-malonic aciduria**. Measurement of the urinary excretion of methylmalonic acid thus is also used to confirm the deficiency of vitamin B_{12}.

Sources and Requirement

Primary source of vitamin B_{12} is its synthesis by the intestinal microbial flora. Besides liver, kidney, egg, fish and milk are good sources. Amongst various vitamins of the B complex group, it has the lowest RDA of 1–3 µg only.

VITAMIN C (ASCORBIC ACID, ANTI-SCORBUTIC FACTOR)

The most important compound with vitamin C activity is **L-ascorbic acid**. The en-diol groups at the

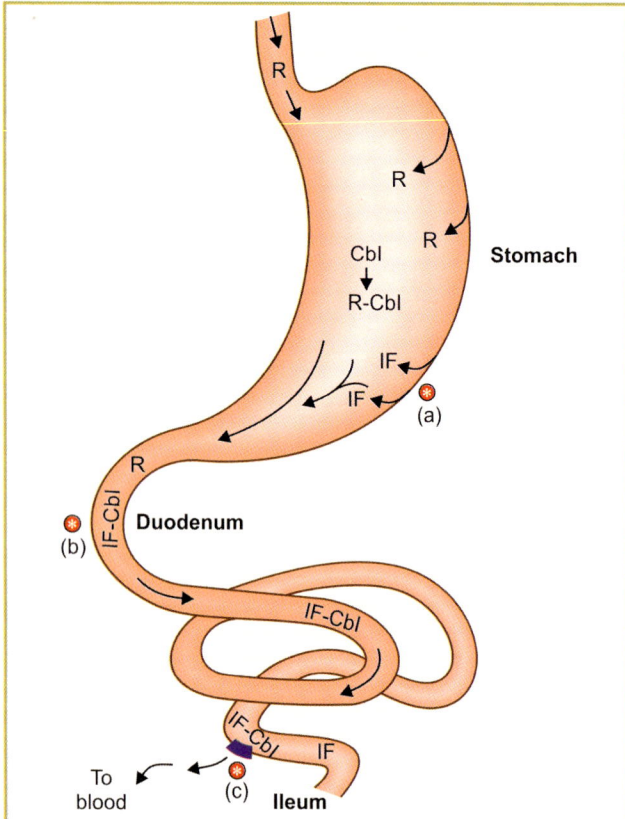

Fig. 28.38: Mechanism of handling of cobalamin (Cbl) in the gastrointestinal tract. ✴Indicates the three types of autoantibodies found in pernicious anemia—(a) antibodies against parietal cells; (b) blocking antibodies prevent formation of IF-Cbl complex; and (c) antibodies against IF-Cbl ileal receptors.

second and the third carbon atoms of the molecule are sensitive to oxidation. The oxidation of ascorbic acid converts it to **dehydroascorbic acid** (Fig. 28.39).

Vitamin C is easily destroyed by heat especially in an alkaline medium.

Majority of the animals can synthesize ascorbic acid from glucuronate but **men, primates and guinea pigs cannot synthesize** it and depend upon its exogenous supply.

Dietary vitamin C is readily absorbed from the intestinal tract. Its absorption is reduced in gastrointestinal infections and in achlorhydria. It is stored in the liver and the adrenals. **Highest concentration is found in the adrenal cortex.**

Biochemical Role

Due to its **oxidation-reduction properties**, ascorbic acid is important for a number of biological functions:
1. Hydroxylation reactions:
   - Hydroxylation of amino acids (particularly aromatic amino acids).
   - Hydroxylation of steroid hormones in the adrenal cortex which are synthesized from cholesterol.
   - Repair of the ground substance present in the tissues, due to its role in the hydroxylation of proline and lysine in the collagens.
2. **Hemopoiesis:** It ensures the availability of iron. As a powerful reducing agent, vitamin C reduces most of the inorganic iron present in the ferric form to the ferrous state which is absorbed more efficiently. Ascorbic acid also helps in the release of iron from ferritin.
3. **Conversion** of FH_4 to folinic acid.
4. **Immunity:** Stimulating effects on the phagocytic activity of the leukocytes and in the formation of antibodies. It thus provides resistance to the body.

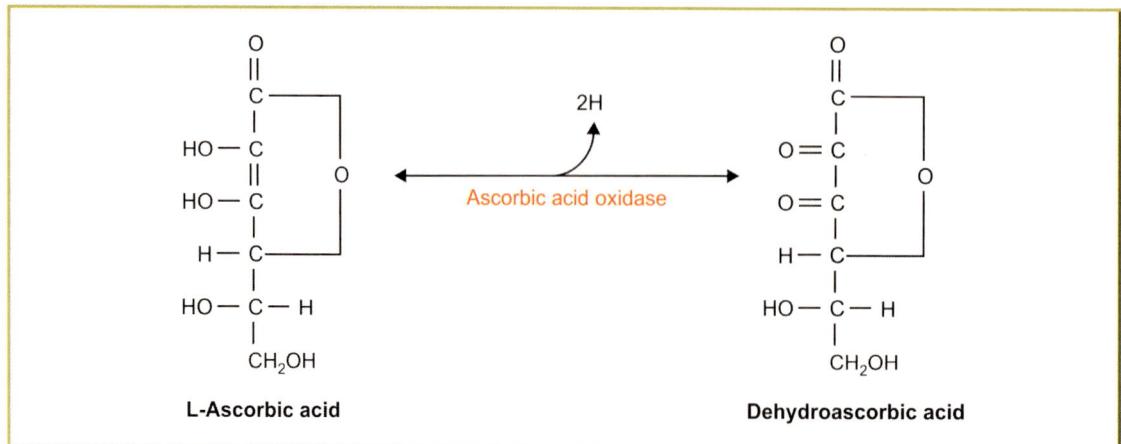

Fig. 28.39: Vitamin C.

5. **Antioxidant** and anticancer agent.
6. **Biosynthesis of bile acids from cholesterol:** Vitamin C thus also helps in lowering blood cholesterol level.

Vitamin C and collagen(s) biosynthesis: The chains of the intracellular precursors of collagens are called **protocollagens** which are synthesized on the ribosomes and are rich in proline and lysine. However, the hydroxylated forms of these amino acids (hydroxyproline and hydroxylysine) are essential components of the collagen fiber. Since there are neither codons nor tRNA molecules for hydroxyproline and hydroxylysine, **proline and lysine are hydroxylated** within the protocollagens to form collagens (**post-translational modifications**).

Ascorbic acid is essentially required for the hydroxylation of these two amino acids and thus plays an important role in collagen biosynthesis (Chapter 37).

Deficiency Disorders

1. **Scurvy:** Prolonged deficiency of vitamin C causes scurvy (Fig. 28.40). It is due to impaired collagen

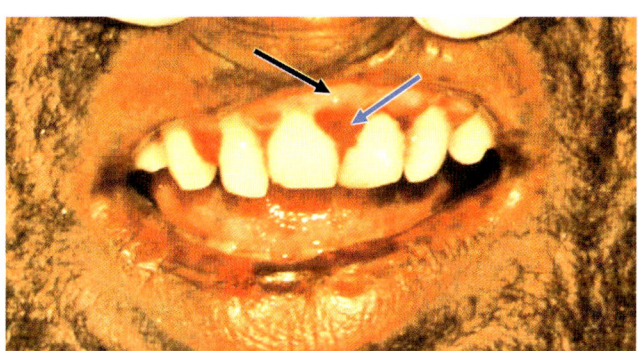

Fig. 28.41: Scurvy: Gingival swelling (black arrow) and hemorrhage (blue arrow).

formation and poor blood vessel support. Bleeding gums are a characteristic feature (Fig. 28.41).

Scurvy may also be observed in infants and is called **infantile scurvy**. Infants loose appetite and weight with painful tenderness of the extremities, and bleeding from gums and mucous membrane. In addition, long bones show cessation of osteogenesis.

2. **Microcytic anemia:** Because of the role of vitamin C in absorption, transport and storage of iron,

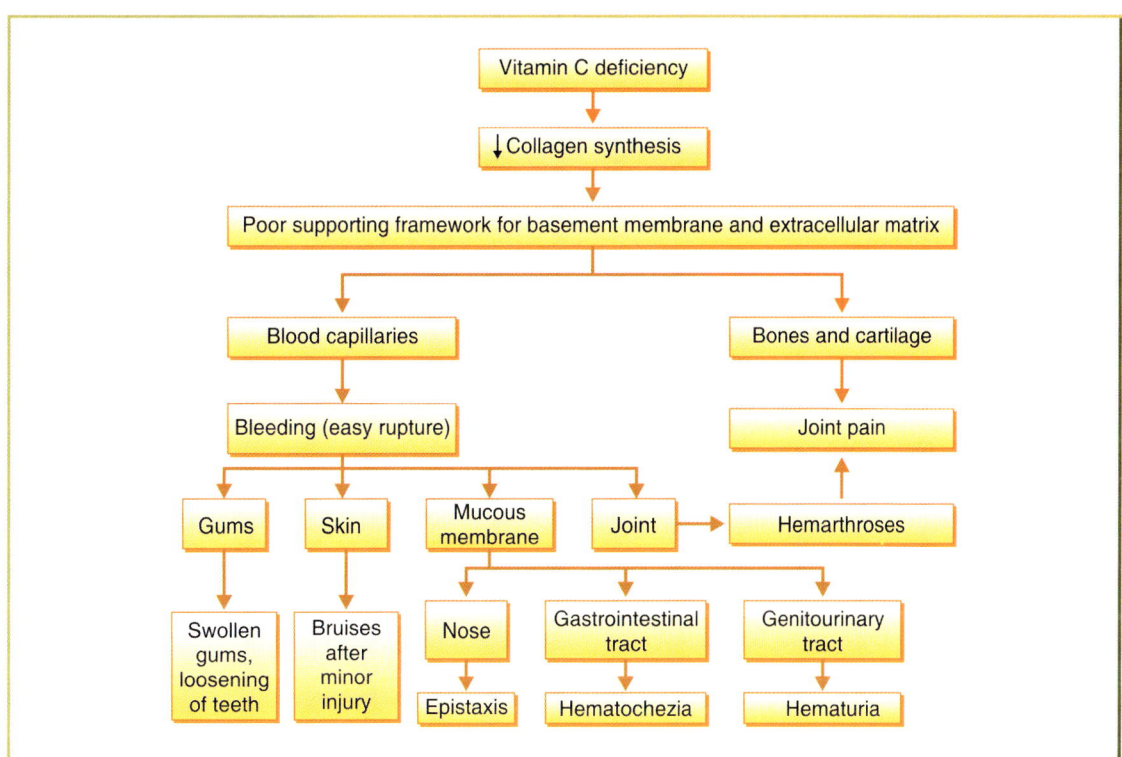

Fig. 28.40: Biochemical-clinical correlations in scurvy.

deficiency of vitamin C may also lead to anemia (microcytic anemia). The accompanying loss of blood may aggravate the anemia.

An early diagnosis of vitamin C deficiency can be made by **ascorbic acid saturation test, in platelets**.

Sources and Requirement

Vitamin C is widely distributed in **citrus fruits**, green chillies, guava and tomato. **Amla (Indian gooseberry) is the richest source** of vitamin C.

Amongst the various water soluble vitamins ascorbic acid has the highest RDA of 40–60 mg.

Hypervitaminosis C

Although vitamin C is water soluble, it may be toxic if taken in megadoses: More than 2 g of vitamin C in a single dose may result in abdominal pain, diarrhea and nausea. As the principal end product of its catabolism is oxalic acid, more than 3 g/day may lead to urolithiasis, i.e. formation of renal oxalate stones.

HEMOPOIETIC VITAMINS

These include methylcobalamin, folate, vitamin C, pyridoxine, biotin, deoxyadenosylcobalamin and pantothenic acid (Fig. 28.42).

Methyl Folate Trap Hypothesis: Megaloblastic Anemia

The metabolism of methylcobalamin and folate is closely linked as far as hemopoiesis is concerned (Fig. 28.36). Therefore, in vitamin B_{12} or folate

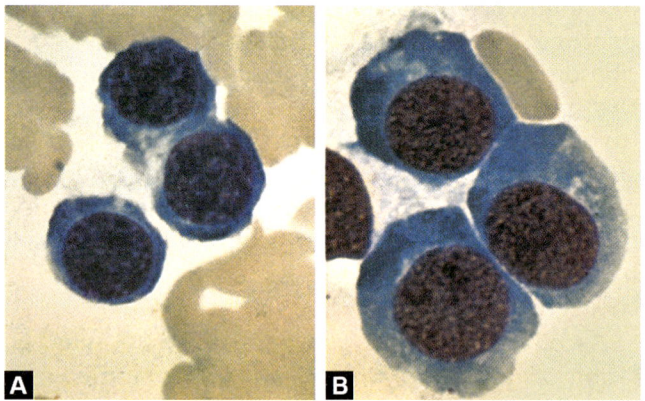

Fig. 28.43: Comparison of normoblasts (A) and megaloblasts (B) in a bone marrow aspirate. The **megaloblast** is an abnormal immature red cell precursor and is the equivalent of the normoblast in normal red cell production (the general term 'erythroblast' covers both normoblasts and megaloblasts). The megaloblast is characterized by its larger size, abundant cytoplasm and the fine reticular nuclear structure in comparison with the very coarse reticular nuclear structure of a normoblast at the same stage of cytoplasmic hemoglobinization. Thus, a megaloblast is characterized by nucleocytoplasmic dissociation.

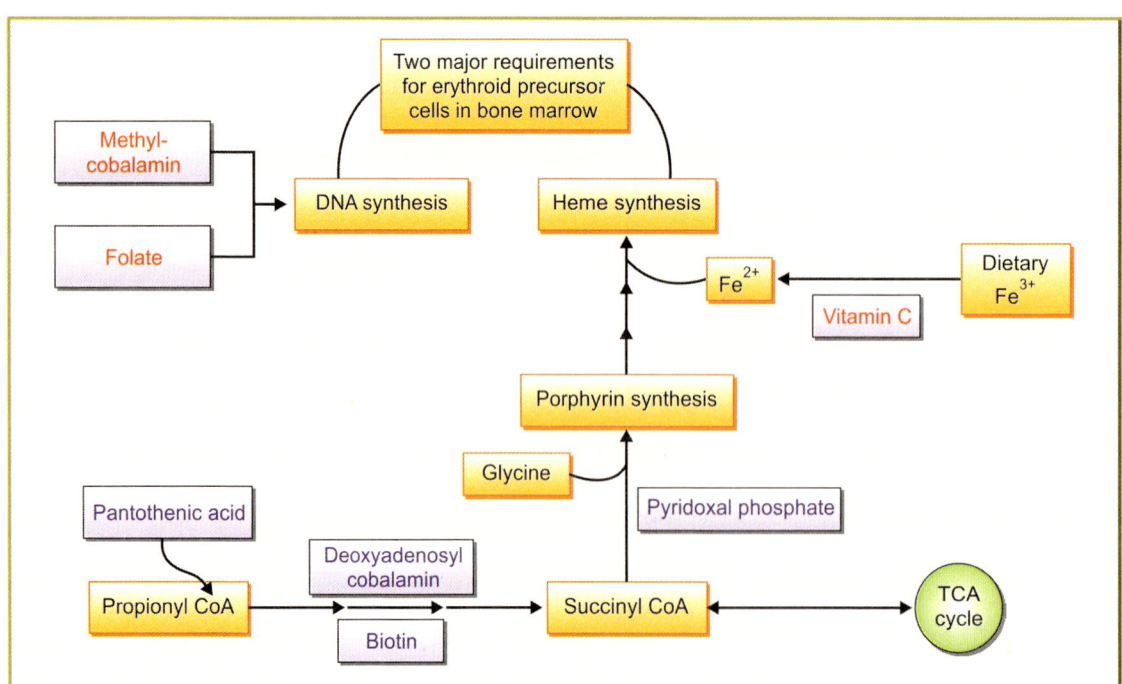

Fig. 28.42: Major (red) and accessory (blue) **hemopoietic** vitamins.

deficiency, folate is 'trapped' in the form of **methyltetrahydrofolate** since it fails to get converted into tetrahydrofolate which is the functionally active form of folate. As a result, deoxythymidylate cannot be synthesized which means that **DNA cannot be synthesized** in the bone marrow erythroid precursor cells. However, **protein synthesis continues** in the cytosol from the pre-existing mRNA so that the cells become enlarged though they fail to divide. These cells are appropriately called '**megaloblasts**' instead of normoblasts (Fig. 28.43) and they mature into large, fragile, short-lived RBC called '**macrocytes**'. The condition is called **megaloblastic or macrocytic anemia** characteristic of vitamin B_{12} or folate deficiency. In addition, an interesting observation is the neurological manifestations of vitamin B_{12} (but not folate) deficiency (Chemistry to Clinics 28.12).

The biochemical diagnosis of vitamin B_{12} or folate deficiency is given in Table 28.4.

Chemistry to Clinics 28.12: Neurological Manifestations of Vitamin B_{12} Deficiency

This is explained by the combined deficiency of both cobamide forms of B_{12}, i.e. deoxyadenosylcobalamin and methylcobalamin:

1. Deficiency of deoxyadenosylcobalamin results in accumulation of methyl malonyl CoA thereby competitively inhibiting the utilization of malonyl CoA in the synthesis of fatty acids with even number of carbon atoms.
2. Propionyl CoA also accumulates and is directed towards the synthesis of fatty acids with odd number of carbon atoms.
3. Lack of methylcobalamin results in decreased formation of methionine from homocysteine. The active form of methionine, S-adenosyl methionine or SAM, is required for the synthesis of choline and hence choline-containing phospholipids.

    The net result of all these factors is an inappropriate synthesis of myelin sheath and subacute combined degeneration of spinal cord that results in neurological manifestations.

Various water soluble vitamins, their coenzyme form, major biochemical role, principal deficiency diseases and daily requirement are given in Table 28.5.

Table 28.4: Biochemical diagnosis of vitamin B_{12} or folate deficiency

Vitamin B_{12} deficiency	*Folate deficiency*
• Low serum B_{12}	• Low RBC folate
• Increased urinary methylmalonic acid	• Increased urinary FIGLU with histidine challenge (FIGLU test)
• Demonstration of serum autoantibodies in case of pernicious anemia	

Table 28.5: Water soluble vitamins, their coenzyme forms, functions, deficiency disorders and RDA

Vitamin	Coenzyme	Biochemical function	Deficiency disorders	RDA
B Complex				
Thiamin (B_1)	TPP	Oxidative decarboxylation	Beriberi	0.4–0.5 mg/1000 kcal
Riboflavin (B_2)	FMN, FAD	Oxidation-reduction with flavoproteins	Cheilosis, lesions on the lips	0.5–0.6 mg/1000 kcal
Niacin	NAD^+, $NADP^+$	Hydrogen acceptor for dehydrogenases	Pellagra	5.5–6.5 mg/1000 kcal
Pyridoxine (B_6)	PLP	Transamination, decarboxylation	Peripheral neuritis	1–2 mg
Pantothenic acid	Coenzyme A	Formation of CoA derivative, component of acyl carrier protein	Muscle cramps, burning feet	5–10 mg
Biotin	Carboxybiocytin	Carrier of CO_2 for carboxylases	Anemia, dermatitis	150–300 μg
Folic acid	FH_4	Carrier of 1-C moiety	Megaloblastic macrocytic anemia	150–300 μg
Cobalamin (B_{12})	Cobamides	Transmethylation with FH_4	Pernicious anemia, megaloblastic anemia, subacute combined degeneration of spinal cord	1–3 μg
Vitamin C				
(Ascorbic acid)	L-Ascorbate	Hydroxylation	Scurvy	40–60 mg

28

SOME IMPORTANT QUESTIONS

1. Name lipid soluble vitamins. Mention their dietary sources, functions and associated deficiency disorders.

2. Describe chemistry, functions and deficiency manifestations of vitamin A.

3. How is vitamin D activated in the body? Describe its biochemical role.

4. Describe sources, functions and deficiency manifestations of folic acid and vitamin B_{12}.

5. Give an account of chemistry, sources, functions and deficiency manifestations of vitamin C.

6. Describe the coenzyme form and biochemical role of:
   - i. Riboflavin
   - ii. Pantothenic acid
   - iii. Biotin
   - iv. Vitamin B_6
   - v. Thiamin
   - vi. Niacin

7. Write notes on:
   - i. Keratomalacia
   - ii. Pellagra
   - iii. Beriberi
   - iv. Scurvy
   - v. Cobamide coenzymes
   - vi. Calcitriol
   - vii. β-Carotene

8. Discuss briefly:
   - i. Role of pyridoxal phosphate in amino acid metabolism
   - ii. Structure and functions of vitamin D
   - iii. Role of vitamin A in vision
   - iv. Methyl folate trap hypothesis
   - v. Megaloblastic anemia
   - vi. Pernicious anemia

MULTIPLE CHOICE QUESTIONS

1. **Vitamin A is stored in the liver as:**
   - A. All *trans*-retinol and 11-*cis*-retinal
   - B. All *trans*-retinal and 11-*cis*-retinol
   - C. β-Carotene
   - D. None of the above

2. **During hypocalcemia, calcitriol:**
   - A. Promotes bone mineralization
   - B. Promotes bone resorption
   - C. Inhibits renal calcium reabsorption
   - D. Inhibits intestinal calcium absorption

3. **The activation of vitamin D sequentially involves:**
   - A. Skin, liver, kidneys
   - B. Liver, skin, kidneys
   - C. Skin, kidneys, liver
   - D. Kidneys, skin, liver

4. **Decreased serum vitamin E may be associated with:**
   - A. Acne
   - B. Abetalipoproteinemia
   - C. Anemia
   - D. Any of the above

5. **Warfarin inhibits:**
   - A. Vitamin K epoxide reductase
   - B. Vitamin K carboxylase
   - C. Factor VIII
   - D. Fibrinogen

28

6. **Thiamin deficiency is confirmed by:**
   A. Increased RBC transketolase, increased plasma pyruvate
   B. Decreased RBC transketolase, decreased plasma pyruvate
   C. Increased RBC transketolase, decreased plasma pyruvate
   D. Decreased RBC transketolase, increased plasma pyruvate

7. **Prolonged consumption of sorghum as staple food may cause:**
   A. Beriberi
   B. Pellagra
   C. Megaloblastic anemia
   D. Burning feet syndrome

8. **Vitamin B_6 deficiency may occur in women using oral contraceptive pills containing:**
   A. No estrogen
   B. Low estrogen
   C. High estrogen
   D. All of the above

9. **The following condition may partly respond to pantothenic acid supplementation:**
   A. Burning feet syndrome
   B. Adrenal insufficiency
   C. Muscle cramps
   D. All of the above

10. **Vitamin B_{12} deficiency may result in:**
   A. Subacute combined degeneration of spinal cord
   B. Megaloblastic anemia
   C. Methylmalonic aciduria
   D. All of the above

5

Immunity and Defence

29

Immunology

All organisms, as we know, are under continuous attack by various pathogens (disease causing microorganisms) such as viruses, bacteria, fungi, protozoa and parasites. In human beings and higher animals, these foreign invaders are destroyed by the **immune system** of the body. If the immune system is disrupted, it can lead to immunodeficiency, hypersensitivity diseases or autoimmune diseases.

IMMUNITY

The **immunologic competence**, i.e. the ability of the body to detect and respond appropriately to the invading microorganisms and other foreign materials that have managed to penetrate the body, is called immunity. **Based on the time of development** of immunity, the latter is classified into innate and acquired/adaptive immunity (Table 29.1) whereas **based on the mode of development**, it is classified into active and passive immunity (Table 29.2).

Figure 29.1 shows both **active** and **passive** immunity may be either natural or artificial. **Natural immunity** is attained by exposure to specific microorganisms or received by the fetus from mother. **Artificial immunity** is otherwise known as **vaccination/immunization**, employing live/killed microorganisms, their products or pre-formed antibodies.

Table 29.1: Innate versus acquired immunity

Innate immunity	Acquired/adaptive immunity
• By virtue of genetic make-up of an individual	• Acquired as the individual grows up
• No prior antigenic stimulus, i.e. immunization or contact with microorganisms is required	• Prior antigenic stimulus is required
• Present since birth, hence no lag phase	• Definite lag phase following antigenic challenge

Table 29.2: Active versus passive immunity

Active immunity	Passive immunity
• **Produced** actively by the host's immune system	• **Received** passively by the host without participation of the immune system
• Requires antigenic challenge	• Introduction of ready-made antibodies
• Effective and durable	• Less effective and transient
• Lag phase is required to generate the immune response	• No lag phase
• Immunological memory present; subsequent challenge serves as booster	• No immunological memory is present; subsequent challenge is less effective
• Not applicable in immunocompromised host	• Applicable in immunocompromised host

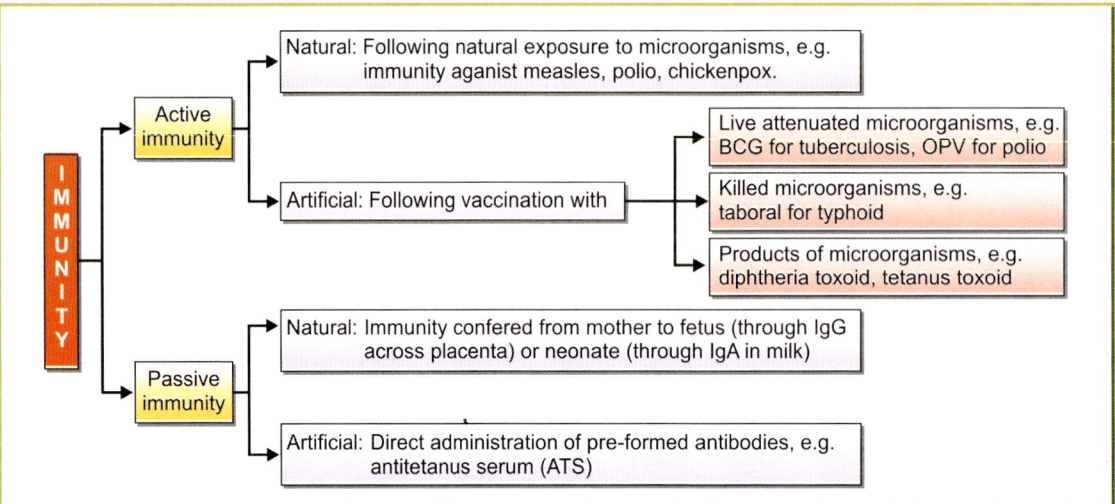

Fig. 29.1: Examples of active and passive immunity.

Cells which Mediate Immunity

These include phagocytes and lymphocytes; phagocytes internalize the pathogens and degrade them while lymphocytes recognize antigens on the pathogens.

Phagocytes

Phagocytic cells such as polymorphonuclear neutrophils (Chemistry to Clinics 29.1) bind to microorganisms, internalize and kill them. They mediate innate immune responses and act as first line of defense against an infection. They also participate in inflammatory responses. They are well supported by monocytes and macrophages. Pro-inflammatory macrophages are called *M1 macrophages* whereas the non-inflammatory ones are designated *M2 macrophages*.

Lymphocytes

Lymphocytes are another set of leukocytes which mediate adaptive immune response and specifically recognize individual pathogens. They fall into two categories, i.e. T lymphocytes (T cells) and B lymphocytes (B cells) (Chemistry to Clinics 29.2).

Chemistry to Clinics 29.1: Hypochlorous Acid

Activated neutrophils secrete hypochlorous acid (HOCl) which is more cytotoxic against microbes compared with H_2O_2. The body lacks direct enzymatic defenses against HOCl. Plasma albumin-SH groups and ascorbic acid protect against HOCl. Neutrophils contain 25 times more ascorbic acid than plasma, avoiding self-destruction.

Chemistry to Clinics 29.2: Cluster of Differentiation (CD)

These refer to specific cell surface proteins with diverse functions. Depending on the cell type, a CD may act as a receptor or ligand or adhesion molecule. The concept was applied for leucocytes (e.g. CD4+ are T helper cells while CD8+ are cytotoxic T cells) but later expanded to include various other cell types (e.g. CD220 for insulin receptor). They are useful in immunophenotyping which identifies alterations in cell types in various disease conditions, e.g. depletion of CD4+ cells in HIV infection.

B lymphocytes: B cells combat extracellular pathogens and their products by releasing antibodies (molecules which specifically recognize and bind to particular target molecules called antigens). These antibody molecules are large glycoproteins found in the blood and tissue fluids. B cells mediate **humoral immunity**.

T lymphocytes: There are several different types of T cells with a variety of functions, such as:
- **Cytotoxic T cells:** They are responsible for the destruction of host cells which have become infected by viruses or other intracellular pathogen.
- **Suppressor T cells:** They inhibit the production of cytotoxic T cells when they are no longer needed. As suppressors of the immune system, they play an important role in maintaining homeostasis.
- **Helper T cells:** Helper CD4+ T cells direct the immune response by secreting chemicals, **effector molecules,** generally referred to as **lymphokines**.
  - One group interacts with mononuclear phagocytes and helps them to destroy intracellular pathogens. They are called **T helper cells type-1** (T_H1).

– Another group interacts with B cells and helps them to divide, differentiate and make antibody. These are called **T helper cells type-2 (T$_H$2)**.

Differentiation of CD4+ T helper cells into T$_H$1 and T$_H$2 cells occurs only after they have been activated during an immune response in the peripheral lymphoid system. Each type of T cell produces a distinct set of effector molecules. For instance, T$_H$1 cells release the macrophage-activating effector molecules interferon-γ and tumor necrosis factor-α, whereas T$_H$2 cells produce B cell-activating effector molecules such as interleukin 4, 5 and 15, among numerous other cytokines.

• **T helper zero cells:** Many T cells express cytokines from both profiles. They are often named T helper zero (**T$_H$0**) cells.

All types of T cells recognize antigen when presented on the surface of the other cell by major histocompatibility complex (**MHC**) molecules.

MAJOR HISTOCOMPATIBILITY COMPLEX

All vertebrate cells express on their surfaces, a sample of peptides derived from the intracellular digestion of specific proteins in their cytosol. This expression, however, requires that the peptides should be bound to a specific class of integral membrane proteins/antigens encoded by a set of genes referred to as the **Major Histocompatibility Complex (MHC) genes**. Initially, MHC encoded antigens were detected on **leukocytes**, hence they were called **Human Leukocyte Antigens (HLA)**.

HLA Loci

Humans express six different **class I genes** (three from each parent) and six different **class II genes** on chromosome 6. The three loci for class I genes are called HLA-A, HLA-B and HLA-C; those for class II genes are called HLA-DP, HLA-DQ and HLA-DR. Because of **high polymorphism** between the HLA loci, it is very rare to find two persons (except monozygotic twins) with identical HLA. This is responsible for

Chemistry to Clinics 29.3: Importance of HLA

• HLA plays a crucial role in **regulating the immune response** (Fig. 29.2). CD8 lymphocytes and their secretory proteins such as perforins and granzymes are responsible for direct killing of target cells recognized via MHC-I. On the other hand, CD4 lymphocytes with the help of B cells combat the targets recognized via MHC-II.

• Specific HLA types are associated with **disease susceptibility**, e.g. ankylosing spondylitis (HLA B27), insulin dependent diabetes mellitus (HLA DR3/4), rheumatoid arthritis (HLA DR4), hemochromatosis (HLA A3), myasthenia gravis (HLA B8), etc.

• HLA **typing** is required before **organ transplantation**.

transplant rejection unless the HLA genotypes of donor and recipient are closely matched. HLA is of physiological and clinical importance (Chemistry to Clinics 29.3).

MHC Classes

The MHC gene encodes **three classes** of MHC proteins/antigens—class I proteins presented to cytotoxic T cells, class II proteins presented to helper T cells (Table 29.3) and class III proteins or complement proteins.

MEMORY CELL

Lymphocytes are stimulated after binding to their specific antigen and express new receptors. These lymphocytes also respond to cytokines which are produced from other cells and signal proliferation. As a result, these cells may also start secreting cytokines themselves as well as through a number of cycles of division before differentiating into mature cells, such as proliferating B cells eventually mature into antibody-producing plasma cells.

Even when the infection has been overcome, some of the newly produced lymphocytes remain **available for restimulation**, in case the antigen is encountered again in future. These cells are called memory cells, since they retain the **immunological memory** of a particular antigen. It is, these memory cells that confer the **lasting immunity** to a particular pathogen.

Table 29.3: Difference between class I and II MHC

Class I MHC	Class II MHC
• Expressed on all cells	• Expressed on antigen-presenting cells (B cells, macrophages, dendritic cells)
• Present cytosolic proteins to cytotoxic T cells	• Present proteins internalized within endosomes to helper T cells
• Assisted by CD8 proteins	• Assisted by CD4 proteins
• Lead to direct killing of target cell	• Lead to enhancement of immune response

29

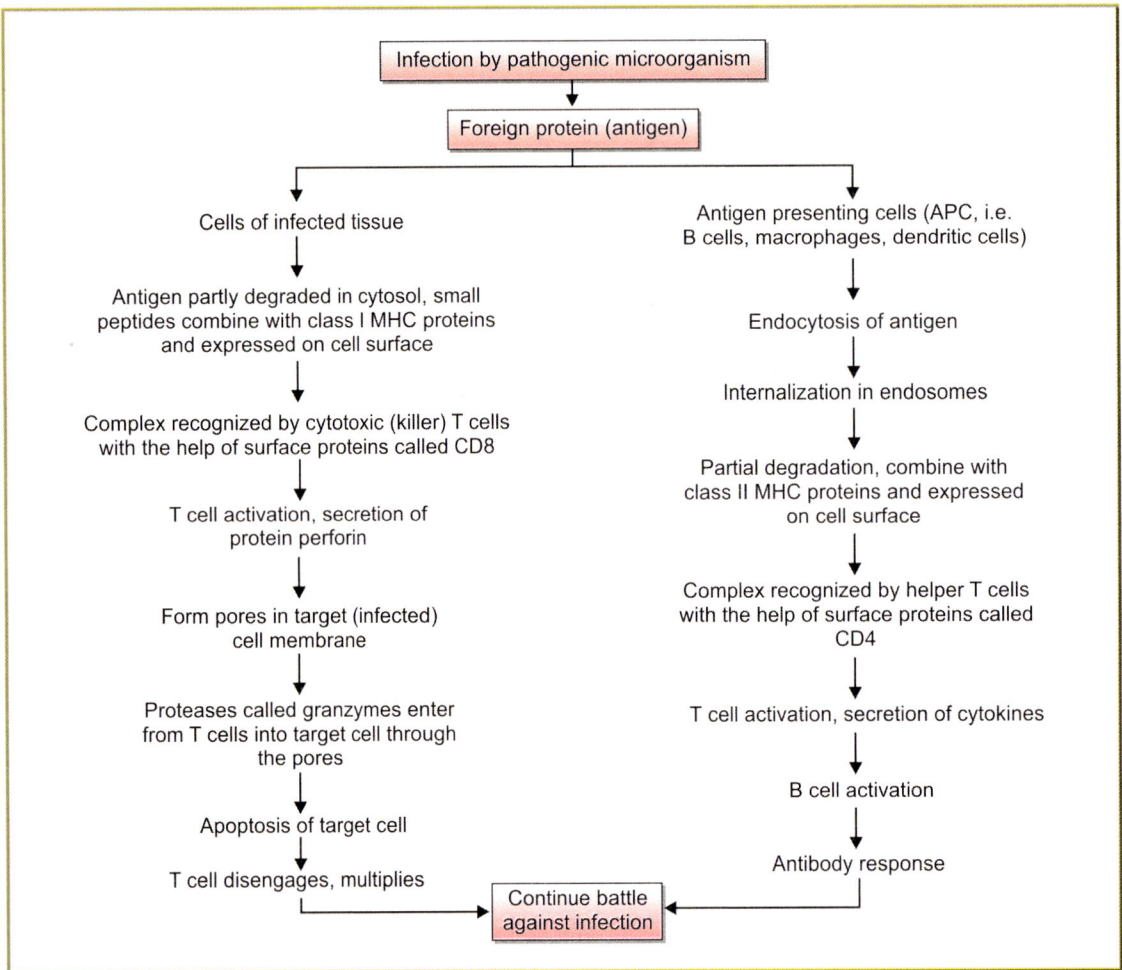

Fig. 29.2: Role of MHC in the generation of immune response.

ANTIGEN

Any molecule that triggers an immune response is called **immunogen**. On the other hand, an **antigen** is a molecule that can bind to its corresponding antibody. An antigen may be a protein, carbohydrate or nucleic acid and can be specifically recognized by the adaptive elements of the immune system, i.e. by B cells or T cells, or both. Thus, **all immunogens are antigens but all antigens may not be immunogenic**, e.g. hapten, antigen inducing immune tolerance, etc.

- Antigen molecules are recognized by receptors on lymphocytes. B lymphocytes usually recognize intact antigen molecules while T lymphocytes recognize antigen fragments on the surface of the cells.
- Each antibody binds to a restricted part of the antigen, called an **antigenic determinant** or **epitope**. A particular antigen can have several different epitopes or repeated epitopes. Antibodies are specific for the epitopes rather than for the whole antigen molecule. In proteins, an antigenic determinant generally comprises only 6 or 7 amino acids.

Hapten

Hapten is a small molecule which can act as an epitope but is **incapable by itself**, of eliciting an antibody response. It can induce synthesis of antibodies only when covalently attached to some large molecule. Though a hapten needs its attachment to a large molecule to elicit antibody production, it retains the ability to bind strongly to the antibody even after it has been detached from the carrier molecule.

Chemistry to Clinics 29.4: Allergies

T$_H$1/T$_H$2 imbalance: A popular hypothesis, often referred to as the hygiene model, proposes that the children who are not exposed to enough antigens or innocuous microorganisms from soil or water early in their childhood, do not adequately develop their T$_H$1 response. This leads to an imbalance toward T$_H$2 responses. Even though this hypothesis is disputed as being grossly oversimplified, it is undisputed that the various manifestations of allergic inflammation are the result of wrongly activated T$_H$2 cells.

Chemical mediators: The symptoms of bronchial asthma ultimately depend on the presence of T$_H$2 cells, which secrete a characteristic cytokine repertoire on antigen challenge. One of the cytokines, interleukin-4, activates B cells to produce IgE antibodies, which bind to mast cells, eosinophils, and other airway cells via receptors that are specific for the Fc portions of the antibodies. On subsequent encounters with the antigen, IgE-cross-linking on mast cells and eosinophils occurs. This leads to their activation, releasing histamine and leukotrienes that cause bronchoconstriction and mucus hypersecretion. These and other inflammatory factors further recruit inflammatory cells including additional T$_H$2 cells to the lung, resulting in a damaging immunological positive feedback cycle. Almost similar biochemical mechanisms operate in other allergies such as food allergies, skin allergies, e.g. urticaria, etc.

Management: Avoidance of allergens (if identified), type 1 antihistaminics, mast cell stabilizers, corticosteroids, and desensitization.

Allergen

An allergen is an antigen that gives rise to **immediate hypersensitivity**. It is an agent, e.g. pollen, dust or animal dander that causes IgE-mediated hypersensitivity reactions popularly called **'allergies'** (Chemistry to Clinics 29.4).

HYPERSENSITIVITY

The adaptive immune response provides specific protection against infection with bacteria, viruses, parasites or fungi. It provides rapid protection against a repeated challenge with the same or similar foreign organism or toxin. Some immune responses, however, give rise to an excessive or inappropriate reaction, referred to as hypersensitivity. It is an exaggerated form of an appropriate response and includes:

- **Type I or immediate hypersensitivity:** It is characterized by the production of **IgE** antibodies against foreign proteins that are commonly present in the environment, e.g. pollens, animal dander or dust mite. These antibodies bind specifically to high affinity receptors on mast cells and basophils which contain histamine. Conditions that are associated with type I hypersensitivity include hay fever, bronchial asthma, atopic dermatitis and anaphylaxis (Chemistry to Clinics 29.5).

- **Type II or antibody mediated hypersensitivity:** These reactions are caused by **IgG or IgM** antibodies against cells surface or extracellular matrix antigens or to intracellular components. Antibodies trigger a cytotoxic reaction and damage cells/tissues by activating the complement system

Chemistry to Clinics 29.5: Anaphylaxis

It is an antigen specific immune reaction mediated primarily by IgE. It results in vasodilation and constriction of smooth muscles including those of the bronchus and may result in death. Anaphylaxis occurs when a patient with immediate hypersensitivity is exposed to a relevant allergen in such a way that antigen enters the circulation rapidly. This can occur after a bee-sting, an injection of penicillin, eating an allergen or even following a therapeutic allergen injection for hyposensitization. It is an emergency and the treatment requires prompt administration of adrenaline.

and by binding and activating effector cells carrying F$_c$ receptors, e.g. autoimmune hemolytic anemia. Damage to tissue may be produced by antibodies to basement membrane, to intracellular adhesion molecules or to receptors, e.g. myasthenia gravis.

- **Type III or immune complex disease:** It occurs when excess **antigen-antibody complexes** are formed in the circulation that cannot be cleared by macrophages or other cells in the reticuloendothelial system. Accumulation of such complexes can trigger either a complement or a cell-mediated local reaction. Systemic lupus erythematosus (SLE) is a classical disease in which immune complexes are involved.

- **Type IV or cell-mediated reactions:** These are reactions in which **specific T cells** are the primary effector cells. Contact sensitivity (e.g. to nickel) and graft rejection are the examples of T cells causing unwanted responses.

INFLAMMATION

Inflammation is a local response of a tissue to damage or infection. It has three principle components:

29

1. An increased blood supply to the area bringing leucocytes and other serum components to the affected site.
2. An increase in capillary permeability allowing exudation of serum proteins (antibody, complement, etc.) required to control the infection.
3. An increase in leukocyte migration into the tissue.

Auxiliary cells including mast cells, basophils and platelets are also important in initiation and development of acute inflammation. They act as a source of vasoactive mediators (such as histamine) which produce vasodilation and increase vascular permeability. Mast cells are also the source of slow reacting inflammatory mediators including leukotrienes and prostaglandins which contribute to a delayed component of acute inflammation. Clinically, an acute inflammation is characterized by the following **classical signs**

- *Rubor* (redness)
- *Calor* (heat)
- *Dolor* (pain)
- *Tumor* (swelling)
- *Functio laesa* (temporary loss of function)

THE COMPLEMENT SYSTEM

Constituents: The complement system consists of approximately 30 protein molecules constituting nearly 10% of total serum proteins and is one of the major defense systems of the body.

Functions
1. Control of inflammatory reactions and chemotaxis.
2. Clearance of immune complexes.
3. Cellular activation and antimicrobial defense.
4. Development of antibody responses.

Activation: Various components of the complement system interact with each other and with other elements of the immune system. Complement activation is a **cascade reaction** with each component sequentially acting on the other. Three principle pathways are involved in complement activation, all of which converge on the activation of the third component (C3, Chemistry to Clinics 29.6). These are:

- The **classical pathway** which is activated by antibody bound to antigen.
- The **lectin pathway** activated by carbohydrates.
- The **alternative pathway** activated in the presence of various microbial pathogens.

Chemistry to Clinics 29.6: Complement System and Disease

1. All three pathways of complement activation generate enzymes which cleave C3 into two fragments, i.e. C3a and C3b. Further, an important role of the complement system is to generate opsonins, proteins that stimulate phagocytosis by neutrophils and macrophages. A major opsonin is C3b. Patients with inherited deficiency of C3 are subjected to repeated bacterial infections.
2. Complement activation is a major effector in immunopathological diseases.

IMMUNOGLOBULINS

Immunoglobulins are a diverse group of glycoproteins synthesized by mature B lymphocytes called **plasma cells**. They are present either in the **free form** in plasma (constituting ≈20% of total plasma proteins, mainly the γ-globulins) and other biological fluids, or **bound** to the surface of B cells where they act as receptors for antigens. Those immunoglobulins which bind to specific antigens are called antibodies. Thus, the term **'immunoglobulin'** is a structural concept while **'antibody'** is a functional one.

They are highly specific for the three-dimensional conformation of the epitope. Certain immunoglobulins (Bence Jones proteins, cryoglobulins, macroglobulins, etc.) have no antibody activity and are found in some diseases and even in some healthy individuals. Therefore, **all antibodies are immunoglobulins while all immunoglobulins may not be antibodies**.

Salient Structural Features of an Immunoglobulin Molecule

- It is a **Y-shaped** molecule having two arms and a stem (Fig. 29.3).
- It has a **quaternary structure** with four polypeptide chains which are bound by disulfide (–S–S–) linkages. They comprise of two small subunits called light (**L**) chains and two large subunits called heavy (**H**) chains.
- Each subunit has a **variable region** towards the N-terminal end and **constant region(s)** towards the C-terminal end.
- The two arms are called the **Fab** fragments (antigen-binding fragments) whereas the stem is called as the **Fc** fragment (crystallizable fragment).
- The arms and the stem are linked together by a flexible region called the **hinge** region.

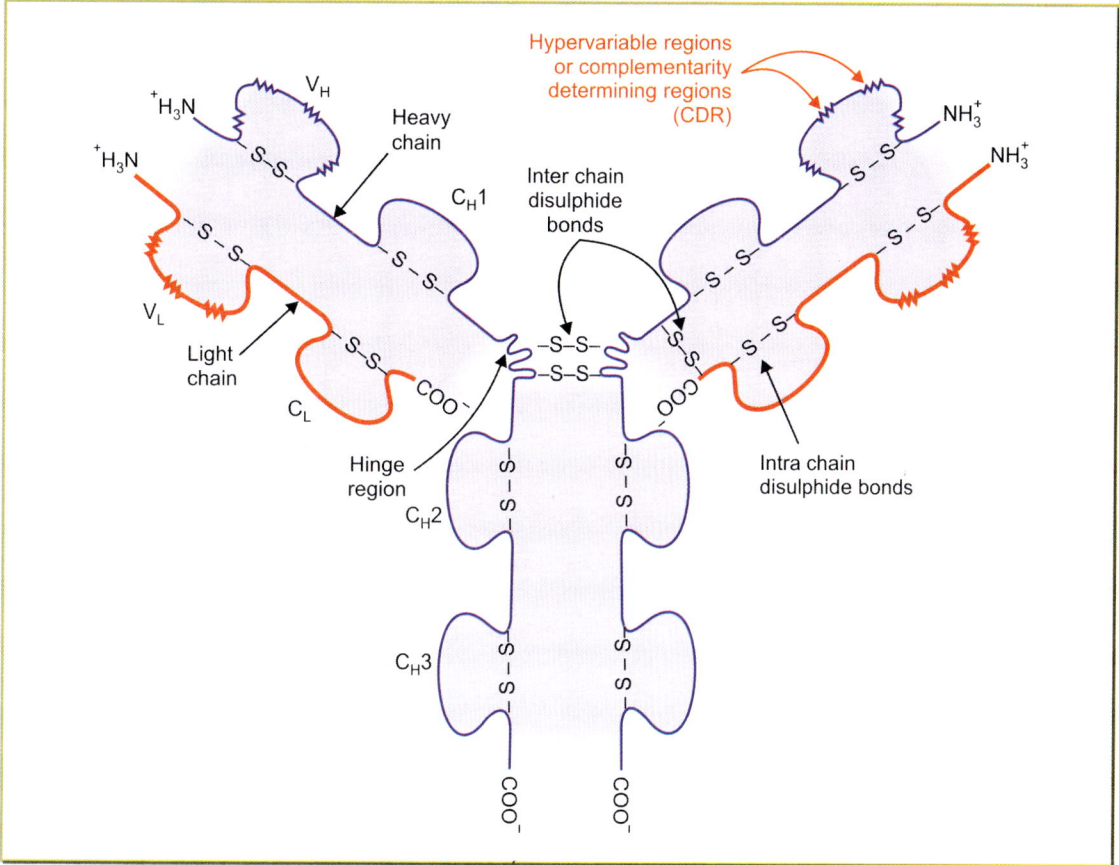

Fig. 29.3: Structure of an immunoglobulin.

Immunoglobulin Light Chains

The smaller polypeptides (≈ 25 kD each) are designated as light chains (**L chains**). Each L chain contains nearly 220 amino acids. Two types of L chains may be found in immunoglobulins. These are designated as **kappa chain (κ chain)** and the **lambda chain (λ chain)**. An immunoglobulin molecule always has **two identical L chains**, i.e. it has either two κ chains (as κ_2) or two λ chains (as λ_2) but **never a mixture** of one κ chain and one λ chain (as $\kappa\lambda$). These are referred to as **isotypes** and are present in all individuals although κ chains are more prevalent than the λ chains.

Immunoglobulin Heavy Chains

The larger subunits (50 to 75 kD) present in an immunoglobulin molecule are called heavy chains (**H chains**). **Five** different types of H chains, each containing 440–450 amino acids, are found in human immunoglobulins. Various H chains are designated as gamma (γ), alpha (α), mu (μ), delta (δ) and epsilon (ε). Each H chain is specific to a class of immunoglobulin and thus depending on it, immunoglobulins are classified as **IgG, IgA, IgM, IgD and IgE**.

L chains and H chains are synthesized as separate proteins and are subsequently assembled to form a mature immunoglobulin tetrameric molecule (L_2H_2), within the plasma cells. During assembly, each one of the two H chains is associated with two L chains as well as with each other, by –S–S–linkages. An L chain is joined to an H chain in such a way that they run parallel to each other. Since L chain is only about half the size of the H chain (as an L chain contains nearly 220 amino acids as compared to 440–450 present in an H chain), complete L chain is therefore associated with only N-terminal half of the H chain.

Various chains are folded into discrete regions called **domains**. There are two domains in the light chain while depending on their class, four or five domains are found in a heavy chain.

29

Variable and Constant Regions

Within each L and H chain of an immunoglobulin molecule, there are regions with sequence homology (constant regions) as well as sequence variability (variable regions).

- **Variable regions:** Amino acid sequences in the N-terminal half of the L chains and one-quarter of the H chains are highly variable, between different immunoglobulin molecules. Therefore, these N-terminal regions are called variable regions (**V regions**). These are **heterogeneous** to the extent that no two V regions, from different humans, have identical amino acid sequences. V regions determine the **antigenic specificity** of the antibody molecule. These regions, in the L chains and the H chains, are designated as V_L and V_H respectively.

- **Constant regions:** The remainder of the molecule, i.e. the C-terminal half of the L chain and the C-terminal three-quarter of the H chain, are **homologous** in sequence with other L or H chains of the same class of immunoglobulin. These regions are called constant regions (**C regions**), which, in the L chains and the H chains are designated as the C_L and C_H respectively. The C_H region is further divided into three homologous sequences of about 110 amino acid residues each, which are designated as $C_H 1$, $C_H 2$ and $C_H 3$ respectively. These three segments of the C_H region are homologous to each other as well as to the C_L region. Each of these homologous segments (sequence repeats) contains an intrachain disulfide bond. The μ and ε types of the H chains have four C_H regions rather than three.

Significance of C_H Region(s)

1. It determines the **antibody class** of an immunoglobulin, i.e. differences in the sequence in the C_H region is responsible for the characteristics of each class of immunoglobulin.
2. It provides site for the **binding of a complement protein**.
3. Sites for the antibodies to **cross the placental membrane**.
4. Depending upon the class of an immunoglobulin, variable amounts of **carbohydrates** (2–15%) are attached to the $C_H 2$ region of the H chain.
5. Amino acid sequences in these C_H regions, **in some cases**, also promote **polymerization** of the basic molecular structure (L_2H_2) of the immunoglobulin molecule, covalently linked with each other around a joining subunit (**J chain**). Generally,

immunoglobulins of the **IgA** class occur as **dimers** while **IgM** as **pentamers** Fig. 29.4.

Hypervariable Sequences

V region of an immunoglobulin molecule, as mentioned above, is involved in recognition and binding of an antigen with it. This ability of an antibody to recognize an antigen, resides in several short sequences which are located in **small loops within the V region**, termed as **hypervariable regions** or **hypervariable sequences**.

Only 5–10 amino acids in each hypervariable sequence, contribute to an antigen binding site (**ab site**), complementary to the topology of an antigen structure and are designated as 'complementarity-determining regions' (**CDR**) or simply as 'complementarity determinants'. Three hypervariable sequences are commonly found in V_L regions while each of the V_H regions may have three or four hypervariable sequences, depending upon the type of the antibody (Fig. 29.3).

Fab and Fc Fragments

Cleavage by the enzyme papain: An immunoglobulin molecule such as IgG, can be **cleaved with the enzyme papain** into three fragments of nearly 50 kD each. Two of these fragments are identical and are obtained from the two arms. These are the fragments where antigen binds and are hence called as **antigen binding fragments (Fab fragments)**. The third fragment is obtained from the stem of the molecule. Since this fragment can be easily crystallized, it is called **Fc fragment** (Fig. 29.5).

- Two Fab fragments (obtained from the two arms) have entire of the L-chain and N-terminal half of the H-chain (comprising of the V_H–$C_H 1$ regions). Each of these two Fab fragments can bind to an antigen, with the affinity similar to that of the intact antibody molecule. Because there are two Fab domains, a molecule of an immunoglobulin can bind two molecules of an antigen simultaneously. An antibody is thus termed as **divalent**.

- The Fc fragment, as mentioned above, is derived from the stem of the antibody molecule. It consists of the C-terminal halves of the two H chains, i.e. the $C_H 2$ and $C_H 3$ regions which are joined together by the disulfide bridges.

Thus, all antibodies are **bifunctional**, i.e. in addition to antigen binding in the Fab region, they also exhibit

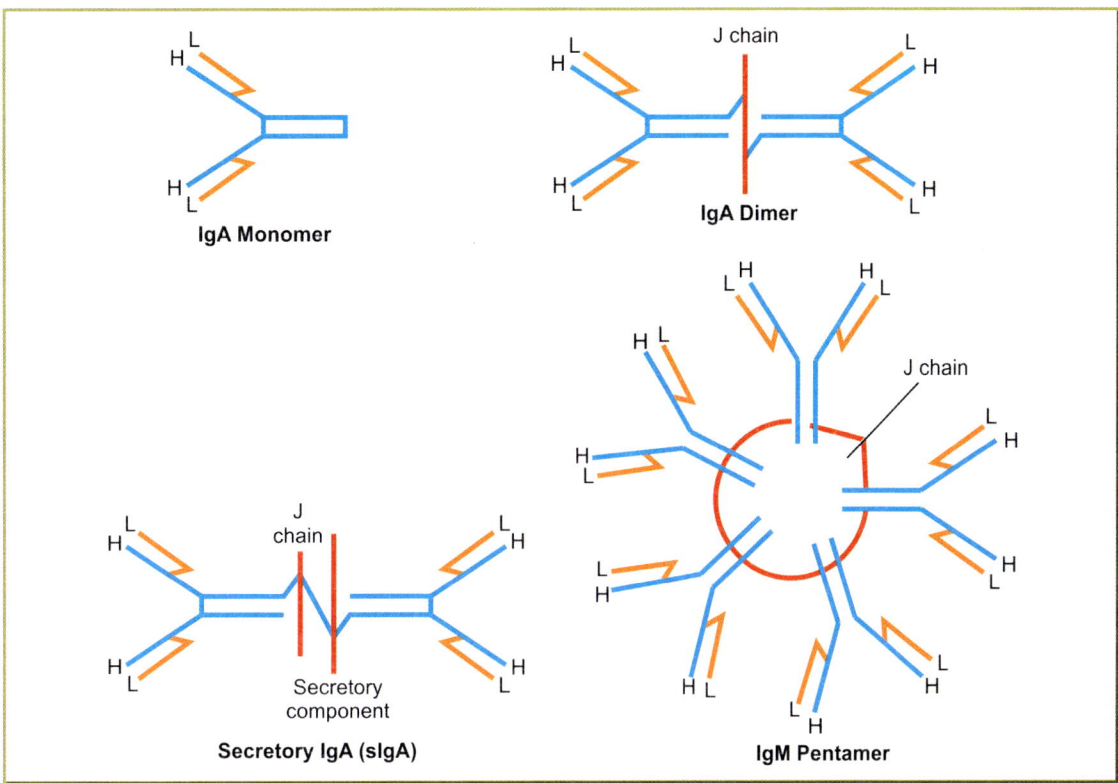

Fig. 29.4: Polymerization of immunoglobulin molecules.

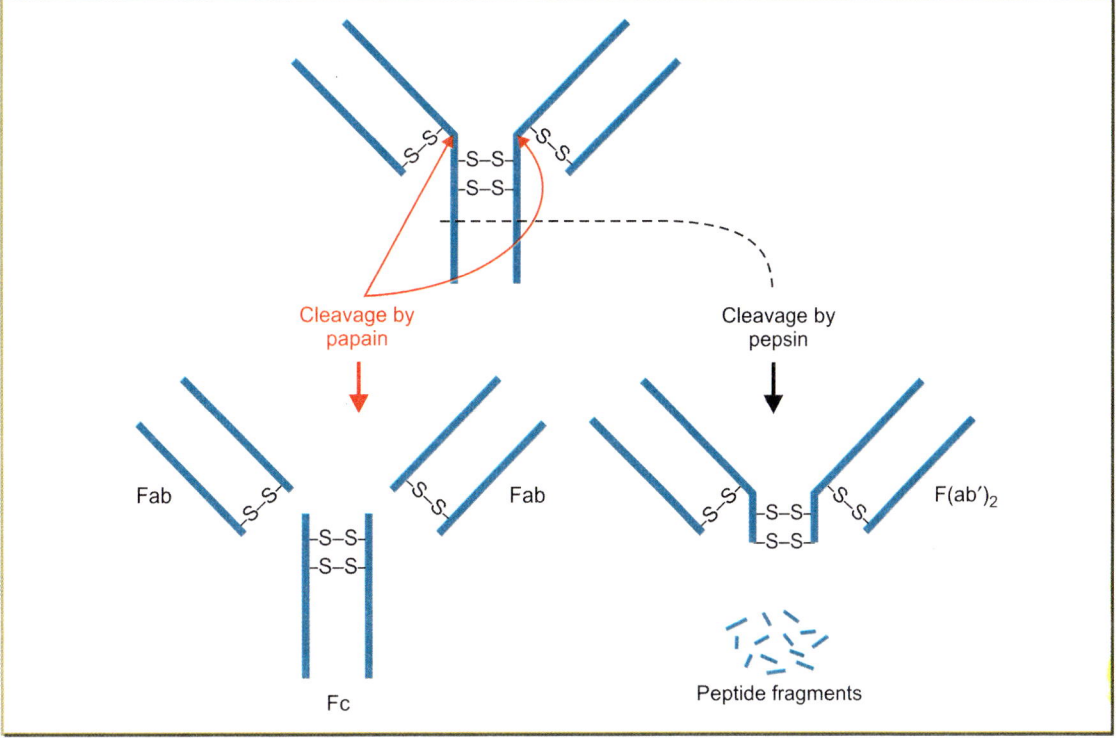

Fig. 29.5: Effects of papain and pepsin on an immunoglobulin molecule.

29

one or more effector functions such as complement activation and cell binding, in the Fc region.

The receptors for immunoglobulins are expressed by mononuclear cells, neutrophils, natural killer (NK) cells, eosinophils and mast cells. These receptors interact with the Fc region of the immunoglobulin and promote various activities such as phagocytosis, tumor cell killing and mast cell degranulation.

Cleavage by the enzyme pepsin: Cleavage by the enzyme **pepsin**, on the other hand, yields a large fragment with the two Fab portions linked together. It is called F(ab')$_2$. The remaining part of the stem is degraded into smaller peptides.

The Hinge Region

Two Fab fragments of an immunoglobulin molecule are connected to the Fc fragment by a flexible region, referred to as hinge region (Figs 29.3 and 29.6). It is present between $C_H 1$ and $C_H 2$, and confers **flexibility** to the antibody molecule. This, in turn, allows two Fab fragments to move independently and thus helps them to bind with two antigens simultaneously, that may be present at different distances apart from each other.

The hinge region contains one or more cysteine residues which provide **interchain disulfide bridges**.

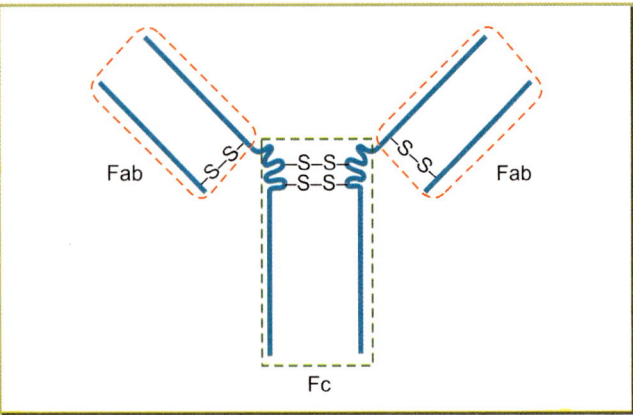

Fig. 29.6: Antigen binding (Fab) and crystallizable (Fc) fragments of immunoglobulin.

It also controls interactions between different parts of the immunoglobulin molecule. Both flexibility and proteolytic digestion are facilitated by **proline** residues present in this part of the molecule.

CLASSIFICATION OF IMMUNOGLOBULINS

There are **five classes** of immunoglobulins, i.e. IgG, IgA, IgM, IgD and IgE, each one of which **differs** from the other with respect to the type of its **H chain**. Various immunoglobulin classes have different physiological functions (Table 29.4).

Ig class	Subclass	M_r (kD)	H chain	Carbohydrate content (%)	Serum concentration (mg/dl)	Distribution	Functions
IgG	IgG$_1$, IgG$_2$, IgG$_3$, IgG$_4$ (differing mainly in the hinge region)	146	γ	2–4	800–1500	Evenly between intravascular and extra-vascular pools	• Placental transfer • Provide immunity to neonate • Secondary immune response • Activation of classical complement pathway
IgA	IgA$_1$, IgA$_2$	160–380; monomer and dimer	α	5–9	150–250	Seromucous secretions	• Mucosal immunity
IgM	–	970; pentamer; presence of J chain	μ	8–12	70–150	Intravascular pool	• Synthesized in neonates • Primary immune response • Activation of classical complement pathway
IgD	–	160	δ	8–12	3–5	Surface of B cells	• B cell receptor
IgE	–	190	ε	10–15	0.01–0.05	Surface of basophils and mast cells	• Allergic reactions • Immunity against parasites • Release of histamine and other vasoactive molecules

Table 29.4: Immunoglobulin (Ig) classes

Secretory IgA (sIgA)

It is the most important form of IgA. It is called secretory IgA since it is the predominant immuno-globulin in **seromucous secretions**, such as tears, nasal secretions, saliva, colostrum, milk, intestinal, tracheobronchial and genitourinary secretions. It exists mainly in the **dimeric** form in association with another protein known as a **secretory component**. It is assembled during an active transport process as locally produced dimeric IgA passes across mucosal epithelium. It provides **mucosal immunity**, i.e. the initial defense against invading viral and bacterial pathogens, prior to their entry into the internal spaces. Its **deficiency** is the commonest disorder which results in **recurrent infections** of the sinuses and the respiratory tract.

IMMUNE RESPONSE: SALIENT FEATURES

Specificity and memory: An immune response consists of **two phases**. In the *first phase*, antigen activates specific lymphocytes that recognize it. In the *second phase* (the effector phase), these lymphocytes coordinate an immune response that eliminates the source of antigen. An adaptive response is highly specific for a particular pathogen. This type of immune response also remembers the infectious agent and prevents it from causing disease at a later stage. Thus, specificity and memory are **two essential features** of the adaptive immune response.

Primary immune response: When the body is exposed to an antigen for the first time, there is a latent phase followed by the generation of antibodies (immuno-globulins, mainly **IgM**) whose levels steadily increase, attain a steady state and **decline** thereafter. This is known as the primary immune response (Fig. 29.7).

Secondary immune response: On subsequent expo-sure to the same antigen, due to **immunologic memory**, the body mounts a stronger and better sustained immune response, mainly constituted by **IgG**. This is the secondary immune response (Fig. 29.7) which forms the basis for all **successful vaccinations (immunizations)**.

ANTIBODY DIVERSITY: BASIC CONCEPTS

Antibody diversity refers to the sum total of all the possible antibody specificities that an organism can make. A human can generate **billions** (10^7–10^8) of different antibody molecules by the mechanisms outlined below (Fig. 29.8):

1. **Limited germline DNA:** The immune system has a potential to produce more than a billion of different antibodies, enough to react with almost every antigen an organism encounters. A human,

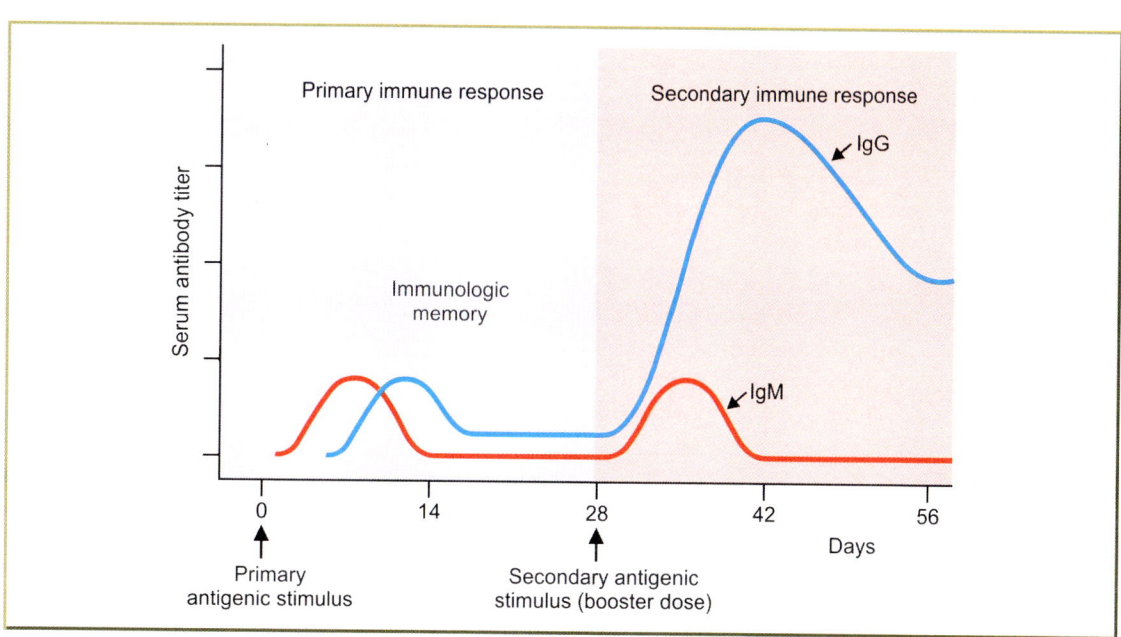

Fig. 29.7: Immune response.

29

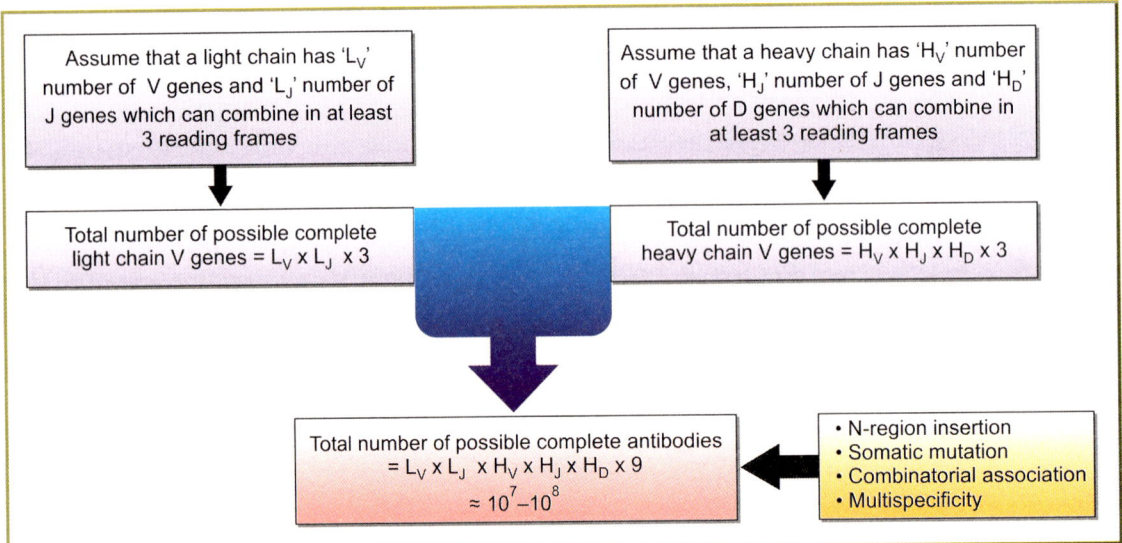

Fig. 29.8: Generation of antibody diversity.

however, does not contain that many numbers of genes so that each one of it can code for an individual immunoglobulin.

2. **Genetic rearrangement and recombination:** The generation of immense antibody diversity is achieved by the rearrangement and recombination of a limited number of gene segments, to produce a vast number of variable domains.

3. **Major structural genes:** A light chain of an immunoglobulin is a product of a cluster of three structural genes referred to as V, J and C gene segments, whereas a heavy chain is a product of the cluster of four structural genes referred to as V, J, C and D (diversity) gene segments.

4. **V genes:** A large number of V genes exist for each of λ, κ and heavy chains.

5. **V–J and V–D–J joining**: The region where the light chain V gene and J region, or the heavy chain V gene and D and J regions come together lies in the third hypervariable region. Since it is random which V and which J or D regions come together, a lot of diversity can be generated by V–J and V–D–J joining.

6. **Junctional diversity:** Additional diversity arises by errors that occur in the recombination event that brings the V region next to the J or D regions or the D region next to the J region (the recombination may occur in at least 3 reading frames).

7. **N-region insertion:** At the junction between D and J segments there is often an insertion of a series of nucleotides which is catalyzed by the enzyme terminal transferase without the need for a template. This leads to further diversity in the third hypervariable region.

8. **Somatic mutation:** It occurs in the V gene, particularly in the sequence encoding the hypervariable regions. It is a favorable mutation enhancing the antigen-antibody binding affinity, hence the phenomenon is also called affinity maturation.

9. **Combinatorial association:** Any B cell has the potential to synthesize any one of the possible heavy chains and any one of the possible light chains. Thus, different combinations of heavy and light chains within an individual B cell adds further diversity.

10. **Multispecificity:** Due to cross reactions between antigenic determinants of similar structure, an antibody may react with more than one antigenic determinant. Thus, multispecificity also contributes to antibody diversity.

CLASS SWITCHING

As mentioned above, B cells produce antibodies of five major classes. In addition, there are also four subclasses of IgG and two of IgA. Whereas all these classes/subclasses of immunoglobulins use the same set of variable region genes, the constant region genes, encoding different heavy chains, are responsible for the generation of antibody classes and subclasses.

These genes are clustered at the 3' end of the **immunoglobulin heavy chain (IGH) locus**, downstream of the J-segment genes, and appear in a determined sequence along chromosome 14. There is one gene for each of the IgM and IgE isotypes, one gene for each of the two IgA isotypes and one gene for each of the four different IgG isotypes.

Initially, B cells transcribe a VDJ gene and a μ gene for heavy chain that is spliced to produce mRNA for IgM. Upstream of the μ genes, there is a switch sequence (S), which is repeated upstream to each of the other constant region genes except δ and class switching occurs under the influence of T cells and cytokines. When class switching occurs, recombination between these regions takes place with the loss of the intervening C genes. After removal of introns during processing, mRNA for secreted IgM is produced. During B cell maturation, class-switch recombination occurs between the Sμ recombination region and a down-stream **switch region**. The intervening region (containing genes for other immunoglobulins) is looped out and then cut with the deletion of the intervening regions and joining of the two switch regions (Fig. 29.9).

Antibody Variants: Isotypes, Allotypes and Idiotypes

Isotypes: Isotypes are variants in molecules seen in all normal persons, e.g. classes and subclasses of immunoglobulins (IgG, IgM, IgA, etc.). Isotypic variation depends upon heavy chain make up such as IgG possesses the γ heavy chain isotype, IgM has μ, IgA has α, and so on. **Allotypes:** Allotypes represent slight differences in the amino acid sequences of heavy or light chains of different individuals (the differences are localized to the constant region of the heavy and light chains). The allotypes have been identified on the γ1, γ2, γ3, and α2 heavy chains, and on the κ light chain. Knowledge of allotypes is important in antibody engineering and development of monoclonal antibodies to improve immunotherapy.

Idiotypes: Idiotypes are the variations in the variable regions, particularly in the highly variable segments, of an antibody. These variations are individually specific to each immunoglobulin molecule and determine the binding specificity of the antigen-recognition site.

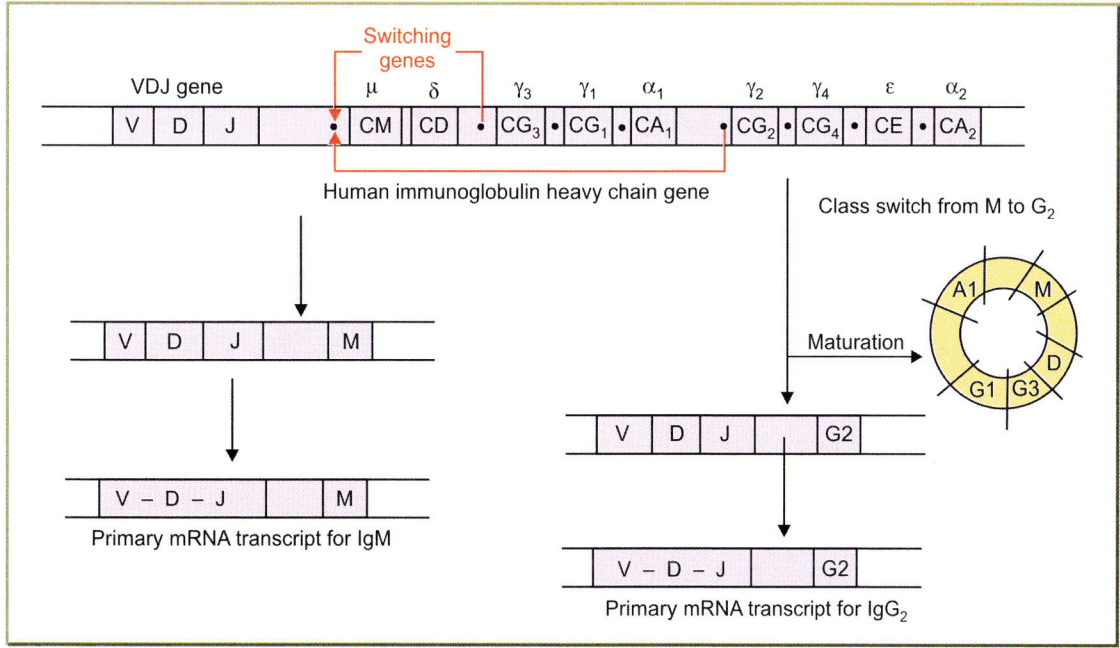

Fig. 29.9: Class switching from IgM to IgG$_2$.

29

POLYCLONAL ANTIBODIES

An antigen stimulates the production of antibodies by a mixture of B cells. These antibodies are called polyclonal antibodies since these are **directed against different epitopes** on the antigen and thus are not monospecific. Various immunoglobulins thus represent a **heterogeneous**, polyclonal mixture of antibodies. These are the products of **different clones of plasma cells**.

MONOCLONAL ANTIBODIES

Monospecificity: Benign or malignant proliferation of a **single clone** produces antibodies which are directed against the binding site for only **a particular epitope** of an antigen. Theses antibodies are called monoclonal antibodies, i.e. the antibodies of defined specificity, produced from an immortal clone of cells and are **homogeneous**.

Production: It is based on the **hybridoma technology** (Fig. 29.10):

- Immortal myeloma cells (B cells with the potential for unlimited replication but unable to produce antibodies) maintained in a tissue culture laboratory are **fused** with B cells isolated from the spleen of animal immunized with a particular antigen (against which monoclonal antibodies are desired to be produced).

- Normally, myeloma cells synthesize purines (required for DNA synthesis) by *de novo* pathway only since they lack the purine salvage pathway enzyme hypoxanthine guanine phosphoribosyl transferase (HGPRTase, hence these **myeloma cells are designated HGPRTase⁻**).

- The fused hybridoma cells are grown in 'HAT' (**h**ypoxanthine-**a**minopterin-**t**hymidine) medium. Aminopterin blocks the *de novo* pathway, therefore hybridoma cells are exclusively dependent on the salvage pathway for which HGPRTase gene is acquired from the splenocytes-derived HGPRTase⁺ B cells. Hypoxanthine and thymidine are the substrates for DNA synthesis.

Applications: Because of their **specificity**, monoclonal antibodies are used for various purposes:

1. To **detect and quantify various proteins** by Western blot or immunohistochemistry.
2. To determine the nature of the **infectious agent**, e.g. types of bacteria.
3. To **subclassify** both, normal and tumor cells, e.g. lymphocytes and leukemic cells.
4. As **immunotherapeutic agents** (Chemistry to Clinics 29.7).

IMMUNODEFICIENCY

An immunodeficiency disorder may affect the cellular and/or the humoral immunity. A **primary immuno-**

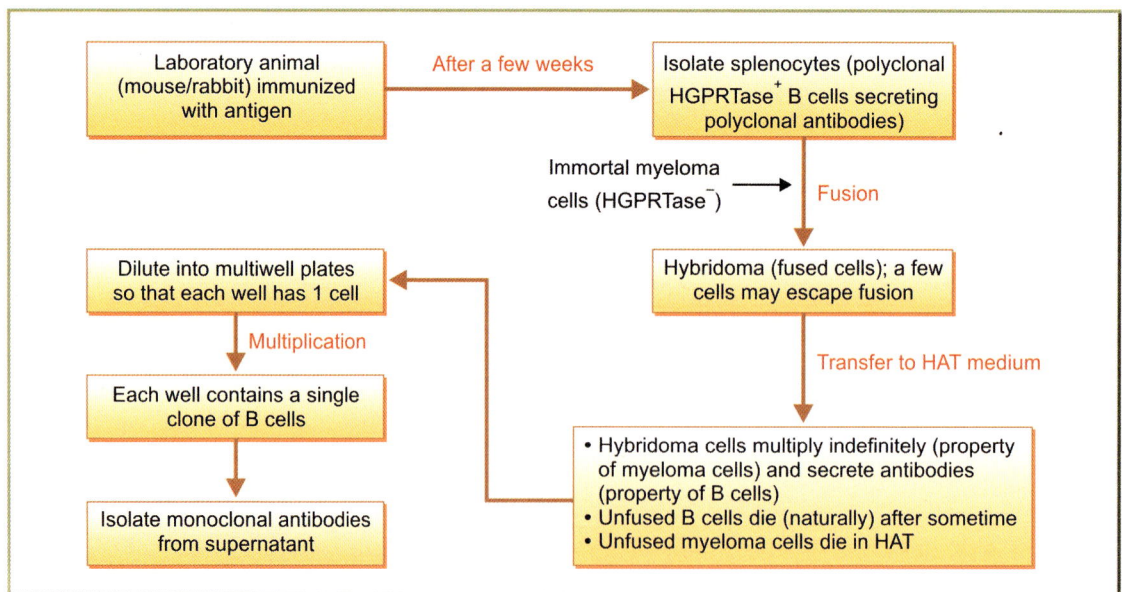

Fig. 29.10: Hybridoma technology.

Monoclonal antibodies target specific epitopes implicated in disease processes and hence are employed as drugs. By convention, the suffix 'mab' (for 'monoclonal antibody') is tagged with the drug. They are useful in the treatment of diverse clinical conditions:

1. Autoimmune diseases: Infliximab for Crohn's disease and rheumatoid arthritis.
2. Age-related macular degeneration: Ranibizumab.
3. Post-menopausal osteoporosis: Denosumab.
4. Allergic bronchial asthma: Omalizumab.
5. Renal transplant rejection: Muromomab.
6. Cancer: Trastuzumab (breast cancer), rituximab (lymphoma, leukemia).

The **advantages** of monoclonal antibodies over conventional drugs include:

1. Higher target specificity.
2. Lower systemic side effects.
3. Longer half-life.
4. Higher barrier for generic competition in the pharmaceutical industry.

deficiency results from an abnormality in the development of the immune mechanisms due to a specific genetic defect (involving lymphopoiesis, phagocytosis or complement) and is usually present **since birth** (Fig. 29.11). On the other hand, a **secondary immuno-deficiency** affects an already developed/mature immune system due to one or more **acquired cause(s)** (Table 29.5).

Table 29.5: Secondary immunodeficiency

- Malnutrition: ↓Ig synthesis
- Infection: Tuberculosis, HIV
- Renal disease: Proteinuria
- Malignancy: ↓Lymphocytes (leukemia), ↑abnormal Igs (multiple myeloma)
- Anticancer drugs: Bone marrow suppression
- Prolonged corticosteroid therapy: Immunosuppression
- Loss of self-regulation and targeting self-antigens: Autoimmunity

AUTOIMMUNE DISEASE

The immune system of the body is geared to detect an antigen that is foreign to the body, i.e. it distinguishes **self from the non-self** antigenic determinants so as to **avoid autoreactivity**. Due to various reasons, such as loss of self-tolerance, genetic mutation, interaction with drugs or certain types of infections, the immunological machinery of an individual sometimes starts forming **antibodies against one's own tissues or cells**. Such a disorder is referred to as an autoimmune disease.

Autoimmune diseases range from **single organ (or cell) type disorder** which involve specific immune reaction directed against only a particular organ or cell type (such as Graves' disease or insulin dependent diabetes mellitus) to **multisystem disease** which are characterized by lesions in many organs and are associated with multiple autoantibodies (e.g. rheumatoid arthritis). Some of the autoimmune diseases are listed in Table 29.6.

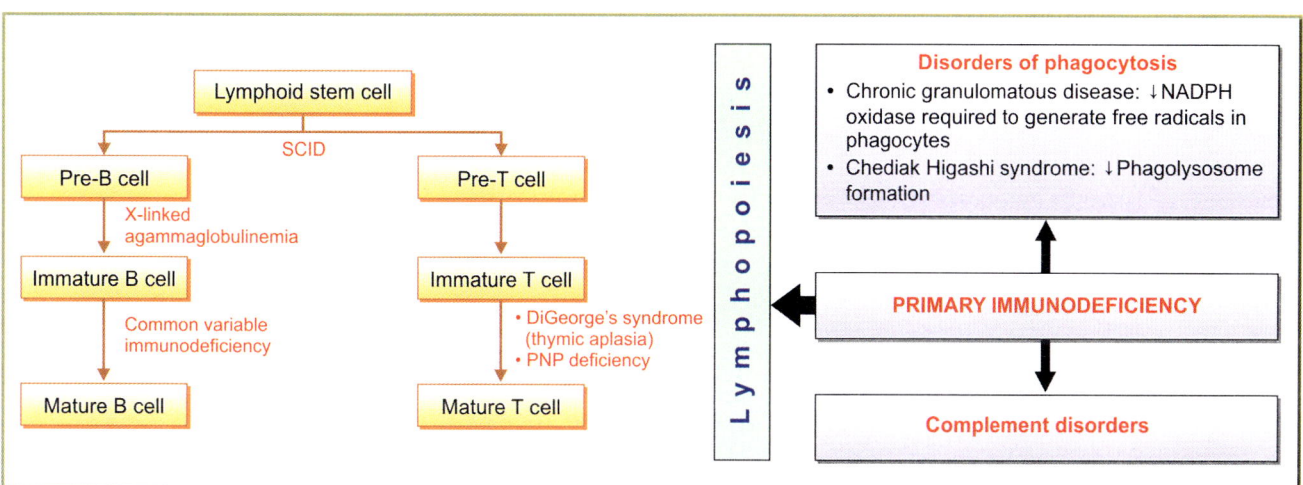

Fig. 29.11: Primary immunodeficiency. **SCID** (severe combined immunodeficiency due to adenosine deaminase deficiency involves both B and T lymphoid precursors) while **PNP** (purine nucleoside phosphorylase) deficiency involves immature T cells in the thymus.

29

Table 29.6: Some autoimmune diseases

Autoimmune disease	Target tissue	Effects
Graves' disease	Thyroid gland	↑ Thyroid hormone secretion
Insulin-dependent diabetes mellitus	Pancreatic β-cells	↓ insulin secretion
Addison's disease	Adrenal cortex	↑ Na$^+$ excretion, K$^+$ retention
Myasthenia gravis	Acetylcholine receptor at neuromuscular junctional synapse	Progressive muscle weakness
Rheumatoid arthritis	Joint connective tissue	Inflammation of joints (arthritis)
Systemic lupus erythematosus	Tissue components, e.g. DNA, phospho-lipids, etc.	Joint and muscle pain, anemia, neurological disturbance, etc.
Pernicious anemia	Gastric parietal cells or intrinsic factor	Megaloblastic anemia

AIDS

Acquired immunodeficiency syndrome (AIDS) is a viral disease caused by human T cell lymphotropic virus, called human immunodeficiency virus (HIV), with severe depletion of **CD4+ T cells** (Chapter 30).

IMMUNIZATION

One important **preventative** measure against the spreading of infectious diseases is immunization or vaccination. Vaccination has eradicated the poliovirus from the Western hemisphere and India. Great effort is currently being undertaken to develop vaccines against AIDS and malaria. The **principle** of vaccination is **to stimulate** the acquired immune system of the body to fight diseases or to provide 'ready-made' immunity.

Types of Immunization

1. **Passive immunization:** It involves the direct administration of antibodies or lymphocytes. These last only a few days and hence provide only transient protection. Nevertheless, it might be a life-saving measure in emergencies, as in the case of a person bitten by an animal with the rabies virus or a person having deep skin injuries with risk of tetanus.

2. **Active immunization:** It is necessary to provide long-term protection because it generates immuno-logical memory. To immunize against viral diseases, the vaccine generally contains an attenuated (weakened) or killed virus. The vaccine for immunization against bacterial diseases often contains only a portion of the bacteria. These vaccines can be generated by recombinant DNA technology, in which the gene coding for the pathogenic epitope of the bacteria is isolated and expressed in an appropriate host cell.

Vaccines

A wide range of antigen preparations are in use as vaccines, from whole organism to simple peptides, sugars and even DNA vaccines (Chapter 30). Living and nonliving vaccines have differences and the living vaccines are generally more effective. Nonspecific immunization, e.g. by cytokines, may be of use in selected conditions when it is desirable to boost general immune activity. Adjuvants, the substances that enhance antibody production, are usually required with nonliving vaccines.

Some of the commonly used vaccines are those against viral hepatitis B, rabies, influenza, pneumococci, measles, mumps, rubella, diphtheria, pertussis, tuberculosis, yellow fever, etc.

SOME IMPORTANT QUESTIONS

1. What are immunoglobulins? Describe the structure of an immunoglobulin.

2. Classify immunoglobulins. Describe the functions of each class of immunoglobulins.

3. Describe:

i. The action of papain and pepsin on an immunoglobulin molecule.
ii. Significance of the C_H regions in an immunoglobulin molecule.
iii. Antibody diversity
iv. Class switching
v. Autoimmune diseases
vi. Immune response

4. Write notes on:

i. Immunity
ii. Antigen
iii. Hapten
iv. Complement system
v. Hypervariable sequences
vi. Hinge region
vii. Monoclonal antibodies
viii. AIDS
ix. Immunization
x. Isotypes
xi. MHC
xii. Cluster of differentiation

MULTIPLE CHOICE QUESTIONS

1. **Administration of antitetanus serum (ATS) is an example of:**
   A. Natural active immunity
   B. Artificial active immunity
   C. Natural passive immunity
   D. Artificial passive immunity

2. **The following is an antigen presenting cell (APC):**
   A. T cell and B cell   B. Macrophage
   C. Dendritic cell   D. All of the above

3. **The following is true for a hapten:**
   A. Small molecule capable of acting as an epitope
   B. Elicits antibody response only when covalently linked to a carrier
   C. Can bind to antibody even after being detached from the carrier
   D. All of the above

4. **The accumulation of immune complexes in SLE is an example of hypersensitivity reaction type:**
   A. I   B. II
   C. III   D. IV

5. **The complement system participates in the following except:**
   A. Regulation of chemotaxis
   B. Clearance of immune complexes

   C. Type I hypersensitivity
   D. Antibody response

6. **Complementarity determining regions (CDR) in an Ig molecule refer to:**
   A. Hypervariable sequences in the V-region
   B. C_H region
   C. J chain
   D. C_L region

7. **The highest serum concentration is of:**
   A. IgE   B. IgD
   C. IgA   D. IgG

8. **The variation in different Ig H and L-chain classes and subclasses is called:**
   A. Isotype   B. Idiotype
   C. Allotype   D. Any of the above

9. **Monoclonal antibodies are used to:**
   A. Quantify proteins
   B. Detect microorganisms
   C. Classify normal and tumor cells
   D. All of the above

10. **The following is an autoimmune disease:**
    A. Folate deficiency anemia
    B. Pernicious anemia
    C. Iron deficiency anemia
    D. Hemorrhagic anemia

Acquired Immunodeficiency Syndrome

Acquired immunodeficiency syndrome (**AIDS**) is a viral disease characterized by profound immunosuppression, associated with opportunistic infections, secondary neoplasms and neurological manifestations. AIDS is caused by **human T cell lymphotropic virus, called human immuno-deficiency virus (HIV)**. There are two main variants, HIV-1 and HIV-2. HIV-2 is endemic is West Africa and appears to be less pathogenic.

HIV is a **retrovirus** (double-stranded RNA virus) possessing reverse transcriptase activity that binds to CD4 and **depletes CD4+ T cells**. Severe depletion of CD4+ cells results from a variety of mechanisms with drastic functional impairment of cell mediated immunity and death from opportunistic infections.

Problem Load

Since its first diagnosis in 1981, nearly 35 million people have died of AIDS.

Mode of Transmission

It is now well established that HIV is transmitted sexually, in blood or blood products, and perinatally. HIV infection cannot be transmitted by casual personal contact in home, workplace or school.

HUMAN IMMUNODEFICIENCY VIRUS

Structural Organization of the Virus

The HIV is roughly spherical with a diameter of 120 nm (Fig. 30.1).
- It is composed of **two copies of single-stranded RNA** enclosed in a protein capsid made of **p24**.

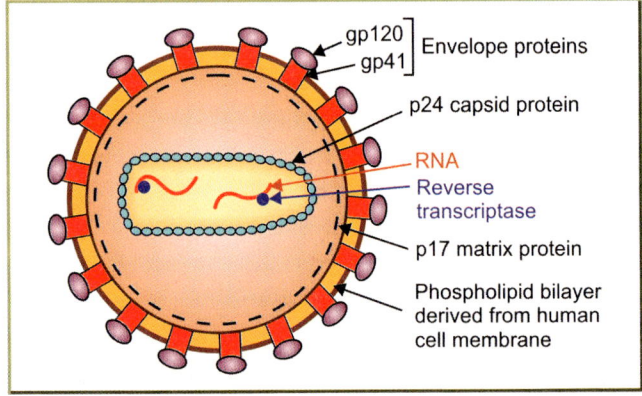

Fig. 30.1: Human immunodeficiency virus (HIV).

- Each RNA strand is associated with the enzymes crucial to the life cycle of the virus such as **reverse transcriptase, integrase, ribonuclease and proteases**.
- The capsid is again surrounded by a protein matrix made of **p17** that is enclosed in a phospholipid bilayer envelope derived from a human host cell membrane.
- Embedded in the viral envelope are Env proteins, each consisting of a cap made of three molecules of glycoprotein 120 (**gp120**) and a stem made up of three molecules of glycoprotein 41 (**gp41**).

Viral Tropism

The term viral tropism refers to which cell types the HIV infects. The virus can infect a variety of immune cells such as **CD4+ T lymphocytes, macrophages and microglial cells**.

- Viral entry into the target cells is mediated through the interaction of gp120 with its receptors, i.e. the CD4+ molecules, besides some co-receptors.
- A commonly employed co-receptor is the β-chemokine receptor **CCR5** (CC chemokine receptor 5). The CC chemokine proteins have 2 adjacent cysteine residues near their amino terminus. Interestingly, people with a specific mutation known as **CCR5-Δ32, are resistant to HIV**.

Viral Replication

- Following the binding of gp120 with its receptors, the viral envelope **fuses** with the host cell membrane with the release of capsid, RNA and associated viral enzymes into the cytosol (Fig. 30.2).
  - The reverse transcriptase liberates the single-stranded RNA from the attached viral proteins and copies it into a **complementary DNA molecule**. The reverse transcription is **extremely error-prone** and the resulting mutations play an important role in allowing the virus to **evade the immune system as well as in the development of drug resistance**.

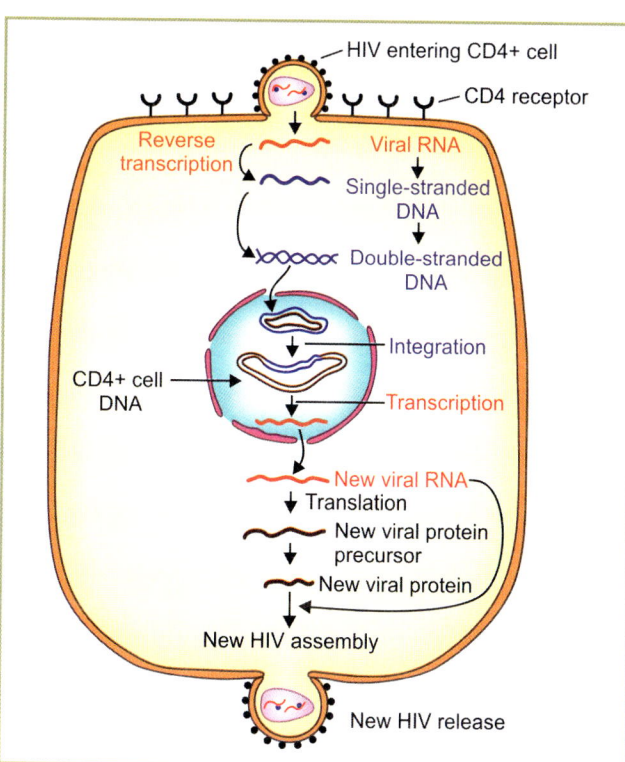

Fig. 30.2: HIV replication.

- The reverse transcriptase also has ribonuclease activity that degrades the viral RNA during the synthesis of cDNA.
  - Further, it possesses DNA-dependent DNA polymerase activity that copies the sense cDNA strand into an antisense DNA.
  - Together, the cDNA and its complement form a double-stranded viral DNA that is then transported to the host cell nucleus. All these events occur during the microtubule-based transport of the viral contents from the host cell membrane to the nucleus.
- The **incorporation of the viral DNA into the host cell genome** is carried out by the viral integrase.
  - This integrated viral DNA may lie **dormant**, explaining the **latent stage** of HIV infection.
  - On the other hand, during **active viral replication**, the integrated viral DNA is transcribed into mRNA which leaves the nucleus and is translated to form viral polyproteins, which are appropriately cleaved by the viral proteases into individual functional proteins, including the viral enzymes.
- Finally, the entire virus is **assembled and released**, ready to infect another cell (Fig. 30.2).

Clinical Presentation

The series of events discussed above may be clinically silent for a long time, known as the HIV latency. However, at one stage the CD4+ cell count is drastically reduced and the individual becomes symptomatic (Chemistry to Clinics 30.1).

Laboratory Diagnosis

- HIV-1 testing consists of **initial screening** with an enzyme-linked immunosorbent assay (ELISA) to detect serum antibodies to HIV-1. 'Non-reactive' results are considered HIV-negative.

Chemistry to Clinics 30.1: Immunosuppression in AIDS

Both the cellular as well as the humoral immune response are compromised in HIV infection. Profound immunosuppression results in opportunistic infections and in some cases, cancer. Microbial and/or tumor antigens trigger an inappropriate immune response which sets up a vicious cycle, completing the full-blown picture of acquired immunodeficiency syndrome (AIDS) (Fig. 30.3).

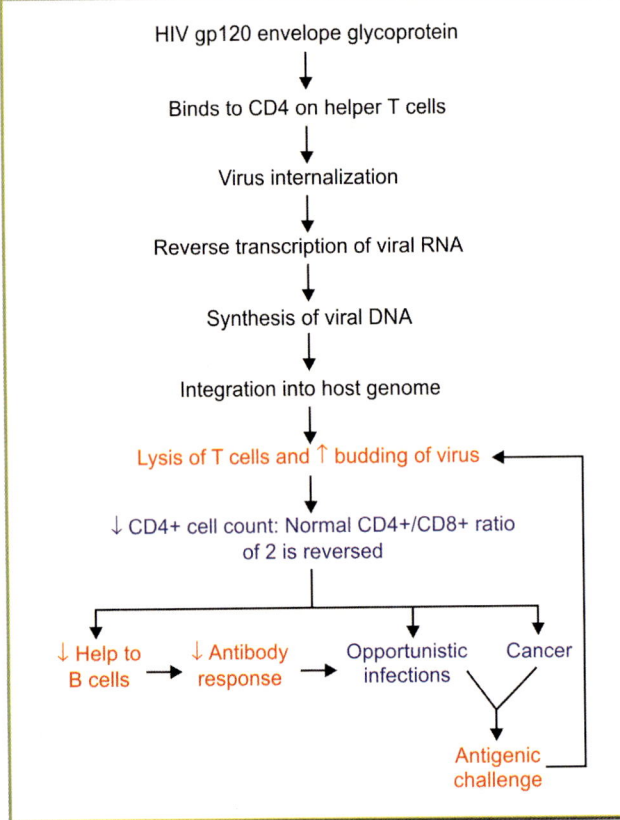

HIV gp120 envelope glycoprotein

↓

Binds to CD4 on helper T cells

↓

Virus internalization

↓

Reverse transcription of viral RNA

↓

Synthesis of viral DNA

↓

Integration into host genome

↓

Lysis of T cells and ↑ budding of virus ←

↓

↓ CD4+ cell count: Normal CD4+/CD8+ ratio of 2 is reversed

↓ Help to B cells → ↓ Antibody response → Opportunistic infections   Cancer

Antigenic challenge

Fig. 30.3: Biochemical-clinical correlations in HIV infection.

- Samples with a 'reactive' ELISA are **re-tested in duplicate**.
- If the result of either duplicate test is reactive, the sample is reported to be '**repeatedly reactive**' and undergoes confirmatory testing with a more specific test such as Western blot.
- **Only when a sample is repeatedly reactive by ELISA and reactive by Western blot, it is considered HIV-positive**.

Sometimes, repeatedly reactive ELISA samples provide inconclusive results on Western blot. This is either due to an incomplete antibody response to HIV in an infected person or non-specific reactions in an uninfected person.

- A repeat ELISA and Western blot is recommended after at least one month.
- Alternatively, more sophisticated tests such as **immunofluorescence assay or nucleic acid extraction/amplification** may provide confirmatory results.

PREVENTION

Role of DNA Vaccines

In the fight against AIDS worldwide, several clinical trials are underway using another type of vaccine, DNA plasmid vaccine. In this case, the gene(s) that encode protein(s) of pathogens (the HIV in this case) are propagated in bacteria as plasmid DNA. When injected in humans, it is taken up by antigen-presenting cells, which then produce the encoded protein. This antigenic protein elicits an immune response just as a conventional vaccine does.

Advantages of DNA Vaccine over Conventional Vaccine

1. **Preferable** for protection against HIV, in which inoculation with a dead or attenuated virus is risky.
2. Activate both **cellular and humoral immune responses**. This is advantageous because live viral vaccines induce the cellular response only, whereas vaccines containing killed microorganisms or their subunits induce the humoral response only.
3. The **stability** of DNA vaccines at ambient temperatures makes them useable in areas where constant refrigeration of the vaccine, i.e. the maintenance of a cold chain, is not possible.
4. **Cheaper and easier to produce** than conventional vaccines.
5. Can be **manipulated** by the tools of recombinant technology.

Drawbacks of DNA Vaccine

1. Risk of **integration into human chromosomal DNA** which could induce cancer as a result of the disruption of a cell division gene or the activation of an oncogene.
2. Risk of **failure to terminate its action**; continuous antigenic stimulation may lead to immune tolerance or autoimmunity.
3. The potential induction of **antibodies** against the plasmid DNA which might lead to autoimmune diseases.

TREATMENT

A suitable vaccine remains elusive despite >30 years of research. The current treatment consists of 'highly active antiretroviral therapy (**HAART**)'. A combination of drugs is used such as:

30

1. Nucleoside analog reverse transcriptase inhibitors.
2. Non-nucleoside reverse transcriptase inhibitors.
3. Protease inhibitors.
4. Virus entry inhibitors.

These drugs intercept the virus at **different stages of its life cycle** (Fig. 30.3). However, drug treatment fails to eradicate the virus from the patient.

Problems in HIV Treatment

The treatment of AIDS is an uphill task because:

1. The **rate of mutation in HIV is higher** than that seen in most living organisms. Thus, new genetic variants emerge rapidly so that different patients with HIV harbor **different strains** of HIV.

2. For the same reason, HIV **rapidly evolves resistance to new treatment** in a given patient.

3. There is a large time interval between an individual getting infected with HIV and the onset of symptoms of AIDS. During this **latent period**, the viral concentration in the blood is low because although huge numbers of viruses are produced, they are destroyed by the host immune system. It means that by the time the clinical symptoms of AIDS appear, the immune system has collapsed and drug resistant viral strains are already prevailing.

4. Treatment-related **side effects** often force patients to discontinue the medications.

5. **Social stigmas** related to the disease.

SOME IMPORTANT QUESTIONS

1. Briefly discuss the biochemical basis of the entry of HIV into the host cell.

2. Briefly discuss the role of DNA vaccines in the prevention of HIV.

3. What are the problems in the development of an effective anti-HIV vaccine?

4. What are the targets in HIV that are exploited for treatment?

MULTIPLE CHOICE QUESTIONS

1. **HIV contains:**
   A. ssRNA
   B. dsRNA
   C. ssDNA
   D. dsDNA

2. **HIV reverse transcriptase has the following activity:**
   A. Transcription of viral RNA to cDNA
   B. Ribonuclease
   C. DNA dependent DNA polymerase
   D. All of the above

3. **Following is an advantage of a DNA vaccine over a conventional vaccine against HIV:**
   A. Stable at high temperature
   B. Cheaper and easy to manipulate by recombinant DNA technology
   C. Induce cellular as well as humoral immunity
   D. All of the above

4. **The following drug classes are employed under 'HAART':**
   A. Reverse transcriptase inhibitors
   B. Protease inhibitors
   C. Virus entry inhibitors
   D. All of the above

5. **The HIV capsid protein is:**
   A. p24
   B. gp120
   C. gp41
   D. p17

Metabolism of Xenobiotics

The term xenobiotic means a foreign substance, excluding antigen, which enters the body by various routes such as by inhalation of the polluted air, e.g. industrial chemicals (Chemistry to Clinics 31.1) and automobile exhaust; ingestion of contaminated food, such as those contaminated with pesticides, insecticides or herbicides; food additives including colors and sweeteners like butter yellow, azo dye or saccharin; cosmetics such as hair dyes, sprays or lipstick and drugs such as aspirin, tranquilizers or oral contraceptives. Besides, these also include some of the toxic metabolites which are formed by the action of bacteria on food in the gastrointestinal tract, such as amines produced by the decarboxylation of the unabsorbed amino acids (Table 31.1).

There are also certain endogenous substances which are produced in the body, i.e. bilirubin produced during normal metabolism of the red blood cells or phenols produced in the large intestine by the action of bacteria on tryptophan. Most of these compounds are highly lipophilic. These may accumulate within the cells and interfere with cellular functions over a period of time.

Biotransformation versus Detoxification

The ability of the body to convert a xenobiotic into its excretory metabolite is called **biotransformation** (Fig. 31.1). It includes all those biochemical changes which convert a xenobiotic (not ordinarily utilized) to the excretory product. Though not always true, majority of these metabolites are **more acidic, less toxic and more water soluble** than the xenobiotics themselves. Because the **toxicity** of the original xenobiotic is **abolished or reduced**, the process of biotransformation is sometimes called **detoxification**.

On the other hand, certain xenobiotics, e.g. some drugs, are administered as a precursor (prodrug) which is **activated** in the body to the active drug. This is an example of biotransformation but not detoxification.

SITES OF METABOLISM OF XENOBIOTICS

The tissues at the portal of entry into or exit from the body are important in the detoxification of xenobiotics, with **liver being the major organ** (Fig. 31.2). Generally, metabolites produced by the liver are relatively more

Table 31.1: Sources of xenobiotics

Sources	Examples
Industrial chemicals	Solvents (benzene, carbon tetrachloride) Detergents Bleaching agents
Air pollutants	Tobacco smoke
Food additives and contaminants	Colors (butter yellow, azo dye) Sweeteners (saccharin) Insecticides
Bacterial metabolites	Bacterial toxins
Cosmetics	Lipstick, hair dyes, body sprays
Drugs	Aspirin, tranquilizers, oral contraceptives

Chemistry to Clinics 31.1: Industrial Chemicals as Xenobiotics
On December 3, 1984, thousands of people died (and even more lie affected till today) in Bhopal (Madhya Pradesh, India) following exposure to the gas methyl isocyanate. The gas, normally used to prepare a pesticide called carbaryl, leaked from a chemical factory in the city. The Bhopal tragedy is known as the 'Hiroshima of the Chemical Industry'.

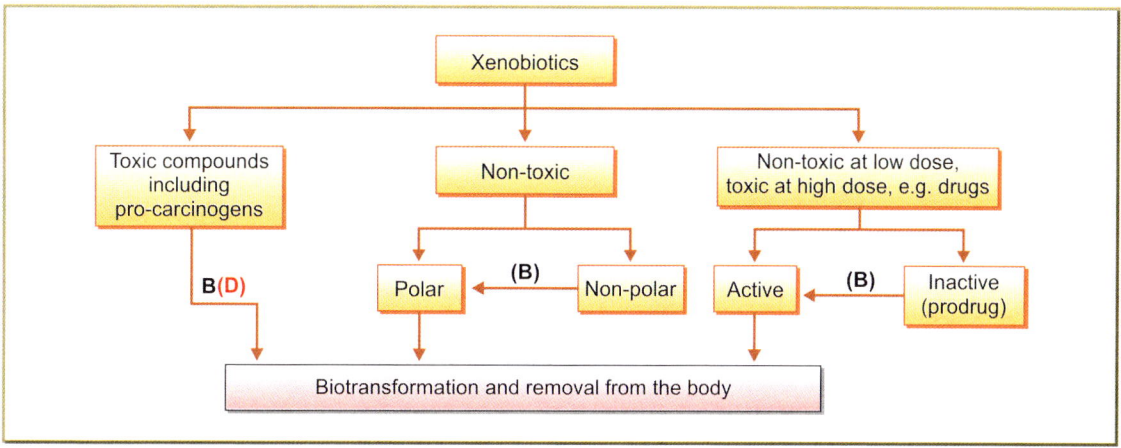

Fig. 31.1: Detoxification (D) is a type of biotransformation (B) of some xenobiotics.

water soluble and pass via blood to the kidney for excretion. Some of the metabolites may also be excreted via feces, bile or the expired air. A small portion of the metabolite may also return to the intestine, by enterohepatic circulation. A xenobiotic or its metabolite may also bind to a cellular macromolecule such as DNA, RNA or protein and may be retained in the tissues. The binding of a xenobiotic or its metabolite, however, can cause serious consequences, such as mutations.

MECHANISMS OF METABOLISM OF XENOBIOTICS

Several biochemical transformations are used by the liver for the detoxification of xenobiotics, and are classified into two groups (Fig. 31.3):

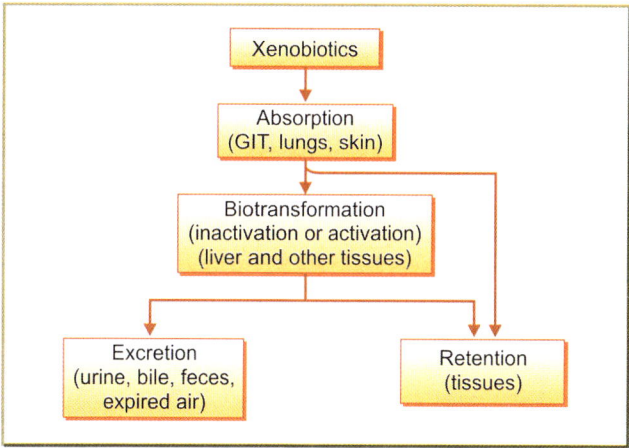

Fig. 31.2: Sites of metabolism of xenobiotics.

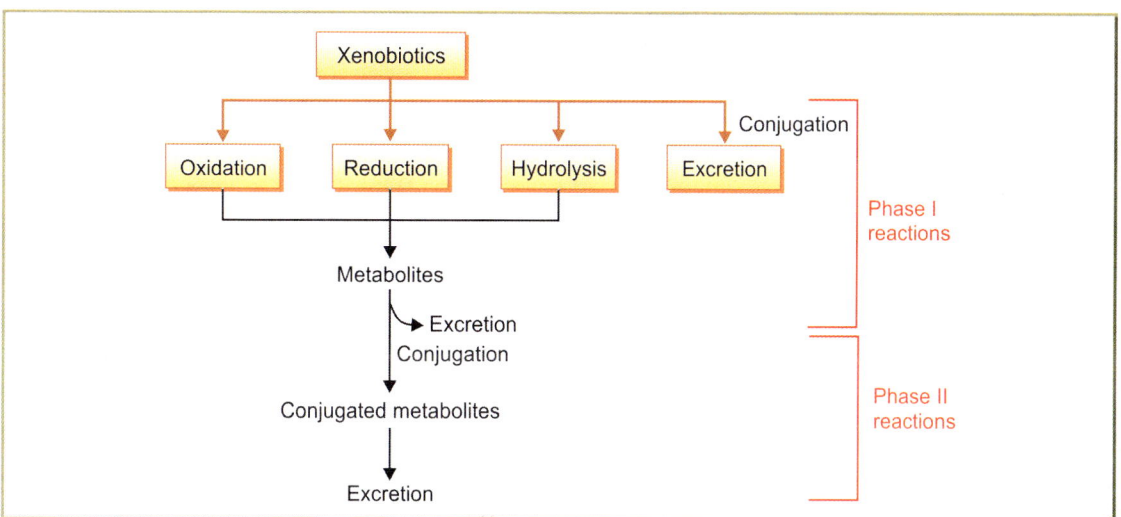

Fig. 31.3: Mechanisms of biotransformation of xenobiotics.

31

1. Phase I reactions: A xenobiotic may undergo oxidation (hydroxylation), reduction or hydrolysis and the metabolite so produced may either be excreted as such or undergoes phase II of the metabolism.

- **Oxidation:** Compounds detoxified by the oxidative processes include alcohols, aldehydes, amines and their derivatives, aromatic hydrocarbons, and certain drugs.
  - **Alcohols:** Aliphatic as well as aromatic alcohols are oxidized to their corresponding acids.
    Methanol → Formic acid
    Ethanol → Acetic acid
    Benzyl alcohol → Benzoic acid (Fig. 31.4).
  - **Aldehydes:** These are also oxidized to their corresponding acids.
    Benzaldehyde → Benzoic acid
    Trichloroaldehyde → Trichloroacetic acid
  - **Amines:** *Primary aliphatic amines* are oxidized to their acids and liberate ammonia.
    $RCH_2 \cdot NH_2 \rightarrow R \cdot COOH$ + Ammonia
  - On the other hand, *aromatic amines* are oxidized to phenols (Fig. 31.5).
  - **Anilides:** These are oxidized to the corresponding phenols, e.g. acetanilide to ρ-acetyl-amino phenol.
  - **Aromatic hydrocarbons:** These are oxidized to phenols, e.g. oxidation of benzene produces several aromatic alcohols such as phenols, quinols and catechols. The process thus involves the introduction of an –OH group (hydroxylation) onto the aromatic ring. This, in turn, provides a site for the attachment of a conjugating group in the phase II reaction.

Some **epoxides** formed during the oxidation of xenobiotics are strong electrophiles and hence are very reactive. These may be converted to relatively inactive hydroxyl compounds by the enzyme epoxide hydrolase, which in turn, provides an –OH group for the conjugating molecule (Fig. 31.6).

  - **Drugs:** Some drugs may be oxidized to their hydroxy derivatives, e.g.
    Meprobamate → Hydroxymeprobamate

Role of Cytochrome P450 in Oxidative Metabolism of Xenobiotics: Oxidation of xenobiotics is mainly dependent upon a special class of cytochromes collectively referred to as cytochrome P450 whose salient features include that:

1. These are **hemoproteins**.
2. The number **450 refers to the absorption peak**, as the enzyme when exposed to carbon monoxide, exhibits a distinct peak at 450 nm.

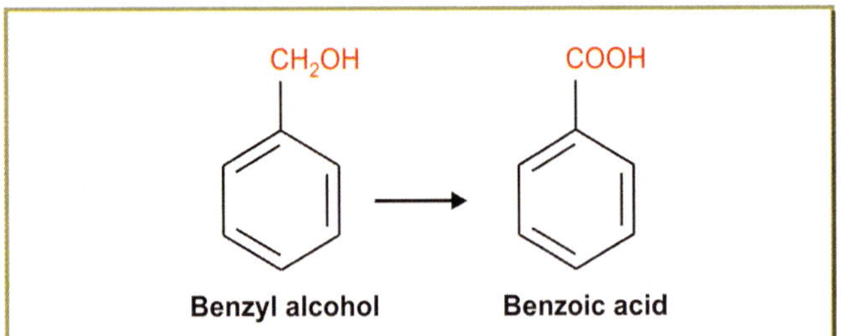

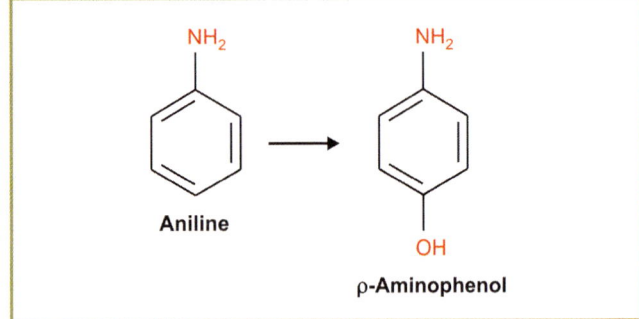

CH$_2$OH → COOH

Benzyl alcohol   Benzoic acid

Fig. 31.4: Oxidation of an aromatic alcohol to acid.

NH$_2$ → NH$_2$

Aniline   OH   ρ-Aminophenol

Fig. 31.5: Oxidation of an aromatic amine to alcohol.

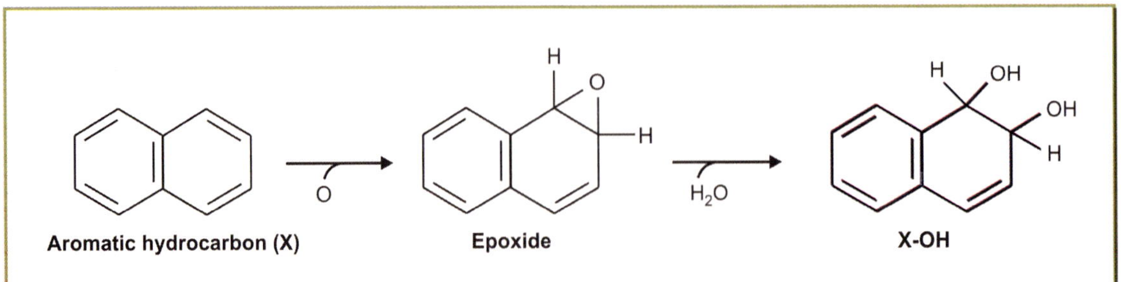

Aromatic hydrocarbon (X) → Epoxide → X-OH (H$_2$O)

Fig. 31.6: Metabolism of an aromatic hydrocarbon (X).

3. Cytochrome P450 **oxidizes a variety of xeno-biotics**, particularly lipophilic compounds such as drugs, carcinogens, pesticides, petroleum products and pollutants.

4. Due to subtle differences in their protein moiety, **multiple forms** of cytochrome P450 are known to exist.

5. All forms of cytochrome P450 are **mono-oxygenases** requiring atmospheric oxygen and NADPH, i.e. the enzyme utilizes one atom of oxygen to form water while the other atom of oxygen is used to form an oxidized derivative of the xenobiotic. Due to their dual function, as well as dual fate of oxygen, these mono-oxygenases are also designated as **mixed function oxidases**. The addition of a hydroxyl group to the substrate makes the compound more polar.

6. Cytochrome P450 is located in the **smooth endoplasmic reticulum** in most of the tissues but **liver** contains it in highest amount.

7. These mono-oxygenases often exhibit **broad substrate specificity** and many of these are **inducible** enzymes, i.e. these are synthesized by cells in response to the nature of a chemical inducing their formation (Chemistry to Clinics 31.2).

8. In addition to hydroxylation, cytochrome P450 is also involved in deamination, desulfuration, epoxidation and peroxygenation of certain xenobiotics.

Cytochrome P448: Metabolism of polycyclic aromatic hydrocarbons and related molecules require another isoform of cytochrome P450 called as cytochrome P448. These enzymes are also designated as aromatic hydrocarbon hydroxylases (Chemistry to Clinics 31.3).

Chemistry to Clinics 31.2: Drug Interactions due to Enzyme Induction

Hydroxylation is the main metabolic pathway for ethinyl estradiol, one of the constituents of oral contraceptive pills (OCPs). Rifampicin, an antitubercular drug, induces cytochrome P450 enzymes in the liver, which results in increased hepatic hydroxylation of estrogens. This reduces plasma estradiol levels and thus its efficacy. It may result in contraceptive failure in female patients suffering from tuberculosis, taking rifampicin and OCPs concomitantly.

Chemistry to Clinics 31.3: Tobacco Smoking and Cytochrome P448
Smokers have higher levels of cytochrome P448 enzymes in some of their tissues particularly the lungs because it is involved in the conversion of an inactive polycyclic aromatic hydrocarbon (procarcinogen) inhaled by smoke, to active carcinogen by the hydroxylation reaction in the lungs.

- **Reduction:** Some of the xenobiotics during the course of their detoxification, undergo reduction, e.g.

    Picric acid → Picramic acid

    Trichloroacetaldehyde → Trichloroethanol

    Sometimes, a reduced metabolite may be more toxic than the original xenobiotic, e.g. prontosil (an azo red dye) is reduced to the more toxic sulfanilamide.

- **Hydrolysis:** Some of the xenobiotics, particularly certain therapeutic compounds, undergo hydrolysis during the course of their detoxification, e.g. aspirin, procaine, etc.

    Aspirin (acetylsalicylic acid) → Acetate + Salicylic acid

    Procaine → ρ-Aminobenzoic acid + Diethyl-aminoethanol

    Aspirin (acetylsalicylic acid) undergoes hydrolysis and produces acetate and salicylic acid. Acetate so formed may be either oxidized or used for the synthesis of various physiological compounds. On the other hand, salicylic acid is excreted by the kidneys after conjugation with glucuronic acid.

    Though some xenobiotics may undergo conjugation directly and the conjugate, so produced, is excreted as such without under-going a preliminary reaction in phase I but conjugation, more often, occurs as a phase II reaction (Fig. 31.3).

2. **Phase II reactions:** A metabolite of the phase I reaction is subsequently conjugated with some other compound (such as glycine) or group (like a methyl group). Conjugation makes the molecule **more polar and highly water soluble** which can be easily excreted from the body. Most of the conjugation reactions are synthetic processes and thus require energy.

    The conjugation of a xenobiotic (X) with the conjugating molecule (Y) can occur via two different pathways, i.e. either the X or the Y gets activated

31

and subsequently conjugates with the other molecule:

$$X \rightarrow X\sim \rightarrow X\sim Y$$
$$Y \rightarrow \sim Y \rightarrow X\sim Y$$

Compounds used for conjugation include readily available reactants such as glutathione, amino acids like glycine or glutamine, glucuronate (as UDP glucuronic acid), a sulfate group, an acetyl group or a methyl group.

- **Conjugation with Glucuronic Acid:** Glucuronic acid is an oxidation product of glucose. It participates in detoxification reactions as UDP glucuronic acid which gets conjugated with a xenobiotic (X-OH) and forms a highly soluble excretory glucuronide (X-O-glucuronide). The reaction is catalyzed by **UDP-glucuronyl transferase** present both in the endoplasmic reticulum as well as cytosol of many tissues but mainly in the liver (Fig. 31.7).

  Various compounds such as benzoic acid, morphine, methanol and camphor are excreted in conjugation with glucuronic acid. Endogenously produced bilirubin is also conjugated in the liver with glucuronic acid.

  Benzoic acid + UDP-glucuronic acid → benzoyl glucuronide + UDP

  Bilirubin + UDP-glucuronic acid → bilirubin monoglucuronide

  Bilirubin monoglucuronide + UDP-glucuronic acid → bilirubin diglucuronide + UDP

- **Conjugation with Glutathione:** A wide range of organic compounds which are toxic electrophiles such as aromatic halogenated compounds, aliphatic halides, sulfates, nitrocompounds and carcinogenic epoxides (formed from polycyclic hydrocarbons) are excreted after conjugation with the cysteinyl moiety of glutathione (a tripeptide of glutamate, cysteine and glycine). A xenobiotic (H-X) after conjugation with glutathione, forms mercapturic acid. The reaction is catalyzed by a group of enzymes referred to as glutathione-S-transferases. These are present in various tissues with high amounts in the liver cytosol.

  – In the initial reaction, reduced glutathione (GSH) reacts with an electrophilic centre on the xenobiotic.

  – The glutamyl- and glycinyl-groups are sequentially removed.

  – Subsequently, an acetyl group is added (from acetyl CoA) to the amino group of the remaining cysteinyl-residue which is bound to the xenobiotic (X-cysteine).

  – The resulting compound, a mercapturic acid, i.e. a conjugate of acetylcysteine, is excreted in the urine (Fig. 31.8).

Due to conjugation with glutathione, large doses of some of the drugs such as paracetamol, leads to depletion of glutathione in the liver (Chemistry to Clinics 31.4).

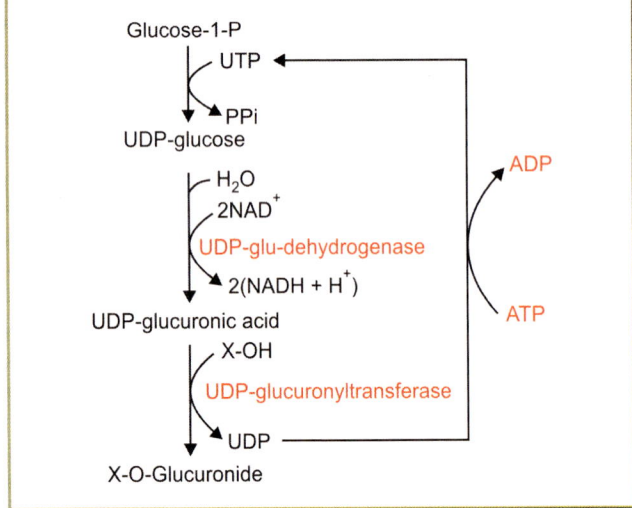

Fig. 31.7: Conjugation of xenobiotic (X-OH) with glucuronic acid.

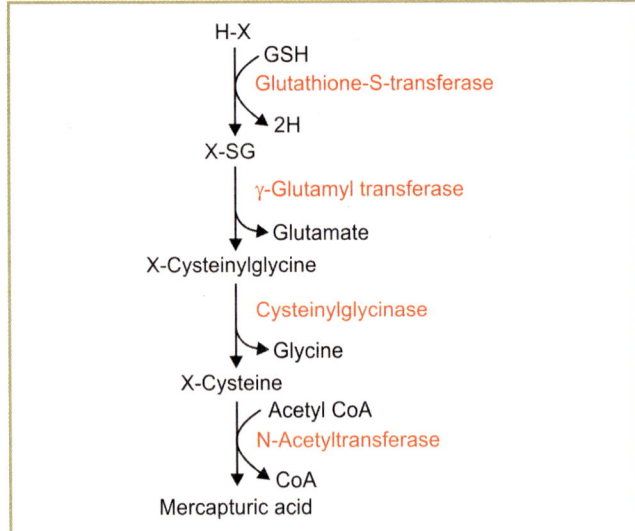

Fig. 31.8: Conjugation of xenobiotic (H-X) with glutathione (GSH).

Chemistry to Clinics 31.4: Paracetamol Poisoning

Paracetamol is the most popular antipyretic (a drug used to treat pyrexia, i.e. fever). It is metabolized mainly in the liver. An overdose of paracetamol generates excess of free radicals in the hepatocytes. Reduced glutathione (GSH), the most important intracellular antioxidant, is depleted in its effort to detoxify the free radicals because it gets oxidized in the process (forming oxidized glutathione, GSSG). The free radicals thus cause widespread cell injury which may be fatal if not timely treated. Prompt administration of N-Acetylcysteine, a sulfhydryl (–SH) donor, replenishes the intracellular pool of GSH thereby restoring the antioxidant capacity of hepatocytes. This helps to recover from paracetamol poisoning.

- **Conjugation with Glycine:** Glycine conjugates with many aromatic carboxylic acids, e.g. benzoic acid, cholic acid, etc. Glycine conjugates are harmless compounds and are excreted in the urine.

  Benzoic acid + Glycine → Benzoyl glycine (Hippuric acid)

  Cholic acid + Glycine → Glycocholic acid

- **Conjugation with Glutamine:** Phenylacetic acid is detoxified by conjugation with glutamine.

  Phenylacetic acid + Glutamine → Phenylacetylglutamine

- **Conjugation with Sulfate:** Biosynthesis of a sulfate ester requires a high energy sulfate donor, i.e. 3'-phosphoadenosine-5'-phosphosulfate (**PAPS** or **active sulfate**). Transfer of sulfate group from active sulfate to various acceptors such a phenol and indole, is catalyzed by specific sulftransferases.

- **Conjugation with Acetate:** As for other acetylation reactions, active acetate (acetyl CoA) is used as an acetyl donor. Acetylation of a xenobiotic is catalyzed by acetyltransferases present in the cytosol of various tissues, mainly in the liver. Many drugs such as sulfanilamide and isoniazid are metabolized by acetylation (Chemistry to Clinics 31.5).

- **Conjugation with a Methyl Group:** The methyl group of S-adenosylmethionine (**SAM or active methionine**) is used by methyltransferases to methylate a xenobiotic, mainly various pyridine derivatives. Many of the methylated products though are less toxic than the parent xenobiotic, some of these however, are more toxic, e.g. excess dose of nicotinamide after methylation is

Chemistry to Clinics 31.5: Acetylation and Drug Toxicity

1. Some of the acetylated products of the drugs such as acetyl sulfanilamide are less soluble than the xenobiotic (sulfanilamide) itself. It gets deposited in the kidney and may cause renal failure.
2. Isoniazid (isonicotinic acid hydrazide, INH), an antitubercular drug, is inactivated in the liver via acetylation. The rate of acetylation is genetically determined. Fast acetylation leads to higher plasma levels of the toxic metabolite acetyl isoniazid and thus to an increase in toxic reactions, e.g. hepatitis which is more common than in slow acetylators. On the other hand, patients with the slow acetylator genotype have higher plasma INH levels and tend to develop neuropathy.

converted to a more toxic product (methylnicotinamide).

LIMITATIONS OF BIOTRANSFORMATION: GLOBAL WARMING

The above discussion does not imply an indefinite capacity of tissues such as the liver, to handle and biotransform xenobiotics such as industrial pollutants, which continue to increase day by day. Global warming refers to the adverse climate change caused by the trapping of **'greenhouse gases'**, affecting the entire ecosystem and posing serious health hazards. Naturally occurring green house gases such as carbon dioxide, water vapor, methane, nitrous oxide and ozone should be present at optimum levels in the atmosphere to keep the earth warm enough to sustain life. This is called the **normal greenhouse effect**. However, certain human activities lead to an **enhanced greenhouse effect** and contribute to **global warming**. These include the burning of fossil fuels (coal, oil and natural gas), solid waste and wood; deforestation; and industrial production of perfluorocarbons and sulfur hexafluoride.

Major health hazards of global warming include:

1. An increase in the incidence of infectious diseases especially those which are vector-borne.
2. Since the cardiovascular system has to work harder to keep the body cool under hot climatic conditions, cardiovascular diseases, heat stroke and renal stones are likely to increase.
3. High air temperature increases the ozone concentration at ground level and ozone is a known respiratory pollutant.
4. Adverse effects on agriculture and rise in sea level may encourage malnutrition and the

31

extinction of those species who fail to adapt to the changing climatic conditions. In fact, the long-term serious consequences to human health may threaten our very existence on this planet.

Countermeasures to facilitate living in hotter temperature actually consume more electricity from power plants that consume fossil fuels. This adds on to the global warming and initiates a vicious cycle. The only **practical remedies** are:

1. To economize the use of fossil fuels.

2. Use energy-efficient products such as compact fluorescent bulbs and solar heaters.
3. Planting more trees.
4. Recycling papers and plastics.
5. Avoid wastage of food and water.

The first global agreement, known as the **Copenhagen Accord**, to comprehensively influence the flow and share of natural resources, was agreed upon by more than 25 countries in December 2009 at Copenhagen, Denmark.

SOME IMPORTANT QUESTIONS

1. What are xenobiotics? Discuss various mechanisms of xenobiotic metabolism.

2. Write notes on:
   i. Biotransformation of xenobiotics.
   ii. Mechanisms of xenobiotic detoxification.
   iii. Role of cytochrome P450 in oxidative metabolism of xenobiotics.
   iv. Cytochrome P448.
   v. Phase II reactions of xenobiotic detoxification.
   vi. Role of glucuronic acid in xenobiotic metabolism.
   vii. Role of glutathione in xenobiotic metabolism.
   viii. Acetylation and drug toxicity.

MULTIPLE CHOICE QUESTIONS

1. **Bhopal gas tragedy is attributed to the inhalation of:**
   A. Hydrogen sulphide
   B. Dichloromethane
   C. Methyl isocyanate
   D. Carbon monoxide

2. **During phase I xenobiotic metabolism, aromatic hydrocarbons are converted to:**
   A. Ketones
   B. Aldehydes
   C. Acids
   D. Phenols

3. **Cytochrome P450 participates in:**
   A. Hydroxylation   B. Deamination
   C. Desulphuration   D. All of the above

4. **The following moiety of GSH is involved in conjugation reactions to form mercapturic acid:**
   A. Cysteine   B. Glutamate
   C. Glycine   D. Any of the above

5. **The following is a hazard of global warming:**
   A. Vector-borne infectious diseases
   B. Renal stones
   C. Heat stroke
   D. All of the above

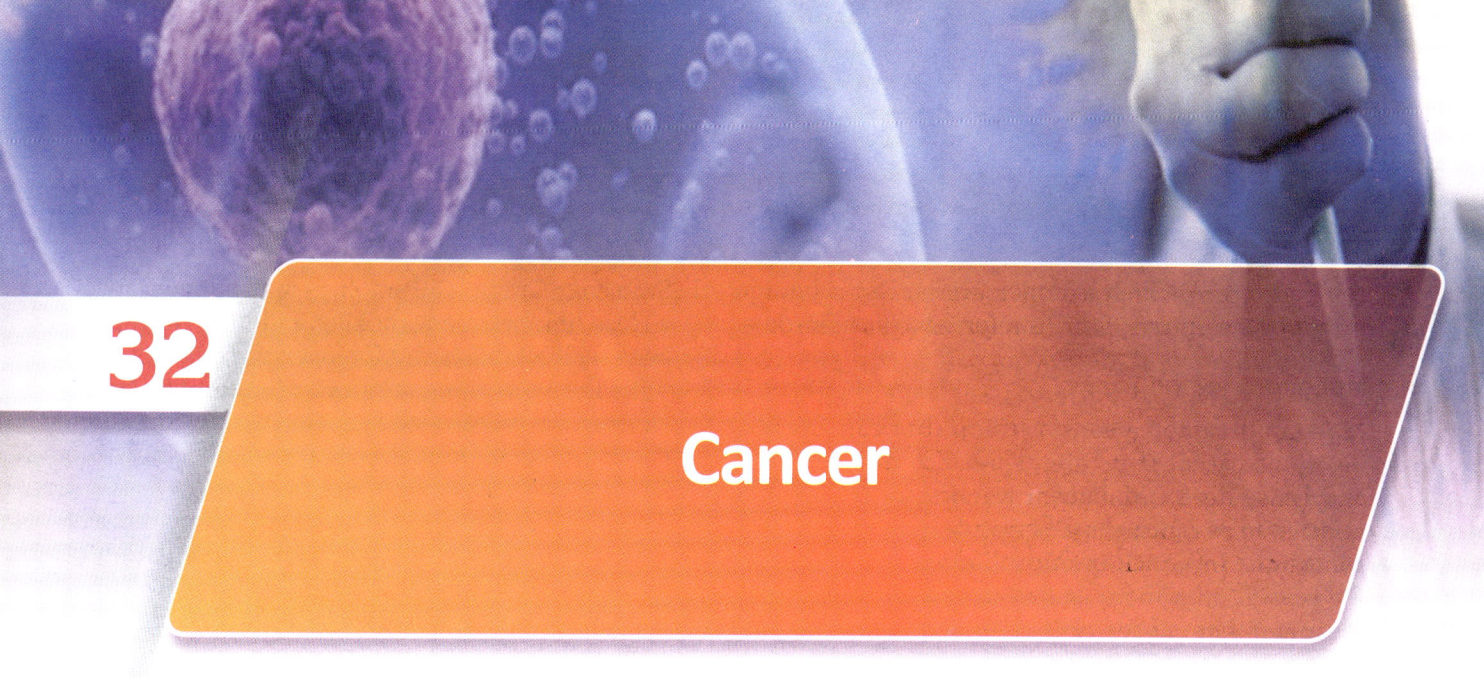

Cancer

Cancer is a most serious disease affecting human beings of all ages, universally. It is the **second most common cause of death**, first being the cardiac diseases.

CELL CYCLE

Cell cycle is a process in which chromosomes appear from 'undistinguishness', line-up with their partners, rejoin and then disperse. Cell cycle is divided into a series of temporally sequential phases consisting of a DNA synthetic phase (**S phase**) and cell division (**M phase** or mitosis) which are separated by the two gaps, referred to as G_1 (the interphase before DNA synthesis when the cell is committed to divide) and G_2 (the gap after DNA synthesis, denoting the period between completion of the S phase and mitosis). This cyclic process results in cell proliferation and is called **proliferative cell cycle** (Fig. 32.1).

Cell Cycle Check Points

The events of the proliferative cell cycle are ordered into dependent pathways in which **initiation of the late events is dependent on the completion of the early events**. These control mechanisms enforcing dependency in the cell cycle are called **check points**. Two major check points have been shown to exist. These are present at the middle to the end of G_1 and G_2, respectively (Fig. 32.1). After completing mitosis, some cells, e.g. hepatocytes enter a prolonged phase, out of the cell cycle, called the quiescent phase (G_0). Concentration of the various regulatory molecules such as growth factors, can divert the cell into G_0 or

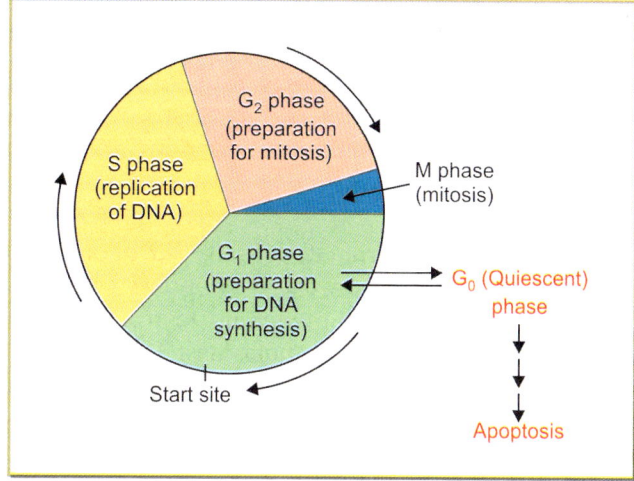

Fig. 32.1: Cell cycle.

stimulate quiescent cells to active cycling. Quiescence can be followed by **apoptosis** if it lasts too long while uncontrolled proliferation can lead to **neoplasm/ tumor**.

NEOPLASM/TUMOR

In common medical usage, a neoplasm ('new growth') is defined as a tumor (an abnormal tissue growth) which may be benign or malignant.

Benign Tumor

A tumor is said to be benign when its microscopic and gross characteristics are relatively **constant**. Further, it remains **localized** within a limited area and normally does not spread to other sites. Benign tumors are generally designated by the suffix '**-oma**', to the

32

cell type from which a tumor arises, e.g. a benign tumor of the fibrous tissue is referred to as a fibroma.

Malignant Tumor/Cancer

Malignant tumor means a lesion that can **invade**, destroy adjacent structures, spread to different sites and cause death. Malignant tumors are collectively referred to as **cancers**, a descriptive term to cover the conditions in which cells proliferate, for whatever the reason, in a more or less **uncontrolled manner** meaning that cancer cells have lost usual growth control. These cells invade adjacent tissues and set up **satellite growth** in other organs. The process, if left undisturbed, may lead to **death** of the host. Malignant neoplasms of epithelial origin are referred to as **carcinomas** while those arising in mesenchymal tissues are termed as **sarcomas**.

A tumor cell is distinguished from a normal cell by its immortality, morphological transformation and ability to undergo metastasis. Comparison of a benign tumor and a malignant tumor is given in Table 32.1.

Metastasis

The spread of cancer from its primary site of origin to other tissues where it grows as a secondary tumor by progressive infiltration, invasion, destruction and penetration is referred to as metastasis. It thus marks the development of secondary implants (simply called **'secondaries'**), discontinuous with the primary tumor, in remote tissues. It is a complex phenomenon, due to a failure in cell-cell interaction and is a major problem presented by the disease.

Epidemiology of Cancer

Epidemiological studies have correlated several environmental, racial and cultural influences to the occurrence of specific neoplasms. For example:

1. **Smoking:** Though all smokers may not get cancer, a close link between smoking and lung cancer has been well established. Moreover, the risk increases with the increasing number of cigarettes/bidis smoked per day as well as the duration of smoking.
2. **Diet:** A high-fat low-fiber diet has been shown to be a causative factor in colon cancer.
3. **Age:** The frequency of occurrence of many types of cancer increases with age, due to accumulation of somatic mutations, a decline in immune competence or age-related hormonal changes (e.g. prostate cancer).
4. **Inherited susceptibility:** It plays a role in the genesis of several types of cancer, such as retinoblastoma.
5. **Pre-neoplastic disorders:** These are conditions which predispose to the development of malignant neoplasia, e.g. leukoplakia of the oral cavity has been shown to increase the risk of squamous cell carcinoma.

CARCINOGENESIS

An agent that causes cancer is termed as a **carcinogen** and the process of cancer development is referred to as **carcinogenesis**. Carcinogens may act **directly or indirectly** to change the genotype of the cell. This transformation may occur spontaneously, may be caused by certain chemical agents or may result from infection with a tumor virus.

Carcinogenesis is a multistep process: Three types of **changes** occur when a cell becomes tumorigenic:
1. *Immortalization*: It is the property of indefinite growth without other changes in the phenotype.
2. *Transformation*: It means failure to observe normal constraints of growth, e.g. transformed cells become independent of growth factors which are usually needed for cell growth.

Table 32.1: Comparison of a benign and a malignant tumor

Benign tumor	Malignant tumor
Usually small in size	Comparatively large in size
Well demarcated	Poorly demarcated
Slow growing	Erratic, slow/rapidly growing with numerous and abnormal mitotic figures
Non-invasive	Locally invasive
No metastasis	Frequent metastasis
Well differentiated	Poorly differentiated
Easily managed by chemotherapy/surgery, mortality low or nil	Treatment is difficult in many cases. May require a combination of chemotherapy/surgery/radiotherapy; mortality moderate to high

3. *Metastasis:* It is the stage at which cancer cells gain the ability to invade normal tissues so that they can move away from the tissue of origin and establish a new colony/colonies elsewhere in the body.

Molecular Events in Carcinogenesis

At the molecular level, **mutations** play an important role in the process of carcinogenesis. A mutation may lead to nonlethal genetic damage and could be a result of the **reactive oxygen/nitrogen species**. As we know that a large number of oxygen-derived free radicals are normally produced within the cell. These radicals participate in a chain-reaction and cause damage to cellular macromolecules including DNA. The **principal targets** of genetic damage are the various **regulatory genes**:

1. Growth promoting proto-oncogenes.
2. Growth inhibiting cancer suppressor genes.
3. Genes which regulate programmed cell death (apoptosis).
4. DNA repair genes, i.e. the genes which regulate repair of the damaged DNA (Fig. 32.2).

CHEMICAL CARCINOGENS

Nearly 80% of human cancers are caused by environmental factors, mainly chemicals. Exposure to such chemicals can be due to a person's occupation, diet, lifestyle or use of therapeutic drugs.

Some carcinogens are direct reacting substances while a majority of them are indirect reacting substances (Table 32.2).

Table 32.2: Some chemical carcinogens

Directly reacting substances
- Cyclophosphamide, nitrosourea
- Alkylating agents
- Acylating agents

Indirectly reacting procarcinogens
- Polycyclic/heterocyclic aromatic hydrocarbons
  - Benzo(a) pyrene
- Aromatic amines, amides, azo dyes
  - 2-Naphthylamine
  - 2-Acetylaminofluorene
  - Dimethylaminoazobenzene
- Plant and microbial products
  - Aflatoxin B_1
  - Griseofulvin
  - Betel nuts
- Others
  - Nitrosoamines and amides
  - Vinyl chloride, nickel, chromium
  - Insecticides, fungicides
  - Polychlorinated biphenyls
  - Arsenic
  - Asbestos

Types of Chemical Carcinogens

- **Direct reacting substances:** These are direct carcinogens, i.e. they do not undergo any metabolic transformation to become a carcinogen. Since such substances enter the body in a mutagenic form, they are also designated as **mutagens**, e.g. cyclophosphamide, nitrosourea, etc. The carcinogenic potential of a mutagen can be tested by the Ames test.

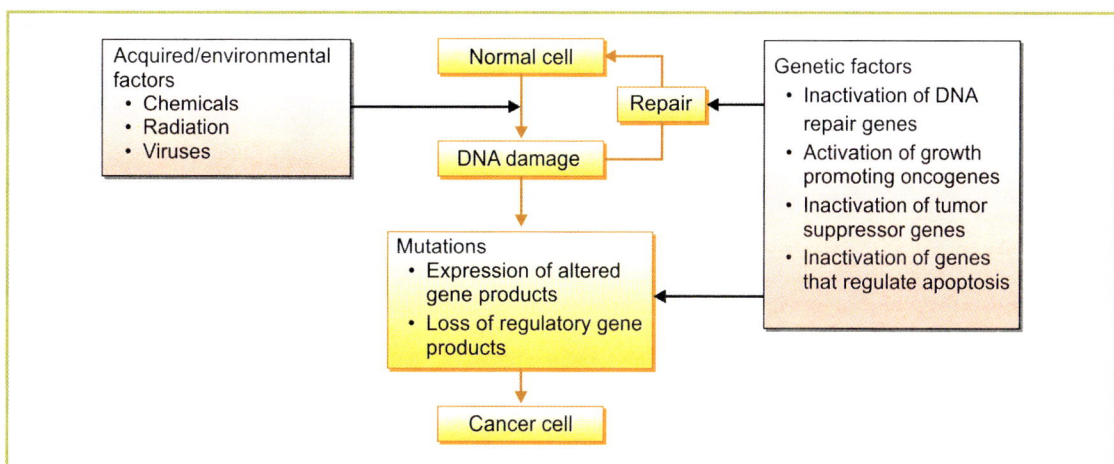

Fig. 32.2: Carcinogenesis: A result of a complex interplay between genetic and environmental factors.

32

Ames test: It is the test for mutagenicity of a compound. A specially constituted strain of *Salmonella typhimurium* (**His⁻**), with a mutation in the gene-encoding one of the enzymes for histidine biosynthesis, is used. Since His⁻ bacteria cannot synthesize histidine, this amino acid has to be added in the medium for optimum growth of the bacteria. Reversion (back conversion) of the mutation, caused by a carcinogen at the same site of the genome (at the His⁻ site), restores its reading sequence and thus **reverts to His⁺**. The progeny of bacteria containing such a **reverse mutation** can now synthesize histidine and grow in a medium lacking histidine. The **conversion proves the mutagenicity** of the test chemical.

Further, indirect carcinogens can also be tested by the Ames test if the medium is supplemented with liver extract which serves as a source of mixed function oxidases.

- **Indirect reacting substances:** These are also called **indirect carcinogens** or **procarcinogens**. These are not mutagenic in the form in which they enter the body. They are converted in the liver to a more reactive form by a family of enzymes referred to as mixed function oxidases through an intermediate

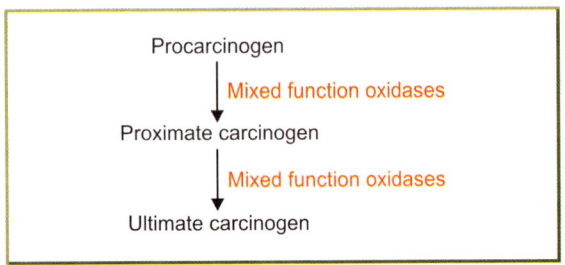

Fig. 32.3: Activation of a procarcinogen.

called **proximate carcinogen**. The final product of the conversion is called **ultimate carcinogen** (Fig. 32.3) which forms adduct with DNA and subsequently mutates it. Such procarcinogens are present in the environment, at the work place or in the food (Chemistry to Clinics 32.1).

Stages of Chemical Carcinogenesis

Sometimes carcinogens are divided into those that initiate and those that promote tumor formation, implying the existence of difference stages in cancer development.

- **Initiation:** It involves mutation, a small but significant change in DNA of the cell. Initiation is an **irreversible** process. Such cells may remain dormant for years within the body without undergoing proliferation. This period is a gap between the exposure to a carcinogen (**initiator**) and the appearance of a full-blown tumor and is referred to as the **latent period** which may vary from 5 to 6 years for the induction of leukemia by radiation to as long as 35–40 years for the asbestos-induced lung cancer. Reasons for this long lag period are not known.

- **Promotion:** Carcinogenicity of an initiator may be **augmented** by the subsequent administration of some of the other agent(s) called a **promoter**, e.g. croton oil (which contains phorbol ester, a promoter of carcinogenesis). A promoter has a **little or no carcinogenic activity of its own**. To be effective, application of a mutagen (an initiator) must follow repeated exposures of the promoter. For example, if skin of a mice is painted with an initiator such as benzo(a)pyrene and no subsequent treatment is

Chemistry to Clinics 32.1: Procarcinogens

Several compounds may act as procarcinogens, e.g:

- **Polycyclic hydrocarbons** such as benzo(a)pyrene are produced during high temperature combustion of tobacco. These substances have been implicated in the causation of lung cancer in smokers as well as in non-smokers exposed to environmental tobacco smoke (passive smokers). Such compounds may also be produced from animal fat (in smoked cheese, meat or fish) and may be risk factors for colon cancer.
- **Aromatic amines, amides** and **azo dyes** are present in dyes and detergents. They increase the incidence of urinary bladder cancer in workers in aniline, dye and rubber industries (an occupational hazard).
- **Food additives** and **toxins** such as colors (butter yellow), sweeteners (saccharin) or certain plant and microbial toxins (aflatoxin B_1) may produce hepatocellular carcinoma.
- **Endogenously** produced substances include **nitrosomines** and **amides** which are formed in the acidic environment of the stomach and may lead to gastric carcinoma.

  Indirect carcinogens can be tested by the Ames test provided the medium is supplemented with liver extract which serves as a source of mixed function oxidases.

given, tumor does not develop. But if this application of the initiator is followed by several applications of the promoter, a tumor subsequently develops. Application of the promoter alone does not cause tumor formation:

An application of Initiator (I) → No tumor

An application of Promoter (P) → No tumor

An application of I followed by several applications of P → Tumor

An application of P followed by several applications of I → No tumor

It is due to the reason that an application of the initiator, as mentioned above, causes mutational activation of some cells and converts them to potential tumor cells. Subsequent applications of the promoter lead to clonal expansion of the initiated (mutated) cells to produce a tumor (Fig. 32.4).

- **Progression:** The mutated cells subsequently acquire many characteristics which make them **autonomous** (free from regulatory controls). For example, these cells acquire the ability to invade and destroy surrounding tissues and to spread to other parts of the body. Their requirement for growth factors is reduced and they become less responsive to growth inhibitory signals. They expand their energy solely for the uncontrolled growth and eventually develop into a malignant tumor.

RADIATION

Radiation, from whatever the source it may be (UV rays of sunlight, X-rays, nuclear fission or radionuclides), is strongly carcinogenic. It causes various **mutagenic effects**, e.g. chromosomal break, translocation or point mutation, etc. Radiation may lead to leukemia, cancer of the skin, lungs, thyroid gland, breast or colon.

Besides, UV rays can also exhibit other biological effects such as that it can cause DNA damage by forming pyrimidine dimers. Apart from its **direct effect** on DNA, radiation also leads to the formation of **free radicals**. Free radicals, in turn, can interact with DNA and other macromolecules thereby leading to their damage which further contribute to the process of carcinogenesis.

ONCOGENIC VIRUSES

Viruses which cause cancer are called oncogenic viruses or tumor viruses. These may be DNA or RNA viruses (Table 32.3).

ONCOGENES AND PROTO-ONCOGENES

Oncogenes: These are the genes carried by viruses that cause transformation of their target (host) cells. They are called oncogenes due to their ability to convert cells to a tumorigenic (oncogenic) state.

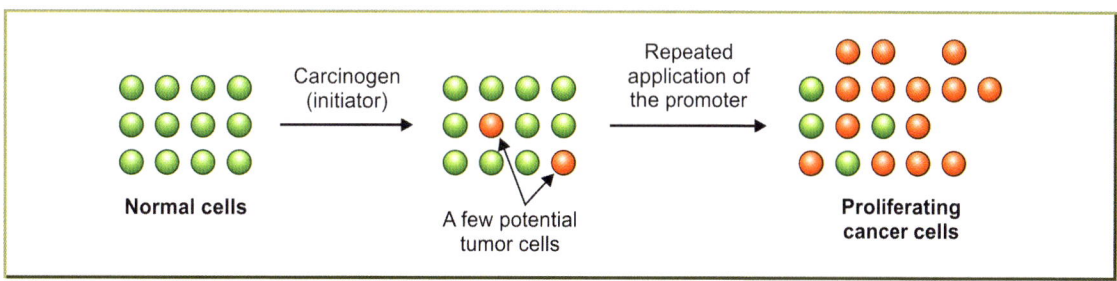

Fig. 32.4: Role of initiator and promoter in tumor development.

Table 32.3: Oncogenic viruses

DNA Virus	Associated tumors
Epstein-Barr virus (EBV)	Nasopharyngeal carcinoma, Burkitt's lymphoma, B cell lymphomas
Hepatitis B virus	Hepatocellular carcinoma
Human papillomavirus	Anogenital cancer
RNA Virus	
Human T cell leukemia-lymphoma virus type 1 (HTLL-1)	Adult T cell leukemia

32

Table 32.4: Examples of proto-oncogenes or oncogenes associated with tumors

Proto-oncogene	Tumor
ras	Carcinoma of colon, lung, pancreas, genito-urinary tract, acute lymphoblastic leukemia
erb	Squamous cell carcinoma
myc	Carcinoma of lung, breast
bcl-2	B cell lymphoma

Proto-oncogenes: The viral oncogenes have their cellular counterparts (in the host) that are involved in normal cell functions. These cellular genes are called proto-oncogenes (Table 32.4).

Nomenclature

The genomes of the acute transforming retroviruses (which cause rapid induction of tumor in animals) contain such unique transforming sequences (genes) referred to as **viral oncogenes** (v-onc). The v-onc sequences are not found in the genome of the non-transforming retroviruses. Each v-onc is designated by three letters that relate a v-onc to the virus from which it was isolated, e.g. v-onc contained in the simian sarcoma virus is referred to as v-sis whereas the v-onc in feline sarcoma virus is called v-fes.

The cellular counterparts of these genes (proto-oncogenes isolated from the host cells) are designated by using the prefix 'c'. For example, the oncogene carried by Rous Sarcoma Virus is called v-src while the proto-oncogene related to it in the cellular genome is called c-src.

Mode of Oncogenesis

During an infection, the transducing virus carries with it the cellular gene(s) that have been obtained by the recombination event. The oncogenes carried by DNA viruses specify proteins that inactivate tumor suppressors so that their action in part mimics **'loss-of-function'** of the tumor suppressors. On the other hand, the oncogenes carried by retroviruses are derived from cellular genes and therefore may mimic the behavior of **'gain-of-function'** in (animal) proto-oncogenes.

Activation of Proto-oncogenes

Any of the following processes can result in the activation of a proto-oncogene:

- **Point mutation:** Substitution in the coding sequence can convert a cellular proto-oncogene into an oncogene. Any mutation at either position 12 or 61 has been shown to convert a c-ras proto-oncogene into an active oncogene. For example, DNA sequences of c-ras proto-oncogenes from normal human cells and that from the human urinary bladder cancer cells have been shown to differ solely in one base. Besides, a large number of other human tumors are also known to carry ras mutations, e.g. carcinoma of the pancreas, colon, lungs and thyroid.

- **Chromosomal translocation:** When a piece of one chromosome is split-off and joins the other chromosome, it is called chromosomal translocation. It is a reciprocal event that exchanges parts of the two chromosomes. Chromosomal translocation results in overexpression of the proto-oncogene such as in certain cases of Burkitt's lymphoma. Translocation has been shown to activate the human c-myc proto-oncogene.

  Translocation in B cell tumors usually involves chromosome 8 which carries c-myc and chromosome 14 which carries immunoglobulin heavy chain locus. There occurs a break of a segment from an end of the q arm of chromosome 8 (containing myc gene) which is translocated to chromosome 14 (containing gene for the heavy chain of IgG). This, in turn, results in transcription of heavy chain of IgG. Synthesis of the increased amounts of DNA-binding protein, coded by the myc gene thus forces the cell towards malignancy (Fig. 32.5).

- **Gene amplification:** Amplification of DNA sequence may result in activation of a proto-oncogene. c-myc Gene in neuroblastoma and c-erb B2 gene in breast cancer are examples of the activation of their proto-oncogenes as a result of amplification of their DNA sequences.

- **Insertion of promoter/enhancer:** Certain retroviruses, e.g. avian leukemia virus, when infect a cell, the DNA copy of their RNA genome (called cDNA) is synthesized by reverse transcriptase and gets integrated into the genome of the host. The integrated double-stranded DNA is called provirus. These cDNA copies of the retroviruses are flanked at both the ends by the sequences termed as long terminal repeats (LTR) which are important in the integration of a provirus.

32

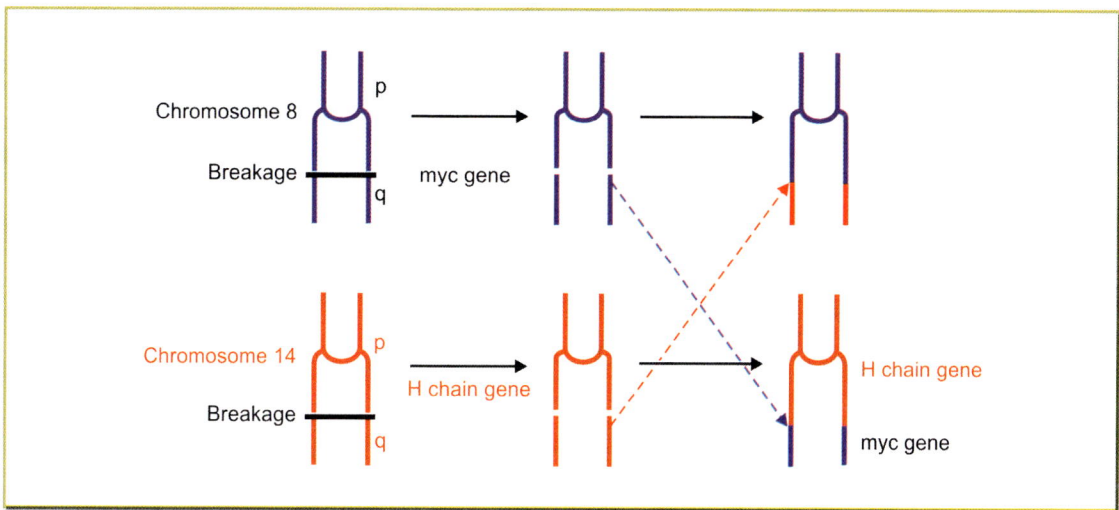

Fig. 32.5: Chromosomal translocation.

Following infection of chicken B lymphocytes by the avian leukemia virus, the provirus becomes integrated near the myc gene and acts as a promoter. This, in turn, promotes transcription of the corresponding myc RNA and subsequent translation of the gene product in such cells (Fig. 32.6).

The transforming potential of the avian leukemia virus (a retrovirus) is due to the ability of LTR of the integrated form to cause expression of cellular gene(s). The provirus may also be inserted downstream, as an enhancer (Fig. 32.6).

Protein Products of Oncogenes/Proto-oncogenes

Protein products of oncogenes are called **oncoproteins** which fall into several groups (Table 32.5). Their common feature is that they trigger general changes

Table 32.5: Oncoproteins (protein products of oncogenes)

Protein function	Example	Result of activation
Growth factor	PDGF-β	Astrocytoma
Growth factor receptor	EGF receptor	Squamous cell lung carcinoma
Regulation of signal transduction	Tyrosine kinase	Leukemia
Regulation of nuclear transcription and cell cycle	Cyclins	Breast cancer

PDGF-β—platelet derived growth factor-β; EGF—epidermal growth factor.

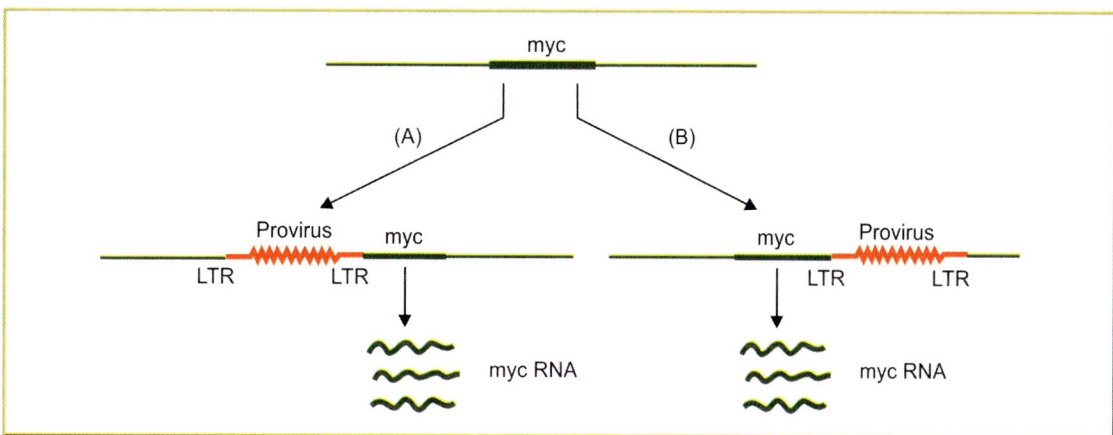

Fig. 32.6: Insertion of a promoter (A) or an enhancer (B).

32

Chemistry to Clinics 32.2: Anti-oncogenes

1. **Retinoblastoma gene (Rb):** Mutation in Rb gene is involved in the genesis of retinoblastoma. It results in inactivation of its protein product, designated as pRb. Loss of the negative regulatory effect of pRb on cell division leads to increased cell multiplication, as seen in tumor originating from retina, bone and connective tissue.

2. **p53:** It is located on the short arm of chromosome 17 and encodes a 53 kD protein, hence the gene is designated as p53. It is a proline-rich phosphoprotein and acts as a **'guardian of the genome'** by:
   - Transcriptional regulation of certain genes involved in cell division.
   - Activation of DNA repair proteins.
   - Participation in the initiation of apoptosis.
   - Interaction with other anti-oncogenes.
     Mutation in p53 gene may result in many tumors, e.g. lung, skin, pancreas, etc.

in cell phenotype either by initiating or responding to changes associated with cell growth or by changing gene expression directly.

Cancer Suppressor Genes

Cancer suppressor genes are also called **anti-oncogenes** or **recessive oncogenes**. They impose some constraint on cell cycle or cell growth. Hence, release of such constraints is tumorigenic (Chemistry to Clinics 32.2).

Protein Products of the Cancer Suppressor Genes

Tumor suppressor genes encode proteins which form various components of the growth inhibitory pathway. These include growth inhibitory factors, molecules that regulate cell adhesion, signal transduction, nuclear transcription and cell cycle (Table 32.6).

Genes that Regulate Apoptosis

Apoptosis (Chapter 33), also called programmed cell death, occurs in many physiological and pathological conditions and is controlled by specific gene regulated events. Cells undergoing apoptosis shrink, their chromatin condenses, DNA gets fragmented and membranes exhibit blebs.

Large families of genes that regulate apoptosis have been identified. These are designated by a series of words which have three letters beginning with b, e.g. bcl-2, bcl-x, bax, bad. Alterations in genes that regulate apoptosis may also result in neoplasia. Over-expression of bcl-2 protects lymphocytes from apoptosis and allows them to survive for longer period. This, in turn, causes steady accumulation of lymphocytes and results in lymphadenopathy and bone marrow infiltration. On the other hand, bax opposes the action of bcl-2 and accelerates cell death. Hence, the relative levels of the two genes regulate cell proliferation.

DNA Repair Genes

There are several inherited disorders in which genes that encode proteins needed in DNA repair are defective. Individuals born with such inherited mutations are at increased risk of developing cancer (Chemistry to Clinics 32.3).

Chemistry to Clinics 32.3: Defective DNA Repair and Cancer

Due to a defect in DNA repair, patients with xeroderma pigmentosum are at increased risk for the development of cancer of the skin due to exposure to ultraviolet light contained in sunrays. Hereditary nonpolyposis colon carcinoma (HNPCC) is another disorder resulting from defects in genes involved in DNA repair.

Table 32.6: Protein products of cancer suppressor genes

Protein function	Example	Result of mutation
Growth inhibition	BRCA-1	Breast cancer
Regulation of cell-cell and cell-matrix adhesion	DCC	Colon cancer
Regulation of signal transduction	NF-1	Neurofibroma
Regulation of nuclear transcription and cell cycle	Rb	Retinoblastoma
	p53	Lung cancer

BRCA-1—breast cancer-1; DCC—deleted in colon carcinoma; NF-1—neurofibromin-1.

BIOCHEMICAL CHANGES DURING TUMOR DEVELOPMENT

The biochemical profile of a malignant cell is different from that of the normal cell as it has a distinct type of metabolism (Table 32.7). Once a cell becomes malignant, its composition and behavior does not remain static and there is always a tendency for the malignancy to increase.

TUMOR MARKERS

Characteristics: A tumor marker is defined as a substance present in or produced by a tumor, or by the host cell in response to a tumor. Such a substance can be used to differentiate a tumor from the normal tissue or to determine the presence of a tumor based upon its measurement in the tissue, cells or body fluids. An **ideal** tumor marker is one which is both **specific** for a given type of cancer as well as **sensitive** enough to help in its early diagnosis.

Classification: Tumor markers can be classified into several groups such as enzymes and isoenzymes, hormones, oncofetal antigens, carbohydrate-epitopes or oncogene products (Table 32.8).

Applications

1. **Detection:** Screening in asymptomatic persons.
2. **Diagnosis:** Differentiate between benign and malignant conditions.

Table 32.7: Biochemical comparison of a normal cell with a tumor cell

Parameter	Normal cell	Tumor cell
1. Ribonucleotide reductase activity	Normal	Enhanced
2. RNA and DNA synthesis	Normal	Enhanced
3. Pyrimidine catabolism	Normal	Suppressed
4. Rate of glycolysis	Normal	Enhanced
5. Isoenzyme profile	Normal	Altered
6. Synthesis of fetal proteins	No	Yes
7. Synthesis of specialized proteins	Yes	No
8. Inappropriate synthesis of growth factors/hormones	No	Yes

Table 32.8: Selected tumor markers with the type of cancer in which these are increased in serum

Tumor marker	Type of cancer
Enzymes	
Alkaline phosphatase	Bone, liver
Heat stable alkaline phosphatase	Uterus, ovary
Acid phosphatase	Prostate
Amylase	Pancreas
Hormones	
ADH	Adrenal cortex, pancreas, small cell lung cancer
Calcitonin	Medullary thyroid carcinoma
Growth hormone	Pituitary adenoma, renal and lung cancers
β-hCG	Testes, trophoblasts
Oncofetal antigens	
α-Fetoprotein (AFP)	Hepatocellular carcinoma
CEA	Colorectal, GIT, lungs, breast
Squamous cell antigen	Head and neck, cervix, lungs, skin
PSA	Prostate

Contd...

32

Contd...

Tumor marker	*Type of cancer*
Carbohydrate markers	
CA 125	Ovary, endometrium
CA 15-3	Breast, ovary
CA 19-9	Pancreas, GIT, liver
Proteins	
β2-microglobulin	Multiple myeloma, B cell lymphoma
C-peptide	Insulinoma
Ferritin	Liver, lungs, breast, leukemias
Immunoglobulins	Multiple myeloma, lymphomas
Oncogenes	
K-ras mutation	Leukemias, lymphomas
c-myc translocation	B and T cell lymphomas, small cell lung cancer
bcl-2	Leukemias, lymphomas
c-erb B2 amplification	Breast, ovary, GIT
Mutations in tumor suppressor genes	
BRCA-1	Breast, melanoma
p53	Breast, colorectal, lungs, liver
Rb1	Retinoblastoma, osteosarcoma
DCC	Colorectal
Others	
Estrogen and progesterone receptors	Breast
Hydroxyproline (in urine)	Bone metastasis, multiple myeloma
Polyamines (in CSF)	Brain

3. **Monitoring/prognosis:** To assess the effect of treatment and predict the clinical outcome.
4. **Classification and staging:** To decide the type of treatment required.
5. **Localization:** Nuclear scanning of injected radioactive marker antibodies.
6. **Therapy:** Directed towards marker-containing cells.

CHEMOPREVENTION

Chemoprevention is defined as the introduction of some of the **natural and/or synthetic substances in the diet, for preventing cancer**. Antioxidant vitamins, e.g. vitamin A and carotenoids, vitamin E and vitamin C have been shown to be the natural dietary inhibitors of carcinogenesis. They work by **various mechanisms**:

- Inhibition of the formation of free radicals as well as increasing their detoxification
- Immune stimulation

Table 32.9: Chemopreventive nutraceuticals

- Vitamins A, C and E ('big three' antioxidants)
- Flavonoids
- Curcumin (major colored component of turmeric)
- Lunasin (a soy peptide)
- Poppy seeds
- Diallyl sulfide (in garlic and onion)
- Aqueous extracts of decaffeinated green or black tea

- Inhibition of nitrosamine formation
- Enhancement of cell-to-cell communication
- Metabolic detoxification of the carcinogen.

Several cancers particularly those of the lungs, stomach, colon, breast, prostate, etc. have been benefited by chemopreventive agents sometimes called **nutraceuticals or nutriceuticals** (Table 32.9). Recent trend is to **encourage enhanced consumption of fruits/vegetables**, which are natural sources of chemopreventive agents, at an early age.

SOME IMPORTANT QUESTIONS

32

1. What is carcinogenesis? Describe in details about chemical carcinogenesis.

2. What are oncogenes? How proto-oncogenes are activated?

3. What are cancer suppressor genes? Outline their protein products.

4. Differentiate between:
   i. A benign tumor and a malignant tumor
   ii. Direct reacting and indirect reacting carcinogens.
   iii. Initiator and promoter.

5. Write notes on:
   i. Metastasis
   ii. Carcinogenesis
   iii. Ames test
   iv. Radiation carcinogenesis
   v. Viral carcinogenesis
   vi. Oncogenes
   vii. Cell cycle
   viii. Apoptosis
   ix. DNA repair genes
   x. Tumor markers
   xi. Chemoprevention

MULTIPLE CHOICE QUESTIONS

1. **High-fat low-fiber diet is associated with cancer of:**
   A. Oral cavity
   B. Esophagus
   C. Stomach
   D. Colon

2. **An increased risk of urinary bladder cancer is an occupational hazard in workers exposed to:**
   A. Azo dyes
   B. Aniline
   C. Rubber
   D. All of the above

3. **An increased risk of hepatocellular carcinoma may be due to exposure to:**
   A. Butter yellow
   B. Saccharin
   C. Aflatoxin B_1
   D. All of the above

4. **Epstein-Barr virus (EBV) is associated with:**
   A. Nasopharyngeal carcinoma
   B. Burkitt's lymphoma
   C. B cell lymphoma
   D. All of the above

5. **The 'guardian of the genome' is:**
   A. pRb
   B. p53
   C. c-erb B1
   D. c-erb B2

6. **The following is an anti-oncogene:**
   A. pRb
   B. hst-1
   C. c-erb B1
   D. c-erb B2

7. **Hereditary non-polyposis colon cancer (HNCC) is mainly attributed to a defect in genes regulating:**
   A. DNA repair
   B. Apoptosis
   C. Nuclear transcription
   D. Cell cycle check points

8. **Serum CEA is a marker for the following tumors *except*:**
   A. Colorectal
   B. Prostate
   C. Lungs
   D. Breast

9. **Serum AFP is a tumor marker for:**
   A. Ovary
   B. Testis
   C. Liver
   D. Tongue

10. **The following hormone may be ectopically produced in paraneoplastic syndrome:**
    A. PTHrP
    B. Calcitriol
    C. Vasopressin
    D. All of the above

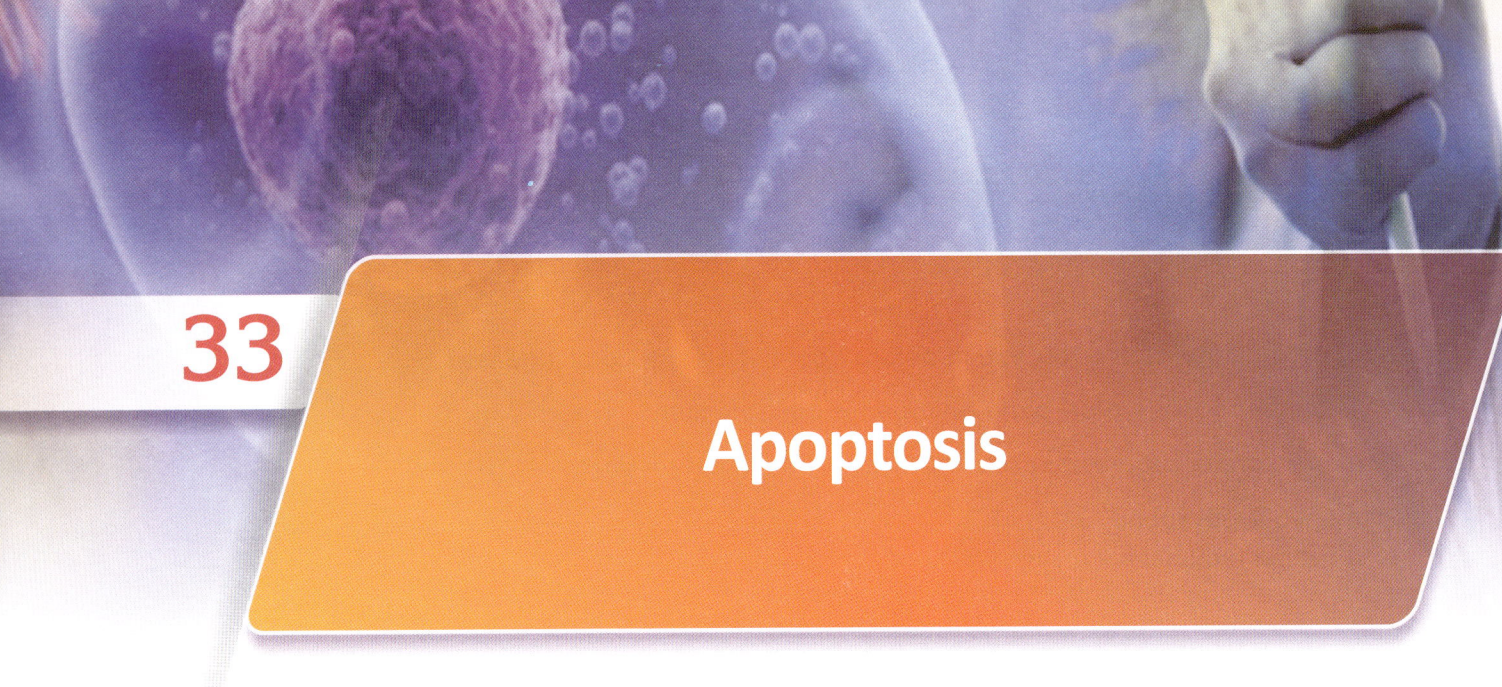

33

Apoptosis

The term **'programmed cell death'** was introduced in 1964, proposing that cell death during development is not of accidental nature but follows a sequence of controlled steps leading to locally and temporally defined self-destruction. Eventually, the term **'apoptosis'** was coined to describe the morphological processes leading to **controlled cellular self-destruction** and was first introduced in a publication by Kerr, Wyllie and Currie in 1972. 'Apoptosis' is of Greek origin, meaning 'falling off or dropping off', in analogy to leaves falling off trees or petals dropping off flowers. It emphasizes that the death of living matter is an integral and necessary part of the life cycle of organisms. **Apoptosis differs from necrosis** in several aspects related to the cell size, membrane changes and inflammatory response.

Biochemical Mechanism of Apoptosis

Apoptosis can be triggered by various stimuli known as **death signals** that may be initiated **outside the cell** (such as the binding of specific 'death' ligands to membrane 'death' receptors, exposure to radiation or cytotoxic drugs) or **within the cell** (such as faulty DNA repair, improper control of the cell cycle check points) (Fig. 33.1).

The death ligand-receptor mediated biochemical mechanisms are said to follow the extrinsic apoptotic pathway; others follow the intrinsic apoptotic pathway. However, death signals of diverse origin eventually activate a common cell death machinery followed by apoptosis.

- *Extrinsic apoptotic pathway*: A hallmark of this pathway is the execution of cells mediated by the enzymes called **caspases**. The term is derived from '**c**ysteine-dependent **a**spartate-**sp**ecific prote**ases**' because they contain a critical cysteine residue at the catalytic site and they cleave their protein substrates after aspartate residues. Many caspases have been identified and all are initially synthesized as the inactive precursors/zymogens called **procaspases**. The activation of **procaspase-8** is a critical event responsible for the serial activation of other caspases in the pathway. By convention, the cells relying on the caspase-dependent activation of apoptosis are called **type I cells**.

- *Intrinsic apoptotic pathway*: A hallmark of this pathway is the release of **cytochrome c** from the mitochondria into the cytosol. The protein cytochrome c is an important mobile component of the electron transport chain located in the inner mitochondrial membrane. Upon release, cytochrome c combines with **procaspase-9** molecules and other proteins to form a complex called **'apoptosome'** with subsequent activation of **caspase-9**. By convention, the cells requiring the mitochondria-dependent activation of caspases and apoptosis are called **type II cells**.

- *Final common pathway*: Ultimately both, the extrinsic and intrinsic pathways, in type I or II cells, **converge** on certain shared series of biochemical events (Fig. 33.1). This includes the activation of procaspases- 3, 6 and 7, and irreversible damage to cellular proteins and DNA. This is aptly referred to as **'death by a thousand tiny cuts'**.

It is interesting to note that apoptosis is an energetically active, i.e. **ATP requiring** process.

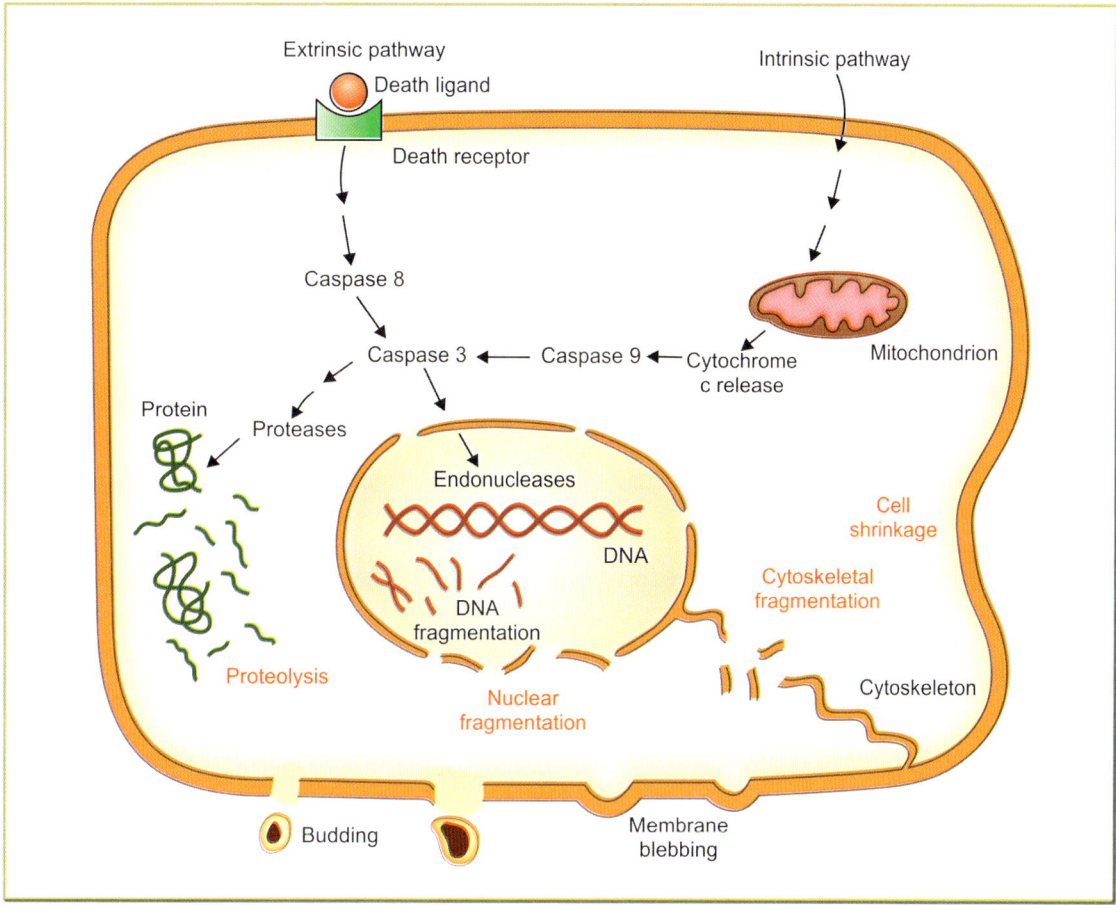

Fig. 33.1: Apoptosis.

Further, **pro-apoptotic** (apoptosis favoring, e.g. p53 tumor suppressor protein) and **anti-apoptotic** (apoptosis inhibiting, e.g. bcl-2 protein family) factors are in **balance** and each is genetically determined and regulated.

Biological Significance of Apoptosis

In the adult human body, early 100,000 cells are produced every second by mitosis and a similar number die by apoptosis. Taken together, apoptotic processes are of widespread biological significance, being involved in embryonic development, proliferation, differentiation, homeostasis, regulation of the immune system, and the removal of defective and harmful cells (Chemistry to Clinics 33.1). For example:

• During the **development of the brain and the reproductive organs**, nearly 50% of the cells that are initially formed die later by the time the systems attain maturity.

Chemistry to Clinics 33.1: Clinical Significance of Apoptosis

1. Failure to correctly initiate apoptosis may result in cancer, autoimmune diseases and spread of infection.
2. Poorly controlled or excessive apoptosis may lead to neurodegenerative disorders such as Alzheimer's disease, Parkinson's disease, Huntington's disease and amyotrophic lateral sclerosis.
3. Gaining insight into the mechanisms and alterations by which components of the apoptotic machinery contribute to pathogenic processes, should allow the development of more effective, specific and better tolerated therapeutic approaches. It may include the targeted activation of pro-apoptotic tumor suppressors or the blockade of anti-apoptotic genes in case of cancer. On the other hand, for the treatment of premature cell death seen in neurodegeneration, the inhibition of key pro-apoptotic molecules, such as caspases, might be promising.

33

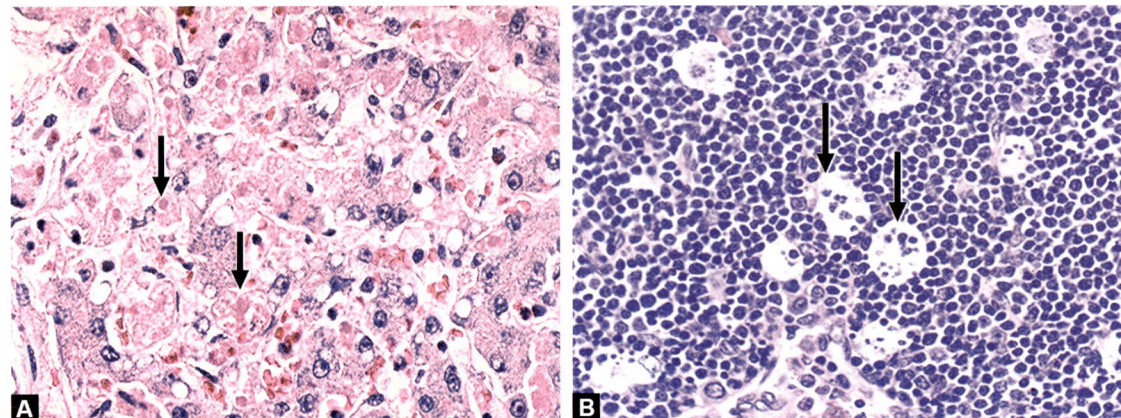

Fig. 33.2: (A) Apoptosis of liver cells (arrows) from injury by viral hepatitis. The cells are pink and without nuclei. (B) Apoptosis of lymphocytes in the fetal thymus. Individual cells fragment and are consumed by phagocytes to give the appearance of clear spaces filled with cellular debris (arrows).

- Several millions of **T and B lymphocytes** are formed daily and nearly 95% die during genetic rearrangement and maturation.
- Cells **infected** by microbes are cleared by apoptosis (Fig. 33.2A).
- Auto-reactive/self-reactive cells of the immune system are destroyed by apoptosis to **prevent autoimmune diseases** (Fig. 33.2B).
- Cells with **extensive DNA damage** that cannot be repaired are removed by apoptosis.

SOME IMPORTANT QUESTIONS

1. What is apoptosis? Briefly discuss the biochemical mechanisms of apoptosis.

2. What is the role of mitochondria in apoptosis?

3. Discuss the biological significance of apoptosis.

MULTIPLE CHOICE QUESTIONS

1. **The critical event in the extrinsic apoptotic pathway is:**
   A. Release of cytochrome c from mitochondria into cytosol
   B. Activation of procaspase-8
   C. Activation of procaspase-9
   D. Formation of apoptosome

2. **The critical event in the intrinsic apoptotic pathway is:**
   A. Release of cytochrome c from mitochondria into cytosol
   B. Activation of procaspase-8
   C. Activation of procaspase-9
   D. Formation of apoptosome

3. **Excessive apoptosis has been linked with:**
   A. Amyotrophic lateral sclerosis
   B. Alzheimer's disease
   C. Huntington's disease
   D. All of the above

Free Radicals and Antioxidants

The elemental oxygen (O_2), as we all know, is essential for life. About 90% of it is used via oxidative phosphorylation while 5–8% in enzymatic hydroxylation and oxygenation reactions. A small fraction of the oxygen, <5%, is converted to inherently toxic forms such as superoxide, hydrogen peroxide, etc. They are a source of chronic damage to biomolecules within the tissues.

REACTIVE OXYGEN SPECIES

In biological redox reactions, oxygen is activated by redox active metal ions such as iron and copper, which are present in metalloenzymes and other proteins, e.g. hemoglobin, myoglobin, etc. These metal ions provide one electron at a time to oxygen and activate it to strong oxidizing forms. A number of reactive oxygen species (ROS), including free radicals and non-radicals, are formed from partial reduction of molecular oxygen (Fig. 34.1). The first product is the superoxide anion free radical (O_2^{-}). Reduction of superoxide yields hydrogen peroxide (**H_2O_2, a non-radical ROS**). Reduction of H_2O_2 causes a cleavage reaction that releases hydroxyl free radical (**OH·**). The end product of complete reduction of oxygen is water.

The major sources of ROS are the mitochondrial electron transport chain, reactions mediated through de-compartmentalized metal ions (Fenton reaction), Haber-Weiss reaction, or by normal enzymatic reactions, e.g. monoamine oxidase (in dopamine metabolism), fatty acid oxidases (in the peroxisomes), etc. Basal levels of ROS are necessary for regulating many physiological processes like phagocytosis, signal transduction, gene expression and apoptosis (Fig. 34.2). Any excess results in a pro-oxidative condition known as **oxidative stress**.

It should be remembered that similar to ROS, nitrogen-based reactive species (reactive nitrogen species or RNS) are also produced in the body. Peroxynitrite ($ONOO^-$) and nitric oxide (NO) are important examples, which in turn, are responsible for **nitrosative stress**.

Oxidative Stress

Various ROS are formed continuously as by-products of aerobic metabolism, through reactions with drugs and environmental toxins. When their level is increased or the level of antioxidants is diminished, it creates a condition called oxidative stress. ROS can

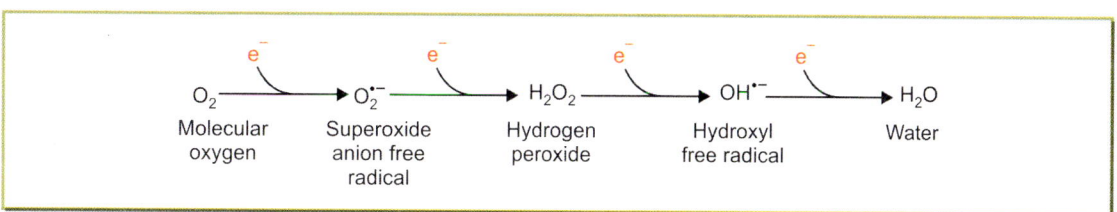

Fig. 34.1: Formation of reactive oxygen species from molecular oxygen (e^- = electron).

34

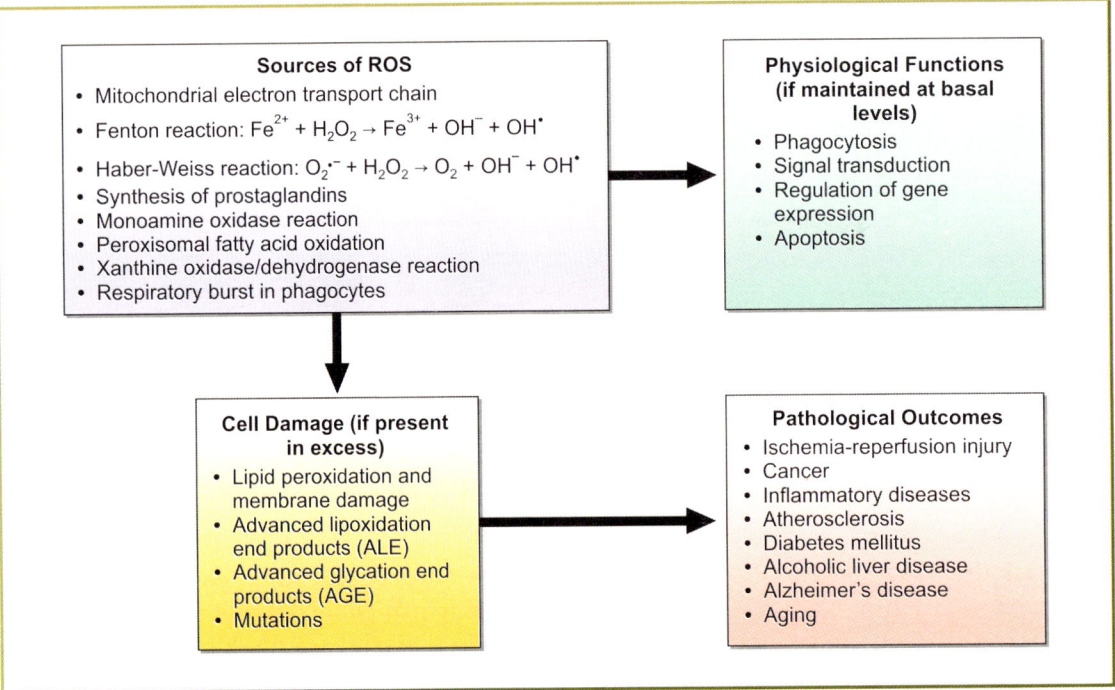

Fig. 34.2: Reactive oxygen species (ROS): Sources, functions and pathological outcomes.

cause serious chemical damage to DNA, proteins, carbohydrates and unsaturated lipids and can eventually lead to cell death. ROS have also been implicated in a number of pathological processes including ischemia-reperfusion injury (Chemistry to Clinics 34.1), cancer, metabolic, degenerative, inflammatory diseases, etc. (Fig. 34.2).

Nature of Oxygen Radical Damage

Among the ROS, hydroxyl free radical **(OH·) is the most reactive and damaging**. Its half-life is measured in nanoseconds. It reacts with biomolecules primarily by hydrogen abstraction and addition reactions.

One of the most sensitive sites of free radical damage is the cell membrane, which is rich in readily oxidizable polyunsaturated fatty acids. The OH· extracts a hydrogen atom from a polyunsaturated fatty acid, setting off a chain of lipid peroxidation reactions. Lipid peroxides formed in this reaction degrade to form characteristics products such as malondialdehyde (MDA). These compounds react with proteins to form adducts and cross links, known as advanced lipoxidation end-products (ALE). Further, ROS also react with carbohydrates to form dicarbonyl compounds that in turn react with proteins to form

cross links and adducts, known as glycoxidation products or advanced glycation end products (AGE). ROS also damage the genome, in the form of mutations in DNA (Fig. 34.2). As a result of oxidative stress, MDA adducts ALE and AGE increase in several chronic conditions such as atherosclerosis, Alzheimer's disease and diabetes mellitus.

ANTIOXIDANT DEFENSE SYSTEM

There are several levels of protection against oxidative damage as discussed below.

Antioxidant Enzymes

There is a group of enzymes that act to detoxify ROS. These include:

- **Catalase:** It is present in peroxisomes and detoxifies H_2O_2 (Fig. 34.3).
- **Superoxide dismutase (SOD):** It detoxifies $O_2^{\cdot-}$ (Fig. 34.4). There are three forms of SOD: SOD1

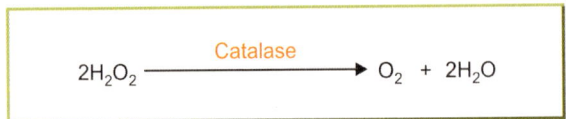

Fig. 34.3: Detoxification of H_2O_2 by catalase.

Chemistry to Clinics 34.1: Ischemia-reperfusion Injury

Ischemia and its consequences

Ischemia is defined as a condition of reduced oxygen availability to a tissue as a result of reduced blood flow, although it can arise from any condition in which the oxygen demand of the tissue is greater than its oxygen supply. In the heart, this most often occurs acutely by the development of an obstruction in one of the major coronary arteries, usually from a blood clot in the area of an advanced or ruptured atherosclerotic plaque. Ischemia cannot be tolerated for long in myocardial tissue. Immediately at the onset of ischemia, the affected myocardial tissue becomes acontractile (unable to contract). Within one hour, the oxygen-dependent cellular ionic and water balance mechanisms fail and the tissues swell, with a further loss of membrane integrity. Calcium extrusion mechanisms fail, and the resultant increase in intracellular Ca^{2+} activates enzymes that destroy myocardial tissue. If acute ischemia involves enough myocardial tissue, the initial loss of contractile ability may be sufficient to cause acute failure of the heart and circulatory collapse (cardiogenic shock). However, even with small ischemic episodes, the resulting tissue damage within hours after the initial insult may be enough to cause death from cardiac failure.

Reperfusion

The best course of action to reduce ischemic damage in the heart is to restore myocardial blood flow as quickly as possible and/or to change hemodynamic variables in such a way as to reduce myocardial oxygen demand. If the ischemia results from a blood clot in a major coronary artery, the physician can inject clot-lysing drugs, such as streptokinase or tissue-type plasminogen activator, through a catheter into the major coronary artery affected by the clot. These drugs dissolve the clot and restore flow. However, in reality, restoration of blood flow is often associated with induction of additional damage to the myocardium instead of restoration of cell viability. This phenomenon is called 'ischemia-reperfusion injury'. It happens because during the ischemic period, the arterioles downstream from the coronary arterial obstruction dilate through myogenic and metabolic mechanisms, lowering vascular resistance. On removal of the obstruction, this lowered resistance allows for a substantial reactive hyperemia, which floods the previously ischemic area with blood-derived inflammatory cells and oxygen. This hyperemia is associated with cell death from necrosis and apoptosis.

Biochemical mediators of ischemia-reperfusion injury

Tissue damage from ischemia-reperfusion injury results from increased generation of oxygen free radicals in the myocardium and endothelium, as well as from infiltrating neutrophils. Myocardial sources may result from ischemic conversion of xanthine dehydrogenase to xanthine oxidase, which produces superoxide anion radical from xanthine. Damaged mitochondria also act as a source of oxygen free radicals. Further, the radicals impair mitochondrial recovery and ATP generation, which leads to cell death. The accompanying neutrophil infiltration sets up a local inflammatory response which produces damaging cytokines, production of additional reactive oxygen species in the tissues and complement activation. Recent studies suggest that nitric oxide (NO) attenuates ischemia-reperfusion injury, perhaps by quenching superoxide produced in the condition.

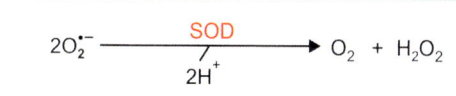

Fig. 34.4: Detoxification of $O_2^{\bullet-}$ by superoxide dismutase (SOD).

(Cu-Zn·SOD, cytoplasm) (Chemistry to Clinics 34.2), SOD2 (Mn·SOD, mitochondria) and SOD3 (Cu-Zn·SOD, extracellular).

- **Glutathione peroxidase (GPx):** It detoxifies H_2O_2 as well as lipid hydroperoxides. GPx is a selenium containing enzyme and requires reduced

glutathione (GSH) as a co-substrate (Fig. 34.5). GSH is a tripeptide-thiol (γ-glutamylcysteinylglycine) containing glutamate, cysteine and glycine. In this reaction, GSH is oxidized to GSSG (oxidized glutathione), which is not protective. The cell

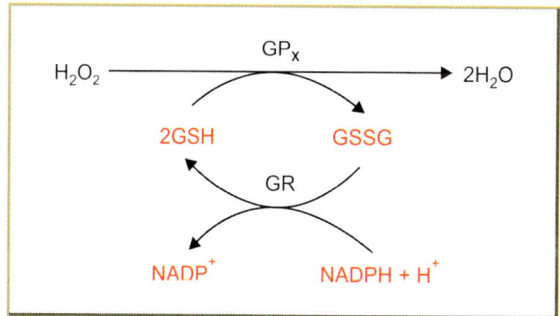

Fig. 34.5: Detoxification of H_2O_2 by glutathione peroxidase (GP$_x$) catalyzed reaction with reduced glutathione (GSH). Oxidized glutathione (GSSG) is reduced by glutathione reductase (GR) to regenerate GSH.

Chemistry to Clinics 34.2: Amyotrophic Lateral Sclerosis

It is the commonest form of motor neuron disease characterized by weakness, atrophy, fasciculation and stiffness of muscles. Besides difficulty in movement, there is compromise in speech, swallowing and breathing. Mutation in SOD1 results in failure to adequately protect against ROS. Aggregation of the abnormal SOD chains also interferes with normal cellular functions.

34

regenerates GSH from GSSG by an NADPH-dependent enzyme called glutathione reductase. NADPH is produced by the pentose phosphate pathway. The erythrocytes are particularly equipped with the GSH-NADPH based antioxidant defense system which prevents membrane lipid peroxidation and hemolysis.

Antioxidant Vitamins

Three vitamins, i.e. **vitamin A, C, and E**, provide the other line of defense against oxidative damage and are called antioxidant vitamins or the **'big three antioxidants'**. Vitamin C (ascorbate) in the aqueous phase while vitamin E (α and γ-tocopherols) in the lipid phase, act as chain-breaking antioxidants. Vitamin C reduces superoxide and lipid peroxyl radicals. It also has a role in reduction and recycling of vitamin E. In response to severe oxidative stress, vitamin E is maintained at constant concentration in the lipid phase until all the vitamin C is consumed. Thus, they do not propagate radical damages and are recycled.

Vitamin A is a lipophilic antioxidant. It is a potent singlet oxygen scavenger and protects against damage from sunlight in the retina and skin. Consumption of food rich in ascorbate, vitamin E, and β-carotene has been correlated with a reduced risk for certain types of cancers and decreased frequency of certain other chronic health problems.

Other Antioxidants

Glutathione (GSH, discussed above) is the **key intracellular non-enzymatic antioxidant**. Besides, lycopene, flavonoids, serum albumin (containing –SH groups), bilirubin, uric acid, etc. are also a part of the antioxidant defense system.

SOME IMPORTANT QUESTION

1. Write notes on:
   i. Reactive oxygen species
   ii. Oxidative stress
   iii. Free radicals
   iv. Antioxidant defenses
   v. Antioxidant vitamins
   vi. Ischemia-reperfusion injury

MULTIPLE CHOICE QUESTIONS

1. **The reactive oxygen species are implicated in the pathogenesis of:**
   A. Ischemia-reperfusion injury
   B. Alzheimer's disease
   C. Diabetes mellitus
   D. All of the above

2. **The following physiological process involves reactive oxygen species:**
   A. Phagocytosis
   B. Regulation of gene expression
   C. Apoptosis
   D. All of the above

3. **The following is not a physiological source of reactive oxygen species:**
   A. Xanthine oxidase reaction
   B. Pyruvate kinase reaction
   C. Oxidative phosphorylation
   D. Peroxisomal fatty acid oxidation

4. **The following detoxifies both H_2O_2 and lipid hydroperoxides:**
   A. Superoxide dismutase
   B. Catalase
   C. Glutathione peroxidase
   D. Vitamin C

5. **The following helps to maintain the levels of vitamin E:**
   A. Vitamin C
   B. Reduced glutathione
   C. β-Carotene
   D. All of the above

6

Special Topics and Clinical Chemistry

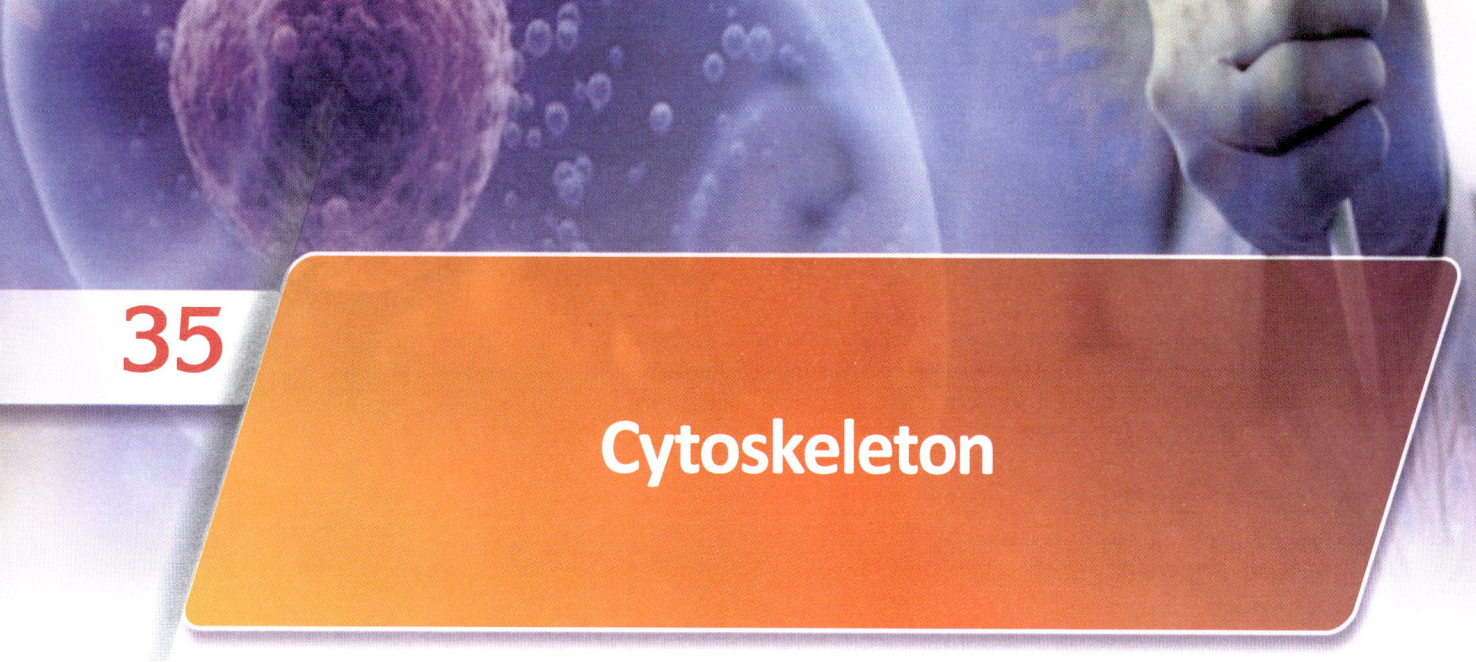

35

Cytoskeleton

The term cytoskeleton is a collective term for **non-membranous sub-cellular cytosolic fractions** that possess a fibrous structure, e.g. **microtubules**, **intermediate filaments** and **microfilaments**. Each of these is a polymer of protein subunits held together by weak, non-covalent bonds. Each cytoskeletal element has distinct properties and performs a variety of functions (Table 35.1).

MICROTUBULES

Microtubules are stiff, hollow, tubular structures, 25 nm in diameter. They are assembled from **αβ-tubulin** heterodimers that are arranged in longitudinal rows called **protofilaments**. Tubulin dimers that are polymerized into a microtubule contain a GTP molecule that is hydrolyzed soon after its incorporation into the polymer. Tubulin, thus, has **GTPase** activity.

Functions of Microtubules

1. Provide structural support that determine **cell shape** and resist forces that tend to deform it.

2. Provide the **internal framework** responsible for positioning various organelles.

3. Provide a network of tracks that direct **movement** of materials and organelles **within cells**, e.g. delivery of mRNA from the nucleus to the ribosomes, movement of molecules destined for exocytose, etc.

4. Form part of the **locomotor machinery** for the movement of cell as a whole, e.g. spermatozoa, WBC, fibroblasts, etc.

5. **Spindle** formation during chromosome segregation and cell division.

Certain *accessory proteins* are required for the proper functioning of microtubules. These include:

- **Microtubule associated proteins (MAP)**, e.g. the **tau** protein (Chemistry to Clinics 35.1).
- **Motor proteins** such as **kinesins** and **dyneins**, that generate the forces required for intracellular movements as well as the movements of the entire cell. To achieve this, the motor proteins convert the chemical energy of ATP into mechanical energy.

Table 35.1: Comparative properties of cytoskeletal elements

Properties	Microtubules	Intermediate filaments	Microfilaments
Structure	Stiff, hollow tube	Tough, rope-like fibers	Flexible, helical
Diameter	25 nm	10 nm	8 nm
Subunits	αβ-tubulin	Globular proteins	Actin monomers
Enzyme activity	GTPase	None	ATPase
Associated proteins	Microtubule-associated proteins, kinesins, dyneins	Plectin	Actin-binding proteins, myosins
Major functions	Structural framework, intracellular transport	Structural framework	Motility, contractility

Chemistry to Clinics 35.1: Tauopathies

Tau proteins influence many properties of microtubules including their flexibility and stability. An abnormally high level of phosphorylation of tau is implicated in several neurodegenerative disorders, e.g. Alzheimer's disease. Non-Alzheimer's tauopathies are grouped together as 'Pick's complex'.

Microtubule Assembly

The assembly of microtubules from αβ-tubulin dimers occurs in two distinct phases. These include a slow phase of nucleation in which a small portion of the microtubule is initially formed, followed by a rapid phase of elongation. The nucleation is controlled by specialized structures called '**microtubules-organizing centers**' that govern the number of microtubules,

their polarity, the number of protofilaments that make up their walls as well as the time and location of their assembly. It should be remembered that the microtubules are dynamic polymers that are constantly subjected to shortening, lengthening, disassembly and reassembly. Some external factors interfere with the functions of microtubules by promoting **disassembly**, e.g. cold temperature, elevated Ca^{2+} concentration, and drugs like colchicine and vincristine (Chemistry to Clinics 35.2 and 35.3).

Chemistry to Clinics 35.3: Cancer and Vincristine

Vincristine, an alkaloid, binds to tubulin dimers, thus inhibiting assembly of microtubules. This arrests mitosis in metaphase. Therefore, vincristine is a useful anticancer drug.

Chemistry to Clinics 35.2: Acute Gouty Arthritis and Colchicine

Persistent high serum uric acid levels trigger an acute attack of gout involving the joints. The initial event is the precipitation of urate crystals in the synovial fluid (known as 'tophi') to initiate an acute inflammatory response. Neutrophils migrate into the joint, phagocytose the urate crystals and release a glycoprotein that adds onto the ongoing inflammation by:

a. Increasing lactic acid production by the inflammatory cells leading to fall in local pH that favors more urate crystallization and sets up a vicious cycle.

b. Releasing lysosomal enzymes which cause joint destruction.

The drug colchicine is very beneficial under these conditions because it binds to the protein tubulin and rapidly leads to disassembly of the microtubules. As a result, neutrophil chemotaxis is halted and the glycoprotein release is also inhibited since both are microtubule-dependent processes. Thus, the vicious cycle gets interrupted. Ironically, colchicine causes metaphase arrest by binding to microtubules in the mitotic spindle (Fig. 35.1). This is detrimental to cells with a high turnover such as the enterocytes and explains the severe gastrointestinal side effects of the drug.

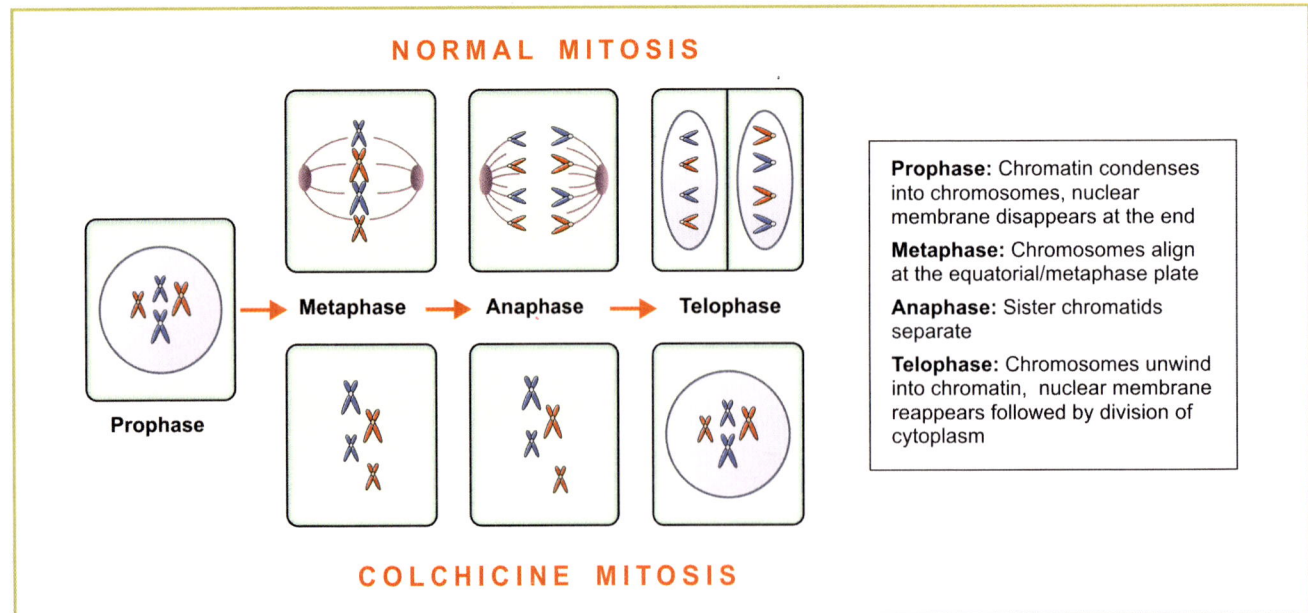

Fig. 35.1: Metaphase arrest by colchicine. Mitosis in presence of colchicine is called '**colchicine mitosis**'.

INTERMEDIATE FILAMENTS

Intermediate filaments are strong rope-like fibers that are approximately 10 nm in diameter. They are often connected by long cross-bridges consisting of the fibrous protein **plectin**. The basic unit of intermediate filaments is a tetramer formed by two dimers, which may be homodimers or heterodimers. Neither ATP nor GTP is required for its assembly. The polypeptide subunits of intermediate filaments can be divided into five major classes based on the type of cell in which they are found as well as certain biochemical, genetic and immunologic criteria. The protein classes are keratin, vimentin (Chemistry to Clinics 35.4), desmin, neurofilaments and lamin. An inherited disease called desmin-related myopathy is caused by a mutation in the gene that encodes desmin.

The assembly and disassembly of intermediate filaments is controlled by phosphorylation and dephosphorylation of its protein subunits. They are relatively insoluble and resistant to tensile forces, a property similar to the extracellular protein collagen. Keratin filaments (note that **'keratin' is different from 'keratan'** which is a glycosaminoglycan found in the extracellular matrix as keratan sulfate) constitute the primary structural proteins of epithelial cells including epidermal cells, hepatocytes and pancreatic acinar

Chemistry to Clinics 35.4: Colorectal Cancer

Stool samples are a rich source of DNA since they always contain exfoliated cells derived from the colonic mucosa. DNA analysis for the *vimentin* gene has revealed that if the gene is hypermethylated, it indicates the loss of gene function. This can be a useful yet non-invasive screening test that predicts the presence of colorectal cancer. The advantage of the technique is that it avoids invasive screening procedures like colonoscopy that can miss very small tumors.

cells. The cytoplasm of neurons contains loosely packed bundles of intermediate filaments called **neurofilaments**, whose long axes are oriented parallel to that of the nerve cell axon.

MICROFILAMENTS

Microfilaments are 8 nm in diameter and composed of a double helical polymer of the protein **actin**, one of the major contractile proteins. In the presence of ATP, actin monomers polymerize to form a flexible, helical filament called actin filament or F-actin. They play a key role in all types of contractility and motility within cells. However, depending on the type of cell and its activity, actin filaments can be organized into highly ordered arrays, tightly held bundles or loose, ill-defined networks.

Before being incorporated into a filament, an actin monomer binds a molecule of ATP that is subsequently hydrolyzed to ADP as the actin filament grows. This is due to the ATPase activity of actin. The bulk of an actin filament thus, consists of ADP-actin subunits. The molecular motors of actin filaments are the **myosin** family of proteins. Myosins are generally divided into two groups:

1. **Type I (unconventional myosins):** Myosin I molecules have a single globular head and a variable tail length and are implicated in cell motility and organelle transport.

2. **Type II (conventional myosins):** These were first identified in muscles and contain a long, rod-shaped tail attached at one end to two globular heads. The head binds the actin filament, hydrolyzes ATP and undergoes conformational changes required for generating force during muscle contraction as well as some non-muscle activities like cytokinesis.

SOME IMPORTANT QUESTIONS

1. What is cytoskeleton? Name various cytoskeletal elements.

2. Briefly discuss the differences between various cytoskeletal elements.

3. Write notes on:
   i. Microtubule assembly
   ii. Myosins

MULTIPLE CHOICE QUESTIONS

35

1. **The following has an associated GTPase activity:**
   - A. Microtubules
   - B. Intermediate filaments
   - C. Microfilaments
   - D. None of the above

2. **The following has an associated ATPase activity:**
   - A. Microtubules
   - B. Intermediate filaments
   - C. Microfilaments
   - D. None of the above

3. **The delivery of mRNA from the nucleus to the ribosomes requires:**
   - A. Microtubules
   - B. Intermediate filaments
   - C. Microfilaments
   - D. None of the above

4. **Hypermethylation of the following gene is linked to colorectal cancer:**
   - A. Keratin
   - B. Vimentin
   - C. Desmin
   - D. Lamin

5. **Microtubules form part of the locomotor machinery in:**
   - A. WBC
   - B. Fibroblasts
   - C. Spermatozoa
   - D. All of the above

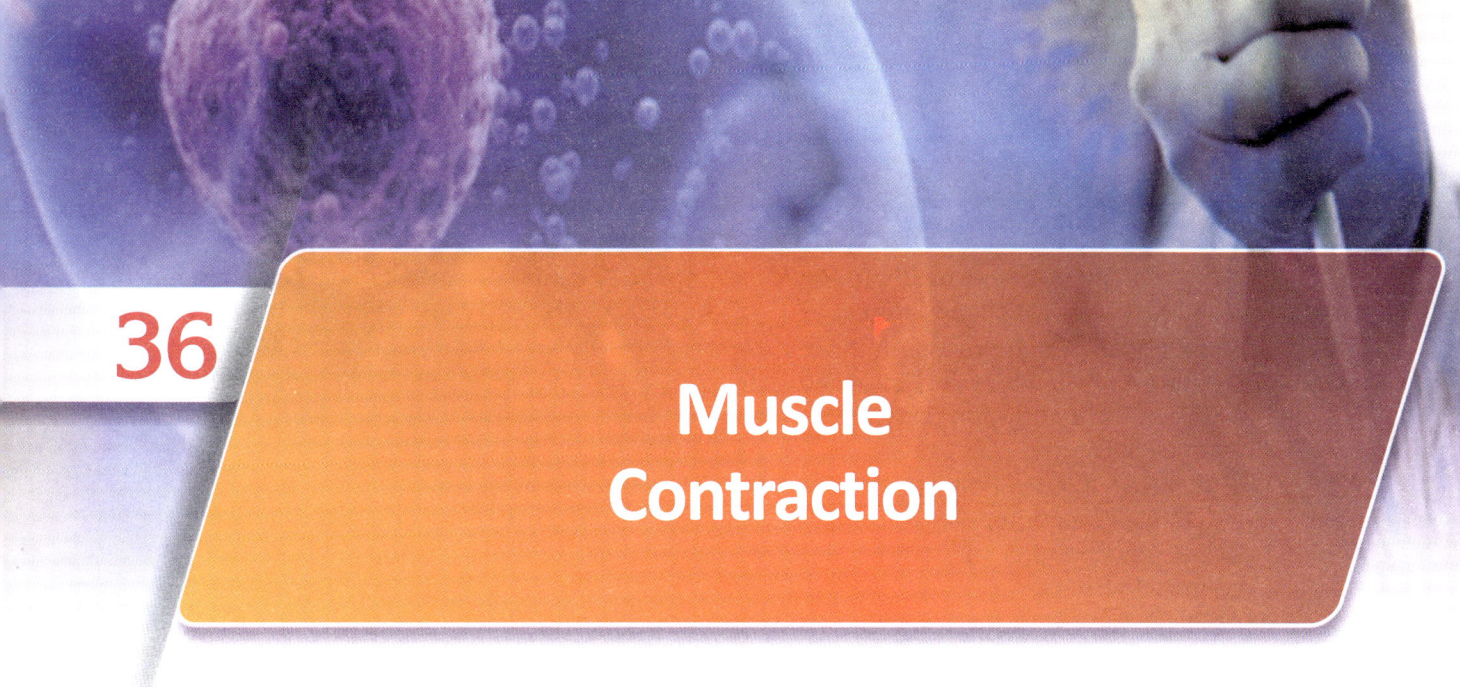

36

Muscle Contraction

In a normal adult, though muscle mass is nearly 40% of the body weight, metabolically it is a highly active tissue and performs more than 50% of the total metabolic activities.

STRUCTURE OF SKELETAL MUSCLE

The voluntary muscles which include the skeletal muscles have a striated (striped) appearance consisting of long, thin, multinucleated cells known as muscle fibers that run along the length of the muscle.

Muscle Fibers

The muscle fibers are 0.01 to 0.1 nm in diameter and 1 to 40 nm in length. A large number of these fibers are bound together by areolar connective tissue and are attached via tendons to the bone or other structures whose movement they control.

- Muscle fiber membrane or **sarcolemma** is an electrically excitable membrane and is important in the transport of motor nerve impulses.
- It also contains a large number of transport ducts called **sarcotubules**.
- Muscle fibers also contain **sarcoplasmic reticulum**, similar in structure and functions to the endoplasmic reticulum found in other cells, and the **sarcoplasm** which may be called muscle plasma. Sarcoplasm contains **myoglobin**, a hemoprotein which stores oxygen derived from hemoglobin in the blood capillaries.

The composition of skeletal muscle is given in Table 36.1.

Table 36.1: Composition of the skeletal muscle

Ingredients	% of total muscle mass
Water	70–80%
Proteins	20
Myosin	
Actin	
Actin cross-linking proteins	
Tropomyosin	
Troponins	
Myoglobin	
Titin, dystrophin	
Lipids	3
Triacylglycerols	
Cholesterol	
Phospholipids	
Glycogen	0.5–1.0
Other organic substances	
Myoinositol	
Creatine phosphate	
Oligopeptides (carnosine, anserine, glutathione)	
Free amino acids	
Enzymes	
Carnitine	
Inorganic ions	
Cations (Na^+, K^+, Mg^{2+}, Ca^{2+})	
Anions (phosphates, sulphates, bicarbonate, chloride)	

Types of muscle fibers: A typical skeletal muscle usually contains a mixture of fiber types out of which a particular type predominates. There are three types of skeletal muscle fibers based on their speed of contraction and ability to withstand fatigue:

- **Type I: Slow twitch**, fatigue resistant; the myosin molecules split ATP slowly; richly supplied with blood vessels, mitochondria and myoglobin, hence called **red muscle fibers**.
- **Type IIA: Fast twitch**, fatigue resistant; the myosin molecules split ATP rapidly; richly supplied with blood vessels, mitochondria and myoglobin, hence called **red muscle fibers**.
- **Type IIB: Fast twitch**, fatiguable; the myosin molecules split ATP rapidly; poorly supplied with blood vessels, mitochondria and myoglobin, hence called **white muscle fibers**.

However, from a practical point of view, a general comparison between fast and slow muscle fibers is shown in Table 36.2.

Myofibrils

Muscle fibers contain parallel bundles of myofibrils (Greek: myos means muscle). Major features of the myofibril are that:

- It has a **light band** called the isotropic band (**I band**) which contains thin filaments and a **dark band**, designated as anisotropic band (**A band**) which has a central **H zone** containing thick filaments and an outer segment with the overlapping thick and thin filaments. The I band is bisected by a dark zone (present in the center of the I band) called the **Z line**.
- The functional unit of a myofibril is known as **sarcomere** (Greek: sarkos means flesh). It is a region between two successive Z lines (present at the center of each I band), i.e. the region comprising of one-half of an I band, the A band and one-half of the next I band.

- The A band is formed of a large number of **thick filaments** whereas I band is composed of a comparable number of **thin filaments** which are interspersed between the thick filaments. Two sets of the filaments, in turn, are linked by cross-bridges in the area where they overlap (Fig. 36.1).
- Thick filaments are composed almost entirely of myosin. Thin filaments consist of chains of the actin molecules with the associated tropomyosin and troponin molecules.
- Thin filaments slide over the thick filaments. Muscle contraction leads to a decrease in length of the sarcomere caused by a reduction in distance between the I band and the H zone. The lengths of the thick filaments and the thin filaments, however, remain constant. A contracted muscle thus is reduced to nearly two-thirds of its fully extended length (Fig. 36.2).

MUSCLE PROTEINS

More than half of the total proteins present in the skeletal muscle are structural proteins including myosin, actin, actin cross-linking proteins, tropomyosin and troponin. Myosin and actin together account for more than two-thirds of the total muscle proteins. Muscle also contains myoglobin and enzymes involved in metabolism, besides the proteins of the extracellular matrix such as collagens.

Myosin

As mentioned above, thick filaments are composed almost entirely of myosin which are placed 'end-to-end' with the light chains, striking out in the form of double heads. Myosin consists of six polypeptide chains which include **two identical heavy chains** and two pairs of **two different types of the light chains**

Parameter	Fast muscle fibers	Slow muscle fibers
• Speed of contraction	Fast	Slow
• Force of contraction	Weak	Powerful
• Duration of contraction	Brief	Sustained
• Response of sarcomeres	No contraction or complete contraction	Partial contraction possible
• Source of ATP	Fermentation (anaerobic glycolysis)	Aerobic glycolysis
• Major fuel	Muscle glycogen	Glucose, fatty acids
• Example	Quadriceps (thigh)	Gluteus maximus (buttocks)

Table 36.2: Comparison between fast and slow muscle fibers

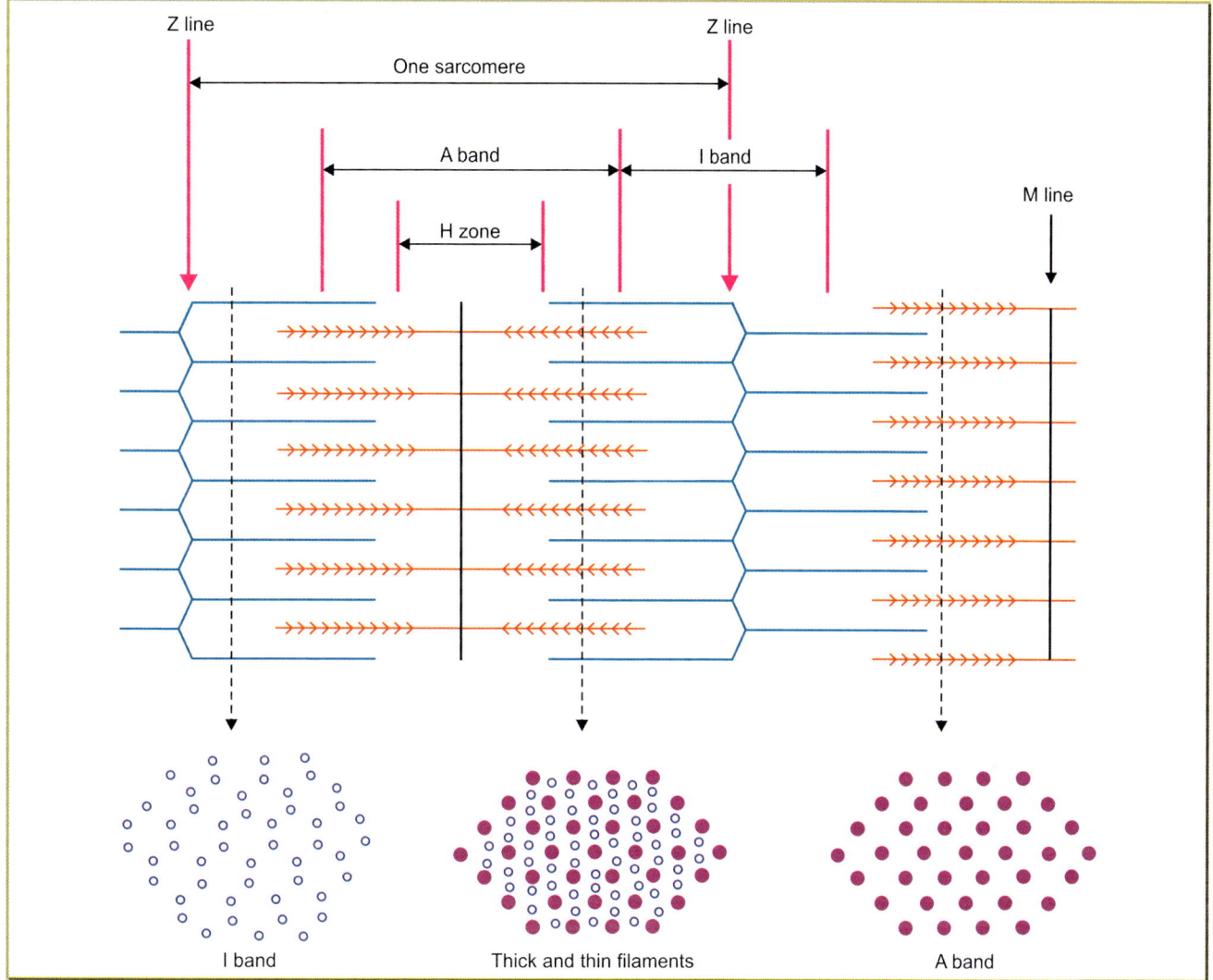

Fig. 36.1: Structure of a sarcomere.

called **regulatory light chains** and **essential light chains**.

- Each myosin head associates with an essential light chain and a regulatory light chain. Regulatory light chains play a role in the control of muscle contraction by Ca^{2+} whereas the essential light chains are required for ATPase activity of the myosin head.

- The N-terminal half of each heavy chain forms an elongated globular head to which two light chains bind.

- The C-terminal half of the heavy chain forms a long fibrous α-helical tail, two of which associate to form a left-handed coil.

- Taken together, a molecule of myosin, thus consists of a long rod-like segment with two globular heads (Fig. 36.3).

Several hundred myosin molecules aggregate to form a thick filament. The rod-like tails pack end-to-end in a regular staggered array, leaving globular heads projecting to the sides on both the ends. These myosin heads form cross-bridges to the thin filaments in the intact myofibril.

Actin

Actin is a globulin and is a major constituent of **thin filaments** of the sarcomere. Actin exists in two forms, i.e. as globular actin (G actin) and filament actin (F actin).

36

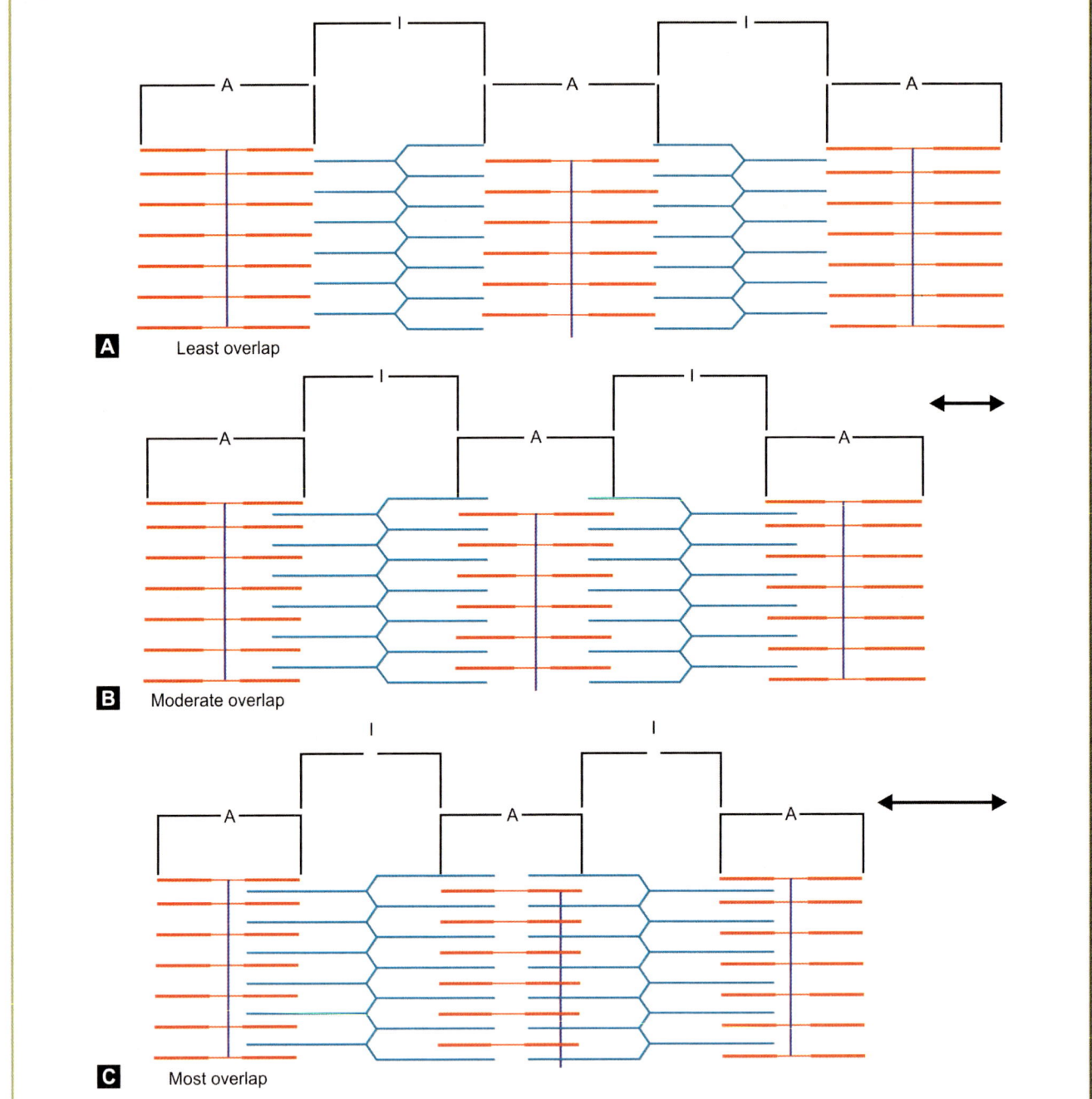

Fig. 36.2: Shortening of a sarcomere.

- **G actin** is a low molecular weight monomeric protein (M_r 42 kD) with a globular conformation. These monomers readily form large, elongated actin filament polymers called **F actin**, for which Mg^{2+} are essential. Besides, monomeric G actin units are oriented in such a way that they acquire a pointed-region (pointed-end) and a barbed-region (barbed-end). Assembly of the monomeric units occurs at the barbed-end.

- A group of proteins called **parafilins** binds to G actin, stabilizes the monomers and prevents their polymerization.

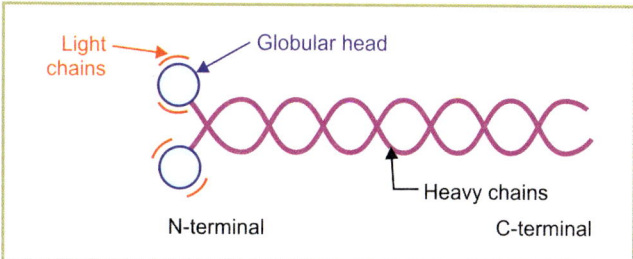

Fig. 36.3: A molecule of myosin.

- F actin contains nearly 1000 monomeric units which are organized as a string of beads. F actin filaments are made up of two strings of the G actin monomers (Fig. 36.4).
- F actin combines with myosin and forms **actomyosin**. Each actin monomer can bind a myosin head by ion-pairing and by association of the hydrophobic patches on each protein. In the presence of ATP, K^+ and Mg^{2+} actomyosin is highly contractile.

Actin is ubiquitous and is usually a most abundant cytoplasmic protein in eukaryotic cells, typically accounting for 5 to 10% of the total proteins. Though actin is most prominent in the muscle, it also exists in other tissues where it is responsible for various motile processes, such as cell locomotion, cytoplasmic streaming and cytokinesis (separation of the daughter cells during cell division). The non-muscle actin forms fibers which are designated as **microfilaments**. Assembly of the actin monomers into the fibers requires ATP. Along with the other proteins fibers, these microfilaments form elements of the cytoskeleton.

Actin Cross-linking Proteins

There are some proteins that cross-link and stabilize actin chains. These include filamin, α-actinin and β-actinin.

- **Filamin:** It is a high molecular weight, flexible protein that usually exists as a dimer. It binds to actin at nearly 40 nm intervals.
- **α-Actinin:** It is mainly located in Z line of the muscle fiber and ensures spacing of the actin filaments.
- **β-Actinin:** It acts as an 'actin capping protein'. It binds to the active site of the G actin monomer, so that the monomer is unable to combine with another monomer. It thus stabilizes G monomers and prevents their polymerization.

Tropomyosin

Tropomyosin is a double-stranded, β-helical protein with a molecular weight of about 70 kD. It is intervened between the two helical strands of F actin, i.e. tropomyosin molecules attach end-to-end and form a thin filament on each strand of the actin molecule. One tropomyosin molecule extends over seven actin molecules whereas 300–400 actin molecules are contained in each filament of the skeletal muscle (which is about 1 μm in length).

Troponin

Thin filaments consist of chains of the actin molecules with the associated tropomyosin and troponin molecules (Fig. 36.5). Troponin is a spherical molecule with a molecular weight of about 70 kD. It is positioned at

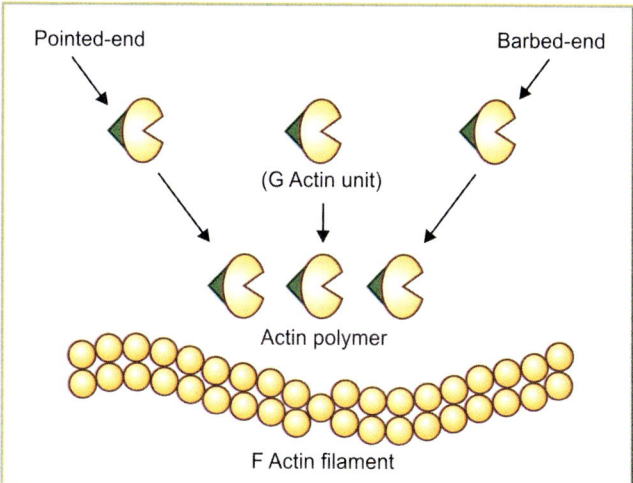

Fig. 36.4: Assembly of F actin filament.

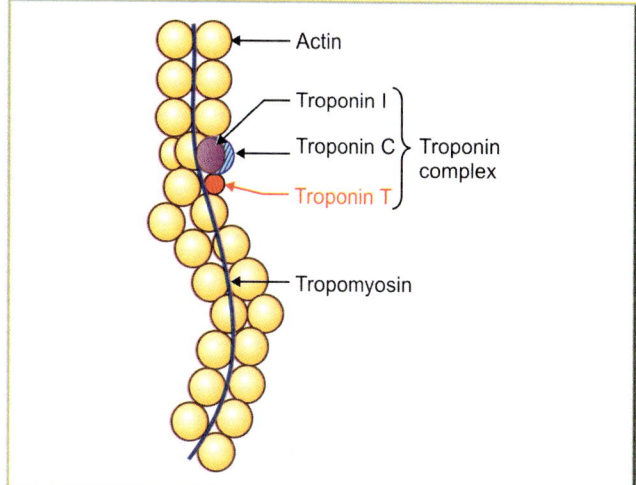

Fig. 36.5: Thin filament.

36

Chemistry to Clinics 36.1: Cardiac Troponins

The skeletal and cardiac isoforms of troponin C are identical. However, the skeletal and cardiac isoforms for troponin I and troponin T are distinct. Measurement of serum cardiac troponins is useful because they are:

1. More sensitive and specific indicators of myocardial infarction (MI) compared with CK-MB.
2. Detectable for a longer time following MI.
3. Able to differentiate between unstable angina and MI in patients with chest pain.
4. Employed in risk stratification of patients following MI.

regular intervals along the actin filaments. Troponin is composed of three different types of subunits called troponin T, troponin I and troponin C (Chemistry to Clinics 36.1).

- **Troponin T:** It binds the other two subunits to the tropomyosin molecule, noncovalently. Tropomyosin-troponin complex, in turn, regulates muscle contraction by controlling access of the myosin heads on the thick filaments to their binding sites on the actin.
- **Troponin I:** It is the inhibitory subunit. Its function is to inhibit the interaction of the head of myosin with actin thereby preventing contraction of myofibrils.
- **Troponin C:** It is a Ca^{2+} binding protein and is rich in aspartate and glutamate. Troponin C can also competitively bind Mg^{2+} ions.

Other Muscle Proteins

- **Titin (connectin):** It is the **largest known single polypeptide**. Titin gene contains the **largest number of introns ever found in any single gene**. The protein participates in muscle contraction and is also a structural protein for chromosomes. Mutations in titin are associated with familial hypertrophic cardiomyopathy and tibial muscular dystrophy. Autoantibodies to titin are found in scleroderma.
- **Dystrophin:** The *dystrophin* gene normally encodes a protein dystrophin localized to the inner surface of the sarcolemma of the muscle fiber. Actually, dystrophin itself is only a part of a more elaborate system of proteins bridging the cytoskeleton (actin filaments) and the extracellular matrix, via a matrix protein laminin. The dystrophin-anchored complex serves the following functions:

Chemistry to Clinics 36.2: Muscular Dystrophy

Presentation: It refers to a group of congenital diseases involving the muscles, characterized by a progressive course in children and death by adolescence. For example, Duchenne muscular dystrophy is an X-linked recessive disorder caused by a mutation in the *dystrophin* gene. Children present with delayed walking, difficulty in climbing stairs and bulky calf muscles.

Complications: Although the child is confined to a wheel chair, the muscle bulk may be maintained because most of the muscle fibers are replaced with fibro-fatty tissue. A common cause of death is lower respiratory tract infections due to non-functioning of respiratory muscles.

Laboratory diagnosis: It is made by raised serum creatinine as well as creatine kinase, particularly the CK-MM isoenzyme. The levels are high at birth and early childhood. Later, the levels may decline due to inactivity and loss of muscle mass (Fig. 36.6). Immunohistochemical staining showing absence of dystrophin or mutation analysis confirm the diagnosis.

Management: Corticosteroids and physiotherapy provide temporary improvement. New approaches to treatment include antisense oligonucleotides (structural analogs of DNA allowing mutated part of dystrophin gene to be skipped when it is transcribed to RNA, permitting the synthesis of a still-truncated but more functional counterpart of the desired protein) and stem cells.

1. It stabilizes the sarcolemmal membrane during contraction/relaxation cycles.
2. It links the contractile force generated in the muscle fiber with the extracellular environment.
3. It maintains the local organization of key membrane proteins called dystroglycans and sarcoglycans.

Abnormal dystrophin results in **Duchenne muscular dystrophy** (Chemistry to Clinics 36.2).

BIOCHEMICAL CHANGES DURING MUSCLE CONTRACTION

- Impulses transmitted via motor nerve (across the neuromuscular junction to the sarcolemma of the muscle fiber), initiates contraction of myofibrils.
- This, in turn, stimulates the **release of Ca^{2+}** which bind to **troponin C** of the thin actin filament and produces a conformational change in it, followed by shift of the tropomyosin and attachment of **crossbridges** of the thick myosin filament to the thin actin filaments.
- **ATP** binds to specific sites on the surface of myosin. The tendency for ATP to bind is so efficient that normally almost every myosin head is bound to ATP.

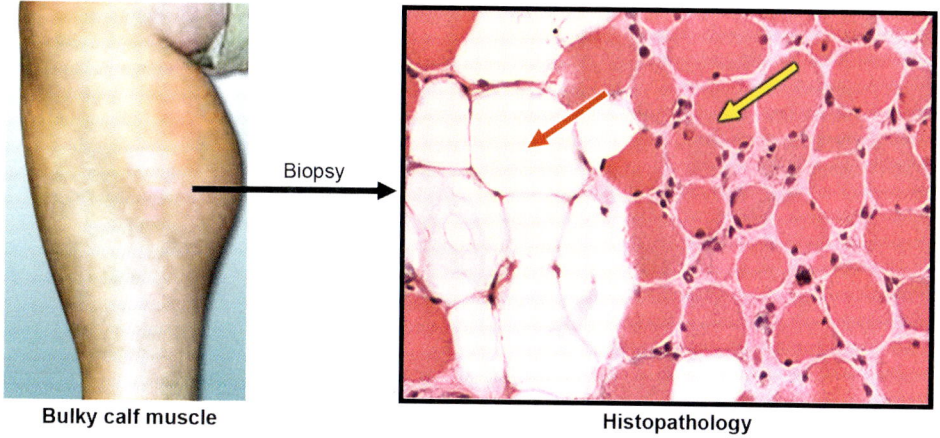

Bulky calf muscle **Histopathology**

Fig. 36.6: Duchenne muscular dystrophy. Muscle (yellow arrow) being replaced by adipocytes (red arrow).

- Formation of the charged **myosin·ATP complex** alters conformation of the protein in a manner that the charged complex shows a greater tendency to bind to an actin molecule.

- After myosin·ATP complex bind to actin, ATP binds to a myosin head whose ATPase action causes hydrolysis of ATP. This puts the myosin head into a high-energy conformation.

- The myosin head is now weak to bind to actin monomer that is closer to the Z line. This results in the **release of inorganic phosphate (Pi),** which further causes a conformational shift and increases the affinity of myosin for actin.

- The resulting transient state is immediately followed by the **power stroke,** causing a further conformational shift that sweeps myosin head's C-terminal tail towards the Z line.

- **ADP is then released,** thereby **completing the cycle** (Fig. 36.7).

- Myosin heads walk or row-up the adjacent thin filaments towards the Z line, with the concomitant **contraction of the muscle,** i.e. the actin filaments slide along the thick myosin filaments (which otherwise were stationary) towards the center of the sarcomere thereby shortening its size. These events occur so rapidly that the whole process of muscle contraction takes only 10–20 milliseconds.

- At the end, **Ca^{2+} are taken-up** into the sarcoplasmic reticulum network and cross-bridges of the myosin retract. As a result, the sarcomeres and the muscle fibers **relax and return to the resting state.**

- In the low-energy state, the complex remains intact until a new molecule of ATP is bound, usually within a very short time (about 1 millisecond).

The sequence continues depending upon the supply of ATP and other components essential for the muscle contraction.

Biochemical Basis of Fatigue

Muscle fatigue is the inability of a muscle to maintain contraction and power output. During maximum exertion, the onset of fatigue takes nearly 20 seconds. It is not the result of depletion of glycogen reserves nor it is due to lactate accumulation as previously thought. It is due to **decreased intramuscular (intracellular) pH** as H^+ are generated during glycolysis. Decreased pH reduces the activity of phosphofructo-kinase-1 (PFK-1), i.e. reduces the rate of glycolysis. Thus, decreased synthesis and availability of ATP result in a feeling of fatigue. Reduced activity of PFK-1 is advantageous because the remaining ATP is not consumed in the PFK-1 reaction.

REGENERATION OF ATP

The energy for muscle contraction, as discussed above, is provided by ATP which is hydrolyzed to ADP and Pi. ATP can be regenerated in the muscle by several routes (Fig. 36.8):

- **Lohmann reaction:** ATP can be regenerated by utilizing high-energy phosphate compound, creatine phosphate. This reaction is catalyzed by

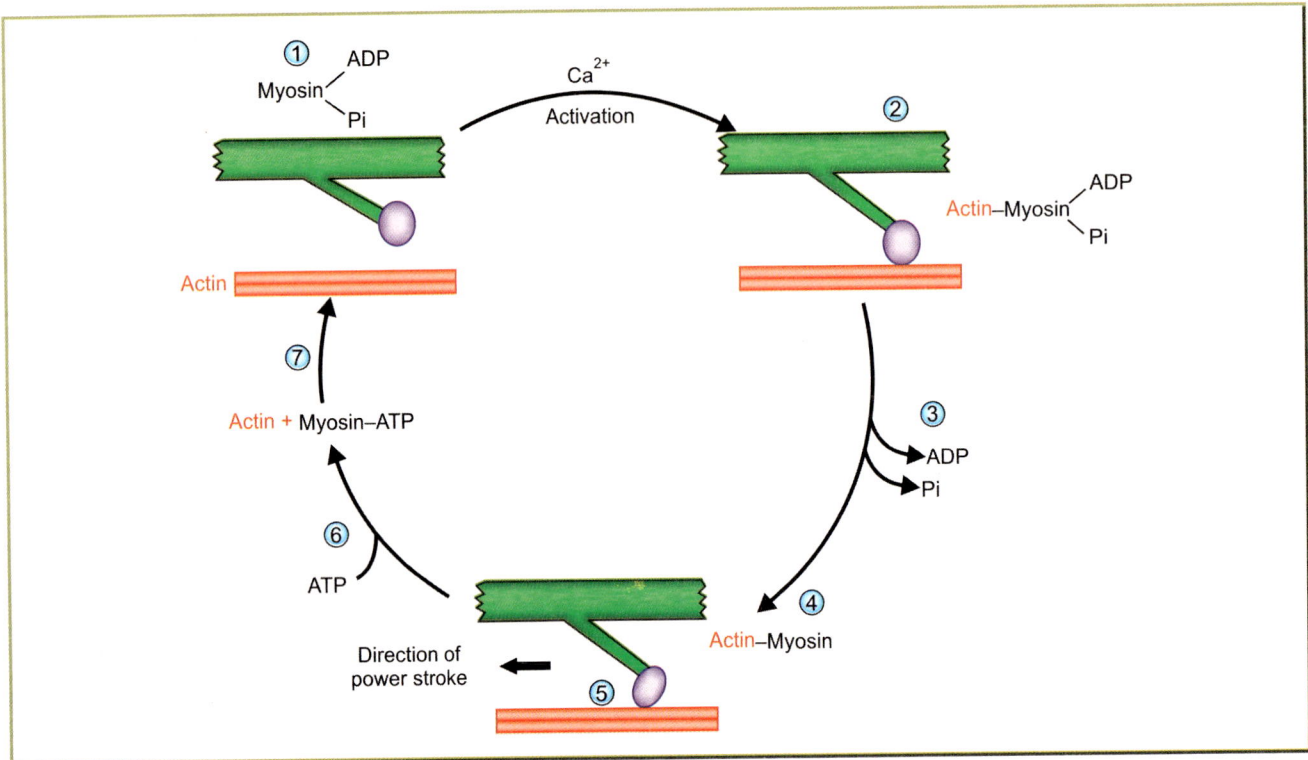

Fig. 36.7: Biochemical changes during muscle contraction. 1. Resting state: Myosin not interacting with actin, hence energy of ATP hydrolysis not released; 2. Activated state: Myosin interacting with actin; 3. Release of products of ATP hydrolysis; 4. Power stroke; 5. Rigor state; 6. Detachment of actin accompanied by binding of new ATP molecule; 7. ATP hydrolysis and return to resting state.

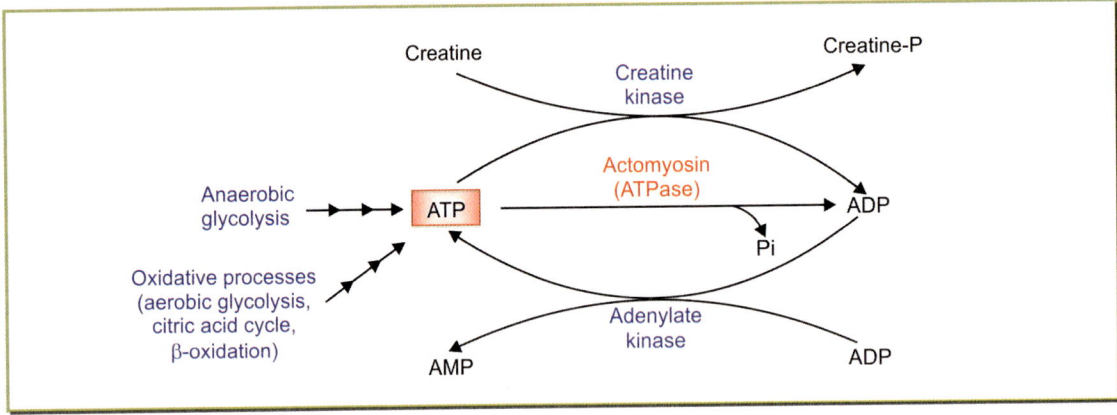

Fig. 36.8: Utilization and resynthesis of ATP in muscle.

creatine kinase (creatine phosphokinase or CPK) and is called the Lohmann reaction (Fig. 36.9).

- **Adenylate kinase reaction:** ATP can also be regenerated from ADP by the enzyme adenylate kinase which is also referred to as myokinase (Fig. 36.10).

- **Anaerobic glycolysis:** Muscles possess the capacity to synthesize ATP under anaerobic conditions by utilizing its glycogen stores. A limited supply of oxygen as may occur during a short period of strenuous exercise, results in the accumulation of lactate in the blood.

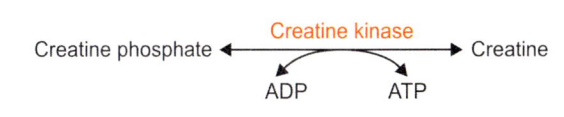

Fig. 36.9: Regeneration of ATP by creatine kinase reaction.

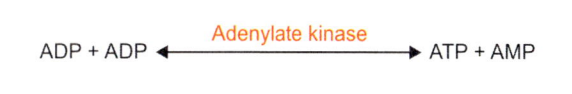

Fig. 36.10: Regeneration of ATP by adenylate kinase reaction.

- **Oxidative processes:** Prolonged exercise gradually increases oxygenation of the muscle to a maximum. Thus, ATP may also be produced by various oxidative processes such as from aerobic glycolysis followed by the citric acid cycle, and from β-oxidation of fatty acids.

SOME IMPORTANT QUESTIONS

1. Describe the structure and composition of skeletal muscle.

2. Describe various functions of proteins present in the skeletal muscle.

3. Describe:
   i. Events during muscle contraction
   ii. Types of muscle fibers.
   iii. Regeneration of ATP in the muscle

4. Write notes on:
   i. Sarcomere
   ii. Actin
   iii. Myosin
   iv. Troponins
   v. Duchenne muscular dystrophy
   vi. Titin

MULTIPLE CHOICE QUESTIONS

1. **The assembly of monomeric G actin into polymeric F actin requires:**
   A. Ca^{2+}
   B. Mg^{2+}
   C. Fe^{2+}
   D. Cu^{2+}

2. **The following is an actin capping protein:**
   A. Filamin
   B. α-Actinin
   C. β-Actinin
   D. Myosin

3. **The following is not true for Duchenne muscular dystrophy:**
   A. Increased serum creatinine in early childhood
   B. Increased serum CK-MB
   C. Muscle bulk maintained due to replacement of muscle fibers by fibro-fatty tissue
   D. LRTI is a common cause of death

4. **The biochemical basis of fatigue is:**
   A. Depletion of Ca^{2+} from the sarcoplasmic reticulum
   B. Inhibition of PFK-1 by accumulation of H^+
   C. Accumulation of lactate
   D. Glycogen depletion

5. **Myokinase is:**
   A. CPK
   B. Adenylate kinase
   C. PFK-1
   D. PFK-2

37

Extracellular Matrix

Various types of connective tissues including tendons, cartilage and the corneal stroma are referred to as the extracellular matrix. Major components of the extracellular matrix including collagens, elastin, proteoglycans and a variety of other proteins form an interconnected network that is bound to the cell surface.

COLLAGENS

Collagens comprise a family of **fibrous glycoproteins** that are present only in extracellular matrices. Collagens are the **most abundant proteins** in the human body. A collagen molecule has a long rigid structure in which three polypeptides called α-chains are wound around one another in a rope-like **triple helix**.

Collagens are found throughout the body. Their types and organization are determined by the structural role collagens play in a particular organ. In some tissues, collagen may be dispersed as gel that gives support to the structure, as in the vitreous humor. In other tissues, collagens may be bundled in tight parallel fibers that provide great **tensile strength** as in tendons (tensile strength means the ability to bear weight/stress without stretching, bending or breaking). In the cornea, collagens are stacked so as to transmit light with a minimum of scattering. Collagens of bone occur as fibers arranged at an angle to each other so as to resist mechanical sheer from any direction.

Types of Collagens

It is a superfamily of proteins which includes **at least 27 distinct types**. Although there are many differences among the members of the collagen family, all share at least two important structural features:

1. All collagen molecules are trimers consisting of three polypeptide chains called α-chains.
2. All three polypeptide chains are wound around each other to form a unique, rod-like triple helix, e.g. collagen type I is $\alpha I_2\alpha 2$ (i.e. it has two αI and one α2 chains). Type II collagen is αI_3 (containing 3 αI chains), etc.

Based on their location and functions in the body, collagens are organized into 3 groups:

1. **Fibril-forming Collagens:** These are linear polymers with characteristic bonding patterns and have rope-like triple-stranded helix, e.g. type I, type II and type III. *Type I collagen fibers* are found in supporting elements of high tensile strength such as in skin, bone, tendon, blood vessels and cornea. *Type II fibres* are found in cartilaginous structures such as cartilage, intervertebral disc and vitreous body. *Type III collagens* occur in more distensible tissues such as blood vessels and fetal skin.

2. **Network-forming Collagens:** They form a three-dimensional mesh, e.g. type IV and VII collagens. *Type IV collagens* are thin, sheet or mesh-like structures that function as semipermeable basement membrane found in the kidney and the lung. *Type VII collagens* are found beneath stratified squamous epithelia.

3. **Fibril-associated Collagens:** These collagens link collagen fibrils to one another as well as to other components in the extracellular matrix, e.g. type IX and type XII collagens. *Type IX collagens* are

found in cartilage whereas *type XII collagens* occur in tendons and ligaments.

Structure and Composition

A collagen molecule is a fibrous protein which has an elongated triple-helical structure (Fig. 37.1)). It is **rich in proline and glycine**, both of which are important in the formation of the triple-stranded helix. Proline facilitates the formation of the helical conformation of each α-chain because of its ring structure that causes kinks in the peptide chain. **Glycine is found in every third position** of the polypeptide chain forming part of a repeating sequence Gly-X-Y. It is due to the reason that glycine is the smallest amino acid and fits into the restricted space where three chains of the helix come together. X is frequently proline while Y may be proline or lysine, which gets hydroxylated and occurs as hydroxyproline or hydroxylysine.

Biosynthesis

1. Polypeptide precursors of the collagens are formed in fibroblasts (or osteoblasts of bone and chondroblasts of cartilage) and secreted into the extracellular matrix. The newly synthesized polypeptide precursors of α-chains (pre-procollagens) contain a special amino acid sequence at the N-terminal end. This signal sequence facilitates the binding of ribosomes to the rough endoplasmic reticulum (RER) and directs the passage of the polypeptide chain into the cisternae of the RER. The signal sequence is rapidly cleaved in the endoplasmic reticulum to yield a precursor called pro-α-chain.

2. The pro-α-chain is processed by a number of enzymes within the lumen of the RER while the polypeptides are still being synthesized. Proline and lysine residues found in the Y-position are hydroxylated by prolyl hydroxylase and lysyl hydroxylase respectively. This is a **post-translational modification** and the hydroxylation reactions require molecular oxygen and **vitamin C. Hydroxyproline is important in stabilizing the triple-helical structure** of collagens because it maximizes interchain hydrogen bond formation. In case of vitamin C deficiency, collagen fibers cannot be cross-linked, greatly decreasing the tensile strength of the assembled fiber, such as in scurvy (Chemistry to Clinics 37.1).

3. Some hydroxylysine residues are enzymatically glycosylated.

4. After hydroxylation and glycosylation, pro-α-chains form procollagen which are translocated to the Golgi apparatus where they are packed in secretory vesicles. The vesicles fuse with the cell membrane causing the release of procollagen into the extracellular space.

5. After their release, the procollagen molecules are cleaved by N- and C-procollagen peptidases, which remove the terminal propeptides, releasing triple-helical molecules.

Chemistry to Clinics 37.1: Scurvy

It is a disease that results from a deficiency of vitamin C and is characterized by inflammed gums and tooth loss, poor wound healing, brittle bones, and weakening of the lining of blood vessels, causing internal bleeding.

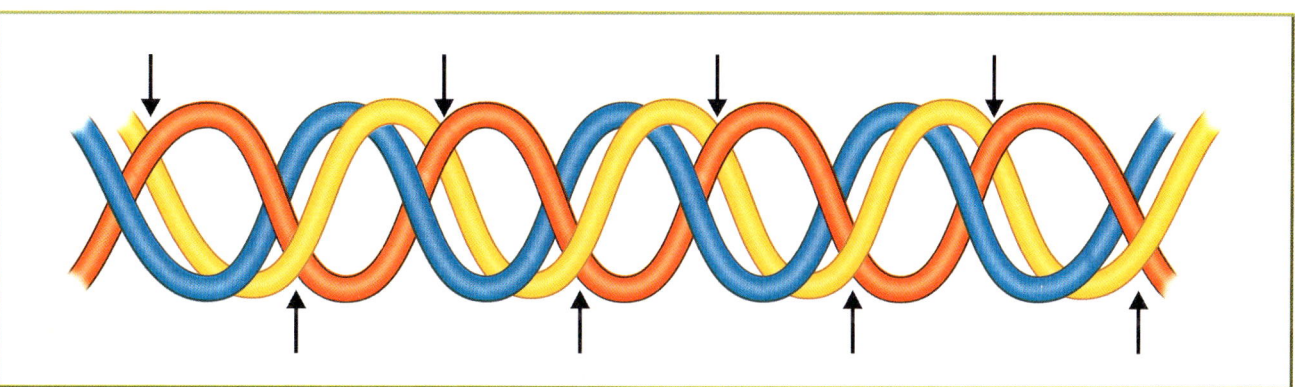

Fig. 37.1: Triple-helical structure of collagen. Arrows indicate the sites where the three chains are very close to each other. Glycine is invariably present at these sites.

37

6. Individual collagen molecules spontaneously associate to form fibrils.
7. Lysyl oxidase oxidatively deaminates some of the lysyl and hydroxylysyl residues resulting in the formation of allysine and hydroxyallysine. These reactive aldehydes condense with lysyl or hydroxylysyl residues in neighboring collagen molecules to form covalent cross-links of mature collagen, called tropocollagen (Fig. 37.2).

Degradation

Normal collagens are highly stable molecules. However, connective tissue is constantly being remodeled, often in response to growth or injury of

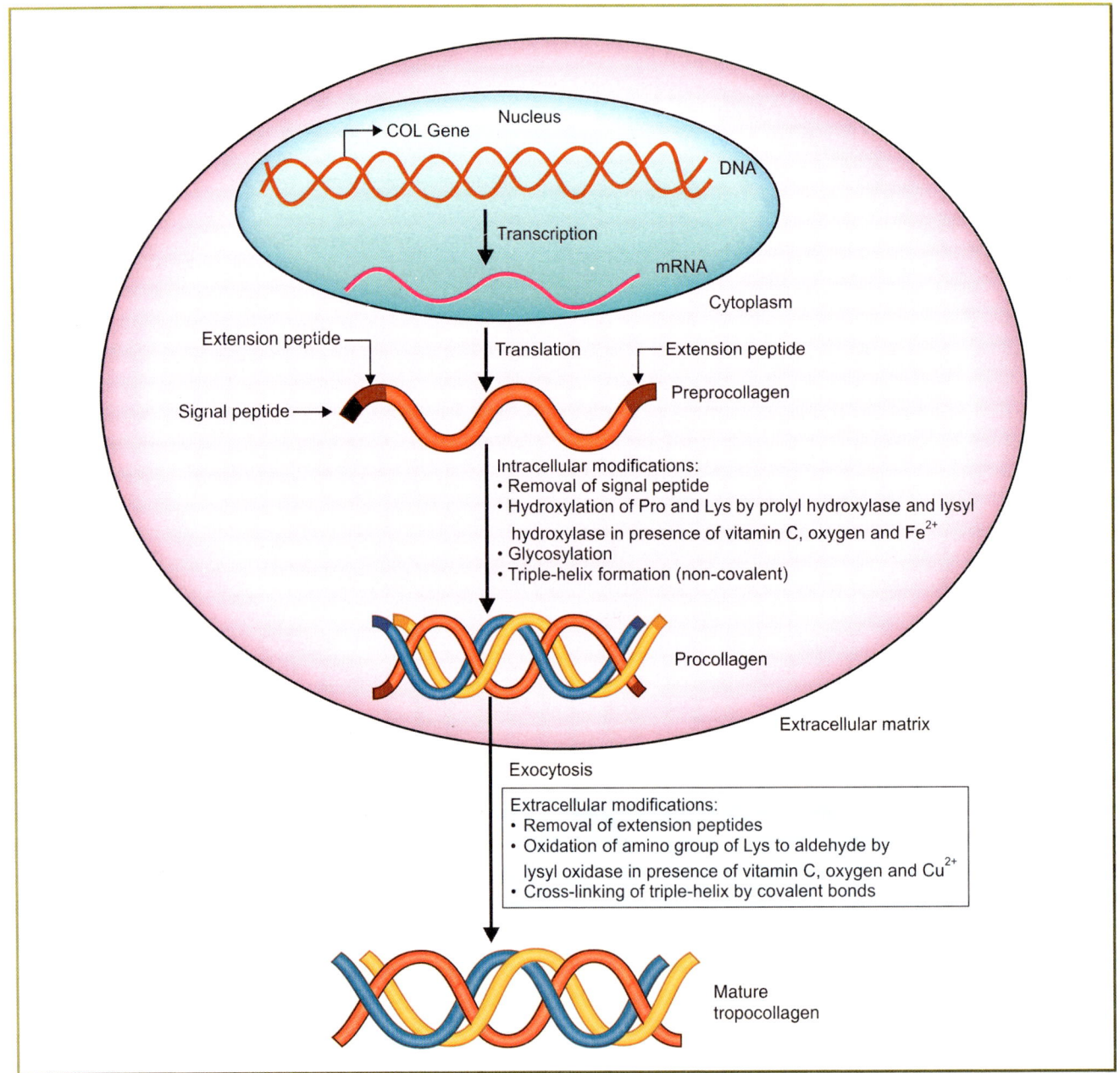

Fig. 37.2: Biosynthesis of collagen by a fibroblast, showing the extensive post-translational modifications.

the tissue. Collagen fibrils are broken down with the help of **specific matrix metalloproteinases called collagenases**. These enzymes cleave the molecules into smaller fragments which are further degraded to the constituent amino acids by other matrix proteinases.

Abnormalities in Synthesis of Collagens

Besides scurvy (an acquired defect in collagen synthesis), a large number of mutations have been identified in genes coding for collagen protein or processing enzymes resulting in reduced synthesis of collagens (Chemistry to Clinics 37.2). On the other hand, abnormally increased synthesis of collagen is observed in healing of open wounds (scar tissue), hepatic cirrhosis and nephrosclerosis.

ELASTIN

Elastin is a connective tissue protein with rubber-like properties. It is the predominant protein of the elastic fibers in the extracellular matrices of blood vessels, lungs, ligaments and spine.

Structure and Synthesis

Elastin is a polymer synthesized from a precursor called tropoelastin which is a linear polypeptide synthesized on the RER and secreted by the cell into the extracellular space. Tropoelastin does not undergo post-translational modification. During the assembly process, some of the lysyl side chains of the tropoelastin polypeptides are oxidatively deaminated by lysyl oxidase, generating **allysine** in specific sequences. The reactive aldehyde of allysine condenses with other allysine or with unmodified lysine from the same or on different tropoelastin polypeptide chains, to form **desmosine** cross-linked heterocyclic structures. As a result, elastin can stretch in any direction giving elasticity to the connective tissue.

Elastin is rich in glycine, proline, lysine and valine. **One in seven of its amino acids is valine**. Its primary structure consists of alternating hydrophilic and hydrophobic lysine and valine-rich domains. Lysines are involved in intermolecular cross-linking while the weak interactions between valine residues in the

Chemistry to Clinics 37.2: Inherited Disorders of Collagen Synthesis

1. **Osteogenesis imperfecta (brittle bone syndrome):** Mutations in the gene for either the pro-1- or pro-2-α chains of type I collagen can result in structurally abnormal pro-α-chains that can prevent folding of the protein into a triple-helical conformation. Extremely fragile bones that easily bend and fracture, thin skin and *weak tendons characterize it. Type I osteogenesis imperfecta, called osteogenesis* imperfecta tarda, presents in early infancy with fractures secondary to minor trauma. *Type II* osteogenesis imperfecta, called *osteogenesis imperfecta congenita*, is more severe and patients die *in utero* or in the neonatal period due to pulmonary hypoplasia.

2. **Ehlers-Danlos syndrome:** It is characterized by a deficiency of any collagen processing enzyme, e.g. lysyl hydroxylase or procollagen peptidase. The defect involves the fibrillar collagen types I and III. The patients have hyper-mobile joints and hyper-extensible skin (Fig. 37.3).

3. **Alport's syndrome:** A renal disease in which the glomerular basement membrane is disrupted due to mutation in type IV collagen gene.

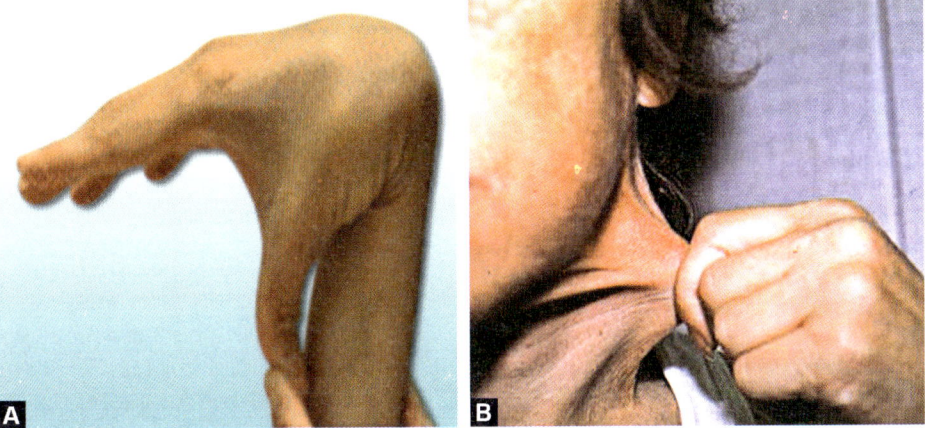

Fig. 37.3: Ehlers-Danlos syndrome: (A) Hyper-mobile joints, (B) Hyper-extensible skin.

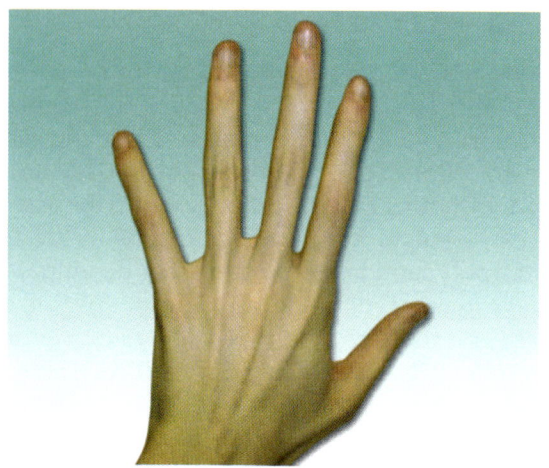

Fig. 37.4: Marfan syndrome: Arachnodactyly (long, slender, **spider-like** fingers).

hydrophobic domains impart elasticity to the molecule.

Elastin is an insoluble, polymeric, amorphous core covered with a sheath of microfibrils, the predominant constituent of which is the glycoprotein fibrillin.

Disorders of Elastin Metabolism

Marfan syndrome: It is due to mutations in the fibrillin gene. Patients have a typically tall stature, long arms and legs, and long spidery fingers (arachnodactyly, Fig. 37.4). The disease in a mild form causes loose joints, deformed spine, floppy mitral valves and lens dislocation. In severely affected individuals, the aortic wall is prone to rupture.

Emphysema: Elastin is degraded by the enzyme elastase. Uncontrolled degradation of elastin in the lungs results in emphysema (Chemistry to Clinics 37.3).

Chemistry to Clinics 37.3: Emphysema

Elastase is a powerful protease that is released from neutrophils (especially during inflammation) into the extracellular space and can degrade elastin of alveolar walls and other structural proteins in a variety of tissues. However, α_1-antitrypsin (α_1-AT), produced primarily by liver and other cells such as monocytes and alveolar macrophages, inhibits a number of proteolytic enzymes including elastase. This, in turn, prevents elastin degradation in the alveolar walls ('elastase/anti-elastase balance').

A deficiency of α_1-AT causes emphysema, which results from the destruction of the connective tissue of alveolar walls ('elastase/anti-elastase imbalance'). Worldwide, it is an important form of chronic obstructive pulmonary disease. The deficiency may be genetic (mutation in α_1-AT gene) or acquired as a result of damage to α_1-AT by reactive oxygen species present in tobacco smoke.

GLYCOSAMINOGLYCANS

Structure, classification and functions of glycosamino-glycans have been discussed in Chapter 4.

Synthesis of Glycosaminoglycans

Glycosaminoglycans are synthesized by a series of glycosyl transferases, epimerases and sulfotrans-ferases, beginning with the synthesis of the core oligosaccharides while the core protein is still in the RER. Synthesis of the repeating oligosaccharides and other modifications take place in the Golgi apparatus.

- Polysaccharide chains are elongated by sequential addition of alternating acidic and amino sugars donated by their UDP-derivatives. UDP-glucuronic acid is produced by oxidation of UDP-glucose.

- After D-glucuronic acid has been incorporated into the carbohydrate chain, some of the D-glucuronic acid residues are converted to L-iduronic acid residues. Epimerization of the D- to the L-sugar is caused by the enzyme uronosyl-5-epimerase.

- Sulfation of the carbohydrate chain occurs after the monosaccharide (to be sulfated) has been incorporated into the growing oligosaccharide chain. 3'-Phosphoadenosyl-5'-phosphosulfate (**PAPS, active sulfate**) is the source of the sulfate, which is transferred at specific sites to cause sulfation of the carbohydrate, by sulfotransferases.

Degradation of Glycosaminoglycans

Glycosaminoglycans are degraded by the sequential action of several lysosomal acid hydrolases including exoglycosidases and sulfatases, beginning from the external end of the glycan chain. This may involve the removal of sulfate by a sulfatase, then removal of the terminal sugar by a specific glycosidase, and so on.

Defects of Glycosaminoglycan Degradation: Mucopolysaccharidoses

- If one of the enzymes involved in the stepwise degradation pathway is missing, the entire degra-dation process is halted at that point. As a result, the undegraded molecule accumulates in the lysosome causing lysosomal storage diseases or mucopolysaccharidoses (Table 37.1; Chemistry to Clinics 37.4).

Table 37.1: The mucopolysaccharidoses

Syndrome	Deficient enzyme	Product (accumulate in lysosomes and excrete in urine)
Hunter syndrome	Iduronate sulfatase	Heparan sulfate and dermatan sulfate
Hurler syndrome	α-L-Iduronidase	- do -
Morquio syndromes		
A	Galactose-6-sulfatase	Keratan sulfate
B	β-Galactosidase	- do -
Sanfilippo syndrome		
A	Heparan sulfamidase	Heparan sulfate
B	N-Acetylglycosaminidase	- do -
C	Acetyl CoA: Glucosaminide N-Acetyl transferase	- do -
D	N-Acetylglucosamine-6-sulfate-sulfatase	- do -
Sly syndrome	β-Glucuronidase	Dermatan sulfate and heparan sulfate

Chemistry to Clinics 37.4: Lysosomal Storage Disorders

Lysosomes are responsible for the intracellular digestion of the extracellular and the intracellular substances. They contain a number of hydrolyzing enzymes (hydrolases) for the hydrolysis of proteins, lipids, carbohydrates and nucleic acids. These hydrolases are most active at acidic pH and split complex molecules into simple low molecular weight compounds that can be reutilized.

In a number of genetic disorders, classified as lysosomal storage diseases, individual lysosomal enzymes are missing leading to accumulation of the substrate of the missing enzyme. The lysosomes become enlarged with undigested material thereby interfering with the normal cell processes. Several lysosomal storage diseases are known to exist, e.g. sphingolipidoses, mucopolysaccharidoses, etc.

- All the deficiencies are autosomal and recessively inherited except Hunter syndrome, which is X-linked.
- They are characterized by the accumulation of GAGs in various tissues, causing varied symptoms such as skeletal and extracellular matrix deformities and mental retardation. Children who are homozygous for one of these diseases are apparently normal at birth and then gradually deteriorate. In most severe cases, death occurs in childhood.
- These diseases can be diagnosed by the identification of the specific glycosaminoglycan chains in the urine, followed by the assay of the specific hydrolases in leukocytes or fibroblasts.

Defects of Sphingolipid Degradation: Sphingolipidoses

This is a group of lipid storage diseases caused by the deficiency of the specific lysosomal hydrolytic enzyme that causes defects in the degradation of sphingolipids (please refer to Chapter 12 for details). Usually, only a single sphingolipid which is the substrate for the deficient enzyme, accumulates in the involved organs in each disease, such as Niemann-Pick disease, Gaucher's disease and Tay-Sach disease. These are autosomal recessive diseases that can be diagnosed by measuring enzyme activity in cultured fibroblasts or peripheral leukocytes.

Niemann-Pick disease: It results from a deficiency of the enzyme sphingomyelinase which leads to accumulation of sphingomyelin in lysosomes. It is characterized by hepatosplenomegaly.

Gaucher's disease: It is a lysosomal storage disease where the enzyme glucocerebrosidase is missing. It is characterized by hepatomegaly, long-bone osteoporosis and neurodegeneration.

Tay-Sach disease: It is due to lack of the enzyme hexosaminidase. It is the most common form of G_{M2} gangliosidosis. Ganglion cells of the cerebral cortex are swollen due to the deposition of G_{M2} gangliosides. The disease is characterized by neurodegeneration, blindness, cherry-red macula, muscular weakness and seizures.

37

SOME IMPORTANT QUESTIONS

1. What are collagens? How they are synthesized? Describe some abnormalities of biosynthesis of collagens.

2. What are glycosaminoglycans? Describe structure, distribution and functions of various types of glycosaminoglycans.

3. Write notes on:

   i. Extracellular matrix
   ii. Collagens
   iii. Osteogenesis imperfecta
   iv. Ehlers-Danlos syndrome
   v. Elastin
   vi. Marfan's syndrome
   vii. Glycosaminoglycans
   viii. Hyaluronic acid
   ix. Heparin
   x. Lysosomal storage disorders
   xi. Tay-Sach disease
   xii. Emphysema

MULTIPLE CHOICE QUESTIONS

1. The following is not true for collagens:
   A. Fibrous proteins
   B. Extracellular
   C. Glycoproteins
   D. Lack quaternary structure

2. The commonest amino acid in collagens is:
   A. Glycine
   B. Proline
   C. Hydroxyproline
   D. Lysine

3. The formation of interchain H-bonds in collagens depends on the presence of:
   A. Glycine
   B. Proline
   C. Hydroxyproline
   D. Lysine

4. The formation of interchain covalent bonds in collagens depends on the presence of:
   A. Glycine
   B. Proline
   C. Hydroxyproline
   D. Hydroxylysine

5. Lysyl hydroxylase requires:
   A. Oxygen
   B. Ferrous ions
   C. Ascorbic acid
   D. All of the above

6. The following is true for extension peptides in procollagen:
   A. Completely retained in mature collagens
   B. Removed intracellularly
   C. Removed extracellularly
   D. Partly retained in mature collagens

7. Osteogenesis imperfecta involves collagen type:
   A. I
   B. II
   C. III
   D. IV

8. Desmosine cross links are found in:
   A. Collagens
   B. Elastin
   C. Fibrillin
   D. Fibronectin

9. The following is true for Marfan's syndrome:
   A. Floppy mitral valves
   B. Arachnodactyly
   C. Fibrillin gene mutation
   D. All of the above

10. The enzyme deficient in Hunter syndrome is:
    A. Iduronate sulphatase
    B. α-L-Iduronidase
    C. Galactose-6-sulphatase
    D. β-Galactosidase

Acid–Base Balance

ACIDS, BASES AND BUFFERS

Acids

An acid is a substance whose dissociation in water releases hydrogen ions (H^+). An H^+ since does not contain any neutron and is essentially equivalent to a proton, an acid, therefore, is often referred to as a **proton donor**. Addition of an acid to a solution thus increases the concentration of free H^+ in the solution and results in a decrease in pH. An acid, e.g. HA in aqueous solution, reversibly dissociates into H^+ and a **conjugate base** (A^-):

$$HA \rightleftharpoons H^+ + A^-$$

This tendency of an acid to give up H^+ depends upon its **strength**. A **strong acid** such as HCl, completely dissociates in an aqueous solution:

$$HCl \rightleftharpoons H^+ + Cl^-$$

On the other hand, a **weak acid** gives up H^+ less rapidly and does not dissociate completely. A solution of a weak acid thus contains both dissociated (ions) as well as the undissociated molecules. Most of the acids produced in living systems are weak acids.

Bases

A base releases hydroxyl ions (OH^-) in an aqueous solution and decreases its H^+ concentration by accepting or binding with the free H^+, resulting in an increase in pH of the solution. A **strong base** such as sodium hydroxide (NaOH), dissociates completely:

$$NaOH \rightarrow Na^+ + OH^-$$

The OH^- so produced accepts H^+ and results in the formation of water. This, in turn, lowers the concentration of H^+ in the solution. A **weak base** such as bicarbonate (HCO_3^-) can also utilize H^+ and thus raises the pH of the solution.

Amphoteric Substances

Some chemical substances such as amino acids and proteins can function both as an acid as well as a base. These substances are referred to as amphoteric substances or **ampholytes**. For example, an amino acid such as glycine, at physiological pH, acts as an acid when the ammonium group (NH_3^+) of glycine donates its H^+ to the OH^- of a base (Fig. 38.1). On the other hand, glycine also acts as a base when its carboxylate group (COO^-) accepts H^+ from an acid.

pH

pH is defined as the negative logarithm to the base 10, of the molar concentration of hydrogen ions (H^+) in a solution:

$$pH = -\log[H^+] = \log(1/[H^+])$$

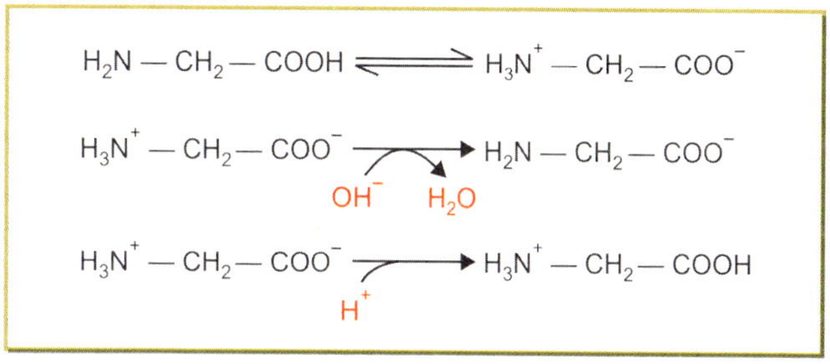

Fig. 38.1: Glycine as an ampholyte.

38

The pH of a solution thus is **inversely related to free H⁺ concentration [H⁺]**. A low pH indicates high H^+ concentration while a high pH indicates low H^+ concentration.

If we add a strong base such as NaOH to water, the OH^- will combine with H^+ supplied by the water. This, in turn, shifts the equilibrium towards the undissociated water and lowers free H^+ ion concentration, thereby resulting in an increase in pH.

The scale of pH measurement varies from 0 to14. If pH of a solution is <7, the solution is said to be **acidic**; if pH of the solution is equal to **7**, it is referred to as **neutral**; and if pH is >7, the solution is said to be **alkaline or basic** in nature.

Ionization Constant

Strong acids dissociate completely, i.e. do not bind H^+, hence they are not effective buffers. Weak acids strongly bind H^+, hence they are also inefficient buffers. Thus, the inherent strength or tendency of an acid to ionize, determines its **buffering capacity**. The **ionization constant** (K_{eq}) is a measure of this strength, expressed as its negative logarithm (pK_a). The most effective buffers have **pK_a close to the physiological pH**.

Henderson-Hasselbalch Equation

Weak acids, when dissolved in water, do not dissociate totally but establish equilibrium between the undissociated compound and the dissociated ions. The concentration of the ionic species can be determined from the equilibrium equation (Fig. 38.2) where K_{eq} is the equilibrium constant, [H⁺], [A⁻] and [HA] indicate the concentrations of the dissociated cations (H^+), anions (A⁻, the conjugate base) and the undissociated weak acid, respectively. K_{eq} is a function of temperature of the system and increases with the increasing temperature. On rearranging the equation, we get:

$$[H^+] = K_{eq} \times ([HA]/[A^-]) = K_{eq} \times ([acid]/[conjugate\ base])$$

$$HA \rightleftharpoons H^+ + A^-$$

$$K'_{eq} = \frac{[H^+][A^-]}{[HA]}$$

Fig. 38.2: Equilibrium constant for the dissociation of a weak acid.

Multiplying the equation by –1, this equation can be written as:

$$-[H^+] = -K_{eq} \times ([acid]/[conjugate\ base])$$

The **logarithmic form** of the above equation is known as Henderson-Hasselbalch equation.

It is derived as follows:

$$-\log[H^+] = -\log K_{eq} + \log ([conjugate\ base]/[acid])$$

Since $-\log[H^+] = pH$, and $-\log K_a = pK_a$, the above equation can be rewritten as:

$$\mathbf{pH = pK_a + \log([conjugate\ base]/[acid])}$$

When half of the acid is present in its dissociated form, i.e. when [A⁻] = [HA], the pH of the solution is equal to its pK_a. Thus, Henderson-Hasselbalch equation is a mathematical rearrangement of the fundamental equilibrium equation which states that there is a direct relationship between pH and ratio of the concentration of conjugate base to the concentration of undissociated weak acid.

Buffers

Something that **tends to resist** a shock and thereby promotes relative stability is defined as a buffer. A pH buffer **minimizes the change in pH** when either an acid or a base is added to a solution. A chemical buffer consists of a weak acid (HA) and its conjugate base (A⁻), or a weak base and its conjugate acid (Fig. 38.3). The **effectiveness of a buffer**, in minimizing changes in pH, depends upon two factors:

1. The **pK_a** of the buffer in relation to the desired pH, e.g. the pK_a of the imidazole group of histidine in hemoglobin is close to 7.4 and thus it is an ideal buffer in the blood.
2. The **amount or concentration** of the buffer. The greater the concentration of a buffer, the greater is its ability to bind or release H^+.

Acid		Conjugate base		
HA	$\rightleftharpoons$	A^-	$+$	H^+
H_2CO_3	$\rightleftharpoons$	HCO_3^-	$+$	H^+
$H_2PO_4^-$	$\rightleftharpoons$	HPO_4^{2-}	$+$	H^+
NH_4^+	$\rightleftharpoons$	NH_3	$+$	H^+

Fig. 38.3: Weak acids and their conjugate bases.

PRODUCTION AND REGULATION OF HYDROGEN IONS IN THE BODY

Acids are continuously produced in the body and threaten the normal pH of the extracellular and intracellular fluids. From a biochemical and clinical perspective, acids fall into two groups:

1. **Volatile acid:** Carbonic acid (H_2CO_3) is in equilibrium with the volatile gas CO_2, which can leave the body via the lungs. A normal adult produces about 300 L of CO_2 daily from the complete oxidation of carbohydrates and lipids. CO_2 from the tissues enters the capillary blood where it reacts with water to form H_2CO_3, which dissociates instantly to yield H^+ and HCO_3^- :

$$CO_2 + H_2O \rightleftharpoons H_2CO_3 \rightleftharpoons H^+ + HCO_3^-$$

Blood pH would rapidly fall to lethal levels if the H_2CO_3 formed from CO_2 is allowed to accumulate in the body. Fortunately, the reactions reverse in the lungs. As long as CO_2 is expired as fast as it is produced, the arterial blood CO_2 tension, H_2CO_3 concentration and pH do not change.

2. **Non-volatile acids:** All other acids (non-carbonic, also called '**fixed' acids**), by contrast, are not directly affected by breathing; they are buffered in the body and then excreted by the kidneys. Examples include:

- Lactic acid, pK_a = 3.9 (incomplete oxidation of carbohydrates)
- Ketone bodies, pK_a = 4–5 (incomplete oxidation of fatty acids)
- Sulfuric acid (oxidation of sulfur-containing amino acids)
- Phosphoric acid (oxidation of phosphoproteins and nucleic acids)

Effect of Diet on pH

A diet containing both meat and vegetables results in a net production of acids, largely from protein oxidation. To some extent, acid-consuming metabolic reactions balance H^+ production. Food also contains basic anions such as citrate, lactate and acetate. When these are oxidized to CO_2 and water, H^+ are consumed (i.e. HCO_3^- is produced). The balance of acid-forming and acid-consuming metabolic reactions results in a net production of about 1 mEq H^+/kg body weight per day in an adult person on a mixed diet. Vegetarians generally have less of a dietary acid burden and a more alkaline urine pH than non-vegetarians because most fruits and vegetables contain large amounts of organic anions that are metabolized to HCO_3^-.

Whether a particular food has an acidifying or an alkalinizing effect depends on whether and how its constituents are metabolized. Cranberry juice has an acidifying effect because of its content of benzoic acid that cannot be broken down in the body. Orange juice has an alkalinizing effect despite its acidic pH of about 3.7, because it contains citrate which is metabolized to HCO_3^-. The citric acid in lemons and pickles is converted to CO_2 and water, hardly affecting blood and urine pH.

BUFFERING MECHANISMS

Despite constant threats to acid–base homeostasis, a healthy person maintains a normal blood pH because of **chemical buffers** along with the role played by **lungs and kidneys** (Fig. 38.4).

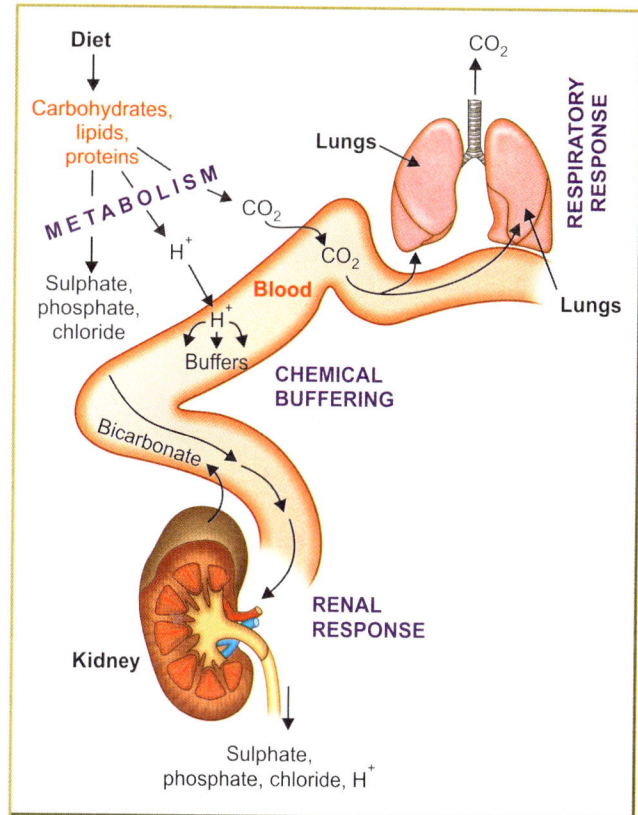

Fig. 38.4: The three major buffering mechanisms.

38

Table 38.1: Major body buffers

Buffer	Reaction
Extracellular fluid	
Bicarbonate/CO_2	$CO_2 + H_2O \rightleftharpoons H_2CO_3 \rightleftharpoons H^+ + HCO_3^-$
Inorganic phosphate	$H_2PO_4^- \rightleftharpoons H^+ + HPO_4^{2-}$
Plasma proteins (Pr)	$HPr \rightleftharpoons H^+ + Pr^-$
Intracellular fluid	
Cell proteins, e.g. hemoglobin (Hb)	$HHb \rightleftharpoons H^+ + Hb^-$
Organic phosphates	$Organic\text{-}HPO_4 \rightleftharpoons H^+ + organic\text{-}PO_4^{2-}$
Bicarbonate/CO_2	$CO_2 + H_2O \rightleftharpoons H_2CO_3 \rightleftharpoons H^+ + HCO_3^-$
Bone	
Mineral phosphates	$H_2PO_4^- \rightleftharpoons H^+ + HPO_4^{2-}$
Mineral carbonates	$HCO_3^- \rightleftharpoons H^+ + CO_3^{2-}$

CHEMICAL BUFFERING—BODY BUFFERS: THE FIRST LINE OF DEFENSE

Chemical buffers in extracellular and intracellular fluids as well as in the bones minimize a change in pH but do not remove acid or base from the body (Table 38.1). In the ECF, the main chemical buffer pair is HCO_3^-/CO_2, while cells are rich in proteins and organic phosphate buffers. Bone contains large buffer stores, specifically salts of phosphate and carbonate. Buffering in ECF occurs rapidly in minutes. Acids or bases also enter cells and bone but this generally occurs more slowly over hours.

Bicarbonate/CO_2 Buffer

For several reasons, the HCO_3^-/CO_2 buffer pair is of **prime importance** in acid–base regulation:

1. **High concentration:** Its components are abundant; the concentration of HCO_3^- in plasma or ECF normally averages 24 mmol/L and metabolism generates an unlimited supply of CO_2.

2. **Open system:** Despite a pKa of 6.10, a little far from the desired plasma pH of 7.40, it is effective because the system is 'open', i.e. its components can be added to or removed from the body at controlled rates as discussed below.

3. **Dual regulation:** It is controlled by the lungs and kidneys. The respiratory system can change the amount of CO_2 in body fluids by hyperventilation or hypoventilation. The kidneys can change the amount of HCO_3^- in the ECF by forming new HCO_3^-

when excess acid has been added to the body or by excreting HCO_3^- when excess base has been added.

Carbon dioxide exists in several forms: CO_2 exists in the body in several different forms—as gaseous CO_2 in the lung alveoli and as dissolved CO_2, H_2CO_3, HCO_3^-, carbonate and carbamino compounds in the body fluids. The solubility coefficient for CO_2 in plasma at 37°C is 0.03 mmol CO_2/L per mmHg. The normal pCO_2 is known to be 40 mm Hg. Therefore, the concentration of dissolved CO_2, represented as $CO_{2(d)}$, is 0.03 × 40 = 1.2 mmol/L.

Carbonic anhydrase: In aqueous solution, the $CO_{2(d)}$ forms carbonic acid:

$$CO_{2(d)} + H_2O \rightleftharpoons H_2CO_3$$

The reaction to the right is called the hydration reaction and the reaction to the left is called the dehydration reaction. These reactions are slow if uncatalyzed. In many tissues such as the kidneys, pancreas, stomach and RBC, the reactions are catalyzed by carbonic anhydrase, a **zinc-containing** enzyme. At equilibrium and at 37°C, the $CO_{2(d)}$ is greatly favored so that the ratio of $CO_{2(d)}$ to H_2CO_3 is 400:1. Therefore, although H_2CO_3 is a fairly strong acid (pKa = 3.5; $H_2CO_3 \rightleftharpoons H^+ + HCO_3^-$), its low concentration in body fluids lessens its impact on acidity. Because plasma H_2CO_3 is so low and difficult to measure and because the ratio $CO_{2(d)}/H_2CO_3$ is 400:1, we can use $CO_{2(d)}$ to represent the acid in the Henderson-Hasselbalch equation.

Phosphate Buffer

The pK_a for phosphate, $H_2PO_4^- \rightleftharpoons H^+ + HPO_4^{2-}$, is 6.8, close to the desired blood pH of 7.4, so phosphate is a good buffer. In the **ECF**, phosphate is present as inorganic phosphate. Its concentration, however, is low so it plays a minor role in extracellular buffering. However, phosphate is an important **intracellular buffer** for two reasons.

- First, cells contain large amounts of phosphate in such organic compounds as adenosine triphosphate (ATP), adenosine diphosphate (ADP) and creatine phosphate. Although these compounds primarily function in energy metabolism, they also act as pH buffers.

- Second, intracellular pH is generally lower than the pH of ECF and is closer to the pK_a of phosphate.

Protein Buffer

Proteins are the **largest buffer pool** in the body and are excellent buffers. Proteins can function as both acids and bases, i.e. they are **amphoteric**. They contain many ionizable groups which can release or bind H^+. Plasma albumin and globulins are the major extracellular protein buffers. Cells also have large protein stores including the **hemoglobin** present in RBC.

Hemoglobin Buffer

Oxyhemoglobin is a stronger acid than deoxy-hemoglobin. Therefore, in the tissues where CO_2 and hence H_2CO_3 are generated, the following reaction occurs in RBC:

$$KHbO_2 + H_2CO_3 \rightarrow HHb + KHCO_3 + O_2$$

HCO_3^- exchanges with Cl^- (chloride shift), while O_2 is delivered to the cells. This reaction is reversed in the lungs.

RESPIRATORY RESPONSE: THE SECOND LINE OF DEFENSE

Normally, CO_2 is expired at the same rate at which it is produced and thus pCO_2 is maintained.

- **If blood becomes acidic** by the addition of fixed acids, pulmonary ventilation is increased and CO_2 is flushed-out at a rate greater than the rate at which it is produced. Consequently, pCO_2 falls and results in a decrease in H^+ concentration of the blood, and the reactions are pulled to the left (Fig. 38.5). This, in turn, lowers the HCO_3^- concentration and reduces acidic shift in the blood.
- On the other hand, **if blood becomes more alkaline**, changes occur in the opposite direction. Accordingly, hypoventilation takes place, CO_2 is not removed at an adequate rate, blood pCO_2 rises and the reactions are pushed to the right (Fig. 38.6).

$$CO_2 + H_2O \rightleftharpoons H_2CO_3 \rightleftharpoons H^+ + HCO_3^-$$

Fig. 38.5: The equilibrium is pulled to the left during hyperventilation.

$$CO_2 + H_2O \rightleftharpoons H_2CO_3 \rightleftharpoons H^+ + HCO_3^-$$

Fig. 38.6: The equilibrium is pushed to the right during hypoventilation.

This results in a higher carbonic acid concentration in the blood and a less alkaline shift in blood pH. Hypoventilation however, is limited because it causes retention of CO_2 which further stimulates ventilation.

Buffering of acid–base disturbances by the respiratory response although is **rapid** but is relatively coarse. It brings blood pH back, close to normal but **cannot eliminate a fixed acid or base** from the body and so it cannot restore pH to normal.

RENAL RESPONSE: THE THIRD LINE OF DEFENSE

Renal responses, in contrast to other buffering mechanisms, are **slow but more complete**; full renal compensation may take 1 to 3 days. The kidney regulates acid–base balance by controlling bicarbonate reabsorption and secreting acid. The kidneys also excrete the anions (phosphate, chloride, sulfate) that are liberated from strong acids.

In the basic ion exchange mechanism, H^+ formed in the reaction is actively secreted into the tubular fluid in exchange for Na^+. Within the tubule cell, Na^+ combines with HCO_3^- and generates sodium bicarbonate which is pumped out of the cell into the interstitial fluid and equilibrates with the plasma (Fig. 38.7). Sodium uptake by the tubular cell is partly passive with Na^+ flowing down the electrochemical gradient and partly active via Na^+/H^+-antiport system, in exchange for H^+.

MECHANISMS OF H⁺ SECRETION

H^+ secreted into the tubular fluid can have one of the three fates, suggesting that three processes are involved in the acidification of urine:

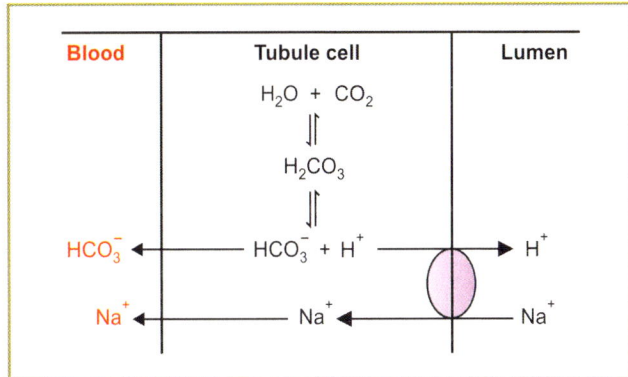

Fig. 38.7: Basic ion exchange mechanism.

38

1. Reabsorption of the filtered bicarbonate.
2. Excretion of the titrable acid.
3. Excretion of ammonia

All the three mechanisms involve H^+ secretion and are associated with the addition of bicarbonate to the peritubular capillary blood by the kidney tubules.

Reabsorption of Filtered Bicarbonate

H^+ that are secreted into the tubules in exchange for Na^+, combine with bicarbonate that has been filtered by the glomeruli. This, in turn, leads to the formation of carbonic acid in the tubular urine. The dissociation of this acid to CO_2 and water is catalyzed in the proximal convoluted tubule lumen by carbonic anhydrase within the brush border membrane. CO_2 rapidly diffuses through the cell membrane where it combines with water and forms carbonic acid, which in turn, gets dissociated into hydrogen and bicarbonate ions. The H^+ are secreted into the lumen while the bicarbonate ions exit from the basolateral membrane along with the sodium ions.

The filtered HCO_3^- thus is not reabsorbed by direct transport out of the tubular urine, rather it is reabsorbed indirectly by the secretion of the hydrogen ions (Fig. 38.8). The overall effect is to move sodium bicarbonate from the tubular fluid, back into the interstitial fluid.

Excretion of Titrable Acid

As reabsorption of sodium bicarbonate proceeds, the tubular fluid becomes depleted of HCO_3^- and the pH drops. At this stage, the H^+ are taken up by the phosphate buffer. Hydrogen ions that are secreted into the tubular urine in exchange for Na^+, titrate phosphate buffer in the urine in the acidic direction:

$$HPO_4^{2-} + H^+ \rightarrow H_2PO_4^-$$

As a result, the basic form of the phosphate (HPO_4^{2-}) is converted to its acidic form $H_2PO_4^-$.

Besides phosphate, which is the most important buffer in the urine, other ions are also significant in the excretion of H^+. For example, in diabetic keto-acidosis, when pH of the urine reaches its minimum ≈ 4.4), acetoacetate and β-hydroxybutyrate pass through the glomerular filtrate and appear in the tubular fluid. Under these conditions these ions also serve as buffers.

Thus, excretion of titrable acids not only eliminates H^+ from the body but also restores the depleted plasma bicarbonate reserves since for each mEq of H^+ excreted as titrable acid, a new HCO_3^- is added to the blood (Fig. 38.9).

Titrable acidity of the urine: The amount of acid excreted (as the acid component of a urinary buffer) can be measured by the titration of urine, back to the normal pH of the plasma (to pH 7.4). The quantity of the base so required is equivalent to the quantity of the acid excreted and is referred to as titrable acidity of the urine. Most of the titrable acid normally, is inorganic phosphate. The formation of titrable acidity accounts for nearly one-third to one-half of our normal daily acid excretion.

Excretion of Ammonia

The third fate of H^+ in the tubular fluid is its neutralization by NH_3 which is mainly synthesized in the proximal tubule from amino acids, predominantly

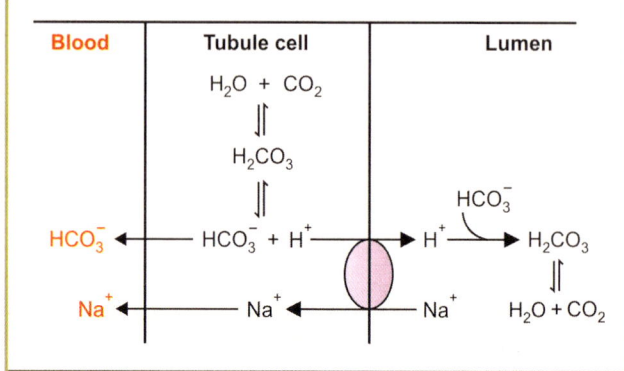

Fig. 38.8: Reabsorption of bicarbonate.

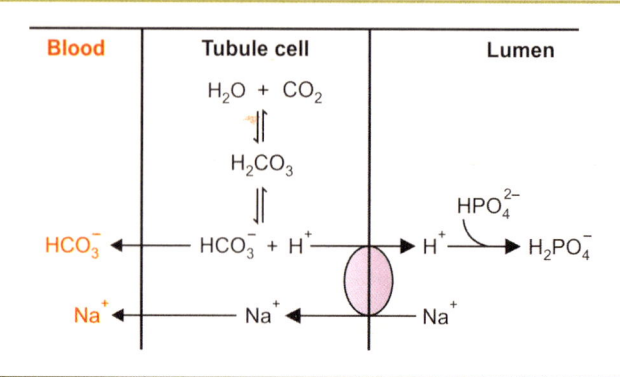

Fig. 38.9: Excretion of titrable acid.

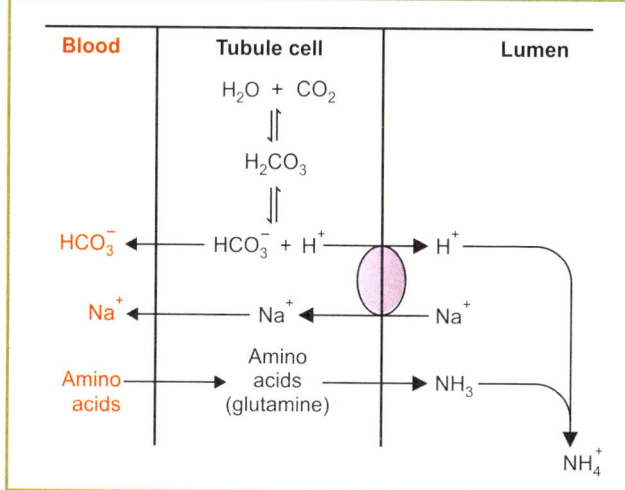

Fig. 38.10: Excretion of ammonia.

from glutamine. The ability of the kidney to synthesize NH_3 from glutamine is increased under conditions of excess acid in the body. Ammonia readily diffuses through the cell membrane and combines with the secreted H^+ and forms NH_4^+, which is usually accompanied by an anion, e.g. chloride, in the urine. For each H^+ excreted in the urine as NH_4^+, an equivalent quantity of HCO_3^- is added to the blood (Fig. 38.10). Nearly, one-half to two-thirds of our daily acid load is excreted as NH_4^+.

Role of Collecting Ducts in Acid–Base Regulation

The intercalated cells of the collecting duct are involved in acid–base transport and are of two types, i.e. **acid-secreting α-intercalated cells** and **bicarbonate-secreting β-intercalated cells**. The α-intercalated cells have vacuolar type of H^+-ATPase (the same kind as is found in lysosomes, endosomes and secretory vesicles) and a H^+/K^+-ATPase (similar to that found in stomach and colon epithelial cells) in the luminal cell membrane. The basolateral cell membrane

contains the Cl^-/HCO_3^- exchanger. The β-intercalated cells have the opposite polarity.

Total acidity of urine: The sum of the titrable acidity and NH_4^+ comprises the total acidity of urine (total acid excretion).

DISTURBANCES OF ACID–BASE BALANCE

General Concepts

1. **Acidemia and alkalemia:** A blood pH below 7.35 (H^+ >45 nmol/L) indicates *'acidemia'* whereas a blood pH above 7.45 (H^+ <35 nmol/L) indicates *'alkalemia'*. The range of pH values compatible with life is approximately 6.8 to 7.8 (H^+ = 160 to 16 nmol/L).

2. **Acidosis and alkalosis:** Four simple acid–base disturbances may lead to an abnormal blood pH: Respiratory acidosis, respiratory alkalosis, metabolic acidosis and metabolic alkalosis. The word 'simple' indicates a single primary cause for the disturbance. *'Acidosis'* is an abnormal process that tends to produce acidemia whereas *'alkalosis'* is an abnormal process that tends to produce alkalemia.

3. **Identifying the primary disturbance:** If there is too much or too little CO_2, then a *respiratory disturbance* is present. If the problem is too much or too little HCO_3^-, then a *metabolic disturbance* (non-respiratory disturbance) is present. Table 38.2 summarizes the various changes that occur in blood in each of the four simple acid–base disturbances.

4. **Compensatory mechanisms:** In considering acid–base disturbances, it is helpful to recall the Henderson-Hasselbalch equation discussed earlier. If the primary problem is a change in HCO_3^- or pCO_2, the pH can be brought closer to normal by changing the other member of the buffer pair in the same direction. For example, if pCO_2 is primarily decreased, a decrease in plasma HCO_3^-

Table 38.2: Changes observed in major acid–base balance disorders

Acid–base disorder	Arterial blood			Compensatory response
	pCO_2	pH	HCO_3^-	
Respiratory acidosis	↑	↓	↑	↑ Renal H^+ excretion increases plasma HCO_3^- concentration
Respiratory alkalosis	↓	↑	↓	↑ Renal HCO_3^- excretion decreases plasma HCO_3^- concentration
Metabolic acidosis	↓	↓	↓	Hyperventilation decreases pCO_2
Metabolic alkalosis	↑	↑	↑	Hypoventilation increases pCO_2

will minimize the change in pH. In various acid–base disturbances, the lungs adjust the blood pCO_2 and the kidneys adjust the plasma HCO_3^- to reduce deviations of pH from normal; these adjustments are called *'compensations'* (Table 38.2). Compensations, however, do not correct the underlying disorder and do not necessarily restore the normal blood pH.

Respiratory Acidosis

Respiratory acidosis is most often due to inadequate ventilation (hypoventilation) of the alveoli. This, in turn, results in the retention of CO_2 and a fall in blood pH. Alveolar hypoventilation occurs when the depth or rate of respiration is diminished, such as airway obstruction or a pulmonary disease. It will result in a rise in pCO_2. As pCO_2 rises, plasma pH drops and HCO_3^- concentration rises.

The kidneys compensate for the respiratory acidosis by increasing the output of H^+ in the urine. The filtered HCO_3^- is reabsorbed and the increased amounts of H^+ combine with the urinary buffers and are excreted in the urine. Thus, by excreting H^+ in the urine, kidneys increase plasma HCO_3^- concentration.

Respiratory Alkalosis

Respiratory alkalosis is produced by hyperventilation which results in the excessive removal of CO_2 from the blood. This, in turn, causes a fall in arterial blood pCO_2, a fall in plasma H^+ concentration, i.e. a rise in pH and a fall in plasma HCO_3^- concentration. Hyperventilation may be caused by anxiety, central nervous system injury involving the respiratory center, salicylate poisoning or fever. At high altitude also, due to decrease in total atmospheric pressure, alveolar pCO_2 falls and results in chronic respiratory alkalosis. The kidneys compensate for the respiratory alkalosis by excreting HCO_3^- in the urine. A low pCO_2 leads to decreased H^+ secretion by the tubular epithelium. This, in turn, results in reduced reabsorption of the filtered bicarbonate and increases its excretion in the urine. This loss of HCO_3^- in the urine results in a further decrease in plasma HCO_3^- and plasma pH towards normal.

Metabolic Acidosis

Metabolic acidosis is characterized by the accumulation of nonvolatile acids (gain of fixed acids other than H_2CO_3) or loss of HCO_3^-. Gain of metabolically produced acid may be due to several reasons, such as:

1. Uncontrolled diabetes mellitus leading to the production of large quantities of ketone bodies (Chemistry to Clinics 38.1).
2. Renal failure leading to reduced excretion of the metabolically produced acids.
3. Inadequate circulation due to cardiogenic or hemorrhagic shock which, in turn, promotes anaerobic glycolysis and increases the production of lactic acid.
4. Heavy exercise resulting in the production of lactic acid.
5. Ingestion of certain acidifying agents, such as ammonium chloride.

Metabolic acidosis may also be due to a loss of HCO_3^- from the body, such as due to diarrhea or abnormal excretion of HCO_3^- in the urine. Thus, an addition of strong organic or inorganic acid, or a loss of HCO_3^- results in a decrease in plasma HCO_3^- concentration in metabolic acidosis.

Two compensatory mechanisms are usually available to deal with the excess acid:

1. Due to the acidic pH, **respiratory system** is stimulated to hyperventilate. This, in turn, lowers the pCO_2 and hence the carbonic acid concentration in the blood. The respiratory compensation though is prompt but usually does not restore the blood pH to normal.
2. The other mechanism which begins almost instantly, is the **renal compensation**. The kidneys increase H^+ excretion. This however, takes time and is not adequate to return HCO_3^- concentration and the pH to normal.

Metabolic Alkalosis

Metabolic alkalosis is characterized by the intake of excess of alkali, i.e. by the gain of strong base or HCO_3^-, or abnormal loss of acid other than H_2CO_3. For example, the ingestion of excess sodium bicarbonate, used in treating gastric ulcer or the oxidation of organic anions, such as citrate, lactate and acetate. A common cause of abnormal loss of acid causing metabolic alkalosis, is prolonged vomiting or gastric lavage since loss of stomach contents results in net addition of HCO_3^- to the blood (Chemistry to Clinics 38.2). It may also be a result of the rapid loss of body water, e.g. in diuresis, which in turn, may result in a temporary rise in HCO_3^- in plasma and extracellular fluid.

38

Chemistry to Clinics 38.1: Diabetic Ketoacidosis

Insulin deficiency leads to decreased glucose utilization, a diversion of metabolism towards the use of fatty acids and an overproduction of ketone bodies (acetoacetic acid and β-hydroxybutyric acid). Ketone bodies, sometimes called ketone body acids, are fairly strong acids (pK$_a$ 4–5). They are neutralized in the body by HCO$_3^-$ and other buffers. Increased production of these acids leads to a fall in plasma HCO$_3^-$, an increase in plasma anion gap and a fall in blood pH (acidemia). This is diabetic ketoacidosis.

Complications: Severe acidemia, whatever its cause, has many adverse effects:

1. Impaired myocardial contractility, decrease in cardiac output, arteriolar dilation, fall in arterial blood pressure, cardiac arrhythmias.
2. Decreased hepatic and renal blood flow.
3. Respiratory muscle fatigue.
4. Activation of the sympathetic nervous system, increased metabolic demands, reduced ATP synthesis, hyperkalemia, protein catabolism.
5. Impaired neuronal metabolism and cell volume regulation leading to progressive obtundation and coma.

Respiratory compensation: Acidemia stimulates pulmonary ventilation resulting in a compensatory lowering of alveolar and arterial blood pCO$_2$. The consequent reduction in blood H$_2$CO$_3$ moves the blood pH back toward normal. The rapid, deep breathing that accompanies severe uncontrolled diabetes is called Kussmaul respiration and the breath gives the fruity smell of acetone, the volatile ketone body.

Renal compensation: The kidneys compensate for metabolic acidosis by reabsorbing all the filtered HCO$_3^-$. They also increase the excretion of titratable acid, part of which is composed of ketone bodies. But these acids can only be partially titrated to their acid form in the urine because the urine pH cannot go below 4.5. Thus, ketone bodies are excreted mostly in their anionic form; because of the requirement of electroneutrality in solutions, increased urinary excretion of Na$^+$ and K$^+$ results.

An important compensation for the acidosis is increased renal synthesis and excretion of ammonia. This adaptive response takes several days to develop fully but it allows the kidneys to dispose of large amounts of H$^+$ in the form NH$_4^+$. The NH$_4^+$ in the urine can replace Na$^+$ and K$^+$ ions thereby helping to conserve these valuable cations.

Treatment: The severe acidemia, electrolyte disturbances and volume depletion that accompany uncontrolled diabetes mellitus may be fatal. Correction of the acid–base disturbance is best achieved by addressing the underlying cause rather than just treating the symptoms. Therefore, the administration of a suitable dose of insulin by intravenous infusion is the key element of therapy. In some patients with marked acidemia (pH < 7.10), NaHCO$_3$ solutions may be infused to speed recovery but this does not correct the underlying metabolic problem. Water and electrolyte corrections should be made.

Chemistry to Clinics 38.2: Vomiting and Metabolic Alkalosis

Vomiting of acidic gastric juice results in metabolic alkalosis and fluid/electrolyte disturbances. The gastric parietal cells have H$^+$/K$^+$-ATPase in their luminal cell membrane and Cl$^-$/HCO$_3^-$ exchanger in the basolateral cell membrane. When HCl is secreted into the stomach lumen and lost to the outside, there is a net gain of HCO$_3^-$ in the blood and no change in the anion gap. The HCO$_3^-$, in effect, replaces lost plasma Cl$^-$.

Respiratory compensation: Ventilation is inhibited by the alkaline blood pH, resulting in a rise in pCO$_2$. This respiratory compensation, however, is limited because hypoventilation-induced hypoxemia stimulates breathing.

Renal compensation: The logical renal compensation for metabolic alkalosis is enhanced excretion of HCO$_3^-$. In people with persistent vomiting, however, the urine is sometimes acidic and renal HCO$_3^-$ reabsorption is enhanced, thereby maintaining the elevated plasma HCO$_3^-$. This situation arises because vomiting is accompanied by losses of extracellular fluid (ECF) and K$^+$ that lead to a decrease in effective arterial blood volume, activation of the renin-angiotensin-aldosterone system and enhanced tubular H$^+$ secretion. With more H$^+$ secretion, more new HCO$_3^-$ is added to the blood. The kidneys reabsorb filtered HCO$_3^-$ completely even though the plasma HCO$_3^-$ level is elevated and thus maintain the metabolic alkalosis.

Hypokalemia: Vomiting results in K$^+$ depletion because of a loss of K$^+$ in the vomitus, decreased food intake and most important quantitatively, enhanced renal K$^+$ excretion. Alkalosis results in a shift of K$^+$ into cells (including renal cells) and thereby promotes K$^+$ secretion and excretion. Elevated plasma aldosterone levels also favor K$^+$ loss in the urine.

Treatment: It primarily depends on eliminating the cause of vomiting. Correction of the alkalosis by administering an organic acid such as lactic acid does not make sense because this acid would simply be converted to CO$_2$ and H$_2$O; this approach also does not address the Cl$^-$ deficit. The ECF volume depletion and the Cl$^-$ and K$^+$ deficits can be corrected by administering isotonic saline and appropriate amounts of KCl. Because replacement of Cl$^-$ is a key component of therapy, this type of metabolic alkalosis is said to be 'chloride-responsive'. After fluid and electrolyte replacement, the excess HCO$_3^-$ (accompanied by surplus Na$^+$) will be excreted in the urine and the kidneys will return blood pH to normal.

38

Characteristic arterial blood changes include a primary increase in plasma HCO_3^- concentration, a rise in pH, and a compensatory rise in pCO_2. Metabolic alkalosis is seldom long lasting. Chemical buffers in the body act to limit the alkaline shift in pH by liberating H^+. As the primary defect is an increase in plasma HCO_3^- concentration, the immediate physiological compensation is hypoventilation followed by increased renal excretion of HCO_3^-.

BIOCHEMICAL ASSESSMENT OF ACID–BASE IMBALANCE

The disturbances of acid–base balance are accompanied by characteristic changes in pH, pCO_2, and HCO_3^-, the normal values for which, in the arterial blood, are as follows:

pH   7.35–7.45
pCO_2 35–45 mm Hg
HCO_3^- 22–26 mmol/L

Besides, base excess and anion gap can also be calculated to give some idea about these imbalances.

Base Excess

Base excess is defined as the amount of acid required to titrate the blood to pH 7.4, at a pCO_2 of 40 mm Hg at 37°C. If a blood sample is acidic, the base excess will be negative. The normal value is –2.0 to +3.0 mmol/L.

Anion Gap

Anion gap is the difference between the sum of Na^+ and K^+ (cations) from the sum of Cl^- and HCO_3^- (anions). Anion gap thus represents plasma anions other than Cl^- and HCO_3^- which are not routinely measured such as lactate, citrate, ketone bodies (acetoacetate and β-hydroxybutyrate), etc.

$$\text{Anion gap} = (Na^+ + K^+) - (Cl^- + HCO_3^-)$$

Normal value for anion gap is in the range of 12–16 mmol/L. This is most commonly used to establish a differential diagnosis for metabolic acidosis. As shown in Table 38.3, certain conditions resulting in metabolic acidosis are characterized by an increased anion gap while others do not lead to any change in the anion gap.

RENAL TUBULAR ACIDOSIS (RTA)

It is a group of kidney disorders characterized by **chronic metabolic acidosis, a normal plasma anion gap and the absence of renal failure**. The kidneys show inadequate H^+ secretion by the distal nephrons, excessive excretion of HCO_3^-, or reduced excretion of NH_4^+. The following types are recognized:

- **Classic type 1 (*distal*) RTA:** The ability of the collecting ducts to lower urine pH is impaired. This condition can be caused by inadequate secretion of H^+ (defective H^+-ATPase or H^+/K^+-ATPase) or abnormal leakiness of the collecting duct epithelium so that the secreted H^+ diffuse back from the lumen into blood. Because the urine pH is inappropriately high, titratable acid excretion is diminished and trapping of ammonia in the urine (as NH_4^+) is decreased. Type 1 RTA may be the result of an inherited defect, autoimmune disease, treatment

Table 38.3: Clinical examples of anion gap

Condition	Explanation
High anion gap metabolic acidosis	
• Ketoacidosis	• Production of acetoacetic and β-hydroxybutyric acids
• Lactacidosis	• H^+ buffered by HCO_3^-, accumulation of lactate
• Uremia	• Sulfuric, phosphoric, uric and hippuric acids retained due to renal failure
• Salicylate intoxication	• Salicylate accumulation, lactacidosis, ketoacidosis
• Methanol intoxication	• Methanol metabolized to formic acid
• Ethylene glycol intoxication	• Ethylene glycol metabolized to glyoxylic, glycolic and oxalic acids
• Paraldehyde intoxication	• Paraldehyde metabolized to acetic and chloroacetic acids
Normal anion gap metabolic acidosis	
• Diarrhea	• Loss of HCO_3^- in stool, renal conservation of Cl^-
• Renal tubular acidosis	• Loss of HCO_3^- in urine/decreased H^+ excretion, renal conservation of Cl^-

38

with lithium or the antibiotic amphotericin B, or diseases of the kidney medulla. The diagnosis is established by challenging the subject with a standard oral dose of NH_4Cl and measuring the urine pH over the next several hours. This results in a urine pH below 5.0 in healthy people. In subjects with type 1 RTA, however, urine pH will not decrease below 5.5. Treatment of type 1 RTA involves the daily administration of modest amounts of alkali (bicarbonate, citrate) sufficient to cover daily metabolic acid production.

- **Type 2 (*proximal*) RTA:** The HCO_3^- reabsorption by the proximal tubule is impaired leading to excessive losses of HCO_3^- in the urine. As a consequence, the plasma HCO_3^- falls and chronic metabolic acidosis ensues. In the new steady state, the tubules are able to reabsorb the filtered HCO_3^- load more completely, because the filtered load is reduced. The distal nephron is no longer over-whelmed by HCO_3^- and the urine pH is acidic. The NH_4Cl challenge results in a urine pH below 5.5. This disorder may be inherited (mutation in genes that code for carbonic anhydrase or Na^+/HCO_3^- cotransporters), may be associated with a number of acquired conditions that result in a generalized disorder of proximal tubule transport or may result from the inhibition of proximal tubule carbonic anhydrase by drugs such as acetazolamide. Treatment requires the daily administration of large amounts of alkali because when the plasma HCO_3^- is raised, excessive urinary excretion of filtered HCO_3^- occurs.

- **Type 3 RTA:** It is rare and shows *mixed features* of types 1 and 2.

- **Type 4 RTA:** It is also known as *hyperkalemic distal RTA*. The collecting duct secretion of both K^+ and H^+ is reduced, explaining the hyperkalemia and metabolic acidosis. Hyperkalemia reduces renal ammonia synthesis resulting in reduced net acid excretion and a fall in plasma HCO_3^-. The urine pH can go below 5.5 after NH_4Cl challenge because there is a little ammonia in the urine to buffer

secreted H^+. The underlying disorder is a result of inadequate production of aldosterone or impaired aldosterone action. Treatment of type 4 RTA requires lowering the plasma K^+ to normal; if this therapy is successful, alkali may not be needed.

REGULATION OF INTRACELLULAR pH

With the help of a combination of ion transport, buffering mechanisms and metabolic reactions, cells ensure a relatively stable intracellular pH as discussed below:

1. The intracellular and extracellular fluids are linked by **exchanges across cell membranes** of H^+, HCO_3^-, CO_2 and various other acids and bases. By stabilizing the ECF pH, the body helps to protect the ICF pH.

2. The protons (H^+) continuously tend to diffuse into cells down their concentration gradient. However, the H^+ is extruded by Na^+/H^+ exchangers (**NHE**) which are present in nearly all body cells. Eight different isoforms of these exchangers (designated NHE1, NHE2, etc.) with different tissue distributions have been identified. These transporters exchange one H^+ for one Na^+ and thus function in an electrically neutral fashion. The activity of the NHE is regulated by the intracellular pH itself as well as a variety of hormones and growth factors.

3. In some cells, various **HCO_3^- transporters** are present in the plasma membrane. These include Na^+-dependent and Na^+-independent Cl^-/HCO_3^- exchangers, and the electrogenic Na^+/HCO_3^- cotransporters.

4. Cells have **large stores of protein and organic phosphate buffers** which can bind or release H^+.

5. Various **chemical reactions** in cells can also use up or release H^+. For example, the conversion of lactic acid to CO_2 and water or to glucose effectively disposes of the acid.

6. Various cell **organelles may sequester H^+**. For example, H^+-ATPases in endosomes and lysosomes pump H^+ out of the cytosol into these organelles.

SOME IMPORTANT QUESTIONS

1. **Define buffer. Name important buffers present in the body. Explain the role of various body buffers in the regulation of blood pH.**

38

2. Explain:

i. Role of kidney in the regulation of blood pH
ii. Various mechanisms of H^+ secretion
iii. Disturbances of acid–base balance
iv. Measures of acid–base imbalance
v. Role of lungs in the regulation of blood pH

3. Write notes on:

i. pH
ii. Henderson-Hasselbalch equation
iii. Chemical buffers in the body
iv. Titratable acidity
v. Respiratory acidosis
vi. Respiratory alkalosis
vii. Metabolic acidosis
viii. Metabolic alkalosis
ix. Base excess
x. Anion gap
xi. Diabetic ketoacidosis

MULTIPLE CHOICE QUESTIONS

1. The following is a correct representation of pH:
   A. $\log_{10}[H^+]$
   B. $\log_{10}[1/H^+]$
   C. $\log_e[H^+]$
   D. $\log_e[1/H^+]$

2. The major buffer system in RBC is:
   A. Bicarbonate
   B. Phosphate
   C. Hemoglobin
   D. Non-heme proteins

3. The following is an 'open' buffer system:
   A. Bicarbonate
   B. Phosphate
   C. Hemoglobin
   D. Plasma proteins

4. The majority of titratable acid in the urine is:
   A. Inorganic phosphate ($H_2PO_4^-$)
   B. Inorganic sulphate (H_2SO_4)
   C. Inorganic chloride (HCl)
   D. Carbonic acid (H_2CO_3)

5. Alkalemia indicates the following H^+ concentration in blood:
   A. <35 mmol/L
   B. <35 nmol/L
   C. <35 mol/L
   D. <35 pmol/L

6. Salicylate poisoning is associated with:
   A. Hyperventilation and respiratory alkalosis
   B. Hypoventilation and respiratory acidosis
   C. Hyperventilation and respiratory acidosis
   D. Hypoventilation and respiratory alkalosis

7. Increased renal HCO_3^- excretion is the main compensation observed in:
   A. Metabolic acidosis
   B. Metabolic alkalosis
   C. Respiratory acidosis
   D. Respiratory alkalosis

8. Increased anion gap is characteristic of:
   A. Uncontrolled diabetes mellitus with metabolic acidosis
   B. Salicylate poisoning with respiratory alkalosis
   C. Status asthmaticus with respiratory acidosis
   D. Prolonged gastric lavage with metabolic alkalosis

9. The sum of all buffering agents in blood is called:
   A. Anion gap
   B. Buffer base
   C. Base excess
   D. Buffering capacity

10. Lithium therapy may be associated with:
    A. Type 1 RTA
    B. Type 2 RTA
    C. Type 3 RTA
    D. Type 4 RTA

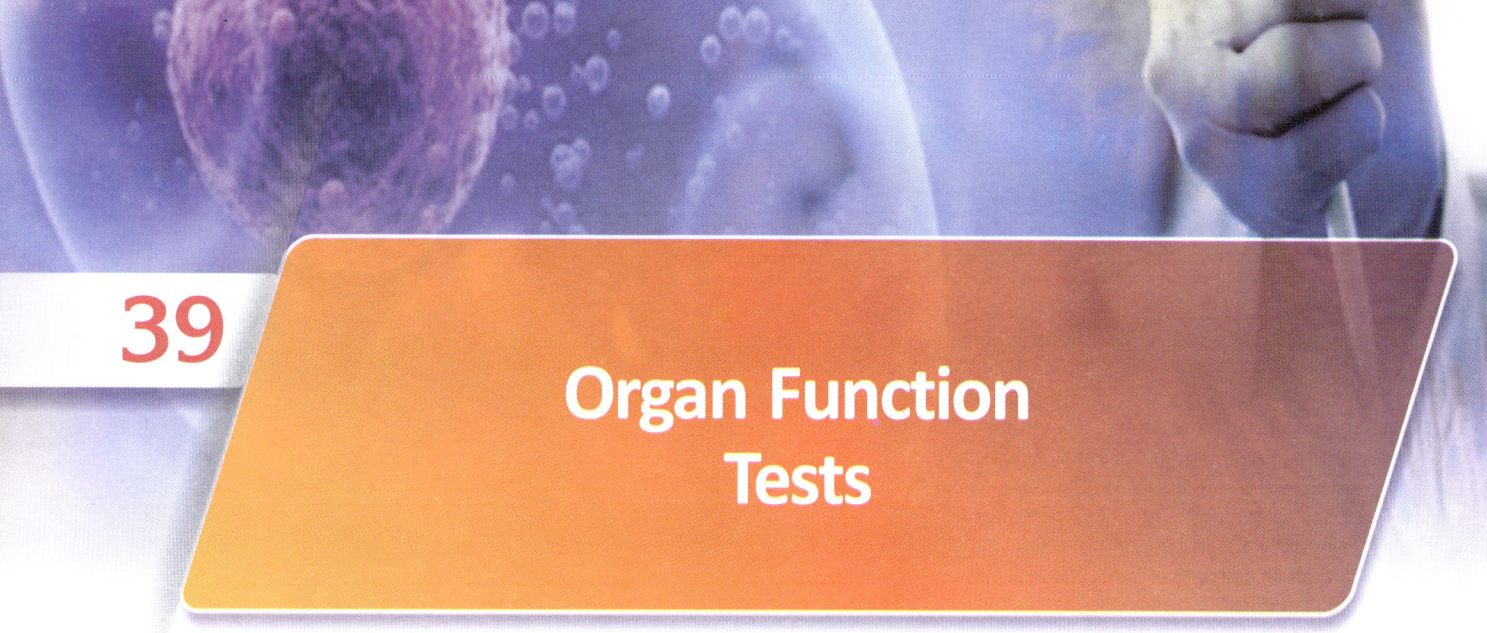

Organ Function Tests

LIVER FUNCTION TESTS

Liver is the **largest organ** of the body, weighing about 1200–1500 g in adults. Traditionally, it is divided into two lobes, i.e. the right lobe and the left lobe. The functional unit of the liver is acinus which comprises of the group of hepatic parenchymal cells called hepatocytes. Liver performs a variety of functions (Fig. 39.1). It is better known as the **chemical workshop** of the body.

A. BIOCHEMICAL TESTS TO ASSESS LIVER FUNCTIONS

Various biochemical tests to assess liver functions for the diagnosis and follow-up of liver disease are briefly described here.

Serum Bilirubin

Bilirubin is an orange yellow pigment derived from the senescent red blood cells in the liver, spleen and bone marrow. Daily bilirubin production in adults averages 250–300 mg. Approximately 85% of this is derived from the heme moiety of hemoglobin which is released from the erythrocytes that are destroyed in the reticuloendothelial cells. The rest of it is formed from catabolism of other hemoproteins such as myoglobin, cytochromes and heme containing enzymes.

Serum contains two different forms of bilirubin, i.e. the **unconjugated (lipid soluble)** form which is bound to albumin and is transported from the

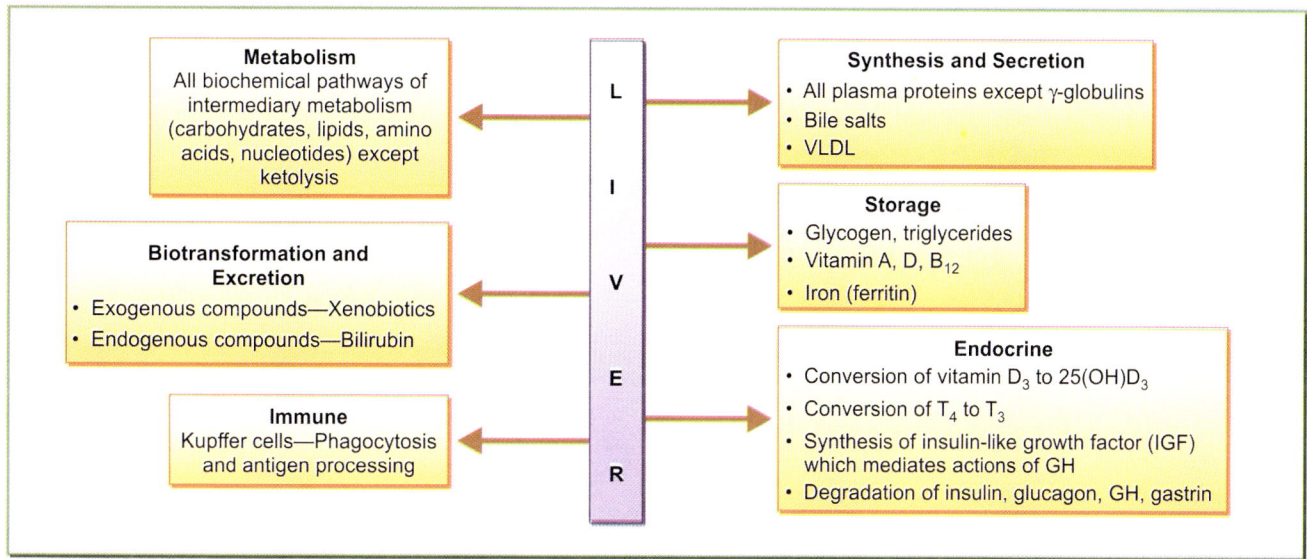

Fig. 39.1: Functions of liver.

39

Chemistry to Clinics 39.1: Delta Bilirubin

Normally, only traces of conjugated bilirubin are non-enzymatically, irreversibly and covalently bound to albumin. Since it is not filtered at the glomerulus, its half-life reflects that of albumin (14 days, i.e. longer than that of the conventional conjugated bilirubin which is easily filtered out at the glomerulus). This is delta bilirubin which is not measured separately in the laboratory. This fraction increases with the duration of biliary outflow obstruction of any cause, i.e. cholestasis. Thus, some patients recovering from cholestatic jaundice continue to have clinical jaundice for about 2 weeks despite biochemical recovery (apparently normal serum conjugated bilirubin and absence of urinary bile pigments.

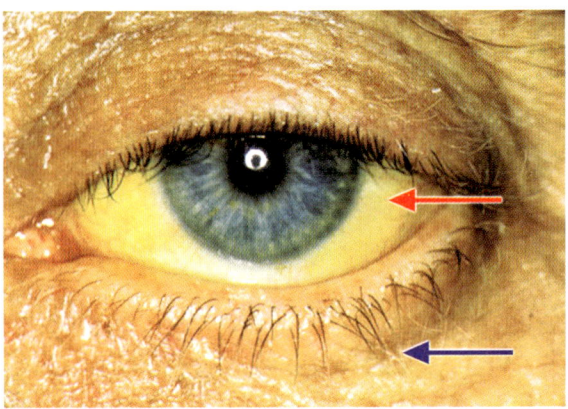

Fig. 39.2: Jaundice: Yellow discoloration of skin (blue arrow) and sclera (red arrow).

reticuloendothelial system to the liver, and the **conjugated (water soluble,** Chemistry to Clinics 39.1) form which has been regurgitated from the liver into the plasma. Majority of the bilirubin in plasma is unconjugated. Disorders of bilirubin metabolism lead to **hyperbilirubinemia** and serial measurement of bilirubin is helpful in knowing severity of liver disease. Bilirubin fractionation is helpful in the differential diagnosis of **jaundice**.

Jaundice

Jaundice is a **physical sign** characterized by yellow appearance of the patient resulting from the deposition of bile pigment (bilirubin) in the skin, mucous membranes and sclera (Fig. 39.2). These tissues are rich in **elastin** which has a high affinity for bilirubin. Jaundice is the most characteristic clinical manifestation of hyperbilirubinemia.

Types of Jaundice

Depending on serum bilirubin levels, jaundice is either clinical or latent. Jaundice is apparent clinically (**clinical jaundice**) when serum bilirubin concentration is >2 mg/dl. If serum bilirubin concentration is <2 mg/dl it is called **latent jaundice (subclinical jaundice)** since at this stage it is not yet detectable, clinically.

Depending on the cause of jaundice, it may be of three types, i.e. **pre-hepatic, hepatic and post-hepatic jaundice**. In this classification, the liver is taken as the reference organ because the key reaction in bilirubin metabolism, i.e. conjugation of bilirubin, occurs in the liver. Biochemical differentiation of three types of jaundice is given in Table 39.1.

Sample	Biochemical parameter	Types of jaundice		
		Pre-hepatic	Hepatic	Post-hepatic
Blood	Serum bilirubin	↑	↑↑	↑↑↑
	Type of bilirubin	Unconjugated	Mixed	Conjugated
	Serum transaminases (especially ALT/SGPT)	N	↑↑↑	↑
	Serum alkaline phosphatase	N	↑	↑↑↑
	Serum 5′-Nucleotidase	N	↑	↑↑↑
	Prothrombin time (PT)	N	↑	↑
	Effect of parental vitamin K on PT	–	Remains ↑	↓ (Normalizes)
Urine	Urobilinogen	↑↑	N/↑	↓/–
	Bilirubin	–	–	↑↑
	Bile salts	–	–	↑
Stool	Stercobilinogen	↑	↓	↓/–

Table 39.1: Biochemical differentiation of three types of jaundice

39

Pre-hepatic jaundice: It is also called **hemolytic jaundice** since it results from excessive hemolysis of RBC as observed in hemolytic anemia. It is characterized by increased serum unconjugated bilirubin which may be due to increased hemolysis, decreased uptake of unconjugated bilirubin across hepatocyte membrane (as in Gilbert syndrome) or decreased biotransformation (as in neonatal jaundice or Criggler-Najjar syndrome).

- **Hemolysis:** In disorders associated with hemolysis, most commonly hemolytic anemia, the rate of bilirubin production is increased which may exceed the amount that can be removed by the liver. This, in turn, results in unconjugated hyperbilirubinemia (Chemistry to Clinics 39.2).

- **Gilbert's syndrome:** This is a heterogeneous group of disorders which is inherited as an autosomal recessive trait. Several defects including the deficiency of bilirubin glucuronyl transferase, defective hepatic uptake of bilirubin and decreased red cell survival have been described. There is a mild unconjugated hyperbilirubinemia.

- **Neonatal jaundice:** It is also called **physiological jaundice of the newborn**. Every infant exhibits some transient unconjugated hyperbilirubinemia between the second and the fifth day of life. Since at this stage the **liver is still immature**, the activity

of the hepatic enzyme glucuronyl transferase may be inadequate to completely conjugate the bilirubin. Hence, unconjugated bilirubin level remains at ≈ 5 mg/dl. The activity of glucuronyl transferase increases within 2 weeks after birth and serum bilirubin returns to normal. Naturally, in a premature infant, physiological jaundice is more pronounced (Chemistry to Clinics 39.3).

- **Criggler-Najjar syndrome:** This disorder is known to exist in two forms. **Type I** is the clinically severe form and is due to complete absence of glucuronyl transferase. **Type II** has moderate clinical findings and is due to partial deficiency of the enzyme. In both the conditions, unconjugated bilirubin is significantly raised.

Hepatic/medical jaundice: In jaundice due to primary liver disease, the serum usually exhibits elevated levels of both conjugated and unconjugated bilirubin. **Hepatitis and cirrhosis** constitute the most common disorders associated with conjugated and unconjugated hyperbilirubinemia.

In most instances of **viral hepatitis**, besides a rise in serum conjugated and unconjugated bilirubin, there is also a variable increase in alanine aminotransferase (ALT, also called serum glutamate pyruvate transaminase or SGPT) and aspartate aminotransferase (AST, also called serum glutamate oxaloacetate transaminase or SGOT).

Besides, inhalation, ingestion or parenteral administration of a number of pharmacological and **chemical agents** such as carbon tetrachloride, acetaminophen, isoniazid and chlorpromazine may also result in liver

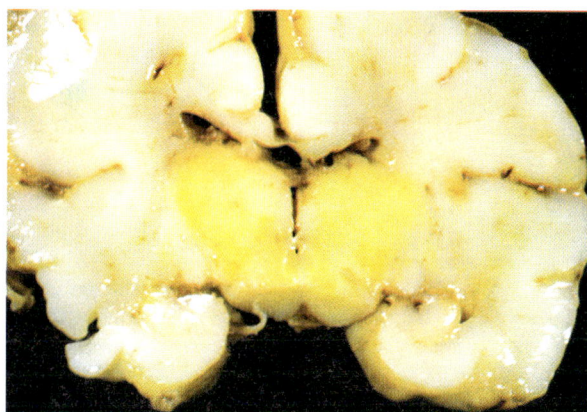

Fig. 39.3: Kernicterus: Cut-section of brain showing permanent yellow staining of **basal ganglia** due to deposition of **unconjugated** bilirubin.

39

injury (called **toxic or drug-induced hepatitis**) leading to hepatic jaundice.

Some other conditions include Dubin-Johnson syndrome and Rotor syndrome.

- **Dubin-Johnson syndrome:** It is a benign, autosomal recessive condition characterized by elevated levels of conjugated as well as unconjugated bilirubin along with dark-brown pigmentation in the liver cells (Fig. 39.4). The defect lies in the secretion of conjugated bilirubin into the bile canaliculi.

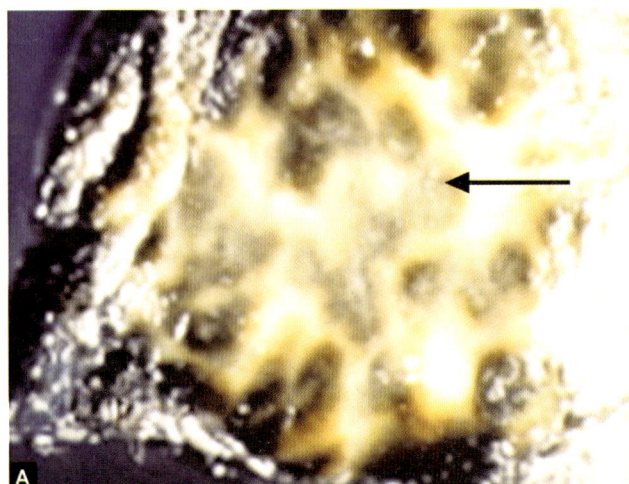
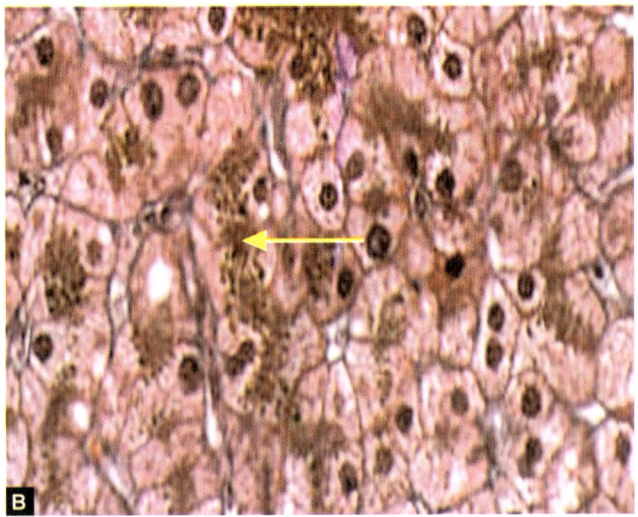

Fig. 39.4: Dubin-Johnson syndrome. (A) Gross liver specimen showing multiple areas of dark pigmentation (black arrow), (B) Light micrograph of a section through liver showing accumulation of large coarse granules of a brown pigment (yellow arrow). The pigment contains a complex association of melanin-like compound, lipofuscin and unidentified bilirubin degradation products. The defect lies in the secretion of conjugated bilirubin from hepatocytes into bile canaliculi and accumulation of the pigment in lysosomes.

- **Rotor syndrome:** Its features are the same as that of Dubin-Johnson syndrome except that no abnormal pigmentation occurs.

Post-hepatic/obstructive/surgical jaundice: It refers to post-hepatic cholestasis caused by **obstruction** of the bile duct outside the liver. Obstructive jaundice, most often, may be due to stones in the common bile duct/hepatic duct (choledocholithiasis), carcinoma of the head of pancreas or carcinoma of the bile duct (cholangiocarcinoma). Serum of such a patient contains excessive amount of the **conjugated bilirubin**. It is also characterized by the presence of excessive amount of bilirubin in the urine.

Since unconjugated bilirubin is not soluble in water, it is not excreted in the urine. Only conjugated bilirubin is excreted in the urine of patients with obstructive jaundice. It is an indirect test for the increased concentration of conjugated bilirubin in the serum.

Urinary Urobilinogen

Normally, 0.5–4 mg of urobilinogen is excreted in the urine in 24 hours. Increased excretion of urobilinogen occurs when hepatocellular function is impaired. Urobilinogen may also increase in the urine if there is an excess of urobilinogen in the gastrointestinal tract that exceeds the capacity of the liver to re-excrete it, e.g. in hemolysis, viral hepatitis and cirrhosis. In contrast, when biliary excretion of bilirubin is impaired, e.g. in cholestasis, urinary excretion of urobilinogen is decreased due to limited delivery of bilirubin to the gut and due to low rate of urobilinogen production. This also results in clay-colored or chalky white stool of patients with cholestatic jaundice.

Fecal Stercobilinogen

Stercobilinogen content of feces of patients with stone obstruction is closer to the lower limit of normal while it is low or absent in those with malignant obstruction. It may thus be of value to distinguish between obstruction due to stone in the bile duct or that due to neoplasm.

Serum Enzymes

In liver diseases, serum levels of several enzymes are elevated. These include:

- **Transaminases (aminotransferases):** These constitute a group of enzymes that catalyze

39

interconversion of amino acids and α-keto acids by the transfer of an amino group. **ALT (SGPT)** and **AST (SGOT)** are the two such enzymes which are liberated into the blood whenever liver cells are damaged. Increased plasma activities of these enzymes are a sensitive index of hepatic damage. In viral hepatitis and other forms of the liver disease associated with hepatic necrosis, serum SGPT and SGOT levels are **elevated even before clinical signs and symptoms of the disease** appear. Peak values occur between day seven and day twelve. Activities thereafter gradually decrease reaching towards normal levels by the third to fifth week of recovery.

Increased levels may also be observed in extrahepatic cholestasis, the increase being comparatively higher with more chronic obstruction. Five to ten folds elevation of both the enzymes occur in patients with primary or metastatic carcinoma of the liver. Although serum levels of both GPT and GOT become elevated whenever a disease process affects the liver, **GPT however, is more liver specific**.

- **Alkaline phosphatase (ALP):** It catalyzes hydrolysis of a variety of substrates at a pH of about 10. The enzyme is present in all tissues of the body, particularly at high levels in intestinal epithelium, kidney tubules, bone (osteoblasts), liver and placenta. Serum ALP measurements are of particular interest in the investigation of hepatobiliary diseases and bone disease associated with increased osteoblastic activity. The response of the liver to any form of **biliary tree obstruction** is to synthesize more ALP, by way of its **induction**. Elevation tends to be **more marked in extrahepatic obstruction** than in intrahepatic obstruction. **Increased ALP in children is a normal finding** due to ongoing bone growth associated with enhanced osteoblastic activity.

- **Glutamate dehydrogenase (GDH):** It is found mainly in the liver, heart, muscle and kidney. GDH is present in normal serum only in traces but increased activities are observed in hepatocellular damage.

- **5'-Nucleotidase (5'-NT):** It is a phosphatase that acts only on nucleoside-5'-phosphate such as AMP and releases inorganic phosphate. Serum 5'-NT activity is increased two to six folds in hepatobiliary diseases. This may be due to extrahepatic causes (such as stone/tumor/fibrosis obstructing the bile

duct) or may arise from intrahepatic conditions (such as cholestasis caused by chlorpromazine, malignant infiltration of the liver, or biliary cirrhosis).

- **Gamma-glutamyl transferase (γ-GT):** It is also called γ-glutamyl transpeptidase. It transfers γ-glutamyl group from peptides and other compounds, to some acceptor. Even though renal tissue has its highest level, the enzyme present in the serum originates primarily from the hepatobiliary system. It is highest in cases of intrahepatic or post-hepatic biliary obstruction. Further, elevated levels of γ-GT occur in sera from people who are heavy alcoholics. Thus, γ-GT is of significance in detecting **alcohol-induced liver disease**.

Prothrombin time (PT)

Increased PT observed in hepatocellular disease (e.g. cirrhosis) is not correctable by vitamin K injections whereas that due to cholestasis is correctable. Thus, serial measurements of PT can be used to **differentiate between cholestasis and severe hepatocellular disease**.

Various liver function tests that are useful in the assessment of liver disease as well as in the differential diagnosis of jaundice are indicated in Table 39.1.

KIDNEY FUNCTION TESTS

Kidneys form a paired organ system. The functional unit of the kidney is called **nephron**. Each kidney has nearly one million nephrons. Each nephron consists of a renal corpuscle and its attached renal tubule.

- **The renal corpuscle** consists of a tuft of capillaries called *glomerulus* surrounded by the *Bowman's capsule*. The glomerulus of the nephron is formed from a specialized capillary network. The resulting structure is relatively impermeable to most proteins >60 kD.

- **The tubule** comprises proximal convoluted tubule, loop of Henle, distal convoluted tubule and collecting ducts. *The proximal tubule* is the most active part of the nephron. It facilitates the reabsorption of 60–80% of the glomerular filtrate volume, ≈70% of the filtered load of Na^+ and Cl^-, most of K^+, glucose, bicarbonate, phosphate and sulfate. Proximal tubules secrete 90% of the H^+ excreted by the kidneys. The main function of the *loop of Henle* is to generate concentrated urine.

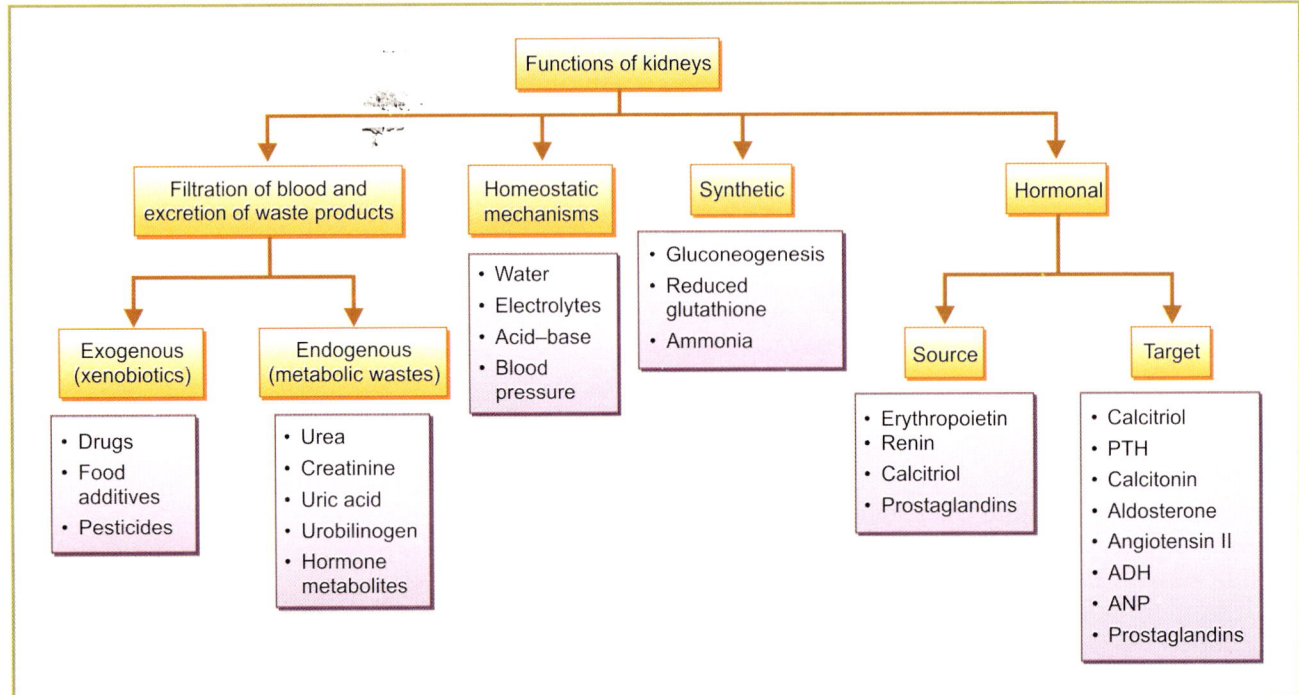

Fig. 39.5: Overview of functions of the kidneys.

B. BIOCHEMICAL FUNCTIONS OF THE KIDNEY

Primary function of the kidneys is the filtration and excretion of waste products, both exogenous and endogenous. Besides, kidneys play a central role in the homeostatic mechanisms of the human body, synthetic and hormonal functions (Fig. 39.5).

Reabsorptive and Excretory Functions

1. **Reabsorption of vital substances:** Substances which are vital to the body are reabsorbed. For example, glucose is normally completely reabsorbed by the proximal tubule. Amino acids are also reabsorbed in the proximal tubule by several specific transport mechanisms. Most of the filtered phosphate is also reabsorbed in the proximal tubule by the processes that are linked to the reabsorption of sodium and water. Reabsorption of phosphate however, is inhibited by parathyroid hormone and increased by vitamin D.

2. **Excretion of waste products:** The excretory function of the kidneys serves to get the body rid of most of the undesirable end products of metabolism including various organic and inorganic substances

along with water in the urine. Only a small amount of protein is normally excreted in the urine. But the end products of metabolism, e.g. urea, creatinine, uric acid, etc. are largely excreted in the urine.

Urine: Urine is defined as a fluid excreted by the kidneys, passed through the ureters, stored in the urinary bladder and discharged through the urethra. In a healthy individual, it is a sterile and clear solution which has amber color, a characteristic odour, pH of about 5.0 to 6.0 and specific gravity of about 1.024. The volume of the urine excreted (about 1.5 L/day or nearly 1 ml/min) is the net effect of two opposing processes, i.e. ultrafiltration of nearly 180 L of fluid per day (nearly 125 ml/min) across glomerular capillaries and the reabsorption of more than 99% of this ultrafiltrate by transport processes operating in the renal tubules.

Glomerular filtration rate: Urine formation begins with the elaboration of a protein free ultrafiltrate of plasma across the walls of the glomerular capillaries. The rate of ultrafiltration is referred to as glomerular filtration rate (**GFR**, Chemistry to Clinics 39.4). It is defined as the **volume of plasma cleared of a**

particular substance by both the kidneys in one minute. GFR is determined by three factors:

1. The balance of pressures acting across the capillary wall.
2. The rate at which plasma flows through the glomeruli.
3. The permeability and the total surface area of the filtering capillaries.

Endocrine Functions

The endocrine functions of the kidney may be regarded as either primary or secondary. In its **primary** endocrine function, kidney **produces** erythropoietin, renin, active vitamin D (calcitriol) and prostaglandins (PGE_2 and PGI_2), both of which are concerned with the control of renal circulation. In the **secondary** endocrine function, kidney is a **target** for the hormones produced either within the kidney itself (e.g. calcitriol) or elsewhere (e.g. aldosterone, ADH, angiotensin II, ANP, PTH, etc).

C. COMMONLY USED BIOCHEMICAL TESTS TO ASSESS KIDNEY FUNCTIONS

Examination of the Urine

Clinical features of renal disease commonly arise from alterations in the chemical composition of the body which may be suspected after detection of abnormalities in the urine:

- **Urine volume:** In temperate climate, 24 hours urine output varies from 800 to 2500 ml with an average of about 1500 ml. **Oliguria** is the failure to produce enough urine (<500 ml/day) to enable solutes to be excreted in adequate amounts. Oliguria develops when renal blood flow and/or GFR are reduced, e.g. reduced blood volume, septicemia, cardiac failure, acute glomerulonephritis and acute tubular

necrosis. If untreated, it results in complete lack of urine output or **anuria**. **Polyuria** is a persistent increase in urinary output (>3000 ml/day) which may be due to an increased osmotic load (diabetes mellitus), disturbances in the concentration mechanism (diabetes insipidus), certain drugs or excessive water intake.

- **Urine pH:** In a healthy individual, urine pH ranges from 4.3 to 8.0. pH >8.0 indicates urinary tract infection with an organism which splits urea and forms ammonia. In certain circumstances, the ability to excrete H^+ is suppressed.

- **Urine proteins:** Routine side room testing of urine for the presence of protein is a part of the clinical examination of a patient. Routine testing for protein is usually carried out on an early morning specimen, as this is normally the most concentrated sample of the urine (Chemistry to Clinics 39.5). **Microalbuminuria** is a useful index of early, pre-clinical renal impairment (Chemistry to Clinics 39.6).

Analysis of the Constituents of Blood

Blood urea: Blood urea level in a normal individual may vary between 15 and 35 mg/dl. Urea is the **major** nitrogen containing metabolic product of protein catabolism in humans, accounting for >75% of the non-protein nitrogen (NPN) which is eventually excreted. Urea is filtered freely by the glomeruli, moderately reabsorbed and secreted by the tubules. In a normal kidney, 40–70% of the highly diffusible urea moves passively out of the renal tubule into the interstitium. Measurement of blood urea is widely used as a test of

39

Chemistry to Clinics 39.6: Microalbuminuria

It was previously thought that plasma albumin is not filtered at the glomerulus. However, the fact is that albumin does cross the filtration barrier but the majority is reabsorbed by the proximal tubules with the help of transport proteins called cubilin and megalin. Values below the lower limit refer to normoalbuminuria while values above the upper limit refer to **macroalbuminuria** (or simply 'albuminuria'). A repeat measurement is suggested after 2–3 months to confirm the diagnosis. **Microalbuminuria** refers to urinary albumin excretion with respect to any one of the following criteria:

1. 30–300 mg/24 h (for 24 h urine sample).
2. 30–300 mg/L (for spot urine sample).
3. 30–300 µg albumin/mg creatinine (called albumin/creatinine ratio [ACR] for spot urine sample).

Microalbuminuria is an indicator of

1. Glomerular endothelial dysfunction.
2. Pre-clinical renal impairment in diabetic nephropathy and hypertensive nephropathy.
3. The need to implement rigorous control of blood glucose and blood pressure.

renal function although it may be raised due to renal or non-renal factors (Chemistry to Clinics 39.7).

Serum creatinine: Normal serum creatinine concentration varies between 0.7 and 1.5 mg/dl. Creatine is synthesized in the kidney, liver and muscles. A portion of free creatine in muscle is spontaneously and irreversibly converted to its anhydride, i.e. creatinine. Free creatinine thus is a waste product of creatine. Its daily production is related to **muscle mass** and does not vary greatly from day to day. The level of creatinine in the blood remains fairly constant. Serum creatinine values are lower in children than in adults, in women than in men (due to lower muscle mass), and during pregnancy. Meal containing meat may slightly increase serum creatinine concentration.

Creatinine is freely filtered by the glomerulus. Although it is not reabsorbed to any great extent by renal tubules, a small amount of creatinine is secreted. Its secretion is increased with the increasing levels of plasma creatinine. In patients with acute renal failure, value may reach 4–6 mg/dl while values >10 mg/dl are seen in untreated chronic renal failure. Determination of serum creatinine thus gives a useful indication of the **degree of renal failure** (Chemistry to Clinics 39.8).

Chemistry to Clinics 39.7: Increased Blood Urea

Pre-renal factors: High protein diet, protein catabolic states, gastrointestinal hemorrhage, treatment with cortisol, some cases of chronic liver disease, decreased renal perfusion due to dehydration (severe diarrhea, vomiting, burns).

Renal factors: Acute and chronic glomerulonephritis, acute and chronic renal failure.

Post-renal factors: Ureteric stones, stricture urethra, ureteric fibrosis, carcinoma of ureters/urinary bladder/prostate.

Chemistry to Clinics 39.8: Increased Serum Creatinine

An increase in serum creatinine is observed in:

1. Any condition in which there is decreased renal perfusion, e.g. reduced blood pressure, fluid deprivation or renal artery stenosis.
2. Most diseases in which there is loss of functioning nephrons, e.g. in acute and chronic glomerulonephritis, acute and chronic renal failure.
3. Diseases where pressure is increased on the tubular side of the nephron, e.g. in urinary tract obstruction due to prostatic enlargement.

Serum cystatin C: Cystatin C is a 13 kD protein constitutively produced by all nucleated cells. Its plasma levels are **independent** of diet, muscle mass or inflammatory conditions. It is freely filtered at the glomerulus, completely reabsorbed and degraded by cells lining the proximal convoluted tubules. It is not secreted by the tubules. Thus, its plasma levels are determined by GFR. It is a **sensitive biomarker to detect kidney disease much earlier** than that possible with the determination of serum creatinine (Chemistry to Clinics 39.9).

Chemistry to Clinics 39.9: Creatinine-blind GFR and Cystatin C

Though creatinine is filtered at the glomerulus, serum creatinine does not rise appreciably until the GFR drops below 60 ml/min. This is because creatinine undergoes tubular secretion and partly compensates for a declining GFR so that serum creatinine rises only when the secretory capacity is saturated. Thus, many patients with mild-moderate decrease in GFR are missed if serum creatinine is used as the sole diagnostic criterion for renal disease. The critical range of GFR, 50–70 ml/min, is called the **'creatinine-blind GFR'**. However, elevation in serum cystatin C occurs in this range as it does not undergo tubular secretion. Therefore, cystatin C provides a superior assessment of renal function.

39

Blood pH, gases and electrolytes: Diminished capacity to excrete H^+ results in metabolic acidosis, the severity of which may be estimated by the measurement of arterial H^+ concentration, HCO_3^- content and pCO_2. Estimations of serum sodium, potassium, calcium and phosphate are also of value in certain conditions, e.g. in chronic renal failure or in metabolic acidosis accompanied by hyponatremia, hyperkalemia, hypocalcemia and hyperphosphatemia.

1. TESTS FOR THE ASSESSMENT OF GLOMERULAR FUNCTIONS

Renal Clearance

Clearance is defined as the volume of plasma from which the substance whose clearance is to be estimated is completely cleared-off by the two kidneys per minute. The clearance of a substance can be calculated by the mathematical relationship shown in Fig. 39.6, where

C_S = Clearance of substance (ml/min, i.e. ml of plasma cleared of a substance in one min)

$$C_S = \frac{U_S \times V}{P_S}$$

Fig. 39.6: Formula for calculating the clearance of a substance (S).

U_S = Urine concentration of the substance (mg/dl)

V = Volumetric flow rate of urine (ml/min)

P_S = Plasma (blood or serum) concentration of the substance (mg/dl).

Measurement of clearance thus requires measurement of plasma and urine concentrations of the marker plus a reliable urine collection. A substance, which can be considered as a suitable marker of glomerular filtration should meet several criteria (Table 39.2). Clearly, in the long-term monitoring of renal function, the **choice is: Cystatin C > Creatinine > Urea.**

Inulin clearance: Inulin is a polymer of fructose. It is filtered by the glomeruli but is neither reabsorbed nor secreted by the tubules. Inulin clearance is nearly equal to GFR. Normal value for GFR as per inulin clearance found in adults is about 125 ml/min. Although inulin meets most of the above criteria for measuring GFR, it is not suitable for routine use as it is not an endogenous substance and has to be administered intravenously.

Urea clearance: Urea clearance depends upon the volume of urine excreted in one min. Urea clearance may be calculated as standard urea clearance or maximum urea clearance.

- **Standard urea clearance:** It is calculated when the urine volume is <2 ml/min. Standard urea clearance is calculated by taking square root of V, i.e. $\sqrt{V}$:

  Standard urea clearance (ml/min) = $U/P \times \sqrt{V}$

  where U and P are the concentrations of urea in urine and blood (mg/100 ml) respectively, while $\sqrt{V}$ is the square root of the volume of urine excreted (ml/min). The mean value for standard urea clearance is 54 ml/min.

- **Maximum urea clearance:** When the volume of urine excreted is ≥2 ml/min, urea clearance is calculated as the maximum urea clearance,

Table 39.2: Desirable characteristics of a substance for determining its clearance and hence glomerular filtration rate (GFR)

Desirable characteristics	Urea	Creatinine	Cystatin C
Blood level independent of diet	No	No	Yes
Blood level independent of muscle mass	Yes	No	Yes
Day-to-day blood level within narrow limits	More variable (15–35 mg/dl)	Less variable (0.7–1.5 mg/dl)	Least variable (0.52–0.95 mg/L)
Freely filtered at the glomerulus	Yes	Yes	Yes
No tubular reabsorption	≈50% reabsorption by passive diffusion	Yes	Yes
No tubular secretion	Moderate secretion	Mild-moderate secretion	Yes
Day-to-day urinary excretion within narrow limits	More variable (25–30 g/day)	Less variable (1–2 g/day)	Yes (minimal excretion)
Blood level or clearance value representative of GFR	≈60%	≈80–90%	≈95%

39

calculated by putting the actual value of V in the above equation, instead of $\sqrt{V}$. The mean value for maximum urea clearance is 75 ml/min.

Since urea clearance depends on urine flow rate and also because urea is affected by dietary protein, urea clearance is not preferred to estimate GFR.

Creatinine clearance: Creatinine, as mentioned above, is generated spontaneously from creatine and gains access to the urine by glomerular filtration. Moreover, creatinine clearance is not affected by the volume of urine excreted or by dietary protein intake. It is, therefore, preferred as a measure of GFR.

Creatinine clearance per 1.73 m^2 surface area is low at birth (35–40 ml/min) but reaches normal adult levels (80–120 ml/min) by 6 months of age. Creatinine clearance declines with age. However, it is increased by 20% during pregnancy.

Plasma Flow

Measurement of renal plasma flow can be done by renal excretion rate of a substance undergoing both glomerular filtration as well as tubular secretion, e.g. ρ-aminohippuric acid (PAH). At low blood levels, PAH clearance is used as a measure of renal plasma flow. Renal plasma flow as determined with PAH in normal adults is about 700 ± 130 ml/min.

Filtration Fraction

Filtration fraction is the fraction of plasma passing through the kidney which is filtered at the glomerulus. It is obtained by dividing the value of inulin clearance by the value of PAH clearance.

2. TESTS FOR THE ASSESSMENT OF TUBULAR FUNCTIONS

Urine Concentration Test

Urine concentration (water deprivation) test can be done by measuring the osmolality of a specimen of the urine which is obtained after water deprivation or after the administration of vasopressin (ADH). Urine osmolality (Osm) is determined by the number of particles of solute per kg water. In normal subjects, restriction of water intake for 8 hours results in maximal stimulation of ADH secretion. Since ADH acts on the collecting tubules and promotes reabsorption of water, it results in concentrated urine.

For water deprivation test, the subject should not take water, coffee or tea and should not smoke but can have light breakfast until the start of the test. No fluids should be given for 8 hours. Thereafter, osmolality of the urine (after 8 hours) should be measured and the value should reach 800 mOsm/kg (or specific gravity of 1.022). If the urine sample has less osmolality or specific gravity, it indicates impaired renal concentrating power either due to tubular defect or due to decreased ADH secretion.

The patient should, however, be weighed at the start and after 5 and 8 hours. The test should be stopped if weight loss is >3% of body weight. The water deprivation test procedure is potentially dangerous when renal concentrating ability is impaired, e.g. in diabetes insipidus.

Urine Dilution Test

Urine dilution (water excretion) test is done to assess the ability of the kidneys to eliminate water. This function is tested by measuring urinary output after ingesting a large volume of water. In normal subjects, at least 750 ml of water is excreted within 4 hours.

After an overnight fast, the subject is asked to empty the bladder. The person is then given 1000 ml of water to drink within 20 minutes. Urine samples are collected at hourly intervals during the next 4 hours. The specific gravity of one of these specimens should fall to at least 1.003, while its osmolality should be <100 mOsm/kg. If renal function is impaired, the quantity eliminated in 4 hours will be less, depending on the degree of impairment. Specific gravity of the urine is often 1.010 or higher in conditions of oliguria.

The test is not advisable in patients with adrenal insufficiency.

Urine Acidification Test

The ability of the kidneys to produce acidic urine is also a function of the tubules. Hence, this test is called urine acidification test and is carried out without any restriction.

The person is asked to empty the bladder. Thereafter, ammonium chloride (0.1 g/kg body weight) is given in a gelatin capsule. Urine samples are collected one hourly for 8 hours. During the test, the patient may eat normally and should drink about 200 ml of water per hour. The pH of the urine is measured. It should be between 4.6 and 5.0. In patients with renal tubular acidosis, pH of the urine does not fall below 5.3 even after a dose of ammonium chloride.

Various renal function tests are summarized in Fig. 39.7.

THYROID FUNCTION TESTS

Main function of the thyroid gland is to synthesize and secrete thyroid hormones. **Hyperthyroidism** is a clinical syndrome which results from exposure of body tissues to excess circulating levels of free thyroid hormones. Females are more affected than males. Main causes include Graves' disease, multinodular goiter and toxic adenoma. **Hypothyroidism** is a deficiency of thyroid activity such as in myxedema and cretinism. *Myxedema* is a form of hypothyroidism in which there is accumulation of mucopolysaccharides in the skin and other tissues in adults. *Cretinism* is the term used to describe hypothyroidism in children.

D. COMMONLY USED BIOCHEMICAL TESTS TO ASSESS THYROID FUNCTIONS

Biochemical tests to establish, if there is any thyroid dysfunction, include the measurements of the thyroid hormones (T_3 and T_4) and TSH in serum. Other tests include radioactive iodine uptake, protein bound iodine, serum cholesterol, etc. (Table 39.3).

Serum Levels of Thyroid Hormones

Measurement of the concentration of T_4 and T_3 in the serum is used in confirming the diagnosis of hyperthyroidism or hypothyroidism.

Table 39.3: Biochemical assessment of thyroid status

Parameter	Hyperthyroidism	Hypothyroidism
Serum T_4	↑	↓
Serum T_3	↑	↓
Serum TSH	↓ (Primary) ↑ (Secondary)	↑ (Primary) ↓ (Secondary)
TRH-stimulation response	Not performed	↑ (Primary) ↓/Delayed (Secondary)
Serum PBI	↑	↓
RAI uptake	↑	↓ (↑ in endemic goiter)
Thyroid stimulating antibodies	↑ (Graves' disease)	–
BMR	↑	↓
Serum cholesterol	↓	↑

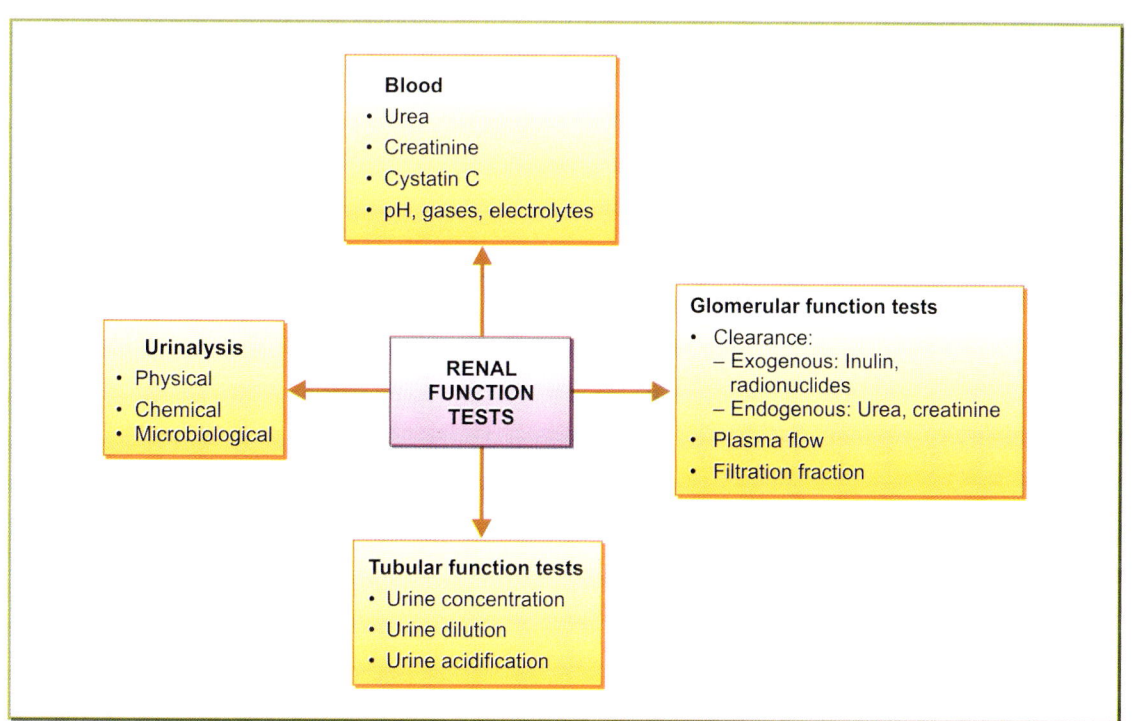

Fig. 39.7: Renal function tests.

39

Chemistry to Clinics 39.10: Low Serum T$_4$

Serum total T$_4$ concentration is low in hypoproteinemia such as in chronic liver disease, nephrotic syndrome and euthyroid patients who are on drugs that block T$_4$ binding to thyroxine-binding globulin (TBG), e.g. salicylates. Treatment with androgens, cortisol and some anticonvulsants, e.g. phenytoin, may produce spuriously low serum total T$_4$ concentration. Free thyroxine (FT$_4$) however, provides more reliable information than does total T$_4$.

Thyroxine: Serum T$_4$ value in a normal person ranges from 5 to 12 μg/dl. In hyperthyroidism, serum T$_4$ concentration is increased to >12 μg/dl whereas in hypothyroidism the value is <5 μg/dl (Chemistry to Clinics 39.10).

Tri-iodothyronine: Normal value for serum T$_3$ varies between 70 and 190 ng/dl. Serum T$_3$ concentration is low at birth. The value rises to near adult level in early childhood and then is maintained up to 30 years of age, after which it again falls (Chemistry to Clinics 39.11).

Chemistry to Clinics 39.11: Serum T$_3$ versus T$_4$

In some conditions, serum T$_3$ concentration is disproportionally high relative to serum T$_4$, e.g. in all types of hyperthyroidism and early thyroid failure in which the gland is exposed to enhanced stimulation by TSH. Serum T$_3$ thus is a superior indicator of hyperthyroidism because thyroidal T$_3$ production is often increased early, such as in Graves' disease where serum T$_3$ becomes abnormal before serum T$_4$. Serum T$_3$ measurement however, is not of diagnostic value in hypothyroidism but is a useful test to monitor the adequacy of therapy. In early hypothyroidism, serum T$_3$ concentration may be normal despite subnormal value for T$_4$.

Measurement of reverse T$_3$ (rT$_3$, a catabolic product of T$_4$) may also be helpful in some cases, e.g. in low T$_3$ syndrome where rT$_3$ concentration is increased.

Thyroid stimulating hormone: Reference value for serum TSH concentration is in the range of 0.3–5.0 mU/L (Chemistry to Clinics 39.12).

Stimulation/Suppression Tests

- **TRH stimulation test:** Thyrotropin releasing hormone (TRH) stimulation test is used to assess

Chemistry to Clinics 39.12: Significance of Serum TSH

Serum TSH measurements are useful:

1. To differentiate between pituitary and hypothalamic cause of hypothyroidism (Table 39.4). Measurement of TSH is most useful and sensitive for primary hypothyroidism. When feedback suppression of the pituitary is reduced by a deficient production of thyroid hormones, TSH rises in an attempt to increase the production of these hormones. Rise in TSH occurs while the patient is still asymptomatic. It is thus an early and sensitive indicator of hypothyroidism. In a hypothyroid patient, the finding of low TSH indicates deficient pituitary secretion of TSH or deficient hypothalamic secretion of TRH.
2. In determining the response to exogenous TRH in the investigation of hypo- and hyperthyroidism
3. To monitor the response to therapy with anti-thyroid drugs (in patients with hyperthyroidism) or thyroid hormone replacement (in patients with hypothyroidism).
4. For the follow-up of patients who have undergone thyroid surgery or developed hypothyroidism following radiation.
5. In the assessment of hyperthyroidism: Serum TSH is subnormal in all patients with hyperthyroidism as a result of feedback suppression except in pituitary TSH secreting adenoma and tertiary hyperthyroidism (Table 39.5).

Table 39.4: Classification of hypothyroidism based on the primary site of defect

	Primary site of defect	*Causes*
Primary hypothyroidism	Thyroid gland	Endemic goiter (iodine deficiency), autoimmune thyroiditis (Hashimoto's disease), following radio-iodine therapy for treating thyrotoxicosis
Secondary hypothyroidism	Pituitary gland	Pituitary tumor (except TSH secreting adenoma), radiation or surgery
Tertiary hypothyroidism	Hypothalamus	Hypothalamic tumor, radiation or surgery

Table 39.5: Classification of hyperthyroidism based on the primary site of defect

	Primary site of defect	*Causes*
Primary hyperthyroidism	Thyroid gland	Autoimmune overstimulation (Graves' disease)
Secondary hyperthyroidism	Pituitary gland	TSH secreting pituitary adenoma
Tertiary hyperthyroidism	Hypothalamus	TRH secreting hypothalamic tumor

39

the functional state of the TSH secretory mechanism. Serum TSH is assayed before and 20, 30 and 60 minutes after a standard dose of TRH. In normal individuals, serum TSH peaks are observed in 30 minutes and values generally range between 5 and 30 mU/L. A normal response excludes the possibility of thyrotoxicosis. In hyperthyroidism, no significant rise in TSH occurs because elevated thyroid hormones inhibit TSH production. In primary hypothyroidism, TSH response to TRH is exaggerated and is of diagnostic significance. It is often useful in differentiating between pituitary and hypothalamic lesion as the cause of secondary hypothyroidism.

- **Thyroid suppression test:** Normally, exogenous thyroid hormone suppresses pituitary TSH secretion, resulting in a decrease in RAIU. An abnormal suppression test is observed in hyperthyroidism, irrespective of the underlying cause. A normal suppression test excludes the diagnosis of hyperthyroidism.

Autoimmune Profile

Antibodies against thyroid peroxidase (**anti-TPO antibodies**) may be detected in the serum of some hypothyroid patients. In Graves' disease, long-acting thyroid stimulator (LATS) is detectable in serum.

Other Tests

- **Radioactive iodine uptake:** As iodine plays an important role in the metabolism of the thyroid gland, radioactive iodine uptake (RAIU) is used for thyroid function studies. Usually 10 µci (microcuries) of sodium or potassium iodide is administered orally (I^{125} delivers low radiation dose, hence it is preferred over I^{131}). The radioactivity mixes uniformly with the endogenous iodide in the extracellular fluid. Percentage of the iodide entering and leaving the extracellular space per unit time, which is accumulated by the thyroid in the steady state, is assessed. RAIU is usually measured 24 hours after the administration of the isotope. Normally, 24 hours RAIU uptake is 5–30% of the administered dose. Values above the normal range indicate hyperfunctioning of the gland and are useful in the diagnosis of hyperthyroidism. RAIU is also used as a part of thyroid suppression test.
- **Protein-bound iodine:** Serum protein-bound iodine (PBI) is an indirect measure for assessing thyroid

function since about 90% of the iodine in serum is bound to thyroxine. PBI value in a normal subject ranges from 4 to 8 µg/100 ml. In hypothyroidism, PBI value varies from 0.2 to 2.5 µg/100 ml whereas in hyperthyroidism PBI value ranges from 9 to 18 µg/100 ml.

- **Basal metabolic rate (BMR):** It is a measurement of oxygen consumption in the basal state. BMR is raised in hyperthyroidism and is reduced in hypothyroidism.
- **Serum cholesterol:** Increase in serum cholesterol is observed in hypothyroidism whereas it is decreased in hyperthyroidism or thyrotoxicosis.
- **Serum calcium:** Hyperthyroidism may result in increased plasma calcium along with increased plasma alkaline phosphatase activity.
- **Glucose tolerance test (GTT):** It is sometimes abnormal in patients with hyperthyroidism who may show a diabetic type of response.

GASTRIC FUNCTION TESTS

The stomach functions as a temporary storage organ for food. It secretes about 2–3 liters of gastric juice everyday. Most of this juice is produced by exocrine glands located in the body and fundus of the stomach. These exocrine secretory glands contain three types of secretory cells, i.e. the chief cells, the parietal cells and the mucous cells.

- **The chief cells**, located in the basal regions of these glands and also in the glands of the antrum, secrete **pepsinogen** (the inactive precursor of pepsin).
- **The parietal cells** secrete **HCl**. In addition to converting pepsinogen to pepsin, HCl provides optimum pH for the activity of this enzyme. The parietal cells also secrete **intrinsic factor** necessary for the intestinal absorption of vitamin B_{12} which is required for formation of normal RBCs.
- **The mucous cells** are located at the necks of these glands, in the glands of the antrum and scattered throughout the gastric epithelial lining. These cells secrete **alkaline mucous containing fluid** which coats the gastric wall and protects against various forms of damage to the gastric mucosa.

E. BIOCHEMICAL FUNCTIONS OF THE STOMACH

- **Secretion of HCl:** The important function of the stomach is that parietal cells secrete an iso-osmotic solution of HCl with a hydrogen ion concentration

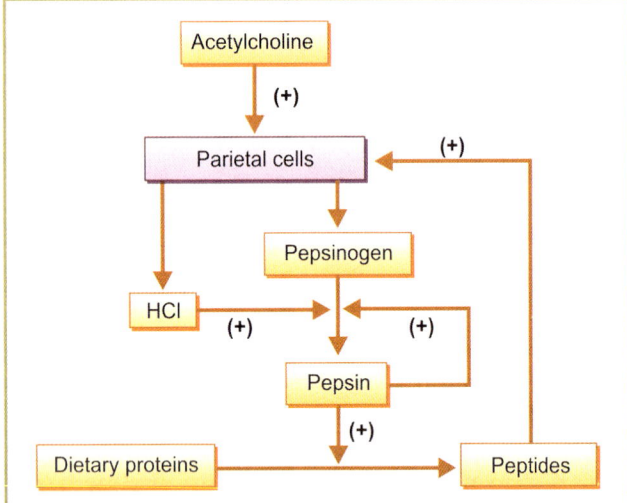

Fig. 39.8: Secretion and activation of pepsinogen.

≈150 mEq/L (pH 0.9–1.0). Both excitatory and inhibitory mechanisms regulate gastric HCl secretion. The gastric mucosa is rich in histamine, a potent stimulus of parietal cell secretion. During the cephalic phase, there is release of acetylcholine as well as gastrin, both of which cause the release of histamine in the vicinity of the parietal cells.

- **Secretion of pepsin:** Pepsinogen, the inactive precursor of pepsin, is synthesized by and stored in the chief cells as zymogen granules. Once pepsinogen enters the gastric lumen, HCl and pre-existing pepsin convert it to pepsin. Both acetylcholine and peptides stimulate secretion of HCl by the parietal cells and thus, in turn, play an important role in the activation of pepsin as well as in the maintenance of the highly acidic environment required for its optimal activity (Fig. 39.8).

F. EXAMINATION OF THE GASTRIC RESIDUE

The content of the stomach after nearly 12 hours of fast is defined as gastric residue (residuum). It is obtained by aspiration through a gastric tube (**Ryle's tube**) and examined for the following:

Physical Characteristics

Volume: Total volume of the resting gastric residue normally varies from 20 to 50 ml. An increase in the volume (>100 ml) may be due to hypersecretion, retention or regurgitation from duodenum and is

Chemistry to Clinics 39.13: Zollinger-Ellison Syndrome
It is due to a gastrin-secreting tumor of the endocrine pancreas. Excess gastrin over-stimulates gastric acid secretion resulting in abdominal pain, mucosal ulceration and diarrhea. It is suspected in patients of acid-peptic disease who fail to respond to conventional treatment with H2-receptor blockers and proton pump inhibitors.

considered abnormal. Various causes include pyloric obstruction, duodenal ulcer or Zollinger-Ellison syndrome (Chemistry to Clinics 39.13).

Consistency: The resting gastric juice is fluid in consistency. It may be viscous in the presence of mucus. Food particles may be present in carcinoma of the stomach.

Color: The resting gastric content is usually colorless. It may be slightly yellow or green due to regurgitation of bile, or red/brown due to the presence of blood.

Chemical Constituents

Bile: It may be found in gastric residuum as a result of intestinal obstruction or ileal stasis.

Mucus: Small amount of mucus is found normally. Increased amounts may be seen in gastritis and gastric carcinoma.

Blood: Accidental trauma to the gastric mucous membrane during the passage of Ryle's tube may result in traces of blood in the gastric juice. Increased amounts of blood may be present due to gastric carcinoma, erosive gastritis or bleeding peptic ulcer.

Organic acids: Lactic and butyric acids may be present in large amounts in hypoacidity, achlorhydria and carcinoma of the stomach. In the absence of free HCl, these organic acids are formed in increased amounts by bacterial fermentation of food, as food is retained in the stomach for longer periods (usually more than 6 hours) at neutral or alkaline pH.

Pepsin: Absence of pepsin is seen in a condition called achylia gastrica. Decreased pepsin levels are seen in diseases associated with chief cell mass, atrophic gastritis and gastric carcinoma. Increased pepsin activity may be observed in disease associated with increased gastric output as in patients with Zollinger-Ellison syndrome, duodenal ulcer, gastritis and after the administration of proton pump inhibitors such as omeprazole.

Chemistry to Clinics 39.14: Gastric Acidity

1. **Hyperchlorhydria:** When free acidity is increased, the condition is called hyperchlorhydria. It occurs in duodenal and gastric ulcers, and in diseases of the gallbladder.

2. **Hypochlorhydria:** Decreased secretion of HCl is called hypochlorhydria. It is observed in gastric carcinoma, chronic gastritis, constipation and anemias.

3. **Achlorhydria:** Complete absence of HCl in the gastric juice is called achlorhydria. It occurs in pernicious anemia. Absence of free HCl in gastric residue is considered abnormal only if the condition persists after maximal stimulation with pentagastrin. In the absence of HCl, bacterial fermentation of food is increased which leads to the formation of lactic acid. A small percentage of the healthy individuals (about 4% of the young ones and 25% at age 60 years) may have no free HCl in the fasting stomach.

Estimation of Free Acidity

The main acid in the gastric juice is HCl which is a strong mineral acid. It accounts for free acidity. HCl is secreted by the parietal cells at a concentration of about 150 mEq/L with pH <1.0. As the parietal secretion gets mixed with other gastric constituents, the concentration of hydrogen ions usually reaches <40 mEq/L with a pH of 1.5–3.5.

Concentration of free acidity in gastric residue in normal individuals varies from 0 to 40 mEq/L (Chemistry to Clinics 39.14).

Estimation of Total Acidity

Total acidity in gastric residue includes hydrogen ions occuring as free HCl, mucoproteins, acid salts and organic acids, such as lactic and butyric acids. The total acid concentration in a normal state is usually 10–50 mEq/L.

G. STIMULATION OF GASTRIC SECRETION

Many compounds or processes such as test meal, alcohol, caffeine, gastrin, pentagastrin or insulin stimulate gastric secretion and, in turn, the secretion of HCl.

- **Test meals:** Stimulation of gastric secretion by administration of a test meal such as toast with water or tea (Ewald's meal) was practiced in the past. This test however, is not used these days.

- **Alcohol:** 50–100 ml of 7% ethyl alcohol (3.5 ml ethanol in 50 ml water) may be administered through the syringe attached to the tube as a stimulant for HCl secretion.

- **Caffeine:** Caffeine sodium benzoate, 500 mg in about 200 ml of water, may be administered into the stomach through a gastric tube as a stimulant of gastric secretion.

- **Histamine:** Histamine is a powerful stimulant for the secretion of gastric juice. It causes secretion of an increased volume of highly acidic gastric juice with low pepsin content. Two types of histamine tests may be carried out.

  In the *'standard histamine test'*, subcutaneous injection of histamine (0.01 mg/kg body weight) is given and the gastric contents are removed. Absence of free HCl in gastric secretion after histamine indicates achylia gastrica.

  A large dose of histamine (0.04 mg/kg body weight) is given for the *'augmented histamine test'*. In pernicious anemia no free HCl is secreted but in other forms of achlorhydria some amount of free HCl may be secreted, after augmented histamine stimulation test is performed (Chemistry to Clinics 39.15).

- **Insulin:** Intravenous injection of 0.1–0.2 U/kg body weight of soluble insulin may also be given for the stimulation of gastric secretion and gastric samples are withdrawn after every 15 min. This is called *Hollander test*. Insulin stimulation is helpful to ascertain the effectiveness of vagotomy in patients with duodenal ulcer. In these patients, concentration of free HCl may be as high as 1200 mEq/L. After successful vagotomy, since there is no response to insulin, gastric acidity remains at a low level of 15–20 mEq/L before as well as after insulin administration.

  As insulin may cause hypoglycemia the test is not preferred.

- **Gastrin and pentagastrin:** *Gastrin* is the most powerful stimulus for gastric HCl secretion. Gastrin is administered in a single subcutaneous dose of 2 µg/kg body weight.

  Pentagastrin, a synthetic pentapeptide with a physiologically active part of the gastrin molecule,

Chemistry to Clinics 39.15: Antihistaminics

Sometimes a high dose of histamine may cause a severe reaction mediated through H1 receptors. Under such a condition, an injection of H1 antihistaminic may be given intramuscularly. This does not interfere in gastric stimulation because the gastric effects of histamine are mediated through H2 receptors.

39

is also a potent stimulus for gastric HCl secretion and is commonly used these days. The fasting content of the stomach is aspirated and its volume is measured. This is termed as the **basal acid output** (BAO). The secretions are collected at 15 minute intervals for 1 hour. Pentagastrin is then given at a dose of 6 µg/kg body weight subcutaneously and post-stimulation secretions are again collected at 15 min intervals for the next one hour. This acid output is termed as the **maximal acid output** (MAO).

This test is useful in differentiating the diagnosis of achlorhydria and hyperchlorhydria. In normal persons, the BAO ranges from 0 to 10 mEq/h. After stimulation with pentagastrin, MAO varies from 0 to 35 mEq/h. A large volume of fasting juice indicates obstruction of gastric outlet. A very high BAO suggests that the patient has Zollinger-Ellison syndrome.

Tests for *Helicobacter pylori*

Helicobacter pylori is a bacteria responsible for some cases of acid-peptic disease. It may be diagnosed by:
1. Serology: Demonstration of serum anti-*Helicobacter pylori* antibodies (IgM, IgG, IgA).
2. Rapid urease test in a gastric biopsy sample obtained by gastroscopy: Based on the conversion of urea present in a medium to NH_3 and CO_2 by bacterial urease. The NH_3 raises the pH which is detected by a suitable indicator.
3. Histological examination and culture of gastric biopsy sample.
4. Stool antigen for *Helicobacter pylori*.
5. Carbon urea breath test: The patient is administered ^{14}C or ^{13}C-labeled urea orally, which is split by the bacterial urease and labeled CO_2 is detected in the expired breath.

PANCREATIC FUNCTION TESTS

The pancreas serves two functions which are carried out by different groups of cells within the organ. These two groups of cells are designated as the endocrine and the exocrine portions of the pancreas.

The Endocrine Pancreas

The endocrine pancreas consists of group of cells known as the **islets of Langerhans**, which are embedded in the exocrine portion of the gland. Islets are composed of four major cell types, each of which synthesize and secrete a different hormone. These include glucagon producing alpha cells, insulin producing beta cells, somatostatin producing delta cells and a pancreatic polypeptide producing F cells.

The Exocrine Pancreas

The exocrine secretory cells are called acinar cells arranged in sac-like clusters called acini. These cells secrete a small volume of juice containing the digestive enzymes of the pancreas. The acini are connected by small intercalated ducts to larger ducts that converge into one duct which delivers the exocrine secretion of the pancreas into the duodenum. The epithelial cells lining the intercalated ducts secrete a relatively large volume of juice with a high concentration of the alkaline salt sodium bicarbonate.

H. BIOCHEMICAL FUNCTIONS OF THE EXOCRINE PANCREAS

Exocrine functions of the pancreas, as described above, include the production and secretion of pancreatic juice which is rich in several enzymes and bicarbonate. Total volume of pancreatic juice secreted in a normal human is 500–800 ml/24 hours. It is strongly alkaline with a pH of about 8.0. Its alkalinity is due to the presence of bicarbonate (HCO_3^-) since pancreatic juice contains nearly 70–100 mEq/L of HCO_3^-. By neutralizing acid that arrives in the duodenum from the stomach, bicarbonate performs two functions:
1. It protects the delicate lining of the upper small intestine from damage by acid.
2. It ensures optimal pH for activity of the pancreatic digestive enzymes (Chemistry to Clinics 39.16).

The pancreas also secretes several digestive enzymes (Table 39.6).

Regulation of exocrine pancreatic secretion: Secretion of the pancreatic juice is controlled by two mechanisms, i.e. by **hormonal control** and **nervous control** (via vagus nerve).

Chemistry to Clinics 39.16: Acuate Pancreatitis
Acute pancreatitis is a condition in which activated proteolytic enzymes are liberated from the pancreatic acinar cells, and in turn, attack the pancreas itself. This self digestion process often results in reduced output of both pancreatic digestive enzymes as well as bicarbonate.

Table 39.6: Digestive enzymes of the pancreatic juice

Enzyme	Substrate	Digestion products
Trypsin	Proteins and peptides	Small peptides
Chymotrypsin	Proteins and peptides	Small peptides
Carboxypeptidase A and B	Proteins and peptides	Peptides and amino acids
Amylase	Starch	Oligosaccharides, maltose
Lipase	Triacylglycerols	Monoacylglycerols and free fatty acids
Phospholipase A_2	Lecithin	Lysolecithin and free fatty acid
Cholesterol esterase	Cholesterol esters	Cholesterol and free fatty acids
RNase	RNA	Ribonucleotides
DNase	DNA	Deoxyribonucleotides

Two hormones, secretin and cholecystokinin, which are released from the duodenal mucosa during the intestinal phase of digestion regulate bicarbonate and enzyme secretion by the pancreas.

- *Secretin* is released into the blood in response to HCl. After its release, the hormone stimulates the intercalated duct cells of the pancreas to secrete bicarbonate-rich juice. The secretion, in turn, neutralizes the acid that causes secretin to be released and so reduces the stimulus for additional secretin release until more acid enters the duodenum from the stomach.

- *Cholecystokinin* is released from duodenal mucosa in response to protein and lipid digestion products. The hormone stimulates the pancreatic acinar cells to secrete digestive enzymes. As a result, more digestion products are produced which further stimulate the pancreas to secrete more enzymes. The process continues as long as food remains in the small intestine to be digested (Fig. 39.9).

Vagus stimulation also helps in the secretion of enzymes.

I. BIOCHEMICAL TESTS TO ASSESS EXOCRINE FUNCTIONS OF THE PANCREAS

Volume and Bicarbonate Concentration of the Pancreatic Juice

The exocrine secretory capacity of the pancreas is assessed by intubating the duodenum and subjecting the pancreas to stimulation with a test meal, secretin or pancreozymin. After the duodenal contents are aspirated, the patient is given secretin (one unit/kg body weight) intravenously and the aspirate is

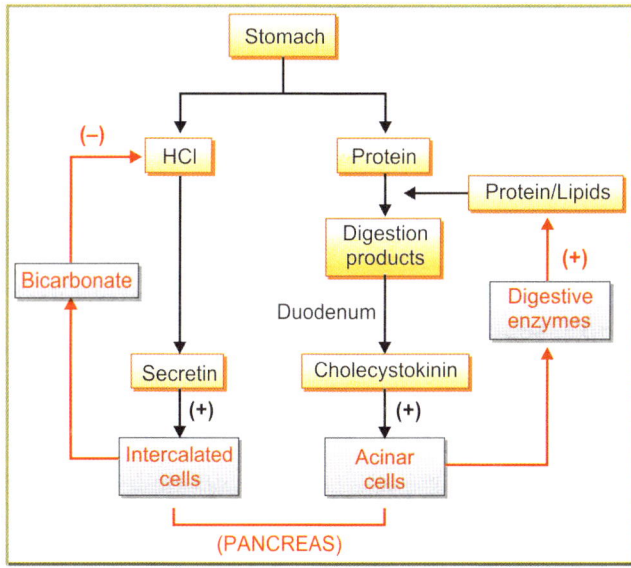

Fig. 39.9: Regulation of exocrine pancreatic secretion.

examined for volume, bicarbonate content and amylase activity.

In pancreatitis, there is usually a reduction in the volume of pancreatic juice as well as its bicarbonate output. In the milder form of pancreatitis, volume of the pancreatic juice and its bicarbonate contents are fairly normal but enzyme activities particularly the activity of amylase is reduced. Patients with chronic pancreatitis are unable to secrete juice of high bicarbonate content (<90 mEq/L). Carcinoma of the head of pancreas obstructs the overall volume flow.

Enzymes in Serum/Urine

- **Serum and urinary amylase:** Serum and urine amylase activities are increased in acute pancreatitis. In early stages of the disease, determination of serum amylase is of great diagnostic

39

importance. Rise starts within 2–12 hours of the onset of pain and usually returns to normal within 3–5 days. There is also an increase in urinary amylase.

- **Serum lipase:** Serum lipase activity rises slower than that of amylase, within 4–8 hours and normalizes by 7–14 days. Thus, it remains elevated for a longer duration than serum amylase. Further, serum lipase as compared to serum amylase is elevated more often in patients with pancreatic carcinoma.

- **Serum elastase:** Elastase-I is a pancreatic proteolytic enzyme that hydrolyzes scleroproteins, a basic ingredient of the connective tissue. It is produced in the acinar portion of the pancreas and appears in the exocrine pancreatic secretion as zymogen (pro-elastase). This, in turn, is activated by trypsin. Serum elastase-I is of significance in the later stages of acute pancreatitis or in patients with relapse or cystic complications of chronic pancreatitis. Elastase-I remains abnormally elevated longer than amylase.

SOME IMPORTANT QUESTIONS

1. Briefly discuss:
  i. Thyroid function tests
  ii. Kidney function tests
  iii. Clearance tests
  iv. Gastric function tests
  v. Differential biochemical diagnosis of jaundice
  vi. Pancreatic function tests

2. Write notes on:
  i. Neonatal jaundice
  ii. GFR
  iii. Tubular function tests
  iv. Cystatin C
  v. Zollinger-Ellison syndrome
  vi. Delta bilirubin

MULTIPLE CHOICE QUESTIONS

1. **The following proteins are not synthesized in the liver:**
   A. α_1-Globulins   B. α_2-Globulins
   C. γ-Globulins   D. β-Globulins

2. **Highest concentration of γ-GT normally occurs in:**
   A. Liver   B. Kidneys
   C. Small intestine   D. Lungs

3. **The maximum urea clearance is:**
   A. 54 ml/min   B. 75 ml/min
   C. 100 ml/min   D. 125 ml/min

4. **The normal inulin clearance is:**
   A. 54 ml/min   B. 75 ml/min
   C. 100 ml/min   D. 125 ml/min

5. **A useful index of renal plasma flow is:**
   A. Inulin clearance   B. PAH clearance
   C. Creatinine clearance   D. Urea clearance

6. **Increased pepsin activity in gastric juice is observed in:**
   A. Zollinger-Ellison syndrome
   B. Achylia gastrica
   C. Atrophic gastritis
   D. Gastric carcinoma

7. **In acute pancreatitis, the following increases in serum:**
   A. Amylase   B. Lipase
   C. Elastase-I   D. All of the above

8. **The total acidity in gastric residue is:**
   A. 10–50 mEq/L   B. 50–90 mEq/L
   C. 90–130 mEq/L   D. 130–170 mEq/L

9. **The most potent stimulus for gastric HCl secretion is:**
   A. Gastrin   B. Histamine
   C. Insulin   D. Caffeine

10. **The normal HCO_3^- content in pancreatic juice is:**
    A. 0.7–1.0 mEq/L   G. 7–10 mEq/L
    C. 70–100 mEq/L   D. 700–1000 mEq/L

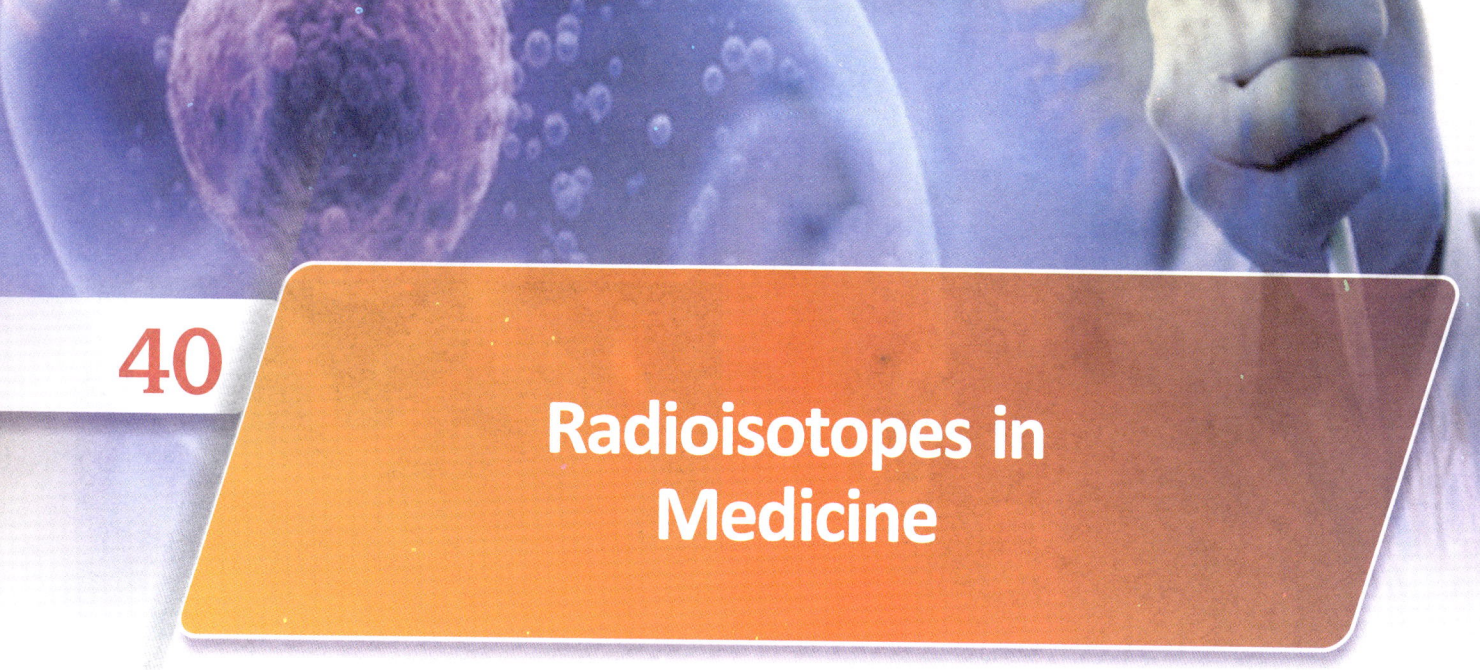

Radioisotopes in Medicine

The **isotopes** of an element have the same number of protons (**same atomic number**) but different masses due to **different number of neutrons**. When a combination of protons and neutrons is produced artificially, the resulting unstable atom is called a **radioisotope**. The nucleus of a radioisotope becomes stable by emitting α or β (positron) particles, with or without γ radiation (electromagnetic waves). This is called **radioactive decay**.

Nuclear medicine is a branch of medicine which employs **radiation** emitted by **radioisotopes** as a diagnostic and therapeutic tool. Radioactive products used in nuclear medicine are **radionuclides** or pharmaceuticals labeled with radionuclides, i.e. **radiopharmaceuticals**. Those which are neutron-rich or result from nuclear fission are prepared in **nuclear reactors** while those which are neutron-deficient are prepared in **cyclotrons**.

Applications of Radioisotopes

1. **Metabolic work-up:** Radioisotope-labeled compounds help in elucidating the origin and fate of various biomolecules in the body as well as in the understanding of metabolic pathways (radioisotope tracer studies).

2. **Diagnostic tool**
   i. **Immunoassay:** In a biological sample, sensitive and accurate identification plus quantification of metabolites, hormones, antigens/antibodies, drugs, etc. can be achieved by radioisotope-based techniques such as radioimmunoassay (RIA).

   ii. **Imaging/scintigraphy:** Radionuclides or radiopharmaceuticals are administered to patients and the radiation emitted is measured, generating an image, with a gamma camera. It is useful to assess:
   - Blood flow to an organ, e.g. thalium 201 for myocardial perfusion scan.
   - Organ function, e.g. iodine 131 for thyroid.
   - Presence of cancer, e.g. fluorine 18 labeled deoxyglucose.
   - Presence of infection, e.g. technetium 99m labeled ciprofloxacin.
   - Response to treatment.
   Advantages of nuclear imaging
   - Reduced uptake of a radionuclide appears as a **'cold spot'** whereas enhanced uptake appears as a **'hot spot'** indicative of organ malfunction (Fig. 40.1).
   - **Both bone and soft tissues** can be imaged.
   - Non-invasive.

3. **Therapeutic tool**
   i. **Cancer:** Rapidly dividing cells such as cancer cells are very sensitive to radiation damage. Thus, radionuclide therapy (RNT) or simply **'radiotherapy'** is employed to target some cancerous growths:
   - *External RNT (teletherapy)*: It uses γ-rays from a cobalt 60 source.
   - *Internal RNT*: It requires planting a small radiation source (α or β emitter) in the body, usually close to the cancer (short-range RNT or **brachytherapy**, e.g. iodine 131 for thyroid cancer). Alternatively, for dispersed cancers,

40

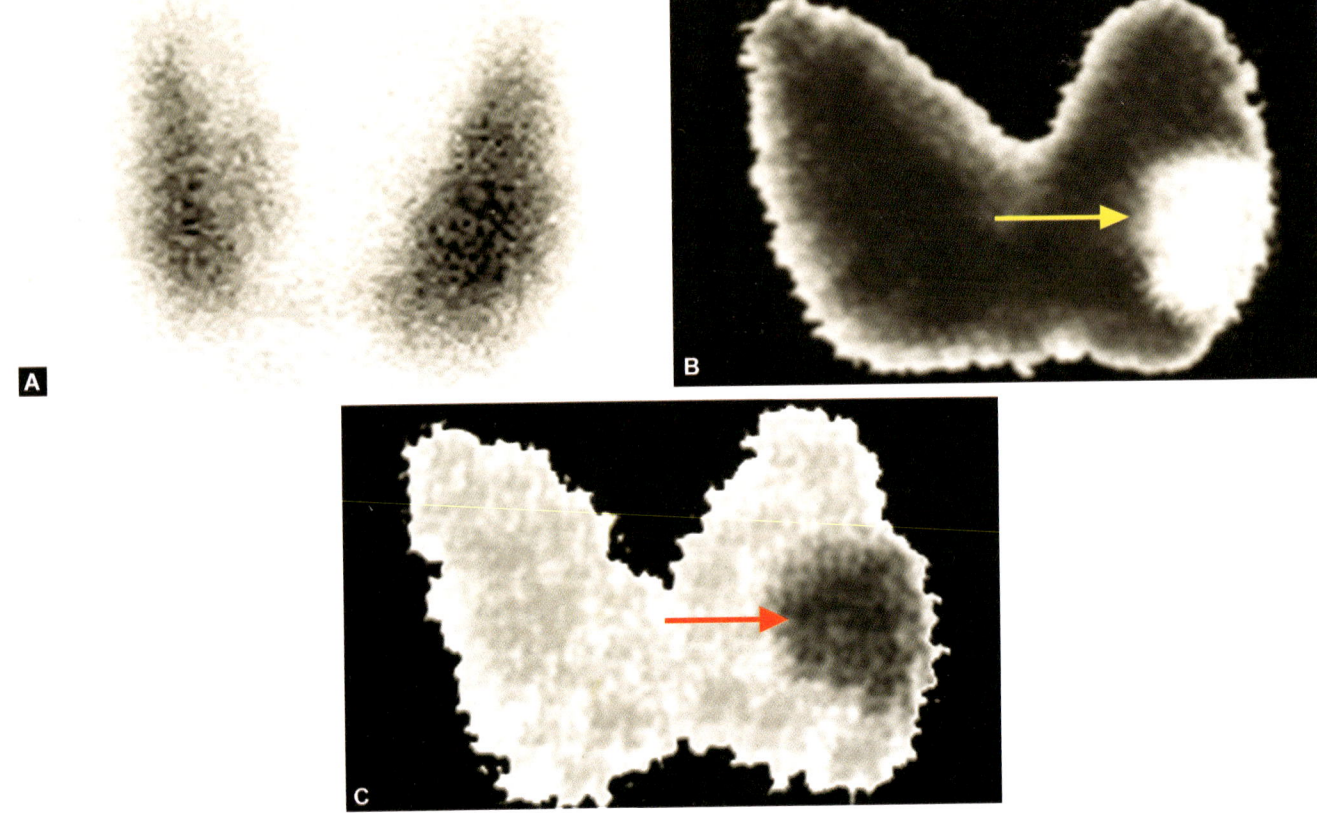

Fig. 40.1: Nuclear imaging of thyroid gland. (A) **Normal scan** showing diffuse, homogeneous radionuclide uptake, (B) A **cold spot** (arrow) in the left lobe due to a degenerated colloid nodule, (C) A **hot spot** (arrow) in the left lobe due to a hyperfunctioning toxic nodule.

tissue-specific monoclonal antibodies attached to α emitters (e.g. bismuth-213) are used as carriers (**targeted alpha therapy**).

ii. **Other conditions:** Radionuclides, e.g. erbium 169, are useful in relieving arthritic pain in synovial joints.

Drawbacks of Nuclear Medicine

Although the radiation exposure is minimum, a specialized infrastructure is required for handling radioactivity and waste disposal.

SOME IMPORTANT QUESTIONS

1. Explain the terms 'radioisotopes' and 'nuclear medicine'.

2. Briefly outline the applications of radioisotopes.

MULTIPLE CHOICE QUESTIONS

1. Medical applications of radioisotopes include:
   - A. Scintigraphy
   - B. Metabolic work-up
   - C. Immunoassay
   - D. All of the above

2. External radionuclide therapy commonly employs:
   - A. Cobalt 60
   - B. Iodine 131
   - C. Bismuth 213
   - D. Erbium 169

Clinical Chemistry Investigations

A 'specimen' is a representative of the 'class of things' to which it belongs. On the other hand, a 'sample' is a part of the 'thing itself', to show the quality of the whole thing. However, the two terms are used interchangeably in medical literature. Commonly used specimen for biochemical investigations include blood and urine.

SPECIMEN COLLECTION

A. Blood

Blood may be obtained from veins, arteries or capillaries. **Venipuncture** is commonly performed through the antecubital vein whereas femoral artery is preferred for obtaining arterial blood. Skin puncture is performed to obtain capillary blood in infants. In order to get accurate results, **hemolysis must be avoided** in all cases. **Pumping of the fist** is sometimes done to make the vein more prominent and easier sampling but may result in **false high serum potassium levels**.

Majority of biochemical investigations are performed in **plasma** or **serum** which are obtained by processing the blood specimen in the presence or absence of an anticoagulant respectively (Fig. 41.1).

Serum is preferred to analyze bilirubin, calcium, cholesterol, creatinine, electrolytes (sodium, potassium, chloride), phosphorus, proteins, triglycerides, uric acid and enzymes such as acid and alkaline phosphatases, amylase, ALT, AST, LDH. etc. For this purpose, blood is collected in a plain vial, allowed to settle and the clear supernatant is collected.

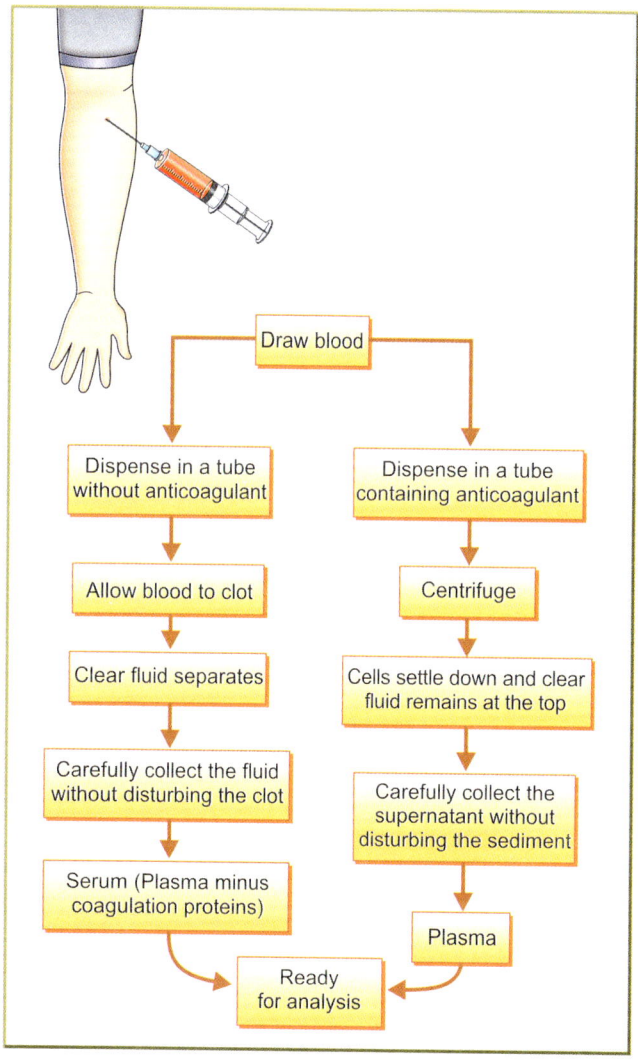

Fig. 41.1: Obtaining serum or plasma from blood.

41

Table 41.1: Normal values of some constituents of blood

Constituent	Normal range
Common constituents	
Bilirubin (total)	0.2–0.8 mg/dl
Calcium (total)	9–11 mg/dl
Cholesterol (total)	140–220 mg/dl
Creatinine	0.8–1.3 mg/dl
Glucose (fasting)	60–100 mg/dl
Phosphorus (inorganic)	3.0–4.5 mg/dl
Urea	15–40 mg/dl
Uric acid	3–7 mg/dl
Proteins	
Total serum proteins	6.0–8.3 g/dL
Serum albumin	3.5–5.2 g/dL
Serum globulins	2.5–3.5 g/dL
A/G Ratio	1.1–1.7
Lipid profile	
Serum triglycerides	50–160 mg/dl
Total cholesterol	140–220 mg/dl
HDL-cholesterol	30–60 mg/dl
LDL-cholesterol	60–160 mg/dl
VLDL-cholesterol	up to 32 mg/dl
Electrolytes	
Sodium	136–145 mEq/L
Potassium	3.5–5.0 mEq/L
Chloride	98–107 mEq/L
Enzymes	
Acid phosphatase	1–3.5 KA Units/dL
Alkaline phosphatase	3–13 KA Units/dL
Amylase	60–180 Somogyi U/dL
LDH	100–190 U/L
SGOT	up to 40 U/L
SGPT	up to 40 U/L
CPK (total)	20–90 U/L
Hormones	
Cortisol	5–25 µg/dl (8 AM)
T_3	70–200 ng/dL
T_4	5–12 µg/dl
TSH	0.3–5 µU/ml
Acid-base analysis and blood gases	
pH	7.35–7.45
Total CO_2	22–28 mmol/L
Bicarbonate	22–26 mmol/L
pCO_2	31–45 mm of Hg
pO_2	85–95 mm of Hg
Oxygen saturation	96–100%
Anion gap $[(Na^+ + K^+) - (Cl^- + HCO_3^-)]$	10–20 mmol/L
Base excess	−2 to +3 mmol/L

On the other hand, for glucose, blood is collected in a vial containing sodium fluoride (which serves the dual purpose of anticoagulation and inhibiting glycolysis); for urea, blood is collected in a vial containing potassium oxalate; for blood gases, 1–2 ml arterial blood drawn in a syringe pre-filled with heparin, avoiding any air bubbles, is kept on ice and sent immediately to the laboratory for analysis.

B. Urine

Many urinary analytes do not require any preservative. However, acidification to pH <3 (with 10 ml of 6 N HCl for 24 h urine) is recommended for calcium, steroids and VMA, whereas alkalinization to pH 8–9 (with small amount of sodium bicarbonate) is required for uric acid and porphyrins. First morning and midstream urine specimen (25–30 ml) is collected for Bence Jones proteins as well as urobilinogen.

Reference Range of Important Analytes

Normal value for any analyte should always be **expressed in a range** in order to cover the average value along with the standard deviation in the human population, which reflects the physiological variation from person to person. The range of normal values of important analytes in various biological fluids are presented in Tables 41.1 to 41.4.

Interconversion of Units

In some cases, it becomes necessary to convert the units of an analyte from mg/dl to mmol/L or *vice versa*. The following formula may be used for this purpose:

Table 41.2: Normal values for some constituents in urine

Constituent	Normal excretion
D-xylose	1–2 g/5 hrs
Total nitrogen	10–20 g/24 hrs
Creatinine	1.0–2.0 g/24 hrs
Calcium	0.1–0.7 g/24 hrs
Chloride	110–250 mEq/24 hrs
Sodium	40–220 mEq/24 hrs
Potassium	25–125 mEq/24 hrs
Phosphorus	0.6–1.5 g/24 hrs
Urea	20–35 g/24 hrs
Uric acid	0.5–1.0 g/24 hrs

Table 41.3: Normal values for some constituents in CSF

Constituent	Normal concentration
Total protein	15–40 mg/dl
Glucose	50–75 mg/dl
Chloride (as NaCl)	700–750 mg/dl (118–132 mmol/L)

$$mmol/L = (mg/dl \times 10)/\text{Molecular weight of the analyte}$$

For example, if we want to express 90 mg/dl of plasma glucose (M_r = 180) in mmol/L, it is calculated as $(90 \times 10)/180$ mmol/L = 5 mmol/L.

Table 41.4: Normal values for some parameters in gastric juice

Parameter	Normal range
Volume	2–3 L/24 hrs
pH	1.6–1.8
Titratable acidity (fasting sample)	15–35 mEq/L
Basal acid output	
Males	1.0–5.0 mEq/hr
Females	0.2–3.8 mEq/hr
Maximal acid output (after histamine/pentagastrin)	
Males	18–28 mEq/hr
Females	11–21 mEq/hr

41

MULTIPLE CHOICE QUESTIONS

1. Pumping of the fist prior to venipuncture may lead to false high serum levels of:
   - A. Vitamin C
   - B. Potassium
   - C. Iodide
   - D. Estradiol

2. Acidification of collected urine specimen is recommended for the analysis of the following *except:*
   - A. Steroids
   - B. VMA
   - C. Porphyrins
   - D. Calcium

Answers to MCQs

CHAPTER 1

1 B   2 A   3 D   4 D   5 A

CHAPTER 2

1 A   2 C   3 D   4 C   5 A   6 C   7 D
8 A   9 B   10 D

CHAPTER 3

1 D   2 A   3 D   4 C   5 D   6 A   7 A
8 A   9 D   10 B

CHAPTER 4

1 B   2 D   3 D   4 A   5 D   6 A   7 C
8 D   9 A   10 D

CHAPTER 5

1 A   2 D   3 B   4 B   5 B   6 D   7 A
8 A   9 D   10 A

CHAPTER 6

1 B   2 A   3 C   4 C   5 A   6 A   7 D
8 D   9 A   10 D

CHAPTER 7

1 A   2 D   3 C   4 B   5 B   6 A   7 B
8 A   9 B   10 B

CHAPTER 8

1 A   2 D   3 B   4 D   5 B   6 D   7 C
8 B   9 C   10 C

CHAPTER 9

1 A   2 A   3 A   4 D   5 C   6 A   7 B
8 A   9 D   10 D

CHAPTER 10

1 A   2 B   3 B   4 B   5 D   6 A   7 D
8 A   9 C   10 D

CHAPTER 11

1 B   2 C   3 C   4 A   5 C   6 C   7 A
8 C   9 A   10 C

CHAPTER 12

1 B   2 B   3 D   4 A   5 C   6 D   7 A
8 D   9 D   10 D

CHAPTER 13

1 D   2 A   3 C   4 C   5 B   6 D   7 B
8 B   9 B   10 C

CHAPTER 14

1 B   2 B   3 A   4 C   5 D

CHAPTER15

1 C   2 D   3 D   4 D   5 A

CHAPTER 16

1 C   2 A   3 C   4 B   5 A

CHAPTER 17

| 1 C | 2 A | 3 B | 4 C | 5 C | 6 A | 7 D |
| 8 D | 9 C | 10 A | | | | |

CHAPTER 18

| 1 C | 2 D | 3 A | 4 B | 5 A | 6 C | 7 C |
| 8 C | 9 C | 10 D | | | | |

CHAPTER 19

| 1 A | 2 A | 3 C | 4 A | 5 A |

CHAPTER 20

| 1 B | 2 C | 3 D | 4 C | 5 C |

CHAPTER 21

| 1 D | 2 D | 3 C | 4 B | 5 D |

CHAPTER 22

| 1 D | 2 C | 3 B | 4 D | 5 D |

CHAPTER 23

| 1 C | 2 D | 3 B | 4 D | 5 C |

CHAPTER 24

| 1 D | 2 B | 3 A | 4 A | 5 B |

CHAPTER 25

| 1 B | 2 B | 3 A | 4 A | 5 D | 6 B | 7 D |
| 8 A | 9 D | 10 A | | | | |

CHAPTER 26

| 1 A | 2 C | 3 B | 4 D | 5 B | 6 B | 7 C |
| 8 C | 9 D | 10 A | | | | |

CHAPTER 27

| 1 A | 2 C | 3 D | 4 A | 5 A | 6 D | 7 D |
| 8 D | 9 A | 10 A | | | | |

CHAPTER 28

| 1 A | 2 B | 3 A | 4 D | 5 A | 6 D | 7 B |
| 8 C | 9 D | 10 D | | | | |

CHAPTER 29

| 1 D | 2 D | 3 D | 4 C | 5 C | 6 A | 7 D |
| 8 A | 9 D | 10 B | | | | |

CHAPTER 30

| 1 B | 2 D | 3 D | 4 D | 5 A |

CHAPTER 31

| 1 C | 2 D | 3 D | 4 A | 5 D |

CHAPTER 32

| 1 D | 2 D | 3 D | 4 D | 5 B | 6 A | 7 A |
| 8 B | 9 C | 10 D | | | | |

CHAPTER 33

| 1 B | 2 A | 3 D |

CHAPTER 34

| 1 D | 2 D | 3 B | 4 C | 5 D |

CHAPTER 35

| 1 A | 2 C | 3 A | 4 B | 5 D |

CHAPTER 36

| 1 B | 2 C | 3 B | 4 B | 5 B |

CHAPTER 37

| 1 D | 2 A | 3 C | 4 D | 5 D | 6 C | 7 A |
| 8 B | 9 D | 10 A | | | | |

CHAPTER 38

| 1 B | 2 C | 3 A | 4 A | 5 B | 6 A | 7 D |
| 8 A | 9 B | 10 A | | | | |

CHAPTER 39

| 1 C | 2 B | 3 B | 4 D | 5 B | 6 A | 7 D |
| 8 A | 9 A | 10 C | | | | |

CHAPTER 40

| 1 D | 2 A |

CHAPTER 41

| 1 B | 2 C |

Glossary

Absolute configuration: The configuration of four different substituent groups around an asymmetric carbon atom, in relation to D- and L-glyceraldehyde.

Acidosis: Diminished capacity of the body to buffer protons in various respiratory/metabolic conditions.

Actin: A protein making up the thin filament of muscles.

Active site: It is the restricted part of a protein (enzyme) to which a substrate binds.

Active transport: Energy-driven, uphill transport of a solute across a membrane.

Adenosine diphosphate (ADP): A nucleotide serving as phosphate group acceptor in cellular respiration.

Adenosine triphosphate (ATP): A nucleotide serving as a phosphate group donor in metabolic reactions.

Aldose: A monosaccharide where terminal carbonyl carbon is an aldehyde.

Alkalosis: Diminished capacity of the body to buffer hydroxyl ions in various respiratory/metabolic conditions.

Allele: One of the several alternative forms of a gene, occupying a given locus on a chromosome.

Allosteric control: Refers to the ability of an interaction at one site of a protein to influence the activity of another site.

Allosteric enzyme: A regulatory enzyme whose catalytic activity is modulated by the noncovalent association with a specific metabolite at a site (other than the active site) known as the allosteric site.

Ame's test: A test for mutagenesis using *Salmonella typhimurium*.

Amino acid: α-Amino substituted carboxylic acid, the monomeric unit of protein.

Amino acid activation: ATP-driven enzymatic esterification of the carboxyl group of an amino acid to the 3′-hydroxyl group of its corresponding tRNA.

Aminotransferases: Transaminases catalyzing the transfer of amino group from α-amino acid to α-keto acid.

Amphibolic pathway: The metabolic pathway used in catabolism as well as anabolism.

Amphipathic molecule: A molecule possessing polar as well as nonpolar domains. Amphipathic structures have two surfaces, one hydrophilic and the other hydrophobic, e.g. a phospholipid.

Amplification: Refers to the production of additional copies of a chromosomal sequence, found as intrachromosomal or extra-chromosomal DNA.

Anabolism: Phase of metabolism concerned with the energy requiring biosynthesis of compounds from smaller precursors.

Anaplerotic reaction: An enzymatic reaction capable of replenishing the supply of intermediates in the TCA cycle.

Annealing: Pairing of complementary single strands of DNA to form a double helix.

Anomers: Stereoisomers of a sugar differing in configuration about the carbonyl (anomeric) carbon atom.

Antibody: A defence protein (immunoglobulin) generated by B lymphocytes and capable of binding specifically to an antigen, to trigger the immune response.

Anticodon: A specific sequence (trinucleotide) in a tRNA, complementary to a codon in an mRNA.

Antigen: A molecule capable of eliciting the synthesis of a specific antibody (immunoglobulin).

Antiport: Cotransport of two solutes across a membrane in opposite directions.

Apoenzyme: The protein portion of an enzyme.

Apolipoprotein (apoprotein): The protein portion of a lipoprotein.

Apoptosis: The capacity of a cell to undergo programmed cell death.

Asymmetric carbon atom: A carbon atom covalently bonded to four different groups and thus capable of existing in two different configurations.

Attenuation: The process of the regulation of termination of transcription that is involved in controlling the expression of some bacterial operons.

Attenuator: A specific RNA sequence functioning as a transcription terminator.

Autoradiography: The process which detects radioactively labeled molecules by their effect in creating an image on photographic film.

Avidin: The raw egg-white factor which can bind to biotin.

Back mutation: It reverses the effect of a mutation that had inactivated a gene.

Bacteriophage: Virus that is capable of replicating in bacteria, often referred to as phage.

Basal metabolic rate (BMR): The rate of oxygen consumption by an animal's body at complete physical and mental rest, 12–14 hrs following the last meal.

Base-pair (bp): A partnership of A with T or G with C, in a DNA double-helix.

Bile salts: Amphipathic steroid derivatives with detergent properties, helping in lipid digestion and absorption.

Biocytin: Active biotin-linked through an amide bond to a lysine residue.

Biopterin: A pterin-derived cofactor involved in some oxido-reduction processes.

Biotin: A water soluble vitamin involved in carboxylation reactions.

B Lymphocytes (B cells): These are the cells responsible for synthesizing antibodies.

Buffer: A system consisting of a conjugate acid–base pair and is capable of resisting change in pH.

CAAT box: A part of a conserved sequence located upstream of the start points of eukaryotic transcription units. It is recognized by a large group of transcription factors.

Capsid: The external protein coat of a virus particle.

Carotenoids: Lipid-soluble pigments made up of isoprene units.

Catabolism: Phase of metabolism concerned with the energy-yielding breakdown of larger molecules.

Catabolite activator protein (CAP): A positive regulatory protein activated by cAMP. It is needed for RNA polymerase to initiate transcription of certain catabolite-sensitive operons of *E. coli*.

Catecholamines: Amino derivatives of catechol acting as transmitters of hormonal or neuronal signals, viz. dopamine, norepinephrine, epinephrine.

Central dogma: Flow of genetic information from DNA to RNA to protein.

Ceramide: Sphingosine derivative containing an acyl group attached to its amino group.

Cerebroside: Ceramide containing one sugar residue as a head group.

Chimeric molecule: A molecule, e.g. DNA, RNA or protein, containing sequences derived from two different species.

Chromatin: The filamentous complex of DNA and histones in the nucleus of interphase cells.

Chromatography: A process of separation of molecules based on partitioning between a mobile phase and a stationary phase.

Chromosome: A discrete unit of the genome carrying many genes, visible as a morphological entity only during cell division.

Chylomicron: A plasma lipoprotein carrying dietary lipids from intestine to the other tissues.

Cistron: The genetic unit of DNA or RNA corresponding to one gene.

Citric acid cycle (Krebs cycle, tricarboxylic acid cycle or TCA cycle): A cyclic system of enzymatic reactions for the oxidation of acetyl residues to carbon dioxide, formation of citrate being the first step.

Cloning: Production of multiple copies of identical cells from a single ancestral cell.

Cloning vector: A plasmid or phage that is used to carry inserted foreign DNA for the purpose of producing more material (a protein product).

Codon: A trinucleotide sequence (triplet) that codes for a specific amino acid or a termination signal.

Coenzyme: An organic cofactor, often containing a vitamin, required for the action of some enzyme.

Coenzyme A (CoA): A pantothenic acid containing coenzyme acting as an acyl group carrier.

Cofactor: An inorganic ion or a coenzyme required for enzyme activity.

Competitive inhibition: An enzyme inhibition reversed by increasing the substrate concentration.

Complementary DNA (cDNA): Single-stranded DNA complementary to an RNA, synthesized from it by reverse transcription *in vitro*.

β-Conformation: An extended, zig-zag arrangement of a polypeptide chain called β-pleated sheet.

Conjugated protein: A protein containing one or more prosthetic group.

Consensus sequence: A sequence of bases consisting of the most commonly occurring residues at each position.

Constitutive enzymes: Enzymes maintained at a constant level and required at all times by a cell.

Cosmids: These are plasmids into which phage λ cos sites have been inserted, as a result of which plasmid DNA can be packaged *in vitro* in the phage coat.

Cotransport: Simultaneous transport of two solutes across a membrane, in the same (uniport) or opposite (antiport) direction.

Coupled reactions: Two reactions having a common intermediate, serving to transfer energy from one to the other.

Cyclic AMP (cAMP): A second messenger formed from ATP by the action of adenylate cyclase in which the phosphate group is joined to both 3′ and 5′ positions of ribose.

Cyclins: Proteins that accumulate continuously throughout the cell cycle and are destroyed by proteolysis during mitosis.

Cytochromes: Hemoproteins serving as electron carriers.

Cytoplasm: Material between the plasma membrane and the nucleus.

Cytoskeleton: Network of fibers in the cytoplasm of the eukaryotic cell.

Cytosol: General volume of cytoplasm in which cell organelles are located.

Dalton: Weight of a single hydrogen atom $(1.66 \times 10^{-24}\,g)$.

Deamination: Enzymatic removal of amino groups from biomolecules.

Degeneracy: Degeneracy in the genetic code refers to the lack of an effect of changes in the third base of the codon, on the represented amino acid.

Dehydrogenases: Enzymes catalyzing the removal of pair of hydrogen atoms from their substrates.

Denaturation: Denaturation of DNA describes its conversion from the double-stranded to the single-stranded state, most often accomplished by heating.

Denaturation of protein describes its conversion from the physiological conformation to an inactive conformation.

De novo pathway: Synthesis of a molecule from simple precursors, distinct from a salvage pathway.

Deoxyribonucleic acid (DNA): The carrier of genetic information containing deoxyribonucleotides linked by 3′,5′-phosphodiester bonds.

Desaturases: Enzymes catalyzing the introduction of double bonds into fatty acids.

Dextrorotatory: A stereoisomer rotating plane-polarized light clockwise.

Diabetes mellitus: A metabolic disease with persistent hyperglycemia due to absolute/relative insulin deficiency.

Diffusion: Net downhill movement of molecules.

Disaccharide: Compound containing two monosaccharides which are linked through a covalent glycosidic bond.

Disulfide bond: A covalent cross-linkage formed by two cysteinyl residues (-cys-cys-).

DNA library: A random collection of cloned DNA fragments including the entire genome of an organism.

DNA ligase: An enzyme catalyzing the formation of a phosphodiester bond between the 3′ end of one DNA segment and the 5′ end of another.

DNA polymerase: An enzyme catalyzing the template-dependent synthesis of DNA from deoxyribonucleotide precursors.

DNA replicase: Complex of all enzymes and proteins required specifically for replication.

DNA supercoiling: Coiling of DNA upon itself due to bending, underwinding or overwinding.

Domain: A distinct structural unit of a molecule.

Double helix: Coiled conformation of two anti-parallel, complementary DNA strands.

Double reciprocal plot: Lineweaver-Burk plot of 1/V versus 1/[S], allowing an accurate determination of V_{max} and K_m.

Electrochemical gradient: The sum of concentration gradient and electrical gradient of an ion across a membrane, the force driving oxidative phosphorylation and photophosphorylation.

Electron carrier: Flavoproteins/cytochromes that can reversibly gain and lose electrons.

Electrophile: A chemical group with a strong affinity for electrons.

Electrophoresis: Movement of charged species in an electric field.

Elongation factors (EF in prokaryotes or eEF in eukaryotes): Specific proteins required in the elongation of polypeptides.

Enantiomers: Stereoisomers that are non-superimposable mirror images of each other.

Endergonic reaction: A reaction that consumes free energy (endothermic for heat consumption).

Endocrine glands: Specialized cells, synthesizing hormones secreted into the blood and acting at distant sites.

Endocytosis: Invagination of plasma membrane leading to the uptake of extracellular material.

Endonuclease: Enzyme hydrolyzing internal phosphodiester bonds of a nucleic acid.

Energy charge: The relative proportion of ATP/ADP/AMP indicating cellular energy status.

Enhancers: DNA sequences facilitating gene expression, located away from the transcribed gene.

Enthalpy: Heat content of a system.

Entropy: Degree of randomness in a system.

Enzyme: A protein/RNA catalyzing a specific reaction without affecting the equilibrium.

Equilibrium: The state of a system with no further net change occurring and has least free energy.

Epimers: Two stereoisomers differing in the configuration at an asymmetric center.

Epitope: The chemical group/antigenic determinant in an antigen to which an antibody binds.

Exergonic reaction: A reaction that releases free energy (exothermic for heat release).

Exocytosis: Fusion of an intracellular vesicle with the plasma membrane for the release of vesicular contents extracellularly.

Exon: A part of the gene that is represented in the mature RNA product.

Exonuclease: An enzyme hydrolyzing the terminal phosphodiester bond of a nucleic acid.

Facilitated diffusion: Diffusion of polar molecules through a membrane, mediated by a protein transporter.

Fatty acids: Long chain aliphatic carboxylic acids found in natural fats and oils.

Feedback inhibition: Inhibition of an enzyme, early in a metabolic sequence, by a product formed later in the sequence.

Fermentation: Exergonic breakdown of a nutrient without net oxidation.

First law of thermodynamics: In all processes, the total energy of the universe remains constant.

Flavin adenine dinucleotide (FAD): Riboflavin-containing coenzyme of some oxidoreductases.

Flavin mononucleotide (FMN): Riboflavin phosphate, a coenzyme for some oxidoreductases.

Flavoprotein: An enzyme with a flavin nucleotide as a tightly bound prosthetic group.

Fluidity: A property of membranes which indicates the ability of lipids to move laterally within their monolayer.

Fluid-mosaic model: Biological membranes having fluid lipid bilayers with embedded proteins.

Frame shift mutation: An insertion/deletion of a base-pair altering the reading frame of codons.

Free energy: That portion of the total energy of a system that can do work at constant temperature and pressure.

Free radical: Highly reactive atom/group of atoms possessing an unpaired electron.

Furanose: A simple sugar having five-membered furan ring.

Gangliosides: Neuronal sphingolipids having complex oligo-saccharides as head groups.

Gene: Gene (cistron) is the segment of DNA encoding a functional RNA or protein.

Gene cluster: A group of adjacent genes that are identical or related.

Genetic code: The correspondence between triplets in DNA (or RNA) and amino acids in protein.

Genome: The entire genetic information contained within a cell/virus.

Genotype: Genetic constitution of an organism.

Geometric isomers: Isomers formed as a result of rotation about a double bond (also called *cis* and *trans* isomers).

Gluconeogenesis (Neoglucogenesis): Synthesis of glucose from noncarbohydrate precursors.

Glycan: Synonym for polysaccharide.

Glycerophospholipid: An amphipathic lipid with a glycerol backbone.

Glycolipid: A lipid containing a carbohydrate group.

Glycolysis: Catabolism of one glucose molecule into two molecules of pyruvate/lactate.

Glycoprotein: A protein containing a carbohydrate group.

Glycosaminoglycan: Synonymous with mucopolysaccharide, a heteropolysaccharide containing alternately repeating amino sugar and uronic acid.

Glycosidic bonds: Bonds between a sugar and another sugar/nonsugar residue through an intervening oxygen/nitrogen atom.

Glyoxylate cycle: Conversion of acetate into succinate (and subsequently carbohydrate) in bacteria and some plant cells (germinating seeds), occurring in glyoxysomes.

G Protein: A guanine nucleotide-binding trimeric protein that resides in the plasma membrane.

Gyrase: A type II topoisomerase of *E. coli* with the ability to introduce negative supercoils into DNA.

Hapten: A small molecule that acts as an antigen when conjugated to a protein.

Helicase: An enzyme catalyzing DNA strand separation.

α-Helix: Right-handed helical conformation of a polypeptide with maximum intrachain hydrogen bonding.

Heme (Haem): The iron-porphyrin prosthetic group of hemoproteins.

Henderson-Hasselbalch equation: An equation relating the pH, pKa and proton-acceptor/donor ratio in a solution.

Heterogeneous nuclear RNA (hnRNA): Transcripts of nuclear genes made by RNA polymerase II.

Heteropolysaccharide: A polysaccharide having more than one type of monosaccharides.

Heterotropic enzyme: An allosteric enzyme modulated by a molecule other than the substrate.

Hexose: A simple sugar with six-carbon backbone.

Histones: Family of conserved DNA-binding proteins of eukaryotes that forms the nucleosome, the basic subunit of chromatin.

Holoenzyme: Complete enzyme with all necessary cofactors.

Homopolysaccharide: Polysaccharide with only one type of sugar (a polymer of same monosaccharides).

Homotropic enzyme: An allosteric enzyme modulated by its substrate.

Hormone: The first messenger secreted in minute amounts from an endocrine gland, carried by blood to a distant tissue and capable of binding with its cognate receptor to generate a cellular response.

Hybridization: Pairing of complementary RNA and DNA strands to give an RNA-DNA hybrid.

Hydrophilic: A polar molecule that easily dissolves in water.

Hydrophobic: A nonpolar molecule that is insoluble in water.

Hyperchromicity: Increase in optical density at 260 nm, after DNA is denatured.

Immunoglobulin: A defense antibody protein generated against and capable of binding specifically to an antigen.

Induced-fit model of enzyme binding site: A conformational change in an enzyme in response to substrate binding, making the enzyme catalytically active.

Induction: Increase in gene expression in the presence of an inducer.

Initiation codon: Triplet of AUG coding for the first amino acid (methionine) in a polypeptide.

Initiation factors (IF in prokaryotes or eIF in eukaryotes): Proteins that associate with the small subunit of the ribosome, specifically at the stage of initiation of protein synthesis.

Insertion: A mutation due to the insertion of an extra base-pair between two successive bases in DNA.

Integral membrane protein: Proteins spanning biological membrane and firmly held by hydrophobic interactions.

Interferon: Specific glycoproteins with antiviral activity.

Intermediary metabolism: Combined activities of all the metabolic pathways that interconvert precursors, metabolites and products (excluding macromolecules, generally after digestion/absorption).

Intron: A nucleotide sequence in a gene that is transcribed but excised before translation. It is also called an intervening sequence.

Inverted repeats: They comprise two copies of the same sequence of DNA, repeated in opposite orientation on the same molecule. Adjacent inverted repeats constitute a palindrome.

Ionophore: A compound that binds one or more metal ions and diffuses across a membrane with the ion.

Isoelectric pH: The pH at which a solute has no net electric charge.

Isoenzymes (Isozymes): Multiple forms of an enzyme catalyzing the same reaction but differing in amino acid sequence, K_m, V_{max} and regulatory properties.

Jaundice: Yellow discoloration of sclera, visible when serum bilirubin exceeds 2 mg/dl.

Keratin: Structural protein consisting of parallel polypeptide chains in α-helical conformation.

Ketogenic amino acid: Amino acid whose carbon skeleton can be a precursor of ketone bodies.

Ketone bodies: Fuel molecules (acetoacetate, β-hydroxybutyrate and acetone) produced by the liver and utilized by the peripheral tissues.

Ketose: A simple monosaccharide with a ketone as the carbonyl group.

Kinase: Enzyme catalyzing substrate phosphorylation by ATP.

Lagging strand: The DNA strand synthesized discontinuously in the form of short fragments, in a direction opposite to the replication fork movement ($5' \rightarrow 3'$ direction).

Leader sequence: A specific short sequence near the N-terminus of a protein for passage into or through a membrane.

Leading strand: The DNA strand synthesized continuously in the direction of replication fork movement ($5' \rightarrow 3'$ direction).

Leucine-zipper: Two interacting α-helices with leucine in every seventh position, a structural motif in many eukaryotic protein-protein interactions.

Leukotrienes: A family of arachidonic acid-derived metabolites involved in inflammatory-allergic responses.

Levorotatory: A stereoisomer rotating the plane of polarized light counter clockwise.

Lineweaver-burk plot (double reciprocal plot): A linear transformation of Michaelis-Menten equation allowing determination of V_{max} and K_m.

Linking number: Number of times the two strands of a closed DNA duplex cross-over each other.

Lipid: Heterogeneous group of water-insoluble compounds soluble in organic solvents.

Lipid bilayer: The form taken by orientation of lipids in which the hydrophobic fatty acids occupy the interior and the polar heads face the exterior.

Lipoate: An intermediate carrier of H-atoms/acyl groups in α-keto acid dehydrogenases.

Lipoprotein: A lipid-protein aggregate carrying water insoluble lipids in the blood, the protein as an apolipoprotein (apoprotein).

Long-terminal repeat (LTR): A sequence directly repeated at both ends of a retroviral DNA.

Lyases: Enzymes catalyzing removal of a group from substrate forming a double bond, or the addition of a group to a double bond.

Lysogeny: The ability of a phage to survive in a bacterium as a part of the host DNA (prophage).

Messenger RNA (mRNA): A class of RNA molecules complementary to one strand of DNA, carrying genetic information from DNA to ribosomes.

Metabolism: The complete set of enzyme-catalyzed transformation of organic molecules in living cells. It includes both anabolism as well as catabolism.

Metalloprotein: A protein with some metal ion as a prosthetic group.

Micelle: An aggregate of amphipathic molecules with the nonpolar part towards the interior, and the polar part exposed to the surrounding aqueous environment.

Michaelis-Menten equation: The hyperbolic dependence of V_o, the initial reaction velocity of an enzymatic reaction, on substrate concentration [S], which is given by the equation:

$$V_0 = V_{max}[S]/K_m + [S]$$

Microbodies: Cytoplasmic organelles containing peroxide-forming and detoxifying enzymes, i.e. lysosomes, peroxisomes and glyoxysomes.

Microfilaments: Thin filaments similar to actin, present in the cytoplasm with a contractile function.

Microsomes: Fragmented pieces of endoplasmic reticulum associated with ribosomes, obtained by ultracentrifugation of homogenized tissue.

Microtubules: Tubulin dimers found in cilia, flagella and centrosomes.

Mixed function oxidases: Enzymes using molecular oxygen to simultaneously oxidize a substrate and a cosubstrate.

Monoclonal antibodies: Antibodies produced by a cloned hybridoma cell, hence identical and directed against the same epitope.

Monosaccharide: A straight-chain carbohydrate with 3 or more carbon atoms.

Mucopolysaccharide: A heteropolysaccharide containing alternately repeating amino sugar and uronic acid.

Mutarotation: Change in specific rotation of a pyranose/furanose glycoside accompanying the equilibration of its α and β anomeric forms.

Mutation: An inheritable alteration in the nucleotide sequence of genomic DNA.

Myosin: The major contractile protein of thick filaments of muscle.

Native conformation: Bioactive conformation of a macromolecule.

Negative feedback: A reaction product inhibiting an earlier step in a metabolic pathway.

Neurotransmitter: A low molecular weight compound secreted from a presynaptic neuron, transmitting nerve impulse by binding to postsynaptic neuron.

Nicotinamide adenine dinucleotide/nicotinamide adenine dinucleotide phosphate (NAD/NADP): Nicotinamide-containing coenzymes functioning as carriers of reducing equivalents during oxidoreduction.

Noncompetitive inhibition: Enzyme inhibition due to the binding of an inhibitor to the enzyme at a site distinct from substrate-binding site and not reversed by increasing the substrate concentration.

Nonessential amino acids: Amino acids synthesized in the human body from simple precursors and not essentially required in the diet.

Non-heme iron proteins: Proteins participating in oxidoreduction, containing iron but no porphyrin ring.

Nonsense codon: A codon that causes the termination of a polypeptide chain.

Nonsense mutation: A mutation resulting in a premature polypeptide chain termination.

Nonsense suppressor: A mutation in a tRNA gene, causing an amino acid to be inserted in a polypeptide in response to a termination codon.

Northern blotting: A technique for transferring RNA from an agarose gel to a nitrocellulose filter on which it can be hybridized to a complementary DNA.

Nucleic acids: Polynucleotides (DNA, RNA) in which monomeric nucleotides are linked in a specific sequence by phosphodiester bonds.

Nucleophile: An electron-rich group with a strong tendency to donate electrons.

Nucleoside: A purine/pyrimidine base linked to a pentose sugar.

Nucleoside diphosphate kinase: An enzyme catalyzing the transfer of a terminal phosphate of a nucleoside 5'-triphosphate to a nucleoside 5'-diphosphate.

Nucleosome: Basic structural subunit of chromatin consisting of about 200 bp of DNA and an octamer of histone proteins.

Nucleotide: A nucleoside phosphorylated at one of its pentose hydroxyl groups.

Okazaki fragments: Short stretches of 1000–2000 bases produced during discontinuous replication which are later joined into a covalently intact strand.

Oligomeric protein: A multisubunit protein having two or more identical polypeptide chains.

Oncogenes: The genes whose products have the ability to transform eukaryotic cells so that they grow in a manner analogous to tumor cells.

Open reading frame: A group of non-overlapping codons that do not include a termination codon.

Operator: The site on DNA at which a repressor protein binds to prevent transcription from initiating at the adjacent promoter.

Operon: A unit of bacterial gene expression consisting of one or more related genes with their operator and promoter sequences.

Optical activity: Ability of a substance to rotate the plane of polarized light.

Origin of replication: The nucleotide sequence where DNA replication is initiated.

β-Oxidation: Successive oxidations at the β-carbon atom of fatty acyl CoA, producing acetyl CoA.

Oxidative phosphorylation: Enzymatic phosphorylation of ADP to ATP coupled to electron flow from a substrate to molecular oxygen.

Oxygenases: Enzymes catalyzing reactions where oxygen is incorporated into an acceptor molecule.

Palindrome: A DNA segment in which the base sequences exhibit two fold rotational symmetry.

Pentose: A simple five-carbon sugar.

Pentose phosphate pathway [hexose monophosphate shunt (HMP shunt)]: A pathway interconverting hexoses and pentoses, and a source of pentoses and NADPH.

Peptide bond: Covalent link between the α-amino group of an amino acid and the α-carboxyl group of another amino acid.

Peptidoglycan: Parallel heteropolysaccharides cross-linked by short peptides in bacterial cell wall.

Peripheral proteins: Proteins loosely bound to a membrane by hydrogen bonds or electrostatic forces.

pH: The negative logarithm of the H^+ concentration in a solution.

Phosphodiester linkage: Two alcohols linked through one phosphoric acid molecule by ester linkage.

Phospholipid: A lipid having one or more phosphate groups.

pK: The negative logarithm of an equilibrium constant.

Plasmalogen: A phospholipid with an ether substituent on the first carbon of glycerol.

Plasma membrane: The continuous membrane defining the boundary of every cell.

Plasmid: An extrachromosomal, self-replicating, circular DNA in bacteria.

Polycistronic mRNA: The coding regions representing more than one gene.

Polyclonal antibodies: A heterogeneous pool of antibodies produced by different B-lymphocytes in response to an antigen, recognizing different epitopes.

Polymerase chain reaction (PCR): A technique in which cycles of denaturation, annealing with primer and extension with DNA polymerase, are used to amplify the number of copies of a target DNA sequence by $>10^6$ times.

Polymorphism: It refers to the simultaneous occurrence in the population of genomes showing allelic variations.

Polyribosome (polysome): An mRNA associated with a series of ribosomes engaged in translation.

Polysaccharide: Polymer of monosaccharide units linked by glycosidic bonds.

Porphyrin: A nitrogenous compound with four substituted pyrroles linked covalently to form a ring, with a central metal ion.

Positive supercoiling: Coiling of the double helix in space, in the same direction as the winding of the two strands of the double helix itself.

Post-transcriptional modification: Enzymatic processing of a primary RNA transcript producing functional RNAs.

Post-translational modification: Enzymatic processing of a polypeptide chain after translation.

Primary structure: The covalent backbone of a polymer including any inter-chain/intra-chain covalent bonds.

Primary transcript: The original unmodified RNA product corresponding to a transcription unit.

Primase: Enzyme catalyzing the synthesis of RNA oligonucleotides used as primer by DNA polymerase.

Primosome: The complex of proteins involved in the primary action that initiates synthesis of each Okazaki fragment during discontinuous replication. It moves along DNA to engage in successive primary events.

Probe: A labelled nucleic acid segment used in hybridization to detect complementary segments.

Promoter: The RNA polymerase binding site of DNA to initiate transcription.

Proofreading: The mechanism for correcting errors in protein or nucleic acid synthesis that involves scrutiny of individual units after they have been added to the chain.

Prophage: A phage genome covalently integrated as a linear part of the bacterial chromosome.

Prostaglandins: A family of arachidonic acid derived metabolites with local hormone-like properties.

Prosthetic group: A metal ion/organic molecule covalently bound to a protein and is essential for its activity.

Protein targeting: Process of sorting of newly synthesized proteins to their respective destinations.

Proteoglycan: A heteropolysaccharide joined to a polypeptide, the latter being a minor component.

Proton-motive force: The electrochemical potential driving ATP synthesis during oxidative phosphorylation.

Proto-oncogenes: Normal counterparts in the eukaryotic genomes, to the oncogenes, carried by some retroviruses. They are given names of the form c-onc.

Provirus: A duplex DNA sequence in the eukaryotic chromosome, corresponding to the genome of an RNA retrovirus.

Pyrimidine dimer: Covalently linked adjacent pyrimidine residues induced by UV light.

Quaternary structure: Three-dimensional assembly of a multisubunit protein.

Racemic mixture: An equimolar mixture of D- and L-stereoisomers of an optically active compound.

Radioimmunoassay (RIA): A sensitive assay for trace amounts of a substance by displacing the radioactive form of the substance from its specific antibody.

Radioisotope: An unstable atom resulting from a combination of protons and neutrons, produced artificially.

Radionuclides: Radioactive products used in nuclear medicine.

Reading frame: One of three possible ways of reading a nucleotide sequence as a series of triplets.

Receptor: A protein located in the plasma membrane or cytosol or nucleus, that binds a specific ligand to generate a cellular response.

Recombinant DNA: DNA formed by the joining of different genes in new combinations.

Reducing end: The end of a polysaccharide with a free anomeric carbon.

Regulatory gene: A gene which codes for an RNA or a protein product whose function is to control the expression of other genes.

Releasing factors: Hypothalamic hormones that stimulate the release of other hormones by the pituitary gland.

Replication: Synthesis of a daughter DNA duplex identical to its parent DNA duplex.

Replication eye: A region in which DNA has been replicated within a longer, unreplicated region.

Replication fork: The point at which strands of parental duplex DNA are separated so that replication can proceed.

Replicon: A unit of the genome in which DNA is replicated. It contains an origin for initiation of replication.

Replisome: A multiprotein structure that assembles at the bacterial replicating fork to undertake synthesis of DNA. It contains DNA polymerase and other enzymes involved in DNA replication at the replication fork.

Repression: Decrease in gene expression in response to altered activity of a regulatory protein. It refers to inhibition of transcription by binding of repressor protein to a specific site on DNA or mRNA.

Restriction endonucleases: Enzymes cleaving both DNA strands at specific points. These are used as an important tool in genetic engineering.

Restriction fragment: A duplex DNA formed by the action of a restriction endonuclease on a larger DNA.

Restriction fragment length polymorphism (RFLP): Inherited differences in sites for restriction enzymes that result in differences in the length of the fragments, produced by cleavage with the relevant restriction enzyme.

Restriction map: A linear array of sites on DNA, cleaved by various restriction enzymes.

Retrovirus: An RNA virus containing reverse transcriptase and propagates via conversion into duplex DNA.

Reverse transcriptase: An RNA-directed DNA polymerase.

Rho factor: A protein involved in assisting *E. coli* RNA polymerase to terminate transcription at certain (rho-dependent) sites.

Rho-independent terminators: Sequences of DNA that cause *E. coli* RNA polymerase to terminate *in vitro*, in the absence of rho factor.

Ribosomal RNA (rRNA): A class of RNA present in ribosomes.

Ribozymes: Catalytic RNA molecules.

RNA polymerase: An enzyme catalyzing the synthesis of RNA from ribonucleoside 5′-triphosphates on a DNA template.

RNA replicase: An enzyme that synthesizes RNA using an RNA template.

RNA splicing: Removal of introns and joining of exons in a primary transcript.

Salvage pathway: A recycling pathway for the synthesis of a compound from metabolites in the catabolic pathway for the compound.

Saponification: Alkaline hydrolysis of neutral fat to release fatty acids as soaps.

Sarcomere: Structural-functional unit of the muscle contractile system.

Satellite DNA (sDNA): It consists of many tendem repeats of a short basic repeating unit.

Secondary structure: Regular, recurring spatial arrangements of adjacent monomers present in a polymer.

Second law of thermodynamics: In any physical/chemical reaction, the entropy of the universe tends to increase.

Second messenger: An intracellular effector molecule synthesized/ activated in response to an extracellular signal, usually a hormone.

Semiconservative replication: It is accomplished by separation of the strands of a parental duplex, each then acting as a template for the synthesis of a complementary strand.

-10 Sequence: The consensus sequence TATAATG, centered about 10 bp before the start point of a bacterial gene. It is involved in the initial melting of DNA by RNA polymerase.

-35 Sequence: The consensus sequence, centered about 35 bp before the startpoint of a bacterial gene. It is involved in the initial recognition by RNA polymerase.

Shine-Dalgarno sequence: A part or all of the poly purine sequence AGGAGG, located on bacterial mRNA, just prior to an AUG initiation codon. It is complementary to the sequence at the 3′-end of 16S rRNA involved in binding of ribosome to mRNA.

Sigma factor (σ factor): A subunit of bacterial RNA polymerase needed for initiation.

Signal sequence: An N-terminal sequence of a protein responsible for co-translational insertion into membranes of the endoplasmic reticulum.

Signal transduction: The process by which a receptor interacts with a ligand at the surface of the cell and then transmits a signal, to trigger a pathway within the cell.

Site-directed mutagenesis: Methods for producing desired gene mutations.

Small nuclear RNA (snRNA): Small nuclear RNAs, found within the nucleus of eukaryotic cells, participating in splicing reactions.

Southern blotting: The procedure for transferring denatured DNA from an agarose gel to a nitrocellulose filter where it can be hybridized with a complementary nucleic acid.

Specific activity: The number of micromoles of a substrate transformed by enzyme/minute/milligram of protein at 25°C, an indicator of enzyme purity.

Sphingolipid: An amphipathic lipid with a sphingosine backbone to which a long-chain fatty acid and an alcohol are attached.

Splicing: The process of removal of introns and joining of axons in a primary RNA transcript.

Standard free energy change ($\Delta G°$): The free energy change for a reaction at standard conditions of 298 K, 1 atmospheric pressure and 1 M reactants.

Stereoisomers: Compounds having the same chemical composition but different spatial arrangements.

Sticky ends (cohesive ends): Short, overhanging, complementary, single-stranded ends of DNA facilitating ligation of the ends.

Structural gene: A gene encoding an RNA or a polypeptide.

Substrate level phosphorylation: ADP/GDP phosphorylation during a dehydrogenation reaction independent of oxidative phosphorylation.

Suicide inhibitor: A compound that is enzymatically activated and then inhibits the same enzyme.

Symport: Cotransport of two solutes across a membrane in the same direction.

TATA Box: A conserved A·T-rich sequence found about 25 bp before the startpoint of each eukaryotic RNA polymerase II transcription unit. It may be involved in positioning the enzyme for correct initiation.

Telomerase: The ribonucleoprotein enzyme that creates repeating units of one strand of the telomere, by adding individual bases.

Telomere: The natural end of a chromosome. Its DNA sequence consists of a simple repeating unit with a protruding single-stranded end that may fold into a hairpin.

Termination codon (stop codon): Codon signaling the termination of a polypeptide chain during translation, usually UAA, UAG or UGA.

Termination factors (release factors, RF in prokaryotes or eRF in eukaryotes): Cytosolic protein factors essential for releasing completed polypeptides from a ribosome.

Tertiary structure: The three-dimensional conformation of a polymer in its native folded state.

Thalassemia: A disease of red blood cells resulting from lack of either α or β globin.

Thromboxanes: A class of arachidonic acid metabolites involved in platelet aggregation.

Thymine dimer: Chemically cross-linked pair of adjacent thymine residues in DNA, due to the damage induced by ultraviolet irradiation.

Topoisomerases: Enzymes introducing positive/negative supercoils in closed, duplex DNA and can change the linking number of DNA.

Topoisomers: DNA isomers differing in linking number.

Transamination: Pyridoxal phosphate dependent enzymatic transfer of an amino group from an α-amino acid to an α-keto acid.

Transcription: Enzymatic transfer of genetic information from a DNA strand to a complementary mRNA.

Transfer RNA (tRNA): A class of RNA molecules binding with a specific amino acid during translation initiation.

Transgenic organism: An organism harboring genes from another organism, produced by genetic engineering.

Transition state: A transient, activated form of a molecule during a chemical reaction.

Translation: Transfer of genetic information from mRNA to a polypeptide.

Translocase: An enzyme catalyzing membrane transport or the movement of ribosome along mRNA during translation.

Transposon: A DNA segment that can move from one genome position to another. It is important in the development of antibiotic-resistance in bacteria.

Tropic hormone: A peptide hormone that stimulates a specific target gland to secrete its hormone.

Turnover number: The number of times an enzyme transforms a substrate molecule per unit time, at saturating substrate concentrations.

Uncoupler: A substance that uncouples ADP phosphorylation from electron transfer (oxidation).

Uniport: A transport system carrying only one solute.

Vector: A self-replicating DNA molecule into which a gene of interest can be inserted to allow its replication, usually plasmid, bacteriophage or cosmid.

Vitamin: An organic compound required in small amounts in the diet of some species, usually serving as a constituent of a coenzyme.

V_{max}: Maximum velocity of an enzymatic reaction at saturating substrate concentration.

Wax: Esters of long chain fatty acids with long chain alcohols, their melting point being higher than that of the triacylglycerols.

Wobble hypothesis: It accounts for the ability of a tRNA to recognize more than one codon, by unusual pairing with the third base of a codon.

X-Linked inheritance: Genetic transmission through X-chromosomes.

X-Ray crystallography: Determination of the three-dimensional structure of a crystal by its characteristic X-ray diffraction pattern.

Y-Protein: A cystolic protein in hepatocytes that binds unconjugated bilirubin.

Zinc finger protein: It has a repeated motif of amino acids with characteristic spacing of cysteines that may be involved in binding zinc. It is characteristic of some proteins that bind DNA and/or RNA.

Zwitterion: A dipolar ion with spatially separate positive and negative charges.

Zymogen: The inactive precursor for some enzymes, activation of which involve selective partial proteolysis.

Index